Maternal-Fetal
Evidence Based Guidelines

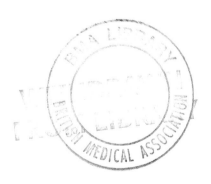

SERIES IN MATERNAL-FETAL MEDICINE

Published in association with the *Journal of Maternal-Fetal & Neonatal Medicine*

Editors in Chief:

Gian Carlo Di Renzo and Dev Maulik

Recent and Forthcoming Titles

Maternal-Fetal Evidence Based Guidelines

Second Edition

Edited by

Vincenzo Berghella, MD, FACOG

Director, Division of Maternal-Fetal Medicine
Professor, Department of Obstetrics and Gynecology
Jefferson Medical College of Thomas Jefferson University
Philadelphia, Pennsylvania
USA

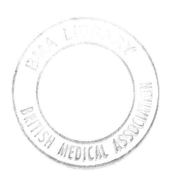

informa

healthcare

New York   London

First published in 2007 by Informa Healthcare, 37–41 Mortimer Street, London W1T 3JH, UK.
This edition published in 2012 by Informa Healthcare, 37–41 Mortimer Street, London W1T 3JH, UK.

Simultaneously published in the USA by Informa Healthcare, 52 Vanderbilt Avenue, 7th Floor, New York, NY 10017, USA

Informa Healthcare is a trading division of Informa UK Ltd. Registered Office: 37–41 Mortimer Street, London W1T 3JH, UK.
Registered in England and Wales number 1072954.

A CIP record for this book is available from the British Library.

ISBN-13: 978-1-84184-822-8
ISSN: 2158-0855

Orders may be sent to: Informa Healthcare, Sheepen Place, Colchester, Essex CO3 3LP, UK
Telephone: +44 (0)20 7017 5540
Email: CSDhealthcarebooks@informa.com
Website: http://informahealthcarebooks.com/

Library of Congress Cataloging-in-Publication Data

Maternal-fetal evidence based guidelines / edited by
Vincenzo Berghella. -- 2nd ed.
    p. ; cm. -- (Series in maternal fetal medicine)

Includes bibliographical references and index.
Summary: ''Maternal-Fetal Medicine Evidence Based Guidelines reviews the evidence for best practice in maternal-fetal medicine. It presents the reader with the right information, in the right format, by summarizing evidence in easy-to-use tables and algorithms. Each guideline is designed to ''make it easy to do it right'', with appropriate use of proven interventions and no use of harmful interventions. Plenty of evidence is available so that well-informed clinicians can reduce errors so that the main aim is ultimately to improve the health of mother and fetus by providing quality care''--Provided by publisher.

  ISBN 978-1-84184-822-8 (hardback : alk. paper) 1. Obstetrics. 2. Evidence-based medicine. I. Berghella, Vincenzo. II. Series: Series in maternal-fetal medicine.

  [DNLM: 1. Pregnancy Complications. 2. Evidence-Based Medicine. 3. Fetal Diseases. WQ 240]
RG101.M36 2012
618.2--dc23

2011025732

For corporate sales please contact: CorporateBooksIHC@informa.com
For foreign rights please contact: RightsIHC@informa.com
For reprint permissions please contact: PermissionsIHC@informa.com

Typeset by MPS Limited, a Macmillan Company
Printed and bound in the United Kingdom

To Paola, Andrea, Pietro, mamma, and papà,
for giving me the serenity, love, and strength at home now, then, and in the future
to fulfill my dreams and spend my talents as best as possible.

To all those who loved the 1st edition

To the health of mothers and babies

And, as I often toast: To the next generation!

Introduction

To me, pregnancy has always been the most fascinating and exciting area of interest, as care involves not one, but at least two persons—the mother and the fetus—and leads to the miracle of a new life. I was a third-year medical student, when, during a lecture, a resident said: "I went into obstetrics because this is the easiest medical field. Pregnancy is a physiologic process, and there isn't much to know. It is simple." I knew from my "classic" background that "obstetrics" means to "stand by, stay near," and that indeed pregnancy used to receive no medical support at all.

After almost 20 years practicing obstetrics, I now know that although physiologic and at times simple, obstetrics and maternal-fetal medicine can be the **most complex of the medical fields**: pregnancy is based on a different physiology than for nonpregnant women, can include any medical disease, require surgery, etc. It is not so simple. In fact, ignorance can kill, in this case with the health of the woman and her baby both at risk. Too often, I have gone to a lecture, journal club, rounds, or other didactic event to hear presented only one or a few articles regarding the subject, without the presenter reviewing the pertinent best review of the total literature and data. It is increasingly difficult to read and acquire knowledge of all that is published, even just in obstetrics, with about 3,000 scientific manuscripts published monthly on this subject. Some residents or even authorities would state at times that "there is no evidence" on a topic. We indeed used to be the field with the worst use of randomized trials (1). As the best way to find something is to look for it, my coauthors and I searched for the best evidence. On careful investigation, indeed there are data on almost everything we do in obstetrics, especially on our interventions. Indeed, **our field is now the pioneer for numbers of meta-analysis and extension of work for evidence-based reviews** (2). Obstetricians are now blessed with lots of data, and should make the best use of it.

The **aims** of this book are to **summarize the best evidence available in the obstetrics and maternal-fetal medicine literature**, and make the results of randomized trials and meta-analyses **easily accessible to guide clinical care**. The intent is to bridge the gap between knowledge (the evidence) and its easy application. To reach these goals, we reviewed all trials on effectiveness of interventions in obstetrics. **Millions of pregnant women have participated in thousands of properly conducted randomized controlled trials (RCT)**. The efforts and sacrifice of mothers and their fetuses for science should be recognized at least by the physicians' awareness and understanding of these studies. Some of the trials have been summarized in almost 400 Cochrane reviews, with hundreds of other meta-analyses also published in obstetrical topics (Table 1). All of the Cochrane reviews, as well as other meta-analyses and trials in obstetrics and maternal-fetal medicine, were reviewed and referenced. The material presented in single trials or meta-analyses is too detailed to be readily translated to advice for the busy clinician who needs to make dozens of clinical decisions a day. Even the Cochrane Library, the undiscussed leader for evidence-based medicine efforts, has been criticized for its lack of flexibility and relevance in failing to be more easily understandable and clinically readily usable (3). It is the gap between research and clinicians that needed to be filled, making sure that proven **interventions** are clearly highlighted, and are included in today's care. Just as all pilots fly planes under similar rules to maximize safety, all obstetricians should manage all aspects of pregnancy with similar, evidenced-based rules. Indeed, **only interventions that have been proven to provide benefit should be used routinely**. On the other hand, **primum non nocere**: interventions that have clearly been shown to be not helpful or indeed harmful to mother and/or baby should be avoided. Another aim of the book is to make sure the pregnant woman and her unborn child are not penalized by the medical community. In most circumstances, medical disorders of pregnant women can be treated as in nonpregnant adults. Moreover, there are several effective interventions for preventing or treating specific pregnancy disorders.

Table 1   Obstetrical Evidence

Over 400 current Cochrane reviews
Hundreds of other current meta-analyses
More than 1000 RCTs
Millions of pregnant women randomized

Evidence-based medicine is the concept of treating patients according to the best available evidence. While George Bernard Shaw said: "I have my own opinion, do not confuse me with the facts," this can be a deadly approach, especially in medicine, and compromise two or more lives at the same time in obstetrics and maternal-fetal medicine. What should be the basis for our interventions in medicine? Meta-analyses provide a comprehensive summary of the best research data available. As such, they provide the best guidance for "effective" clinical care (4). It is unscientific and unethical to practice medicine, teach, or conduct research without first knowing all that has already been proven (4). In the absence of trials or meta-analyses, lower level evidence is reviewed. This book aims at providing a current systematic review of the evidence, **so that current practice and education, as well as future research can be based on the full story from the best-conducted research, not just the latest data or someone's opinion** (Table 2). These evidence-based guidelines cannot be used as a "cookbook," or a document dictating the best care. The knowledge from the best evidence presented in the guidelines needs to be integrated with other knowledge gained from clinical judgment, individual patient circumstances, and patient preferences, to lead to best medical practice. These are guidelines, not rules. Even the best scientific studies are not always perfectly related to any given individual, and clinical judgment must still be applied to allow the best "particularization" of the best knowledge for the individual, unique patient. Evidence-based medicine informs clinical judgment, but does not substitute it. It is important to understand though that greater clinical experience by the physician actually correlates with inferior quality of care, if not integrated with knowledge of the best evidence (5). The appropriate treatment is given in only 50% of visits to general physicians (5). At times, limitations in resources may also limit the applicability of the guidelines, but should not limit the physician's knowledge. Guidelines and clinical pathways based on evidence not only point to the right management, but also can decrease medicolegal risk (6).

We aimed for brevity and clarity. Suggested management of the healthy or sick mother and child is stated as straightforwardly as possible, **for everyone to easily understand and implement** (Table 3). If you find the Cochrane reviews, scientific manuscripts, and other publications difficult to "translate" into care of your patients, this book is for you. We wanted to prevent information overload.

Table 2   Aims of This Book

- Improve the health of women and their children
- "Make it easy to do it right"
- Implement the best clinical care based on science (evidence), not opinion
- Research ideas
- Education
- Develop lectures
- Decrease disease, use of detrimental interventions, and therefore costs
- Reduce medicolegal risks

Table 3   This Book Is For

- Obstetricians
- Midwives
- Family medicine and others (practicing obstetrics)
- Residents
- Nurses
- Medical students
- Maternal-fetal medicine attendings
- Maternal-fetal medicine fellows
- Other consultants on pregnancy
- Lay public who wants to know "the evidence"
- Politicians responsible for health care

On the other hand, "everything should be made as simple as possible, but not simpler" (A. Einstein). Key management points are highlighted at the beginning of each guideline, and in bold in the text. The chapters are divided in two volumes, one on obstetrics and one on maternal-fetal medicine; cross-references to chapters in *Obstetric Evidence Based Guidelines* have been noted in the text where applicable. Please contact us (vincenzo.berghella@jefferson.edu) for any comments, criticisms, corrections, missing evidence, etc.

I have the most fun discovering the best ways to alleviate discomfort and disease. The search for the best evidence for these guidelines has been a wonderful, stimulating journey. Keeping up with evidence-based medicine is exciting. The most rewarding part, as a teacher, is the dissemination of knowledge. I hope, truly, that this effort will be helpful to you, too.

REFERENCES

1. Cochrane AL. 1931–1971: a critical review, with particular reference to the medical profession. In: Medicines for the Year 2000. London: Office of Health Economics, 1979:1–11. [Review]
2. Dickersin K, Manheimer E. The Cochrane Collaboration: evaluation of health care and services using systematic reviews of the results of randomized controlled trials. Clinic Obstet Gynecol 1998; 41:315–331. [Review]
3. Summerskill W. Cochrane Collaboration and the evolution of evidence. Lancet 2005; 366:1760. [Review]
4. Chalmers I. Academia's failure to support systematic reviews. Lancet 2005; 365:469. [III]
5. Arky RA. The family business—to educate. NEJM 2006; 354:1922–1926. [Review]
6. Ransom SB, Studdert DM, Dombrowski MP, et al. Reduced medico-legal risk by compliance with obstetric clinical pathways: a case-control study. Obstet Gynecol 2003; 101:751–755. [II-2]

How to "Read" This Book

The knowledge from randomized controlled trials (RCTs) and meta-analyses is summarized and easily available for clinical implementation. Key management points are highlighted at the beginning of each guideline, and in bold in the text. Relative risks and 95% confidence intervals from studies are generally not quoted, unless trends were evident. Instead, the straight recommendation for care is made if one intervention is superior to the other, with the percent improvement often quoted to assess degree of benefit. If there is insufficient evidence to compare to interventions or managements, this is clearly stated.

References: Cochrane reviews with 0 RCT are not referenced, and, instead of referencing a meta-analysis with only one RCT, the actual RCT is usually referenced. RCTs that are already included in meta-analyses are not referenced, for brevity and because they can be easily accessed by reviewing the meta-analysis. If new RCTs are not included in meta-analysis, they are obviously referenced. Each reference was reviewed and evaluated for quality according to a modified method as outlined by the U.S. Preventive Services Task Force (http://www.ahrq.gov):

I	Evidence obtained from at least one properly designed randomized controlled trial.
II-1	Evidence obtained from well-designed controlled trials without randomization.
II-2	Evidence obtained from well-designed cohort or case-control analytic studies, preferably from more than one center or research group.
II-3	Evidence obtained from multiple time series with or without the intervention. Dramatic results in uncontrolled experiments could also be regarded as this type of evidence.
III (Review)	Opinions of respected authorities, based on clinical experience, descriptive studies, or reports of expert committees.

These levels are quoted after each reference. For RCTs and meta-analyses, the number of subjects studied is stated, and, sometimes, more details are provided to aid the reader to understand the study better.

Contents

Part I: Maternal Medical Complications

Cardiology

Endocrinology and Metabolism

Gastroenterology

Hematology

Nephrology

Neurology

Psychiatry and Abuse

Pulmonology

Rheumatology

Thromboembolic Disease

Infectious Diseases

Contributors

James A. Airoldi MD, MPH Division of Maternal Fetal Medicine, St. Luke's Hospital and Health Network, Bethlehem, Pennsylvania, U.S.A.

Vincent T. Armenti MD, PhD Department of Surgery, Jefferson Medical College of Thomas Jefferson University, Philadelphia, Pennsylvania, U.S.A.

Joshua H. Barash MD Department of Family and Community Medicine, Jefferson Medical College of Thomas Jefferson University, Philadelphia, Pennsylvania, U.S.A.

Jason K. Baxter MD, MSCP, FACOG Division of Maternal-Fetal Medicine, Jefferson Medical College of Thomas Jefferson University, Philadelphia, Pennsylvania, U.S.A.

Madeleine Becker MD Department of Psychiatry, Thomas Jefferson University Hospital, Philadelphia, Pennsylvania, U.S.A.

Meriem Bensalem-Owen MD Department of Neurology, University of Kentucky, Lexington, Kentucky, U.S.A.

Vincenzo Berghella MD, FACOG Division of Maternal-Fetal Medicine, Jefferson Medical College of Thomas Jefferson University, Philadelphia, Pennsylvania, U.S.A.

Michelle Broetzman MD Division of Pediatrics, Aurora Bay Care Medical Center, Green Bay, Wisconsin, U.S.A.

Edward M. Buchanan MD Department of Family and Community Medicine, Jefferson Medical College of Thomas Jefferson University, Philadelphia, Pennsylvania, U.S.A.

Elyce Cardonick MD Division of Maternal-Fetal Medicine, Robert Wood Johnson Medical School, New Brunswick, New Jersey, U.S.A.

Suneet P. Chauhan MD Division of Maternal-Fetal Medicine, Eastern Virginia Medical School, Norfolk, Virginia, U.S.A.

Cuckoo Choudhary MD Division of Gastroenterology, Department of Internal Medicine, Jefferson Medical College of Thomas Jefferson University, Philadelphia, Pennsylvania, U.S.A.

Geeta Chhibber MD Holy Redeemer Hospital and Medical Center, Meadowbrook, Pennsylvania, U.S.A.

Dana Correale MD Private Practice, Cheshire, Connecticut, U.S.A.

Amanda Cotter MD Department of Obstetrics and Gynaecology, Graduate Entry Medical School, University of Limerick, Limerick, Ireland.

Lex Denysenko MD Psychosomatic Medicine, Thomas Jefferson University, Philadelphia, Pennsylvania, U.S.A.

Cataldo Doria MD, PhD Department of Surgery, Jefferson Medical College of Thomas Jefferson University, Philadelphia, Pennsylvania, U.S.A.

Jeffrey Ecker MD Vincent Memorial Obstetric Service, Massachusetts General Hospital, Harvard Medical School, Boston, Massachusetts, U.S.A.

Henry L. Galan MD Division of Maternal Fetal Medicine, University of Colorado, Aurora, Colorado, U.S.A.

Alessandro Ghidini MD The Brock Family Perinatal Diagnostic Center, Alexandria, Virginia, U.S.A.

Maria A. Giraldo-Isaza MD Division of Maternal-Fetal Medicine, Jefferson Medical College of Thomas Jefferson University, Philadelphia, Pennsylvania, U.S.A.

Ricardo Gómez MD Center for Perinatal Diagnosis and Research (CEDIP), Pedro Hurtado Hospital, Universidad del Desarrollo; and Chief of Ultrasound, Clinica Santa Maria, Santiago, Chile.

Christopher R. Harman MD Division of Maternal-Fetal Medicine, University of Maryland Medical Center, Baltimore, Maryland, U.S.A.

Laura A. Hart MD Department of Obstetrics and Gynecology, Drexel University College of Medicine, Philadelphia, Pennsylvania, U.S.A.

Edward J. Hayes MD, MSCP Division of Maternal-Fetal Medicine, Aurora Bay Care Medical Center, Green Bay, Wisconsin, U.S.A.

Steven K. Herrine MD Division of Gastroenterology and Hepatology, Thomas Jefferson University, Philadelphia, Pennsylvania, U.S.A.

Christina M. Hillson MD Department of Family and Community Medicine, Jefferson Medical College of Thomas Jefferson University, Philadelphia, Pennsylvania, U.S.A.

Priyadarshini Koduri MD Division of Maternal-Fetal Medicine, Jefferson Medical College of Thomas Jefferson University, Philadelphia, Pennsylvania, U.S.A.

Elisabeth J. S. Kunkel MD Department of Psychiatry, Thomas Jefferson University Hospital, Philadelphia, Pennsylvania, U.S.A.

Juan Pedro Kusanovic MD Perinatal Research Center, Sótero del Rió Hospital, Universidad Católica del Chile, Santiago, Chile

Jason B. Lee MD Department of Dermatology and Cutaneous Biology at Thomas Jefferson University Hospital and Jefferson Dermatology Associates, Philadelphia, Pennsylvania, U.S.A.

Cassie Leonard MD Department of Obstetrics and Gynecology, West Virginia University Hospital, Morgantown, West Virginia, U.S.A.

Keren Lerner MD Department of Obstetrics and Gynecology, Drexel University College of Medicine, Philadelphia, Pennsylvania, U.S.A.

Dawnette Lewis MD, MPH Division Maternal-Fetal Medicine, SUNY Downstate Medical Center, and University Hospital of Brooklyn, Long Island College Hospital, Brooklyn, New York, U.S.A.

A. Dhanya Mackeen MD, MPH Division of Maternal Fetal Medicine, Jefferson Medical College of Thomas Jefferson University, Philadelphia, Pennsylvania, U.S.A.

Everett F. Magann MD Maternal Fetal Medicine, University of Arkansas for the Medical Sciences, Little Rock, Arkansas, U.S.A.

Melissa I. March MD Division of Maternal-Fetal Medicine, Beth Israel Deaconess Medical Center, Boston, Massachusetts, U.S.A.

Giancarlo Mari MD Division of Maternal-Fetal Medicine, University of Tennessee Health Science Center, Memphis, Tennessee, U.S.A.

Luis Medina MD Center for Perinatal Diagnosis and Research (CEDIP), Sótero del Rió Hospital, Universidad Católica del Chile, Santiago, Chile

Maria Teresa Mella MD Department of Obstetrics and Gynecology, Jefferson Medical College of Thomas Jefferson University, Philadelphia, Pennsylvania, U.S.A.

M. Kathryn Menard MD, MPH Division of Maternal and Fetal Medicine, and Center for Maternal and Infant Health, University of North Carolina School of Medicine, Chapel Hill, North Carolina, U.S.A.

Michael J. Moritz MD Department of Surgery, Lehigh Valley Health Network, Allentown, Pennsylvania, U.S.A.

Sara Nicholas MD Division of Maternal-Fetal Medicine, Jefferson Medical College of Thomas Jefferson University, Philadelphia, Pennsylvania, U.S.A.

Aisha Nnoli MD People's Community Health Center/University of Maryland Affiliated Hospitals, and Department of Obstetrics and Gynecology, Harbor Hospitals, Baltimore, Maryland, U.S.A.

A. Marie O'Neill MD Division of Maternal-Fetal Medicine, Cooper Hospital Camden, New Jersey, U.S.A.

Britta Panda MD, PhD Vincent Memorial Obstetric Service, Massachusetts General Hospital, Harvard Medical School, Boston, Massachusetts, U.S.A.

Leonardo Pereira MD, MCR Division of Maternal-Fetal Medicine, Oregon Health & Science University, Portland, Oregon, U.S.A.

Lauren A. Plante MD Departments of Obstetrics and Gynecology and Anesthesiology, Drexel University College of Medicine, Philadelphia, Pennsylvania, U.S.A.

Sarah Poggi MD The Brock Perinatal Diagnostic Center, Alexandria, Virginia, U.S.A.

Sushma Potti MD Division of Maternal-Fetal Medicine, Jefferson Medical College of Thomas Jefferson University, Philadelphia, Pennsylvania, U.S.A.

Timothy J. Rafael MD Division of Maternal-Fetal Medicine, Department of Obstetrics and Gynecology, Winthrop University Hospital, Mineola, New York, U.S.A.

Carlo B. Ramirez MD Department of Surgery, Jefferson Medical College of Thomas Jefferson University, Philadelphia, Pennsylvania, U.S.A.

Uma M. Reddy MD, MPH Pregnancy and Perinatology Branch, NICHD, NIH, Bethesda, Maryland, U.S.A.

Shane Reeves MD Division of Maternal Fetal Medicine, University of Colorado, Aurora, Colorado, U.S.A.

Sharon Rubin MD Advanced Heart Failure and Transplant Center, Jefferson Heart Institute, Thomas Jefferson University, Philadelphia, Pennsylvania, U.S.A.

Joya Sahu MD Jefferson Dermatology Associates, Philadelphia, Pennsylvania, U.S.A.

Jacques E. Samson MD Division of Maternal-Fetal Medicine, University of Tennessee Health Science Center, Memphis, Tennessee, U.S.A.

Neil S. Seligman MD Division of Maternal-Fetal Medicine, University of Rochester Medical Center, Rochester, New York, U.S.A.

Viola Seravalli MD Department of Woman and Child Health, Section of Gynecology and Obstetrics, Careggi University Hospital, Florence, Italy

Shailen Shah MD Virtua Maternal Fetal Medicine Unit, Voorhees, New Jersey, and Thomas Jefferson University Hospital, Philadelphia, Pennsylvania, U.S.A.

William R. Short MD Division of Infectious Diseases, Jefferson Medical College of Thomas Jefferson University, Philadelphia, Pennsylvania, U.S.A.

Stephen Silberstein MD Jefferson Headache Center, Thomas Jefferson University Philadelphia, Pennsylvania, U.S.A.

Neil Silverman MD Division of Maternal-Fetal Medicine, David Geffen School of Medicine at UCLA, Los Angeles, California, U.S.A.

Robert A. Strauss MD Division of Maternal and Fetal Medicine, University of North Carolina School of Medicine, Chapel Hill, North Carolina, U.S.A.

Jorge E. Tolosa MD, MSCE Division of Maternal-Fetal Medicine, Department of Obstetrics and Gynecology, Oregon Health and Science University, Portland, Oregon, U.S.A.

Patrice M. L. Trauffer MD Mercer Perinatal Group, Capital Health Systems, Mercer Campus, Trenton, New Jersey, U.S.A.

Jeroen Vanderhoeven MD Division of Maternal-Fetal Medicine, Department of Obstetrics and Gynecology, University of Washington, Seattle, Washington, DC, U.S.A.

Tal Weinberger MD Department of Psychiatry, Thomas Jefferson University Hospital, Philadelphia, Pennsylvania, U.S.A.

List of Abbreviations

Ab	antibody
AC	abdominal circumference
ACA	anticardiolipin antibody
ACOG	American College of Obstetricians and Gynecologists
ACS	acute chest syndrome
ADR	autosomic dysreflexia
AF	amniotic fluid
AFI	amniotic fluid index
AFP	alpha-fetoprotein
AFV	amniotic fluid volume
Ag	antigen
AIDS	acquired immune deficiency syndrome
ALT	alanine aminotransferase
ANA	antinuclear antibodies
aPT	activated prothrombin time
APS	antiphospholipid syndrome
aPTT	activated partial thromboplastin time
AROM	artificial rupture of membranes
ART	assisted reproductive technologies
ARV	antiretroviral therapy
ASA	aspirin
ASD	atrial septal defect
AST	aspartate aminotransferase
AT III	antithrombin III
AZT	ziduvudine
bid	"bis in die," i.e., twice per day
BPD	biparietal diameter
BPD	bronchopulmonary dysplasia
BPP	biophysical profile
BMI	body mass index
BP	blood pressure
CAP	community-acquired pneumonia
CBC	complete blood count
CDC	Center for Disease Control
CF	cystic fibrosis
CHD	congenital heart defect
CL	cervical length
CMV	cytomegalovirus
CNS	central nervous system
CRL	crown-rump length
CSE	combined spinal epidural
CSF	cerebrospinal fluid
CT	computerized tomography
CVS	chorionic villus sampling
DES	diethylstilbestrol
DIC	disseminated intravascular coagulation
DM	diabetes mellitus
DNA	deoxyribonucleic acid
DRVVT	dilute Russell's viper venom time
DV	ductus venosus
DVP	deepest vertical pocket
DVT	deep vein thrombosis
ECV	external cephalic version
EDC	estimated date of confinement
EDD	estimated date of delivery (synonym of EDC)

EKG	electrocardiogram
FBS	fetal blood sampling
FDA	Food and Drug Administration
FFN	fetal fibronectin
FGR	fetal growth restriction
FHR	fetal heart rate
FISH	fluorescent in situ hybridization
FLM	fetal lung maturity
FOB	father of baby
FPR	false positive rate
FTS	first-trimester screening
FVL	factor V Leiden
g	grams
GA	gestational age
GBS	group B streptococcus
GDM	gestational diabetes
GI	gastrointestinal
HAART	highly active antiretroviral therapy
HAV	hepatitis A virus
HBV	hepatitis B virus
HBsAg	hepatitis B surface antigen
HCG	human chorionic gonadotroponin
Hct	hematocrit
HCV	hepatitis C virus
HG	hyperemesis gravidarum
Hgb	hemoglobin
HIE	hypoxic-ischemic encephalopathy
HIV	human immunodeficiency virus
HR	heart rate
HSV	herpes simplex virus
HTN	hypertension
ICU	intensive care unit
IUGR	intrauterine growth restriction (synonym of FGR)
IV	intravenous
IVH	intraventricular hemorrhage
L&D	labor and delivery floor
LA	lupus anticoagulant
Lab	laboratory
LFT	liver function tests
LMP	last menstrual period
LBW	low birth weight (infants)
LMW	low molecular weight
LMWH	low-molecular-weight heparin
LR	likelihood ratio
MAS	meconium aspiration syndrome
MCA	middle cerebral artery
MCV	mean corpuscular volume
MOM	multiple of the median
MRI	magnetic resonance imaging
MTHFR	methylenetetrahydrofolate reductase
MVP	maximum vertical pocket
NA	not available
NAIT	neonatal alloimmune thrombocytopenia
NEC	necrotizing enterocolitis
NIH	National Institute of Health
NIH	nonimmune hydrops
NRFS	nonreassuring fetal status
NRFHR	nonreassuring fetal heart rate
NRFHT	nonreassuring fetal heart testing
NSAIDS	nonsteroidal anti-inflammatory drugs
NT	nuchal translucency
NTD	neural tube defects
NST	nonstress test
n/v	nausea and/or vomiting

OR	operating room
PC	protein C
PCR	polymerase chain reaction
PE	pulmonary embolus
PFT	pulmonary function tests
PGM	prothrombin gene mutation
PID	pelvic inflammatory disease
PL	pregnancy loss
PNC	prenatal care
po	"per os," i.e., by mouth
PPH	postpartum hemorrhage
PRCD	planned repeat cesarean delivery
PS	protein S
PT	prothrombin time
PTB	preterm birth
PTT	partial thromboplastin time
PPROM	preterm premature rupture of membranes
pRBC	packed red blood cells
PROM	preterm rupture of membranes
PSV	peak systolic velocity
PTL	preterm labor
PTU	propylthiouracil
PUBS	percutaneous umbilical blood sampling
qd	once a day
qid	four times per day
qhs	before bedtime
QS	quadruple screen
RBC	red blood cell
RCT	randomized controlled study
RDS	respiratory distress syndrome
RNA	ribonucleic acid
ROM	rupture of membranes
RPR	rapid plasma reagin
RR	respiratory rate
Rx	treatment
SAB	spontaneous abortion
SC	subcutaneous
SCI	spinal cord injury
SDP	single deepest pocket
SIDS	sudden infant death syndrome
SLE	systemic lupus erythematosus
SPTB	spontaneous preterm birth
STD	sexually transmitted diseases (synonym of STI)
STI	sexually transmitted infections
STS	second-trimester screening
TB	tuberculosis
TG	*Toxoplasma gondii*
tid	three times per day
TOL	trial of labor
TRAP	twin reversal arterial perfusion
TSH	thyroid-stimulating hormone
TSI	thyroid-stimulating immune globulins
TTTS	twin-twin transfusion syndrome
TVU	transvaginal ultrasound
UA	umbilical artery
UFH	unfractionated heparin
U/S (or u/s)	ultrasound
VBAC	vaginal birth after cesarean
VDRL	venereal disease research laboratory
VSD	ventricular septal defect
VTE	venous thromboembolism
WHO	World Health Organization

Hypertensive disorders[a]

Viola Seravalli and Jason K. Baxter

CHRONIC HYPERTENSION
Key Points

- Chronic hypertension (HTN) is defined as either a **history of hypertension preceding the pregnancy** or a **blood pressure (BP) ≥140/90 prior to 20 weeks' gestation.**
- **Severe HTN** has been defined as systolic blood pressure (SBP) ≥160 mmHg or diastolic blood pressure (DBP) ≥110 mmHg. **High-risk** HTN has been defined in pregnancy as that associated with **secondary hypertension, target organ damage (left ventricular dysfunction, retinopathy, dyslipidemia, microvascular disease, prior stroke), maternal age >40, previous pregnancy loss, SBP ≥180, or DBP ≥110 mmHg.**
- **Complications** of chronic HTN include (maternal) **worsening HTN; superimposed preeclampsia; severe preeclampsia; eclampsia, HELLP** (Hemolysis, Elevated Liver enzymes and Low Platelet count) **syndrome; cesarean delivery,** and (uncommonly) **pulmonary edema, hypertensive encephalopathy, retinopathy, cerebral hemorrhage, and acute renal failure,** and (fetal) **growth restriction (FGR); oligohydramnios; placental abruption; preterm birth (PTB); and perinatal death.**
- **Prevention** (mostly prepregnancy) consists of **exercise, weight reduction, proper diet,** and **restriction of sodium intake.**
- In addition to **history** and **physical examination, initial evaluation** may include **liver function tests (LFTs), platelet count, creatinine, urine analysis, 24-hour urine for total protein (and creatinine clearance).** Women with high-risk, severe, or long-standing HTN may need an electrocardiogram (EKG) and echocardiogram, as well. If hypertension is newly diagnosed and has not been evaluated previously, a medical consult may be indicated to assess for possible etiologic factors (renal artery stenosis, pheochromocytoma, hyperaldosteronism, etc.).
- There is **insufficient evidence** to assess **bed rest** for managing HTN in pregnancy.
- Blood pressure decreases physiologically in the first and second trimester in pregnancy, especially in women with HTN. **As blood pressure is usually <140/90 mmHg at the first visit for hypertensive women, often antihypertensive drugs do not need to be increased.** BP will usually increase again in the third trimester, leading to workup for preeclampsia and, if absent, restarting of antihypertensive drugs. **So antihypertensive medications should probably be started (or increased, modified) in pregnancy only** when SBP ≥160 or DBP ≥100 on two occasions. **The goal is usually to maintain a BP of around 140–150/90–100 mmHg. With end-organ damage such as renal disease, diabetes with vascular disease, or left ventricular dysfunction, these thresholds should probably be lowered to <140/90.**
- On the basis of limited trial data, **labetalol** is considered **the current antihypertensive drug of choice** by many experts. Dosing can start at 100 mg twice a day, with a maximum dose of 1200 mg twice a day. **Nifedipine** is a reasonable **alternative,** started at 10 mg twice a day, with a maximum dose of 120 mg/day. Angiotensin-converting enzyme **(ACE) inhibitors are contraindicated** in pregnancy.

Diagnosis/Definition (Table 1.1)

Chronic hypertension in pregnancy is defined as either a **history of hypertension preceding the pregnancy** or a **blood pressure ≥140/90 prior to 20 weeks' gestation.** Though controversial, the 5th Korotkoff sound is used for the diastolic reading. Blood pressure measurements can be obtained using a manual or an automated cuff with the patient in the sitting position. Severe hypertension is defined as SBP ≥160 mmHg or DBP ≥110 mmHg. In **nonpregnant** adults, BP < 120/80 mmHg is normal, BP 120–139/80–89 mmHg is prehypertension, BP 140–159/90–99 is stage 1 hypertension, and BP ≥160/100 mmHg is stage 2 hypertension.

Epidemiology/Incidence

Hypertension occurs in about **1% to 5%** of pregnant women. Hypertension in pregnancy is the second leading cause of maternal mortality in the United States, accounting for about 15% of such deaths. Hypertensive disorders such as hypertension, gestational hypertension, preeclampsia, or HELLP syndrome occur in 12% to 22% of pregnancies.

Etiology/Basic Pathophysiology

Hypertension mostly develops as a complex quantitative trait affected by both genetic and environmental factors.

Classification

Severe HTN has been defined as SBP ≥160 mmHg, or DBP ≥110 mmHg (1). **High-risk** HTN has been defined in pregnancy as that associated with **secondary hypertension, target organ damage (left ventricular dysfunction, retinopathy, dyslipidemia, maternal age >40 years, microvascular disease, prior stroke), previous loss, SBP ≥180 mmHg or DBP ≥110 mmHg.** For gestational HTN, see below.

---

[a]Hypertensive disorders of pregnancy include chronic hypertension, gestational hypertension, preeclampsia, HELLP syndrome, and eclampsia.

Table 1.1 Definitions and Diagnostic Criteria for Hypertensive Disorders of Pregnancy

Chronic hypertension in pregnancy

Either a history of hypertension (HTN) preceding the pregnancy or a blood pressure ≥140/90 prior to 20 weeks' gestation

Gestational Hypertension

Sustained (on at least two occasions, 6 hr apart) BP ≥140/90 after 20 wk, without proteinuria, other signs or symptoms of preeclampsia, or a prior history of HTN.

Preeclampsia

Sustained (at least twice, 6 hr but not >7 days apart) BP ≥ 140/90 mmHg and proteinuria (≥300 mg in 24 hr in a woman without prior proteinuria) after 20 wk of gestation in a woman with previously normal blood pressure

Superimposed preeclampsia

One or more of the following criteria:
- Proteinuria (≥300 mg in 24 hr in a woman without prior proteinuria) after 20 wk in a woman with chronic HTN.
- If hypertension and proteinuria present before 20 weeks' gestation,
  - a sudden increase in proteinuria
  - a sudden increase in hypertension
  - platelet count <100,000/mm^3
  - increased hepatic transaminases (AST and/or ALT ≥70 IU/L)

Severe preeclampsia

Preeclampsia, with any one of the following criteria:
- BP ≥ 160/110 mmHg (two occasions, ≥6 hr apart)
- Proteinuria ≥5 g in a 24-hr urine specimen (some use also ≥3+ on two random urine samples collected at least 4 hr apart)
- Platelets <100,000/mm^3 (and/or evidence of microangiopathic hemolytic anemia)
- Increased hepatic transaminases (AST and/or ALT ≥70 IU/L)
- Persistent headache or other cerebral or visual disturbances (including grand mal seizures)
- Persistent epigastric (or right upper quadrant) pain
- Pulmonary edema or cyanosis
- Oliguria (<500 mL urine in 24 hr)

HELLP syndrome

Tennessee Classification (most commonly used)
- **Hemolysis** as evidenced by an abnormal peripheral smear in addition to either serum LDH >600 IU/L, or total bilirubin ≥1.2 mg/dL (≥20.52 μmol/L)
- Elevated liver enzymes, as evidenced by an **AST** or **ALT** **≥70 IU/L**
- **Platelets <100,000 cells/mm^3**.

If all the criteria are met, the syndrome is defined "complete"; if only one or two criteria are present, the term "partial HELLP" is preferred.

Subclassification: Mississippi HELLP Classification System
- Class 1: HELLP syndrome (severe thrombocytopenia): platelet count ≤50,000 cells/mm^3 + LDH >600 IU/L and AST or ALT ≥70 IU/L
- Class 2: HELLP syndrome (moderate thrombocytopenia): platelet count >50,000 but ≤100,000 cells/mm^3 + LDH >600 IU/L and AST or ALT ≥70 IU/L
- Class 3: HELLP syndrome (mild thrombocytopenia): platelet count >100,000 but ≤150,000 cells/mm^3 + LDH >600 IU/L and AST or ALT ≥40 IU/L

Eclampsia

- Seizures in the presence of preeclampsia and/or HELLP syndrome.

Abbreviations: ALT, alanine aminotransferase; AST, aspartate aminotransferase; BP, blood pressure; HELLP, hemolysis, elevated liver enzymes, low platelets; LDH, lactase dehydrogenase; wk, weeks.

Risk Factors/Associations

Renal disease; collagen vascular disease; antiphospholipid syndrome; diabetes; and other disorders such as thyrotoxicosis, Cushing's disease, hyperaldosteronism, pheochromocytoma, or coarctation of the aorta.

Complications

Maternal

Worsening HTN, superimposed preeclampsia (20%), severe preeclampsia, eclampsia, HELLP syndrome, and cesarean delivery. Pulmonary edema, hypertensive encephalopathy,

retinopathy, cerebral hemorrhage, and acute renal failure are uncommon, but more common with severe HTN (2).

Fetal
Growth restriction (8–15%); **oligohydramnios, placental abruption** (0.7–1.5%, about a twofold increase), **PTB** (12–34%), and **perinatal death** (two- to fourfold increase). All of these complications have higher incidences with severe or high-risk hypertension.

Management
Principles
Pregnancy is characterized by increased blood volume, decreased colloid oncotic pressure (see also chap. 3, *Obstetric Evidence-Based Guidelines*). Physiologic BP decrease in first and second trimester may mask chronic HTN.

Initial Evaluation/Workup
　　History. Antihypertensive drugs, prior workup, end-organ damage, prior obstetrical history.
　　Physical examination. Blood pressure, edema.
　　Laboratory tests. Baseline values may be useful to be able to compare in cases of possible later preeclampsia, **LFTs, platelets, creatinine, urine analysis, 24-hour urine for total protein (and creatinine clearance),** antinuclear antibodies (ANA), anticardiolipin antibody (ACA), and lupus anticoagulant (LA) (see also chap. 23). An early glucose challenge test may be indicated. Coagulation studies (especially fibrinogen) are usually not indicated, except in specific severe cases. Creatinine clearance (mL/min) is calculated as follows:

$$\frac{\text{Urine creatinine}(\text{mg/dL}) \times \text{Total urine volume (mL)}}{\text{Serum}(\text{mg/dL}) \times 1440 \text{ minutes}}$$

　　Other tests. Maternal **EKG, echocardiogram, and ophthalmological examination** are suggested, especially in women with long-standing, high-risk, or severe hypertension.

Workup
It is important to identify cardiovascular risk factors or any reversible cause of hypertension, and assess for target organ damage or cardiovascular disease. Reversible causes include chronic kidney disease, coarctation of the aorta, Cushing's syndrome, drug-induced/related causes, pheochromocytoma, hyperaldosteronism, renovascular hypertension (renal artery stenosis), thyroid/parathyroid disease, and sleep apnea. If hypertension is newly diagnosed and has not been evaluated previously, a medical consult may be indicated to assess for any of these factors. Secondary hypertension, target organ damage (left ventricular dysfunction, retinopathy, dyslipidemia, maternal age >40 years, microvascular disease, prior stroke), previous loss, SBP ≥180 or DBP ≥110 mmHg are associated with higher risks in pregnancy.

Prevention
In women with mild hypertension, gestational hypertensive disorders, or a family history of hypertensive disorders, 30 minutes of **exercise** three times a week may decrease DBP, as per a very small trial (3). **Weight reduction** preconception is recommended if overweight or obese. A **proper diet** should be rich in fruits, vegetables, and low-fat dairy foods, with reduced saturated and total fats. **Restriction of sodium intake**

to <2.4-g sodium daily intake, recommended for essential hypertension, is beneficial in nonpregnant adults. Use of alcohol and tobacco is strongly discouraged.

Screening/Diagnosis
Initial BP evaluation may help to identify women with chronic hypertension, while third-trimester blood pressure readings aid in preeclampsia screening. **A BP of ≥120/80 mmHg in the first or second trimester is not normal,** and associated with later risks of preeclampsia. **Blood pressure should be taken properly.** Appropriate measurement of BP includes using Korotkoff phase V, appropriate cuff size (length 1.5 × upper-arm circumference, or a cuff with a bladder that encircles ≥80% of the arm), and position, so that the woman's arm is at the level of the heart (sitting up), at rest.

Preconception Counseling
There are significant risks associated with hypertension and preeclampsia in pregnancy. All women should be counseled appropriately regarding the possible complications and preventive and management strategies for hypertensive disorders in pregnancy. ACE inhibitors and angiotensin type II (AII) receptor antagonists should be discontinued. A complete evaluation and workup, as described above, should be done, especially if she has a several-year history of hypertension and/or hypertension never fully evaluated. Baseline tests can also be obtained for later comparison. Abnormalities should be addressed and managed appropriately (see specific chapters). If, for example, serum creatinine (Cr) is >1.4 mg/dL, the woman should be aware of increased risks in pregnancy (pregnancy/fetal loss, reduced birth weight, preterm delivery, and accelerated deterioration of maternal renal disease). Even mild renal disease (Cr = 1.1–1.4 mg/dL) with uncontrolled HTN is associated with 10 times higher risk of fetal loss (see chap. 17).

Prenatal Care
Often BP monitoring at home is suggested in pregnancies with HTN. At present, the possible advantages and risks of ambulatory blood pressure monitoring during pregnancy, in particular in hypertensive pregnant women, cannot be defined, since there is no randomized controlled trial (RCT) evidence to support the use of ambulatory BP monitoring during pregnancy (4).

Therapy
　　Lifestyle changes and bed rest. There are no trials to assess lifestyle changes other than bed rest in pregnancy. Weight reduction is not recommended. The diet should be rich in fruits, vegetables, low-fat dairy foods, with reduced saturated and total fats and with sodium intake restricted to <2.4-g sodium daily.
　　There is **insufficient evidence** to demonstrate any differences between bed rest (in or out of the hospital) for reported outcomes overall. Compared with routine activity at home, some bed rest in hospital for **nonproteinuric hypertension** is associated with a 42% reduced risk of severe hypertension and a borderline 47% reduction in risk of PTB in one trial (5). The trial did not address possible adverse effects of bed rest. Three times more women in the bed rest group opted **not** to have the same management in future pregnancies, if the choice is given. There are no significant differences for any other outcomes (5).

Antihypertensive drugs.
Common types

- *Methyldopa (Aldomet)*: This drug was the preferred first-line agent historically, since it is associated with stable uteroplacental blood flow and fetal hemodynamics, and no long-term adverse effects are seen in exposed children (up to 7.5 years; best documentation of fetal safety of any antihypertensive drug). Liver disease is a contraindication. Initial dose is usually 250 mg two to three times a day, with highest dose 500 mg four times a day (2 g/day). Side effects include dry mouth and drowsiness/somnolence.

- *Labetalol (alpha- and beta-blocker)*: On the basis of limited trial data (see below), labetalol is the **current drug of choice** of many experts (1). Dosing can start at 100 mg twice a day, with maximum dose of 1200 mg twice a day. As with other drugs, generally a different agent should not be added until maximum doses of the first drug are achieved.

- *Beta-blockers*: Atenolol has been associated with FGR in pregnancy compared to placebo, and with higher mortality in nonpregnant adults compared to other agents, and should probably be avoided. There is insufficient evidence to assess if other drugs in this class (or even other classes) are associated with the same effect (see below).

- *Calcium channel blockers (especially nifedipine)*: There is no known association with birth defects, with reassuring long-term follow-up of babies up to 1.5 years. Nifedipine can be started at 10 mg twice a day, with maximum dose 120 mg/day. Long-acting nifedipine XL can be started at 30 mg, with 120 mg as maximum dose. Very rare cases of neuromuscular blockade have been reported when nifedipine is used simultaneously with magnesium sulfate. This blockade is reversible with 10% solution of calcium gluconate.

- *Diuretics*: Women who use diuretics from early in pregnancy do not have the physiologic increase in plasma volume, which poses a theoretical concern since preeclampsia is associated with reduced plasma volume. Nonetheless, the reduction in plasma volume associated with diuretics has not been associated with adverse effects on outcomes. Diuretics are not contraindicated in pregnancy, except in settings where uteroplacental perfusion is already reduced (i.e., preeclampsia and FGR). This is usually the drug of first choice for some nonpregnant adults. The initial dose is usually 12.5 mg twice a day, with maximum dose 50 mg/day.

- *ACE inhibitor (or AII receptor antagonists)*: These drugs are contraindicated in the first trimester because they might be associated with a twofold increase in malformations, and later because they are associated with FGR, oligohydramnios, neonatal renal failure, and neonatal death.

Effectiveness
Mild-to-moderate HTN Mild-to-moderate HTN is usually defined in the trials as a SBP of 140 to 169 mmHg or a DBP of 90 to 109 mmHg. In pregnant women with **mild-to-moderate hypertension**, antihypertensive drugs are associated with a **50% reduction in the risk of developing severe hypertension**, which is expected given their effects in nonpregnant adults. There is **no difference in preeclampsia, PTB, small for gestational age (SGA), perinatal death** (nonsignificant 27% reduction), **or any other outcomes** (6). Improvement in control of maternal blood pressure with use of drugs would be worth-

while only if it were reflected in substantive benefits for mother and/or baby, and none have been clearly demonstrated.

Compared to placebo/no beta-blocker, oral beta-blockers decrease by 63% the risk of severe hypertension and by 56% the need for additional antihypertensives. Maternal hospital admission may be decreased, neonatal bradycardia increased, and respiratory distress syndrome decreased, but these outcomes are reported in only a small proportion of trials (7). There are insufficient data for conclusions about the effect on perinatal mortality or PTB (7). Compared to controls not taking antihypertensives, women receiving **beta-blockers** had a significant 38% increase in SGA birth weight and a threefold **increase** in **birth weight** <**5th percentile** (6,7). These data are partly dependent on one small outlying trial (6). **The woman's natural BP may be necessary for adequate placental perfusion, so that artificial lowering of the blood pressure may then impair fetal growth**. There is insufficient evidence to assess if beta-blockers are more detrimental in this respect than other antihypertensive regimes. Compared to methyldopa, beta-blockers appear to be more effective in reducing the risk of severe hypertension, without any clear difference in the risk of proteinuria/preeclampsia, and seem to be better tolerated by women than methyldopa (6). However, concerns remain about their possible role in the risk of having SGA babies. Single small trials have compared beta-blockers with hydralazine, nicardipine, or isradipine. It is unusual for women to change drugs because of side effects (7). Other outcomes are only reported by a small proportion of studies, and there are no clear differences. **There is insufficient evidence to conclude that one antihypertensive is better than another** (6).

As blood pressure is usually <**140/90 at the first visit for hypertensive women, antihypertensive drugs usually do not need to be increased, and can also be stopped.** Often BP will increase again in the third trimester, leading to workup for preeclampsia, and, if preeclampsia is absent, restarting of antihypertensive drugs. **So antihypertensive medications should probably be started (or increased, modified) in pregnancy only when SBP ≥160 mmHg or DBP ≥100 mmHg** on two occasions. This is to decrease the risk of cerebrovascular accidents, and cardiovascular (e.g., congestive heart failure) and renal complications. **The goal is to maintain BP around 140–150/90–100 mmHg. With end-organ damage (high-risk HTN), for example, renal disease, diabetes with vascular disease, or left ventricular dysfunction, these thresholds should probably be lowered to <140/90 mmHg.**

Severe HTN. Severe HTN is usually defined in the trials as **SBP ≥160 mmHg or DBP ≥110 mmHg**. There is insufficient evidence to assess benefits and risks of different antihypertensive drugs for severe HTN, as shown in a meta-analysis of 24 trials (8). Hydralazine is the most common drug evaluated in trials. Women allocated calcium channel blockers (nifedipine, nimodipine, nicardipine, or isradipine) rather than hydralazine are less likely to have persistent high BP. Compared with hydralazine, ketanserin is associated with more persistent high BP but less side effects and a lower risk of HELLP syndrome. The risk of persistent high BP is lower for nimodipine compared to magnesium sulfate, although nimodipine is associated with a higher risk of eclampsia. Labetalol is associated with a lower risk of hypotension and cesarean section than diazoxide (8). In a more recent trial not included in the meta-analysis, diazoxide is as safe and effective as hydralazine, and the mini-bolus doses of 15 mg of diazoxide does not precipitate maternal hypotension as previously described (9). There is **no clear evidence that one antihypertensive is preferable to the others for improving outcome for women with very high blood pressure during pregnancy.** Therefore, **the choice of antihypertensive should depend on the experience and familiarity of an individual clinician with a particular drug, and on what is known about adverse maternal and fetal side effects.** Three drugs **(high-dose diazoxide, ketanserin, and nimodipine) have serious disadvantages and so should probably be avoided** for women with very high blood pressure during pregnancy (8).

Antepartum Testing

Increased perinatal morbidity and mortality is mainly attributed to superimposed preeclampsia and/or FGR; therefore, look to detect these early. Initial **dating ultrasound,** preferably in the first trimester (FTS at 11–14 weeks), **anatomy ultrasound** at around 18 to 20 weeks, and **ultrasound for growth** at 28 to 32 weeks are suggested (see also chap. 4, *Obstetric Evidence-Based Guidelines*).

Antenatal testing (usually with weekly nonstress tests) is suggested starting around 32 weeks, especially if poorly controlled or severe HTN, FGR, or preeclampsia is indicated. Umbilical artery Doppler is recommended in cases of FGR (see chap. 44). For uterine artery Doppler, see section "Preeclampsia."

Delivery

Often PTB (either spontaneous or iatrogenic) occurs because of complications. In the uncomplicated pregnancy with hypertension, the pregnancy should probably be delivered by the estimated date of confinement (EDC). Unfortunately, there are no RCT evaluating timing of delivery for women with chronic HTN. In a large population-based cohort study, among women with otherwise uncomplicated chronic hypertension, **delivery at 38 or 39 weeks** appears to provide the optimal trade-off between the risk of adverse fetal and adverse neonatal outcomes. The risk of stillbirth is significantly higher at 41 weeks (10).

Anesthesia

See section "Preeclampsia," and also chap. 11, *Obstetric Evidence-Based Guidelines*.

Postpartum/Breast-feeding

Methyldopa, labetalol, beta-blockers, calcium channel blockers, and most other agents are safe with breast-feeding, with the possible exception of ACE inhibitors, because even low concentrations in breast milk could affect neonatal renal function.

GESTATIONAL HYPERTENSION
Definition (Table 1.1)

Gestational HTN, formerly known as pregnancy-induced hypertension, is defined as sustained (on at least two occasions, 6 hours apart) BP ≥140/90 after 20 weeks, without proteinuria, other signs or symptoms of preeclampsia, or a prior history of HTN. Severe gestational HTN is defined similarly, except that the cutoffs are ≥160/110 mmHg.

Incidence

About 6% to 17% healthy nulliparous women.

Complications and Management

This condition is usually associated with good outcomes, similar to low-risk pregnant women (11), so that **close surveillance for development of preeclampsia,** but no other intervention, is usually needed. Severe gestational HTN is associated with higher morbidities than mild preeclampsia, with incidences of abruption, PTB, and SGA, similar to severe preeclampsia. If gestational HTN develops before 30 weeks or is severe, there is a high (50%) rate of progression to preeclampsia. Before 37 weeks, in **the absence of severe HTN,** or preterm labor, and in the presence of reassuring fetal testing, expectant management is suggested, with delivery for development of any severe preeclampsia criteria (see below).

Compared to expectant management, induction of labor in women with mostly (about 66%) gestational hypertension (or mild preeclampsia) at 36 to 41 weeks' gestation is associated with a trend for lower incidence of maternal complications (e.g., HELLP, severe HTN, and pulmonary edema) (RR 0.81, 95% CI 0.63–1.03), and lower incidence of neonatal pH <7.05 with induction of labor ≥37 weeks (12). Trends were seen for benefit of induction associated with less cesarean delivery and maternal ICU admission. Therefore, **delivery (usually by induction) even with just gestational HTN at about ≥37 weeks may be considered.**

PREECLAMPSIA
Key Points

- Preeclampsia is defined as sustained (at least twice, 6 hours but not >7 days apart) **BP ≥ 140/90** mmHg and **proteinuria (≥300 mg in 24 hours, without prior proteinuria) after 20 weeks of gestation in a woman with previously normal blood pressure.**
- **Superimposed preeclampsia** is defined as proteinuria (**≥300 mg in 24 hours, without prior proteinuria)** after 20 weeks in a woman with **chronic HTN.** In a woman with hypertension and proteinuria before 20 weeks' gestation, the criteria for the diagnosis are a sudden increase in proteinuria, a sudden increase in hypertension, or the development of HELLP syndrome.
- **Severe preeclampsia** is defined as preeclampsia with any of the following: BP ≥160/110 mmHg, proteinuria ≥5 g in 24 hours, platelets <100,000/mm³, aspartate aminotransferase (AST) and/or alanine aminotransferase (ALT) ≥70 IU/L, persistent headache or other cerebral or visual disturbances (including grand mal seizures), persistent epigastric (or right upper quadrant) pain, pulmonary edema, or oliguria (<500-mL urine/24 hr).
- **HELLP syndrome** is defined as **hemolysis, AST or ALT ≥70 IU/L, or platelets <100,000/mm³.**
- **Eclampsia** is defined as seizures in the presence of preeclampsia and/or HELLP syndrome.
- **Complications** of preeclampsia include (maternal) **HELLP syndrome,** disseminated intravascular coagulation **(DIC), pulmonary edema, abruptio placentae, renal failure, seizures** (eclampsia), **cerebral hemorrhage, liver hemorrhage,** and **PTB** (fetal/neonatal), **FGR, perinatal death, hypoxemia, or neurologic injury.**
- **Low-dose aspirin (75–150 mg/day)** given to women with **risk factors for preeclampsia** is associated with a **17% reduction** in the risk of **preeclampsia,** a small (8%) **reduction** in the risk of **PTB < 37 weeks,** a **10% reduction** in **SGA** babies, and a **14% reduction** in **perinatal deaths.**

- If low-dose aspirin is given anyway because of a history of preeclampsia, then uterine artery Doppler screening may not be necessary or beneficial. **Low-dose aspirin started early (≤16 weeks) in women with abnormal uterine Doppler is associated with a 90% reduction in severe preeclampsia, a 69% reduction in gestational hypertension, and a 49% reduction in intrauterine growth restriction (IUGR).** Aspirin treatment started after 16 weeks is not associated with a significant decrease in the incidence of preeclampsia or IUGR.
- **Calcium supplementation** is associated with a 35% **reduction in the incidence of high blood pressure** and a 55% **reduction in the risk of preeclampsia.** This effect is greatest in women with low baseline calcium intake or high risk of preeclampsia, in which calcium supplementation (1.5–2 g/day) may be indicated.
- **Antioxidant therapy with vitamin C** 1000 mg/day and **vitamin E** 400 IU/day starting in the early second trimester is not associated with a **reduction** in risk of **preeclampsia.** Given also the facts that the four largest most recent trials do not show any maternal or fetal benefit, and that in one of them the intervention is associated with an increased risk of fetal loss, perinatal death, premature rupture of membranes (PROM) and preterm premature rupture of membranes (PPROM), antioxidant therapy is **not recommended for prevention of preeclampsia.**
- Workup for preeclampsia should include, apart from history and physical examination (BP), **AST** and **ALT**, **platelets**, creatinine, and **24-hour urine for total protein** (and creatinine clearance). It is **important to know the baseline values;** hence, these tests should be obtained **at first prenatal visit** in women with risk factors.
- **Magnesium is the drug of choice for prevention of eclampsia,** as it is associated with a 59% **reduction in** the risk of **eclampsia,** a 36% reduction in **abruption,** and a nonstatistically significant but clinically important 46% reduction in **maternal death. The reduction is similar regardless of severity of preeclampsia,** with about 400 women who need to be treated to prevent eclampsia for mild preeclampsia, 71 for severe preeclampsia, and 36 for preeclampsia with central nervous system (CNS) symptoms. The **intravenous** route at **1 g/ hr is preferable, usually given at least in active labor and for 12 to 24 hours postpartum, but for a shorter or longer period depending on the severity of preeclampsia,** without mandatory serum monitoring.
- **Antihypertensive drugs** for the treatment of **severe HTN with preeclampsia** are usually **labetalol, nifedipine, or hydralazine. Severe preeclampsia at ≥34 weeks** warrants **expeditious delivery. Before 34 weeks, delivery within 48 hours after completion of corticosteroid administration** is suggested **for uncontrollable BP** in spite of continuing increase in antihypertensive drugs, **persistent headache and/or visual/CNS symptoms, epigastric pain, vaginal bleeding, persistent oliguria, preterm labor, PPROM, platelets <100,000/mm³ or elevated liver enzymes >70 IU/L (partial or complete HELLP syndrome), nonreassuring fetal heart rate, or reversed umbilical artery end-diastolic flow ≥ 32 weeks. Immediate delivery** even before completion of steroids is recommended in case of **eclampsia, pulmonary edema, acute renal failure, DIC, suspected abruptio placentae, or nonreassuring fetal status.**

- There is **insufficient evidence to recommend the use of dexamethasone or other steroids for therapy specific for HELLP syndrome.**
- In **about 15% of cases, hypertension or proteinuria** may be **absent before eclampsia. A high index of suspicion for eclampsia** should be maintained in **all cases of hypertensive disorders in pregnancy,** in particular those with **CNS symptoms (e.g., headache and visual disturbances).**
- In **eclampsia,** the first priorities are **airway, breathing, and circulation.**
- **Magnesium sulfate is the drug of choice for preventing recurrence of eclampsia,** as it is also associated with maternal and fetal/neonatal benefits compared to placebo, no treatment, or other treatments.
- Women with **prior preeclampsia or its complications** are not only at **increased risk of recurrence,** but also at **increased risk of cardiovascular disease in the future.**

Diagnoses/Definitions (Table 1.1)

Preeclampsia

Sustained (at least twice, 6 hours but not >7 days apart) **BP ≥140/90 mmHg and proteinuria (≥300 mg in 24 hours, without prior proteinuria) after 20 weeks of gestation in a woman with previously normal blood pressure** (13,14). BP should be measured with adequate cuff size, position of the heart at arm level, and with calibrated equipment. The accuracy of dipstick urinalysis with a 1+ (0.1 g/L) threshold as well as random protein-to-creatinine ratios in the prediction of significant proteinuria by 24-hour urine is poor (15). **Mild** preeclampsia is usually defined as preeclampsia not meeting severe criteria (see below). "Toxemia" is a lay term. The "30–15 rule" and edema have been eliminated as criteria to diagnose preeclampsia.

Superimposed Preeclampsia

One or more of the following criteria:

- Proteinuria (**≥300 mg in 24 hours, without prior proteinuria**) after 20 weeks in a woman with chronic HTN.
- If hypertension and proteinuria present before 20 weeks' gestation:
  - A sudden increase in proteinuria
  - A sudden increase in hypertension
  - Platelet count <100,000/mm³
  - Increased hepatic transaminases (AST and/or ALT ≥70 IU/L)

Severe Preeclampsia

Preeclampsia, with any one of the following criteria:

- BP ≥160/110 mmHg (two occasions, ≥6 hours apart)
- Proteinuria ≥5 g in a 24-hour urine specimen (some also use ≥3+ on two random urine samples collected at least 4 hours apart)
- Platelets <100,000/mm³ (and/or evidence of microangiopathic hemolytic anemia)
- Increased hepatic transaminases (AST and/or ALT ≥70 IU/L)
- Persistent headache or other cerebral or visual disturbances (including grand mal seizures)
- Persistent epigastric (or right upper quadrant) pain
- Pulmonary edema or cyanosis
- Oliguria (<500 mL urine in 24 hours)

An increased serum creatinine >1.2 mg/dL or other conditions are associated with worse outcomes with preeclampsia, but are not always considered criteria for severe preeclampsia.

HELLP Syndrome

For HELLP syndrome to be diagnosed, there must be microangiopathic hemolysis, thrombocytopenia, and abnormalities of liver function. There is no consensus, however, on the classification criteria and the specific thresholds of hematologic and biochemical values to use in establishing the diagnosis of HELLP syndrome. The following criteria are most commonly used (*Tennessee Classification*): **hemolysis** as evidenced by an abnormal peripheral smear in addition to either serum lactate dehydrogenase (LDH) >600 IU/L, or total bilirubin ≥1.2 mg/dL (≥20.52 μmol/L); elevated liver enzymes, as evidenced by an **AST** or **ALT** ≥**70 IU/L**, and **platelets** <**100,000 cells/mm**^{3} (16). If all the criteria are met, the syndrome can be also called "complete"; if only one or two criteria are present, the term "partial HELLP" is preferred.

A further subclassification, known as the *Mississippi HELLP Classification System*, classifies the disorder by the lowest platelet count (16):

- Class 1 HELLP syndrome (severe thrombocytopenia): platelet count ≤50,000 cells/mm^3 + LDH >600 IU/L and AST or ALT ≥70 IU/L
- Class 2 HELLP syndrome (moderate thrombocytopenia): platelet count >50,000 but ≤100,000 cells/mm^3 + LDH >600 IU/L and AST or ALT ≥70 IU/L
- Class 3 HELLP syndrome (mild thrombocytopenia): platelet count >100,000 but ≤150,000 cells/mm^3 + LDH >600 IU/L and AST or ALT ≥40 IU/L

Peripheral smear findings and bilirubin abnormalities are not considered in this classification.

Eclampsia

Seizures in the presence of preeclampsia and/or HELLP syndrome.

Symptoms

Persistent headache or other cerebral or visual disturbances (including grand mal seizures), and persistent epigastric (or right upper quadrant) pain are criteria for severe preeclampsia. Edema, especially central, should prompt evaluation of preeclampsia.

Epidemiology/Incidence

In healthy nulliparous women, about 7% (most occur at term and are mild).

Etiology/Basic Pathophysiology

Preeclampsia is a **systemic** disease of unknown etiology. It is associated with **endothelial disease**, with **vasospasm** and **sympathetic overactivity**. **Trophoblastic invasion** by the placenta into the spiral arteries of the uterus is **incomplete**, resulting in **reduced perfusion**. Hypoxia, free radicals, oxidative stress, and activation of endothelium are characteristic. Thromboxane (which is associated with vasoconstriction, platelet aggregation, and decreased uteroplacental blood flow) is increased, while prostacyclin (which has opposite effects) is decreased. FGR is also theorized to develop as a result of

defective placentation and the imbalance between prostacyclin and thromboxane.

- Alterations of the immune response.
- *Vascular*: vasospasm and subsequent hemoconcentration are associated with contraction of intravascular space; capillary leak and decreased colloid oncotic pressure may predispose to pulmonary edema.
- *Cardiac*: usually reduced cardiac output, decreased plasma volume, increased systemic vascular resistance.
- *Hematological*: thrombocytopenia and hemolysis with HELLP syndrome (also elevated LDH).
- *Hepatic*: elevated AST, ALT; subcapsular hematoma.
- *CNS*: eclampsia, intracranial hemorrhage, headache, blurred vision, scotomata, hyperreflexia, temporary blindness.
- *Rena*: vasospasm, hemoconcentration, and decreased renal blood flow resulting in oliguria (rarely leading to acute tubular necrosis, possibly leading to acute renal failure).
- *Fetal*: impaired uteroplacental blood flow [FGR, oligohydramnios, abruption, and nonreassuring fetal heart rate testing (NRFHT)].

Despite an abundance of early predictive tests for preeclampsia, with significant associations, the statistical accuracy and positive predictive value of these tests is often poor.

Classification

See "mild" versus severe, discussed above.

Risk Factors/Associations

Nulliparity, limited sperm exposure, primipaternity, "dangerous father" (for preeclampsia), donor eggs and/or sperm, multifetal gestation, prior preeclampsia, chronic HTN, diabetes, vascular and connective tissue disease, nephropathy, antiphospholipid syndrome (APS), obesity, insulin resistance, young maternal age or advanced maternal age, African-American race, family history of preeclampsia, maternal low birth weight, low socioeconomic status, increased soluble fms-like tyrosine kinase 1 (sFlt-1), reduced placental growth factor, and higher fetal cells in maternal circulation. A change in partner is usually associated with a protective effect if prior pregnancy had preeclampsia. Previous pregnancy with same partner seems to be protective, albeit for a short (one to three years) time. Smoking is associated with decreased incidence of preeclampsia. The presence of inherited thrombophilias such as factor V Leiden, prothrombin 20210, and MTHFR has not been associated with preeclampsia when the best studies (prospective, large, etc.) are evaluated (see chap. 27 and Table 27.3). While antiphospholipid antibodies, in particular ACA, are associated with an increased risk of preeclampsia, screening is not suggested as no therapy has been evaluated in these cases (see chap. 26).

Prediction

Despite the variety of methods studied, there are still no sensitive prediction tests for preeclampsia. Doppler ultrasonography of uterine arteries seems to be the most useful method, especially in pregnant women who are at high risk for preeclampsia (17). Abnormal **uterine Doppler** findings in the second trimester have a sensitivity of 20% to 60%, and a positive predictive value of 6% to 40%, depending on prevalence of preeclampsia. According to recent meta-analyses, an increased pulsatility index alone or combined with notching is the best predictor of preeclampsia in women with risk factors (positive likelihood ratios = 21.0 in high-risk women), but it is not so predictive in low-risk population (positive likelihood ratio = 7.5) (18). Furthermore, the studies included in the meta-analysis are heterogeneous in severity of disease and outcomes, timing of Doppler assessment, and inclusion of other screening tests.

A variety of blood tests to predict the risk of preeclampsia have been studied. Some of the metabolites that have been proposed as early biochemical markers of preeclampsia are beta–human chorionic gonadotropin (β-hCG), α-fetoprotein; first-trimester serum levels of the biomarkers placental protein-13 (PP-13), pregnancy-associated plasma protein-A (PAPP-A), soluble Flt-1 (soluble vascular endothelial growth factor receptor-1), and soluble endoglin. Currently, there is no reliable predictive test for the condition.

Further research is needed to identify the ideal timing of uterine artery Doppler and the possible combination with other predictors of preeclampsia, such as measurement of maternal serum biomarkers, to improve perinatal outcomes.

Complications

Complications depend on gestational age at time of diagnosis, severity of disease, presence of other medical conditions, and, of course, management. Most cases of mild preeclampsia, at term, do not convey significant risks. Rates of complications **for severe preeclampsia** are given in the following subsections in parenthesis (19).

Maternal
HELLP syndrome (20%), **DIC** (10%), **pulmonary edema** (2–5%), **abruptio placentae** (1–4%), **renal failure** (1–2%), **seizures** (eclampsia) (<1%), **cerebral hemorrhage** (<1%), **liver hemorrhage** (<1%), death (rare).

Fetal/Neonatal
PTB (15–60%), **FGR** (10–25%), **perinatal death** (1–2%), **hypoxemia-neurologic injury** (<1%), long-term cardiovascular morbidity (rate unknown—fetal origin of adult disease).

Management
(Figs. 1.1 and 1.2) (19–22)

Principles
Preeclampsia is one of the most common, and perhaps most typical, obstetric complications. The only interventions associated with significant prevention of preeclampsia are antiplatelet agents, primarily low-dose aspirin, and calcium supplementation. It is important to understand that preeclampsia's **only cure is delivery**. As such, preeclampsia is a temporary disease, which resolves usually 24 to 48 hours after delivery. Remember that there are two patients: delivery is always good for the mother, but not always for the baby, especially if very premature. In general, most patients with preeclampsia are otherwise healthy.

Prevention
Aspirin
Aspirin acts to inhibit thromboxane synthesis, which could theoretically improve uteroplacental blood flow and fetal growth.

Compared to placebo or no treatment, antiplatelet agents such as **low-dose aspirin (75–150 mg/day)** given to women **with risk factors for preeclampsia** (especially severe preeclampsia in previous pregnancies) are associated with a **17%**

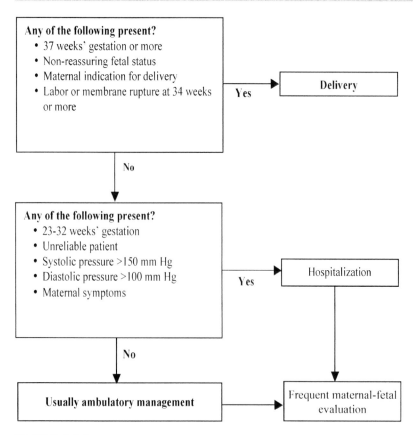

Any of the following present?
- 37 weeks' gestation or more
- Non-reassuring fetal status
- Maternal indication for delivery
- Labor or membrane rupture at 34 weeks or more

Yes → **Delivery**

No ↓

Any of the following present?
- 23-32 weeks' gestation
- Unreliable patient
- Systolic pressure >150 mm Hg
- Diastolic pressure >100 mm Hg
- Maternal symptoms

Yes → Hospitalization

No ↓

Usually ambulatory management → Frequent maternal-fetal evaluation

Figure 1.1 Suggested management of mild preeclampsia. *Source:* Adapted from Ref. 21.

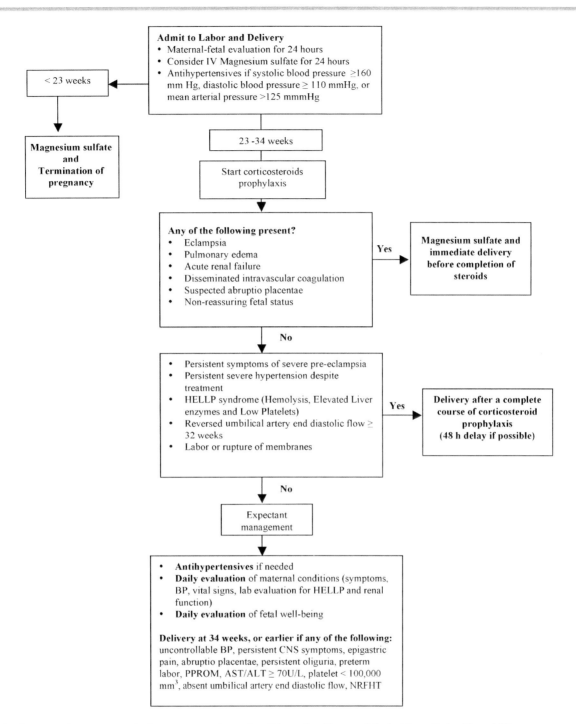

Figure 1.2 Suggested management of severe preeclampsia <34 weeks. *Source*: Adapted from Refs. 20 and 22.

reduction in the risk of **preeclampsia** (23). Low-dose aspirin is also associated with a small **(8%) reduction** in the risk of **PTB** <**37 weeks**, a **10% reduction** in **SGA** babies, and a **14% reduction** in **perinatal deaths** (23).

Compared with trials using 75 mg or less of aspirin, there is a significant reduction in the risk of preeclampsia in trials using higher doses (e.g., 81 mg). Although there is evidence that higher doses of aspirin may be more effective, this requires careful evaluation as risks may also be increased (23). Low-dose aspirin use has been shown to be safe for the fetus, even in the first trimester (24).

There is some evidence that **the earlier low-dose aspirin is started in pregnancy, the greater the benefits are**, as shown in a recent meta-analysis of 34 RCTs (25). Low-dose aspirin initiated **before 16 weeks** is associated with a significant decrease in the incidence of preeclampsia (53%), severe preeclampsia (90%), IUGR (54%), and PTB (78%) in women identified to be at risk for preeclampsia, whereas such results are not observed when aspirin is started after 16 weeks.

Aspirin prophylaxis should be discontinued before delivery, by 37 to 38 weeks.

Prevention with abnormal uterine Doppler ultrasound
Abnormal uterine artery Doppler in the second trimester has been associated with an increased risk of preeclampsia. The only intervention studied if this screening test is abnormal is low-dose aspirin. **If low-dose aspirin is given anyway because of a history of preeclampsia (see above), then uterine artery Doppler screening may not be necessary or beneficial**.

A meta-analysis of 9 RCTs (*n* = 1317) comparing **low-dose** (50–150 mg/day) **aspirin** to placebo or no treatment in women **with abnormal uterine Doppler ultrasound at 14 to 24 weeks** reveals that **preeclampsia is decreased by 52% when aspirin treatment starts before 16 weeks**, with no significant reduction when started later in pregnancy. Early start of the treatment in women with abnormal uterine Doppler also significantly **reduces the incidence of severe preeclampsia by 90%, gestational hypertension by 69%, and IUGR by 49% (26)**. There are **insufficient data to assess other important outcomes**, such as abruption and perinatal death.

The largest trial (27) trying to assess this intervention had a different study design from the others, and is not included in the meta-analysis. Women in this trial are randomized to having the uterine Doppler examination between 22 and 24 week of gestation and always getting aspirin if abnormal, or not receiving the Doppler screening. There are no differences in these two groups in any of the outcomes (27). The late initiation of treatment reported in this trial may explain the negative results obtained, confirming that aspirin treatment may be not effective in preventing preeclampsia if started late in pregnancy.

Heparin. One RCT investigates the use of prophylactic low-molecular-weight heparin (LMWH) to prevent the recurrence of preeclampsia and IUGR in women without thrombophilia. Compared to no use, LMWH is associated with a significant 85% reduction in the primary outcome (a composite of one or more of: severe preeclampsia, newborn weight ≤5th percentile, or major abruptio placentae) (28). Further trials are needed to evaluate the potential benefits of heparin in preventing preeclampsia. Therefore, LMWH is not recommended at this time as prophylaxis for recurrence for women with a history of preeclampsia (29).

Calcium. Compared with placebo or no treatment, calcium supplementation is associated with a 35% **reduction in the incidence of high blood pressure and a 55% reduction in the risk of preeclampsia**, as shown in a meta-analysis of 13 studies (30). The reduction is greater among women at high risk of developing hypertension (78%), and in those with low baseline calcium intake (64%). Although the risk of preeclampsia is reduced, this is not clearly reflected in any reduction in severe preeclampsia, eclampsia, or admission to intensive care. One of the largest trials reported no reduction in the rate or severity of preeclampsia, and no delay in its onset (31). Optimum dosage and the effect on some substantive outcomes require further investigation.

Calcium supplementation is also associated with a 24% reduction in the risk of PTB overall, and by 55% in women at high risk of preeclampsia. There is no evidence of any effect on fetal death or death before discharge from hospital. The risk ratio of the composite outcome "maternal death or severe morbidity" is reduced by 20% for women receiving calcium supplementation. In one study, childhood systolic blood pressure >95th percentile is reduced by 41%.

Overall, these results support the use of calcium supplementation during pregnancy, especially for women at high risk of developing preeclampsia and for those with low dietary intake (30). For most studies the intervention was 1.5 to 2 g/day of calcium. Nonetheless, some experts still doubt calcium benefit in this settings, as the data and the selection factors are not homogeneous (e.g., several different risk factors for preeclampsia included) and final results are mostly due to influence of smaller and lower quality studies (32).

Antioxidant therapy. Preeclampsia has been associated in some studies (but not in others) with oxidative stress. Antioxidative therapy (e.g., vitamins C and E) has been tested as a preventative intervention. Evidence from a meta-analysis of 10 trials does not support routine antioxidant supplementation during pregnancy to reduce the risk of preeclampsia and its complications (33). Comparing antioxidant use with placebo or no treatment, **there is no significant difference in the risk of preeclampsia**, PTB, SGA infants, or fetal or neonatal death. These results are confirmed in four additional large most recent trials (34–37), which do not show any maternal or fetal benefit, including no reduction in preeclampsia, eclampsia, or gestational hypertension, among high- and low-risk women receiving daily supplementation with 1000 mg of vitamin C and 400 IU of vitamin E, starting in the early second trimester. In one of the trials (37) the intervention is associated with an increased risk of fetal loss or perinatal death, PROM, and PPROM (an increased risk of PPROM is observed in another previous trial) (38). Given these results, antioxidant therapy should **not be recommended for prevention of preeclampsia**.

Magnesium. There is insufficient evidence to assess magnesium as a preventive intervention for preeclampsia.

Diuretics. There is insufficient evidence to support the use of diuretics on prevention of preeclampsia and its complications. Diuretics for preventing preeclampsia are not associated with benefits, but have adverse effects and so their use for this purpose cannot be recommended (39).

Salt intake. Compared to advice to continue a normal diet, advice to reduce dietary salt intake is associated with similar outcomes, including incidence of preeclampsia (40). In the absence of evidence that advice to alter salt intake during pregnancy has any beneficial effect for prevention of preeclampsia or any other outcome, either reliance on the nonpregnancy data on beneficial salt restricted diet or personal preference can guide salt intake.

Fish oil. The use of omega-3 fatty acids contained in fish oil is not associated with significant prevention of preeclampsia (41).

Garlic. There is not enough evidence to recommend increased garlic intake for preventing preeclampsia and its complications (42).

Rest/exercise. There is insufficient evidence to support recommending rest or reduced activity to women for preventing preeclampsia and its complications (43). It has been suggested that exercise may help prevent preeclampsia in women at moderate-to-high risk, but current evidence is insufficient to draw reliable conclusions about this effect (44).

Progesterone. There is insufficient evidence for reliable conclusions about the effects of progesterone for preventing preeclampsia and its complications. Therefore, progesterone should not be used for this purpose in clinical practice at present (45).

Nitric oxide. There is insufficient evidence to draw reliable conclusions about whether nitric oxide donors and precursors prevent preeclampsia or its complications (46).

Preconception Counseling
Preventive measures are as per chronic hypertension, as described above, plus avoidance of risk factors, if feasible.

Diagnosis
Diagnosis is described above.

History
Headache; blurry vision, "spots in front of eyes"; abdominal pain.

Physical Examination
BP, edema (especially if hands, face; excessive quick weight gain), increased reflexes. Period when hypertension is first documented (before or after 20 weeks) is important.

Workup
Laboratory tests: **AST** and **ALT, platelets,** creatinine, 24-**hour urine for total protein** (and creatinine clearance). It is **important to know the baseline values** of these tests in the woman when either not pregnant or at least in the beginning of the pregnancy to be able to compare in women being evaluated for preeclampsia or its complications. Therefore, these tests should be obtained **at first prenatal visit** in women with significant risk factors (e.g., chronic hypertension, diabetes, collagen disorders, APS, prior preeclampsia, and HELLP). Coagulation studies (especially fibrinogen) can be obtained only in severe cases. Uric acid is neither sensitive nor specific, and has not been shown to be helpful in management. **Repeat** laboratory tests can be performed as clinically indicated.

Evaluate for symptoms and laboratory tests to distinguish preeclampsia from chronic HTN, and to assess disease progression and severity.

Counseling
Delivery (the only definite treatment) is always appropriate for the mother, but may not be so for the fetus. The woman should be instructed on the signs and symptoms of preeclampsia and severe preeclampsia. The management plan should always consider gestational age, maternal and fetal status, and presence of labor or PPROM. Expectant management aims to palliate the maternal condition to allow fetal maturation and cervical ripening. Consider **corticosteroid administration** to accelerate fetal lung maturity between 24 and 33 6/7 weeks. BP (several times a day), urine for protein, fluid input and output, weight, laboratory tests (as above), and fetal status should be closely monitored.

Admission
Management of proteinuric and nonproteinuric hypertension in **day care units** has **similar clinical outcomes** and costs but **greater maternal satisfaction** compared to hospital admission (47–49). Hospitalization may be indicated in cases in which the woman is unreliable, two or more SBPs >150 mmHg or DBP >100 mmHg, or persistent maternal symptoms.

Magnesium Prophylaxis
Magnesium is the drug of choice for prevention of eclampsia. Compared with placebo or no anticonvulsant, magnesium sulfate is associated with a **59% reduction in** the risk of **eclampsia** (number needed to treat for an additional beneficial outcome: 100), a 36% reduction in **abruption**, and a nonstatistically significant but clinically important 46% reduction in **maternal death** (50).

Table 1.2 Maternal Serum Magnesium Concentrations Associated with Toxicity

	mmol/L	mEq/L	mg/dL
Loss of patellar reflexes	3.5–5	7–10	8.5–12
Respiratory depression	5–6.5	10–13	12–16
Altered cardiac conduction	>7.5	>15	>18
Cardiac arrest	>12.5	>25	>30

The **reduction of the risk of eclampsia** is consistent across the subgroups. In particular, **the reduction is similar regardless of severity of preeclampsia**. As eclampsia is more common among women with severe preeclampsia than among those with mild preeclampsia, the number of women who would need to be treated to prevent one case of eclampsia is greater for nonsevere (mild) preeclampsia (i.e., 400 for mild preeclampsia, 71 for severe preeclampsia, and 36 in those with CNS symptoms) (51). In women with **mild preeclampsia**, the incidence of eclampsia may be only <1/200, and magnesium has not been shown to affect perinatal outcome, possibly because too few ($n = 357$) women with mild preeclampsia have been enrolled in the two specific trials (51). In women with **severe preeclampsia** the incidence of eclampsia decreases 61%, **from 2% in the placebo group to 0.6% in the magnesium group** (four trials) (50,51).

Magnesium is also associated with trend for a 33% decrease in abruption in women with severe preeclampsia. Women allocated to magnesium sulfate have a **small increase (5%) in the risk of cesarean section**. There is no overall difference in the risk of fetal or neonatal death.

Side effects, in particular flushing, occur in 24% of women on magnesium, compared to 5% of controls. Almost all the data on side effects and safety come from studies that used either the intramuscular (IM) regimen for maintenance therapy, or the **intravenous** (IV) route with **1 g/hr**, and for around 24 hours. One trial compared a low-dose regimen with a standard-dose regimen over 24 hours. This study was too small for any reliable conclusions about the comparative effects (52). Other toxicities and their associated magnesium serum levels are shown in Table 1.2.

Intravenous administration is preferable, where there are appropriate resources, as side effects and injection site problems are lower. Magnesium is **usually given at least in active labor and for 12 to 24 hours postpartum, but can be given for a shorter or longer period depending on the severity of preeclampsia** (monitored for this purpose in particular with maternal urine output). Three trials compared short maintenance regimens postpartum (e.g., 12 hours) with continuing for 24 hours after the birth, but even taken together these trials were too small for any reliable conclusions (52). Most trials managed magnesium **without serum monitoring**, but with clinical monitoring of respiration, tendon reflexes, and urine output. If serum levels are used, Table 1.2 shows the correlations with side effects. Monitoring of patellar reflexes can be used to avoid toxicity. The use of higher doses and longer duration cannot be supported by trial data. Magnesium sulfate for preeclampsia prophylaxis does not significantly affect labor but is associated with higher use of oxytocin (53).

Compared to **phenytoin**, magnesium sulfate is associated with a **92% better reduction in the risk of eclampsia,** with a 21% increased risk of cesarean section (50).

Compared to **nimodipine**, magnesium sulfate is associated with a **67% better reduction in the risk of eclampsia.**

There is insufficient evidence on other agents, such as diazepam or methyldopa (50).

Plasma Volume Expansion
Blood plasma volume increases gradually in women during pregnancy. The increase is usually greater for women with multiple pregnancies and less for those with small babies. Plasma volume is reduced in women with preeclampsia. There is insufficient data to assess any effect of plasma volume expansion on outcomes in women with preeclampsia. Three small trials compared a colloid solution with no plasma volume expansion. For every outcome reported, the confidence intervals are very wide and cross the no-effect line (54).

Antihypertensive Therapy
Patients with SBP consistently ≥160 mmHg and/or DBP ≥ 110 (severe HTN) should be placed on antihypertensive medication; this includes those women with preeclampsia or its complications (HELLP, etc.). As stated above, it is appropriate to initiate therapy at lower blood pressures in patients with evidence of end-organ damage (renal, cardiovascular, etc.) and diabetes. Target BP should be 140 to 150 mmHg systolic and about 90 mmHg diastolic. ACE inhibitors are contraindicated in pregnancy. Any patient requiring antihypertensive agents may be placed on home BP monitoring if managed as an outpatient. There are no trials on this intervention in preeclampsia.

Most antihypertensive drugs are effective at reducing blood pressure, with little evidence that one is any better or worse than another (8). Types of medications include the following:

- *Labetalol*: 20-mg IV bolus, then 40, 80, 80 mg as needed, every 10 minutes (maximum 220 mg total dose).
- *Hydralazine*: 5 to 10 mg IV (or IM) every 20 minutes. Change to another drug if no success by 30 mg (maximum dose). Hydralazine may be associated with more maternal side effects and NRFHT than IV labetalol or oral nifedipine (55).
- *Nifedipine*: 10 to 20 mg orally, may repeat in 30 minutes. This drug is associated with diuresis when used postpartum. Nifedipine and magnesium sulfate can probably be used simultaneously.
- *Sodium nitroprusside* (rarely needed): start at 0.25 μ/kg/min to a maximum of 5 μ/kg/min.

Antiplatelet Agents
Five trials compared antiplatelet agents with placebo or no antiplatelet agent for the **treatment** of preeclampsia. There are insufficient data for any firm conclusions about the possible effects of these agents when used for treatment of preeclampsia (56) (meta-analysis, now withdrawn).

Antepartum Testing
Antenatal testing (usually with nonstress tests) is done at diagnosis and repeated once or twice weekly; twice weekly for FGR or oligohydramnios. Umbilical artery Doppler ultrasound is recommended at least weekly if FGR is present. Ultrasound for fetal growth and amniotic fluid assessment should be performed at diagnosis and every three weeks if still pregnant.

Anesthesia
(See also chapter 11 of *Obstetric Evidence-Based Guidelines*.) Regional anesthesia is preferred, but contraindicated with coagulopathy or platelets <75,000/mm³. Patients with hypertension may benefit from epidural analgesia, as it may improve uterine perfusion through several pathways (localized neuraxial vasodilatory effect, reduced catecholamine release). **Epidural analgesia is the analgesia of choice in hypertensive pregnant women**. Patients with hypertension, preeclampsia, and eclampsia are at increased risk for hemodynamic instability during both labor and surgical anesthesia. Some, but not all studies, have found a higher incidence of hypotension in parturients receiving a spinal versus epidural. Methods to prevent hypotension should be employed. The prevention, rather than treatment, of hypotension has been associated with better outcomes for the fetus. In women with severe preeclampsia, a careful approach is necessary for either regional or general anesthesia. Provided this is followed, they are associated with similar, good outcomes in a small trial (57). Women with severe preeclampsia who must undergo **general anesthesia** are **at risk for an extremely exaggerated hypertensive response to intubation** and often benefit from pretreatment with an antihypertensive, such as labetalol, immediately prior to induction. Prophylaxis with magnesium sulfate for preeclampsia/eclampsia can potentiate neuromuscular blockade in patients receiving general anesthesia, so care must be taken in using intermediate- to long-acting nondepolarizing muscle relaxants.

Delivery (Figs. 1.1 and 1.2)
Timing
Before 37 weeks, in **the absence of severe criteria**, or preterm labor, and in the presence of reassuring fetal testing, expectant management is suggested, with delivery for development of any severe criteria (see below).

Compared to expectant management, induction of labor in women with gestational hypertension or mild preeclampsia at 36 to 41 weeks' gestation is associated with an improved maternal outcome (e.g., HELLP, severe HTN, and pulmonary edema) and lower incidence of neonatal pH <7.05 with induction of labor ≥37 weeks (12). Trends were seen for benefit of induction associated with less cesarean delivery and maternal ICU admission.

Therefore, **even with "mild" preeclampsia delivery (usually by induction) at ≥37 weeks is recommended**.

Mode
Vaginal delivery is preferred, with induction of labor if necessary. With severe preeclampsia, the chances of a successful induction vary from 34% to over 90% in different studies (58–64). Table 1.3 shows the rate of cesarean delivery in induced labors at different gestational ages, and should be helpful with counseling and management. If the woman is stable and accepts this low incidence of success, induction may be reasonable, especially in a woman desiring a large family, if management includes a clear end point for delivery (e.g., within 24 hours).

Table 1.3 Rate of Cesarean Delivery in Induced Labors in Women with Severe Preeclampsia at 24 to 34 Weeks' Gestation

Author	24–28 wk % (n)	28–32 wk % (n)	32–34 wk % (n)
Nassar (64)	68 (13/19)	55 (47/86)	38 (15/40)
Blackwell (61)	96 (26/27)	65 (33/51)	31 (23/73)
Alanis (58)	93 (14/15)	53 (84/158)	31 (34/109)
Mashiloane (63)		35 (14/40)	
OVERALL	**87** (53/61)	**53** (178/335)	**32** (72/222)

Hemodynamic Monitoring

Invasive hemodynamic monitoring in preeclamptic women, even with severe cardiac disease, renal disease, refractory HTN, pulmonary edema, or unexplained oliguria, is usually unnecessary, especially since Swan–Ganz catheters have been associated with complications and no improvements in outcomes in nonpregnant critically ill adults. There are no trials on this intervention in pregnancy.

PREECLAMPSIA COMPLICATIONS
Superimposed Preeclampsia

Prognosis may be much worse for mother and fetus than with either diagnosis (chronic hypertension or preeclampsia) alone. Complications are similar to preeclampsia, but more common and severe (e.g., PTB 50–60%, FGR 15%, abruption 2–5%, perinatal death 5%). There are no specific trials to guide management, therefore management should follow as per preeclampsia (Figs. 1.1 and 1.2), with even more caution given the higher morbidity and mortality.

Severe Preeclampsia

See section "Preeclampsia."

Management (Fig. 1.2)

Magnesium sulfate. See section "Preeclampsia."

Plasma volume expansion. The addition of **plasma volume expansion** as a temporizing treatment does not improve maternal or fetal outcome in women with early preterm severe preeclampsia (65).

Timing of delivery (Fig. 1.2). In the presence of severe preeclampsia at ≥**34 weeks, expeditious delivery** is recommended, given the high maternal incidence of complications with expectant management. Timing the delivery of a very premature infant <34 weeks in the presence of severe preeclampsia is a difficult clinical decision. When the mother's life is in danger, there is no doubt that delivery is the only correct course of action. This situation is rare. More usually, the risks of maternal morbidity if the pregnancy is continued have to be constantly balanced against the hazards of prematurity to the fetus if it is delivered too early. The **options are expeditious delivery or expectant management** to improve perinatal outcome, but there are only two small trials comparing these approaches at 28 to 32–34 weeks (66,67). In general, an interventionist approach with **delivery within 48 hours after completion of corticosteroid administration ("aggressive management")** is suggested **for uncontrollable BP** in spite of continuing increase in antihypertensive drugs, **persistent headache and/or visual/CNS symptoms, epigastric pain, vaginal bleeding, persistent oliguria, preterm labor, PROM, AST/ALT >70 IU/L, platelets <100,000/mm³ (partial or complete HELLP syndrome)**, or **reversed umbilical artery end-diastolic flow ≥32 weeks** (20,68).

Immediate delivery before 48 hours (even before completion of steroids) is recommended in case of eclampsia, pulmonary edema, acute renal failure, DIC, suspected abruptio placentae, or nonreassuring fetal status (Fig. 1.2).

There are insufficient data for reliable conclusions comparing these policies for outcome for the mother. For the baby, there is insufficient evidence for reliable conclusions about the effects on fetal or neonatal death. Babies whose mothers are allocated to **interventionist** group have 2.3-fold **more hyaline membrane disease** and 5.5-fold **more necrotizing enterocolitis**, and are 32% **more likely to need admission to neonatal**

intensive care unit (NICU) than those allocated to an expectant policy (68). Nevertheless, babies allocated to the interventionist policy are 64% less likely to be SGA. There are no statistically significant differences between the two strategies for any other outcomes.

In observational studies expectant care of severe preeclampsia <34 weeks is associated with pregnancy prolongation of 7 to 14 days, and few serious maternal complications (<5%), similar to interventionist care (69).

Expectant management. **Expectant management (prolonging pregnancy beyond 48 hours)** is possible only if none of the conditions described above is present. At any time during expectant management, the development of any sign described above necessitates delivery (Fig. 1.2) (20). Expectant management is not recommended beyond 34 weeks, because maternal risks outweigh perinatal benefits.

Expectant management of severe preeclampsia remote from term warrants hospitalization at a tertiary facility, daily antenatal testing, and laboratory studies at frequent intervals, with the decision to prolong pregnancy determined day to day.

In cases of severe HTN, such as those with severe preeclampsia, in which expectant management is appropriate, we suggest adding labetalol 200 to 800 mg orally every eight hours to the antihypertensive therapy described above. An alternative is nifedipine 10 to 20 mg orally every four to six hours.

Women with renal disease, systemic lupus erythematosus, insulin-dependent diabetes, or multiple gestations require very careful management if expectantly managed. Massive proteinuria, even >10 g in 24 hours, is not associated per se with worse maternal or neonatal outcomes compared with proteinuria of <10 or even <5 g, and so should probably not be a criterion for delivery by itself. The presence of FGR requires even closer monitoring, is associated with worse outcomes, but is usually not in itself a criterion for delivery.

HELLP Syndrome
Epidemiology

HELLP syndrome is a severe manifestation of preeclampsia and complicates approximately 0.5% to 0.9% of all pregnancies and 10% to 20% of cases with severe preeclampsia (70). Approximately 72% of cases are diagnosed antepartum, and 28% postpartum (of which 80% <48 hours, and 20% ≥48 hours postpartum). Of the antepartum cases, about 70% occur 28 to 36 weeks, 20% >37 weeks, and about 10% <28 weeks. HELLP syndrome detected before fetal viability may identify a pregnancy complicated by partial mole/triploidy, trisomy 13, antiphospholipid syndrome, autoantibodies to angiotensin AT(1)-receptor or severe preterm preeclampsia with "mirror" syndrome (16).

Diagnosis

See above and Table 1.1. Patients presumptively diagnosed with HELLP syndrome can have other disorders concurrent with HELLP syndrome or other disorders altogether. The diseases that may imitate HELLP syndrome and that have to be considered in the differential diagnosis are shown in Table 1.4 (16).

Signs and Symptoms

The presenting symptoms are usually right upper abdominal quadrant or epigastric pain, nausea, and vomiting. Headache and visual symptoms can occur. Malaise or viral syndrome–like symptoms may be present with advanced HELLP

Table 1.4 Differential Diagnosis of HELLP Syndrome

Acute fatty liver of pregnancy (AFLP)
Lupus flare: Exacerbation of systemic lupus erythematosus
Thrombotic thrombocytopenic purpura (TTP)
Hemolytic uremic syndrome (HUS)
Immune thrombocytopenic purpura (ITP)
Thrombophilias (e.g., antiphospholipid syndrome)
Severe folate deficiency
Cholangitis/cholecystitis/pancreatitis/ruptured bile duct
Gastric ulcer
Cardiomyopathy
Dissecting aortic aneurysm
Systemic viral sepsis (herpes, cytomegalovirus)
SIRS/sepsis
Hemorrhagic or hypotensive shock
Stroke in pregnancy or puerperium
Paroxysmal nocturnal hemoglobinuria
Pheochromocytoma
Advanced embryonal cell carcinoma of the liver
Acute cocaine intoxication
Myasthenia gravis
Pseudocholinesterase deficiency

Source: Adapted from Ref. 16.

Table 1.5 Signs and Symptoms of HELLP Syndrome

Condition	Frequency (%)
Hypertension	85
Proteinuria	87
Right upper quadrant or epigastric pain	40–90
Nausea or vomiting	30–85
Headaches	35–60
Visual changes	10–20
Mucosal bleeding	10
Jaundice	5

Abbreviation: HELLP, Hemolysis, Elevated Liver enzymes and a Low Platelet count.
Source: Adapted from Ref. 71.

syndrome. It is important to note that 15% have no hypertension, and 13% no proteinuria (Table 1.5) (71).

Complications
Complications (Table 1.6) of HELLP syndrome are somewhat similar in incidence and severity to those of severe preeclampsia, once gestational age is controlled (71). If profound hypovolemic shock occurs, suspect liver hematoma. If confirmed, liver hematoma is best managed conservatively. Contributing factors to deaths of women with HELLP syndrome are, in order of decreasing frequency, stroke, cardiac arrest, DIC, adult respiratory distress syndrome, renal failure, sepsis, hepatic rupture, hypoxic encephalopathy (16).

Management
See Figure 1.3 for management (72).
   Workup. Laboratory tests as per severe preeclampsia, plus peripheral smear evaluation.
   Corticosteroids. Eleven trials (550 women) have assessed corticosteroids versus placebo/no treatment and are summarized in a meta-analysis (73). The dose of dexamethasone was usually 10-mg IV every 6 to 12 hours for two to three doses, followed by 5- to 6-mg IV 6 to 12 hours later for two to three more doses. There is **no difference in the risk of maternal**

Table 1.6 Complications of HELLP Syndrome

Complication	Frequency (%)
Maternal death	1
Adult respiratory distress syndrome (ARDS)	1
Laryngeal edema	1–2
Liver failure or hemorrhage	1–2
Acute renal failure	3
Pulmonary edema	6–8
Pleural effusions	10–15
Abruptio placentae	10–15
Disseminated intravascular coagulopathy	10–15
Marked ascites	10–15
Perinatal death	7–20
PTB	70

Abbreviations: HELLP, Hemolysis, Elevated Liver enzymes and Low Platelets; PTB, preterm birth.
Source: Adapted from Ref. 71.

death, maternal death or severe maternal morbidity, or perinatal/infant death. The only significant effect of treatment on individual outcomes is improved platelet count: This effect is strongest if the treatment is started antenatally.

In two trials comparing dexamethasone with betamethasone, there is no clear evidence of a difference between groups in respect to perinatal morbidity or mortality. Maternal death and severe maternal morbidity is not reported. Regarding platelet count, dexamethasone is superior to betamethasone, when treatment is commenced both antenatally and postnatally (74,75).

The two largest and only placebo-controlled trials (76,77) failed to show any significant difference between dexamethasone and placebo with respect to duration of hospitalization, recovery time for laboratory or clinical parameters, complications, or need for blood transfusion. These results remained unchanged, even following analysis stratified according to whether the patients were still pregnant or postpartum. A subgroup analysis according to the severity of disease shows a shorter platelet recovery and duration of hospitalization in the subgroup with class 1 HELLP who received dexamethasone (51).

There is only one randomized placebo-controlled trial evaluating the effect of prolonged administration of high-dose prednisolone in 31 pregnant women with early-onset (<30 weeks) HELLP syndrome, during expectant management (mean prolongation of about 7 days) (78). The results show a reduced risk of recurrent HELLP syndrome exacerbations (presence of at least two of the following three criteria: right upper abdominal or epigastrical pain, a platelet count decrease below 100,000/mm^3, and an increase of AST activity over 50 IU/L) in the prednisolone group as compared to the placebo group (hazard ratio 0.3, 95% CI 0.3–0.9). Nevertheless, expectant management for >48 hours in women with HELLP syndrome, even with early onset, is not recommended.

Given no significant improvements in important maternal and fetal outcomes, there is still **insufficient evidence to recommend the routine use steroids for therapy specific for HELLP syndrome**, and this approach should be considered experimental. The use of corticosteroids may be justified in clinical situations in which increased rate of recovery in platelet count is considered clinically worthwhile.

Anesthesia
Regional anesthesia is usually allowed by anesthesiologists in cases with platelet counts ≥75,000/mm^3. General anesthesia may be safer in cases with lower platelet counts.

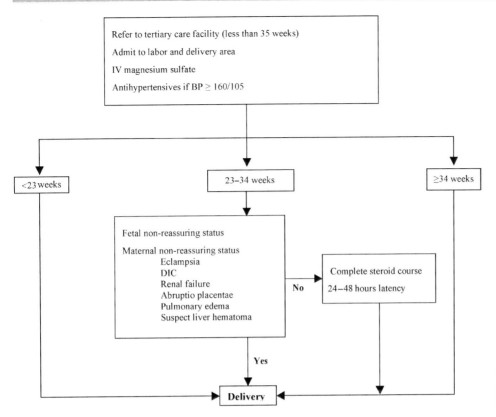

Refer to tertiary care facility (less than 35 weeks)

Admit to labor and delivery area

IV magnesium sulfate

Antihypertensives if BP ≥ 160/105

<23 weeks

23–34 weeks

≥34 weeks

Fetal non-reassuring status

Maternal non-reassuring status
    Eclampsia
    DIC
    Renal failure
    Abruptio placentae
    Pulmonary edema
    Suspect liver hematoma

No

Complete steroid course

24–48 hours latency

Yes

Delivery

Figure 1.3 Suggested management of HELLP syndrome. *Source*: Adapted from Ref. 72.

Delivery

Timing (Fig. 1.3). Prompt delivery is indicated if HELLP is diagnosed at ≥34 weeks, or even earlier if multiorgan dysfunction, DIC, liver failure or hemorrhage, renal failure, possible abruption, or NRFHT are present. Delivery can only be delayed for a maximum of 48 hours between 24 and 33 6/7 weeks to give steroids for fetal maturity, but even this management is not tested in trials. Although some women may have improvement in laboratory values in these 48 hours, delivery is still indicated in most cases.

Mode. Mode of delivery should generally follow obstetrical indications, with HELLP syndrome not being an indication for cesarean per se. No randomized trial compared maternal and neonatal outcome after vaginal delivery or cesarean section in women with HELLP syndrome. Counseling and management should include the information that the incidence of cesarean delivery in trial of labor of nulliparous women or those with Bishop <5 with HELLP at <30 weeks is high.

With platelet count <100,000/mm^3, a drain may be indicated under and/or over the fascia in cases of cesarean delivery.

Eclampsia

Incidence

The incidence is about 2 to 3 cases per 10,000 births in Europe and other developed countries, and 16 to 69 cases per 10,000 births in developing countries (79). The onset can be antepartum (40–50%), intrapartum (20–35%), or postpartum (10–40%). Late postpartum eclampsia (>48 hours but <4 weeks after delivery) is rare, but can occur.

Definition

Eclampsia is the occurrence of ≥1 seizure(s) in association with preeclampsia.

Complications

The risk of **maternal death** is around **1% to 2%** in the developed world and up to **10%** in developing countries. An estimated 50,000 women die each year worldwide having had an eclamptic convulsion. **Perinatal mortality** is 6% to 12% in the developed world and up to 25% in developing countries. Other complications are similar and possibly more severe than severe preeclampsia cases (maternal—abruption 7–10%, DIC 7–11%, HELLP 10–15%, pulmonary edema 3–5%, renal failure 5–9%, aspiration pneumonia 2–3%, cardiopulmonary arrest 2–5%; perinatal—PTB 50%) (51).

Management

Principles. **In about 15% of cases, hypertension or proteinuria may be absent before eclampsia. A high index of suspicion for eclampsia should be maintained in all cases of hypertensive disorders in pregnancy, in particular those with CNS symptoms (headache, visual disturbances).** Up to 50% or more of cases of eclampsia, occurring in women with no diagnosis of preeclampsia, or only mild disease, preterm or before hospitalization, may not be preventable.

The first priorities are **airway, breathing, and circulation**. Multidisciplinary care is essential, as several people are needed for immediate stabilization. Interventions include airway assessment and placing the patient in the lateral decubitus position (to avoid aspiration). Maintain oxygenation with supplemental oxygen via 8 to 10 L/min mask. Obtain vital signs and assess pulse oximetry. Supportive care includes inserting a tongue blade between the teeth (avoiding inducing a gag reflex), and preventing maternal injury.

Workup. Cerebral imaging is usually not necessary for the diagnosis and management of most women with eclampsia. It might be helpful in cases complicated by neurologic deficits, coma, refractory to magnesium, or seizures >48 hours after delivery.

Therapy. **Magnesium sulfate is the drug of choice to treat eclampsia and prevent recurrent convulsions,** as it is associated with maternal and fetal/neonatal benefits compared to all interventions against which it has been tested. The standard intravenous regimen widely used in many countries consists in a loading dose of 4 g, followed by an infusion of 1 g/hr (52). Increasing the loading dose to 6 g and the infusion rate to 2 g/hr has also been suggested (51).

Trials comparing alternative treatment regimens (loading dose alone vs. loading dose plus maintenance therapy for 24 hours or low-dose regimen vs. a standard-dose regimen over 24 hours) are too small for reliable conclusions (52).

Serum monitoring of magnesium levels is not absolutely necessary. The effectiveness and safety of magnesium sulfate has been demonstrated with clinical monitoring alone (52).

Trials comparing magnesium sulfate with other anticonvulsants for treating eclampsia demonstrate that it is more effective than diazepam, phenytoin, or lytic cocktail (80–82).

Magnesium vs. diazepam Compared with diazepam, magnesium sulfate is associated with **reductions** in **maternal death** by 41%, in **further convulsions** from eclampsia by 57%, in **Apgar scores <7 at 5 minutes** by 30%, in the need of intubation at the place of birth by 33%, and in **length of stay in special care baby unit >7 days** by 34% (80). There was no clear difference in perinatal deaths.

Magnesium vs. phenytoin Compared with phenytoin, magnesium sulfate is associated with **reduction** in maternal complications such as the **recurrence of convulsions** by 66%, **maternal death** by 50% (nonsignificant because of small numbers: RR 0.50, 95% CI 0.24 to 1.05), **pneumonia** by 56%, ventilation by 32%, and **admission to the intensive care unit** by 33%. For the baby, magnesium sulfate is associated with 27% **fewer admissions to a special care baby unit** and 23% **fewer babies who died or were in special baby care unit for >7 days** (81).

Magnesium vs. lytic cocktail Lytic cocktail is usually a mixture of Thorazine (chlorpromazine), Phenergan (promethazine), and Demerol (meperidine). Compared to a lytic cocktail, magnesium sulfate is associated with a **86% reduction in maternal death** and a **94% reduction in subsequent convulsions.** Magnesium sulfate is also associated with **88% less maternal respiratory depression** and **94% less coma, without any clear difference in the risk of neonatal death** (82).

Other issues About 10% of women will have a **second seizure** even after receiving magnesium sulfate. In that case, another bolus of 2 g of magnesium sulfate can be then given intravenously over three to five minutes, and, rarely, if another convulsion occurs, sodium amobarbital 250-mg IV over three to five minutes is necessary (51).

Blood pressure should be maintained at about 140–159/90–109 by antihypertensive agents, as described for preeclampsia.

Antepartum Testing
NRFHT occurs in many cases of eclampsia, but usually resolves spontaneously in 3 to 10 minutes by **fetal in utero resuscitation** with maternal support. Therefore, **NRFHT is not an indication for immediate cesarean delivery in case of** eclampsia, unless it continues >10 to 15 minutes despite normal maternal oxygenation.

Delivery
Delivery should occur expeditiously, but only **when the mother is stable.** This requires a **multidisciplinary, efficient, and timely** effort.

Postpartum Management
Eclampsia prophylaxis. **Magnesium** should be continued for at least 12 hours, and often for about 24 hours or at least improvement in maternal urinary output (e.g., >100 mL/hr). In some cases of severe preeclampsia, eclampsia, HELLP or continuing oliguria, or other complications, magnesium may need to be continued for >24 hours. Preeclampsia can worsen postpartum. Edema always worsens, and the woman should be aware of this. Eclampsia can still occur, especially in the first 48 hours postdelivery, but even up to ≥14 days postpartum.

Management of hypertension. There are no reliable data to guide management of women who are hypertensive postpartum or at increased risk of becoming so. Women should be informed that they will require long-term surveillance (and possible therapy) for hypertension at their postpartum visit.

For prevention in women who had antenatal preeclampsia, there is **insufficient data** to assess outcomes comparing furosemide or nifedipine with placebo/no therapy (83). Compared to no therapy, postpartum **furosemide** 20 mg orally for five days does not affect any outcomes in women with mild or superimposed preeclampsia (84). In women with severe preeclampsia, this intervention normalizes blood pressure more rapidly and reduces the need for antihypertensive therapy, but does not affect the incidence of delayed complications or the length of hospitalization (84). L-**Arginine** therapy does hasten recovery in postpartum preeclampsia (85). Therefore, **for women with antenatal hypertension, even that of preeclampsia, it is unclear whether or not they should routinely receive postpartum antihypertensive therapy.** Although blood pressure peaks on day 3 to 6 postpartum, whether or not routine postpartum treatment can prevent transient severe maternal hypertension and/or prolongation of maternal hospital stay has not been established (83).

For treatment, there is insufficient data to assess the antihypertensive studied: these are oral timolol or hydralazine compared with oral methyldopa for treatment of mild-to-moderate postpartum hypertension, and oral hydralazine plus sublingual nifedipine compared with sublingual nifedipine (83). Oral **nifedipine** (10 mg every 8 hours short-acting or 30 mg daily long-acting; maximum dose 120 mg/day) is a reasonable choice, with **ACE inhibitors for women with diabetes or nephropathy. If a clinician feels that hypertension is severe enough to treat, the agent used should be based on his/her familiarity with the drug.**

Long-term counseling

Since a history of early-onset hypertensive disorders of pregnancy increases the risk of recurrence in subsequent pregnancies, long-term counseling should involve review of recurrence, and preventive measures (see above). The risk of complications in the subsequent pregnancy depends on how early in gestation and how severe the complications were, other underlying medical conditions, age of the woman at future pregnancy, same versus different partner, and many other variables (see section "Risk Factors" above). Several studies tried to identify prediction tests for recurrent hypertensive disease in pregnancy, but there is insufficient evidence to assess the clinical usefulness of these tests (86).

In a large cohort study the **recurrence risk** of preeclampsia is around **15%** in the second pregnancy for women who had had preeclampsia in their first pregnancy and 30% for women who had preeclampsia in the previous two pregnancies (87). In a systematic review of seven studies, the pooled risk of recurrence of hypertension, preeclampsia, or HELLP syndrome resulting in a delivery before 34 weeks is 7.8% (88). In two recent large cohort studies, the recurrence rate of preeclampsia associated with delivery before 34 weeks' gestation is 6.8% and 17%, respectively (87,89).

Women with a history of the HELLP syndrome have an increased risk of at least 20% (range 5–52%) that some form of hypertension will recur in a subsequent gestation (70), about 5% for recurrence of HELLP, 30% to 40% of PTB, 25% of SGA, and up to 5% to 10% of perinatal death (90).

Moreover, **women with prior preeclampsia and related hypertensive disorders are at increased risk of cardiovascular disease in the future**, even premenopause if the preeclampsia occurred early in pregnancy or as a multipara, or in menopause if it happened at term in a primipara. For prevention of this cardiovascular disease and its complications, early intervention is suggested (91).

REFERENCES

1. Sibai BM. Chronic hypertension in pregnancy. Obstet Gynecol 2002; 100(2):369–377. [Review; III]
2. ACOG Practice Bulletin. Chronic hypertension in pregnancy. ACOG Committee on Practice Bulletins. Obstet Gynecol 2001; 98(1):suppl 177–185. [Review III]
3. Yeo S, Steele NM, Chang MC, Effect of exercise on blood pressure in pregnant women with a high risk of gestational hypertensive disorders. J Reprod Med 2000; 45(4):293–298. [RCT, *n* = 16; I]
4. Bergel E, Carroli G, Althabe F. Ambulatory versus conventional methods for monitoring blood pressure during pregnancy. Cochrane Database Syst Rev 2002; (2):CD001231. [Review; III]
5. Meher S, Abalos E, Carroli G. Bed rest with or without hospitalisation for hypertension during pregnancy. Cochrane Database Syst Rev 2005;(4):CD003514. [Meta-analysis; 4 RCTs, *n* = 449; I]
6. Abalos E, Duley L, Steyn DW, Antihypertensive drug therapy for mild to moderate hypertension during pregnancy. Cochrane Database Syst Rev 2007; (1):CD002252. [Meta-analysis; 46 RCTs, *n* = 4282; 28 of which compared an antihypertensive drug with placebo/no antihypertensive drug (*n* = 3200); I]
7. Magee LA, Duley L. Oral beta-blockers for mild to moderate hypertension during pregnancy. Cochrane Database Syst Rev 2003; (3):CD002863. [Meta-analysis; 29 RCTs, *n* = 2500; I]
8. Duley L, Henderson-Smart DJ, Meher S. Drugs for treatment of very high blood pressure during pregnancy. Cochrane Database Syst Rev 2006; 3:CD001449. [Meta-analysis; 24 RCTs, *n* = 2949]
9. Hennessy A, Thornton CE, Makris A, A randomised comparison of hydralazine and mini-bolus diazoxide for hypertensive emergencies in pregnancy: the PIVOT trial. Aust N Z J Obstet Gynaecol 2007; 47(4):279–285. [RCT, *n* = 124, hydralazine vs mini-bolus diazoxide; not included in Cochrane by Duley; I]
10. Hutcheon JA, Lisonkova S, Magee LA, Optimal timing of delivery in pregnancies with pre-existing hypertension. BJOG 2011; 118 (1):49–54. [Population-based cohort study, *n* = 171,669; II-2]
11. Sibai BM. Diagnosis and management of gestational hypertension and preeclampsia. Obstet Gynecol 2003; 102(1):181–192. [Review; III]
12. Koopmans CM, Bijlenga D, Groen H, Induction of labour versus expectant monitoring for gestational hypertension or mild preeclampsia after 36 weeks' gestation (HYPITAT): a multicentre, open-label randomised controlled trial. Lancet 2009; 374 (9694):979–988. [RCT, *n* = 756; I]
13. ACOG practice bulletin. Diagnosis and management of preeclampsia and eclampsia. Number 33, January 2002. Obstet Gynecol 2002; 99(1):159–167. [Review III]
14. Report of the National High Blood Pressure Education Program Working Group on High Blood Pressure in Pregnancy. Am J Obstet Gynecol 2000; 183(1):S1–S22. [Guideline]
15. Waugh JJ, Clark TJ, Divakaran TG, Accuracy of urinalysis dipstick techniques in predicting significant proteinuria in pregnancy. Obstet Gynecol 2004; 103(4):769–777. [Review; III]
16. Martin JN Jr., Rose CH, Briery CM. Understanding and managing HELLP syndrome: the integral role of aggressive glucocorticoids for mother and child. Am J Obstet Gynecol 2006; 195(4):914–934. [Review; III]
17. Rath W, Fischer T. The diagnosis and treatment of hypertensive disorders of pregnancy: new findings for antenatal and inpatient care. Dtsch Arztebl Int 2009; 106(45):733–738. [Review; III]
18. Cnossen JS, Morris RK, ter Riet G, Use of uterine artery Doppler ultrasonography to predict pre-eclampsia and intrauterine growth restriction: a systematic review and bivariable meta-analysis. CMAJ 2008; 178(6):701–711. [Meta-analysis, 74 studies, *n* = 79,547; I]
19. Sibai B, Dekker G, Kupferminc M. Pre-eclampsia. Lancet 2005; 365(9461):785–799. [Review; III]
20. Haddad B, Sibai BM. Expectant management in pregnancies with severe pre-eclampsia. Semin Perinatol 2009; 33(3):143–151. [Review; III]
21. Sibai BM. Expectant management of preeclampsia. OBG Management 2005; 3:18–36. [Review; III]
22. Sibai BM, Barton JR. Expectant management of severe preeclampsia remote from term: patient selection, treatment, and delivery indications. Am J Obstet Gynecol 2007; 196(6):514–519. [Review; III]
23. Duley L, Henderson-Smart DJ, Meher S, Antiplatelet agents for preventing pre-eclampsia and its complications. Cochrane Database Syst Rev 2007; (2):CD004659. [Meta-analysis; 59 RCTs, *n* = 37,560; I]
24. Kozer E, Nikfar S, Costei A, Aspirin consumption during the first trimester of pregnancy and congenital anomalies: a meta-analysis. Am J Obstet Gynecol 2002; 187(6):1623–1630. [Meta-analysis; 22 RCTs; I]
25. Bujold E, Roberge S, Lacasse Y, Prevention of preeclampsia and intrauterine growth restriction with aspirin started in early pregnancy: a meta-analysis. Obstet Gynecol 2010; 116(2 pt 1):402–414. [Meta-analysis; 34 RCTs, *n* = 11,348; I]
26. Bujold E, Morency AM, Roberge S, Acetylsalicylic acid for the prevention of preeclampsia and intra-uterine growth restriction in women with abnormal uterine artery Doppler: a systematic review and meta-analysis. J Obstet Gynaecol Can 2009; 31(9):818–826. [Meta-analysis; 9 RCTs, *n* = 1317; I]
27. Subtil D, Goeusse P, Houfflin-Debarge V, Randomised comparison of uterine artery Doppler and aspirin (100 mg) with placebo in nulliparous women: the Essai Regional Aspirine Mere-Enfant study (Part 2). BJOG 2003; 110(5):485–491. [RCT, *n* = 1253; I]
28. Rey E, Garneau P, David M, Dalteparin for the prevention of recurrence of placental-mediated complications of pregnancy in women without thrombophilia: a pilot randomized controlled trial. J Thromb Haemost 2009; 7(1):58–64. [RCT, *n* = 116; I]
29. Bates SM, Greer IA, Pabinger I, Venous thromboembolism, thrombophilia, antithrombotic therapy, and pregnancy: American College of Chest Physicians Evidence-Based Clinical Practice Guidelines (8th Edition). Chest 2008; 133(6 suppl):844S–886S. [Guidelines]
30. Hofmeyr GJ, Lawrie TA, Atallah AN, Calcium supplementation during pregnancy for preventing hypertensive disorders and related problems. Cochrane Database Syst Rev 2010; (8): CD001059. [Meta-analysis; 13 RCTs, *n* = 15,730; I]
31. Levine RJ, Hauth JC, Curet LB, Trial of calcium to prevent preeclampsia. N Engl J Med 1997; 337(2):69–76.
32. Sibai BM. Calcium supplementation during pregnancy reduces risk of high blood pressure, pre-eclampsia and premature birth compared with placebo? Evid Based Med 2011; 16(2):40–41. [Review; III]
33. Rumbold A, Duley L, Crowther CA, Antioxidants for preventing pre-eclampsia. Cochrane Database Syst Rev 2008; (1):CD004227. [Meta-analysis; 10 RCTs, *n* = 6533; I]

34. Villar J, Purwar M, Merialdi M, World Health Organisation multicentre randomised trial of supplementation with vitamins C and E among pregnant women at high risk for pre-eclampsia in populations of low nutritional status from developing countries. BJOG 2009; 116(6):780–788. [RCTs, n = 1365; I]

35. Roberts JM, Myatt L, Spong CY, Vitamins C and E to prevent complications of pregnancy-associated hypertension. N Engl J Med 2010; 362(14):1282–1291. [RCT, n = 10,154; I]

36. McCance DR, Holmes VA, Maresh MJ, Vitamins C and E for prevention of pre-eclampsia in women with type 1 diabetes (DAPIT): a randomised placebo-controlled trial. Lancet 2010; 376(9737):259–266. [RCT, n = 762; I]

37. Xu H, Perez-Cuevas R, Xiong X, An international trial of anti-oxidants in the prevention of preeclampsia (INTAPP). Am J Obstet Gynecol 2010; 202(3):239. [RCT, n = 2363; I]

38. Spinnato JA, Freire S, Pinto e Silva JL, Antioxidant supplementation and premature rupture of the membranes: a planned secondary analysis. Am J Obstet Gynecol 2008; 199(4):433–438. [RCT, n = 697; I]

39. Churchill D, Beevers GD, Meher S, Diuretics for preventing pre-eclampsia. Cochrane Database Syst Rev 2007; (1):CD004451. [Meta-analysis; 5 RCTs, n = 1836; I]

40. Duley L, Henderson-Smart D, Meher S. Altered dietary salt for preventing pre-eclampsia, and its complications. Cochrane Database Syst Rev 2005; (4):CD005548. [Meta-analysis; 2 RCTs, n = 603; I]

41. Makrides M, Duley L, Olsen SF. Marine oil, and other prostaglandin precursor, supplementation for pregnancy uncomplicated by pre-eclampsia or intrauterine growth restriction. Cochrane Database Syst Rev 2006; 3:CD003402. [Meta-analysis; 6 RCTs, n = 2783; I]

42. Meher S, Duley L. Garlic for preventing pre-eclampsia and its complications. Cochrane Database Syst Rev 2006; 3:CD006065. [Meta-analysis; 1 RCT, n = 100; I]

43. Meher S, Duley L. Rest during pregnancy for preventing pre-eclampsia and its complications in women with normal blood pressure. Cochrane Database Syst Rev 2006; (2):CD005939. [Meta-analysis; 2 RCT, n = 106; I]

44. Meher S, Duley L. Exercise or other physical activity for preventing pre-eclampsia and its complications. Cochrane Database Syst Rev 2006; (2):CD005942. [Meta-analysis; 2 RCTs, n = 45]

45. Meher S, Duley L. Progesterone for preventing pre-eclampsia and its complications. Cochrane Database Syst Rev 2006; (4):CD006175. [Meta-analysis; 2 RCTs, n = 296; I]

46. Meher S, Duley L. Nitric oxide for preventing pre-eclampsia and its complications. Cochrane Database Syst Rev 2007; (2):CD006490. [Meta-analysis, 6 RCTs, n = 310]

47. Kroner C, Turnbull D, Wilkinson C. Antenatal day care units versus hospital admission for women with complicated pregnancy. Cochrane Database Syst Rev 2001; (4):CD001803. [Meta-analysis; 1 RCT, n = 54]

48. Tuffnell DJ, Lilford RJ, Buchan PC, Randomised controlled trial of day care for hypertension in pregnancy. Lancet 1992; 339 (8787):224–227. [RCT, n = 54; included in Cochrane by Kroner; I]

49. Turnbull DA, Wilkinson C, Gerard K, Clinical, psychosocial, and economic effects of antenatal day care for three medical complications of pregnancy: a randomised controlled trial of 395 women. Lancet 2004; 363(9415):1104–1109. [RCT, n = 395; not included in Cochrane by Kroner; I]

50. Duley L, Gulmezoglu AM, Henderson-Smart DJ, Magnesium sulphate and other anticonvulsants for women with pre-eclampsia. Cochrane Database Syst Rev 2010; 11:CD000025. [Meta-analysis; 15 RCTs, n = 11,444; I]

51. Sibai BM. Diagnosis, prevention, and management of eclampsia. Obstet Gynecol 2005; 105(2):402–410. [Review; III]

52. Duley L, Matar HE, Almerie MQ, Alternative magnesium sulphate regimens for women with pre-eclampsia and eclampsia. Cochrane Database Syst Rev 2010; (8):CD007388. [Meta-analysis; 6 RCTs, n = 866; of which 2 compared regimens for women with eclampsia and 4 for women with pre-eclampsia; I]

53. Witlin AG, Friedman SA, Sibai BM. The effect of magnesium sulfate therapy on the duration of labor in women with mild preeclampsia at term: a randomized, double-blind, placebo-controlled trial. Am J Obstet Gynecol 1997; 176(3):623–627. [RCT, n = 135; I]

54. Duley L, Williams J, Henderson-Smart DJ. Plasma volume expansion for treatment of women with pre-eclampsia. Cochrane Database Syst Rev 2000; (2):CD001805. [Meta-analysis; 3 RCTs, n = 61; I]

55. Magee LA, Cham C, Waterman EJ, Hydralazine for treatment of severe hypertension in pregnancy: meta-analysis. BMJ 2003; 327 (7421):955–960. [Meta-analysis; 1 RCTs, n = 893, of which eight compared hydralazine with nifedipine and five with labetalol; I]

56. Knight M, Duley L, Henderson-Smart DJ, Withdrawn: antiplatelet agents for preventing and treating pre-eclampsia. Cochrane Database Syst Rev 2007; (2):CD000492. [Meta-analysis; 42 RCTs, n = 32,000; I]

57. Wallace DH, Leveno KJ, Cunningham FG, Randomized comparison of general and regional anesthesia for cesarean delivery in pregnancies complicated by severe preeclampsia. Obstet Gynecol 1995; 86(2):193–199. [RCT, n = 80; I]

58. Alanis MC, Robinson CJ, Hulsey TC, Early-onset severe preeclampsia: induction of labor vs. elective cesarean delivery and neonatal outcomes. Am J Obstet Gynecol 2008; 199(3):262–266. [Level II-3]

59. Alexander JM, Bloom SL, McIntire DD, Severe preeclampsia and the very low birth weight infant: is induction of labor harmful? Obstet Gynecol 1999; 93(4):485–488. [Level III]

60. Berkley E, Meng C, Rayburn WF. Success rates with low dose misoprostol before induction of labor for nulliparas with severe preeclampsia at various gestational ages. J Matern Fetal Neonatal Med 2007; 20(11):825–831. [Level III]

61. Blackwell SC, Redman ME, Tomlinson M, Labor induction for the preterm severe pre-eclamptic patient: is it worth the effort? J Matern Fetal Med 2001; 10(5):305–311. [Level III]

62. Hall DR, Odendaal HJ, Steyn DW. Delivery of patients with early onset, severe pre-eclampsia. Int J Gynaecol Obstet 2001; 74 (2):143–150. [Level III]

63. Mashiloane CD, Moodley J. Induction or caesarean section for preterm pre-eclampsia? J Obstet Gynaecol 2002; 22(4):353–356. [Level III]

64. Nassar AH, Adra AM, Chakhtoura N, Severe preeclampsia remote from term: labor induction or elective cesarean delivery? Am J Obstet Gynecol 1998; 179(5):1210–1213. [Level III]

65. Ganzevoort W, Rep A, Bonsel GJ, A randomised controlled trial comparing two temporising management strategies, one with and one without plasma volume expansion, for severe and early onset pre-eclampsia. BJOG 2005; 112(10):1358–1368. [Meta-analysis; 2 RCTs, n = 216; I]

66. Odendaal HJ, Pattinson RC, Bam R, Aggressive or expectant management for patients with severe preeclampsia between 28–34 weeks' gestation: a randomized controlled trial. Obstet Gynecol 1990; 76(6):1070–1075. [RCT, n = 28; included in Cochrane by Churchill, 2002; I]

67. Sibai BM, Mercer BM, Schiff E, Aggressive versus expectant management of severe preeclampsia at 28 to 32 weeks' gestation: a randomized controlled trial. Am J Obstet Gynecol 1994; 171 (3):818–822. [RCT, n = 95; included in Cochrane by Churchill, 2002; I]

68. Churchill D, Duley L. Interventionist versus expectant care for severe pre-eclampsia before term. Cochrane Database Syst Rev 2002; (3):CD003106. [Meta-analysis; 2 RCTs, n = 133; I]

69. Magee LA, Yong PJ, Espinosa V, Expectant management of severe preeclampsia remote from term: a structured systematic review. Hypertens Pregnancy 2009; 28(3):312–347. [Review; 72 studies; III]

70. Haram K, Svendsen E, Abildgaard U. The HELLP syndrome: clinical issues and management. A review. BMC Pregnancy Childbirth 2009; 9:8. [Review; III]

71. Sibai BM. A practical plan to detect and manage HELLP syndrome. OBG Management 2005; 4:52–69. [Review; III]

72. Sibai BM. Diagnosis, controversies, and management of the syndrome of hemolysis, elevated liver enzymes, and low platelet count. Obstet Gynecol 2004; 103(5 pt 1):981–991. [Review; III]

73. Woudstra DM, Chandra S, Hofmeyr GJ, Corticosteroids for HELLP (hemolysis, elevated liver enzymes, low platelets) syndrome in pregnancy. Cochrane Database Syst Rev 2010; (9): CD008148. [Meta-analysis; 11 RCTs, n = 550; I]

74. Isler CM, Barrilleaux PS, Magann EF, A prospective, randomized trial comparing the efficacy of dexamethasone and betamethasone for the treatment of antepartum HELLP (hemolysis, elevated liver enzymes, and low platelet count) syndrome. Am J Obstet Gynecol 2001; 184(7):1332–1337. [RCT, n = 40. Dexamethasone versus betamethasone; I]

75. Isler CM, Magann EF, Rinehart BK, Dexamethasone compared with betamethasone for glucocorticoid treatment of postpartum HELLP syndrome. Int J Gynaecol Obstet 2003; 80(3):291–297. [RCT, n = 36; Dexamethasone versus betamethasone I]

76. Fonseca JE, Mendez F, Catano C, Dexamethasone treatment does not improve the outcome of women with HELLP syndrome: a double-blind, placebo-controlled, randomized clinical trial. Am J Obstet Gynecol 2005; 193(5):1591–1598. [RCT, n = 132; I]

77. Katz L, de Amorim MM, Figueiroa JN, Postpartum dexamethasone for women with hemolysis, elevated liver enzymes, and low platelets (HELLP) syndrome: a double-blind, placebo-controlled, randomized clinical trial. Am J Obstet Gynecol 2008; 198(3):283–288. [RCT, n = 105;I]

78. van Runnard Heimel PJ, Huisjes AJ, Franx A, A randomised placebo-controlled trial of prolonged prednisolone administration to patients with HELLP syndrome remote from term. Eur J Obstet Gynecol Reprod Biol 2006; 128(1–2):187–193. [RCT, n = 31; I]

79. Duley L. The global impact of pre-eclampsia and eclampsia. Semin Perinatol 2009; 33(3):130–137. [Review; III]

80. Duley L, Henderson-Smart DJ, Walker GJ, Magnesium sulphate versus diazepam for eclampsia. Cochrane Database Syst Rev 2010; 12:CD000127. [Meta-analysis; 7 RCTs, n = 1396; I]

81. Duley L, Henderson-Smart DJ, Chou D. Magnesium sulphate versus phenytoin for eclampsia. Cochrane Database Syst Rev 2010; (10):CD000128. [Meta-analysis; 7 RCTs, n = 972; I]

82. Duley L, Gulmezoglu AM, Chou D. Magnesium sulphate versus lytic cocktail for eclampsia. Cochrane Database Syst Rev 2010; (9): CD002960.

83. Magee L, Sadeghi S. Prevention and treatment of postpartum hypertension. Cochrane Database Syst Rev 2005; (1):CD004351. [Meta-analysis; 6 RCTs: 3 RCTs on prevention, n = 315; 3 RCTs on treatment, n = 144; I]

84. Ascarelli MH, Johnson V, McCreary H, Postpartum preeclampsia management with furosemide: a randomized clinical trial. Obstet Gynecol 2005; 105(1):29–33. [RCT, n = 264; I]

85. Hladunewich MA, Derby GC, Lafayette RA, Effect of L-arginine therapy on the glomerular injury of preeclampsia: a randomized controlled trial. Obstet Gynecol 2006; 107(4):886–895. [RCT, n = 45;I]

86. Sep S, Smits L, Prins M, Prediction tests for recurrent hypertensive disease in pregnancy, a systematic review. Hypertens Pregnancy 2010; 29(2):206–230. [Review, 33 studies; III]

87. Hernandez-Diaz S, Toh S, Cnattingius S. Risk of pre-eclampsia in first and subsequent pregnancies: prospective cohort study. BMJ 2009; 338:b2255. [Cohort analytic study, n = 763,795; II-2]

88. Langenveld J, Jansen S, van der Post J, Recurrence risk of a delivery before 34 weeks of pregnancy due to an early onset hypertensive disorder: a systematic review. Am J Perinatol 2010; 27(7):565–571. [Meta-analysis; 7 RCTs, n = 2188; I]

89. Langenveld J, Buttinger A, van der Post J, Recurrence risk and prediction of a delivery under 34 weeks of gestation after a history of a severe hypertensive disorder. BJOG 2011; 118 (5):589–595. [Cohort analytic study, n = 211; II-2]

90. Chames MC, Haddad B, Barton JR, Subsequent pregnancy outcome in women with a history of HELLP syndrome at < or = 28 weeks of gestation. Am J Obstet Gynecol 2003; 188(6):1504–1507. [II-2]

91. Magnussen EB, Vatten LJ, Smith GD, Hypertensive disorders in pregnancy and subsequently measured cardiovascular risk factors. Obstet Gynecol 2009; 114(5):961–970. [Observational study, n = 15,065; II-3]

2

Cardiac disease

Shailen Shah and Sharon Rubin

KEY POINTS

- Normal pregnancy physiology—particularly increased intravascular volume, hypercoagulability, and decreased systemic vascular resistance—can severely exacerbate cardiac disease during pregnancy.
- **For many cardiac conditions**, especially pulmonary hypertension and aortic stenosis, **relative hypervolemia**, rather than fluid restriction, and **avoidance of hypotension** are the **key intrapartum management principles**. Mitral stenosis and some cases of cardiomyopathy are the main exceptions to this principle.
- Women with congenital heart disease should have a **fetal echocardiogram** at around 22 weeks.
- Most cardiac diseases in pregnancy do *not* benefit from cesarean delivery, and this can be reserved for usual obstetrical indications.
- Pulmonary hypertension, Marfan syndrome with aortic root >4 cm, and severe cardiomyopathy are associated with high maternal mortality, and should be counseled prepregnancy of this risk and provided alternatives to their own pregnancy.

BACKGROUND

For "cardiac disease in pregnancy," this guideline reviews *maternal* cardiac disease. These women are at higher risk for cardiovascular complications, neonatal complications, and even maternal death (1,2). Concern for cardiac decompensation occurs when the heart, either from acquired or congenital physiologic or structural defects, is unable to accommodate pregnancy physiology or dynamics of parturition. There are no trials of intervention for cardiac disease in pregnancy.

SYMPTOMS/SIGNS

Symptoms can include fatigue, limitation of physical activity, palpitations, tachycardia, shortness of breath, chest pain, dyspnea on exertion, and cyanosis. These symptoms and signs of cardiac disease can often be confused with common pregnancy complaints.

EPIDEMIOLOGY/INCIDENCE

Cardiac disease complicates 1% to 4% of pregnancies, but accounts for 10% to 25% of maternal mortality (3–5). In the United States, congenital heart disease (CHD) is more common than rheumatic heart disease as a result of medical care and surgical advances. Despite significant medical and surgical advances over the past two decades, cardiac disease remains a significant cause of maternal mortality.

GENETICS

When the mother has a congenital heart defect, the fetus is at increased risk for a congenital heart defect (generally 3–5%, but ranges from 1% to 15%). Therefore, **fetal echocardiography** (best if done at around 22 weeks) is recommended. DiGeorge syndrome (chromosomal deletion in 22q11), Marfan syndrome, and hypertrophic obstructive cardiomyopathy are all autosomal dominant.

ETIOLOGY/BASIC PATHOPHYSIOLOGY/ PREGNANCY CONSIDERATIONS

The main function of the heart is to provide oxygen (and other nutrients), and remove carbon dioxide (and other wastes) to and from all end organs of the body, which include the uterus and fetus during pregnancy. The chief determinants of oxygen delivery include the amount carried by the blood (determined by the amount of hemoglobin and degree of saturation) and the delivery of that blood: primarily cardiac output (determined by preload, afterload, cardiac contractility, and heart rate). Any disease process or pregnancy physiology that interferes with this main function of the heart can result in maternal and fetal morbidity and mortality.

Five principal physiologic changes of pregnancy can complicate cardiac disease during pregnancy. See also chap. 3, *Obstetric Evidence Based Guidelines* (6):

1. *Decreased systemic vascular resistance (SVR).* For example, ventricular septal defects (VSDs) result in the shunting of blood from the left ventricle to the right ventricle because the systemic blood pressure is greater than the pulmonary blood pressure. Over time, this will result in pulmonary hypertension (PHTN) that can approach systemic blood pressures. Pregnancy, with its associated 20% decrease in SVR, can allow pulmonary pressures to equal or exceed systemic pressures resulting in a reversal, or right to left shunting of blood. This would result in deoxygenated right ventricular blood entering the left ventricle, resulting in decreased oxygen delivery to the body and even cyanosis and death (7).
2. *Increase in intravascular volume.* This occurs throughout pregnancy (50% increase), and is maximal by 32 weeks gestation. Women with severe myocardial dysfunction, such as cardiomyopathy, may not be able to accommodate this physiologic demand and may experience congestive heart failure and pulmonary edema.
3. *Postpartum increase in intravascular volume from "autotransfusion" of blood from the contracted uterus and mobilization of third spaced fluid.* Women with mitral stenosis have restricted left ventricular filling. This postpartum vascular load could result in pulmonary edema (8).
4. *Hypercoagulability.* This well characterized pregnancy adaptation can dramatically heighten the risk for thromboembolism in at-risk patients. Pregnant women with

artificial mechanical heart valves, for example, can develop fatal thromboses despite adequate heparin anticoagulation as a result of this physiology (9,10).

5. *Marked increase in cardiac output during parturition* (11). This increase occurs during pregnancy, and is both necessary for and partly "worsened" by labor and delivery and the postpartum volume shift described above. In women whose cardiac output is fixed and very dependent on preload, like aortic stenosis, these volume shifts are poorly tolerated. A negative volume shift from postpartum hemorrhage can result in a precipitous drop in cardiac output and lead to inadequate coronary and cerebral perfusion (12).

Understanding these pathophysiologic interactions forms the basis for understanding, anticipating, and managing patients with cardiac disease during pregnancy.

CLASSIFICATION

Patients with heart disease are symptomatically classified by their clinical functional class [New York Heart Association (NYHA) system]. Pregnant women who are NYHA III or IV have a poor prognosis for pregnancy, but even less symptomatic women are at risk during pregnancy because up to 40% of those who develop congestive heart failure during gestation begin their pregnancy without symptoms (class I) (13) (Table 2.1), and 15% to 55% of pregnant women with heart disease show deterioration by this system. Contemporary classification categorizes women according to an estimate of risk for mortality because of pregnancy and cardiac disease (Table 2.2) (14).

RISK FACTORS

Predictors of maternal complications include prior cardiac events, NYHA class III or IV (Table 2.1), lesions classified as group II or, especially, III (Table 2.2), left heart obstruction (mitral stenosis, aortic stenosis), mechanical heart valve, Marfan syndrome, and significant left ventricular systolic dysfunction [ejection fraction (EF) $\leq$40%] (15–17).

Table 2.1 New York Heart Association Classification

Class I
    No symptoms or limitations.
    Ordinary physical activity does not cause undue
      fatigue, dyspnea, palpitations, or angina
Class II
    Slight limitation of physical activity.
    Comfortable at rest.
    Ordinary physical activity (e.g., carrying heavy
      packages) may result in fatigue, palpitations,
      or angina
Class III
    Marked limitation of physical activity.
    Comfortable at rest.
    Less than ordinary physical activity
      (e.g., getting dressed) leads to symptoms
Class IV
    Severe limitation of physical activity.
    Symptoms of heart failure or angina are present
      at rest and worsen with any activity

Table 2.2 Maternal Risk Associated with Pregnancy

Group I: Minimal risk of mortality (<1%)
    Atrial septal defect (ASD)
    Ventricular septal defect (VSD)
    Pulmonic or tricuspid valvular disease
    Corrected tetralogy of Fallot
    Bioprosthetic heart valve
    Mitral stenosis, NYHA classes I and II
    Marfan syndrome, normal aorta
    Aortic or mitral insufficiency
    Hypertrophic cardiomyopathy
Group II: Moderate risk of mortality (5–15%)
    Mitral stenosis, NYHA classes III and IV
    Artificial mechanical heart valve, if anticoagulation
      with heparin
    Aortic stenosis
    Coarctation of the aorta, uncomplicated
    Uncorrected tetralogy of Fallot
    Myocardial infarction
Group III: Major risk of mortality (>25%)
    Pulmonary hypertension (PHTN)
    Coarctation of aorta, complicated
    Marfan syndrome, with aortic root >4 cm
    Severe dilated cardiomyopathy

COMPLICATIONS

Today, with proper modern management, maternal mortality is predominantly restricted to patients with severe PHTN, coronary artery disease (CAD), cardiomyopathy, endocarditis, and sudden arrhythmia (4,18). These groups can be used to determine general treatment principles. Neonatal complications mostly derive from preterm birth, miscarriage, and growth restriction.

MANAGEMENT
Preconception Counseling

Women with **cardiac diseases that can be ameliorated** (invasively or noninvasively) **should be advised to do so before pregnancy** to decrease their pregnancy-related morbidity and mortality. These include severe mitral, aortic, or pulmonic stenosis, uncorrected tetralogy of Fallot, CAD, coarctation of the aorta, large intracardiac shunt from atrial septal defect (ASD) or VSD with mild or moderate PHTN (19). Coexisting disorders such as anemia, thyroid disease, or hypertension should be treated and controlled before pregnancy.

On the other hand, certain women should be advised to complete their childbearing before their cardiac condition requires repair, which could further complicate pregnancy management. For example, a woman with moderately severe valvular disease may ultimately require a prosthetic valve in the future. During pregnancy, some of these valves carry very high thromboembolic and anticoagulant risk (9,10).

Counseling should include diet and activity modifications, infection prevention and control, and review of prognosis, possible complications, and management in a future pregnancy.

Patients with group III lesions or significant dilated cardiomyopathy (including peripartum cardiomyopathy with residual left ventricular dysfunction) should be advised *not* to conceive because they have an unacceptable risk of mortality. Contraception and sterilization counseling should be offered. If such patients present postconception, pregnancy termination should be offered (19).

Table 2.3 Cardiac Conditions for Which Antibiotics Prophylaxis for Bacterial Endocarditis is Reasonable

Prosthetic cardiac valve or prosthetic material used for cardiac valve repair
Previous infective endocarditis
Congenital heart disease (CHD):
    Unrepaired cyanotic CHD, including palliative shunts and conduits
    Completely repaired CHD with prosthetic material or conduits (where placed by surgery or catheter intervention
    within six months of procedure)
    Incompletely repaired CHD with residual defects at or near the site of prosthetic patch or device

Source: Adapted from Ref. 28.

Prenatal Care/Antepartum Testing

The patient should be questioned and examined during frequent prenatal visits for cardiac failure. **Maternal echocardiogram** allows assessment of heart function. PHTN is often unreliable when estimated noninvasively by echocardiogram, and so may need to be confirmed by cardiac catheterization. EKG shows physiologic changes such as QRS axis shift to left (because of elevated diaphragm), and minor ST and T-wave changes in lead III. Fetal growth ultrasounds should be performed every four to six weeks when there is concern for developing intrauterine growth restriction. This can be coupled with serial antenatal testing at 34 weeks (20). Postdatism is often best avoided. Finally, future contraceptive plans, including sterilization, should be reviewed (14,21).

General Management

Certain general principles apply to most women with cardiac disease:

1. *Antepartum bed rest.* This can be used to minimize maternal exertion and oxygen demand in the pregnant patient with limited cardiac output or cyanotic heart disease (14). Strict bed rest should be avoided to prevent thromboembolism.
2. *Treat coexisting medical conditions.* The morbidity of cardiac disease can be compounded by medical conditions such as anemia, hypertension, or thyroid disease. Therefore, these conditions should be optimized to minimize their comorbidity (19).
3. *Collaborative care by multiple specialists.* Pregnant patients with cardiac disease are very complex, and should be **managed by a multidisciplinary team of specialists from a variety of areas**, including obstetrics, maternal-fetal medicine, cardiology, and anesthesiology (22).
4. *Labor in the lateral decubitus position.* This maximizes blood return to the heart by decreasing vena caval compression by the gravid uterus, and therefore, maximizes cardiac output (23,24). This preload preservation can be critical to the women with cardiac compromise (14,21).
5. *Epidural anesthesia.* This minimizes pain, sympathetic stress, oxygen utilization, and fluctuations in cardiac output. Sometimes "just" a narcotic epidural should be used, avoiding the sympathetic blockade (and consequent hypotension) of local anesthetics. Spinal anesthesia should be avoided, and epidural should be dosed slowly with adequate prehydration (intravenous fluids) to minimize risk of hypotension and its consequent drop in preload leading to decreased cardiac output (14,25–27).
6. *Oxygen, particularly during labor and delivery, as necessary.* Keeping maternal $PaO_2 \geq 70$ mmHg allows for adequate maternal and fetal hemoglobin oxygen saturation (21,27).
7. *Bacterial endocarditis prophylaxis.* **Antibiotics are recommended only for** those patients deemed to be at *highest*

risk for infective endocarditis: **prosthetic heart valve, unrepaired CHD, repaired CHD with prosthetic material during the first six months after the procedure (during endothelialization), and repaired CHD with residual defect(s)** (Table 2.3) (28). Some experts have even suggested that no prophylaxis is needed at all (29). The usual recommended antibiotic regimen for cardiac prophylaxis is a single dose of ampicillin 2.0 g IV preprocedure. Cefazolin, or ceftriaxone, or clindamycin can be substituted in the penicillin allergic patient (30).

8. *Cesarean delivery is usually reserved for obstetrical indications.* Operative delivery is associated with greater blood loss, increased pain, and prolonged bed rest compared to vaginal delivery, and therefore can complicate the gravida with heart disease. While labor induction and/or assisted second stage may be necessary for certain maternal or fetal indications, **cesarean delivery should be used for usual obstetrical reasons** (20,21,26). Contraindications to trial of labor to be considered are Marfan syndrome with root >4 cm, aortopathy, and maternal therapeutic anticoagulation with Coumadin®, which cannot be interrupted.

9. *Invasive hemodynamic monitoring with a pulmonary artery catheter (PAC).* While the safety and utility of PACs in critically ill nonpregnant patients have been recently questioned (31–33), they may be helpful in managing certain high-risk conditions that are preload dependent, such as critical aortic stenosis or PHTN (14,21).

10. *Most patients benefit from avoiding hypotension during labor and delivery.* While not true for all patients, most with group II and III cardiac lesions will benefit from avoiding hypotension or hypovolemia. **To avoid hypotension, keep woman on "wetter" side, avoid hemorrhage, replenish blood loss adequately, avoid spinal anesthesia, hydrate at least 1 L of intravenous fluids before "slow" epidural, and avoid supine hypotension.**

Pregnancy Management of Specific Diseases

Palpitations

Workup should be similar to the nonpregnant patient, and include thyroid function, and ruling out drugs, alcohol, caffeine, or smoking, as well as an EKG and echocardiogram. The woman can be counseled that premature atrial and ventricular contractions are increased in pregnancy, and usually benign.

VSD

Pregnancy outcome is usually good. Rule out PHTN, especially in large, long-standing cases. In the absence of PHTN, mortality is unlikely (34). Intrapartum, avoid fluid overload (14).

PHTN

It is important to avoid false positive diagnosis of PHTN by echocardiogram, as up to 30% of women with this diagnosis (pulmonary artery systolic pressure >30–40 mmHg) by echocardiography have normal pulmonary pressures by pulmonary artery catheterization. While not all patients require pulmonary catheterization confirmation, it is a useful test when the diagnosis is in doubt or mild, and can be done either antepartum or just before induction (the latter timing allows the catheter to remain in place for labor management).

Over time, in women with unrepaired VSD, ASD, or patent ductus arteriosus (PDA), the congenital left to right shunt leads to PHTN, right to left shunt, and consequently decreased pulmonary perfusion, and hypoxemia. Even with modern management, high risk of maternal death remains (35). Some of this mortality is secondary to thromboembolic events (36). Delayed postpartum death can be seen four to six weeks after delivery, possibly secondary to loss of pregnancy-associated hormones and increased pulmonary vascular resistance (PVR) (14,36).

The main physiologic difficulty in PHTN is maintenance of adequate pulmonary blood flow. Any situation that decreases venous return to the heart decreases right ventricular preload and consequently pulmonary blood flow. Therefore, as hypovolemia and **hypotension** can fatally precipitate decreased pulmonary perfusion and oxygenation (and reverse the left to right cardiac shunt in cases of Eisenmenger's syndrome; see section "Etiology/Basic Pathophysiology/Pregnancy Considerations"), leading to sudden death, it **must be avoided**. Such situations are common intrapartum (vasodilation from regional anesthesia or pooling of blood in the lower extremities from vena caval compression) and sometimes unanticipated (hemorrhage). As such, patients are better managed on the "wet" side, even at the expense of mild pulmonary edema. This allows a margin of safety against unexpected hemorrhage or drug-induced hypotension (36). PAC may be useful in this regard (14). Avoid increase in PVR and myocardial depressants. Anticoagulant prophylaxis may be useful in preventing thromboembolic risk, and intravenous prostacyclin (or its analogues) or inhaled nitric oxide may be helpful in reducing PVR while sparing the SVR (37,38).

Coarctation of the Aorta

If surgically corrected, maternal outcome is good. There is increased risk for maternal mortality when associated with aneurysmal dilation or associated cardiac lesions (VSD, PDA) (39). Avoid hypotension, myocardial depression, and bradycardia (40).

Tetralogy of Fallot

It consists of VSD, pulmonary stenosis, hypertrophy of right ventricle, and overriding aorta. Corrected lesions do well, but uncorrected ones are still associated with high maternal mortality (41). Because of the VSD-associated shunting in uncorrected cases, **hypotension**, myocardial depressants, and bradycardia **should be avoided** (14).

Mitral Stenosis

Women with >1.5 cm² mitral valve area, usually have good outcomes. When significant (valve area < 1.5 cm²) mitral stenosis is present, left ventricular filling is limited, which leads to fixed cardiac output. If the pregnant patient is unable to accommodate the volume shifts that occur during gestation and puerperium, pulmonary edema can result (see pathophysiology above). Antenatally, this risk is greatest at 30 to

32 weeks when maternal blood volume peaks. In that scenario, percutaneous balloon valvuloplasty may be relatively safely performed in certain patients (42). While it appears safer for the fetus than open mitral commissurotomy, it should be reserved for women who are unresponsive to aggressive medical therapy (43,44). As cardiac output is dependent on adequate diastolic filling time, **tachycardia** can result in hemodynamic decompensation (hypotension and fall in cardiac output) and should be **avoided**. Intrapartum, therefore, short-acting beta-blockers should be considered when pulse exceeds 90 to 100 bpm (14,45). While inadequate preload will decrease cardiac output, too much will result in pulmonary edema, particularly postpartum when pulmonary capillary wedge pressure (PCWP) can rise up to 16 mmHg (8). PAC and cautious, individualized intrapartum diuresis to a predelivery target of 14 mmHg (while normal is 6 to 9 mmHg, mitral stenosis patients often need elevated wedge pressures to maintain left ventricular filling) are desirable in some patients (14). Patients with moderate stenosis with only mild fluid overload can often be managed with just fluid restriction to complement their insensible loss during labor (14). Avoid decrease in SVR and increase in PVR.

Aortic Stenosis

The major issue is fixed and limited cardiac output through a restricted valve area. Mortality is related to degree of stenosis, with >100 mmHg of mean shunt gradient associated with 15% to 20% mortality. CHF (congestive heart failure), syncope, and previous cardiac arrest are other contraindications to pregnancy. Hypotension and decreased preload can lead to a precipitous drop in cardiac output. Consequently, **hypotension should be avoided** (46). Intrapartum, PAC monitoring may be helpful to increase the PCWP to the range of 15 to 17 mmHg to maintain a margin of safety against unexpected blood loss or hypotension (although the data is insufficient for an evidence-based recommendation) (14,21). This range of PCWP minimizes risk of frank pulmonary edema even with normal postpartum fluid shifts, and furthermore, hypovolemia is potentially more dangerous in these patients than pulmonary edema. Avoid decrease in venous return, and tachycardia.

Mitral and Aortic Insufficiency

These lesions are usually well tolerated in pregnancy unless associated with NYHA III or IV symptoms at baseline. Avoid arrhythmia, bradycardia, increase in SVR, and myocardial depressants.

Mechanical Heart Valves

Women who anticipate ultimately needing valve replacement surgery should be encouraged to complete childbearing before valve replacement. For women with mechanical heart valves, optimal anticoagulation during pregnancy is controversial. The highest risk is with first-generation mechanical valves (Starr–Edwards, Bjork–Shiley) in the mitral position, followed by second-generation valves (St. Jude) in the aortic position. These women need to be **therapeutically anticoagulated throughout pregnancy and postpartum, with blood levels frequently (usually weekly) checked to ensure therapeutic levels of anticoagulation**. With unfractionated heparin, mid-interval activated partial thromboplastin time (PTT) should be maintained at about 60 to 80 seconds. With warfarin, international normalized ratio (INR) should be maintained at 2.0 to 3.0. With low-molecular-weight heparin, peak anti-Xa level should be about 0.8 to 1.2 and trough 0.6 to 0.7. Warfarin throughout pregnancy and postpartum is probably the regimen associated with the least maternal risks of thromboembolism, but in the first trimester warfarin is associated with a 10% to 15% teratogenic risk (nasal hypoplasia, optic atrophy, digital anomalies, mental impairment). On the other hand, heparin throughout can be ineffective (9,10). A common option recommended by many authorities utilizes unfractionated **heparin during the first trimester to minimize teratogenesis, warfarin for the majority of pregnancy (12–36 weeks), and unfractionated heparin again in the last month to prepare for delivery and allow for epidural anesthesia** (47–50). For high-risk valves, this staged approach is considered by many as the best option, given very high risk for thromboembolic complication with just heparin or Lovenox[R]. While this may be efficacious, fetal risk is not completely eliminated (51). Low-molecular-weight heparin in this setting has been associated with reports of valve thrombosis, with an FDA warning against its use in this setting (although this decision was criticized) (52,53). Regarding delivery, therapeutic anticoagulation should be stopped during active labor and for delivery, with therapeutic heparin restarted about 6 to 12 hours after delivery, and warfarin restarted in an overlapping fashion (to avoid paradoxical thrombosis) 24 to 36 hours after delivery (the night after delivery). Extensive counseling on all these options and risks is required.

Marfan Syndrome
Marfan syndrome is an autosomal dominant generalized connective tissue disorder, with 80% of affected women having a family history of this condition. Its main risk in pregnancy is aortic aneurysm, leading to rupture and dissection. Women with personal or family history of Marfan syndrome should have an **echocardiogram**, possibly a slit lamp examination to look for ectopia lentis and **genetic counseling**. Prognosis is reasonable when there is no aortic root involvement (<5% mortality), although mortality can still occur. There is a risk of aortic rupture, dissection, and mortality (up to 50%) in pregnancy **when the aortic root is dilated beyond 4 cm**, such that pregnancy is contraindicated in these women before repair. This may result from the "shearing force" of normal pregnancy because of increase in blood volume and cardiac output (54–56). Prenatally, serial maternal echocardiograms to follow the cardiac root should be performed (55). **Hypertension should be avoided**, and **beta-blockade therapy** should be considered. While pregnancy data are limited for this last recommendation, long-term use in nonpregnant patients has been shown to slow the progression of aortic root dilation (57). Avoid positive inotropic drugs, and plan epidural (watch for dural ectasia, present in about 90% of patients with Marfan syndrome) to reduce cardiovascular stress. If cesarean delivery is required, retention sutures should be considered because of generalized connective tissue weakness (14).

Hypertrophic Cardiomyopathy
(Previously called idiopathic hypertrophic subaortic stenosis.) It can be inherited as autosomal dominant, with variable penetrance. It can result in left ventricular hypertrophy, leading to obstruction of the left ventricular outflow. The decrease in SVR of pregnancy can worsen outflow obstruction. Also, tachycardia decreases diastolic filling time, compromising cardiac output. Peripartum management focuses on avoiding tachycardia (treatment with beta-blockade), hypovolemia, and hypotension (58,59).

Dilated Cardiomyopathy
The left ventricle is hypokinetic, cardiac output falls, and can be associated with arrhythmia and possible CHF. Etiology includes autoimmune, alcohol, infection, and genetic. When severe, ideal treatment is prepregnancy transplantation.

Peripartum Cardiomyopathy
This is defined as cardiomyopathy (with EF <45%) occurring during last four weeks of pregnancy or within five months postpartum (peaks at 2 months postpartum), without other cause. The incidence is 1/3000 to 4000 live births. Risk factors are older maternal age, multiparity, African-American race, multiple gestations, and hypertensive disorders of pregnancy. Serial echocardiography, medical management (**digoxin, diuretics**, afterload reduction—**hydralazine** and/or **beta-blockers** in pregnancy, ACE inhibitors postpartum), anticoagulation if EF is <35%, and possible intrapartum PAC in severe patients are useful for management (14,60–63). The addition of bromocriptine to standard heart failure therapy appears to improve left ventricular EF and a composite clinical outcome in women with acute severe peripartum cardiomyopathy, but the number of patients studied was too small to make any recommendation (64).

Regarding future pregnancies after a diagnosis of peripartum cardiomyopathy, persistent dilated cardiomyopathy with abnormal EF predicts a high risk (19%) of mortality and symptoms of cardiac failure (44%) with subsequent gestation, and should be discouraged. Even women with "normal" echocardiograms (EF ≥ 45–50%) after recovering from peripartum cardiomyopathy can have persistent "subclinical" low contractile reserve (61), with up to 21% risk of developing symptoms of CHF, but no mortality reported in one study (63). Of women with EF < 25%, 57% require a cardiac transplant or are on a transplant list because of progressive symptoms of heart failure at a mean of 3.4 years of follow-up postpartum (65).

Coronary Artery Disease
Underlying risks factors, such as diabetes, obesity, hypercholesterolemia, smoking, hypertension, and stress, should be individually addressed and treated, ideally before conception. Stable angina can be treated with nitrates, calcium channel blockers, and/or beta-blockers in pregnancy. With unstable angina, the woman should be counseled regarding severe risks, and offered termination if early enough in pregnancy. Myocardial infarction (MI) is rare in reproductive age women, with a 1/10,000 incidence in the pregnancy. When it occurs in the third trimester or within two weeks of labor, there is a high (20%) maternal mortality risk (66). Women with prior MI with recovered heart function and optimally controlled CAD can anticipate a successful pregnancy (67). Management of MI during pregnancy is similar to management principles in nonpregnant patients including coronary angioplasty (or stent), although thrombolytic therapy is a relative contraindication (21,66,68). Heparin and beta-blockers are recommended. If labor occurs within four days of an MI, cesarean delivery is often advocated (69). Women with a prior MI should wait at least one year and ensure normal cardiac function before pregnancy. In such circumstances, a future pregnancy is associated with low risk of maternal or fetal morbidity or mortality.

CONCLUSION
With medical and surgical advances, and advancing maternal age, heart disease complicating pregnancy is increasingly common. Understanding the physiologic changes of pregnancy and their effect on specific cardiac conditions forms the basis for management during pregnancy. Optimizing

cardiac function and decreasing risk of cardiac decompensation by proper management and close prenatal surveillance will allow most pregnant women with heart disease to enjoy favorable maternal and fetal outcome.

REFERENCES

1. Siu S, Colman J, Sorenson S. Adverse neonatal and cardiac outcomes are more common in pregnant women with cardiac disease. Circulation 2002; 105:2179. [II-3]
2. Berg C, Callaghan W, Syverson C, et al. Pregnancy-related mortality in the United States, 1998 to 2005. Obstet Gynecol 2010; 116:1302–1309. [II-3]
3. Koonin LM, Atrash HK, Lawson HW, et al. Maternal mortality surveillance, United States 1979–1986. MMWR CDC Surveill Summ 1991; 40:1–13. [II-3]
4. DeSweit M. Maternal mortality from heart disease in pregnancy. Br Heart J 1993; 69:524. [II-3]
5. Berg CJ, Atrash HK, Koonin LM, et al. Pregnancy-related mortality in the United States, 1987–1990. Obstet Gynecol 1996; 88:161–167. [II-3]
6. American College of Obstetricians and Gynecologists. Cardiac Disease in Pregnancy. ACOG Technical Bulletin No. 168—June 1992. Int J Gynaecol Obstet. 1993; 41(3):298–306. [III]
7. Sinnenberg RJ. Pulmonary hypertension in pregnancy. South Med J 1980; 73:1529–1531. [III]
8. Clark SL, Phelan JP, Greenspoon J, et al. Labor and delivery in the presence of mitral stenosis: central hemodynamic observations. Am J Obstet Gynecol 1985; 152:984–988. [II-3]
9. Oakley CM, Doherty P. Pregnancy in patients after heart valve replacement. Br Heart J 1976; 38:1140–1148. [II-3]
10. Golby AJ, Bush EC, DeRook FA, et al. Failure of high-dose heparin to prevent recurrent cardioembolic strokes in a pregnancy patient with a mechanical heart valve. Neurology 1992; 42:2204–2206. [III]
11. van Oppen ACC, Stigter RH, Bruinse HW. Cardiac output in normal pregnancy: a critical review. Obstet Gynecol 1996; 87:310–318. [III]
12. Arias F, Pineda J. Aortic stenosis and pregnancy. J Reprod Med 1978; 20:229–232. [II-3]
13. Sciscione AC, Callen NA. Pregnancy and contraception: congenital heart disease in adolescents and adults. Cardiol Clin 1993; 11:701–709. [III]
14. Foley MR. Cardiac disease. In: Dildy GA, Belfort MA, Saade GR, et al. eds. Critical Care Obstetrics. 4th ed. Molden, MA: Blackwell Publishing Company, 2004; 252–274. [II-3]
15. Siu S, Sermer M, Colman J, et al. Prospective multicenter study of pregnancy outcomes in women with heart disease. Circulation 2001; 104(5):515–521. [II-2]
16. Bonow R, Carabello B, Chatterjee K, et al. 2008 Focused update incorporated into the ACC/AHA 2006 guidelines for the management of patients with valvular heart disease: a report of the American College of Cardiology/American Heart Association Task Force on Practice Guidelines (Writing Committee to Revise the 1998 Guidelines for the Management of Patients With Valvular Heart Disease): endorsed by the Society of Cardiovascular Anesthesiologists, Society for Cardiovascular Angiography and Interventions, and Society of Thoracic Surgeons. Circulation 2008; 118(15):e523–e661. [III]
17. Vahanian A, Baumgartner H, Bax J, et al. Guidelines on the management of valvular heart disease: The Task Force on the Management of Valvular Heart Disease of the European Society of Cardiology. Eur Heart J 2007; 28:230. [III]
18. Jacob S, Bloebaum L, Shah G, et al. Maternal mortality in Utah. Obstet Gynecol 1998; 91:187–191. [II-3]
19. Blanchard DG, Shabetai R. Cardiac diseases. In: Creasy RK, Resnik R, Iams JD, eds. Maternal Fetal Medicine Principles and Practice. 5th ed. Philadelphia, PA: Saunders, 2004; 815–844. [III]
20. McFaul PB, Dornan JC, Lamki H, et al. Pregnancy complicated by maternal heart disease: a review of 519 women. BJOG 1988; 95:861–867. [III]
21. Tomlinson MW. Cardiac disease. In: James DK, Steer PJ, Weiner CP, et al. eds. High Risk Pregnancy Management Options. 3rd ed. Philadelphia, PA: Saunders, 2006. [III]
22. Surgue D, Blake S, MacDonald D. Pregnancy complicated by maternal heart disease at the National Maternity Hospital, Dublin, Ireland, 1969–1978. Am J Obstet Gynecol 1981; 139:1–6. [III]
23. Ueland K, Novy MJ, Peterson EN, et al. Maternal cardiovascular dynamics IV. The influence of gestational age on maternal cardiovascular response to posture and exercise. Am J Obstet Gynecol 1969; 104:856. [II-3]
24. Clark SL, Cotton DB, Pivarnik JM, et al. Position change and hemodynamic profiling during normal third-trimester pregnancy and postpartum. Am J Obstet Gynecol 1991; 164:883. [II-3]
25. Vadhera RB. Anesthesia for the critically ill parturient with cardiac disease and pregnancy induced hypertension. In: Dildy GA, Belfort MA, Saade GR, et al. eds. Critical Care Obstetrics. 4th ed. Malden, MA: Blackwell Publishing, 2004. [III]
26. Siu S, Sermer M, Colman J, et al. Prospective multicenter study of pregnancy outcome in women with heart disease. Circulation 2001; 104:515–521. [II-3]
27. Sobrevilla LA, Cassinella MT, Carcelen A, et al. Human fetal and maternal oxygen tension and acid–base status during delivery at high altitude. Am J Obstet Gynecol 1971; 111:1111–1118. [III]
28. Antibiotic prophylaxis for infective endocarditis. ACOG Committee Opinion No. 421. American College of Obstetricians and Gynecologists. Obstet Gynecol 2008; 112:1193–1194. [Review]
29. Tower C, Nallapena S, Vause S. Prophylaxis against endocarditis in obstetrics: new NICE guideline: a commentary. BJOG 2008; 115:1601–1604. [III]
30. Wilson W, Taubert K, Gewitz M, et al. Prevention of infective endocarditis: guidelines from the AHA. Circulation 2007; 116:1736–1754. [III]
31. Bernard G, Sopko G, Cerra F, et al. Pulmonary artery catheterization and clinical outcomes: National Heart, Lung, and Blood Institute and Food and Drug Administration Workshop Report. JAMA 2000; 283:2568–2572. [III]
32. Sandham JD, Hull RD, Brant RF, et al. A randomized, controlled trial of the use of pulmonary-artery catheters in high-risk surgical patients. N Engl J Med 2003; 348:5–14. [I]
33. Parson PE. Progress in research on pulmonary-artery catheters. N Engl J Med 2003; 348:66–68. [III]
34. Schaefer G, Arditi LI, Solomon HA, et al. Congenital heart disease and pregnancy. Clin Obstet Gynecol 1968; 11:1048–1063. [III]
35. Avila WS, Grinberg M, Snitcowsky R, et al. Maternal and fetal outcome in pregnant women with Eisenmenger's syndrome. Eur Heart J 1995; 16:460–464. [III]
36. Weiss BM, Zemp L, Seifert B, et al. Outcome of pulmonary vascular disease in pregnancy: a systematic overview from 1978–1996. J Am Coll Cardiol 1998; 31:1650–1657. [III]
37. Stewart R, Tuazon D, Olson G, et al. Pregnancy and primary pulmonary hypertension. Chest 2001; 119:973–975. [III]
38. Lam JK, Stafford RE, Thorp J, et al. Inhaled nitric oxide for primary pulmonary hypertension in pregnancy. Obstet Gynecol 2001; 98:895–898. [II-3]
39. Deal K, Wooley CF. Coarctation of the aorta and pregnancy. Ann Intern Med 1973; 78:706–710. [III]
40. Koszalka, MF. Cardiac disease in pregnancy. In: Foley MR, Strong TH. Obstetric Intensive Care: A Practical Manual. Philadelphia, PA: Saunders, 1997. [III]
41. Shime J, Mocarski EJM, Hastings D, et al. Congenital heart disease in pregnancy: short and long term implications. Am J Obstet Gynecol 1987; 156:313–322. [III]
42. Iung B, Cormier B, Elias J, et al. Usefulness of percutaneous balloon commissurotomy for mitral stenosis during pregnancy. Am J Cardiol 1994; 73:398–400. [III]
43. Elkayam U, Bitar F. Valvular heart disease in pregnancy. Part I: native valves. J Am Coll Cardiol 2005; 46:223. [III]
44. de Souza J, Martinez E, Ambrose J, et al. Percutaneous balloon mitral valvuloplasty in comparison with open mitral valve commissurotomy for mitral stenosis during pregnancy. J Am Coll Vardiol 2001; 37(3):900–903. [II-3]

45. Al Kasab SM, Sabag T, Al Zailbag M, et al. β-Adrenergic receptor blockade in the management of pregnant women with mitral stenosis. Am J Obstet Gynecol 1990; 163:37–40. [III]

46. Lao TT, Stemmer M, Magee L, et al. Congenital aortic stenosis and pregnancy: a reappraisal. Am J Obstet Gynecol 1993; 169:540–545. [III]

47. Vongpatanasin W, Hillis LD, Lange RA. Prosthetic heart valves. N Eng J Med 1996; 335:407–416. [III]

48. Gohlke-Barwolf C, Acar J, Burckhardt D, et al. Guidelines for prevention of thromboembolic events in valvular heart disease. Ad Hoc Committee of the Working Group on Valvular Heart Disease, European Society of Cardiology: J Heart Valve Dis 1993; 2:398–410. [III]

49. Elkayam U, Bitar F. Valvular heart disease in pregnancy. Part II: Prosthetic valves. J Am Coll Cardiol 2005; 46:403. [III]

50. Bates S, Greer I, Hirsh J, et al. Use of antithrombotic agents during pregnancy: the seventh ACCP conference on antithrombotic and thrombolytic therapy. Chest 2004; 126:627S. [III]

51. Briggs GG, Freeman RK, Yaffe SJ. Drugs in Pregnancy and Lactation. Baltimore: Williams and Wilkins, 1994. [Review]

52. Ginsberg JS, Chan WS, Bates SM, et al. Anticoagulation of pregnant women with mechanical heart valves. Arch Intern Med 2003; 163:694–698. [III]

53. The Anticoagulation in Prosthetic Valves and Pregnancy Consensus Report Panel and Scientific Roundtable. Anticoagulation and enoxaparin use in patients with prosthetic heart valves and/or pregnancy. Fetal–Maternal Medicine Consensus Reports 2002; 3:1–20. [III]

54. Pyeritz RE. Maternal and fetal complications of pregnancy in the Marfan syndrome. Am J Med 1981; 71:784–790. [III]

55. Rossiter JP, Repke JT, Morales AJ, et al. A prospective longitudinal evaluation of pregnancy in the Marfan syndrome. Am J Obstet Gynecol 1995; 173:1599–1606. [III]

56. Lipscomb KJ, Smith JC, Clarke B, et al. Outcome of pregnancy in women with Marfan's syndrome. BJOG 1997; 104:201–206.

57. Shores J, Berger KR, Murphy EA, et al. Progression of aortic dilatation and the benefit of long term β-adrenergic blockade in Marfan's syndrome. N Eng J Med 1994; 330:1335–1341. [II-3]

58. Maron BJ. Hypertrophic cardiomyopathy: a systematic review. JAMA 2002; 287:1308–1320. [III]

59. Fairley CJ, Clarke JT. Use of esmolol in a parturient with hypertrophic obstructive cardiomyopathy. Br J Anaesth 1995; 74:801–804. [III]

60. Demakis JG, Rahimtoola SH, Sutton GC, et al. Natural course of peripartum cardiomyopathy. Circulation 1971; 44:1053–1061. [III]

61. Lampert MB, Weinert L, Hibbard J, et al. Contractile reserve in patients with peripartum cardiomyopathy and recovered left ventricular function. Am J Obstet Gynecol 1997; 176:189–195. [II-3]

62. Witlin AG, Mabie WC, Sibai BM. Peripartum cardiomyopathy: an ominous diagnosis. Am J Obstet Gynecol 1997; 176:182–188. [III]

63. Elkayam U, Tummala PP, Rao K, et al. Maternal and fetal outcomes of subsequent pregnancies in women with peripartum cardiomyopathy. N Eng J Med 2001; 344:1567–1571. [II-3]

64. Sliwa K, Blauwet L, Tibazarwa K, et al. Evaluation of bromocriptine in the treatment of acute severe peripartum cardiomyopathy: a proof-of-concept pilot study. Circulation 2010; 121 (13):1465–1473. [RCT, *n* = 20]

65. Habli M, O'Brien T, Nowack E, et al. Peripartum cardiomyopathy: prognostic factors for long-term outcome. Am J Obstet Gynecol 2008; 199(4):415.e1–415.e5. [II-2]

66. Roth A, Elkayam RA. Acute myocardial infarction associated with pregnancy. Ann Intern Med 1996; 125:751–762. [III]

67. Vinatier D, Virelizier S, Depret-Mosser S, et al. Pregnancy after myocardial infarction. Eur J Obstet Gynecol Reprod Biol 1994; 56:89–93. [III]

68. Garry D, Leikin E, Fleisher AG, et al. Acute myocardial infarction in pregnancy with subsequent medical and surgical management. Obstet Gynecol 1996; 87:802–804. [III]

69. Mabie WC, Anderson GD, Addington MB, et al. The benefit of cesarean section in acute myocardial infarction complicated by premature labor. Obstet Gynecol 1988; 71:503–506. [III]

3

Obesity

Geeta Chhibber

KEY POINTS

- **The preconception visit may be the single most important health care visit when viewed in the context of its effect on pregnancy. Height in meters and weight in kilograms should be recorded for all women at each doctor visit to allow for calculation of BMI. The BMI category should be reviewed with the patient, making sure she understands that her category is not normal.**

- Obesity is a risk factor for cardiovascular disease; diabetes; hypertension; stroke; osteoarthritis; gall stones; increased incidence of endometrial, breast, or colon cancer; cardiomyopathy; fatty liver; obstructive sleep apnea; urinary tract infections; other complications; and, most importantly, mortality. Prepregnancy obesity and excessive gestational weight gain are associated with increased risk of childhood obesity.

- **Preconception weight loss with diet, exercise, behavior change**, and, if necessary, pharmacotherapy is recommended. Weight loss of at least 5% to 10% will help reduce the incidence of obesity-related comorbidities.

- Preconception (and at first prenatal visit), check **BP with a large cuff, fasting lipid profile and blood sugar, thyroid function tests**, and **overnight polysomnogram**. In obese patients with chronic hypertension or type 2 diabetes, it is advisable to obtain an **EKG** and an **echocardiogram**.

- Women with BMI ≥40 or ≥35 with comorbidities are candidates for **bariatric surgery** in the preconception or interconception period. Incidences of gestational diabetes and hypertension are reduced after gastric bypass surgery, especially if BMI is back to less than obese levels. Pregnant patients with bariatric surgery can be started on **vitamin B12, folate, iron, and calcium if deficient.**

- Obesity is strongly correlated with impaired fertility, miscarriage, congenital malformations, gestational diabetes, hypertension, preeclampsia, stillbirth, cesarean birth, labor abnormalities, macrosomia, anesthesia complications, wound infection, and thromboembolism.

- **Discussion and education about obesity and its comorbidities and poor perinatal outcomes are recommended.**

- Optimal gestational weight gain in the obese remains unclear. Some data **suggest no weight gain or even some weight loss in obese (especially class III obesity) gravidas for optimal obstetric outcomes.**

- **At cesarean, the subcutaneous layer should be closed with sutures if depth is >2 cm to reduce wound infection and separation.**

- **Early mobilization** after delivery, and **graduated compression stocking** during and after cesarean are recommended.

- Postpartum, women should be strongly encouraged and helped to **return to a normal BMI**, through **counseling, diet, exercise, and breast-feeding**.

DEFINITION AND CLASSIFICATION

Obesity is defined as **BMI ≥ 30 kg/m²** (Table 3.1) (1). BMI is defined as weight in kilograms divided by height in meters squared. BMI correlates best with body fat mass. It is a simple clinical tool, with online calculators available (http://www.nhlbisupport.com/bmi/). Increasing severity of class of obesity in pregnancy is associated with greater risks of adverse perinatal outcomes (Table 3.2) and other health risks (Table 3.3) (2). A waist circumference >88 cm or 35 in. measured at the level of the iliac crest in expiration is an indicator of central obesity that identifies obese women at higher risk for cardiovascular disease and metabolic disorders.

EPIDEMIOLOGY/INCIDENCE

WHO describes **obesity** as "one of the most blatantly visible, yet neglected, public-health problems that threatens to overwhelm both more and less developed countries." The International Obesity Taskforce estimates that there are presently **at least 1.1 billion overweight adults worldwide**, including 312 million who are obese. At all ages and throughout the world, women are generally found to have higher mean BMI and higher rates of obesity than men for biological reasons (49). These numbers are increasing as the obesity epidemic explodes on the public health stage. WHO further projects that by 2015 approximately 2.3 billion adults will be overweight and **700 million will be obese** (50). In the United States, there has been a recent 40% increase in prepregnancy prevalence of overweight and obesity in women, and 36% increase in obesity at time of delivery in the course of a decade. As a consequence, 1 in 7 cesarean deliveries in 2001 were because of the problem of overweight and obesity in women (51).

Morbid obesity (BMI > 40 kg/m², class III obesity) has almost doubled from 1990 to 2000 (51).

A U.S. National 2007–2008 survey has noted the **prevalence of obesity** as **36%**, class II obesity as 18%, and class III obesity as 7% of all women >20 years of age (52). About 63% of these women are in their reproductive years. There are racial differences with **non-Hispanic black women** at greatest risk for all levels of obesity, **50% with BMI > 30**, 28% with BMI > 35, and 14% with BMI > 40, followed by the Hispanic population including Mexican Americans (52).

GENETICS

A heritability of about 50% to 90% has been shown in adoptive and biological relationships (53). Role of chromosome 2 p 21 with serum leptin levels in human pregnancies has been identified in some ethnic groups (53). The risk of childhood obesity is significantly increased if one parent is obese, but the risk is even higher if both parents are affected (adjusted odds ratio 10.4, 95% confidence interval 5.1–21.3) (54). Many other single mutations in different genes have been identified (55).

Table 3.1 The International Classification of Adult Underweight, Overweight, and Obesity According to BMI, WHO

Classification	BMI (kg/m^2)
Underweight	<18.5
Normal range	18.5–24.9
Overweight	25.0–30.0
Obese	≥30.0
Obese class I	30.0–34.9
Obese class II	35.0–39.9
Obese class III	≥40.0

Source: From Ref. 1.

Maternal obesity results in in-utero programming and childhood obesity. Additionally, environmental factors such as diet play a role in obesity (55).

ETIOLOGY/BASIC PATHOPHYSIOLOGY

White adipose tissue produces proteins with endocrine function called adipokines. A state of relative hypoxia occurs in the adipocytes in obesity, which sets a chronic inflammatory response, causing the release of adipokines. Leptin, adiponectin, resistin, and ghrelin are the most studied adipokines (56).

Table 3.2 Complications of Obesity Related to Pregnancy (see also text)

	Risk (%) or OR	Comments	Ref.
Infertility	OR 1.7–2	Smoking is a risk factor in the obese	3–5
Miscarriage	OR 2–3		3,6,7
Prenatal/Medical			
Chronic hypertension	OR 2–3		3,8,9
Gestational hypertension	OR 2.5–3.2		10
Preeclampsia	OR 1.6–3.3	OR 4.8 class III	10–14
Gestational diabetes	OR 1.4–20		3,8,15,16
Venous thromboembolism	OR 2		3
Obstructive sleep apnea	OR 1.12		17–20
Respiratory problems (e.g., asthma exacerbations)	OR 1.3		21
Depression	OR 1.12	OR 4.9 class III	22,23
Urinary tract infections	OR 1.4		4
Obstetric			
Spontaneous pregnancy loss	OR 1.7		6,15
Indicated preterm birth	OR 1.3	Includes overweight	24
Spontaneous preterm birth	OR 1.24		24
Lower accuracy of ultrasound	25–48% detection—residual anomaly risk after ultrasound in obese 1%	Progressively worse with increasing BMI	25
Difficulty with fetal testing (e.g., FH monitoring)		No definite recommendation for invasive monitoring	26
Failure to progress	OR 2.6	Class II	27
Induction of labor	OR 2.2		8,13
Fetal distress	OR 1.3	Class II (BMI >35)	27
Lower success of TOLAC	OR 0.53–2.0	Excessive weight gain lowers success—Class III	28,29
Rupture/dehiscence after TOLAC	OR 5.6		29
Postterm birth (less likely to go into spontaneous labor)	OR 1.7		30
Lower rates of breast-feeding (Failure to start and sustain)	OR 2.6	Class III	4
Late prenatal care	OR 1.56		8
Fetus/Neonate			
Congenital fetal defects			
NTD	OR 1.7–2.2	OR 3–4 class II–III	31,32
CHD	OR 1.3–1.5		32–36
Cleft lip/palate	OR 1.2–1.9		32,36
Anorectal atresia	OR 1.5		32,36
Hydrocephalus	OR 1.7		36
Limb reduction defects	OR 1.3		32
Gastroschisis	OR 0.17	Reduced risk in the obese	32
Macrosomia (>4000 g)	OR 2.1		4,8,37,38
Birth injury, shoulder dystocia	OR 3.1	Associated most with macrosomia	12,38
Low Apgar scores	OR 1.6		4
Fetal death	OR 2.0–3.6		12,39,40–42
Neonatal mortality	OR 1.3	OR 3.4 class III	12,32
Childhood obesity BMI >95 percentile and metabolic syndrome	OR 1.9–2.2	Increases with increasing levels of obesity and GWG	4
NICU admission	OR 1.34		8,9

Table 3.2 Complications of Obesity Related to Pregnancy (see also text) (*Continued*)

	Risk (%) or OR	Comments	Ref.
Intrapartum			
Earlier admission			
Longer labor	7 hr (obese) vs. 5.4 hr (normal)	Slow labor to 7 cm	43
Anesthesia complications	8.4% composite morbidity	6/8 maternal deaths were in obese gravida (45)	44–46
Difficult regional anesthesia placement	OR 19.4		47
Difficult intubations (general anesthesia)	OR 2.1		47
Cesarean delivery (incidence)	OR 3.0	47% in class II–III (especially failure to progress)	10
Increase operative time >60 min;	OR 9.3		12,45,47
Emergency cesarean	OR 4.7		47
Wound infections/disruptions	OR 2.2		8
Hemorrhage	OR 5.2	Morbid obesity >300 lb	47
Postpartum hemorrhage	OR 1.4		8,43
Longer hospitalization	OR 1.48		8
ICU admissions	OR 3.8	BMI >50	14
Hormonal contraceptive failure	OR 1.91	BMI > 25; limited studies, may still be the best if used properly	48

Abbreviations: OR, odds ratio; NTD, neural tube defect; CHD, congenital heart disease; TOLAC, trial of labor after cesarean; GWG, gestational weight gain; BMI, body mass index

Table 3.3 Health Risks Associated with Obesity

- Premature death
- Type 2 diabetes
- Metabolic syndrome
- Heart disease
- Stroke
- Hypertension
- Gallbladder disease
- Sleep apnea
- Depression
- Cancer
- High cholesterol
- Hirsutism
- Stress incontinence
- Surgical risk
- Osteoarthritis
- Asthma
- Social stigma

Source: Adapted from Ref. 2.

The name "leptin" is derived from the Greek, which means the "thinning factor." Leptin is a neuroendocrine hormone. It suppresses hunger and thereby food intake and may stimulate energy expenditure. Leptin is produced by the adipocytes, placenta, and fetal adipose tissue. Endometrium and ovarian follicles have leptin receptors.

Maternal leptin levels increase throughout pregnancy from six weeks onward and decrease rapidly after parturition. High levels of serum leptin in pregnancy are similar to that seen in obesity (57). Leptin appears to be an independent regulator of fetal growth. Fetal leptin levels are a marker for fetal fat mass. Majority of leptin (95%) produced by the placenta is released into maternal circulation. This increased level stimulates increased production of cytokines such as interleukin-6, interleukin-1, and alpha tumor necrosis factor that lead to a chronic inflammatory state, further resulting in structural and vascular damage (58). Epigenetic modification in the preimplantation stage, alteration in very early metabolism of the embryo, and endometrial abnormalities seen on biopsy in obese patients could result in low implantation rates, birth defects, and fetal growth aberrations (59).

RISK FACTORS

Older, multiparous women from lower socioeconomic background, limited resource environment especially for good nutrition, unsafe neighborhoods for unrestricted physical activity, lack of access to medical care, minority status, family history, all are risk factors for obesity in general and for its associated complications in pregnancy (60).

PREGNANCY COMPLICATIONS

Table 3.2 summarizes the long list of pregnancy complications associated with obesity in pregnancy. **The higher is the patient's BMI, the higher is the chance of complications. Regarding congenital birth defects**, neural tube defects (NTDs) may be due to folate deficiency or local endometrial and placental factors, leading to altered angiogenesis related to leptin or altered carbohydrate metabolism with undetected hyperglycemia. Prepregnancy BMI > 25 and increasing levels of obesity are associated with several phenotypes of congenital heart defects such as conotruncal defects, total anomalous pulmonary venous return, hypoplastic left heart syndrome, right ventricular outflow tract defects, and septal defects (33,34). The use of periconception multivitamins did not reduce this risk of congenital heart disease (CHD) in the overweight and obese population (35). Maternal obesity (BMI ≥30) significantly increased the risk of other defects such as hypospadias, cystic kidney, pes equinovarus, omphalocele, and diaphragmatic hernia (36). This higher rate of anomalies persists in obese women even after controlling for diabetes.

Excluding women with hypertension, the risk of **preeclampsia** is doubled with each 5 to 7 kg/m^2 increase in prepregnancy BMI (11). Women with class III obesity had higher incidence of preeclampsia, antepartum stillbirth, cesarean delivery, instrumental delivery, shoulder dystocia, meconium aspiration, fetal distress, early neonatal death, and large babies as compared to normal-weight women (12).

Increased BMI is a risk factor for **impairment of carbohydrate tolerance**. Fasting and postprandial plasma insulin concentrations are higher in obese pregnant women than in those who are not obese.

Each 1-unit increase in pregravid BMI (5 lb) increases the risk of **cesarean delivery** by about 7% (61). Success rates of vaginal birth are low in the obese population and infectious morbidity increased particularly after labor (28,29,62). Antepartum complications of obesity largely account for this higher cesarean delivery rate, as well as macrosomia-associated cephalopelvic disproportion, nonreassuring fetal testing, and failed induction. Operative risks are also high in obese patients, including **increased total operative time, blood loss, endometritis, and wound disruptions and infections** (3).

Fetal deaths are mostly unexplained or secondary to placental dysfunction and related comorbidities (39,40).

Prepregnancy obesity and excessive gestational weight gain are associated with **indicated preterm birth**, while obesity seems to protect against spontaneous preterm birth (24,30,63–66). Nulligravid obese women are likely at greater risk than the multiparous women.

Obstructive sleep apnea (OSA) has a higher incidence in obese women especially with neck circumference >38 cm. It is associated with fetal heart rate decelerations during periods of maternal hypoxia. Hypertension is commonly associated with OSA and preeclampsia can be seen in pregnancy. Lower Apgar scores, low birth weight, and increased admission to neonatal intensive care unit are seen in infants of obese women with OSA. OSA may complicate anesthesia and postoperative care (17–19).

Prepregnancy obesity is an independent risk factor for large for gestational age (LGA) fetuses and **macrosomia** and is correlated with increasing categories of obesity and gestational weight gain. Macrosomic fetuses are at high risk for childhood obesity and adult metabolic syndrome. Excessive weight gain during pregnancy can increase the risk of macrosomia by 30%. Incidence of shoulder dystocia remains undefined, with some reporting a higher incidence and others no difference in the obese population versus the nonobese. Shoulder dystocia is associated with birth weight rather than increasing levels of obesity (37,38).

In the obese gravida, **labor is longer**, use of oxytocin is increased, and risk of postpartum hemorrhage is high (43).

Multiple attempts at placement of epidural and spinal have to be made in the obese population as compared to the nonobese. The initial failure rate of epidural catheter placement can be as high as 42% in the morbidly obese. Obese women can be a challenge because of related OSA and asthma. Positioning and placement of panniculus can impair respiratory function (44). In morbidly obese patient (BMI > 40 kg/m^2) undergoing planned cesarean delivery, overall conductive anesthesia complication rate is about 8%. Complications of difficult catheter placement, inability to obtain adequate anesthetic levels, and duration are more common in increasing degrees of obesity. **General anesthesia** is used more frequently in morbidly obese patients and intraoperative hypotension can be a problem (45). Of about 1% maternal deaths that were anesthesia related, 75% were noted to be obese (46). The incidence of partially obliterated oropharyngeal anatomy among obese parturients is double that among nonobese parturients. This leads to an increased risk of **difficult intubations, gastric aspiration, and difficulty in maintaining adequate mask ventilation** (44). Mask ventilation tends to be difficult because of low chest wall compliance and increased intra-abdominal pressure.

Wound infections after cesarean are more common in the obese gravida than women with normal BMI (47). Tissue oxygenation is poor in the obese population. Increased oxygen supplementation perioperatively may enhance wound healing (67). There is not sufficient data to assess which is the best surgical incision for cesarean in the obese gravida, as this may differ depending on the category and type (e.g., central) of obesity. Placing the incision above the panniculus adiposus, which at times means above the umbilicus, may be necessary in the woman with extreme obesity (68). The use of the Mobius retractor during cesarean delivery of obese gravidas has not been associated with benefit or harm (69). During cesarean delivery, the subcutaneous fat should be closed with sutures in any woman in which this thickness is >2 cm (68) (see chap. 13, *Obstetric Evidence Based Guidelines*).

Some studies have shown increased incidence of **depression** in the obese population. Eating disorders and arthritic pain together with psychosocial factors (e.g., social stigmatization) could account for this increase (22).

Obesity is associated with **greater health care usage** with more prenatal visits with physicians, fetal testing, obstetrical ultrasound, medications, telephone calls, longer length of stay, increased cesarean deliveries, and medical conditions associated with obesity (70). It is estimated that 5.7% of the total U.S. health expenditure is from obesity-related illness (71).

Close to 300,000 deaths annually are attributed to a diagnosis of obesity (2). About 24% deaths in adult women aged 25 to 64 years are due to obesity (72).

PRECONCEPTION CARE/PREVENTION

The preconception visit may be the single most important health care visit when viewed in the context of its effect on pregnancy (chapter 1, *Obstetric Evidence Based Guidelines*). **Height in meters and weight in kilograms should be recorded for all women at each doctor visit to allow for calculation of BMI** (http://www.nhlbisupport.com/bmi) (Fig. 3.1). Identification and awareness by both patient (especially) and health care worker of obesity is the first step in prevention of complications and appropriate management. **The BMI category should be reviewed with the patient, making sure she understands that her category is not normal.**

Once obesity is confirmed, a **waist circumference** can be measured at the end of expiration, at the level of the iliac crest. This, as well as the exact BMI, should be documented. A risk assessment of cardiovascular disease by taking **BP with a large cuff**, dyslipidemia by obtaining a **fasting lipid profile** and diabetes evaluation with a **fasting blood sugar**, thyroid disease with **thyroid function tests**, and OSA requiring a standard **overnight polysomnogram** should be initiated. In obese patients with chronic hypertension or type 2 diabetes, it is advisable to obtain an **EKG** and an **echocardiogram** (73). Obese women are more likely to experience congestive heart failure and cardiomyopathy. Family history should be elicited. History of weight cycling is important and indicates poor compliance and may be associated with increased risk of comorbidities.

Discussion and education about obesity and its comorbidities and poor perinatal outcomes should be provided (e. g., give a copy of Tables 3.2 and 3.3). An assessment should be made to see if the patient is ready for intervention with diet and exercise. **Motivational interviewing** is defined as a "directive, client-centered counseling style for eliciting behavior change by helping clients explore and resolve ambivalence" (Table 3.4) (74,75).

The most effective intervention in the adult obese population is diet, physical activity, and behavior modification (http://www.nhlbi.nih.gov/guidelines/obesity/ob_home. htm). **The most important interventions in the management of obesity in reproductive age women are weight reduction prior to conception, and prevention of excessive gestational weight gain** (Table 3.5) (37,76).

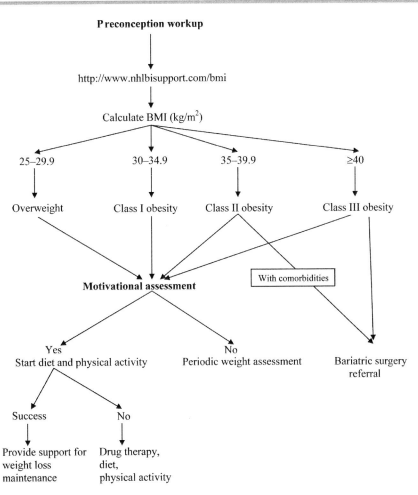

Figure 3.1 Algorithm.

Table 3.4 Stages of Change Model to Assess Readiness for Weight Loss

Stage	Characteristic	Appropriate intervention	Sample dialogue
Precontemplation	Unaware of problem, no interest in change	Provide information about health risks and benefit of weight loss	"Would you like to read some information about the health aspects of obesity"
Contemplation	Aware of problem, beginning to think of changing	Help resolve ambivalence; discuss barriers	"Let's look at the benefits of weight loss, as well what you may need to change"
Preparation	Realizes benefits of making changes and thinking about how to change	Teach behavior modification; provide education	"Let's take a closer look at how you can reduce some of the calories you eat and how to increase your activity during the day"
Action	Actively taking steps toward change	Provide support and guidance, with a focus on the long term	"It's terrific that you are working so hard. What problems have you had? How have you solved them?"
Maintenance	Initial treatment goals reached	Relapse control	"What situations continue to tempt you to overeat? What can be helpful for the next time you face the situation?"

Source: Modified from ACOG Committee Opinion No.319 (73) and from American Medical Association—Roadmaps for Clinical Practice series: Assessment and management of adult obesity. Available at: http://www.ama-assn.org/ama/pub/category/10931.html.

Prepregnancy Weight Reduction

Diet

Use of a low-calorie diet that creates a deficit of 500 to 1000 kcal/day will cause a weight loss of 1 to 2 lb/wk and a 10% weight loss over six months (74). There is good evidence that such a weight loss can be sustained over long periods of time, at least one year. This level of weight loss will improve the BP, lipid profile, and blood glucose levels. Patients can be referred to nutritionist or can visit websites such as http://www.mypyramid.gov.

Table 3.5 Suggested Management of the Obese Gravida

Preconception

Calculate and record BMI and category

Review history and comorbidities

Counseling of pregnancy complications (show, review, and give a copy of Table 3.2)

Counseling of medical long-term complications (show, review, and give a copy of Table 3.3)

Glucose screen

Counsel and plan regarding weight loss and exercise before considering pregnancy—behavior modification

Nutrition counseling

Exercise counseling

Baseline 24-hr urine for proteinuria; LFTs, platelets

Evaluation for possible long-term complications (especially if BMI ≥ 35)

    Echocardiogram

    EKG

    Sleep apnea evaluation

Pregnancy

First trimester

    All recommendations as **Preconception**, except weight loss

    Confirm pregnancy with first-trimester ultrasound for dating

    Review weight gain goals (Table 3.7)

Second/third trimester

    Counsel regarding limitations of fetal ultrasound

    Consider fetal echocardiogram, especially if poorly controlled diabetes

    Consider fetal growth ultrasound in third trimester (e.g., 32 wk)

    Repeat as needed if suspected macrosomia

    Repeat 1-hr glucose screen if negative (tight glucose control if DM)

    Begin antepartum testing ≥32 wk

    Anesthesia consult in third trimester

Intrapartum

Closure of subcutaneous fat ≥2 cm with sutures during cesarean

Graduated compression stockings

Postpartum

Graduated compression stockings and prophylactic heparin until ambulation

Early mobilization and hydration

Compression boots and/or prophylactic heparin during prolonged bed rest

75-mg, 2-hr glucose challenge test >6 wk postpartum

Referral to nutritional and behavioral counselors for weight loss

---

Routine screening offered to all pregnant women (e.g., sequential screening) not included.

Abbreviations: BMI, body mass index; LFT, liver function test; DM, diabetes mellitus. *Source*: Adapted From Ref. 76.

Physical Activity

Exercise contributes only modestly to weight loss, but it may decrease visceral fat; it increases cardiorespiratory fitness and helps with all weight loss maintenance programs. **Moderate exercise for 30 to 45 minutes for at least 3 to 5 days initially and followed by accumulation of at least 30 minutes daily on most days** should be an integral part of weight loss and weight maintenance (74).

Behavior Therapy

Specific strategies include self-monitoring of eating habits and physical activity, stress management, stimulus control, problem solving, contingency management, cognitive restructuring, and social support (74).

Pharmacotherapy

Weight loss drugs should only be used when concomitant lifestyle modifications have not obtained sufficient results. Indications for use are BMI >30 or BMI >27 with comorbidities despite maximal efforts at diet, exercise, and behavior therapy. Weight loss produced by antiobesity drugs has not been shown to be any better than weight loss through lifestyle modification in reducing related comorbidities. The average weight loss with drugs is about 5 kg, and the safety of use has not been established beyond one year of use. There are two classes of weight loss drugs—the appetite suppressants and the lipase inhibitors (74,77,78).

Orlistat (Xenical) is a lipase inhibitor that prevents the absorption of fat from the gut. It is associated with about 6% weight loss over baseline weight. The dose is 120 mg three times a day. It can cause diarrhea, fecal urgency, and oily spotting. It interferes with the absorption of fat-soluble vitamins. It is generally well tolerated by most (77,78). Orlistat can be associated with severe liver failure.

Sibutramine (Meridia) selectively inhibits reuptake of serotonin and is used to reduce food intake. The dose is 10 to 20 mg daily. Its weight loss profile is similar to orlistat. It causes headaches, palpitations, and hypertension. On October 8, 2010, Abbott Laboratories and the U.S. Food and Drug Administration (FDA) withdrew Meridia (sibutramine) voluntarily from the U.S. market because of an increased risk of heart attack and stroke.

Chitosin is a deacetylated chitin, a dietary supplement, available over the counter and used for weight loss. RCTs of chitosin use for at least four weeks were analyzed, which demonstrated significant weight loss (weighted mean difference −1.7 kg; 95% confidence interval (CI) −2.1 to −1.3 kg, $P < 0.00001$). However, larger trials did not demonstrate this effectively and some studies were of suboptimal quality (79).

Other pharmacotherapies, including other Chinese herbal medicines, are currently being studied and undergoing assessment.

Bariatric Surgery

Women with BMI >40 or BMI >35 with comorbidities are candidates for bariatric surgery when diet, physical activity, and behavior modification (and possible drug therapy) have failed (Table 3.6). The weight loss following surgery is in the range of 10 to 105 kg and is sustained for as long as eight years. More than 50,000 women of reproductive age underwent bariatric surgery inpatient procedures annually between 2003 and 2005.

There are two general types of surgery—the restrictive and the malabsorptive. There are two commonly performed procedures. They can be done by laparoscopy or laparotomy.

The **Roux-en-Y gastric bypass** is a combination of both malabsorptive and restrictive type.

The **vertical banded gastroplasty,** adjustable gastric band procedure, or intragastric banding are restrictive procedures. Recently, it has been noted that intragastric balloon appears to have little benefit in weight loss therapy over diet, behavior modification, and motivation (80). Adjustable gastric band management during pregnancy is not well defined, but almost 20% may need adjustment or removal of band for nausea and vomiting (81).

The biliopancreatic and the jejunoileal bypass (both malabsorptive) are rarely performed today because of nutritional problems and internal hernias.

A weight maintenance program consisting of diet, physical activity, and behavior therapy should be a priority after

Table 3.6 Special Considerations for Preconception and Prenatal Care after Bariatric Surgery

- Preconception
  - Fertility often resumes after bariatric surgery
  - Bariatric surgery should not be considered a treatment for infertility
  - Oral contraception is often ineffective because of potential malabsorption; consider injectable forms of hormonal contraception as needed. Use reliable contraception until period of maximal weight loss (at least 12 months) is over
  - Consider waiting 12 months or more after bariatric surgery before conception
  - Evaluate and treat comorbidities

- Prenatal
- Monitor for nutritional deficiencies (especially after Roux-en-Y) such as
  - Vitamin B12 (if needed, 500–1000 μg daily)
  - Folate (up to 5 mg daily)
  - Iron (check ferritin) (if needed, ferrous fumarate)
  - Vitamin D (if needed, do not exceed pregnancy RDA of 400 IU maximum)
  - Calcium (if needed, 1200 mg calcium citrate)
- Be aware that nausea, vomiting, abdominal pain, etc., may be signs of bariatric surgery complications such as intestinal obstruction, GI hemorrhage, anastomic leaks, hernias, band erosions and migrations, and even maternal death. Early consultation with bariatric surgeon is suggested.
- Avoid glucola screening given risk of dumping syndrome. Use fasting and 2-hr postprandial blood sugar monitoring as an alternative.
- If BMI is still 30 kg/m², risks remain as in Table 3.2 and 3.3, and management in general as in Table 3.5.
- Bariatric surgery is not an indication for cesarean delivery

the initial 6 to 12 months of weight loss therapy. Lifelong medical surveillance after surgical therapy is a necessity. Almost 20% of patients who undergo bariatric surgery experience some complication, although they are usually minor and the postoperative mortality is <1%. There is 5% failure rate from use of OCP following bariatric surgery (82). Patients should be advised to **delay pregnancy for at least 12 months** (15,82). There is little evidence to support the duration of delay for conception with regard to birth weight, cesarean delivery, or congenital malformation. Weight loss usually plateaus after 12 to 18 months.

Prognosis for a future pregnancy depends mostly on the BMI that has been attained. There is **significant decrease in incidence of gestational diabetes, preeclampsia and hypertension, and macrosomia following bariatric surgery**, especially for women capable of starting the pregnancy with a BMI < 30 kg/m², compared to before bariatric surgery or to obese (often morbidly) women who have not had bariatric surgery (81–83). Often the studies are not matched for BMI, a major shortcoming.

Nutritional supplementation should be recommended because there is good evidence of increased incidences of maternal and neonatal deficiencies of **vitamin B12, vitamin D, iron, and calcium** in women post bariatric surgery (84) (Table 3.6).

Other Preconception Preparations
Proper preconception care should be provided (chapter 1, *Obstetric Evidence Based Guidelines*). Since almost 50%

pregnancies are unplanned, all patients capable of childbearing should be placed on folic acid 0.4 to 0.8 mg (400–800 μg) supplementation at least one month before conception, and continue daily supplements through the first two to three months of pregnancy (85). Folate levels have been noted to be low in the obese population (86). Although obesity is considered a risk factor for NTD, the **folic acid supplementation** in the United States has remained the same (85). However, both the Royal College of Obstetricians and Gynaecologists (RCOG) (87) and the Society of Obstetricians and Gynaecologists of Canada (SOGC) (26) have recommended a dose of **5 mg daily** for the obese population (BMI ≥ 35) starting from one to three months preconception through the first trimester. Drug history should be reviewed to identify any potential teratogens.

PRENATAL CARE
Preconception management, except for large weight loss, should be followed (Table 3.5).

Prevention of Excessive Weight Gain
There is limited evidence to make recommendations regarding weight changes in the obese gravida. One should remember that the total weight of an average fetus, placenta, and amniotic fluid at term is about 4 to 5 kg. In the past more than 20 years, both the Institute of Medicine (IOM) and American College of Obstetricians and Gynaecologists (ACOG) have suggested 5 to 9 kg (11–20 lb) as total weight gain in pregnancy for obese women (88). This suggestion does not account for differences in class of obesity. Significant weight loss during pregnancy is not recommended by ACOG and IOM.

More recent data suggest that lower weight gain in the obese gravida is associated with maternal and fetal benefits (37,89–93). For obese women, weight gain has no benefit. The lowest risks for mother and baby seem to occur with weight gain of 0 to 9 lb for class II obese women, and weight loss of 0 to 9 lb for class III obese women (13,27,89,91). On the basis of these data, new guidelines should be considered for obese women (Table 3.7).

Nutritional consult may be sought to prevent excessive gestational weight gain. Charts to outline the patient's progress should be a permanent part of the prenatal record. Excessive weight retention self-perpetuates the obesity cycle for subsequent pregnancies (37). Almost three-fourths of all women will weigh more at a subsequent pregnancy (94). Excessive gestational weight gain is associated with childhood obesity (95).

Diet
A balanced diet, rich in high fiber and complex carbohydrates, with low glycemic intake, is suggested. Up to 5 mg of folic acid should be continued from the prepregnancy period until at least 10 weeks' gestation (26,87). Education about weight gain, healthy eating, and exercise decreases the percentage of women who exceed weight gain recommendations (96). The evidence for antenatal dietary and lifestyle interventions in overweight and obese pregnant women to decrease complications is still insufficient to make recommendations (97).

Exercise
Physical activity during pregnancy is successful in restricting gestational weight gain (98). Physical activity should be encouraged as per ACOG recommendations (99). During pregnancy, women can be encouraged to maintain an active lifestyle as long as there are no risks to the pregnancy. Class III obesity is considered a relative contraindication to aerobic exercise during pregnancy (99).

Table 3.7 Weight Gain Suggestions for Overweight and Obese Women

Prepregnancy weight category	Our suggested total weight gain range (lb)	IOM recommendations (lb)
Overweight (BMI 25–29.9 kg/m^2)	6–20 (2.7–9.0 kg)	15–25 (6.8–11.4 kg)
Class I Obesity (BMI 30–34.9 kg/m^2)	5–15 (2.3–6.8 kg)	11–20 (5–9.1 kg)
Class II Obesity (BMI 35–39.9 kg/m^2)	−9 to 9 (−4.0 to 4.0 kg)	11–20 (5–9.1 kg)
Class III Obesity (BMI > 40 kg/m^2)	−15 to 0 (−6.8 to 0 kg)	11–20 (5–9.1 kg)

Source: From Refs. 27, 37, 88–93.

Other Antepartum Issues

Gestational age should be established with early (e.g., **first trimester** is optimal) **ultrasound** (chapter 4, *Obstetric Evidence Based Guidelines*). **Diabetic screen should be done at the first visit.** If this is negative, it should be repeated at 24 to 28 weeks (100). Baseline data to evaluate renal function and liver status, such as liver function tests (**LFTs), 24-hour urine for protein and creatinine clearance** can be obtained. Reassessment of risk and the need for **EKG and echocardiogram** can be made. Excess weight has an effect on biochemical serum aneuploidy screening, so adjustment has to be made according to maternal weight to achieve similar detection rates as in other women.

Equipment in the office or clinic to accommodate the needs of this population, such as wide chairs, sit-on weighing scales, tables, and large BP cuffs, should be available. The professional team should undertake discussion of pregnancy, maternal and fetal outcomes. Educational materials should be provided. Pharmacotherapy for obesity is contraindicated in pregnancy. While the RCOG recommends more frequent prenatal visit every 3 weeks from 24 to 32 weeks and then every 2 weeks till delivery, there is insufficient level I data to make this an evidence-based recommendation (87).

Ultrasonography for detection of anomalies can be limited with increasing severity of obesity. For normal BMI, overweight, and class I, II, and III obesity, detection with standard ultrasonography was 66%, 49%, 48%, 42%, and 25%, respectively, and with targeted ultrasonography 97%, 91%, 75%, 88%, and 75%, respectively (25). Ultrasound should be used to **monitor fetal growth** since this may be difficult to assess clinically.

Bariatric Surgery: Prenatal Care Issues

Preconception issues mentioned above should be reviewed (Table 3.6). Patients with bariatric surgery should be started on **vitamin B12, folate, iron, and calcium if deficient** (82). **Vitamin D supplement 10 µg daily** during pregnancy and breast-feeding can be recommended as per the RCOG guidelines (87). Bariatric surgeon should be involved during prenatal care, should gastric band need some adjustments. During pregnancy, patients who present with signs and symptoms of intestinal obstruction, perforation, or hemorrhage should have a CT scan done to establish diagnosis since this can be associated with 20% maternal mortality.

Antepartum Fetal Testing

There is insufficient evidence that fetal heart rate testing would benefit the perinatal outcomes in the obese population. These women should be encouraged to monitor fetal movements, as in the case of the general obstetrical patients. Since the risk of fetal demise is high, antepartum fetal testing may be considered.

INTRAPARTUM CARE

The hospital facility should be notified so that appropriate equipment, graduated compression stockings (teds), beds, transfer equipment, hoists, wide corridors, and stretchers are available. Early venous access is suggested.

There may be limitations to monitoring uterine contractions and fetal heart rate in active labor. Invasive tocomonitoring may become necessary if there are no other contraindications. Oxytocin use is high in this population. A scheduled cesarean at 39 weeks should be planned if the estimated fetal weight is >4500 in a diabetic patient and >5000 in a nondiabetic obese patient (15). Active management of the third stage would help reduce the incidence of postpartum hemorrhage.

Prophylactic antibiotics (e.g., with cefazolin 2 g IV) at least 30 minutes prior to cesarean delivery is recommended (chapter 13, *Obstetric Evidence Based Guidelines*). **A subcutaneous layer should be closed with sutures if depth is >2 cm to reduce wound infection and separation**. It remains unclear which abdominal incision would be most appropriate in the obese gravida. ACOG has recommended early mobilization, **graduated compression stocking,** and hydration for thromboprophylaxis after cesarean section (15). RCOG recommends low-molecular-weight heparin for thromboprophylaxis post cesarean in the morbidly obese (BMI > 40) for one week postoperatively (87).

ANESTHESIA

If anesthesia consult was not obtained antepartum, then it should be obtained early in labor. Conductive regional anesthesia is the anesthetic of choice. However, it has limitations in this population as noted above. It is often necessary to have long epidural needles, and equipments such as laryngeal mask ventilation available in case of difficult intubation.

POSTPARTUM

Immediately postoperatively, **continue pneumatic compression devises until walking is established should be routine**. Encourage **early ambulation** and hydration. The additional use of prophylactic anticoagulation, for example, with heparin, has not been sufficiently studied to make a recommendation (101).

Women should be strongly encouraged and helped to **return to a normal BMI**, through **counseling, diet, exercise, and breast-feeding**. Breast-feeding is encouraged (chapter 27, *Obstetric Evidence Based Guidelines*). It benefits both the mother and infant. In particular, it helps to return faster to prepregnancy weight and helps avoid weight retention and decreases risk of chronic diseases such as type 2 diabetes, and breast and ovarian cancer. For the infant, breast-feeding reduces the risk of obesity. To increase the rates of breast-feeding, consultation with a lactation specialist is often beneficial.

CONTRACEPTION

Hormonal contraception may not be as effective as in the nonobese, but a Cochrane review has determined that it may still be the best (48). Pregnancy rates are high after weight loss surgery; therefore, effective contraception should be discussed prior to the procedure.

FUTURE

Future research should assess the degree of intensiveness and contact with health care provider during management with diet and exercise, drug therapy to target different biological pathways to obesity, the mechanisms of fetal macrosomia, fetal demise secondary to obesity, and childhood obesity, among many others. Controlling maternal prepregnancy obesity and excessive gestational weight retention will help control the obesity epidemic. Food industry companies, insurance companies, public education, school education, tax breaks, premium breaks, fitness programs, and many others should work together to end this vicious cycle, leading to now earlier mortality than previous generations because of obesity.

RESOURCES

ACOG Committee Opinion # 315 (73)
American Medical Association. Roadmaps for Clinical Practice Series: Assessment and management of adult obesity.
http://www.ama-assn.org/ama/pub/category/10931.html

American Society for Bariatric Surgery
http://www.asbs.org

ACOG Clinical Updates in Women's Health Care—Weight control: assessment and management
http://www.clinicalupdates.org

National Heart, Lung, and Blood Institute—Clinical guidelines on the identification, evaluation, and treatment of overweight and obesity in adults
http://www.nhlbi.nih.gov/guidelines/obesity/ob_home.htm

The Surgeon General's call to action to prevent and decrease overweight and obesity
http://www.surgeongeneral.gov/topics/obesity

U.S. Preventive Services Task Force—Screening for obesity in adults
http://www.ahrq.gov/clinic/uspstf/uspobes.htm

Patient Resources from ACOG Committee Opinion #315 (73)
American Obesity Association
http://www.obesity.org

American Society of Bariatric Physicians
http://www.asbp.org

MedlinePlus: Weight loss and dieting
http://www.nlm.nih.gov/medlineplus/weightlossanddieting.html

National Heart, Lung, and Blood Institute. Obesity education initiative
http://www.nhlbi.nih.gov/about/oei/index.htm

Overeaters Anonymous
http://www.overeatersanonymous.org

TOPS—Take Off Pounds Sensibly
http://www.tops.org

Weight-control Information Network
http://www.win.niddk.nih.gov

REFERENCES

1. World Health Organization. Obesity: preventing and managing the global epidemic. Geneva, Switzerland: World Health Organisation: 2000. WHO Technical Report Series 894:1–253. [Review]
2. U.S. Department of Health and Human Services. The Surgeon General's Call to Action to Prevent and Decrease Overweight and Obesity. Rockville, MD: U.S. Department of Health and Human Services, Public Health Service, Office of the Surgeon General, 2001. [Review]
3. Yogev Y, Catalano P. Pregnancy and obesity. Obstet Gynecol Clin North Am 2009; 36:285–300. [Review]
4. Nohr EA, Timpson NJ, Anderson CS, et al. Severe obesity in young women and reproductive health: the Danish National Birth Cohort. PloS One 2009; 4(12):e8444. [II-2:Danish National Birth Cohort, prospective cohort, $n = 4901$, obese BMI > 30 kg/m^2, $n = 2451$]
5. Bolumar F, Olsen J, Rebagliato M, et al. Body mass index and delayed conception: a European Multicenter Study on Infertility and Subfecundity. Am J Epidemiol 2000; 151:1072–1079. [II-2: European multicenter prospective study, $n = 4.035$]
6. Metwally M, Ong KJ, Ledger WL, et al. Does high body mass index increase the risk of miscarriage after spontaneous and assisted conception? A meta-analysis of the evidence. Fertil Steril 2008; 90:714–726. [II-2: 16 studies meta-analysis $n = 5545$, BMI > 25]
7. Lashen H, Fear K, Sturdee DW. Obesity is associated with increased risk of first trimester and recurrent miscarriage: matched case-control study. Hum Reprod 2004; 19:1644–1646. [II-2: BMI > 30 kg/m^2, $n = 1644$]
8. Sebire NJ, Jolly M, Harris JP, et al. Maternal obesity and pregnancy outcome: a study of 287,213 pregnancies in London. Int J Obes 2001; 25:1175–1182. [II-3: UK observational study 1989–1997, $n = 287,213$; BMI > 30 kg/m^2, $n = 31,276$]
9. Kumari A. Pregnancy outcome in women with morbid obesity. Int J Gynaecol Obstet 2001; 73:101–107. [II-2: United Arab Emirates, retrospective case control study, $n = 488$, BMI > 40 kg/m^2, $n = 180$]
10. Weiss JL, Malone FD, Emig D, et al., Obesity, obstetric complications and cesarean delivery rate—a population-based screening study. FASTER Research Consortium. Am J Obstet Gynecol 2004; 190:1091–1097. [II-1: Prospective multicenter population-based screening study, $n = 16,102$; BMI 30–35 kg/m^2, $n = 1473$; BMI > 35 kg/m^2, $n = 877$]
11. O'Brien TE, Ray JG, Chan W-S. Maternal body mass index and the risk of preeclampsia: a systematic overview. Epidemiology 2003; 14:368–374. [II-2: 13 studies, 4 prospective cohort, 9 retrospective cohort, $n = 1,390,226$]
12. Cedergren MI. Maternal morbid obesity and the risk of adverse pregnancy outcome. Obstet Gynecol 2004; 103:219–224. [II-2: Prospective population cohort study, $n = 3480$ with BMI > 40]
13. Jensen DM, Damm P, Sørensen B, et al. Pregnancy outcome and prepregnancy body mass index in 2459 glucose-tolerant Danish women. Am J Obstet Gynecol 2003; 189:239–244. [II-2: Retrospective cohort study, $n = 2459$]
14. Knight M, Kurinczuk JJ, Spark P, et al., on behalf of the UK Obstetric Surveillance System Extreme Obesity in Pregnancy in the United Kingdom. Extreme obesity in pregnancy in the United Kingdom. Obstet Gynecol 2010; 115:989–997. [II-2: Population-based cohort study, BMI > 50 kg/m^2, $n = 665$]
15. American College of Obstetricians and Gynecologists. Obesity in pregnancy. ACOG Committee Opinion No. 315, Sept. 2005. Obstet Gynecol 2005; 106:671–675. [Review]
16. Baeten JM, Bukusi EA, Lambe M. Pregnancy complications and outcomes among overweight and obese nulliparous women. Am J Public Health 2001; 91:436–440. [II-2: Population-based cohort study $n = 96,801$]
17. Sahin FK, Koken G, Cosar E, et al. Obstructive sleep apnea in pregnancy and fetal outcome. Int J Gynaecol Obstet 2008; 100:141–146. [II: Prospective observational study, $n = 35$]
18. Lefcourt LA, Rodis JF. Obstructive sleep apnea in pregnancy. Obstet Gynecol Surv 1996; 51:503–506. [Review]

19. Louis JM, Auckley D, Sokol RJ, et al. Maternal and neonatal morbidities associated with obstructive sleep apnea complicating pregnancy. Am J Obstet Gynecol 2010; 202(3):261.e1–261.e5. [II-3: Retrospective cohort, n = 114]

20. Olivarez SA, Maheshwari B, McCarthy M, et al. Prospective trial on obstructive sleep apnea in pregnancy and fetal heart rate monitoring. Am J Obstet Gynecol 2010; 202(6):552.e1–552.e7. [II-3, Prospective study, n = 100]

21. Hendler I, Schatz M, Momirova V, et al., for the National Institute of Child Health and Human Development Maternal–Fetal Medicine Units Network. Association of obesity with pulmonary and nonpulmonary complications of pregnancy in asthmatic women. Obstet Gynecol 2006; 108:77–82. [II-1]

22. Atlantis E, Baker M. Obesity effects on depression: systematic review of epidemiological studies. Int J Obes (Lond) 2008; 32:881–891. [Systematic review, 4 prospective cohort studies, 20 cross-sectional, 10 from the US]

23. Ma J, Xiao L. Obesity and depression in US women: results from the 2005–2006 National Health and Nutritional Examination Survey. Obesity (Silver Spring) 2010; 18:347–353. [II: Population-based study, n = 1875, average age 48 years]

24. McDonald SD, Han Z, Mulla S, et al., on behalf of the Knowledge Synthesis Group. Overweight and obesity in mothers and risk of preterm birth and low birth weight infants: systematic review and metaanalyses. BMJ 2010; 341:c3428. doi:10.1136/bmj.c3428. [Systematic review and meta-analysis, cohort studies, n = 64, case control studies, n = 20]

25. Dashe JS, McIntire DD, Twickler DM. Effect of maternal obesity on the ultrasound detection of anomalous fetuses. Obstet Gynecol 2009; 113:1001–1007. [II-2: Retrospective cohort study]

26. Davies GAL, Maxwell C, McLeod L, et al. Obesity in pregnancy. SOGC Clinical Practice Guidelines. Int J Gynaecol Obstet 2010; 110(2):165–173. [Clinical guideline, 79 references]

27. Bianco AT, Smilen SW, Davis Y, et al. Pregnancy outcome and weight gain recommendations for the morbidly obese woman. Obstet Gynecol 1998; 91:97–102. [II-2, U.S. retrospective cohort study, n = 11,926]

28. Gabor J, Gyamfi C, Gyamfi P, et al. Effect of body mass index and excessive weight gain on success of vaginal birth after cesarean delivery. Obstet Gynecol 2005; 106:741–746. [II-2 : Retrospective study, n = 1213]

29. Hibbard JU, Gilbert S, Landon MB, et al., for the National Institute of Child Health and Human Development Maternal–Fetal Medicine Units Network. Trial of labor or repeat cesarean delivery in women with morbid obesity and previous cesarean delivery. Obstet Gynecol 2006; 108(1):125–133. [II-2: Multicenter, prospective study, n = 28,442]

30. Stotland NE, Washington AE, Caughey AB. Prepregnancy body mass index and the length of gestation at term. Am J Obstet Gynecol 2007; 197(4):378.e371–378.e375. [II-2: Retrospective study, US, one center, n = 9336]

31. Rasmussen SA, Chu SY, Kim SY, et al. Maternal obesity and risk of neural tube defects: a metaanalysis. Am J Obstet Gynecol 2008; 198:611–619. [II-2: 4 cohort studies, 8 case control studies]

32. Stothard KJ, Tennant PWG, Bell R, et al. Maternal overweight and obesity and risk of congenital anomalies a systematic review and meta-analysis. JAMA 2009; 301:636–650. [II-2: Systematic review 39 studies mostly from the US, meta-analysis 18 studies]

33. Gilboa SM, Correa A, Botto LD, et al., and the National Birth Defects Prevention Study. Association between prepregnancy body mass index and congenital heart defects. Am J Obstet Gynecol 2010; 202(1):51.e1–51.e10. [II-2: US population-based observational study, n = 11,113]

34. Waller DK, Shaw GM, Rasmussen SA, et al. Prepregnancy obesity as a risk factor for structural birth defects. Arch Pediatr Adolesc Med 2007; 161:745–750. [II-2: Case-control, National Birth Defects Prevention Study, n = 10,249]

35. Watkins ML, Botto LD. Maternal prepregnancy weight and congenital heart defects in the offspring. Epidemiology 2001; 11:439–446. [II-2: Atlanta Birth Defects Case-Control Study, n = 1049]

36. Blomberg MI, Källén B. Maternal obesity and morbid obesity: the risk for birth defects in the offspring. Birth Defects Res A Clin Mol Teratol 2010; 88(1):35–40. [II-2: Swedish Medical Health Registries, n = 1,049,582]

37. Siega-Riz AM, Viswanathan M, Moos MK, et al. A systematic review of outcomes of maternal weight gain according to the Institute of Medicine recommendations: birthweight, fetal growth, and postpartum weight retention. Am J Obstet Gynecol 2009; 201 (4):339.e1–e14. [Systematic review of 35 studies from 1990 to 2007]

38. Robinson H, Tkatch S, Mayes DC, et al. Is maternal obesity a predictor of shoulder dystocia? Obstet Gynecol 2003; 101(1):24–27. [II-2: Canada, case control study, n = 45,877]

39. Nohr EA, Bech BH, Davies MJ, et al. Prepregnancy obesity and fetal death: a study within the Danish National Birth Cohort. Obstet Gynecol 2005; 106(2):250–259. [II-2: Retrospective, population-based cohort study, n = 54,505]

40. Chu SY, Kim SY, Lau J, et al. Maternal obesity and risk of stillbirth: a meta-analysis. Am J Obstet Gynecol 2007; 197(3):223–228. [Meta-analysis of 9 observational studies]

41. Salihu HM, Alio AP, Wilson RE, et al. Obesity and extreme obesity: new insights into the black–white disparity in neonatal mortality. Obstet Gynecol 2008; 111:1410–1416. [II: Missouri state 1978–1997 population-based cohort study, n = 1,405,698]

42. Cnattingius S, Bergstrom R, Lipworth L, et al. Pregnancy weight and the risk of adverse pregnancy outcome. N Engl J Med 1998; 338(3):147–152. [II-2: Sweden 1992–1993, population-based cohort study, n = 167,750]

43. Vahratian A, Zhang J, Troendle JF, et al. Maternal prepregnancy overweight and obesity and the pattern of labor progression in term nulliparous women. Obstet Gynecol 2004; 104(5 pt 1):943–951. [II-2: US prospective cohort study, n = 612]

44. Saravanakumar K, Rao SG, Cooper GM. The challenges of obesity and obstetric anaesthesia. Curr Opin Obstet Gynecol 2006; 18:631–635. [Review]

45. Vricella LK, Louis JM, Mercer BM, et al. Anesthesia complications during scheduled cesarean delivery for morbidly obese women. Am J Obstet Gynecol 2010; 203(3):276.e1–e5. [II-2: Retrospective cohort study, n = 578]

46. Mhyre JM, Riesner MN, Polley LS, et al. A series of anesthesia-related maternal deaths in Michigan, 1985–2003. Anesthesiology 2007; 106:1096–1104. [II-2: Michigan Maternal Mortality Surveillance 1985–2003, retrospective study]

47. Perlow JH, Morgan MA. Massive maternal obesity and perioperative cesarean morbidity. Am J Obstet Gynecol 1994; 170:560–565. [II-2: n = 43 patients >300 lb]

48. Lopez LM, Grimes DA, Chen-Mok M, et al. Hormonal contraceptives for contraception in overweight or obese women. Cochrane Database Syst Rev 2010; 7:CD008452. [Reviews: 11 trials, n = 39,531]

49. James WPT, Jackson-Leach R, Ni Mhurchu C. Overweight and obesity (high body mass index). In: Ezzati TM, ed. Comparative Quantification of Health Risks Global and Regional Burden of Disease Attributable to Selected Major Risk Factors. Vol 1. Geneva: World Health Organization 2004:497–596. [Review]

50. WHO fact sheet #311, 2006. Accessed 10/18/10. [Epidemiology data]

51. LaCoursiere DY, Bloebaum L, Duncan JD, et al. Population-based trends and correlates of maternal overweight and obesity, Utah 1991–2001. Am J Obstet Gynecol 2005; 192:832–839. [II-3: Retrospective, population-based cohort, n = 229,483]

52. Flegal KM, Carroll MD, Ogden CL, et al. Prevalence and trends in obesity among US adults, 1999–2008. JAMA 2010; 303(3):235–241. [II-3: Population based, n = 2805 nonpregnant adult women]

53. Barsh GS, Farooqi IS, O'Rahilly S. Genetics of body-weight regulation. Nature 2000; 404:644–651. [Review]

54. Reilly JJ, Armstrong J, Dorosty AR, et al., for the Avon Longitudinal Study of Parents and Children Study Team. Early life risk factors for obesity in childhood: cohort study. BMJ 2005; 330 (7504):1357. [II-2: Prospective cohort observational study, n = 8234]

55. Centers for Disease Control and Prevention. Obesity and genomics. Available at: http://www.cdc.gov/genomics/resources/diseases/obesity/obesedit.htm. Accessed 02/07/11.

56. Metwally M, Ledger WL, Li TC. Reproductive endocrinology and clinical aspects of obesity. Ann N Y Acad Sci 2008; 1127:140–146. [Review]

57. Kratzsch J, Hockel M, Kiess W. Leptin and pregnancy outcome. Curr Opin Obstet Gynecol 2000; 12:501–505. [Review]

58. Hauguel-de Mouzon S, Lepercq J, Catalano P. The known and unknown of leptin in pregnancy. Am J Obstet Gynecol 2006; 194 (6):1537–1545. [Review]

59. Jungheim ES, Moley KH. Current knowledge of obesity's effects in the pre- and periconceptional periods and avenues for future research. Am J Obstet Gynecol 2010; 203(6):525–530. [Review]

60. American College of Obstetricians and Gynecologists. Challenges for overweight and obese urban women. ACOG Committee Opinion No. 470. Obstet Gynecol 2010; 116(4):1011–1014. [Review]

61. Brost BC, Goldenberg RL, Mercer BM, et al. The Preterm Prediction Study: association of cesarean section with increases in maternal weight and body mass index. Am J Obstet Gynecol 1997; 177(2):333–337. [II-2: Prospective study, $n = 2809$]

62. Chauhan SP, Magann EF, Carroll CS, et al. Mode of delivery for the morbidly obese with prior cesarean delivery: vaginal versus repeat cesarean section. Am J Obstet Gynecol 2001; 185:349–354. [II-2: Prospective study, $n = 69$, maternal weight >300 lb]

63. Hendler I, Goldenberg RL, Mercer BM, et al., for the National Institute of Child Health and Human Development, Maternal–Fetal Medicine Units Network, National Institutes of Health. The Preterm Prediction Study: Association between maternal body mass index and spontaneous and indicated preterm birth. Am J Obstet Gynecol 2005; 192(3):882–886. [II-1: US 10 centers, prospective observational study, $n = 2910$, BMI >30 kg/m^2, $n = 597$]

64. Salihu HM, Lynch O, Alio AP, et al. Obesity subtypes and risk of spontaneous versus medically indicated preterm births in singletons and twins. Am J Epidemiol 2008; 168(1):13–20. [II-2: US population cohort study, $n = 459,913$]

65. Dietz PM, Callaghan WM, Cogswell ME, et al. Combined effects of prepregnancy body mass index and weight gain during pregnancy on the risk of preterm delivery. Epidemiology 2006; 17:170–177. [II: Prospective observational cohort (PRAMS) US study 21 states, $n = 113,019$]

66. Ehrenberg HM, Iams JD, Goldenberg RL, et al., for the Eunice Kennedy Shriver National Institute of Child Health and Human Development (NICHD), Maternal–Fetal Medicine Units Network. Maternal obesity, uterine activity, and the risk of spontaneous preterm birth. Obstet Gynecol 2009; 113:48–52. [II: US multicenter, case control, $n = 253$]

67. Kabon B, Nagele A, Reddy D, et al. Obesity decreases perioperative tissue oxygenation. Anesthesiology 2004; 100:274–280. [Clinical investigation, $n = 46$]

68. Berghella V, Baxter JK, Chauhan SP. Evidence-based surgery for cesarean delivery. Am J Obstet Gynecol 2005; 193(5):1607–1617. [II-2]

69. Moroz L, Bowers G, Hayes EJ, et al. Self-retained vs. traditional retractors for cesarean delivery in obese women: a randomized controlled trial. Am J Obstet Gynecol 2008; 111:101S–102S. [RCT, $n = 60$]

70. Chu SY, Bachman DJ, Callaghan WM, et al. Association between obesity during pregnancy and increased use of health care. N Engl J Med 2008; 358(14):1444–1453. [II-3]

71. Available at: nhlbi.nih.gov/guidelines/obesity. Accessed 02/07/11.

72. Flegal KM, Williamson DF, Pamuk ER, et al. Estimating deaths attributable to obesity in the United States. Am J Public Health 2004; 94:1486–1489. [Overview]

73. ACOG Committee on Gynecologic Practice. The role of the obstetrician–gynecologist in the assessment and management of obesity. ACOG Committee Opinion No. 319. Obstet Gynecol 2005; 106(4):895–899. [Review]

74. National Institutes of Health. Clinical guidelines on the identification, evaluation, and treatment of overweight and obesity in adults—the Evidence Report 1998. Obes Res 1998:6(suppl 2):51S–209S. [Review]

75. American College of Obstetricians and Gynecologists. Motivational interviewing: a tool for behaviour change. ACOG Committee Opinion No.423. Obstet Gynecol 2009; 113:234–236. [Review]

76. Di Lillo M, Hendrix N, O'Neill M, et al. Pregnancy in obese women: what you need to know. Cont Obstet Gynecol 2008; 11:48–53. [Review]

77. Bray GA, Tartaglia LA. Medicinal strategies in the treatment of obesity. Nature 2000; 404:672–677. [Review]

78. Perrio MJ, Wilton LV, Shakir SAW. The safety profiles of orlistat and sibutramine: results of prescription-event monitoring studies in England. Obesity (Silver Spring) 2007; 15(11):2712–2722. [II-2: Observational cohort study]

79. Jull AB, Ni Mhurchu C, Bennett DA, et al. Chitosan for overweight or obesity. Cochrane Database of Systematic Reviews 2008, Issue 3. Art. No.: CD003892. DOI: 10.1002/14651858. CD003892.pub3.

80. Fernandes MAP, Atallah AN, Soares BG, et al. Intragastric balloon for obesity. Cochrane Database Syst Rev 2007; (1): CD004931. [Meta-analysis, 9 RCTs, $n = 395$, high level of bias, nonpregnant participants]

81. Maggard M, Li Z, Yermilov I, et al. Bariatric surgery in women of reproductive age: special concerns for pregnancy. Evid Rep Technol Assess (Full Rep) 2008; (169):1–51. [57 studies; 23 case reports, 21 case series, 12 cohort, 1 case control]

82. American College of Obstetricians and Gynecologists. Bariatric surgery and pregnancy. ACOG Practice Bulletin No. 105. Obstet Gynecol 2009; 113:1405–1413. [Review]

83. Catalano PM. Management of obesity in pregnancy. Obstet Gynecol 2007; 109:419–433. [Review]

84. Shekelle PG, Morton SC, Maglione MA, et al. Pharmacological and surgical treatment of obesity. Evid Rep Technol Assess (Summ) 2004; (103):1–6. [Meta-analysis: 28 trials of orlistat; 147 total studies for surgery, 89 for weight loss analysis, 134 for mortality analysis, 128 for complication analysis]

85. U.S. Preventive Services Task Force. Folic acid for the prevention of neural tube defects: U.S. Preventive Services Task Force recommendation statement. Ann Intern Med 2009; 150(9):626–631. [5 studies from 1995-2008; RCT = 1]

86. Mojtabai R. Body mass index and serum folate in childbearing women. Eur J Epidemiol 2004; 19:1029–1036. [II-1: US population based cohort study National Health and Nutrition Examination Survey (NHANES) from 1988 to 1994 and 1999 to 2000]

87. Centre for Maternal and Child Enquiries/Royal College of Obstetricians and Gynaecologists. Management of women with obesity in pregnancy. RCOG Guidelines. 2010. [Clinical guideline, 77 references]

88. Rasmussen KM, Yaktine AL, for Institute for Medicine and National Research Council (US) Committee to Reexamine IOM Pregnancy Weight Guidelines. Weight gain during pregnancy: reexamining the guidelines. Washington, DC: National Academic Press 2009. [Consensus Report]

89. Oken E, Kleinman KP, Belfort MB, et al. Association of gestational weight gain with short- and longer-term maternal and child health outcomes. Am J Epidemiol 2009; 170:173–180. [II-2: Project Viva, Massachusetts 1999–2002 US observational study, $n = 2012$]

90. Cedergren MI. Optimal gestational weight gain for body mass index categories. Obstet Gynecol 2007; 110(4):759–764. [II-2: Swedish Medical Birth Register, population-based cohort study, $n = 298,648$]

91. Kiel DW, Dodson EA, Artal R, et al. Gestational weight gain and pregnancy outcomes in obese women. How much is enough? Obstet Gynecol 2007; 110:752–758. [II-2: Population-based cohort, $n = 120,251$]

92. Nohr EA, Vaeth M, Baker JL, et al. Pregnancy outcomes related to gestational weight gain in women defined by their body mass index, parity, height, and smoking status. Am J Clin Nutr 2009;

90:1288–1294. [II-2: Danish population based observational study, *n* = 59,147]

93. Dietz PM, Callaghan WM, Smith R, et al. Low pregnancy weight gain and small for gestational age: a comparison of the association using 3 different measures of small for gestational age. Am J Obstet Gynecol 2009; 201:53.e1–e7. [II-2: Retrospective cohort study, Pregnancy Risk Assessment Monitoring System (PRAMS), *n* = 104,980]

94. Gore S, Brown DM, Smith-West D. The role of postpartum weight retention in obesity among women: a review of evidence. Ann Behav Med 2003; 26:149–159. [Review]

95. Oken E, Taveras EM, Kleinman KP, et al. Gestational weight gain and child adiposity at age 3 years. Am J Obstet Gynecol 2007; 196:322. [II-2: Prospective cohort study]

96. Polley BA, Wing RR, Sims CJ. Randomized controlled trial to prevent excessive weight gain in pregnant women. Int J Obesity Relat Metab Disord 2002; 26:1494–1502. [RCT, *n* = 120]

97. Dodd JM, Grivell RM, Crowther CA, et al. Antenatal interventions for overweight or obese pregnant women: a systematic review of randomized trials. BJOG 2010; 117:1316–1326. [Meta-analysis; 9 RCTs, *n* = 743]

98. Streuling I, Beyerlein A, Rosenfeld E, et al. Physical activity and gestational weight gain: a meta-analysis of intervention trials. BJOG 2011; 118:278–284. [Meta-analysis; 12 RCTs, *n* = 1073]

99. American College of Obstetricians and Gynecologists. Exercise during pregnancy and the postpartum period. ACOG Committee Opinion No.267. Ostet Gynecol 2002; 99:171–173. [Review]

100. American Academy of Pediatrics and the American College of Obstetrics and Gynecologists. Guidelines for Perinatal Care. 6th ed. October 2007:191–192.

101. Marik PE, Plante LA. Pregnancy and venous thromboembolic disease: a clinical review. N Engl J Med 2008; 359:2025–2033. [Review]

4

Pregestational diabetes

A. Dhanya Mackeen and Patrice M. L. Trauffer

KEY POINTS

- **Poorly controlled** diabetes in pregnancy is associated with **increased risks** of first-trimester miscarriage, congenital malformations (especially cardiac defects and CNS anomalies), intrauterine fetal demise, preterm birth, pre-eclampsia, ketoacidosis, polyhydramnios, macrosomia, operative (both vaginal and cesarean) delivery, birth injury (including brachial plexus), delayed lung maturity, respiratory distress syndrome, jaundice, hypoglycemia, hypocalcemia, perinatal mortality, long-term obesity, type II diabetes, and lower IQ.
- **Preconception counseling should include weight loss, exercise, appropriate diet, and optimization of blood sugar control.** Normalization of glucose levels (**hemoglobin A_{1c} <6%) prevents most, if not all, of the complications of diabetes in pregnancy.**
- In pregestational diabetics, **fasting glucose <95 mg/dL and two-hour postprandial ≤120 mg/dL** should be achieved and maintained at all times with diet, exercise, and insulin therapy as necessary.
- There is insufficient evidence to assess the safety and efficacy of oral hypoglycemic agents in pregestational diabetes.
- **Diabetic ketoacidosis is treated with aggressive hydration and intravenous insulin.**
- In pregestational diabetics, timing of delivery is about 39 weeks; cesarean delivery may be offered if estimated fetal weight is ≥4500 g.

PREGESTATIONAL DIABETES
Diagnosis/Definition

Diabetes mellitus (DM) is defined as a metabolic abnormality characterized by elevated circulating glucose. **The diagnoses of diabetes and impaired glucose tolerance outside of pregnancy are established on the basis of formal laboratory criteria** (Table 4.1) (1–3). As different countries use either mmol/L or mg/dL for glucose values, a comparison is provided (Table 4.2).

Symptoms

Often asymptomatic, but classic symptoms of uncontrolled diabetes are polydipsia, polyuria, and polyphagia.

Epidemiology/Incidence

Pregestational DM complicates approximately 1.8% of all pregnancies (4).

Basic Pathophysiology

The etiology of the disease varies and includes a primary insulin production defect, insulin receptor abnormalities, end-organ insulin resistance, and diabetes secondary to another disease process, such as cystic fibrosis (3). *Type I* diabetics are insulin deficient, secondary to the autoimmune destruction of the pancreatic islet beta-cells (3). These individuals develop disease early in life, require insulin replacement, and become acutely symptomatic with ketoacidosis if no therapy is initiated. In contrast, *type II* diabetics continue to produce insulin, but do so at diminished levels. They are often hyperinsulinemic, at least in the early stages; relative hypoinsulinemia may (or may not) develop later (3). Insulin resistance is the cardinal feature and many exhibit insulin resistance at the level of the end-organ receptor. The onset of disease is usually later in life, the course is gradual but progressive, and the disease is linked to obesity (3). This is rapidly changing: type II diabetes is now being seen at earlier ages, including childhood and adolescence. Both groups can be further subclassified on the basis of the presence of vascular complications, such as hypertension, renal disease, and retinopathy. The same physiologic changes of pregnancy that cause gestational diabetes (see chap. 5) also complicate the achievement of optimal glucose control in the pregestational diabetic.

Classification

To facilitate the management of these patients, the classification of diabetes has undergone recent revisions to reflect the physiology and implications of the disease process. Classification as type I and type II diabetes as defined above is still commonly used, especially in nonpregnant patients. Presence of vascular disease, defined as chronic hypertension (HTN), renal insufficiency, retinopathy, coronary artery disease, or prior cerebrovascular accident, is a better predictor of adverse pregnancy outcome than is White's classification (5,6).

Risk Factors/Associations

Obesity, hypertension, advanced maternal age, non-white race, family history (type II diabetes), metabolic syndrome, among others.

Complications

Incidence of complications is **inversely proportional to glucose control**, with minimal complications if glucose control is optimal (7). Pedersen first proposed that the exaggerated fetal response to insulin is provoked by fetal hyperglycemia that results from maternal hyperglycemia (8). Poorly controlled DM is associated with increased risks of the following: *first-trimester miscarriage*; *congenital malformations* (most common malformations are cardiac defects and CNS anomalies, especially neural tube defects (9); most pathognomonic are sacral

Table 4.1 Criteria for the Diagnosis of Diabetes Mellitus in the Nonpregnant State

Normal values	Impaired fasting glucose or impaired glucose tolerance	Diabetes mellitus (3)
FPG: <110 mg/dL 75-g, 2-hr OGTT: 2-hr PG <140 mg/dL	FPG: 110–125 mg/dL 75-g, 2-hr OGTT: 2-hr PG 140–199 mg/dL	FPG: ≥126 mg/dL (7.0 mmol/L)[a] 75-g, 2-hr OGTT: 2-hr PG ≥200 mg/dL (11.1 mmol/L)[a] Hemoglobin A$_{1C}$ ≥ 6.5%[a] Symptoms of hyperglycemia and PG (without regard to time since last meal) ≥200 mg/dL (11.1 mmol/L)

The diagnosis of diabetes mellitus should be confirmed on a separate day by any of these three tests.
[a]Repeat testing to confirm result unless unequivocal hyperglycemia is present (3). *Abbreviations*: FPG, fasting plasma glucose; OGTT, oral glucose tolerance test; PG, plasma glucose. *Source*: From Refs. 1, 2.

Table 4.2 Glucose Equivalents

mmol/L	mg/dL
5.9	105
6.7	120
7.8	140
8.0	144
11.0	198

agenesis/caudal regression); *intrauterine fetal demise; preterm birth* (both iatrogenic and spontaneous); *preeclampsia; ketoacidosis;* polyhydramnios; *macrosomia* (increased fetal insulin acts as growth factor; the degree of macrosomia is correlated with postprandial blood glucose values outside of the suggested parameters); *operative delivery* (both vaginal and cesarean) and *birth injury* (including brachial plexus) (both related to macrosomia); *delayed lung maturity; respiratory distress syndrome; jaundice* (because of polycythemia), *hypoglycemia, hypocalcemia* and *polycythemia* in the neonate, all related to elevated glucose levels and consequent hyperinsulinemia antenatally; and *perinatal mortality* (10,11). Long-term follow-up has shown higher rates of *obesity, type II DM,* and *lower IQ* with poorly controlled DM in pregnancy (10–15).

Pregnancy Considerations

It is always important to consider the effect of maternal disease on pregnancy, and conversely, the effect of pregnancy on maternal end organs (Table 4.3). Because pregestational diabetes affects the micro- and macrovascular system, these considerations must include the effect pregnancy may have on end organs. Diabetic **retinopathy** is the leading cause of blindness in reproductive years. Background retinopathy is characterized by retinal microaneurysms and dot-blot hemorrhages, and proliferative retinopathy by neovascularization. Proliferative diabetic retinopathy may progress as tightened glycemic control is achieved (16). However, clinicians should not be deterred from achieving optimal glucose control as the risk of subsequent progression of retinopathy is overall decreased as compared to patients not managed with intensive therapy (16). Diabetic **nephropathy** occurs in 5% to 10% of pregestational diabetics and can progress to end-stage renal disease especially in women with creatinine of ≥1.4 mg/dL or 24-hour proteinuria of ≥3 g (see chap. 17). Proteinuria increases in diabetic patients as they approach term, particularly in those who have baseline nephropathy. Women with baseline nephropathy are at increased risk of iatrogenic preterm birth and uteroplacental insufficiency. Progression of renal insufficiency is not clearly linked to the physiologically increased glomerular

filtration rate of pregnancy, although those with nephrotic range proteinuria and moderate to severe renal insufficiency may progress to end-stage renal disease. Diabetic **neuropathy** is not worsened, per se, in pregnancy, although decreased gastrointestinal motility related to progesterone and mechanical factors may exacerbate underlying gastroparesis. The presence of **hypertension** (in 5–10% of women with pregestational DM) further increases the risks of preeclampsia, fetal growth restriction, and fetal death. Progression of **cardiovascular** disease in the diabetic pregnant patient has not been reported, but symptomatic coronary artery disease is a contraindication to pregnancy in these diabetic women.

Management (Fig. 4.1)

Principles
Strict glycemic control, aiming for HgbA$_{1C}$ of <6%.

Workup
See Table 4.3.

Prevention
Weight loss, exercise, and optimization of blood sugar control can prevent most, if not all, of the complications of DM in pregnancy.

Preconception Counseling

The care of the pregestational diabetic is best instituted in the preconception period. The objectives of prepregnancy care are shown in Table 4.4. The frequency of maternal hospitalizations, length of NICU admission, congenital malformations, and perinatal mortality are reduced in women with DM who seek consultation in preparation for pregnancy; unfortunately, only about one third of these women receive such consultation (17).

Table 4.3 Diabetes Workup in Pregnancy

Workup

- Careful history (review of glucose control and therapy; history of end-organ disease)
- Laboratory tests (preconceptionally or first trimester if feasible):
  - Hemoglobin A$_{1c}$
  - Metabolic profile (glucose, creatinine)
  - Urine culture: repeat each trimester
  - 24-hr urine collection for protein and creatinine clearance
  - TSH for type I diabetics
- Consider EKG, especially if concomitant HTN
- Consider ophthalmologic consult to assess for any retinopathy, especially if long-standing or poorly controlled DM

Figure 4.1 Management of the pregestational diabetic.

Preconception counseling
- Weight loss
- Exercise
- Glucose testing
- Treatment of hyperglycemia as appropriate
- Strict glucose control

Preconception evaluation (Table 4.4)
- Normalization of the hemoglobin A_{1C} to within 1% of normal (<7%)
- Evaluate the presence of vascular disease
  - Ophthalmologic exam with retinal evaluation
  - 24-hr urine for protein and creatinine clearance
  - EKG
- Nutritional counseling (Table 4.6)
  - 30–35 kcal/kg/day if normal weight
- Institute glucose testing to include fasting and 2-hr postprandial values (Table 4.7)
- Incorporate exercise regimen
- Start or refine insulin regimen (Figs. 4.2 and 4.3)

Antepartum management
- Insulin therapy adjusted by weight and pregnancy trimester as guided by glucose monitoring (Tables 4.7 and 4.9, Figs. 4.2 and 4.3)
- Viability/dating scan
- Fetal surveillance and antepartum testing (Table 4.11)
  - Alpha-fetoprotein screening at 16–20 weeks
  - Detailed anatomic survey at 18–20 weeks
  - Fetal echocardiogram at 20–22 weeks
  - Serial ultrasounds for growth in the second and third trimester
  - Antenatal assessments with NST or BPP weekly from 32 to 36 weeks, then twice weekly until delivery. Start earlier if diabetes is poorly controlled

Intrapartum management (Fig. 4.4)
- Trial of labor unless clinical or ultrasound estimated fetal weight greater than 4500 g
- Delivery at 39 weeks or prior to 39 wk if pulmonary maturity documented by amniocentesis
- IV insulin therapy to maintain blood sugar between 70 and 110 mg/dL
- IV dextrose solution if blood sugars fall <70 mg/dL or with development of ketonuria
- For scheduled cesarean section, administer the dose of long-acting insulin in PM and withhold the AM short-acting dose
- Monitor blood glucose hourly

Postpartum management
- Reduce the antepartum insulin dose by half and administer it with the resumption of oral intake
- Supplement breastfeeding mothers with extra 500 kcal compared to nonpregnant levels

Abbreviations: BPP, biophysical profile; EKG, electrocardiogram; NST, non-stress test.

Table 4.4 The Objectives of Diabetes Prepregnancy Care

- Patient education
- Assessment of patient's medical condition
- Optimize glycemic control (hemoglobin A_{1c} <6%) *prior to* conception
- Folic acid supplementation (at least 400 μg) for at least 1 mo *prior to* conception

Table 4.5 Risk of Congenital Malformations Based on Hemoglobin A_{1c}

HbA_{1c} (%)	Risk
<7	No increased risk
7–10	3–7%
10–11	8–10%
≥11	10–20% or more

Source: From Ref. 18.

The evaluation should emphasize the importance of tight glycemic control, with **normalization of the hemoglobin A_{1c} (aim for <6%)** (Table 4.5) (5). Decreased spontaneous miscarriage, congenital anomalies, and other complications have been demonstrated in multiple studies, including RCTs, when optimal glucose control is attained via multiple daily insulin doses adjusted to glucose monitoring ≥4 times per day (19,20). Given the long-term complications of poorly controlled pregestational DM, optimal glucose control also prevents future obesity, DM, and its complications in the offspring. In addition to advocating the use of at least 400 μg of folic acid for at least one month prior to conception, this consultation affords the opportunity to screen for end-organ damage (Table 4.3). Ophthalmologic evaluation, EKG, and renal evaluation via a 24-hour urine collection for total protein and creatinine clearance will ascertain end-organ damage and determine ancillary pregnancy risks. As 40% of young women with type 1 diabetes have hypothyroidism, thyroid-stimulating hormone (TSH) should be checked. Proliferative retinopathy should be treated with laser before pregnancy. Women compliant with insulin pumps may continue this regimen. Sexually active diabetic adolescents benefit from preconception counseling (21,22).

Prenatal Care

Optimizing health outcomes can be achieved by a combination of diet, exercise, glucose monitoring, and insulin therapy. Women with type I DM and glucose levels of >200 mg/dL should check their urine ketones. A glass of milk is preferable to juice for hypoglycemia. Glucagon should be immediately available.

Diet

Nutritional requirements are adjusted on the basis of maternal body mass index (BMI); women with normal BMI require 30 to 35 kcal/kg/day (Table 4.6) (5). Individuals <90% of their ideal body weight (IBW) may increase this by an additional 5 kcal/kg/day, while those >120% of their IBW should decrease this value to 24 kcal/kg/day (5). The content should be distributed as 45% complex, high-fiber carbohydrates, 20% protein, and 35% primarily unsaturated fats (Table 4.6) (5,17). The calories are distributed over three meals and three snacks with breakfast receiving the smallest allotment at 15%, and the other two meals receiving near equal distribution. Saccharin, aspartame, acesulfame-K, maltodextin, and sucralose may be used safely in moderate amounts. Carbohydrate counting and help of a

Table 4.6 Diabetic Diet

30–35 kcal/kg/day (usually 2000–2400 kcal/day)	
3 Meals, 3 snacks	
Composition	
Carbohydrate (complex)	45%
Protein	20%
Fat (<10% saturated)	35%

Source: From Ref. 5.

Table 4.7   Target Venous Plasma Glucose Levels

Fasting	60–90 mg/dL
Preprandial	60–100 mg/dL
One-hour postprandial	≤140 mg/dL
Two-hour postprandial	≤120 mg/dL
3 AM	60–90 mg/dL

Source: From Ref. 23.

Table 4.8   Types of Insulin and Their Pharmacokinetics

Type	Onset	Peak	Duration
Lispro/aspart	1–15 min	1–2 hr	4–5 hr
Regular	30–60 min	2–4 hr	6–8 hr
NPH	1–3 hr	5–7 hr	13–18 hr
Lente	1–3 hr	4–8 hr	13–20 hr
Ultralente	2–4 hr	8–14 hr	18–30 hr
Glargine	1 hr	none	24 hr

registered dietitian may provide benefit, but these two interventions have been insufficiently studied in pregnancy.

Exercise
Moderate exercise decreases the need for insulin therapy in type II diabetics by increasing the glucose uptake in skeletal muscle, and therefore, should be strongly encouraged for any diabetic patient.

Glucose Monitoring
Frequent home glucose monitoring, both pre- and postprandially, has been associated with enhanced glucose control and shorter interval to achieve target blood sugars. Capillary blood glucose ("fingerstick") measurements using a glucometer should be obtained at least four times a day—fasting and two hours postprandial. Target levels are in Table 4.7 (23). Some women will require another assessment at 3 AM for prevention of hypoglycemic episodes.

Glycosylated hemoglobin A_{1c} <6% is normal (5). Hemoglobin A_{1c} of 6% reflects a mean glucose level of 120 mg/dL; each 1% increment in hemoglobin A_{1c} is equal to a change in mean glucose level of 30 mg/dL. There is no evidence that serial glycosylated hemoglobin A_{1c} measurements after the first trimester affect outcomes (25).

Though not in widespread use, randomized controlled trials in pregnant women have shown that continuous glucose monitoring (e.g., with 288 glucose values per day) is associated with decreased birth weight and incidence of macrosomia (26,27).

Oral Hypoglycemic Agents
There is insufficient evidence to assess the safety of oral hypoglycemic agents in pregestational diabetes (28,29). There is also insufficient evidence to assess their effectiveness on glucose control in these patients. Therefore, even in women on oral hypoglycemic control before pregnancy, insulin therapy is suggested for glucose control. Occasionally, a woman well controlled on either glyburide or metformin prepregnancy, and a normal hemoglobin A_{1c}, can be managed by continuing these medications, as long as glycemic control remains optimal (20,28,30).

Insulin
Insulin therapy is the mainstay in the management of pregestational diabetics. All subcutaneous insulin types have been approved during pregnancy.

A review of the types of insulin, their onset, and duration of action are listed in Table 4.8. Human insulin is preferred to animal insulin (31). Women, particularly those new to insulin therapy, need to be counseled about the differences in the various insulins in order to use them to their greatest efficacy. Close monitoring with **at least weekly contact with a provider** is suggested to maximize insulin adjustment. The goal of therapy is as shown in Table 4.7 (23). The postprandial blood sugar has been found to have the greatest correlation with fetal macrosomia (see chap. 5). While it has not been

associated with adverse fetal outcomes, hypoglycemia can cause significant maternal morbidities. *Glucagon* should be available for home use in emergency situations.

Though satisfactory glucose control may be obtained solely with an intermediate-acting insulin rather than a short-acting insulin (32), we suggest optimizing metabolic control with one evening injection of **long-acting (e.g., insulin glargine)** insulin, and meal-time (three daily) injections of **short-acting (e.g., lispro or aspart) insulin** (Figs. 4.2 and 4.3). Intermediate-acting insulin (e.g., Neutral Protamine Hagedorn [NPH]) twice daily can also be used, instead of insulin glargine.

Studies have shown that short-acting insulin is as effective as regular insulin and may result in improved postprandial glucose control and less preterm deliveries (33,34). Insulin lispro should be given immediately before eating. As compared to two daily insulin injections, additional doses are associated with improved glycemic control (35).

A meta-analysis of cohort studies comparing insulin glargine to NPH did not reveal any significant differences in outcomes including infant birth weight, congenital anomalies, and respiratory distress (36). However, a randomized controlled trial has not yet been done. Glargine cannot be mixed in the same syringe with other insulins.

Subcutaneous insulin pump therapy (continuous insulin infusion therapy) may be continued in women already compliant with this mode of therapy. In nonpregnant adults, women compliant with insulin pumps have increased satisfaction, decreased episodes of severe hypoglycemia, and better control of hyperglycemia (5). There is insufficient evidence to recommend subcutaneous insulin infusion versus multiple daily injections in pregnancy in women not already on pumps (37,38). Inhaled insulin has been tested in nonpregnant adults, but there are yet insufficient data for pregnancy management (39).

Carbohydrate counting and the use of an insulin-to-carbohydrate ratio of 1 unit of insulin for every 15 g of carbohydrate in early gestation can allow for greater flexibility in eating, but has not been studied in a trial. As pregnancy advances with its concomitant increased insulin resistance, an increased ratio is required with 1 unit covering a lower amount of carbohydrates, for example, 1 unit/10 g of carbohydrate.

Useful sample calculations for the total daily insulin requirement and insulin regimen are in Table 4.9 (5,7,40) and Figures 4.2 and 4.3.

Very Tight vs. Tight Control
There are limited data to assess the effect of tight versus very tight glycemic control in pregestational diabetic women. Compared to tight control (either fasting and 2 hour postprandial (pp) 5.6–6.7 mmol/L or fasting <5.6 mmol/L and 1.5 hour pp <7.8 mmol/L), **very tight control** (either fasting and 2 hour pp <5.6 mmol/L or fasting <4.4 mmol/L and 1.5 hour pp <6.7 mmol/L) is associated with similar incidence of preeclampsia and CD, but **lower incidence of neonatal hypoglycemia**, and

Table 4.9 Total Insulin Requirements

Trimester	Units/kg/day
1	0.7–0.8
2	0.8–1.0
3	0.9–1.2

Patients with multifetal gestations or who have received steroids or betamimetics often require higher doses. *Source*: From Refs. 5,7,40.

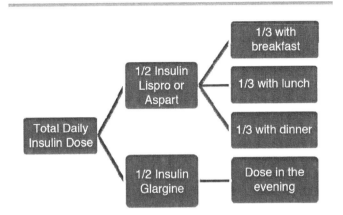

Figure 4.2 Distribution of insulin dose throughout the day if using insulin glargine and lispro/aspart.

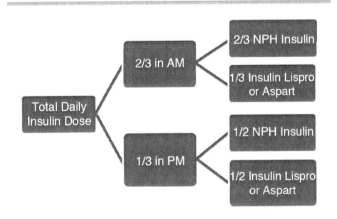

Figure 4.3 Distribution of insulin dose throughout the day if using NPH and insulin lispro/aspart.

trends for improvements in other neonatal metabolic outcomes, with **increased incidence of maternal hypoglycemia** based on limited trial numbers (41). There was no difference detected in perinatal outcome between the groups. Suboptimal ("loose") control (above 6.7 mmol/L or 120 mg/dL) is associated with increased incidence of preeclampsia, cesarean deliveries, and infants that were large for gestational age (42). There are no data to assess the clinical value with respect to prevention of significant long-term neonatal morbidity.

Diabetic Ketoacidosis

Diabetic ketoacidosis occurs in 5% to 10% of women with pregestational type I diabetes. It is defined by elevated glucose (usually >250 mg/dL), positive serum ketones, and acidosis.

Risk factors include type I diabetes, new onset diabetes, infections (e.g., urinary or respiratory tract infections), poor compliance, insulin pump failure, and treatment with betamimetics or steroids (5). Symptoms include abdominal pain, nausea, vomiting, and altered sensorium. Laboratory tests should include an arterial blood gas (pH <7.3), electrolytes (serum bicarbonate <15 mEq/L and elevated anion gap), serum, and urinary ketones (elevated). **Aggressive hydration, intravenous insulin, and correction of the underlying etiology are the most important interventions**, with close electrolyte (especially glucose and potassium) monitoring (Table 4.10) (5,43). Fetal mortality may be up to 10%, even with aggressive management.

Antepartum Testing

Fetal surveillance is required to determine whether congenital anomalies are present and to minimize perinatal mortality (Table 4.11). The nature of this surveillance is by convention and expert consensus rather than supported by well-performed trials. Because of the increased risk of birth defects, particularly cardiac and neural tube defects, patients should be offered alpha-fetoprotein screening at 16 to 18 weeks gestation, targeted ultrasonography at 18 to 20 weeks, and **fetal echocardiography at 20 to 22 weeks**. Some suggest an earlier first

Table 4.10 Management of Diabetic Ketoacidosis in Pregnancy

IV hydration: Use isotonic saline (0.9% NS)

- First hour: Give 1 L NS
- Hours 2–4: 0.5–1 L NS/hr
- Thereafter (24 hr): Give 250 mL/hr 0.45% NS until 80% deficit corrected
- Body water deficit = {[0.6 body weight (kg)] + [1−(140/serum sodium)]} ≈ 100 mL deficit/kg body weight

Insulin: Mix 50 units of regular insulin in 500 mL of NS and flush IV tubing prior to infusion

- Loading: 0.2–0.4 units/kg
- Maintenance: 2–10 units/hr
- Continue insulin therapy until bicarbonate and anion gap normalize

Potassium replacement: Maintain serum K$^+$ at 4–5 mEq/L

- If K$^+$ is initially normal or reduced, consider an infusion of up to 15–20 mEq/hr
- If K$^+$ is elevated, do not add supplemental potassium until levels are within normal range, then add 20–30 mEq/L

Phosphate: Consider replacement if serum phosphate <1.0 mg/dL or if cardiac dysfunction present or patient obtunded

Bicarbonate: If pH is <7.1, add one ampule (44 mEq) of bicarbonate to 1 L of 0.45% NS

Laboratory tests: Check arterial blood gas on admission; check serum glucose, ketones, and electrolytes every 1 to 2 hrs until normal

- Consider doubling insulin infusion rate if serum glucose does not decrease by 20% within the first two hours
- When blood glucose reaches 250 mg/dL, change IVF to D5NS
- Continue insulin drip until ketosis resolves and the first subcutaneous dose of insulin is administered

Abbreviation: NS, normal saline; IVF, intravenous fluids; K+, potassium; kg, kilograms. *Source*: Adapted from Refs. 5, 43.

Table 4.11 Antepartum Testing

A. Assessment of viability and exact GA: first-trimester ultrasound
B. Detection of congenital malformations
  a. If hemoglobin A_{1C} is elevated, consider transvaginal ultrasound at about 14 wks to rule out structural defects, including cardiac
  b. Maternal serum alpha-fetoprotein level at 16 wk
  c. Level II ultrasound at 18–20 wk
  d. Fetal echocardiogram at 20–22 wk
C. Assessment of fetal growth
  a. Serial growth ultrasounds in third trimester every 3–4 wk
D. Assessment of fetal well-being
  a. Maternal assessment of fetal activity ("fetal kick counts")
  b. Nonstress tests weekly from 32 wks until 36 wks, then twice weekly until delivery. Begin at 32 wk if maternal glycemic control is satisfactory, fetal growth is appropriate, and there are no coexisting maternal medical or obstetric complications. Begin earlier (~28 wks) and increase frequency if the above conditions are not met

anatomic fetal sonographic survey, at around 14 to 16 weeks, as well early fetal echocardiography at this time, especially in women with poor glycemic control in the first trimester (e.g., hemoglobin A_{1c} >10 mg/dL). Serial ultrasounds in the third trimester to evaluate fetal growth and frequent prenatal visits

to review glucose control are also advocated. The use of fetal surveillance with nonstress test (NST) and/or biophysical profile is recommended by expert opinion (17), but the frequency and nature of the testing cannot be determined, since there is no randomized trial to direct effective screening. For women with good glycemic control, antepartum testing can start at 32 weeks with weekly NSTs (5). More frequent testing in the form of NST or biophysical profile occurs after 36 weeks, with twice weekly testing usually employed. For women with poor glycemic control, antepartum testing may need to begin earlier (5).

Delivery
Timing
Timing of delivery is usually delayed to the 39th week, unless maternal or fetal factors dictate earlier intervention; but should be accomplished by the estimated date of delivery, as perinatal mortality increases after this gestational age. In general, indicated delivery before 39 weeks, if truly indicated, should not require assessment of fetal maturity. If assessment of fetal lung maturity is done, laboratory tests are interpreted as in nondiabetic patients, with phosphatidylglycerol ≥3% accepted by most authorities as the lab value indicating the least risk for fetal respiratory insufficiency in diabetic women; patients should be cautioned that a positive test does not preclude infant morbidities (see chap. 57).

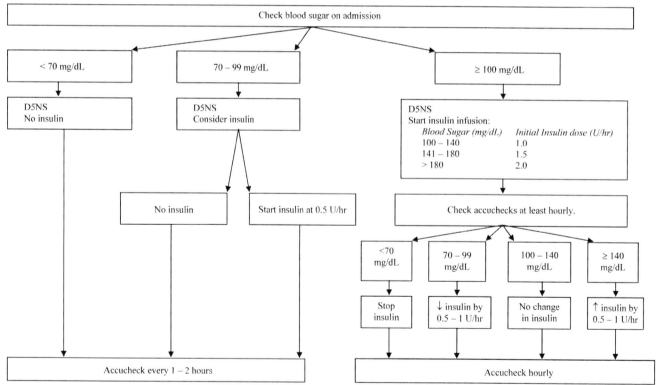

Please note:
- These are suggestions and patients should be managed on a case by case basis
- Insulin should be mixed as follows: mix 10 units of short-acting insulin in 1000 mL of D5NS
- Intravenous fluids should be infused at a rate of 100–150 cc/h (2.5 mg/kg/min)
- If patient persistently has blood sugars > 180 mg/dL, consider Normal Saline (NS) instead of D5NS and evaluate for DKA
- We suggest having two lines, one running NS and one running D5NS, so that rate of NS infusion can be changed as per L&D needs and D5NS can be consistently infused

Figure 4.4 Intrapartum management evidence of diabetes (GDMA2 and pregestational). Adapted from References 5 and 23. *Abbreviations*: DKA, diabetic ketoacidosis; L&D, labor and delivery; NS, normal saline.

Mode

Mode of delivery is generally vaginal. **Cesarean** is indicated if estimated **fetal weight is** $\geq$**4500 g** (see chap. 45). The diagnosis of macrosomia is inexact by ultrasound and clinical estimation, confounding the ability to make a clear recommendation. Induction for macrosomia increases the rate of cesarean, but may not reduce birth trauma (44).

Intrapartum Glucose Management

Intrapartum management (Fig. 4.4) (5,23) is targeted to maintain maternal glucose levels between 70 and 110 mg/dL. Often the insulin requirement is decreased because of the energy requirements of labor. The usual subcutaneous long-acting (e.g., glargine) or intermediate-acting insulin (e.g., NPH) is given at bedtime, while the usual subcutaneous morning insulin is withheld. Intravenous insulin, dextrose solution, frequent (usually every one hour) glucose monitoring, and evaluation of urinary ketones are required to prevent a catabolic state and the development of ketoacidosis. Once active labor begins or glucose is <70 mg/dL, IV 5% dextrose at 125 cc/hr can be started. Once glucose level is $\geq$100 mg/dL, short-acting (e.g., lispro or regular) IV insulin should be started. IV 5% dextrose and insulin infusions should be separate, and often should occur at the same time, to prevent ketonuria. Adjustments to the basal infusion rates are based on hourly fingerstick blood sugars while in labor. The use of the insulin pump, maintaining the basal rate, rather than using an IV insulin infusion, is an accepted alternative.

With cesarean delivery, use of a single injection of long-acting insulin, an IV insulin infusion, or subcutaneous pump at a low basal rate are equal alternatives, until oral intake is assured and more standard dosing can be reinstituted. Insulin requirements are diminished postpartum and are generally half of the antepartum requirement.

Anesthesia

No specific adjustments necessary.

Postpartum/Breast-feeding

Usual diabetic diet should be restarted after delivery, with one half of the predelivery dose or the prepregnancy dose (if this achieved euglycemia) restarted (23). If food intake cannot be restarted soon, then glucose levels of >140 mg/dL should be treated with proper coverage. Breast-feeding has increased maternal caloric demands and an additional 500 kcal/day needs to be added to the diet to avoid hypoglycemia. All forms of contraception are available to diabetics, providing they have no contraindications such as hypertension or vascular disease (see chap. 27, *Obstetrics Evidence Based Guidelines*).

Future

New therapeutic approaches include pancreatic islet cell transplant.

REFERENCES

1. Galernau F, Inzucchi SE. Diabetes mellitus in pregnancy. Obstet Gynecol Clin North Am 2004; 31:907–933. [Review]
2. Expert Committee on the Diagnosis and Classification of Diabetes Mellitus. Report of the expert committee on the diagnosis and classification of diabetes mellitus. Diabetes Care 2003; 26(suppl 1):S5–S20. [Review, guideline]
3. American Diabetes Association. Diagnosis and classification of diabetes mellitus. Diabetes Care 2010; 33(suppl 1):S62–S69. [Review, guideline]
4. D'Angelo D, Williams L, Morrow B, et al. Preconception and interconception health status of women who recently gave birth to a live-born infant—pregnancy risk assessment monitoring system (PRAMS), United States, 26 Reporting Areas, 2004—December 14, 2007; 56(SS10):1–35. Available at: http://www.cdc.gov/mmwr/preview/mmwrhtml/ss5610a1.htm. Accessed February 21, 2011. [II-3]
5. ACOG Practice Bulletin. Pregestational diabetes mellitus. Clinical Management Guidelines for Obstetrician–Gynecologists No. 60. Obstet Gynecol 2005; 105(3):675–685. [Review, guideline]
6. Cormier CM, Martinez CA, Refuerzo JS, et al. White's classification of diabetes in pregnancy in the 21st century: is it still valid? Am J Perinatol 2010; 27(5):349–352. [II-2]
7. Jovanovic L, Druzin M, Peterson CM. Effect of euglycemia on the outcome of pregnancy in insulin-dependent diabetic women as compared with normal control subjects. Am J Med 1981; 71 (6):921–927. [II-2]
8. Pedersen J. Diabetes and pregnancy: blood sugar of newborn infants during fasting and glucose administration. Nord Med 1952; 2:1049. [Level III]
9. Yazdy MM, Liu S, Mitchell AA, et al. Maternal dietary glycemic intake and the risk of neural tube defects. Am J Epidemiol 2010; 171(4):407–414. [Case control, n = 1394]
10. Tyrala EE. The infant of the diabetic mother. Obstet Gynecol Clin North Am 1996; 23(1):221–241. [Review]
11. Boulet SL, Alexander GR, Salihu HM, et al. Macrosomic births in the United States: determinants, outcomes, and proposed grades of risk. Am J Obstet Gynecol 2003; 188(5):1372–1378. [Case control, n = 8.2 million]
12. Murtaugh MA, Jacobs DR Jr., Moran A, et al. Relation of birth weight to fasting insulin, insulin resistance, and body size in adolescence. Diabetes Care 2003; 26(1):187–192. [Descriptive, n = 296]
13. Van Assche FA, Holemans K, Aerts L. Fetal growth and consequences for later life. J Perinat Med 1998; 26(5):337–346. [Review]
14. Rizzo T, Metzger BE, Burns WJ, et al. Correlations between antepartum maternal metabolism and child intelligence. N Engl J Med 1991; 325(13):911–916. [Observational, n = 223]
15. Dabelea D, Knowler WC, Pettitt DJ. Effect of diabetes in pregnancy on offspring: follow-up research in the Pima Indians. J Matern Fetal Med 2000; 9(1):83–88. [II-3]
16. The effect of intensive treatment of diabetes on the development and progression of long-term complications in insulin-dependent diabetes mellitus. The Diabetes Control and Complications Trial Research Group. N Engl J Med 1993; 329(14):977–986. [RCT, n = 1441]
17. Koerenbrot CC, Steinberg A, Bender C, et al. Preconception care: a systematic review. Matern Child Health J 2002; 6:75–88. [Review of seven studies addressing the value of preconceptional care in the diabetic patient]
18. Guerin A, Nisenbaum R, Ray JG. Use of maternal GHb concentration to estimate the risk of congenital anomalies in the offspring of women with prepregnancy diabetes. Diabetes Care 2007; 30(7):1920–1925. [II-2]
19. Pregnancy outcomes in the Diabetes Control and Complications Trial. Am J Obstet Gynecol 1996; 174(4):1343–1353. [RCT, n = 180]
20. Tieu J, Middleton P, Crowther CA. Preconception care for diabetic women for improving maternal and infant health. Cochrane Database Syst Rev 2010; 12:CD007776. [1 RCT, n = 53]
21. Fischl AF, Herman WH, Sereika SM, et al. Impact of a preconception counseling program for teens with type 1 diabetes (READY-Girls) on patient–provider interaction, resource utilization, and cost. Diabetes Care 2010; 33(4):701–705. [RCT, n = 88]
22. Charron-Prochownik D, Ferons-Hannan M, Sereika S, et al. Randomized efficacy trial of early preconception counseling for diabetic teens (READY-girls). Diabetes Care 2008; 31(7):1327–1330. [RCT, n = 53]
23. Landon MB, Catalano PM, Gabbe SG. Diabetes mellitus complicating pregnancy. In: Gabbe SG, Niebyl JR, Simpson JL, eds.

Obstetrics: Normal and Problem Pregnancies. 5th ed. Elsevier, 2007:976–1005. [Review]

24. Gabbe SG, Graves CR. Management of diabetes mellitus complicating pregnancy. Obstet Gynecol 2003; 102(4):857–868. [III]

25. National Institute for Health and Clinical Excellence. Diabetes in pregnancy: management of diabetes and its complications from preconception to the postnatal period. Available at: http://www.nice.org.uk/nicemedia/pdf/DiabetesFullGuidelineRevised-JULY2008.pdf. Updated London: NICE, 2008. [Level III]. Accessed 1/17/2011.

26. Murphy HR, Rayman G, Lewis K, et al. Effectiveness of continuous glucose monitoring in pregnant women with diabetes: randomised clinical trial. BMJ 2008; 337:a1680. [RCT, *n* = 71]

27. McLachlan K, Jenkins A, O'Neal D. The role of continuous glucose monitoring in clinical decision-making in diabetes in pregnancy. Aust N Z J Obstet Gynaecol 2007; 47(3):186–190. [Descriptive study, *n* = 68]

28. Tieu J, Coat S, Hague W, et al. Oral anti-diabetic agents for women with pre-existing diabetes mellitus/impaired glucose tolerance or previous gestational diabetes mellitus. Cochrane Database Syst Rev 2010; (10):CD007724. [Meta-analysis, RCTs = 0]

29. Feig DS, Briggs GG, Koren G. Oral antidiabetic agents in pregnancy and lactation: a paradigm shift? Ann Pharmacother 2007; 41(7):1174–1180. [Review]

30. Tieu J, Crowther CA, Middleton P. Dietary advice in pregnancy for preventing gestational diabetes mellitus. Cochrane Database Syst Rev 2008; (2):CD006674. [Meta-analysis, 2 RCTs, *n* =82]

31. Jovanovic-Peterson L, Kitzmiller JL, Peterson CM. Randomized trial of human versus animal species insulin in diabetic pregnant women: improved glycemic control, not fewer antibodies to insulin, influences birth weight. Am J Obstet Gynecol 1992; 167 (5):1325–1330. [RCT, *n* = 43]

32. Nor Azlin MI, Nor NA, Sufian SS, et al. Comparative study of two insulin regimes in pregnancy complicated by diabetes mellitus. Acta Obstet Gynecol Scand 2007; 86(4):407–408. [RCT, *n* = 68]

33. Hod M, Damm P, Kaaja R, et al. Fetal and perinatal outcomes in type 1 diabetes pregnancy: a randomized study comparing insulin aspart with human insulin in 322 subjects. Am J Obstet Gynecol 2008; 198(2):186.e1–186.e7. [RCT, *n* = 322]

34. Mathiesen ER, Kinsley B, Amiel SA, et al. Maternal glycemic control and hypoglycemia in type 1 diabetic pregnancy: a random-

ized trial of insulin aspart versus human insulin in 322 pregnant women. Diabetes Care 2007; 30(4):771–776. [RCT, *n* = 322]

35. Nachum Z, Ben-Shlomo I, Weiner E, et al. Twice daily versus four times daily insulin dose regimens for diabetes in pregnancy: randomised controlled trial. BMJ 1999; 319(7219):1223–1227. [RCT, *n* = 392]

36. Pollex E, Moretti ME, Koren G, et al. Safety of insulin glargine use in pregnancy: a systematic review and meta-analysis. Ann Pharmacother 2011; 45(1):9–16. [Meta-analysis, *n* = 702]

37. Farrar D, Tuffnell DJ, West J. Continuous subcutaneous insulin infusion versus multiple daily injections of insulin for pregnant women with diabetes. Cochrane Database Syst Rev 2007; (3): CD005542. [Meta-analysis, RCT 2, *n* =60]

38. Mukhopadhyay A, Farrell T, Fraser RB, et al. Continuous subcutaneous insulin infusion vs. intensive conventional insulin therapy in pregnant diabetic women: a systematic review and metaanalysis of randomized, controlled trials. Am J Obstet Gynecol 2007; 197(5):447–456. [Meta-analysis, 6 RCTs or quasi-RCTs, *n* = 213]

39. Hollander PA, Blonde L, Rowe R, et al. Efficacy and safety of inhaled insulin (exubera) compared with subcutaneous insulin therapy in patients with type 2 diabetes: results of a 6-month, randomized, comparative trial. Diabetes Care 2004; 27(10):2356–2362. [RCT, *n* = 299]

40. Langer O, Anyaegbunam A, Brustman L, et al. Pregestational diabetes: insulin requirements throughout pregnancy. Am J Obstet Gynecol 1988; 159(3):616–621. [II-2]

41. Walkinshaw SA. Very tight versus tight control for diabetes in pregnancy. Cochrane Database of Syst Rev 2007; (2):CD000226. [Meta-analysis; 2 RCTs, *n* = 182]

42. Middleton P, Crowther CA, Simmonds L, et al. Different intensities of glycaemic control for pregnant women with pre-existing diabetes. Cochrane Database Syst Rev 2010; (9):CD008540. [Meta-analysis, 3 RCTs, *n* = 223]

43. Carroll MA, Yeomans ER. Diabetic ketoacidosis in pregnancy. Crit Care Med 2005; 33(10 suppl):S347–S353. [Review]

44. Sanchez-Ramos L, Bernstein S, Kaunitz AM. Expectant management versus labor induction for suspected fetal macrosomia: a systematic review. Obstet Gynecol 2002; 100(5(1)):997–1102. [Meta-analysis, 9 observational studies, 2 RCTs, 3751 subjects]

5

Gestational diabetes

A. Dhanya Mackeen and Patrice M. L. Trauffer

KEY POINTS

- **Poorly controlled** gestational diabetes (GDM) in pregnancy is associated with **increased risks of** fetal death, preterm birth, preeclampsia, polyhydramnios, macrosomia, operative (both vaginal and cesarean) delivery and birth injury (including brachial plexus), delayed lung maturity, respiratory distress syndrome, jaundice, hypoglycemia, hypocalcemia, and perinatal mortality.
- Prevention of GDM can be achieved with weight loss and exercise before pregnancy.
- **Optimization of blood glucose control with diet and insulin to achieve fasting glucose <95 mg/dL and two-hour postprandial <120 mg/dL is associated with reduced macrosomia, perinatal morbidity and maternal comorbidities including preeclampsia and depression.**
- Compared to insulin therapy, **glyburide and metformin are as efficacious in glucose control and result in similar pregnancy outcomes** [including incidences of macrosomia, cesarean delivery (CD), neonatal hypoglycemia, neonatal intensive care unit (NICU) admission, and other neonatal outcomes] **for gestational diabetics** in the second and third trimester. Glyburide is associated with lower failure rates than metformin.
- In GDM, **exercise** is associated with similar rate of macrosomia compared to insulin, improvement in glycemic control when done with diet compared to diet only, and improvement in cardiovascular fitness.
- Women with GDM should be **screened for diabetes six to eight weeks postpartum.**

SCREENING/DIAGNOSIS

Gestational diabetes (GDM) is hyperglycemia that is first recognized or diagnosed during pregnancy (1). If hyperglycemia is detected before 20 weeks, pregestational diabetes is probably present. The importance of screening for GDM, and treatment to optimize glycemic control to reduce complications associated with hyperglycemia, has been established (2–6). Who, when, and how to screen, and the diagnostic glucose cutoffs for GDM are controversial.

Who to Screen

The population who should be offered screening has not been uniformly identified (1). **Low-risk individuals in whom screening may not be necessary must meet all of the following criteria: age <25 years; ethnic origin of low risk (not Hispanic, African, native American, south or east Asian, or Pacific Islander); BMI <25; no previous personal or family history of impaired glucose tolerance; no previous history of adverse obstetric outcomes associated with GDM** (1,7). However, universal screening is most commonly adopted and more

cases of GDM would remain undiagnosed with selective screening. The risk of developing GDM is directly associated with prepregnancy BMI (8).

When to Screen

To balance sensitivity and specificity with adequate treatment duration, screen women at **24 to 28 weeks**. However, the incidence of GDM (related to placental mass and hormone production) increases with GA. **Women with risk factors (Table 5.1) should be screened preconception or at first prenatal visit** (7). About 5% to 10% of women with these risk factors will have early GDM, and these represent 40% of all GDM diagnosed later at 24 to 28 weeks (9). If the early screen is negative, a repeat screen should be performed at 24 to 28 weeks gestation.

How to Screen

While studies have compared different GDM screening approaches including glucose polymer, glucose monomer, candy bar, and food, there is insufficient evidence to compare the effects of these different ways to glucose load, and the subsequent management of GDM, thereafter (10).

One-Step Process

In most countries, the World Health Organization (WHO) **75-gram, one-step** screening process is employed in women with risk factors, using two abnormal values as criteria for diagnosis: fasting > 5.3 mmol/L (95 mg/dL), 1 hour > 10.0 mmol/L (180 mg/dL), 2 hour > 8.6 mmol/L (155 mg/dL) (5). This approach diagnoses twice as many women as having GDM than the two-step process generally employed in North America (11).

Although the need for treatment has not been established for women with screening values less than those noted above for the 75-g glucose test, one multicenter study of 23,316 women revealed increased incidence of large for gestational age (LGA) infants, premature delivery, shoulder dystocia/birth injury, NICU admission, hyperbilirubinemia, and preeclampsia in women with glucose levels >75 mg/dL (fasting), 133 mg/dL (1 hour), or 109 mg/dL (2 hours) (12). As such, on the basis of the results of the HAPO study (12), the following criteria have been suggested as diagnostic of GDM after a 75-g glucose load: fasting ≥92 mg/dL or 1 hour ≥180 mg/dL or 2 hour ≥153 mg/dL; but these have not been systematically reviewed (5,13). Unfortunately, no trial has evaluated the efficacy of any therapy based on these values, and so they cannot be used yet for clinical care.

Two-Step Process

The first (screening) step involves a **50-g, 1-hour oral glucose load** (*glucose challenge test*), applied in the nonfasting state (14), with a venous glucose value obtained one hour after consumption. Glucose polymer solutions are better tolerated than

Table 5.1   Risk Factors for GDM

- Prior unexplained stillbirth
- Prior infant with congenital anomaly (if not screened in that pregnancy)
- Prior macrosomic infant
- History of gestational diabetes
- Family history of diabetes
- Obesity
- Chronic use of steroids
- Age >35 yr
- Glycosuria

monomeric solutions (15). Jelly beans have not been sufficiently tested to be a valid alternative (16).

A positive result on the first part of the screening test is defined as 130, 135, or 140 mg/dL. The lower threshold identifies 90% of gestational diabetics, but subjects 20% to 25% of those screened to the second diagnostic test. In contrast, the higher value has a lower sensitivity of 80%, but subjects fewer women, 14% to 18%, to further testing. Any of these thresholds is acceptable (1). We use **135 mg/dL**. Over 80% of women with values ≥200 mg/dL will fail the three-hour glucose tolerance test (GTT), so some use this cutoff as meeting the diagnosis of GDM (17).

Definitive diagnosis of GDM is then made on the basis of the results of a **100-g, three-hour oral GTT**, administered after an overnight fast (8–14 hours), ideally following three days of unrestricted diet and activity, while the patient remains seated and refrains from smoking.

Unfortunately the criteria to establish diagnosis by this test are not universally accepted. The two competing criteria and their diagnostic levels are listed in Table 5.2. Two or more abnormal values on these tests establish the diagnosis of GDM. The Carpenter–Coustan stricter criteria increase by about 50% the number of women with a diagnosis of GDM compared to the NDDG criteria, and these pregnancies have elevated incidences of macrosomia and neonatal insulinemia (18). Therefore, we **suggest using Carpenter–Coustan criteria** as opposed to those of NDDG. In fact, there is evidence to suggest that hyperglycemia below the cutoff of even the Carpenter–Coustan criteria result in poor outcomes (12). Table 5.3 (6,19–24) shows the characteristics of the randomized studies comparing intervention with no intervention for women with GDM.

If GDM is diagnosed <20 weeks, counseling and management should be as for pregestational diabetes. The presence or absence of fasting hyperglycemia further subdivides this category.

If **one abnormal value** in the three-hour GTT is present, the patient is counseled to avoid excess glucose consumption; fasting and two-hour postprandial glucose samples or a repeat three-hour GTT can be obtained three to four weeks later. In

one randomized controlled trial (RCT) in these women with one abnormal value, **strict glycemic control with diet and insulin** was associated with less neonatal complications and decreased incidence of LGA, when compared with no such therapies (25).

One large trial has shown that **two-step screening is more cost-effective** than the one-step screening (24).

INCIDENCE

There is a **7%** incidence of GDM (5), representing one of the most common medical complications facing obstetricians. Of cases of DM in pregnancy, 88% are GDM (1,26). Incidence obviously depends on the screening strategy used, with some suggesting that stricter criteria would result in 18% of pregnant women being diagnosed with GDM (12,13).

PATHOPHYSIOLOGY

The pathophysiology of GDM is insulin resistance caused by circulating hormonal factors: increased maternal and placental production of human placental lactogen, progesterone, growth hormone, cortisol, and prolactin. Increased body weight and caloric intake also contribute to the insulin resistance associated with pregnancy, and may offset the normally increased insulin production in the pregnant woman (26). Women with GDM have been found to have lower basal islet cell function, in addition to insulin resistance, when compared to a nondiabetic cohort. The combination of the two factors contributes to the development of GDM. This insulin resistance and decreased insulin production persists in the postpartum state and leads to the development of type II diabetes in this population.

RISK FACTORS/ASSOCIATIONS

Pregnancy, obesity, hypertension, age greater than or equal to 35 years at delivery, metabolic syndrome, family history of type II DM, nonwhite ethnicity, previous macrosomia.

COMPLICATIONS

Incidence of complications is inversely proportional to glucose control. In poorly controlled DM, increased glucose in the mother causes abnormal metabolism, while in the fetus it causes hyperinsulinemia, and its consequences.

Other complications are hypertensive disorders and preeclampsia, macrosomia, operative delivery, and birth injury (confounded by maternal obesity; both related to macrosomia) (6,12,23).

Apart from transient neonatal hypoglycemia, no other metabolic derangement has been reported in the infant of the GDM mother. Long-term adult disorders, such as glucose intolerance and obesity, have been postulated to occur as frequently in these neonates as in neonates of women with pregestational diabetes, but this has not been verified by observational studies. Approximately 50% of women identified as having GDM will develop frank diabetes within 10 years, if followed longitudinally (27).

PREVENTION

Low-glycemic diet (28), a diet with adequate (not excessive) caloric intake, achieving and maintaining a normal BMI, and exercise are probably beneficial, especially preconception, in preventing GDM, but have been insufficiently studied in RCTs so far.

Table 5.2   Criteria for Standard 100-g Glucose Load to Diagnose Gestational Diabetes

	National Diabetes Data Group		Carpenter–Coustan criteria	
	mg/dL	mmol/L	mg/dL	mmol/L
Fasting	105	5.8	95	5.3
1 hr	190	10.6	180	10.0
2 hr	165	9.2	155	8.6
3 hr	145	8.0	140	7.8

Table 5.3 Randomized Studies of Intervention for GDM: Comparing Therapy to No Therapy

Study	Sample size	Gestational age at screening	Screening test & threshold for performing diagnostic test	Diagnostic test	Cases (intervention) group	Control group	Outcomes
Landon (23)	958	24–30 6/7 wks	50-g glucose load: blood glucose level 135–200 mg/dL 1 hr post glucose load	**3-hr, 100-g screen.** Included if mild GDM, i.e., fasting < 95 mg/dL and 2 abnormal serum values: **180 mg/dL (at 1 hr), 155 mg/dL (at 2 hrs), 140 mg/dL (at 3 hrs)**	Nutrition counseling, self-monitoring of glucose and diet therapy. Insulin could be added to either group to minimize hyperglycemia.	Usual prenatal care. Insulin could be added to either group to minimize hyperglycemia.	Primary outcome: composite of perinatal mortality, hypoglycemia, hyperbilirubinemia, neonatal hyperinsulinemia and birth trauma. There were no significant differences between the groups with respect to the primary outcome. **Birth weight, birth weight > 4000g, LGA, and, neonatal fat mass were greater in the control group. Cesarean, shoulder dystocia, preeclampsia (with or without gestational hypertension), and BMI at delivery were also higher in the control group.**
Crowther (6)	1000	16–30 wks	Risk factors or blood glucose level >140 mg/dL 1-hr post 50-g glucose load	**75-g test** at 24–34 weeks. Diagnosed if **fasting** <**140 mg/dL and 2 hr 140–198 mg/dL.**	Dietary counseling, self-monitoring of glucose and insulin for optimization of blood sugars.	Usual prenatal care as if the patient did not have GDM screening performed.	Primary neonatal outcome: composite of serious complications (death, shoulder dystocia, bone fracture, and nerve palsy), admission to NICU and phototherapy for jaundice. Primary maternal outcome: IOL and CS. The rate of **serious neonatal outcomes was lower in the intervention group,** though these babies had more NICU admissions. Induction was higher in the intervention group. **Infants were less likely to be LGA or macrosomic and had smaller birth weights in the intervention group.**
Garner (22)	300	24–28 wks	75-g glucose load: blood glucose level > 144 mg/dL 1-hr post glucose load	75-g glucose load. If the 2 hr value exceeded 136 mg/dL (2nd trimester) or 175 mg/dL (3rd trimester), they were randomized	Calorie restricted diet, biophysical profiles at each visit, daily self-glucose monitoring, and insulin as necessary to optimize blood sugar control.	Usual prenatal care, unrestricted healthy diet and self-glucose monitoring twice/week. If women in this group persistently had fasting blood sugars > 140 mg/dL or 1-hr postprandial values > 200 mg/dL, they were transferred to the treatment arm.	Primary outcome: birth weight > 4500 grams. There were no differences in primary outcome between the groups. There were no stillbirths, neonatal deaths, or congenital anomalies. Frequency of neonatal hyperglycemia, hypocalcemia and hyperbilirubinemia did not differ between the groups. 16 women had to be transferred to the treatment group.

(Continued)

Table 5.3   Randomized Studies of Intervention for GDM: Comparing Therapy to No Therapy (Continued)

Study	Sample size	Gestational age at screening	Screening test & threshold for performing diagnostic test	Diagnostic test	Cases (intervention) group	Control group	Outcomes
Persson (20)	202	N/A	N/A	Women were offered inclusion if the area under the curve was 2 SD above normal after a 3-hr, 50-g oral glucose load	Diet + insulin versus diet. Self-monitoring was performed by all subjects before and 1 hr after each meal 3 days/week.	Diet. Insulin could be added to the control group to minimize hyperglycemia. Self-monitoring was performed by all subjects before and 1 hr after each meal 3 days/week.	Primary outcome: to compare the effect of the 2 regimens on maternal blood glucose control, fetal beta-cell function and neonatal outcome. There were no differences in neonatal complications, infant birth weight, LGA, SGA, or maternal hemoglobin A_{1c}. 15 women in the diet arm needed insulin added for blood sugar control.
Bancroft (21)	68	N/A	N/A	Inclusion if impaired glucose tolerance after 75-g glucose load (fasting < 126 mg/dL and 2-hr postprandial 140–198 mg/dL)	Monitoring of capillary glucose samples 1–2 hrs after meals 5 times per week with the addition of insulin as necessary. Both groups received dietary advice and monthly hemoglobin A_{1c}.	No monitoring of blood sugars. Both groups received dietary advice and monthly hemoglobin A_{1c}.	Primary outcome: frequency of admission to the special care baby unit. No differences in frequency of admission to the special care baby unit, hypoglycemia, gestational age at delivery, birth weight, LGA, or delivery mode.
Thompson (19)	108	≤28 wks	50-g load: fasting ≥ 105 mg/dL or 1 hr ≥ 140 mg/dL post glucose load	3-hr, 100-g load and diagnosis of GDM if 2 abnormal values, i.e., >105 mg/dL (fasting), 190 mg/dL (1 hr), 165 mg/dL (2 hr), 145 mg/dL (3hr)	Diabetic diet + NPH insulin.	Diabetic diet. Insulin could be added for subjects in the control group if necessary.	Primary outcome: perinatal morbidity (trauma at delivery, birth weight > 4000 g, hypoglycemia, hyperbilirubinemia, and hypocalcemia) and mortality. There were no cases of perinatal death. Infants in the control group had greater birth weights, ponderal indices and were more likely to be > 4000g.

Abbreviations: GDM, gestational diabetes; IOL, induction of labor; CS, cesarean section; NICU, neonatal intensive care unit; LGA, large for gestational age; SGA, small for gestational age; BMI, body mass index; N/A, not available.

TREATMENT OF GDM (FIG. 5.1)

Treatment of GDM consists of **diet, exercise, and glucose monitoring**; medications such as **oral hypoglycemic agents and/or insulin** are reserved for use when glycemic control is not achieved with diet and exercise.

Compared to usual prenatal care, treatment as described above is associated with significantly decreased incidences of **birth weight > 4000 g, perinatal morbidity (death, shoulder dystocia, bone fracture, and nerve palsy), and preeclampsia in women with GDM** (3,29). Incidence of CD is not significantly affected (3).

Diet

Dietary therapy consists of approximately 30 kcal/kg/day for the average patient and ±5 kcal/kg/day for underweight and overweight women, respectively (17). Calories should be divided between three meals and three snacks: 45% carbohydrate, 20% protein, and 35% unsaturated fat. Since about 30% to 40% of gestational diabetics fail to achieve glucose control with diet alone, other interventions may be necessary. If two glucose levels are >99 mg/dL (fasting), or ≥126 at ≤ 35 weeks or ≥144 after 35 weeks (2-hour postprandial), or ever ≥162 mg/dL (2-hour postprandial), despite diet and exercise, medical therapy should be considered (6). Once diagnosed with GDM, a diet with a low-glycemic index (e.g., decreased

Figure 5.1 Management of the Gestational Diabetic

Preconception prevention

* Weight loss
* Exercise

Antepartum management

* Nutritional counseling for dietary control
* Fingerstick blood sugar assessments: fasting values should be <95 mg/dL and 2-hr postprandial values should be <120 mg/dL
* Exercise program
* Insulin or oral hypoglycemic agent, if diet not sufficient to optimize blood sugars
* Fetal surveillance
  * Diet controlled: NSTs weekly from 40 wk until delivery
  * Medication controlled: NSTs weekly from 32–36 wk; twice weekly from 36 wk until delivery, which is usually accomplished between 39 and 40 wk

Intrapartum management (see Fig. 4.4)

* Induction of labor
  * Diet controlled: at 41 wks
  * Medication controlled: by EDC (40 wk)
* Cesarean section if EFW >4500 g
* Frequent glucose assessment
  * Q 1 hr if required medication
  * Q 4 hr if diet controlled
* Target blood sugars 70–110 mg/dL
* IV insulin therapy if blood sugars greater than target blood sugars or with ketonuria
  * IV saline infusion at 125cc/hr unless ketonuric, then add 5% dextrose solution at rate to keep blood sugar in target range

Postpartum management

* Standard 75-g glucose challenge test at 6 wk postpartum visit (see Fig. 5.2 and Table 4.1)

Abbreviations: NSTs, non-stress tests; EDC, estimated date of confinement.

consumption of white bread, processed cereals and potatoes) can decrease the need for insulin for glycemic control in women with GDM (30).

Exercise

Exercising three times a week for 20 to 45 minutes is probably beneficial for women with GDM. In small RCTs, in women with GDM, exercise (as defined by 30 minutes of non-weight-bearing activity at 50% of aerobic capacity) has been associated with **similar rate of macrosomia compared to insulin** (31), **improvement in glycemic control when done with diet compared to diet only** (32), **and improvement in cardiovascular fitness** (33). Overall, there is insufficient evidence (total of 114 women in four RCTs) to definitively prove that exercise programs for women with GDM affect maternal or neonatal outcomes (4).

Glucose Monitoring

With a glucometer, **fasting and two-hour postprandial glucose levels should be followed daily**. Although not in widespread use, studies have shown that continuous glucose monitoring may reveal more postprandial hyperglycemia than is detected by checking 2-hour postprandial values (34,35). Compared to preprandial monitoring, **postprandial monitoring is associated with improvement in glycosylated hemoglobin, less CD for dystocia, smaller birth weights, and less neonatal hypoglycemia** (36). Since the risk of macrosomia appears to be linked with postprandial hyperglycemia, following these values appear to be reasonable, and is what trials have tested (6,21,25,37). Target goals (euglycemia) are **fasting glucose between 60 and 95 mg/dL and two-hour postprandial <120 mg/dL**. Achieving euglycemia decreases neonatal complications. If all values are within normal limits for extended periods, less frequent monitoring can be considered.

Oral Hypoglycemic Agents

Concerns regarding the safety of oral hypoglycemic agents in pregnancy initially precluded their use during pregnancy.

The second-generation sulfonylurea agents have been demonstrated to have less transplacental passage in both in vitro and in vivo models, although glyburide has been detected in cord blood (38).

Glyburide

Compared to insulin therapy, **glyburide is as efficacious in controlling glucose levels and results in similar pregnancy outcomes (including incidences of macrosomia, CD, neonatal hypoglycemia, admission to NICU, and other neonatal outcomes) for gestational diabetics in the second and third trimester** (in trial, women were started as early as 11 weeks) (39,40). **Glyburide is started at 2.5 mg orally in the morning, with a maximum dose of 20 mg daily.** Approximately 10% to 20% of women on this regimen do not achieve euglycemia, especially women with a BMI >30. Obese women with GDM requiring medication to achieve euglycemia should probably be treated with insulin rather than with oral agents (41).

Metformin

Metformin (Glucophage) is commonly used in women with polycystic ovarian syndrome to treat infertility related to anovulation. The incidence of miscarriage and GDM is decreased in women who are continued on this therapy throughout pregnancy. No attributable birth defects or adverse outcomes in this patient population have been reported.

Compared to insulin therapy, metformin (± insulin, if necessary) is associated with similar neonatal morbidity and mortality, increased patient satisfaction and increased preterm birth in women with GDM (42). Women with GDM who are obese, have a high fasting glucose, or need pharmacologic therapy early (e.g., <24 weeks) in pregnancy may be more suitable for insulin therapy (43).

Compared to glyburide, those treated with metformin are twice as likely to fail glycemic control (i.e., they will need the addition of insulin), and are more likely to be delivered by cesarean and have smaller infants (44).

One meta-analysis showed a significant reduction in cesarean rates when women were treated with oral hypogly-cemics as compared to insulin (3).

The use of these two medications can be supported during pregnancy, in view of their safety and efficacy. This is, however, not true for the other oral medications. Glyburide may be preferred when starting oral hypoglycemics. If the patient is already on metformin and therapy is effective, it can safely be continued.

Insulin
As in pregestational DM, Neutral Protamine Hagedorn (NPH) and Lispro can be used for glucose control (see Figure 4.2). Compared to regular insulin, Lispro is associated with a lower incidence of maternal hypoglycemic episodes in women with GDM (45).

In women with GDM, compared to no treatment or diet only, **diet and glucose monitoring with insulin,** if needed, is associated with reduced macrosomia and shoulder dystocia; similar incidences of cesarean, NICU admission, and neonatal hypoglycemia; and **no birth trauma** (bone fracture, nerve palsy) (vs. 1%) or **perinatal death** (vs. 1%) (3,6). **Mood and quality of life are improved**, and the incidence of **depression decreases** with the above interventions and the optimization of glycemic control (6).

Antepartum Testing
Antepartum fetal testing and ultrasound evaluations have not been standardly applied to the management of gestational diabetics, as there is no clear literature to provide direction.

* *Euglycemia with diet only*: No special testing is necessary. Consider weekly nonstress tests (NSTs) starting at 40 weeks.
* *Hyperglycemia or medication necessary*: Consider management similar to pregestational diabetics: weekly NSTs from 32 to 35 6/7 weeks, then twice weekly NSTs from 36 weeks until delivery, which is usually accomplished between 39 and 40 weeks (see chap. 4).

Ultrasound assessment of fetal weight is commonly employed, but because of the inherent inaccuracy of predicting macrosomia, it has not been supported by any studies.

Delivery
Timing, Mode, and Lung Maturity
There is insufficient evidence to assess the timing and mode of delivery in gestational diabetics, as there is only one small trial on this subject. **Compared to expectant management until 42 weeks, induction of labor at 38 completed weeks in women with insulin-dependent diabetes (of which >90% were gestational) is associated with reduced incidences of** macrosomia and shoulder dystocia and a similar incidence of CD (2,46). However, the sample size was too small to evaluate the impact on perinatal mortality (2).

In women requiring medication, management is usually similar to that of the pregestational diabetic, and delivery is advocated in the 39th week. Assessment of fetal lung maturity is not necessary if delivery occurs ≥39 weeks in a well-dated, well-controlled patient. If delivery occurs prior to this time unrelated to maternal or obstetric indications, documentation through amniocentesis of mature lung indices is advocated, using a phosphatidylglycerol level of ≥3%. While recognizing that macrosomia remains a difficult antenatal diagnosis both clinically and by ultrasound, delivery via cesarean section is suggested for fetuses estimated to be >4500 g (1) (see chap. 45). Operative deliveries should be avoided in women with fetuses estimated to be >4000 g and prolonged second stage of labor.

Intrapartum Glucose Management
Intrapartum management requires frequent assessment of blood glucose levels during labor (see Figure 4.3). For patients who have required insulin therapy, perform hourly assessments of blood sugars to maintain them between 70 and 120 mg/dL. Intravenous insulin may need to be instituted to maintain the above glucose levels, but is seldom required in these patients. Patients managed with diet alone may not need as frequent evaluations during labor, and can have assessments every four hours.

Anesthesia
No specific adjustments necessary, unless woman is obese.

Postpartum/Breast-feeding
In the postpartum period, women with GDM do not, in general, require medication to control their blood sugars. Checking a fasting and postprandial value prior to discharge can be employed, especially if pregestational diabetes is suspected. Because these women have an increased risk of developing frank diabetes, **screening with a 75-g glucose challenge or other nonpregnant tests** (see Table 4.1) is advocated when the woman is **six to eight weeks postpartum (Fig. 5.2)** (47) **and every two to three years, thereafter** (27,48–50). This can be accomplished by either the obstetrician with referral if values are abnormal, or by referral for the screening to a medicine specialist. Breast-feeding, diet, and exercise should be encouraged in these women, particularly if they are obese. All forms of contraception are available to diabetics, providing they have no contraindications, such as hypertension or vascular disease.

Patients should be informed that they are at increased risk for developing diabetes during their lifetime, up to 50% over the next 10 years (27). Women who are obese, diagnosed with GDM early in gestation, and have significantly abnormal screening results during and after pregnancy have the highest chance of adult onset diabetes. Prepregnancy BMI and fasting glucose >87 mg/dL after 100-g glucose load are associated with increased risk of development of metabolic syndrome (51). Some suggest that women with an abnormal 1-hour result are also at increased risk of metabolic derangements later in life, despite a normal three-hour GTT (52). Counseling regarding diet and exercise, maintenance of normal BMI, and surveillance with periodic screening are indicated.

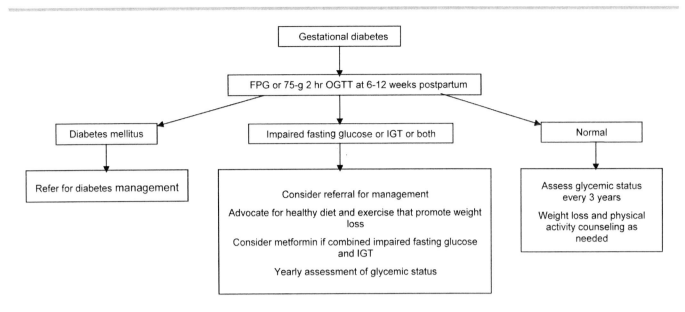

Figure 5.2 Postpartum screening of patients who had GDM. *Abbreviations*: FPG, fasting plasma glucose; OGTT, oral glucose tolerance test; IGT, impaired glucose tolerance. *Source*: Adapted from Ref. 47.

REFERENCES

1. ACOG Practice Bulletin. Gestational diabetes. Clinical Management Guidelines for Obstetricians–Gynecologists No. 30. Obstet Gynecol 2001; 98(3):525–538. [Review]
2. Boulvain M, Stan C, Irion O. Elective delivery in diabetic pregnant women. Cochrane Database Syst Rev 2001; (2):CD001997. [Meta-analysis, 1 RCT, $n = 200$]
3. Alwan N, Tuffnell DJ, West J. Treatments for gestational diabetes. Cochrane Database Syst Rev 2009; (3):CD003395. [Meta-analysis, 8 RCTs, $n = 1418$]
4. Ceysens G, Rouiller D, Boulvain M. Exercise for diabetic pregnant women. Cochrane Database Syst Rev 2006; 3:CD004225. [Meta-analysis, 4 RCTs, $n = 114$]
5. American Diabetes Association. Diagnosis and classification of diabetes mellitus. Diabetes Care 2011; 34(supp 1):S62–S69. [Review, guideline]
6. Crowther CA, Hiller JE, Moss JR, et al. Effect of treatment of gestational diabetes mellitus on pregnancy outcomes. N Engl J Med 2005; 352(24):2477–2486. [RCT, $n = 1000$. Impaired glucose tolerance (defined following 75-g OGTT as fasting <7.0 mmol/L, 2-hour between 7.8 mmol/L and 11.0 mmol/L). Diet, glucose monitoring and insulin as needed vs. routine care]
7. Metzger BE, Buchanan TA, Coustan DR, et al. Summary and recommendations of the Fifth International Workshop-Conference on Gestational Diabetes Mellitus. Diabetes Care 2007; 30(suppl 2): S251–S260. [Review]
8. Torloni MR, Betran AP, Horta BL, et al. Prepregnancy BMI and the risk of gestational diabetes: a systematic review of the literature with meta-analysis. Obes Rev 2009; 10(2):194–203. [Meta-analysis of 59 cohorts and 11 case-controls with 671,945 women]
9. Meyer WJ, Carbone J, Gauthier DW, et al. Early gestational glucose screening and gestational diabetes. J Reprod Med 1996; 41:675–679. [II-3]
10. Tieu J, Middleton P, McPhee AJ, et al. Screening and subsequent management for gestational diabetes for improving maternal and infant health. Cochrane Database Syst Rev 2010; (7):CD007222. [Meta-analysis of 3 RCTs and 1 quasi-RCT, $n = 3972$]
11. Brody SC, Harris R, Lohr K. Screening for gestational diabetes: a summary of the evidence for the U. S. preventive services task force. Obstet Gynecol 2003; 101:380–392. [Review]
12. Metzger BE, Lowe LP, et al., for HAPO Study Cooperative Research Group. Hyperglycemia and adverse pregnancy outcomes. N Engl J Med 2008; 358(19):1991–2002. [Prospective, $n = 25,505$]
13. Coustan DR, Lowe LP, Metzger BE, et al., for International Association of Diabetes and Pregnancy Study Groups. The Hyperglycemia and Adverse Pregnancy Outcome (HAPO) study: paving the way for new diagnostic criteria for gestational diabetes mellitus. Am J Obstet Gynecol 2010; 202(6):654.e1–654.e6. [III]
14. Coustan DR, Widness JA, Carpenter MW, et al. Should the 50-gram, one-hour plasma glucose screening test for gestational diabetes be administered in the fasting or fed state? Am J Obstet Gynecol 1986; 154:1031–1035. [II-2, $n = 72$]
15. Murphy NJ, Meyer BA, O'Kell RT, et al. Carbohydrate sources for gestational diabetes mellitus screening. J Reprod Med 1994; 39:977–981. [RCT, $n = 108$]
16. Lamar ME, Kuehl TJ, Cooney AT, et al. Jelly beans as an alternative to a fifty-gram glucose beverage for gestational diabetes screening. Am J Obstet Gynecol 1999; 181(5 pt 1):1154–1157. [RCT, $n = 160$]
17. Gabbe SG, Graves CR. Management of diabetes mellitus complicating pregnancy. Obstet Gynecol 2003; 102(4):857–868. [III]
18. Magee MS, Walden CE, Benedetti TJ, et al. Influence of diagnostic criteria on the incidence of gestational diabetes and perinatal morbidity. JAMA 1993; 269(5):609–615. [Observational study, $n = 2015$]
19. Thompson DJ, Porter KB, Gunnells DJ, et al. Prophylactic insulin in the management of gestational diabetes. Obstet Gynecol 1990; 7(6):960–964. [RCT, $n = 108$]
20. Persson S, Stangenberg M, Hansson U, et al. Gestational diabetes mellitus (GDM). Comparative evaluation of two treatment regimens, diet versus insulin and diet. Diabetes 1985; 34(suppl 2):101–105. [RCT, $n = 202$]
21. Bancroft K, Tuffnell DJ, Mason GC, et al. A randomised controlled pilot study of the management of gestational impaired glucose tolerance. BJOG 2000; 107(8):959–963. [RCT, $n = 68$. Impaired glucose tolerance (defined following 75-g OGTT as fasting <7.0 mmol/L, 2-hour between 7.8 mmol/L and 11.0 mmol/L-same as Crowther). Monitored group was given standard dietary advice, glucose metabolism was **monitored by capillary glucose** series five days a week, HbA1c was measured monthly (**insulin** was introduced if 5 or more capillary measurements >7.0 mmol/L in 1 week), serial ultrasound for growth and amniotic fluid, Doppler studies,

CTG monitoring. Unmonitored group received *dietary* advice, HbA1c monthly but no capillary glucose measurements.]

22. Garner P, Okun N, Keeley E, et al. A randomized controlled trial of strict glycemia control and tertiary level obstetric care versus routine obstetric care in the management of gestational diabetes: a pilot study. Am J Obstet Gynecol 1997; 177(1):190–195. [RCT, *n* = 300]

23. Landon MB, Spong CY, Thom E, et al. A multicenter, randomized trial of treatment for mild gestational diabetes. N Engl J Med 2009; 361(14):1339–1348. [RCT, *n* = 958]

24. Meltzer SJ, Snyder J, Penrod JR, et al. Gestational diabetes mellitus screening and diagnosis: a prospective randomised controlled trial comparing costs of one-step and two-step methods. BJOG 2010; 117(4):407–415. [RCT, *n* = 1500]

25. Langer O, Anyaegbunan A, Brustman L, et al. Management of women with one abnormal oral glucose tolerance test value reduces adverse outcome in pregnancy. Am J Obstet Gynecol 1989; 161:593–599. [RCT, *n* = 272]

26. American Diabetes Association. Gestational diabetes mellitus. Diabetes Care 2004; 27(suppl 1):S88—S90. [Review]

27. Kim C, Newton KM, Knopp RH. Gestational diabetes and the incidence of type 2 diabetes: a systematic review. Diabetes Care 2002; 25(10):1862–1868. [Review]

28. Tieu J, Crowther CA, Middleton P. Dietary advice in pregnancy for preventing gestational diabetes mellitus. Cochrane Database Syst Rev 2008; 2:CD006674 [Meta-analysis, 3 RCTs, *n* = 107]

29. Horvath K, Koch K, Jeitler K, et al. Effects of treatment in women with gestational diabetes mellitus: systematic review and meta-analysis. BMJ 2010; 340:c1395. [Meta-analysis, 5 RCTs, *n* = 2999]

30. Moses RG, Barker M, Winter M, et al. Can a low-glycemic index diet reduce the need for insulin in gestational diabetes mellitus? A randomized trial. Diabetes Care 2009; 32(6):996–1000. [RCT, *n* = 63]

31. Bung P, Bung C, Artal R, et al. Therapeutic exercise for insulin-requiring gestational diabetics: effects on fetus—results of a randomized prospective longitudinal study. J Perinat Med 1993; 21:125–137. [RCT]

32. Jovanovich-Peterson L, Durak EP, Peterson CM. Randomized trial of diet versus diet plus cardiovascular conditioning on glucose levels in gestational diabetes. Am J Obstet Gynecol 1989; 161(2):415–419. [RCT, *n* = 19]

33. Avery MD, Leon AS, Kopher RA. Effects of a partially home-based exercise program for women with gestational diabetes. Obstet Gynecol 1997; 89:10–15. [RCT, *n* = 33]

34. Kestila KK, Ekblad UU, Ronnemaa T. Continuous glucose monitoring versus self-monitoring of blood glucose in the treatment of gestational diabetes mellitus. Diabetes Res Clin Pract 2007; 77 (2):174–179. [RCT, *n* = 71]

35. McLachlan K, Jenkins A, O'Neal D. The role of continuous glucose monitoring in clinical decision-making in diabetes in pregnancy. Aust N Z J Obstet Gynaecol 2007; 47(3):186–190. [Descriptive study, *n* = 68]

36. de Veciana M, Major CA, Morgan MA, et al. Postprandial versus preprandial blood glucose monitoring in women with gestational diabetes mellitus requiring insulin therapy. N Engl J Med 1195; 333:1237–1241. [RCT, *n* = 66]

37. Ford FA, Bruce CB, Fraser RB. Preliminary report of a randomised trial of dietary advice in women with mild abnormalities of glucose tolerance in pregnancy. Personal Communication, 1997. [RCT, *n* = 29. Impaired glucose tolerance (defined following a 75-g OGTT as 2-hour plasma glucose level between 8 mmol/L and 11 mmol/L-similar to Crowther. **Dietary** treatment group

was given specific "diabetic type" advice (i.e., "high fiber, high carbohydrate, low fat, and appropriate energy"). No mention of insulin therapy. The control group received *no specific dietary* advice. Both groups attended clinic weekly and performed plasma glucose profiles.]

38. Hebert MF, Ma X, Naraharisetti SB, et al. Are we optimizing gestational diabetes treatment with glyburide? The pharmacologic basis for better clinical practice. Clin Pharmacol Ther 2009; 85(6):607–614. [Assessed steady-state PK of glyburide, insulin sensitivity, and β-cell responsivity after a mixed-meal tolerance test in women with GDM (*n* = 40), healthy pregnant women (*n* = 40) and nonpregnant women with DM (*n* = 26)]

39. Lain KY, Garabedian MJ, Daftary A, et al. Neonatal adiposity following maternal treatment of gestational diabetes with glyburide compared with insulin. Am J Obstet Gynecol 2009; 200:501.e1–501.e6. [RCT of 83 neonates]

40. Langer O, Conway DL, Berkus MD, et al. A comparison of glyburide and insulin in women with gestational diabetes mellitus. N Engl J Med 2000; 343(16):1134–1138. [RCT, *n* = 404]

41. Langer O, Yogev Y, Xenakis EMJ, et al. Overweight and obese in gestational diabetes: the impact on pregnancy outcomes. Am J Obstet Gynecol 2005; 192:1768–1776. [II-2]

42. Rowan JA, Hague WM, Gao W, et al, for MiG Trial Investigators. Metformin versus insulin for the treatment of gestational diabetes. N Engl J Med 2008; 358(19):2003–2015. [RCT, *n* = 751]

43. Ijas H, Vaarasmaki M, Morin-Papunen L, et al. Metformin should be considered in the treatment of gestational diabetes: a prospective randomized trial. BJOG 2011; 118(7):880–885. [RCT, *n* = 100]

44. Moore LE, Clokey D, Rappaport VJ, et al. Metformin compared with glyburide in gestational diabetes: a randomized controlled trial. Obstet Gynecol 2010; 115(1):55–59. [RCT, *n* = 149]

45. Jovanovic L, Ilic S, Pettitt DJ, et al. Metabolism and immunologic effects of insulin lispro in gestational diabetes. Diabetes Care 1999; 22:1422–1427. [RCT, *n* = 42]

46. Kjos SL, Henry OA, Montoro M, et al. Insulin-requiring diabetes in pregnancy: a randomized trial of active induction of labor and expectant management. Am J Obstet Gynecol 1993; 169:611–615. [RCT, *n* = 200]

47. American College of Obstetricians and Gynecologists. Postpartum screening for abnormal glucose tolerance in women who had gestational diabetes mellitus. ACOG Committee Opinion No 435. Obstet Gynecol 2009; 113:1419–1421. [Review]

48. Bellamy L, Casas JP, Hingorani AD, et al. Type 2 diabetes mellitus after gestational diabetes: a systematic review and meta-analysis. Lancet 2009; 373(9677):1773–1779. [20 cohort studies (retrospective and prospective), *n* = 675,455]

49. Expert Committee on the Diagnosis and Classification of Diabetes Mellitus. Report of the expert committee on the diagnosis and classification of diabetes mellitus. Diabetes Care 2003; 26(suppl 1):S5–S20. [Review, guideline]

50. The Royal Australian and New Zealand College of Obstetricians and Gynaecologists. College Statement. Diagnosis of gestational diabetes mellitus. 2008. Available at: http://www.ranzcog.edu.au/publications/statements/C-obs7.pdf. [III]

51. Akinci B, Celtik A, Yener S, et al. Prediction of developing metabolic syndrome after gestational diabetes mellitus. Fertil Steril 2010; 93(4):1248–1254. [Prospective, *n* = 164]

52. Retnakaran R, Qi Y, Sermer M, et al. An abnormal screening glucose challenge test in pregnancy predicts postpartum metabolic dysfunction, even when the antepartum oral glucose tolerance test is normal. Clin Endocrinol (Oxf) 2009; 71(2):208–214. [Observational study, *n* = 259]

6

Hypothyroidism

Sushma Potti

KEY POINTS

- **Hypothyroidism** is characterized by inadequate thyroid hormone production, and usually requires for diagnosis **elevated thyroid-stimulating hormone (TSH) and low free thyroxine (FT4)** [or free triiodothyronine (FT3)].
- **Subclinical hypothyroidism** requires for diagnosis **elevated TSH but normal FT4.**
- **Hashimoto's thyroiditis** is the most common cause of hypothyroidism in pregnancy, with thyroid peroxidase antibodies in >90% of these women.
- Untreated or partially treated hypothyroidism is associated with increased risk of **preeclampsia, abruption, preterm birth, low birth weight, fetal death,** and long-term **impaired psychomotor function.**
- All physiologic changes and placental transfer should be known by the physician caring for thyroid disease in pregnancy (Table 6.1).
- **Women at high risk for hypothyroidism** should be **screened** with TSH and FT4.
- **Goal of** levothyroxine **treatment** in pregnancy is **maternal serum TSH 0.5 to 2.0 µU/mL,** and FT4 in upper third of normal range. **Most women with hypothyroidism need an increase in thyroxine replacement dose.**
- **Iodine supplementation** in a population with high levels of endemic cretinism results in a reduction in deaths during infancy and early childhood, with decreased endemic cretinism at 4 years of age and better psychomotor development scores between 4 and 25 months of age.
- **TSH and FT4 levels** should be checked **preconceptionally, at first prenatal visit in first trimester,** 4 weeks after altering the doses, (therefore, **every 4 weeks until TSH is normal,** especially in the first 20 weeks), **and at least every trimester in pregnancy.**
- Every woman with a thyroid nodule should have fine-needle aspiration and TSH checked.

CLINICAL HYPOTHYROIDISM
Definitions

Clinical (or overt) hypothyroidism: Inadequate thyroid hormone production of any cause. Usually requires **elevated TSH and low FT4 (or FT3).**

Subclinical hypothyroidism: Elevated TSH and normal FT4. Elevated TSH reflects the sensitivity of the hypothalamic-pituitary axis to small decreases in thyroid hormone; as the thyroid gland fails, the TSH level may rise above the upper limit of normal while the FT4 is still within the normal range.

Hypothyroxinemia: Normal TSH and low FT4.

TSH is also called thyrotropin, T4 is also called thyroxine, T3 is also called triiodothyronine; FT4 stands for free T4.

Incidence

1% in general population; 0.3% in pregnant women (1,2). General screening of obstetric patients reveals an incidence of 2.5% of elevated serum TSH (2). There is an increased incidence with concurrent autoimmune disease, that is, 5% to 8% incidence in patients with type 1 diabetes (3). Up to 25% of patients with type I diabetes develop postpartum thyroid dysfunction (3). In the United States, 10% to 15% of pregnant women are iodine deficient (urinary iodine concentration <5 µg/dL) (4).

Signs/Symptoms

May be masked by hypermetabolic state of pregnancy. The most common signs include dry skin, weakness, facial puffiness, and mild-to-moderate weight gain (5). Fatigue, constipation, cold intolerance, muscle cramps, insomnia, hair loss, goiter, prolonged relaxation phase of deep tendon reflexes, carpal tunnel syndrome, intellectual slowness, voice changes, myxedema, and (extremely rarely) coma are less common.

Pathophysiology

The thyroid maintains the metabolism in cells by stimulating transcription and translation. It also stimulates oxygen consumption and regulates lipid and carbohydrate metabolism, and is necessary for normal growth and maturation. The thyroid is under the control of TSH from the anterior pituitary. TSH induces thyroid growth, differentiation, and iodine metabolism.

Majority (>99%) of cases of hypothyroidism are due to primary thyroid abnormality. Secondary hypothyroidism is pituitary in origin following irradiation or hypophysectomy or Sheehan's syndrome (postpartum pituitary necrosis). Tertiary hypothyroidism (hypothalamic) is rare.

Hashimoto's thyroiditis is the most common cause of hypothyroidism in pregnancy. It is a chronic autoimmune lymphocytic thyroiditis, characterized by antithyroid antibodies [thyroid peroxidase (TPO) antibodies 90%, thyroglobulin antibodies 20–50%], and usually firm, painless goiter as presenting symptom (6). TPO antibodies are present in 6% of the general population. Less common causes are subacute viral thyroiditis; iodine deficiency (median urinary iodine level <100 µg/L); "burned-out" Graves' disease, after radioiodine therapy, thyroidectomy, or antithyroid drugs; other head and neck surgery; other radiation therapy to the head, neck, or chest area; medications—lithium, iodine, amiodarone; rarely hypothalamic dysfunction, that is, Sheehan's syndrome.

Complications

Untreated or partially treated clinical hypothyroidism is associated with increased risk of **infertility, miscarriage, preeclampsia** (44%), **abruption** (19%), **preterm birth, low birth weight** (31%), or **fetal death** (12%) (7–9). Fetal goiter does not develop in women with hypothyroidism, unless they had

Table 6.1 Thyroid Physiology Changes in Pregnancy and Transplacental Passage

	Change in pregnancy	Placental transfer
Thyroid-binding globulin (TBG)	↑	+
Total thyroxine (TT4)	↑	− (minimal)
Total triiodothyronine (TT3)	↑	−
Resin triiodothyronine uptake (RT3U)	↓	−
Thyroid-stimulating hormone (TSH)	−	−
Free thyroxine (FT4)	−	++
Free triiodothyronine (FT3)	−	++
TRH	−	− (<1%)
Iodide	↓	++
Thyroid-stimulating immunoglobulin (TSI)	−	++
Antithyroid peroxidase antibody	↓	++
Levothyroxine replacement	NA	− (minimal)
Thioamide (PTU or methimazole) therapy	NA	++
Free thyroxine index (FTI)	−	NA

previous hyperthyroidism and thyroid-stimulating immuno-globulins (TSIs) are still >200%. Infants whose mothers had serum FT4 below 10th percentile may have a high incidence of **impaired psychomotor function** (10). Untreated subclinical hypothyroidism may be associated with a significantly lower IQ in children compared to normal controls (11).

Management

Prevention

Recently, trace element selenium has been shown to reduce the incidence of hypothyroidism during pregnancy and post-partum periods (12). Selenoproteins act as antioxidants and decrease thyroid inflammation in autoimmune thyroiditis by reducing TPO antibody titers. Up to 30% of women with TPO antibodies develop permanent hypothyroidism following postpartum thyroid dysfunction (13). This may suggest a preventive role of selenomethionine supplementation in autoimmune thyroid dysfunction.

Preconception

In a small RCT, it was shown that preconception adjustment with increased dosage of levothyroxine supplementation in hypothyroid women of reproductive age results in better control by TSH and FT4 at first prenatal visit (14).

Pregnancy Considerations

Anatomy/Radiology

In pregnancy, moderate glandular hyperplasia, and increased vascularity in the thyroid are physiologic. Thyroid volume by ultrasound increases a mean of 18% during pregnancy and returns to normal size in the postpartum period (4,15). **Any significant goiter should be worked up**.

Physiology

Several changes occur, as shown in Table 6.1 (chap. 3, *Obstetric Evidence Based Guidelines*). **Thyroid-binding globulin** (TBG) increases about 200% secondary to estrogen-stimulated hep-atocyte production and altered glycosylation, which inhibits degradation. **High levels of HCG**, which peak at 10 to 12 weeks, have some TSH-like activity and stimulate thyroid

Table 6.2 Thyroid-Stimulating Hormone Percentiles According to Gestational Age in Singleton Pregnancies

Gestational age (wk)	2.5th percentile	50th percentile	97.5th percentile
6	0.23	1.36	4.94
7	0.14	1.21	5.09
8	0.09	1.01	4.93
9	0.03	0.84	4.04
10	0.02	0.74	3.12
11	0.01	0.76	3.65
12	0.01	0.79	3.32
13	0.01	0.78	4.05
14	0.01	0.85	3.33
15	0.02	0.92	3.40
16	0.04	0.92	2.74
17	0.02	0.98	3.32
18	0.17	1.07	3.48
19	0.22	1.07	3.03
20	0.25	1.11	3.20
21	0.28	1.21	3.04
22	0.26	1.15	4.09
23	0.25	1.08	3.02
24	0.34	1.13	2.99
25	0.30	1.11	2.82
26	0.20	1.07	2.89
27	0.36	1.11	2.84
28	0.30	1.03	2.78
29	0.31	1.07	3.14
30	0.20	1.07	3.27
31	0.23	1.06	2.81
32	0.31	1.07	2.98
33	0.31	1.20	5.25
34	0.20	1.18	3.18
35	0.30	1.20	3.41
36	0.33	1.31	4.59
37	0.37	1.35	6.40
38	0.23	1.16	4.33
39	0.57	1.59	5.14
≥40	0.38	1.68	5.43

Source: Adapted from Ref. 16.

hormone secretion, which in turn **suppresses TSH**. Normal TSH levels in pregnancy are shown in Table 6.2. TSH suppres-sion is even more marked for twins (16). Peripheral metabo-lism of thyroid hormones is also altered by placental deiodinases, more in second half of pregnancy (17).

Throughout pregnancy there is an approximately 30% to 50% increase in T4 requirement (18,19). Plasma iodide levels decrease during pregnancy because of fetal use of iodide and increased maternal renal clearance of iodide (20). Pregnancy does not appear to alter the course of thyroid cancer (21).

Fetal Thyroid Physiology

In the fetus, the small amount of thyroxine that crosses the placenta provides all the thyroid hormone until 10 to 12 weeks. Before 12 weeks (time period for initiation of fetal brain development), the fetus is entirely dependent on maternal transfer of thyroid hormones. Upon beginning of activation of the fetal hypothalamic/pituitary-thyroid axis at this gesta-tional age, the fetal thyroid begins to concentrate iodine and synthesize iodothyronines. At 18 to 20 weeks, the fetal thyroid is controlled by fetal pituitary TSH and mature hormone synthesis begins. TSH, T4, and T3 all begin to increase throughout gestation, as there seems to be minimal negative feedback mechanism (20).

Table 6.3 Screening for Hypothyroidism in Pregnancy

Symptomatic (see Signs/symptoms)
Previous therapy for hyperthyroidism
History of high-dose neck irradiation
Goiter/palpable thyroid nodules
Family history of thyroid disease
Suspected hypopituitarism
Type 1 DM (3)
Hyperlipidemia
Medications (iodine, amiodarone, lithium, dilantin, rifampin)

Source: From Ref. 6.

Placenta Physiology
It is important to be aware of which molecules cross the placenta and can affect the fetus. FT4, FT3, thyrotropin-releasing hormone, iodine, TSI, and anti-TPO cross placenta (22) (Table 6.1). TSH does not cross. The placenta rapidly deiodinates maternal T4 and T3 to the inactive reverse-T3.

Screening/Diagnosis
Universal screening for maternal hypothyroidism is not usually recommended (23) even if some have proposed it (11). **Women at high risk for hypothyroidism** should be **screened** (Table 6.3) (24). Tests used for screening and diagnosis include **TSH** (most sensitive) (25,26) and **FT4**. Elevated TSH, and either low FT4 or low FT3, is consistent with clinical hypothyroidism (Table 6.4). In the first trimester, even a TSH level >2.5 is abnormal. Hypothyroidism in pregnancy is mainly (>99%) primary. Elevated TSH and normal FT4 are consistent with **subclinical hypothyroidism.**

TPO antibody is present in not only 90% women with Hashimoto's thyroiditis but also 10% women with euthyroid at 12 weeks. It crosses the placenta, may increase incidence of spontaneous abortion (27), and increases the incidence of postpartum thyroid dysfunction (28). TPO antibody levels >50 IU/mL have been shown to be associated with increased risk of abruption (29). Measuring TPO or thyroglobulin antibodies is important for diagnosis, but serial levels are usually not indicated since treatment does not alter them. At present, routine testing of TPO antibodies during pregnancy is not recommended.

Treatment
Goal
Maternal serum TSH 0.5 to 2.0 μU/mL, and FT4 in upper third of normal range.

Thyroxine Replacement
  Dose.
  Preexisting hypothyroidism Approximately **45% to 85% of women need** up to 45% **increase in thyroxine replacement dose** during pregnancy because of increased metabolism of

Table 6.4 Primary vs. Secondary Hypothyroidism

Primary hypothyroidism	
TSH	↑
FT4	↓
Antithyroglobulin	+/−
Antithyroid peroxidase	+/−
Secondary hypothyroidism	
TSH	↓
FT4	↓

Abbreviations: TSH, thyroid-stimulating hormone; FT4, free thyroxine.

thyroxine, weight gain, increased T4 pool, high serum TBG, placental deiodinase activity, and transfer of T4 to fetus (30,31). Some advocate increasing replacement by 30% as soon as pregnancy is confirmed, but outcome data are not available (18).

New diagnosis Levothyroxine can be started at 0.1 to 0.15 mg/day, and adjusted by monitoring TSH levels. Thyroxine replacement will need to be increased as in preexisting disease.

Ferrous sulfate and calcium carbonate interfere with T4 absorption and should be taken at a different time of day from thyroxine therapy (32). Therefore, **pregnant women should space their levothyroxine and prenatal vitamin by at least two to three hours**. Carbamazepine, phenytoin, and rifampin can increase the clearance of T4. It takes approximately four weeks for thyroxine therapy to alter TSH level. Not only under replacement (see above) but also over replacement (pregnancy loss, low birth weight) should be avoided (33).

  Type.
  Levothyroxine Levothyroxine is the recommended thyroid replacement. Desiccated thyroid preparation such as Armour Thyroid at 30 mg/day initial dose, then increased incrementally by 15 mg every two to three weeks until maintenance dose of 60 to 120 mg/day, is an alternative if levothyroxine is unavailable.

Iodine supplement **Iodine supplementation in a population with high levels of endemic cretinism results in a reduction of the condition** with no apparent adverse effects (34). Iodine supplementation is associated with **a reduction in deaths during infancy and early childhood**, with decreased endemic cretinism at 4 years of age, and better psychomotor development scores between 4 and 25 months of age. About 10% to 15% of the U.S. population has iodine deficiency, which can manifest as subclinical hypothyroidism, or with normal TSH and low T4. A daily dose of **250 μg of iodine is recommended during pregnancy and breast-feeding** (35).

Antepartum Management
- **TSH and FT4 levels** should be checked **preconception, at first prenatal visit in first trimester, 4 weeks after altering the doses, (therefore, every 4 weeks until TSH is normal, especially in first 20 weeks), and at least every trimester in pregnancy.**
- Fetal heart rate should be assessed at each visit by doptone to rule out fetal bradycardia <120.
- Antepartum testing is not recommended if euthyroid; weekly nonstress tests beginning at 32 to 34 weeks can be considered for clinically hypothyroid patients.
- Ultrasound is not recommended if euthyroid; monthly ultrasound can be considered for fetal growth, thyroid circumference (36), and fetal heart rate if clinically hypothyroid.
- Important to inform pediatrician at time of delivery.

Neonatal
The incidence of iodine-deficient congenital hypothyroidism is 1/4000 births, 5% identified at birth by clinical symptoms, others by newborn screening. The United States screens all newborns. If discovered and treated in first few weeks of life, near-normal growth and intelligence are expected (37,38). The majority of cases are due to agenesis/dysgenesis of fetal thyroid, dyshormonogenesis, or iodine deficiency. Fetuses are protected in utero by small quantity of maternal T4 that crosses placenta. Neonatal issues include neuropsychological abnormalities, deafness, respiratory difficulties, growth failure, lethargy, and hypotonia and myxedema of the larynx and epiglottis.

Postpartum
Immediately post delivery, the dosage of levothyroxine should be reduced to the prepregnancy dose, and TSH levels should be measured six to eight weeks postpartum, with follow-up with medical doctor/endocrinologist.

SUBCLINICAL HYPOTHYROIDISM
Incidence
2.2% in first or second trimester (39).

Diagnosis
Elevated TSH and normal FT4.

Screening and Management
Screening or treatment for subclinical hypothyroidism is controversial, at present recommended by endocrinologists (40), but not obstetricians (23). Routine screening for subclinical hypothyroidism is currently not recommended since treatment of subclinical hypothyroidism has not yet been demonstrated to improve maternal or fetal outcomes (41). Maternal subclinical hypothyroidism may be associated with a 19% incidence of IQ <85 at seven to nine years, versus 5% in children of euthyroid mothers (11). Subclinical hypothyroidism has been associated with an increased incidence of preterm birth, abruption, respiratory distress syndrome, and admission to intensive care nursery (42), but not consistently (39). **There is insufficient evidence (no large trials) to assess whether treatment of maternal subclinical hypothyroidism with thyroid hormone replacement affects any outcome of the offspring.** A small trial reported lower incidence of preterm birth when euthyroid women with TPO antibodies were treated with levothyroxine compared to controls (7,43). Women with subclinical hypothyroidism and thyroid antibodies (e.g., TPO) frequently progress to overt hypothyroidism, and may develop hyperlipidemia and atherosclerotic heart disease (44).

HYPOTHYROXINEMIA
Incidence
1.3% (45).

Diagnosis
Normal TSH and low FT4.

Screening and Management
Since isolated maternal hypothyroxinemia is not associated with adverse effects on perinatal outcome (45), there is no need to screen or treat for this condition.

THYROID NODULE
Incidence
5% to 10% of thyroid tumors are neoplastic. Thyroid cancer occurs in 1/1000 pregnant women with palpable thyroid nodule.

Diagnosis
Ultrasound to define dominant nodule, followed by **fine-needle aspiration for nodules >1 cm,** which has a 95% diagnostic accuracy in pregnancy (46). Radioisotope scanning is contraindicated in pregnancy. Serum TSH and FT4 should be checked.

Thyroid Surgery
For malignancy diagnosed on fine-needle aspiration, neck exploration should be performed ideally either in the second trimester or postpartum (46). Neck irradiation for malignancy should be deferred until after pregnancy.

POSTPARTUM THYROIDITIS
Definition
Autoimmune inflammation of the thyroid gland that presents as new-onset painless hypothyroidism, transient thyrotoxicosis, or thyrotoxicosis followed by hypothyroidism **within one year postpartum**.

Incidence
Occurs in 5% of women in United States who do not have a history of thyroid disease (47), and may occur after delivery or pregnancy loss.

Risk Factors
Postpartum depression, high serum TPO antibody concentration, history of Graves's disease, or type 1 diabetes.

Etiology
Subacute lymphocytic thyroiditis or postpartum exacerbation of chronic lymphocytic thyroiditis.

Diagnosis
Documentation of new-onset abnormal levels of TSH and/or FT4 within the first postpartum year. All women with symptoms of thyroid dysfunction or who develop a goiter postpartum should be evaluated with TSH, FT4. If the diagnosis is unclear, an anti-TPO antibody level should be measured. Women with highest levels of TSH and anti-TPO antibodies have the highest risk for developing permanent hypothyroidism (48).

Three Clinical Presentations
1. Transient hyperthyroidism followed by recovery—28%
2. Transient hyperthyroidism, followed by transient or rarely permanent hypothyroidism—28%
3. Transient or permanent hypothyroidism—44%

Management
Most women do not require treatment. Treatment is based on symptoms.

   If symptomatic, thyrotoxicosis should be treated with a beta-adrenergic antagonist drug. Transient hypothyroidism is treated with thyroxine, with attempts made to wean the patient off of thyroid replacement within six months.

Recurrence Risk
Risk of recurrence is 70% (49).

   Risk of developing permanent primary hypothyroidism in the 5- to 10-year period following an episode of postpartum thyroiditis is markedly increased. Annual TSH level should be performed in them (50).

REFERENCES

1. Montoro MN. Management of hypothyroidism during pregnancy. Clin Obstet Gynecol 1997; 40(1):65–80. [II-2]
2. Klein RZ, Haddow JE, Faix JD, et al. Prevalence of thyroid deficiency in pregnant women. Clin Endocrinol (Oxf) 1991; 35(1):41–46. [II-2]
3. Alvarez-Marfany M, Roman SH, Drexler AJ, et al. Long-term prospective study of postpartum thyroid dysfunction in women with insulin dependent diabetes mellitus. J Clin Endocrinol Metab 1994; 79(1):10–16. [II-2]
4. Hollowell JG, Staehling NW, Hannon WH, et al. Iodine nutrition in the United States. Trends and public health implications: Iodine excretion data from national health and nutrition examination surveys I and III (1971–1974 and 1988–1994). J Clin Endocrinol Metab 1998; 83(10):3401–3408. [II-2]
5. Rakel RE. Textbook of Family Practice. 6th ed. Philadelphia: WB Saunders, 2002. [Review]
6. Weetman AP, McGregor AM. Autoimmune thyroid disease: developments in our understanding. Endocr Rev 1984; 5(2):309–355. [III]
7. Reid SM, Middleton P, Cossich MC, et al. Interventions for clinical and subclinical hypothyroidism in pregnancy. Cochrane Database Syst Rev 2010; (7):CD007752. [Review]
8. Leung AS, Millar LK, Koonings PP, et al. Perinatal outcome in hypothyroid pregnancies. Obstet Gynecol 1993; 81(3):349–353. [II-2]
9. Davis LE, Leveno KJ, Cunningham FG. Hypothyroidism complicating pregnancy. Obstet Gynecol 1988; 72(1):108–112. [II-3]
10. Pop VJ, Kuijpens JL, van Baar AL, et al. Low maternal free thyroxine concentrations during early pregnancy are associated with impaired psychomotor development in infancy. Clin Endocrinol (Oxf) 1999; 50(2):149–155. [II-2]
11. Haddow JE, Palomaki GE, Allan WC, et al. Maternal thyroid deficiency during pregnancy and subsequent neuropsychological development of the child. N Engl J Med 1999; 341(8):549–555. [II-2]
12. Negro R, Greco G, Mangieri T, et al. The influence of selenium supplementation on postpartum thyroid status in pregnant women with thyroid peroxidase autoantibodies. J Clin Endocrinol Metab 2007; 92(4):1263–1268. [RCT, *n* = 2143]
13. Premawardhana LD, Parkes AB, Ammari F, et al. Postpartum thyroiditis and long-term thyroid status: prognostic influence of thyroid peroxidase antibodies and ultrasound echogenicity. J Clin Endocrinol Metab 2000; 85(1):71–75. [II-2]
14. Rotondi M, Mazziotti G, Sorvillo F, et al. Effects of increased thyroxine dosage pre-conception on thyroid function during early pregnancy. Eur J Endocrinol 2004; 151(6):695–700. [RCT, *n* = 25]
15. Rasmussen NG, Hornnes PJ, Hegedus L. Ultrasonographically determined thyroid size in pregnancy and post partum: the goitrogenic effect of pregnancy. Am J Obstet Gynecol 1989; 160(5 pt 1):1216–1220. [II-3]
16. Dashe JS, Casey BM, Wells CE, et al. Thyroid-stimulating hormone in singleton and twin pregnancy: importance of gestational age-specific reference ranges. Obstet Gynecol 2005; 106(4):753–757. [II-3]
17. Glinoer D, de Nayer P, Bourdoux P, et al. Regulation of maternal thyroid during pregnancy. J Clin Endocrinol Metab 1990; 71(2):276–287. [II-3]
18. Alexander EK, Marqusee E, Lawrence J, et al. Timing and magnitude of increases in levothyroxine requirements during pregnancy in women with hypothyroidism. N Engl J Med 2004; 351(3):241–249. [II-2, *n* = 19]
19. Glinoer D. The regulation of thyroid function in pregnancy: pathways of endocrine adaptation from physiology to pathology. Endocr Rev 1997; 18(3):404–433. [III]
20. Burrow GN, Fisher DA, Larsen PR. Maternal and fetal thyroid function. N Engl J Med 1994; 331(16):1072–1078. [III]
21. Moosa M, Mazzaferri EL. Outcome of differentiated thyroid cancer diagnosed in pregnant women. J Clin Endocrinol Metab 1997; 82(9):2862–2866. [II-2]
22. Bajoria R, Fisk NM. Permeability of human placenta and fetal membranes to thyrotropin-stimulating hormone in vitro. Pediatr Res 1998; 43(5):621–628.[II-3]
23. ACOG. Thyroid disease in pregnancy. ACOG Practice Bulletin No. 37. Int J Gynaecol Obstet 2002; 79(2):171–180. [Review]
24. Gharib H, Cobin RH, Dickey RA. Subclinical hypothyroidism during pregnancy: position statement from the American Association of Clinical Endocrinologists. Endocr Pract 1999; 5(6):367–368. [Review, guideline]
25. American Association of Clinical Endocrinologists. AACE Clinical Practice Guidelines for Evaluation and Treatment of Hyperthyroidism and Hypothyroidism. Jackonville, Florida: AACE; 1996. [Review, guideline]
26. Ladenson PW, Singer PA, Ain KB, et al. American Thyroid Association guidelines for detection of thyroid dysfunction. Arch Intern Med 2000; 160(11):1573–1575. [Review, guideline]
27. Stagnaro-Green A, Roman SH, Cobin RH, et al. Detection of at-risk pregnancy by means of highly sensitive assays for thyroid autoantibodies. JAMA 1990; 264(11):1422–1425. [II-3]
28. Kuijpens JL, Pop VJ, Vader HL, et al. Prediction of post partum thyroid dysfunction: can it be improved? Eur J Endocrinol 1998; 139(1):36–43. [II-2]
29. Haddow JE, McClain MR, Palomaki GE, et al., First and Second Trimester Risk of Aneuploidy (FaSTER) Research Consortium. Thyroperoxidase and thyroglobulin antibodies in early pregnancy and placental abruption. Obstet Gynecol 2011; 117(2 pt 1):287–292. [II-2]
30. Mandel SJ, Larsen PR, Seely EW, et al. Increased need for thyroxine during pregnancy in women with primary hypothyroidism. N Engl J Med 1990; 323(2):91–96. [II-2]
31. Kaplan MM. Management of thyroxine therapy during pregnancy. Endocr Pract 1996; 2(4):281–286. [III]
32. Brent GA. Maternal hypothyroidism: recognition and management. Thyroid 1999; 9(7):661–665. [III]
33. Anselmo J, Cao D, Karrison T, et al. Fetal loss associated with excess thyroid hormone exposure. JAMA 2004; 292(6):691–695. [II-3]
34. Mahomed K, Gulmezoglu AM. Maternal iodine supplements in areas of deficiency. Cochrane Database Syst Rev 2006; 1. [Meta-analysis: 3 RCTs, *n* = 1551]
35. Andersson M, de Benoist B, Delange F, et al., WHO Secretariat. Prevention and control of iodine deficiency in pregnant and lactating women and in children less than 2-years-old: conclusions and recommendations of the technical consultation. Public Health Nutr 2007; 10(12A):1606–1611. [Review]
36. Ranzini AC, Ananth CV, Smulian JC, et al. Ultrasonography of the fetal thyroid: nomograms based on biparietal diameter and gestational age. J Ultrasound Med 2001; 20(6):613–617. [II-2]
37. Glorieux J, Dussault J, Van Vliet G. Intellectual development at age 12 years of children with congenital hypothyroidism diagnosed by neonatal screening. J Pediatr 1992; 121(4):581–584. [II-2]
38. Rovet JF, Ehrlich RM, Sorbara DL. Neurodevelopment in infants and preschool children with congenital hypothyroidism: etiological and treatment factors affecting outcome. J Pediatr Psychol 1992; 17(2):187–213. [II-2]
39. Cleary-Goldman J, Malone FD, Lambert-Messerlian G, et al. Maternal thyroid hypofunction and pregnancy outcome. Obstet Gynecol 2008; 112(1):85–92. [II-1]
40. Gharib H, Tuttle RM, Baskin HJ, et al. Consensus statement #1: subclinical thyroid dysfunction; a joint statement on management from the American Association of Clinical Endocrinologists, the American Thyroid Association, and the Endocrine Society. Thyroid 2005; 15(1):24–28. [III]
41. ACOG. Subclinical hypothyroidism in pregnancy. ACOG Committee Opinion No. 381. Obstet Gynecol 2007; 110(4):959–960. [Review]
42. Casey BM, Dashe JS, Wells CE, et al. Subclinical hypothyroidism and pregnancy outcomes. Obstet Gynecol 2005; 105(2):239–245. [II-2]

43. Negro R, Formoso G, Mangieri T, et al. Levothyroxine treatment in euthyroid pregnant women with autoimmune thyroid disease: effects on obstetrical complications. J Clin Endocrinol Metab 2006; 91(7):2587–2591. [RCT, *n* = 115]

44. Pearce EN, Farwell AP, Braverman LE. Thyroiditis. N Engl J Med 2003; 348(26):2646–2655. [III]

45. Casey BM, Dashe JS, Spong CY, et al. Perinatal significance of isolated maternal hypothyroxinemia identified in the first half of pregnancy. Obstet Gynecol 2007; 109(5):1129–1135. [II-2]

46. Tan GH, Gharib H, Goellner JR, et al. Management of thyroid nodules in pregnancy. Arch Intern Med 1996; 156(20):2317–2320. [II-2]

47. Gerstein HC. How common is postpartum thyroiditis? A methodologic overview of the literature. Arch Intern Med 1990; 150 (7):1397–1400. [III]

48. Lucas A, Pizarro E, Granada ML, et al. Postpartum thyroiditis: epidemiology and clinical evolution in a nonselected population. Thyroid 2000; 10(1):71–77. [II-2]

49. Lazarus JH, Ammari F, Oretti R, et al. Clinical aspects of recurrent postpartum thyroiditis. Br J Gen Pract 1997; 47(418):305–308. [II-3]

50. Azizi F. The occurrence of permanent thyroid failure in patients with subclinical postpartum thyroiditis. Eur J Endocrinol 2005; 153(3):367–371. [II-2]

7

Hyperthyroidism

Sushma Potti

KEY POINTS

- **Hyperthyroidism occurs in 0.1% to 0.4% of pregnancies.**
- **Graves' disease accounts for 95% of women with hyperthyroidism.**
- Untreated hyperthyroidism is associated with increased risks of **spontaneous pregnancy loss, preterm birth, preeclampsia, fetal death, abruption, fetal growth restriction (FGR), neonatal Graves' disease, as well as** maternal **congestive heart failure,** and **thyroid storm.**
- **Hyperemesis gravidarum (HG)** can be associated with **gestational transient biochemical thyrotoxicosis** [low, usually undetectable thyroid-stimulating hormone (TSH), and/or elevated T4], but this biochemical change always resolves spontaneously. Therefore, there should be **no testing, follow-up, or treatment for biochemical thyrotoxicosis in women with HG.**
- Clinical hyperthyroidism is **diagnosed** by **suppressed TSH** and **elevated serum** free thyroxine **(FT4)**. Thyroid-stimulating immunoglobulin (TSI) can be obtained, as positive TSI is consistent with Graves' disease, and values ≥200% to 500% indicate higher risk for fetal/neonatal hyperthyroidism.
- Goal of treatment is to keep FT4 in high normal range. **Measure TSH and FT4** every four weeks until FT4 is consistently in the high normal range, and then every trimester.
- Main treatment is with **either propylthiouracil (PTU) or methimazole.** Because of the very rare teratogenic effects of methimazole, and the dual mechanism of action of PTU, PTU has been suggested as the thionamide of choice in pregnancy, but methimazole is an effective alternative.
- Radioiodine is absolutely contraindicated in pregnancy.
- **Thyroid storm** is initially diagnosed clinically and treated aggressively with PTU, saturated solution of potassium iodide (SSKI), dexamethasone, and propranolol.

DEFINITIONS

Hyperthyroidism

Hyperfunctioning thyroid gland resulting in thyrotoxicosis. It usually implies low TSH and high T4 (or T3).

Graves' Disease

An autoimmune disease causing hyperthyroidism, characterized by production of thyroid-stimulating immunoglobulins (TSIs) or thyroid-stimulating hormone-binding inhibitory immunoglobulins (TBIIs). TSI coexists with TBII 30% of the time (1). TSIs stimulate thyrotropin receptor. Instead, TBII can stimulate or inhibit TSH receptor (2). TBIIs are seen in 30% of patients with Graves' disease and in 10% of patients with autoimmune Hashimoto's thyroiditis. TBII disappear and

patients achieve euthyroidism in 40% of the cases. Therefore, TBII assays have not been developed for clinical use because of higher costs involved in developing TBII assays as compared to the number of patients who would benefit from them.

TRAb (TSH receptor antibodies) is a broader term used to include both TSI and TBII. TRAb assays, in general, measure TSIs as TBII assays have not been established so far (3).

Thyrotoxicosis

Clinical and biochemical state that results from an excess production or exposure to thyroid hormone, from any etiology.

Gestational Thyrotoxicosis

Biochemical tests consistent with hyperthyroidism during pregnancy, but not a disease.

Thyroid Storm

Severe, acute, life-threatening exacerbation of the signs/symptoms of hyperthyroidism.

Subclinical Hyperthyroidism

Sustained TSH <0.1 mU/L with normal FT4 and free triiodothyronine (FT3), in the absence of nonthyroidal illness.

SIGNS/SYMPTOMS

Symptoms (may mimic hypermetabolic state of pregnancy): nervousness, tremor, frequent stools, excessive sweating, heat intolerance, insomnia, palpitations, decreased appetite, pruritus, decreased exercise tolerance, shortness of breath, eye symptoms of frequent lacrimation, double vision, and retro-orbital pain.

Physical Examination

Hypertension, goiter, tachycardia (>100 bpm, that does not decrease with Valsalva), wide pulse pressure, weight loss, ophthalmopathy (lid lag, lid retraction), and dermopathy (localized, pretibial myxedema). Goiter occurs only with iodine deficiency or thyroid disease, and must be considered pathological.

INCIDENCE

0.1% to 0.4% of pregnancies (4,5).

ETIOLOGY

Graves' disease accounts for 95% of women with hyperthyroidism. It can be associated with diffuse thyromegaly or infiltrative ophthalmopathy. Non-Graves' hyperthyroidism accounts for 5% of women with hyperthyroidism, and can be associated with gestational trophoblastic neoplasia (4,6), toxic nodular and multinodular goiter (5), hyperfunctioning thyroid adenoma, subacute thyroiditis, extrathyroid source of thyroid hormone (e.g., struma ovarii), iodine-induced hyperthyroidism, thyrotropin receptor activation (7), or viral thyroiditis.

BASIC PHYSIOLOGY/PATHOPHYSIOLOGY

See also hypothyroid guideline (see chap. 6). Ninety-five percent of cases are due to TSIs (7) stimulating excess thyroid hormone production from thyroid gland (Graves' disease). These IgG antibodies bind to and activate the G-protein-coupled thyrotropin receptor, which then stimulates follicular hypertrophy and hyperplasia, as well as increases thyroid hormones production, T3 more than T4 (2). Of women with Graves' disease, 40% to 50% have remission of the disease in 12 to 18 months (8).

COMPLICATIONS

Untreated hyperthyroidism preconception or in pregnancy is associated with increased risks of **spontaneous pregnancy loss, preterm birth, preeclampsia, abruption, fetal death, FGR, low birth weight,** maternal **congestive heart failure,** and **thyroid storm** (4,5,7,9–13). **Neonatal Graves' disease** can affect neonates of women with Graves' disease. Fetal thyrotoxicosis is a possibility in women with Graves' disease. Long-term uncontrolled hyperthyroidism, even subclinical, is associated with increased maternal risk for atrial fibrillation, dementia, Alzheimer's, and hip fractures.

MANAGEMENT
Pregnancy Considerations

See also hypothyroid guideline in chap. 6, including tables. **High levels of HCG,** which peak at 10 to 12 weeks, have some TSH-like activity, and stimulate thyroid hormone secretion, which in turn **suppress TSH.** Normal TSH levels in pregnancy are shown in Table 6.2. TSH suppression is even more marked for twins.

Hyperemesis gravidarum (HG) is diagnosed by severe nausea and vomiting associated with ketonuria and 5% weight loss (see chap. 9). **Gestational transient biochemical thyrotoxicosis** (low, usually undetectable TSH, and/or elevated T4) may be related to high serum HCG, and can occur in 3% to 11% of normal pregnancies especially during the period of highest serum HCG concentrations (10–12 weeks) (14). Therefore, **no testing, follow-up, or treatment for thyroid disease in women with HG should be initiated,** since there is no true thyroid disease, and the biochemical hyperthyroidism always spontaneously resolves (9). Women with signs or symptoms of hyperthyroidism from before pregnancy can be tested, regardless of HG.

Gestational Trophoblastic Disease

In women with hydatidiform mole or choriocarcinoma, 50% to 60% may have severe hyperthyroidism, which is primarily treated with evacuation of the mole or therapy directed against the choriocarcinoma.

Women with thyroid surgery/ablation in past who continue to produce antibodies (i.e., TSI) warrant assessment of maternal TSI level as these antibodies are associated with fetal/neonatal Graves' disease (15). Because of pregnancy physiologic changes, **hyperthyroidism typically ameliorates during third trimester, but may worsen postpartum.**

Women of childbearing age should have an average iodine intake of 150 μg/day. During pregnancy and breast-feeding, women should increase their daily iodine intake to 250 μg on average (16–18). Most prenatal vitamins have at least 200 μg in them. In the United States, 10% to 15% of pregnant women are iodine deficient.

SCREENING/DIAGNOSIS

Women with signs/symptoms consistent with hyperthyroidism should be screened with serum **TSH and FT4** (19,20). **Clinical hyperthyroidism is diagnosed by suppressed TSH and elevated serum FT4.** FT3 is measured in thyrotoxic patients with suppressed TSH but normal FT4 measurements (5% of hyperthyroid women). FT3 elevation indicates T3 thyrotoxicosis.

TSI can be obtained in women with clinical hyperthyroidism at the first visit and/or at 28 to 30 weeks (15–21). A positive TSI is consistent with Graves' disease. **Values ≥200% to 500% indicate higher risk for fetal/neonatal hyperthyroidism, and can help fetal and neonatal management.** Unfortunately, there is no standard test for TSI, often making comparisons between different laboratories or studies impossible. Presence of TSI differentiates Graves' disease from gestational thyrotoxicosis (biochemical tests consistent with hyperthyroidism during pregnancy, but no disease) and HG (5,10,12,22–24). In patients with HG, routine measurements of thyroid function are **not** recommended unless other overt signs of hyperthyroidism are evident (see chap. 9).

TREATMENT

Goal is to control symptoms of hyperthyroidism without causing fetal hypothyroidism, keeping **FT4 in high normal range,** TSH in low normal range, with lowest possible dose of thionamide. Propylthiouracil (PTU) >200 mg/day may result in fetal goiter (25), while keeping the FT4 in upper nonpregnant reference range (26,27) minimizes the risk of fetal hypothyroidism. **It may be helpful to measure TSH and FT4 every four weeks until FT4 is consistently in the high normal range.** Then measurements every trimester may be obtained. Dosing may need to be decreased as pregnancy advances, and about 30% can discontinue antithyroid therapy and still remain euthyroid.

Pregnancy outcomes have not been shown to improve with treatment of maternal subclinical hyperthyroidism and may result in unnecessary exposure of the fetus to antithyroid drugs (4,22,28). Identification and treatment of subclinical hyperthyroidism during pregnancy are unwarranted (28).

Thionamides
Propylthiouracil
PTU can be started at 100 mg every eight hours, and dose adjusted according to laboratory values and symptoms. It might take six to eight weeks to get adequate effect, with initial clinical response in as little as two to three weeks. Usual doses are 50 to 150 mg every eight hours, with requirements usually inversely proportional to gestational age (decrease as pregnancy advances).

Methimazole
Can be started at 20 mg once a day, and modified as needed according to laboratory values and symptoms. It is an acceptable alternative as it is equally effective. In fact, in nonpregnant

women, methimazole is often preferred to PTU, as the longer half-life often allows once-daily dosing (compared to three times a day for PTU). Efficacy of methimazole may be superior to PTU with fewer side effects (2). The teratologic risks of aplasia cutis and esophageal and choanal atresia (nine cases in literature) are extremely rare (4,8,29–32). There is no significant difference between PTU and methimazole in normalizing maternal TSH or on neonatal thyroid function, which might imply that transplacental transfer is similar (30). **Because of the very rare teratogenic effects of methimazole, and the dual mechanism of action of PTU, PTU has been recommended as the thionamide of choice in pregnancy** (8). There is no trial comparing the two in pregnancy, and methimazole may be preferred because of once-daily dosing. **Methimazole is a very reasonable alternative**, and can also be used also when there is an allergic reaction to PTU.

Mode of Action
Both compete for peroxidase, blocking organification of iodide, and so decreasing thyroid hormone synthesis. PTU also inhibits peripheral T4 to T3 conversion, and is therefore thought to work faster than methimazole.

Side Effects
   Maternal. **Agranulocytosis** (granulocytes <250/mL) is the most serious side effect, and occurs in 0.1% to 0.4% of cases. Risk factors are older gravidas and higher doses. It presents with fever, sore throat, malaise, gingivitis. If hyperthyroid women treated with thionamides present with sore throat and fever, discontinue therapy and check a white blood count (8). Other side effects (all with incidence of <5%) are thrombocytopenia, hepatitis, lupus-like syndrome, vasculitis, rash, hives, pruritus, nausea, vomiting, arthritis, anorexia, drug fever, and loss of taste or smell (8,33).
   Fetal/neonatal. As PTU and methimazole both cross the placenta, they may cause **fetal hypothyroidism**. Transient hypothyroidism may cause goiter secondary to suppression of fetal pituitary-thyroid axis. This, however, rarely requires therapy. IQ scores of children exposed to thionamide in utero are normal compared to nonexposed siblings (34,35).

Radioiodine

Radioiodine therapy is often used in the United States as the first- or second-line (after thionamides) therapy. The goal of radioiodine therapy is induced hypothyroidism in order to prevent a recurrence of Graves' disease. This goal is achieved in about 80% of patients (2). All women of reproductive age should have a pregnancy test immediately before this treatment. It is generally recommended that women do not attempt conception for 6 to 12 months after radioiodine treatment (2). As the half-life for radioiodine is eight days, reassurance can be provided to women who present with conception more than four weeks from therapy.
   This therapy **is absolutely contraindicated** in pregnancy. Fetal thyroid tissue will be ablated after 10 weeks. If given after 10 weeks, termination should be presented as an option. If given prior to 10 weeks, radioiodine does not appear to cause congenital hypothyroidism (36,37). Breast-feeding should be avoided for 120 days after this therapy.

Beta-Blocker

Propranolol 20 to 40 mg orally every 8 to 12 hours, or atenolol 50 to 100 mg orally once a day, are useful for rapid control of adrenergic symptoms of thyrotoxicosis, until thionamide takes effect (four to six weeks). This therapy does **not** alter synthesis or secretion of thyroid hormone. The goal is to keep maternal heart rate at 80 to 90 bpm, without palpitations. Prolonged therapy can lead to fetal side effects such as FGR, fetal bradycardia, hypoglycemia, and subnormal response to hypoxemic stress.

Surgery

This is the least-often used treatment. Thyroidectomy may be indicated for women who (*i*) cannot tolerate thionamide; (*ii*) need persistently high doses of antithyroid drugs; (*iii*) are noncompliant with antithyroid drugs; or (*iv*) have other indications similar to nonpregnant women. Second trimester is the optimal time for surgery (38–40).

Iodine

Short-term use is safe for symptomatic relief (41), while use for longer than two weeks may cause fetal goiter (42).

ANTEPARTUM TESTING

- The **fetal heart rate** can be assessed for at least one minute at each visit by doptone to rule out fetal tachycardia >180.
- Thyroid function testing with **TSH and FT4** should be performed at least every trimester.
- Weekly **NSTs** can begin at 32 to 34 weeks, especially in women with uncontrolled hyperthyroidism or elevated TSIs.
- **Ultrasound** can assess fetal heart rate, thyroid (for goiter), and growth. If clinically hyperthyroid, ultrasounds every four weeks for growth may be indicated. If FGR or fetal tachycardia is present, fetal thyroid circumference can be assessed (43). The sensitivity and specificity of fetal thyroid ultrasound at 32 weeks are 92% and 100%, respectively, for the diagnosis of clinically relevant fetal thyroid dysfunction (44).
- The fetus is at risk from either hypothyroidism from transplacental passage of antithyroid drugs, or from hyperthyroidism from TSI. The presence of a fetal goiter would point to fetal thyroid dysfunction, but not distinguish between these two possibilities. **Fetal blood sampling** is rarely indicated, but can be considered if high maternal TSI (200–500% normal), and fetal signs suggestive of severe thyroid disease, that is, fetal hydrops, goiter, tachycardia, cardiomegaly, FGR, or history of prior fetus with hyperthyroidism (45,46). Fetal hyperthyroidism should not be feared or tested for if TSIs are <130% (normal range). If the fetus is hypothyroid, injection of thyroxine in amniotic fluid is a possible intervention (47). If fetus is hyperthyroid, maternal treatment with thionamide to prevent fetal effects may be indicated even if maternal T4 is low or normal (48).
- It is important to **inform pediatrician** at time of delivery of maternal diagnosis and drug therapy.

NEONATE

Neonates born to mothers with Graves' disease should be followed closely by a pediatrician for the possibility of transient neonatal hyperthyroidism (44,49,50). **Neonatal Graves' disease** can affect 2% to 5% neonates of women with Graves', unrelated to maternal thyroid function, secondary to transplacental transfer of TSI or TBII. The risk is high if the TSI index is ≥ 5, or $\geq 200\%$ to 500% (51). Signs are tachycardia (>160 bpm), goiter, FGR, advanced bone age, craniosynostosis, hydrops, later motor difficulties, hyperactivity, or failure to thrive (51). Neonates of women who have been treated surgically or with radioactive iodine before pregnancy and still gave TSI are at highest risk for neonatal Graves' disease since thionamide therapy is not present to counteract this effect. On the other hand, fetal and neonatal complications can also arise from thionamide treatment of the disease, as, when this is excessive, signs of hypothyroidism can occur.

POSTPARTUM

Both PTU and methimazole are considered safe (52). Only small amounts of PTU cross into breast milk, while higher amounts of methimazole are present in breast milk (53,54). Of pregnant patients in remission from Graves' disease, 75% will either relapse postpartum or develop postpartum thyroiditis (8).

TSH should be performed three and six months postpartum in women known to have thyroid peroxidase antibodies (TPO-Ab) (55,56). Annual TSH level should be performed in women with history of postpartum thyroiditis as they have a markedly increased risk of developing permanent primary hypothyroidism in the next 5- to 10-year period following the episode of postpartum thyroiditis (57–60).

THYROID STORM
Incidence
Rare hypermetabolic state, which occurs in 1% of hyperthyroid women.

Precipitating Factors
Labor, infection, preeclampsia, surgery.

Signs/Symptoms
Fever, tachycardia disproportionate to fever, mental status change, vomiting, diarrhea, dehydration, cardiac arrhythmia, congestive heart failure (5), and rarely seizures, shock, stupor and coma.

Diagnosis
It initially should be made **clinically** with a combination of signs and symptoms. Confirmatory labs include increased FT4 (or increased FT3) and very low TSH.

Treatment
PTU, SSKI, dexamethasone, and propranolol should be given as shown in Figure 7.1 (53). The saturated solution of potassium iodide and sodium iodide block the release of thyroid hormone from the gland. Dexamethasone decreases thyroid hormone release and peripheral conversion of T4 to T3. Propanolol inhibits the adrenergic effects of excessive thyroid hormone. Supportive measures include IV fluids with glucose, acetaminophen (as antipyretic), and oxygen, as needed. Fetal monitoring and maternal cardiac monitoring are recommended (21). Delivery in the presence of thyroid storm should be avoided if possible, with maternal treatment leading to in utero fetal resuscitation. The underlying cause, for example, infection, should be treated.

Figure 7.1 Treatment of thyroid storm in pregnant women. *Source*: Adapted from Ref. 53.

1. *Propylthiouracil* (PTU), 600–800 mg orally, immediately, even before labs are back; then 150–200 mg orally every 4–6 hours. If oral administration is not possible, use methimazole rectal suppositories.
2. Starting 1–2 hr after PTU administration, saturated solution of *potassium iodide* (SSKI), 2–5 drops orally every 8 hours; or sodium iodide, 0.5–1.0 g intravenously every 8 hours; or Lugol's solution, 8 drops every 6 hours; or Lithium carbonate, 300 mg orally every 6 hr.
3. *Dexamethasone*, 2 mg intravenously or intramuscularly every 6 hr for four doses.
4. *Propranolol*, 20–80 mg orally every 4–6 hours; or propranolol, 1–2 mg intravenously every 5 min for a total of 6 mg, then 1–10 mg intravenously every 4 hours.
5. If the patient has a history of severe bronchospasm:
   - Reserpine, 1–5 mg intramuscularly every 4–6 hours.
   - Guanethidine, 1mg/kg orally every 12 hours.
   - Diltiazem, 60 mg orally every 6–8 hours.
6. Phenobarbital, 30–60 mg orally every 6–8 hours as needed for extreme restlessness.

RESOURCES
- National Graves' Disease Foundation (http://www.ngdf.org)
- American Thyroid Association Alliance for Patient Education (http://www.thyroid.org/patients/patients.html)
- Thyroid Foundation of Canada (http://www.thyroid.ca)

REFERENCES

1. Amino N, Izumi Y, Hidaka Y, et al. No increase of blocking type anti-thyrotropin receptor antibodies during pregnancy in patients with Graves' disease. J Clin Endocrinol Metab 2003; 88(12):5871–5874. [II-3]
2. Brent GA. Clinical practice. Graves' disease. N Engl J Med 2008; 358(24):2594–2605. [III]
3. Zophel K, Roggenbuck D, Schott M. Clinical review about TRAb assay's history. Autoimmun Rev 2010; 9(10):695–700. [III, review]
4. Abalovich M, Amino N, Barbour LA, et al. Management of thyroid dysfunction during pregnancy and postpartum: an Endocrine Society Clinical Practice Guideline. J Clin Endocrinol Metab 2007; 92(8 suppl):S1–S47. [Review]
5. Mestman JH. Hyperthyroidism in pregnancy. Best Pract Res Clin Endocrinol Metab 2004; 18(2):267–288. [Review]
6. Palmieri C, Fisher RA, Sebire NJ, et al. Placental-site trophoblastic tumour: an unusual presentation with bilateral ovarian involvement. Lancet Oncol 2005; 6(1):59–61. [III]
7. Marx H, Amin P, Lazarus JH. Hyperthyroidism and pregnancy. BMJ 2008; 336(7645):663–667. [Review]
8. Cooper DS. Antithyroid drugs. N Engl J Med 2005; 352(9):905–917. [III, review]
9. LeBeau SO, Mandel SJ. Thyroid disorders during pregnancy. Endocrinol Metab Clin North Am 2006; 35(1):117–136, vii. [Review]
10. Davis LE, Lucas MJ, Hankins GD, et al. Thyrotoxicosis complicating pregnancy. Am J Obstet Gynecol 1989; 160(1):63–70. [II-2]
11. Mestman JH. Diagnosis and management of maternal and fetal thyroid disorders. Curr Opin Obstet Gynecol 1999; 11(2):167–175. [III, review]

12. Millar LK, Wing DA, Leung AS, et al. Low birth weight and preeclampsia in pregnancies complicated by hyperthyroidism. Obstet Gynecol 1994; 84(6):946–949. [II-2]

13. Phoojaroenchanachai M, Sriussadaporn S, Peerapatdit T, et al. Effect of maternal hyperthyroidism during late pregnancy on the risk of neonatal low birth weight. Clin Endocrinol (Oxf) 2001; 54 (3):365–370. [II-3]

14. Yeo CP, Khoo DH, Eng PH, et al. Prevalence of gestational thyrotoxicosis in Asian women evaluated in the 8th to 14th weeks of pregnancy: correlations with total and free beta human chorionic gonadotrophin. Clin Endocrinol (Oxf) 2001; 55 (3):391–398. [II-2]

15. Weetman AP. Graves' disease. N Engl J Med 2000; 343(17):1236–1248. [III, review]

16. Glinoer D. Pregnancy and iodine. Thyroid 2001; 11(5):471–481. [Review]

17. Glinoer D. Feto-maternal repercussions of iodine deficiency during pregnancy. An update. Ann Endocrinol (Paris) 2003; 64(1):37–44. [Review]

18. Hollowell JG, Staehling NW, Hannon WH, et al. Iodine nutrition in the United States. Trends and public health implications: iodine excretion data from national health and nutrition examination surveys I and III (1971–1974 and 1988–1994). J Clin Endocrinol Metab 1998; 83(10):3401–3408. [II-2]

19. American Association of Clinical Endocrinologists. AACE clinical practice guidelines for evaluation and treatment of hyperthyroidism and hypothyroidism. Jacksonville, Florida, 1996. [Review]

20. Ladenson PW, Singer PA, Ain KB, et al. American Thyroid Association Guidelines for detection of thyroid dysfunction. Arch Intern Med 2000; 160(11):1573–1575. [III]

21. Ecker JL. Thyroid function and disease in pregnancy. Curr Probl Obstet Gynecol Fertil 2000; (23):109–122. [III]

22. Tan JY, Loh KC, Yeo GS, et al. Transient hyperthyroidism of hyperemesis gravidarum. BJOG 2002; 109(6):683–688. [III]

23. Goodwin TM, Montoro M, Mestman JH. Transient hyperthyroidism and hyperemesis gravidarum: clinical aspects. Am J Obstet Gynecol 1992; 167(3):648–652. [III]

24. Goodwin TM, Montoro M, Mestman JH, et al. The role of chorionic gonadotropin in transient hyperthyroidism of hyperemesis gravidarum. J Clin Endocrinol Metab 1992; 75(5):1333–1337. [II-2]

25. Hamburger JI. Thyroid nodules in pregnancy. Thyroid 1992; 2 (2):165–168. [III]

26. Momotani N, Noh J, Oyanagi H, et al. Antithyroid drug therapy for Graves' disease during pregnancy. Optimal regimen for fetal thyroid status. N Engl J Med 1986; 315(1):24–28. [II-2]

27. Mortimer RH, Tyack SA, Galligan JP, et al. Graves' disease in pregnancy: TSH receptor binding inhibiting immunoglobulins and maternal and neonatal thyroid function. Clin Endocrinol (Oxf) 1990; 32(2):141–152. [II-3]

28. Casey BM, Dashe JS, Wells CE, et al. Subclinical hyperthyroidism and pregnancy outcomes. Obstet Gynecol 2006; 107(2 pt 1):337–341. [II-2]

29. Wing DA, Millar LK, Koonings PP, et al. A comparison of propylthiouracil versus methimazole in the treatment of hyperthyroidism in pregnancy. Am J Obstet Gynecol 1994; 170(1 pt 1):90–95. [II-2]

30. Momotani N, Noh JY, Ishikawa N, et al. Effects of propylthiouracil and methimazole on fetal thyroid status in mothers with Graves' hyperthyroidism. J Clin Endocrinol Metab 1997; 82 (11):3633–3636. [II-2]

31. Clementi M, Di Gianantonio E, Pelo E, et al. Methimazole embryopathy: delineation of the phenotype. Am J Med Genet 1999; 83(1):43–46. [III]

32. Di Gianantonio E, Schaefer C, Mastroiacovo PP, et al. Adverse effects of prenatal methimazole exposure. Teratology 2001; 64 (5):262–266. [II-2]

33. Abraham P, Avenell A, Watson WA, et al. Antithyroid drug regimen for treating Graves' hyperthyroidism. Cochrane Database Syst Rev 2005; (2):CD003420. [Meta-analysis, review]

34. Burrow GN, Klatskin EH, Genel M. Intellectual development in children whose mothers received propylthiouracil during pregnancy. Yale J Biol Med 1978; 51(2):151–156. [II-2]

35. Eisenstein Z, Weiss M, Katz Y, et al. Intellectual capacity of subjects exposed to methimazole or propylthiouracil in utero. Eur J Pediatr 1992; 151(8):558–559. [II-2]

36. Berg GE, Nystrom EH, Jacobsson L, et al. Radioiodine treatment of hyperthyroidism in a pregnant women. J Nucl Med 1998; 39 (2):357–361. [II-3]

37. Evans PM, Webster J, Evans WD, et al. Radioiodine treatment in unsuspected pregnancy. Clin Endocrinol (Oxf) 1998; 48(3):281–283. [II-3]

38. Stice RC, Grant CS, Gharib H, et al. The management of Graves' disease during pregnancy. Surg Gynecol Obstet 1984; 158(2):157–160. [II-3]

39. Burrow GN. The management of thyrotoxicosis in pregnancy. N Engl J Med 1985; 313(9):562–565. [Review]

40. Brodsky JB, Cohen EN, Brown BW Jr., et al. Surgery during pregnancy and fetal outcome. Am J Obstet Gynecol 1980; 138 (8):1165–1167. [II-2]

41. Nohr SB, Jorgensen A, Pedersen KM, et al. Postpartum thyroid dysfunction in pregnant thyroid peroxidase antibody-positive women living in an area with mild to moderate iodine deficiency: is iodine supplementation safe? J Clin Endocrinol Metab 2000; 85 (9):3191–3198. [II-2]

42. Momotani N, Hisaoka T, Noh J, et al. Effects of iodine on thyroid status of fetus versus mother in treatment of Graves' disease complicated by pregnancy. J Clin Endocrinol Metab 1992; 75 (3):738–744. [II-2]

43. Ranzini AC, Ananth CV, Smulian JC, et al. Ultrasonography of the fetal thyroid: nomograms based on biparietal diameter and gestational age. J Ultrasound Med 2001; 20(6):613–617. [II-2]

44. Luton D, Le Gac I, Vuillard E, et al. Management of Graves' disease during pregnancy: the key role of fetal thyroid gland monitoring. J Clin Endocrinol Metab 2005; 90(11):6093–6098. [II-3]

45. Nachum Z, Rakover Y, Weiner E, et al. Graves' disease in pregnancy: prospective evaluation of a selective invasive treatment protocol. Am J Obstet Gynecol 2003; 189(1):159–165. [II-2]

46. Kilpatrick S. Umbilical blood sampling in women with thyroid disease in pregnancy: is it necessary? Am J Obstet Gynecol 2003; 189(1):1–2. [III]

47. Hanono A, Shah B, David R, et al. Antenatal treatment of fetal goiter: a therapeutic challenge. J Matern Fetal Neonatal Med 2009; 22(1):76–80. [11-3]

48. Peleg D, Cada S, Peleg A, et al. The relationship between maternal serum thyroid-stimulating immunoglobulin and fetal and neonatal thyrotoxicosis. Obstet Gynecol 2002; 99(6):1040–1043. [II-2]

49. McKenzie JM, Zakarija M. Fetal and neonatal hyperthyroidism and hypothyroidism due to maternal TSH receptor antibodies. Thyroid 1992; 2(2):155–159. [Review]

50. Mitsuda N, Tamaki H, Amino N, et al. Risk factors for developmental disorders in infants born to women with Graves' disease. Obstet Gynecol 1992; 80(3 pt 1):359–364. [III]

51. Becks GP, Burrow GN. Thyroid disease and pregnancy. Med Clin North Am 1991; 75(1):121–150. [III, review]

52. American Academy of Pediatrics Committee on Drugs. Transfer of drugs and other chemicals into human milk. Pediatrics 2001; 108(3):776–789. [Review]

53. American College of Obstetricians and Gynecologists. Thyroid disease in pregnancy. ACOG Practice Bulletin No. 37. Obstet Gynecol 2002; 100(2):387–396. [Review]

54. Briggs GG, Freeman RK, Yaffe SJ, eds. Drugs in Pregnancy and Lactation: A Reference Guide to Fetal and Neonatal Risk. 6th ed. Philadelphia, PA: Lippincott Williams & Wilkins 2001. [II-2]

55. Premawardhana LD, Parkes AB, John R, et al. Thyroid peroxidase antibodies in early pregnancy: utility for prediction of postpartum thyroid dysfunction and implications for screening. Thyroid 2004; 14(8):610–615. [II-2]

56. Stagnaro-Green A. Clinical review 152: postpartum thyroiditis. J Clin Endocrinol Metab 2002; 87(9):4042–4047. [Review]

57. Azizi F. The occurrence of permanent thyroid failure in patients with subclinical postpartum thyroiditis. Eur J Endocrinol 2005; 153(3):367–371. [II-3]

58. Premawardhana LD, Parkes AB, Ammari F, et al. Postpartum thyroiditis and long-term thyroid status: prognostic influence of thyroid peroxidase antibodies and ultrasound echogenicity. J Clin Endocrinol Metab 2000; 85(1):71–75. [II-1]

59. Othman S, Phillips DI, Parkes AB, et al. A long-term follow-up of postpartum thyroiditis. Clin Endocrinol (Oxf) 1990; 32(5):559–564. [II-2]

60. Tachi J, Amino N, Tamaki H, et al. Long term follow-up and HLA association in patients with postpartum hypothyroidism. J Clin Endocrinol Metab 1988; 66(3):480–484. [II-2]

8

Prolactinoma

Vincenzo Berghella

KEY POINTS

- **Diagnosis: elevated prolactin and MRI-proven pituitary adenoma.**
- **Preconception: treat with dopamine agonist** (bromocriptine or cabergoline) aiming to normalize prolactin and decrease size of adenoma, continuing therapy up to positive pregnancy test. Discourage pregnancy until those aims have been achieved, and any neurologic or visual symptoms or suprasellar involvement have been resolved.
- **Maternal risk is adenoma enlargement**; this occurs in pregnancy in 1% to 5% of microadenomas and about 15% to 36% of macroadenomas.
- **Bromocriptine** (and probably cabergoline) has been shown to **be safe for the fetus.**
- Compared to cabergoline, bromocriptine has the following advantages: cheaper, more pregnancy safety data, no association with cardiac-valve disease; but its disadvantages include twice daily (versus twice weekly) dosing, and more side effects.
- **Management depends on the size of adenoma:**
  - **Microadenoma (<1 cm):** Consider stopping dopamine agonist in pregnancy, especially if normal prolactin and stable microadenoma ≥2 years. During the pregnancy, the woman should be **asked about headaches and changes in vision at each visit (at least every three months). The decision to treat with dopamine agonist is based on symptoms (e.g., headache) and signs (e.g., abnormal visual field examination) only.** Prolactin levels should not be checked since they physiologically (10-fold) increase in pregnancy.
  - **Macroadenoma (≥1 cm): Dopamine agonist should be continued.** Monitoring as per microadenoma, plus **formal visual field testing every three months.** Transsphenoidal surgery suggested usually only if maximal dopamine agonist therapy is ineffective.

DIAGNOSIS/DEFINITION

Pituitary adenomas producing prolactin (prolactinomas, or lactotroph adenomas) are diagnosed by sustained **elevation of serum prolactin** (usually >40 µg/L × 2; normal prolactin nonpregnant: <20 µg/L) *and* radiographic (best is MRI) evidence of **pituitary adenoma**. Rule out other causes of prolactinemia (1).

SYMPTOMS
Before Pregnancy

Galactorrhea in 80% of women and irregular menses (e.g., oligomenorrhea).

EPIDEMIOLOGY/INCIDENCE

Prolactinomas account for about 40% of pituitary tumors. They are the most common type of secretory pituitary tumor.

ETIOLOGY/BASIC PATHOPHYSIOLOGY

These adenomas produce prolactin. Outside of pregnancy, prolactin levels parallel tumor size fairly closely. Increased prolactin usually causes **infertility** because of the inhibitory effect of prolactin on secretion of GNRH, which in turn inhibits the release of LH and FSH, thus impairing gonadal steroidogenesis and ovulation, and thereby conception. Sometimes the mass effect of a macroadenoma can also lead to infertility. Prolactinomas are usually benign and nonhereditary.

CLASSIFICATION

Microadenoma: <10 mm; macroadenoma: ≥10 mm.

COMPLICATIONS
Mother

The principal risk is the **increase in adenoma size** sufficient to cause neurologic symptoms, most importantly **visual impairment** or also headaches. In women with lactotroph adenomas who become pregnant, the hyperestrogenemia of pregnancy may increase the size of the adenoma. This should be distinguished from increase in pituitary (overall) size (physiologic in pregnancy). **The risk that the adenoma increase will be clinically important depends on the size of the adenoma before pregnancy.** The risk of a clinically important increase in the size of a lactotroph microadenoma during pregnancy is small. Because of enlargement, about 1% to 5% of pregnant women with **microadenomas** develop neurologic symptoms, such as headaches and/or a visual field abnormality, and about 1% diabetes insipidus. With **macroadenomas**, neurologic symptoms occur in about 13% to 36% or higher of pregnant women, and diabetes insipidus in about 1% to 2% (2–4). Long-term hyperprolactinemia may lead to **decrease in bone density**, which again increases (not back to normal levels) after normal prolactin levels are reestablished (1).

Fetus

Main potential risk to the fetus is from dopamine agonist treatment of hyperprolactinemia. Administration of bromocriptine during the first month of pregnancy does not harm the fetus (over 1000 pregnancies reported) (5,6). Data available about the use of bromocriptine later in pregnancy are less, but no adverse events have been reported. Cabergoline use in pregnancy is probably safe too (about 300 pregnancies reported), but less experience is reported (7,8).

PREGNANCY CONSIDERATIONS

The ability to treat prolactinomas successfully with dopamine agonists in >90% of patients allows most women with this disorder to become pregnant. The theoretical basis for an **increase in size of the pituitary** during pregnancy is that hyperestrogenemia causes lactotroph hyperplasia. Secondary to estrogen causing lactotroph hyperplasia, there is a progressive increase in pituitary size, as assessed by MR imaging, throughout pregnancy, so that the volume during the third trimester is more than double of that in nonpregnant women (9).

PREGNANCY-RELATED MANAGEMENT
Principles
Effect of Pregnancy on Disease
The whole pituitary enlarges in pregnancy. The prolactinoma can enlarge. Prolactin levels are physiologically elevated, and cannot be used for management. Serum levels of prolactin in nonpregnant patients with prolactinomas are usually proportional to the tumor mass, but this relation is lost in pregnancy. Prolactin levels do not correlate well with symptoms in both nonpregnant and pregnant patients with prolactinomas (10).

Effect of Disease on Pregnancy
No obstetrical effects unless major surgery is needed.

Workup
In Pregnancy (Fig. 8.1)

- **Prolactin** levels are not helpful in pregnancy.
- **MRI** is more effective in revealing small tumors and the extension of large tumors compared to CT scan (1).
- **Visual field testing** is indicated in women with **macroadenomas.**

In Nonpregnant Woman
If an elevated prolactin is detected, this should be repeated. If still elevated, then head MRI is performed, even in cases of mild hyperprolactinemia. At initial diagnosis, thyroid-stimulating hormone and free T4, renal and hepatic function should be assessed (10).

Treatment (Fig. 8.1; Tables 8.1, 8.2)
The primary therapy for all prolactinomas is a dopamine agonist. The dopamine agonists approved in the United States are bromocriptine and cabergoline. Dose recommendations and side effects are listed in Table 8.1 (10).

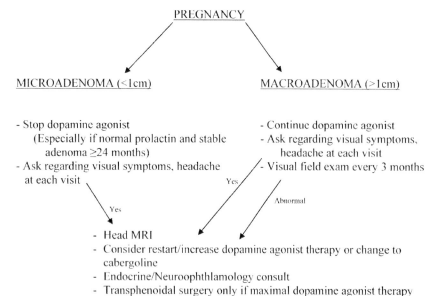

PRECONCEPTION

- Dopamine agonist therapy aiming to normalize prolactin and shrink adenoma
- Discourage pregnancy until neurologic/visual symptoms have resolved
- MRI (gadolinium-enhanced) before pregnancy

PREGNANCY

MICROADENOMA (<1cm)

- Stop dopamine agonist
  (Especially if normal prolactin and stable adenoma ≥24 months)
- Ask regarding visual symptoms, headache at each visit

Yes

MACROADENOMA (>1cm)

- Continue dopamine agonist
- Ask regarding visual symptoms, headache at each visit
- Visual field exam every 3 months

Yes

Abnormal

- Head MRI
- Consider restart/increase dopamine agonist therapy or change to cabergoline
- Endocrine/Neuroophthlamology consult
- Transphenoidal surgery only if maximal dopamine agonist therapy ineffective (Table 8.3)

Figure 8.1 Management of prolactinoma in pregnancy (see also Table 8.2).

Table 8.1 Dose and Side Effect Profiles for Dopamine Agonists Approved for Use in the United States

Medication	Dose	Side effects of both drugs[a]
Bromocriptine	Initial: 0.625–1.25 mg daily; usual range for maintenance dose: 2.5–10.0 mg daily	Nausea, headaches, dizziness (postural hypotension), nasal congestion, constipation Infrequent: fatigue, anxiety, depression, alcohol intolerance Rare: cold-sensitive vasospasm, psychosis
Cabergoline	Initial: 0.25–0.5 mg weekly; usual range for maintenance dose: 0.25–3.0 mg weekly	Possible: cardiac-valve abnormalities (reported with cabergoline)

[a]More common with bromocriptine. *Source*: Modified from Ref. 10.

Table 8.2 Indications for Therapy in Patients with Prolactinomas

Main indication in pregnancy
  Macroadenoma
Pregnant and nonpregnant
  Enlarging microadenoma
  Bothersome galactorrhea
  Gynecomastia
  Acne and hirsutism
Nonpregnant
  Infertility
  Oligomenorrhea or amenorrhea

Source: Modified from Ref. 10.

Bromocriptine (Parlodel)

Dose: Started at **0.625 mg po qhs** with snack for one week. Then add 1.25 mg qam for one week, and increase by 1.25 mg. So at four weeks, a total of 5 mg total dose (split **2.5 mg** q12h) is reached and prolactin rechecked. Usually a total of 5 to 7.5 mg (split q12h) total dose is required. *It can also be used intravaginally* (same dose, less side effects, minimal vaginal irritation).

Mechanism of Action: Dopamine agonist (dopamine inhibits lactotroph receptors, so less prolactin is produced, and the size of tumors is decreased); ergot derivative.

Evidence for effectiveness: See below.

Safety in pregnancy: Safe (FDA category B); breast-feeding is contraindicated.

Side effects: Nausea, hypotension, and depression (less if therapy initiated at night).

Cabergoline (Dostinex)

Dose: Start at 0.25 mg twice weekly, increase monthly to normal prolactin. Usual required dose is 0.25 to 0.5 mg twice weekly; maximum dose should be 1 mg twice weekly.

Mechanism of action: Dopamine agonist (see above); non-ergot; high affinity for lactotroph dopamine receptors.

Evidence for effectiveness: See below.

Safety in pregnancy: Safe (FDA category B); breast-feeding is contraindicated.

Side effects: Associated with heart-valve disease in very high doses.

Preconception Counseling

Treatment of women with lactotroph adenomas outside of pregnancy is based on the size of the tumor, presence/absence of gonadal dysfunction, and woman's desire regarding fertility (1). Indications for therapy in adults with prolactinoma are listed in Table 8.2 (10). Treatment should begin before conception with advice to the woman and her partner about the risks of pregnancy to her and the fetus. When a **dopamine** agonist is needed to lower the serum prolactin concentration to permit ovulation, counseling should include the fact that **bromocriptine** has larger safety data, while **cabergoline** (Dostinex) has less data in pregnancy (all reassuring so far). Bromocriptine normalizes prolactin levels in >80% of women with microadenomas, restoring menses and fertility in >90%. **Compared to cabergoline, bromocriptine** has the following advantages: it is cheaper, there are more pregnancy safety data, and there is no association with heart-valve disease; but its disadvantages include twice daily (vs. twice weekly) dosing, less effective at

normalizing prolactin levels, and more side effects (10). If a woman cannot tolerate bromocriptine, cabergoline should be recommended; 70% of patients who do not have a response to bromocriptine respond to cabergoline. Quinagolide (Pergolide) should not be recommended because it is not FDA approved to treat hyperprolactinemia, has not been well studied during pregnancy, and has been associated with cardiac valvular defects (11). In nonpregnant adults with prolactinomas, prolactin levels and MRI should be checked after diagnosis and stabilization once a year for three years, and then about every two years if the patient's condition is stable. In patients with normal prolactin for ≥2 years on low-dose therapy, some consider stopping the dopamine agonist therapy. The risk of enlargement over time in untreated patients is about 20% (10).

Microadenomas

A woman who has a lactotroph microadenoma should be told that the risk of clinically important enlargement of her adenoma during pregnancy is very small (1–5%) and that it **should not be a deterrent to becoming pregnant**. She should also be told that bromocriptine or cabergoline will likely be effective if symptoms do occur. If she is willing to take this small risk of enlargement, she should be given bromocriptine or cabergoline before pregnancy in whatever dosage is necessary to lower her serum prolactin concentration to normal. Bromocriptine is the drug associated with the greater experience. When the serum prolactin concentration is normal and menses have occurred regularly for a few months, the woman can attempt to become pregnant. Before pregnancy, the dopamine agonist should be tapered to lowest effective dose, and can be discontinued before pregnancy if used for ≥24 months with normal prolactin levels, as about 25% of patients maintain normal levels even off medication; most need to restart it, though.

Macroadenomas

A woman who has a lactotroph macroadenoma should be advised of the relatively higher risk of clinically important tumor enlargement during pregnancy (2–4). A macroadenoma is an **absolute indication for therapy** (dopamine agonist, followed together with endocrinologist), in nonpregnant or pregnant women. Doses of dopamine agonists sufficient to control the macroadenoma are usually higher (bromocriptine 7.5–10 mg/daily; cabergoline 0.5–1 mg twice weekly) than with microadenomas. The goals of treatment are not only to decrease prolactin levels and symptoms, but also to decrease and stabilize the tumor mass and prevent headaches and cranial nerve compression (10). Before pregnancy, the dopamine agonist should be carefully tapered to lowest effective dose. This may take weeks to years. Advice and monitoring depend on how large the adenoma is.

- If the macroadenoma does not elevate the optic chiasm or extend behind the sella, treatment with bromocriptine or cabergoline for a sufficient period to shrink it substantially should reduce the chance of clinically important enlargement during pregnancy (2,12). Once this has occurred, the woman can attempt to become pregnant.

- If the adenoma is very large or elevates the optic chiasm, pregnancy should be strongly discouraged until the adenoma has been adequately treated. If the macroadenoma extends behind the sella, the woman should undergo visual field examination and testing of anterior pituitary function. Transsphenoidal surgery may be necessary, and perhaps postoperatively radiation. Postoperative treatment with bromocriptine or cabergoline may also be helpful in reducing adenoma size further and lowering the serum prolactin concentration to normal. Such a regimen reduces the chance that symptomatic expansion will occur during pregnancy (2,3), but it may still occur.

- **Pregnancy should also be discouraged in a woman whose macroadenoma is unresponsive to bromocriptine and cabergoline**, even if it is not elevating the optic chiasm, until the size has been greatly reduced by transsphenoidal surgery, because medical treatment would not likely be effective if the adenoma enlarges during pregnancy.

PRENATAL CARE
See also section "Preconception Counseling."

Microadenoma
Bromocriptine, and probably cabergoline, are safe in pregnancy. They can be discontinued as soon as pregnancy has been confirmed if the patient who has a normal prolactin and a recent reassuring (adenoma <1 cm) MRI so desires. The risk of clinically significant tumor enlargement during pregnancy is about 3% for microprolactinomas (10).

During the pregnancy, the woman should be asked about headaches and changes in vision at each visit (or at least every three months). Formal visual field test every three months can be performed, but are not absolutely necessary. The decision to treat with dopamine agonist is based on symptoms (e.g., headache) and signs (e.g., abnormal visual filed examination) only. It should not be based on prolactin levels. In fact, **prolactin levels should not be checked** since they physiologically increase (about 10-fold) in pregnancy. If no symptoms occur, serum prolactin can be measured about two months after delivery or cessation of nursing, and if it is similar to the pretreatment value, the drug can be resumed.

Macroadenoma
The **dopamine agonist should be continued during pregnancy** in most cases. In these patients, discontinuation of the drug usually leads to expansion of the adenoma (1). Monitoring during pregnancy should be similar to that described above for women with microadenomas, except for the fact that **formal visual field testing every three months should be performed**. The risk of clinically significant tumor enlargement during pregnancy is about 30% for macroprolactinomas. The risk of clinically significant tumor enlargement during pregnancy is about 3% for microprolactinomas (10).

A perceived a change in vision should be assessed by a neuro-ophthalmologist, and an MRI (gadolinium-enhanced; more effective than CT scan) (1) should be performed if an abnormality consistent with a pituitary adenoma is confirmed. If the adenoma has enlarged to a degree that could account for the symptoms, the woman should be treated with higher doses of bromocriptine throughout the remainder of the pregnancy, which will usually decrease the size of the adenoma and alleviate the symptoms (13,14). If the adenoma does not respond to bromocriptine, cabergoline may be successful (15). If cabergoline is not successful, transsphenoidal surgery could be considered in the second trimester if vision is severely

Table 8.3 Indication for Neurosurgery in Patients with Prolactinomas

Pregnant or nonpregnant
   Increasing tumor size despite optimal medical therapy
   Dopamine agonist-resistant macroadenoma
   Pituitary apoplexy
   Inability to tolerate necessary dopamine agonist therapy
   Persistent chiasmal compression despite optimal medical
      therapy
   Medically unresponsive cystic prolactinoma
   Cerebrospinal fluid leak during administration of dopamine
      agonist
   Macroadenoma in a patient with a psychiatric condition for which
      dopamine agonists are contraindicated
Infertility patient
   Dopamine agonist-resistant microadenoma, if ovulation induction
      is not appropriate
   Macroadenoma in proximity to optic chiasm despite optimal
      medical therapy (prepregnancy debulking recommended)

Source: Modified from Ref. 10.

compromised; in comparison, surgery for persistent visual symptoms in the third trimester should be deferred until delivery if possible. **Surgery is recommended *only* if medical therapy is ineffective**. Indications for neurosurgery in a patient with prolactinoma are listed in Table 8.3 (10). Surgical cure rates are <50% with macroadenomas, with up to 80% of these patients experiencing recurrent hyperprolactinemia (10).

ANTEPARTUM TESTING
None needed (except if other indications present).

DELIVERY
No special precautions.

ANESTHESIA
No special precautions.

POSTPARTUM
A prolactin level and a gadolinium-enhanced MRI can be performed six to eight weeks postpartum. Prolactin levels may not normalize until six months postpartum (10). All women with macroadenomas and those with microadenomas and elevated prolactin should be continued/started on dopamine agonist therapy, with endocrine follow-up. In women stable for over two years with microadenoma with normal prolactin and low dose of therapy, consideration can be given to stopping therapy (10). If therapy is stopped, close follow-up is necessary, as even in stable patients with normal prolactin, recurrence hyperprolactinemia is over 30% for microprolactinomas and >50% for macroprolactinomas (10). Other methods of contraception can be used, but oral estrogen-containing pills are also probably safe (10).

BREAST-FEEDING
A microadenoma is not a contraindication to nursing. If the woman has no neurologic symptoms at the time of delivery, nursing should not be of substantial risk. If she does have neurologic symptoms at the time of delivery or if they develop during nursing, she should be treated with a dopamine agonist.

Since the dopamine agonists suppress lactation, the woman on these drugs should be advised against breast-feeding.

REFERENCES

1. Schlechte JA. Prolactinoma. N Engl J Med 2003; 349:2035–2041. [III; review]
2. Gemzell C, Wang CF. Outcome of pregnancy in women with pituitary adenoma. Fertil Steril 1979; 31:363. [A survey of 25 physicians in 1979 revealed that they had seen a total of 91 pregnancies in 85 women with lactotroph microadenomas and 46 women with lactotroph macroadenomas were followed during 56 pregnancies]
3. Molitch ME. Management of prolactinomas during pregnancy. J Reprod Med 1999; 44:1121. [III; review]
4. Kupersmith MJ, Rosenberg C, Kleinberg D. Visual loss in pregnant women with pituitary adenomas. Ann Intern Med 1994; 121:473. [II-3]
5. Turkalj I, Braun P, Krupp P. Surveillance of bromocriptine in pregnancy. JAMA 1982; 247:1589. [The manufacturer of bromocriptine, surveyed physicians known to prescribe bromocriptine. The survey evaluated 1410 pregnancies in 1335 women who took the drug during pregnancy, primarily during the first month [5]. The incidence of spontaneous abortions (11.1 percent) and major (1%) and minor (2.5%) congenital malformations was similar to that in the general population. Only eight women had taken bromocriptine after the second month of pregnancy]
6. Molitch M. Pregnancy and the hyperprolactinemic woman. N Engl J Med 1985; 23:1364–1370. [II-c; safety of bromocriptine]
7. Robert E, Musatti L, Piscitelli G, et al. Pregnancy outcome after treatment with the ergot derivative, cabergoline. Reprod Toxicol 1996; 10:333. [II-3; $n = 226$]
8. Ricci E, Parazzini F, Motta T, et al. Pregnancy outcome after cabergoline treatment in early weeks of gestation. Reprod Toxicol 2002; 16:791–793. [II-3; cabergoline safety proven in 61 pregnancies]
9. Gonzalez JG, Elizondo G, Saldivar D, et al. Pituitary gland growth during normal pregnancy: an in vivo study using magnetic resonance imaging. Am J Med 1988; 85:217. [II-3]
10. Klibanski A. Prolactinomas. N Engl J Med 2010; 362:1219–1226. [III]
11. Flowers CM, Racoosin JA, Lu SL, et al. The US Food and Drug Administration's registry of patients with Pergolide-associated valvular heart disease. Mayo Clin Proc 2003; 78:730. [II-3]
12. Ahmed M, Al-Dossary E, Woodhouse NJY. Macroprolactinomas with suprasellar extension: effect of bromocriptine withdrawal during one or more pregnancies. Fertil Steril 1992; 58:492. [II-2]
13. Konopka P, Raymond JP, Merceron RE, et al. Continuous administration of bromocriptine in the prevention of neurological complications in pregnant women with prolactinomas. Am J Obstet Gynecol 1983; 146:935. [II-3]
14. Van Roon E, van der Vijver JC, Gerretsen G, et al. Rapid regression of a suprasellar extending prolactinoma after bromocriptine treatment during pregnancy. Fertil Steril 1981; 36:173. [II-3]
15. Liu C, Tyrrell JB. Successful treatment of a large macroprolactinoma with cabergoline during pregnancy. Pituitary 2001; 4:179. [II-3]

9

Nausea/vomiting of pregnancy and hyperemesis gravidarum

Maria Teresa Mella

KEY POINTS

- **Diagnosis of hyperemesis gravidarum is nausea and vomiting ≥3 times a day**, with **large ketones in urine** or acetone in blood (dehydration, fluid, and electrolytes changes), *and* **weight loss of >3 kg or >5% prepregnancy weight**, having excluded other diagnoses.
- Do not test for thyroid-stimulating hormone (TSH) in women with nausea/vomiting or hyperemesis gravidarum, unless they have a preexisting history/symptoms of hyperthyroidism.
- **For prevention, start prenatal vitamins before conception.**
- Start treating nausea and vomiting early, to prevent hyperemesis gravidarum.
- **Therapies proven to improve nausea, vomiting, and hyperemesis gravidarum are** (in approximate order of increasing risk/invasiveness/potency):
  - ○ Acupuncture
  - ○ Acupressure
  - ○ **Ginger capsules**
  - ○ **Vitamin B$_6$ with doxylamine in combination**
  - ○ **Metoclopramide**
  - ○ **Ondansetron**

DIAGNOSIS/DEFINITION
Hyperemesis Gravidarum

Severe **nausea and vomiting (n/v) ≥3 times a day, with large ketones in urine** or acetone in blood (dehydration—high urine specific gravity; fluid and electrolytes changes—hypokalemia), *and* **weight loss of >3 kg or >5% prepregnancy weight**, having excluded other diagnoses (diagnosis of exclusion).

N/v of pregnancy can be quite variable and symptoms can range from mild to severe (hyperemesis gravidarum, HG). Mild symptoms include intermittent nausea, odor and food aversion, retching, and occasional vomiting.

EPIDEMIOLOGY/INCIDENCE

About 75% of pregnant women have nausea and/or vomiting (25% are unaffected): 50% have both nausea and vomiting, while 25% have nausea only; 18% have more than once a day vomiting; **0.5% to 1% have true HG** (1,2). The onset is about 4 to 6 weeks, peak 8 to 12 weeks, resolution <20 weeks. HG is the most common indication for hospital admission in the first trimester of pregnancy and second to preterm labor throughout the entire pregnancy. Of the cases, 60% resolve by the end of the first trimester, and 91% have complete resolution by 20 weeks (2). Doubt diagnosis if symptoms start after 9 weeks. Not usually just "morning sickness" (3).

GENETICS

More common in first-degree relatives (daughters, sisters, monozygotic more than dizygotic twins). Daughters born to mothers with HG have a three times higher risk of future development (4).

ETIOLOGY

Hypotheses:

1. Gastrointestinal (GI) motility decreases in pregnancy because of increasing levels of progesterone (but not particularly in HG; probably secondary phenomenon).
2. Hormones (hCG, thyroxine, cortisol, etc.) trigger chemoreceptor trigger zone (CTZ), in brainstem-vomiting center.
3. CTZ more sensitive to hormones.
4. Abnormalities in vestibulo-ocular reflex pathway (5).
5. N/v correlates with the rise and fall of hCG. It has been theorized that hCG stimulates the ovary to produce more estrogen, which is known to increase n/v (2).
6. *Helicobacter pylori* (IgG 90.5% in HG patients, 47.5% in controls (6); no randomized controlled trials (RCTs) exist for treatment of *H. pylori* in HG) (7).
7. Possible psychologic predisposition, associated with unwanted, unplanned pregnancies, or excessive life stressors (and conversion disorder) (8). Of women with HG report, 85% have poor support by partner.

Some have also postulated that n/v is evolutionary, to protect the fetus from teratogenic exposures since time frame correlates with the period of organogenesis.

CLASSIFICATION

A pregnancy-unique quantification of emesis/nausea (PUQE) index has been proposed, validated, and recently slightly modified (9,10) (Table 9.1). Management is based mostly on woman's perception of severity and desire for treatment.

RISK FACTORS/ASSOCIATIONS

Young maternal age; nulliparity; prior HG (recurrence in about 67%); female fetus; history of motion sickness, migraines, or psychiatric illness; preexisting hyperthyroidism, diabetes, GI disorders, or asthma (11). Associated with high hCG levels (larger placental mass as in multiple pregnancy, molar pregnancy, Trisomy 21 [T21]); high estradiol levels (if n/v on oral contraceptive pills, woman will probably get n/v in pregnancy). Smoking is associated with lower levels of hCG and estradiol, and therefore smokers have lower incidence of HG (11).

Very little is known regarding **ptyalism** (aka sialorrhea, excessive salivation). Diagnosis: salivation >1900 mL/day;

Table 9.1 PUQE Score

1. On an average day, for how long do you feel nauseated or sick to your stomach?				
>6 hr	4–6 hr	2–3 hr	≤1 hr	Not at all
(5 points)	(4 points)	(3 points)	(2 points)	(1 point)
2. On an average day, how many times do you vomit or throw up?				
≥7	5–6	3–4	1–2	None
(5 points)	(4 points)	(3 points)	(2 points)	(1 point)
3. On an average day, how many times do you have retching or dry heaves without bringing anything up?				
≥7	5–6	3–4	1–2	None
(5 points)	(4 points)	(3 points)	(2 points)	(1 point)

Modified Pregnancy-Unique Quantification of Emesis/Nausea (PUQE) index. Total score is sum of replies to each of the items of the three questions. **Mild NVP, ≤6; moderate NVP, 7–12; severe NVP, ≥13.** *Source:* Adapted from Ref. 10.

etiologic hypothesis: stimulation by starch (possibly pica). It is characterized by inability to swallow, not excessive production. No therapy (gum, lozengers, small meals, anticholinergics, ganglion-blocking agents, oxyphenonium bromide, etc.) has been studied appropriately or shown to be efficacious in pregnancy. Check hydration, nutrition, psychologic status, and other issues as per n/v (12).

COMPLICATIONS
Maternal
Minimal complications in mild cases of n/v. For HG, diminished quality of life may lead to decision for termination [2.9% in Sweden (13) or depression. Rare: Wernicke's encephalopathy (vitamin B1 deficiency; permanent neurologic disability or maternal death), peripheral neuropathies (vitamin B_6 and B_{12} deficiency), central pontine myelinolysis, splenic avulsion, esophageal rupture, pneumothorax, or acute tubular necrosis. In extreme and very rare cases of HG, maternal death can occur.

Fetal/Neonatal
Minimal complications in mild cases of n/v; no increased fetal growth restriction (FGR) and no higher incidence of congenital anomalies. Severe HG, usually necessitating parental nutrition, is associated with FGR and fetal death.

N/v and HG are also associated with lower incidence of pregnancy loss (secondary to robust placental synthesis) and high health care costs (time lost from work).

PREGNANCY MANAGEMENT
Principles
Prevention is better than treatment, that is, **intervening early in nausea/vomiting is helpful in preventing worsening symptoms** (14). HG is a diagnosis of exclusion. N/v tends to be undertreated by both some physicians and some patients, while there are many safe and effective therapies that exist. Approximately 10% of patients with n/v during pregnancy will require medication (2).

Workup
Differential diagnostic possibilities should be ruled out, such as gastrointestinal (gastroenteritis, gallbladder disease, hepatitis, pancreatitis, appendicitis, inflammatory bowel disease), genitourinary, ovarian torsion, thyrotoxicosis, diabetic ketoacidosis, Addison's disease, brain tumor, migraine, vestibular lesion, pseudotumor cerebri, food/drug poisoning/toxicity, acute fatty liver/preeclampsia, and others (Table 9.2) (15).

Table 9.2 Differential Diagnosis of Nausea and Vomiting of Pregnancy

Gastrointestinal conditions
- Gastroparesis/Ileus
- Gastroenteritis
- Cyclic vomiting syndrome
- Achalasia
- Biliary tract disease
- Hepatitis
- Intestinal obstruction
- Peptic ulcer disease/*H. pylori*
- Pancreatitis
- Appendicitis
- Inflammatory bowel disease

Genitourinary tract conditions
- Pyelonephritis
- Uremia
- Ovarian torsion
- Fibroid degeneration
- Kidney stones
- Degenerating uterine fibroids

Metabolic diseases
- Diabetic ketoacidosis
- Porphyria
- Addison's disease
- Hyperthyroidism

Neurologic disorders
- Pseudotumor cerebri
- Vestibular lesions
- Migraines
- Tumors of the central nervous system

Miscellaneous
- Drug toxicity or intolerance
- Psychologic
- Neoplasia

Pregnancy-related conditions
- Acute fatty livery of pregnancy
- Preeclampsia
- Trophoblastic disease
- Multiple gestations

Source: Adapted from Ref. 15.

History and Review of Systems
Special attention to severity of n/v, weight loss, prior GI diagnosis, and stressors—dietary, physical, and psychologic. Abdominal pain, fever, headache/migraine are atypical complaints of a patient with n/v of pregnancy.

Physical Exam
Special attention to vital signs, signs of dehydration, goiter, and abdominal and neurologic examinations.

Labs
> *Serum* (especially for severe cases): Electrolytes, BUN, creatinine, glucose, LFTs, amylase, lipase, acetone (quantitative hCG not helpful in management)
> *Urine*: ketones, specific gravity
> *Thyroid-stimulating hormone (TSH)*: **No need to send TSH** (60–70% of HG have "transient biochemical hyperthyroidism of pregnancy" with decreased TSH and increased free thyroid index; this is secondary to hCG-stimulating thyroxine synthesis from pituitary; always resolves spontaneously in 1 to 10 weeks (16,17); only test if pregnant woman has a history of thyroid disease or goiter).

Radiologic
Fetal ultrasound (to assess for molar pregnancy, multiple gestation, etc.)

Consults
Occasionally consider psychiatry consult, nutrition, or gastroenterology involvement depending on history.

Therapy
Prevention
Prenatal multivitamin (MVI) before/at conception. Vitamin B$_6$ found in MVI has been shown to reduce the incidence of n/v (18).

Suggested Stepwise Therapeutic Approach (Fig. 9.1)
Several interventions are available for treatment of n/v and HG (19) (Table 9.3). It is suggested to intervene early on n/v. A combination of interventions is often necessary. We suggest moving sequentially on the PUQE index assessment score if n/v persists. For HG, consider starting at least at step 3, but still consider implementing steps 1 and 2 as appropriate. Any underlining/concomitant GI disorder (reflux, ulcer, anorexia, etc.) should be treated appropriately.

STEP 1
Lifestyle/Dietary Changes
Avoid odor/food triggers. Stop medications (e.g., iron, large vitamins) producing n/v. Counsel regarding safety and efficacy of treatment; provide reassurance regarding outcomes (see above). There is no evidence that rest improves n/v. Diet includes frequent, small meals: eat only one spoonful, wait, eat again, and so on; avoid an empty stomach; eat crackers in the morning upon waking; avoid fatty greasy spicy foods; ginger ale; prefer protein, but prolonged high-protein diet is associated with higher incidences of preterm birth and fetal death.

STEP 2
Drugs/Interventions
The drugs/interventions in the following subsections have been evaluated in at least one RCT showing efficacy (19):

Nonpharmacologic
Acupressure Wrist Bands
Acupressure at P6 "Neiguan" point (20–29) (Brands: Seaband; Bioband) has been associated with benefit in several RCTs, but not in one of the largest, placebo-controlled ones (26). An RCT showed no significant difference between P6 acupressure versus vitamin B$_6$ therapy (29). There are no pregnancy safety or

breast-feeding concerns. This intervention therefore can be reserved for women who decline pharmaceutical interventions.

Acustimulation Wrist Bands
Acustimulation at P6 Neiguan point (30,31) (Brand: Relief Band Device, Woodside Biomedical—http://www.reliefband.com). This device for noninvasive nerve electric stimulation was associated with less n/v and higher weight gain compared to placebo (30,31), but in the largest RCT the assessment of the outcomes was not blinded and the study was industry-sponsored by the makers of the device (31). There are limited pregnancy safety or breast-feeding concerns.

Auricular Acupressure
Auricular acupressure has shown effectiveness, but with limited data available (32).
> There are no pregnancy safety or breast-feeding concerns.

Acupuncture
One trial of **acupuncture** was as effective in treating nausea of pregnancy as a sham procedure (33), but a larger trial showed that acupuncture is an **effective treatment** for women with n/v in pregnancy (34).

Ginger
Several RCTs demonstrate benefit of ginger compared to placebo (35–39), and better efficacy for decrease in nausea compared to vitamin B$_6$ therapy (40–44). An RCT showed that ginger is as effective as dimenhydrate (45). Ginger use has been suggested as early therapy in outpatients (42,46). Side effects include reflux and heartburn.

> **In summary, ginger is the only nonpharmacologic intervention shown to be consistently beneficial for n/v in multiple RCTs, and so should be used** (Fig. 9.1). Acupressure and/or acupuncture can be considered, but evidence of effectiveness is still insufficient. Several other nonpharmacologic alternatives such as hypnotherapy, behavioral therapy, chamomile, peppermint, and raspberry leaf have not been assessed in RCTs. Hypnosis decreased vomiting in one nonrandomized study (47).

Pharmacologic

STEP 3
> *Vitamin B$_6$ (pyridoxine).* Associated with decrease in nausea, not in vomiting (48,49). When used in women hospitalized for HG, it does not seem to affect n/v (50). So, for women with vomiting, it is best to use in combination with doxylamine.
> *Doxylamine and vitamin B$_6$.* This combination (formerly known as Bendectin and available as Unisom Sleeptabs in the United States, Diclectin in Canada, Debendox in the United Kingdom) is safe, with no evidence of teratogenicity (proven with over 200,000 exposures, by far the most for any other drug in pregnancy), and effective (>70% decrease in n/v) (2,15). Doxylamine and vitamin B$_6$ are associated with decrease in both nausea and vomiting when used together compared to no therapy or placebo (51–54). A double-blind RCT showed Diclectin (a doxylamine-pyridoxine delayed-release preparation available) to significantly improve n/v and quality of life compared to placebo (54).
> **In summary, if n/v persist even after step 1 and 2, add vitamin B$_6$ and doxylamine orally.**

STEP 4
> *Other antihistamines (histamine-1 receptor antagonists).* Other antihistamines are safe (Table 9.3) and often used.

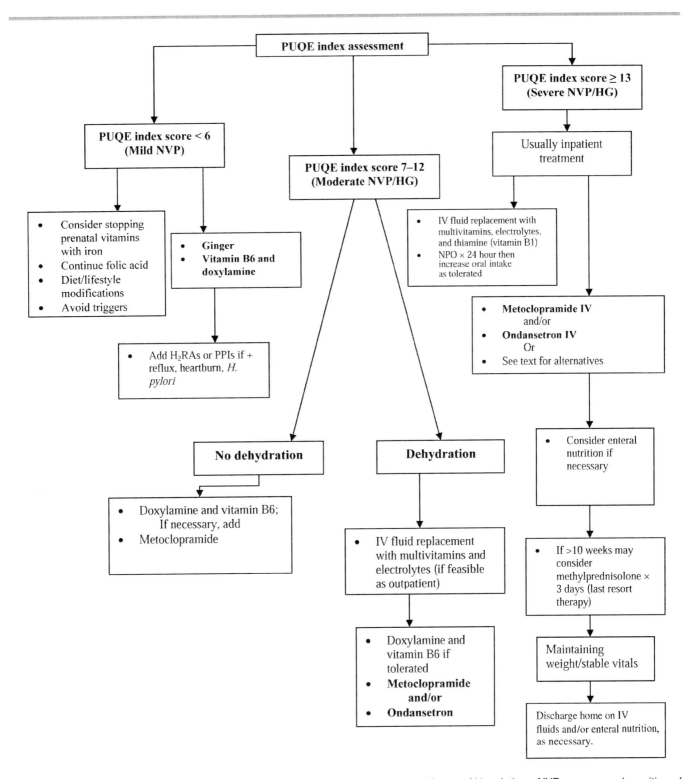

Figure 9.1 Management of nausea, vomiting of pregnancy, and hyperemesis gravidarum. *Abbreviations*: NVP, nausea and vomiting of pregnancy; HG, hyperemesis gravidarum; IV, intravenous; NPO, nil per os or nothing by mouth; H₂RAs, histamine₂ receptor antagonists; PPIs, proton pump inhibitors. *Source*: Adapted from Ref. 46

These include diphenhydramine, meclizine, hydroxizine, and dimenhydrinate, used mostly for relief of vestibular-type symptoms. An RCT showed that dimenhydrinate is as effective as ginger in the treatment of n/v with fewer side effects (45). No RCTs exist for the other histamine-1 receptor antagonists (H₁RAs) to assess their effectiveness for n/v in preg-nancy or HG. Do *not* use diazepam, a category D drug, because of possible fetal effects, despite one trial on its efficacy (55).

Histamine-2 receptor antagonists. Cimetidine, famotidine, ranitidine, and nizatidine are approved for use in pregnancy to treat symptoms of heartburn, acid reflux, and *H. pylori*, which can exacerbate n/v. They may be added if symptoms are

Table 9.3 Selected Treatment of Nausea and Vomiting and HG in Pregnancy

Agent	Oral dose	Side effects	FDA category	Comments
Ginger extract				
Vitamin B$_6$ (pyridoxine)	125–250 mg tid/qid, po	Reflux, heartburn	C	Step 2; OTC availability, food supplement
	10–25 mg q8h po, do not exceed 100 mg qd		A	Step 3; recommended as first-line pharmacologic intervention
Doxylamine (Unisom sleep tabs); Antihistamine	12.5–25 mg q8h		A	Step 3
Vitamin B$_6$–doxylamine combination	Pyridoxine, 10–25 mg q8h, po; doxylamine, 25 mg qhs, 12.5 mg bid prn, po	Sedation	A	Step 3; take before onset of symptoms, taper dose; Dicletin (extended release form)
Other Antihistamines (H$_1$-receptor antagonists)		Sedation, dizziness, drowsiness, anticholinergic effects	Step 4; good for acute relief of vestibular-type symptoms	
• Diphenhydramine (Benadryl)	25–50 mg q4–6h prn; po, IV, IM Maximum: 100 mg/dose, 400 mg/day		B	
• Meclizine (Bonine, Antivert)	25–50 mg q6h, po; maximum: 100 mg/24 hr		B	
• Hydroxyzine (Atarax, Vistaril)	25–100 mg q6–8h prn, po/IM; maximum: 600 mg/24 h		C	
• Dimenhydrinate (Dramamine)	50–100 mg q4–6h, po/pr/IM or 50 mg IV (in 50cc saline over 20 min) q4–6h IV (not to exceed 400 mg/day, or 200 mg/day if also doxylamine)		B	
H$_2$ receptor antagonists			B	Step 4; for patients with reflux, *H. pylori*
• Cimetidine (Tagamet)	1600 mg qd divided bid/qid			
• Famotidine (Pepcid)	20–40 mg bid, po/IV			
• Ranitidine (Zantac)	75–150 mg prn, po (maximum 2 tabs/24 hr); 50 mg q6h IM/IV			
Proton Pump Inhibitors (PPIs)			B	Step 4; Second line for reflux symptoms
• Omeprazole (Prilosec)	20–40 mg qd, po (maximum 80 mg/day)			
• Pantoprazole (Protonix)	40 mg bid, po			
• Esomeprazole (Nexium)	20–40 mg qd, po/NG/IV (maximum: 80 mg/day)			
• Lansoprazole (Prevacid)	15–30 mg qd, po			
Phenothiazines (D$_2$-receptor antagonists)		Sedation; ↓BP if given too quickly, Parkinsons' tremors, rash, anticholinergic side effects, tardive dyskinesia		Step 4
• Promethazine (Phenergan)	12.5–25 mg q4–6h, po/pr/IM/IV (maximum: 50 mg/dose po/IM; 25 mg/dose IV)	Severe tissue injury with undiluted IV use	C	
• Prochlorperazine maleate (Compazine; Bukatel)	5–10 mg q4–6h; po/IM/IV/ buccal, 10–25 mg q6h pr (maximum:10 mg/dose, 40 mg/day)	D/c if unexplained decrease in WBCs	C	Buccal form is costly
Dopamine$_2$–antagonists				
• Trimethobenzamide (Tigan)	300 mg tid/qid, po; 200 mg tid/qid, IM	Sedation, anticholinergic effects	C	Step 4/5 Dopamine antagonist directly to emetic center CTZ
• **Metoclopramide (Reglan)**	10–20 mg q6–8 h, po/IM/IV; 1–2 mg/kg IV continuous subQ pump available	Tardive dyskinesia with increased duration of use (>12 wk) and high total cumulative dose.	B	Second-line therapy. Also available for pump therapy. Stimulates GI tract motility.

Table 9.3 Selected Treatment of Nausea and Vomiting and HG in Pregnancy (Continued)

Drug	Dose	Category	Side effects	Notes
● Droperidol (Inapsine)	0.625–2.5 mg over 15 min, then 1.25 or 2.5 mg IM q3–4h prn, IM or continuous IV at 1–1.25 mg/hr (maximum: 2.5 mg/dose, slow push over 2–5 min, repeat doses with caution)	C	Black box warning of torsades	Give with benadryl to prevent extrapyramidal symptoms
5-hydroxytryptamine3 (5-HT3) receptor antagonist				
● Odansetron (Zofran)	4–8 mg tid/qid po; 4–8 mg over 15 min q12h IV; or 1 mg/hr continuous for 24 hr	B	Constipation, diarrhea, headache, fatigue, mild sedation.	Step 5 Also available for pump therapy. Comes as oral dissolving tablet→$$
Glucocorticoid				
● Methylprednisolone (Medrol)	125–250 mg q6h	C	Increased risk of cleft lip if used before 10 wk gestation	6 wk for maximum duration, when other therapies have failed. If no improvement after 72 hr, stop. May be tapered over 1–2 wk

Bold: therapies with best level I evidence for efficacy; underline: at least 1 RCT in pregnancy. So therapies listed with no bolding or underlining have no RCT(s) consistently proving efficacy in pregnancy. Food and Drug Administration (FDA) categories are as follows: A, controlled studies show no risk; B, no evidence of risk in humans; C, risk cannot be ruled out; D, positive evidence of risk; and X, contraindicated in pregnancy (http://www.fda.gov/). *Abbreviations*: po, per os; IV, intravenous; IM, intramuscular; pr, per rectum; NG, nasogastric; buccal, cheek; qd, once daily; bid, twice a day; tid, three times a day; qid, four times a day; qhs, quaque hora somni or given at bedtime; q4h, given every four hours; q6h, given every 6 hours; q8h, given every eight hours; /24hr, every 24 hours; prn, pro re nata or take as needed; OTC, over the counter medication; min, minute; divd, divided; BP, blood pressure; WBCs, white blood cells; SubQ, subcutaneous; GI, gastrointestinal; CTZ, chemoreceptor trigger zone; D/c, discontinue; $$, expensive.

present. No RCTs exist regarding their effectiveness for n/v or HG. A meta-analysis showed no increased risk of congenital malformations, risk of spontaneous abortions, or preterm delivery compared to controls (56). In intractable cases of n/v with positive *H. pylori* serology, a nonrandomized study suggested benefit with triple therapy with ranitidine/flagyl/ampicillin (57).

Proton-pump inhibitors. Common proton-pump inhibitors (PPIs) used in pregnancy are omeprazole, pantoprazole, esomeprazole, and lansoprazole. These can be used in conjunction with or separately from histamine-2 receptor antagonists (H2RAs) for heartburn and reflux, and *H. pylori* infections. A recent meta-analysis (58) and separate cohort study (59) showed that there is no evidence to suggest that the use of PPIs anytime during pregnancy increases the overall risk of birth defects, preterm delivery, or spontaneous abortion. There are no RCTs on this intervention for n/v of pregnancy or HG.

Dopamine-2 antagonist. **Metoclopramide** (Reglan) is safe in pregnancy without increased risk of teratogenicity, preterm birth, low birth weight, or perinatal mortality (60,61). An RCT showed that metoclopramide (with one IM shot of 50 mg of pyridoxine) is superior in decreasing vomiting and subjective improvement compared to monotherapy with either prochlorperazine or promethazine (62). A recent RCT of inpatient HG patients showed that **metoclopramide** 10-mg IV q8h had similar efficacy and decreased drowsiness/dizziness when compared to IV promethazine (63). A subcutaneous Reglan pump is an alternative mode of administering the drug, not yet tested in any pregnancy RCT (64).

Phenothiazines. Phenothiazines [prochlorperazine, promethazine (Phenergan)] are safe (Table 9.3). A case-control study of promethazine showed no evidence of increase risk/rate of congenital anomalies in humans (65). Phenothiazines are often used in addition to or instead of antihistamines. The level 1 evidence for effectiveness is limited. As said above, metoclopramide (with one IM shot of 50 mg of pyridoxine) is superior in decreasing vomiting and subjective improvement compared to monotherapy with either prochlorperazine or promethazine (62). Compared to prednisolone, promethazine has a more rapid effect on decreasing symptoms of HG (66).

In summary, if n/v persist even with steps 1 to 3, metoclopramide can be added. Phenergan can also be considered, with limited evidence of effectiveness. If symptoms of reflux, heartburn, or *H. pylori* are present, H2RAs and PPIs can also be considered.

STEP 5
5-HT3 receptor antagonist
Ondansetron (Zofran) Serotonin 5-hydroxytryptamine-3 receptor antagonist. Safe in pregnancy (67). At least as effective as Phenergan 50 mg q8h, but probably better (68). Used in refractory cases. No RCTs for Zofran pump, very costly.

Corticosteroids. In general, do *not* use steroids to treat HG or just n/v of pregnancy, or use only as last resort for maximum of three days. Usual dosing is methylprednisolone 16 mg po/IV tid, prednisolone 20 mg po bid, or hydrocortisone 300 mg IV qd. Safety data include possible increased incidence of oral cleft if used <10 weeks (2). There are significant maternal side effects. Adrenocorticoticotropic hormone (ACTH) is not beneficial (69); IV then po methylprednisolone is not better than placebo (70); methylprednisolone is more effective than promethazine in one RCT (71) but not in another (66); prednisone is not beneficial (72); IV hydrocortisone is better than IV metoclopramide for symptom relief and decreased readmission in a small RCT (73).

In summary, if n/v persists despite steps 1 to 4, consider ondansetron therapy. In refractory cases, consider combination of effective therapies described above. Use corticosteroids as last resort after 10 weeks' gestation.

STEP 6
Inpatient management. Admit only if HG diagnosis is confirmed, woman is not tolerating oral intake, and failed outpatient management. Some suggest just brief ER visits for severe cases needing emergent hydration. Home infusion services should be used as much as safely possible. Admission by itself does not improve HG, and should be limited.

Diet. Nothing per mouth (NPO) at first; with improvement, advance to small dry meals (see above).

Intravenous fluid (IVF) hydration. IV fluids can be used if dehydration is present. Volume should be adequate to replenish loss and ongoing loss through vomiting. Normal saline or lactated ringers solution recommended over dextrose containing fluids. The dextrose in IVFs increases the body's requirements for thiamine and therefore increases the likelihood of Wernicke's encephalopathy in thiamine-deficient patients (74). Add thiamine 100 mg qd for two to three days, then multivitamins to IV fluids. Hypertonic solutions should be avoided; rapid overcorrection of hyponatremia may cause central pontine myelinolysis. Can also add potassium (20–40 mmol/L).

Pharmacologic therapy. A combination antiemetic therapy as above, especially steps 3 to 5, can be used. First IV/IM therapy around the clock, then IV only prn, then oral therapy when tolerated. Acupressure is not effective for inpatient treatment of HG (75).

Disposition. Woman can be discharged home on IV fluids and/or parenteral nutrition (PN) as long as stable, not losing weight, or other factors. If persistent weight loss or dehydration (e.g., over five to seven days despite aggressive inpatient therapy), consider consulting gastroenterology, and either enteral or parenteral nutrition.

ENTERAL NUTRITION: NASOGASTRIC TUBE
These are of several types (e.g., 8 French Dobbhoff).

Mechanism
Avoid contact/smell of food. This intervention is best used for persistent n/v, with no response to antiemetic therapy. There are no trials of comparison between nasogastric (NG) tube or PN. Since PN is associated with several possible complications, NG tube should be tried first, as tolerated (15).

Nutrition (Harris–Benedict Equation)
$$655 + [9.6 \times wt(kg)] + [1.8 \times ht(cm)] - [4.7 - age(yr)]$$

Order enteric nutrition in consultation with nutrition service. Basal energy expenditure plus 300 cal (pregnancy); divide by 24 hour. Start at 25 mL/hr, increase by 25 mL/hr until goal. Then give over 8 to 12 hours overnight (76).

Complications
Poorly tolerated by some women; NG tube occlusion.

PARENTERAL NUTRITION
Several catheters and regimens are possible [peripherally inserted central catheter (PICC), midline IV, etc.]; individualize and consult nutrition.

Generally PN is associated with high incidence of catheter complications, for example, infection, leading to sepsis, (about 25%) thrombosis/occlusion, and dislodgement/mechanical failure, with no effect on neonatal outcome (77–80). Peripheral catheters have high morbidity, and central catheters have central access complications. Other complications include pneumothorax, cholestasis, preterm birth, and fetal death. This is an expensive therapy, to be used only when HG is refractory to treatment, with significant weight loss (>5%), and failure of enteral nutrition.

OTHER ISSUES

Consider psychiatric consult in severe, refractory-to-therapy cases. Psychotherapy has not been evaluated in any trial.

Postpartum

The risk of recurrence of HG (2,4,15) is about 15% (vs. 0.7% in controls without prior HG). The risk is reduced by change in paternity (81).

REFERENCES

1. Askling J, Erlandsson G, Kaijser M, et al. Sickness in pregnancy and sex of child. Lancet 1999; 354:2053. [II-3]
2. Niebyl JR. Nausea and vomiting in pregnancy. N Engl J Med 2010; 363:1544–1550. [Review]
3. Lacroix R, Eason E, Melzack R. Nausea and vomiting during pregnancy: a prospective study of its frequency, intensity, and patterns of change. Am J Obstet Gynecol 2000; 182:931–937. [II-3]
4. Vikanes A, Skjaerven R, Grijbovski AM, et al. Recurrence of hyperemesis gravidarum across generations: a population based cohort study. BMJ 2010; 340:c2050. [II-2]
5. Goodwin TM, Nwankwo OA, O'Leary LD, et al. The first demonstration that a subset of women with hyperemesis gravidarum has abnormalities in the vestibuloocular reflex pathway. Am J Obstet Gynecol 2008; 199:417.e1–417.e9. [II-3]
6. Frigo P, Lang C, Reisenberger K, et al. Hyperemesis gravidarum associated with *Helicobacter pylori* seropositivity. Obstet Gynecol 1998; 91:615–617. [II-3]
7. Sandven I, Abdelnoor M, Nesheim BI, et al. *Helicobacter pylori* infection and hyperemesis gravidarum: a systematic review and meta-analysis of case–control studies. Acta Obstet Gynecol Scand 2009; 88:1190–1200. [Meta-analysis, 25 case-control studies, 3425pts total, 1970 controls]
8. El-Mallakh RS, Liebowitz NR, Hale MS. Hypermesesis gravidarum as conversion disorder. J Nerv Ment Dis 1990; 178(10):655–659. [II-3]
9. Koren G, Boskovic R, Hard M, et al. Motherisk–PUQE (pregnancy-unique quantification of emesis and nausea) scoring system for nausea and vomiting of pregnancy. Am J Obstet Gynecol 2002; 186(5 suppl):s228–s231. [II-3]
10. Lacasse A, Rey E, Ferreira E, et al. Validity of a modified Pregnancy-Unique Quantification of Emesis and Nausea (PUQE) scoring index to assess severity of nausea and vomiting of pregnancy. Am J Obstet Gynecol 2008; 198(1):71.e1–71.e7. [II-3]
11. Fell DB, Dodds L, Joseph KS, et al. Risk factors for hyperemesis gravidarum requiring hospital admission during pregnancy. Obstet Gynecol 2006; 107(2 pt1):277–284. [II-2]
12. Van Dinter MC. Ptyalism in pregnant women. J Obstet Gynecol Neonatal Nurs 1991; 20:206–209. [Review]
13. Jarnfelt-Samsioe A, Eriksson B, Waldenström J, et al. Some new aspects on emesis gravidarum. Relations to clinical data, serum electrolytes, total protein and creatinine. Gynecol Obstet Invest 1985; 19:174–186. [II-2]
14. Brent R. Medical, social, and legal implications of treating nausea and vomiting of pregnancy. Am J Obstet Gynecol 2002; 186:s262–s266. [Review]
15. American College of Obstetrics and Gynecology. Nausea and vomiting of pregnancy. ACOG Practice Bulletin No. 52. Obstet Gynecol 2004; 103:803–815. [Review]
16. Goodwin TM, Montoro M, Mestman JH. Transient hyperthyroidism and hyperemesis gravidarum: clinical aspects. Am J Obstet Gynecol 1992; 167:648–652. [II-3]
17. Goodwin TM, Mestman J. Transient hyperthyroidism of hyperemesis gravidarum. Contemp Obstet Gynecol 1996; 6:65–78. [II-3, and review]
18. Czeizel AE, Dudas I, Fritz G, et al. The effect of periconceptional multivitamin-mineral supplementation on vertigo, nausea and vomiting. Arch Gynecol Obstet 1992; 251:181–185. [RCT, n = 48]
19. Matthews A, Dowswell T, Haas DM, et al. Interventions for nausea and vomiting in early pregnancy. Cochrane Database Syst Rev 2010; 9:CD007575. [Meta-analysis: n = 4041pts, 27 RCTs]
20. Murphy PA. Alternative therapies for nausea and vomiting of pregnancy. Obstet Gynecol 1998; 91:149–155. [Meta-analysis; 10 RCTs; 7 RCTs on acupressure]
21. Dundee JW, Sourial FB, Ghaly RG, et al. P6 acupressure reduces morning sickness. J Royal Soc Med 1988; 81(8):456–457. [RCT]
22. Hyde E. Acupressure therapy for morning sickness. A controlled clinical trial. J Nurse Midwifery 1989; 34(4):171–178. [RCT]
23. de Aloysio D, Penacchioni P. Morning sickness control in early pregnancy by Neiguan point acupressure. Obstet Gynecol 1992; 80(5):852–854. [RCT]
24. Bayreuther J, Lewith GT, Pickering R. A double-blind cross-over study to evaluate the effectiveness of acupressure at pericardium 6 (P6) in the treatment of early morning sickness (EMS). Complem Ther Med 1994; 2:70–76. [RCT, n = 23]
25. Belluomini J, Litt RC, Lee KA, et al. Acupressure for nausea and vomiting of pregnancy: a randomized, blinded study. Obstet Gynecol 1994; 84(2):245–248. [RCT]
26. O'Brien B, Relyea MJ, Taerum T. Efficacy of P6 acupressure in the treatment of nausea and vomiting during pregnancy. Am J Obstet Gynecol 1996; 174:708–715. [RCT]
27. Werntoft E, Dykes AK. Effect of acupressure on nausea and vomiting during pregnancy. J Reprod Med 2001; 46:835–839. [RCT, n = 60]
28. Shin HS, Song YA, Seo S. Effect of Neiguan point (P6) acupressure on ketonuria, nausea, and vomiting in women with hyperemesis gravidarum. J Adv Nurs 2007; 59:510–519. [RCT, n = 66]
29. Jamigorn M, Phupong V. Acupressure and vitamin B_6 to relieve nausea and vomiting in pregnancy: a randomized study. Archives Gynecol Obstet 2007; 276(3):245–249. [RCT, n = 66]
30. Evans AT, Samuels SN, Marshall C, et al. Suppression of pregnancy-induced nausea and vomiting with sensory afferent stimulation. J Repro Med 1993; 38:603–606. [RCT, n = 23]
31. Rosen T, de Veciana M, Miller HS, et al. A randomized controlled trial of nerve stimulation for relief of nausea and vomiting in pregnancy. Obstet Gynecol 2003; 102:129–135. [RCT, n = 230]
32. Puangsricharern A, Mahasukhon S. Effectiveness of auricular acupressure in the treatment of nausea and vomiting in early pregnancy. J Med Assoc Thai 2008; 91(11):1633–1638. [RCT, n = 98]
33. Knight B, Mudge C, Openshaw S, et al. Effect of acupuncture on nausea of pregnancy: a randomized, controlled trial. Obstet Gynecol 2001; 97:184–188. [RCT, n = 55]
34. Smith C, Crowther C, Beilby J. Acupuncture to treat nausea and vomiting in early pregnancy: a randomized controlled trial. Birth 2002; 29:1–9. [RCT, n = 593]
35. Fischer-Rasmussen W, Kjaer SK, Dahl C, et al. Ginger treatment of hyperemesis gravidarum. Eur J Obstet Gynecol Reprod Biol 1991; 38:19–24. [RCT, n = 27]
36. Vutyavanich T, Kraisarin T, Ruangsri R. Ginger for nausea and vomiting in pregnancy: randomized, double-masked, placebo-controlled trial. Obstet Gynecol 2001; 97:577–582. [RCT, n = 70]
37. Keating A, Chez RA. Ginger syrup as an antiemetic in early pregnancy. Altern Ther Health Med 2002; 8:89–91. [RCT, n = 26]
38. Willetts C, Ekanganki A, Eden JA. Effect of a ginger extract on pregnancy-induced nausea: a randomized trial. Austr N Z J Obstet Gynaecol 2003; 43:139–144. [RCT, n = 120]

39. Ozgoli G, Goli M, Simbar M. Effects of ginger capsules on pregnancy, nausea, and vomiting. J Altern Complement Med 2009; 15(3):243–246. [RCT, n = 70]

40. Sripramote M, Lekhyananda N. A randomized comparison of ginger and vitamin B6 in the treatment of nausea and vomiting in pregnancy. J Med Assoc Thai 2003; 86:846–853. [RCT, n = 128]

41. Smith C, Crowther C, Willson K, et al. A randomized controlled trial of ginger to treat nausea and vomiting in pregnancy. Obstet Gynecol 2004; 103:639–645. [RCT, n = 291]

42. Borrelli F, Capasso R, Aviello G, et al. Effectiveness and safety of ginger in the treatment of pregnancy-induced nausea and vomiting. Obstet Gynecol 2005; 105:849–856. [Meta-analysis; 6 RCTs, n = 675]

43. Chittumma P, Kaewkiattikun K, Wiriyasiriwach B. Comparison of the effectiveness of ginger and vitamin B6 for treatment of nausea and vomiting in early pregnancy: a randomized double-blind controlled trial. J Med Assoc Thai 2007; 90(1):15–20. [RCT, n = 126]

44. Ensiyeh J, Sakineh MAC. Comparing ginger and vitamin B6 for the treatment of nausea and vomiting in pregnancy: a randomized controlled trial. Midwifery 2009; 25(6):649–653. [RCT, n = 70]

45. Pongrojpaw D, Somprasit C, Chanthasenanont A. A randomized comparison of ginger and dimenhydrinate in the treatment of nausea and vomiting in pregnancy. J Med Assoc Thai 2007; 90 (9):1703–1709. [RCT, n = 170]

46. King TL, Murphy PA. Evidence-based approaches to managing nausea and vomiting in early pregnancy. J Midwifery Womens Health 2009; 54:430–444. [Meta-analysis review]

47. Apfel RJ, Kelly SF, Frankel FH. The role of hypnotazibility in the pathogenesis and treatment of nausea and vomiting of pregnancy. J Psychosom Obstet Gynecol 1986; 5:179–186. [II-3]

48. Sahakian V, Rouse D, Sipes S, et al. Vitamin B6 is effective therapy for nausea and vomiting of pregnancy: a randomized double-blind placebo-controlled study. Obstet Gynecol 1991; 78:33. [RCT, n = 59; vitamin B6 25-mg orally q8h × 72hr versus placebo]

49. Vutyavanich T, Wongtrangan S, Ruangsri RA. Pyridoxine for nausea and vomiting of pregnancy: a randomized, double-blind, placebo-controlled trial. Am J Obstet Gynecol 1995; 173:881–884. [RCT, n = 342; vitamin B6 30-mg orally q8h versus placebo]

50. Tan PC, Yow CM, Omar ST. A placebo-controlled trial of oral pyridoxine in hyperemesis gravidarum. Gynecol Obstet Invest 2009; 77:151–157. [RCT, n = 92]

51. Geiger CJ, Fahrenbach DM, Healey FJ. Bendectin in the treatment of nausea and vomiting in pregnancy. Obstet Gynecol 1959; 14:688–690. [RCT, n = 110]

52. McGuiness BW, Binns DT. "Debendox" in pregnancy sickness. J R Coll Gen Pract 1971; 21:500–503. [RCT, n = 81]

53. Wheatley D. Treatment of pregnancy sickness. Br J Obstet Gynecol 1977; 84:444–447. [RCT, n = 56]

54. Koren G, Clark S, Hankins GDV, et al. Effectiveness of delayed-release doxylamine and pyridoxine for nausea and vomiting of pregnancy: a randomized placebo controlled trial. Am J Obstet Gynecol 2010; 203:571.e1–571.e7. [RCT, n = 256]

55. Ditto A, Morgante G, la Marca A, et al. Evaluation of treatment of hyperemesis gravidarum using parenteral fluid with or without diazepam. A randomized study. Gynecol Obstet Invest 1999; 48:232–236. [RCT, n = 50]

56. Gill SK, O'Brien L, Koren G. The safety of histamine 2 (H2) blockers in pregnancy: a meta-analysis. Dig Dis Sci 2009; 54 (9):1835–1838. [II-3, n = 2398 patients]

57. Mansour GM, Nashaat EH. Role of Helicobacter pylori in the pathogenesis of hyperemesis gravidarum. Arch Gynecol Obstet 2010. DOI 10.1007/s00404-010-1759-8. [II-1, n = 160]

58. Gill SK, O'Brien L, Einarson TR, et al. The safety of proton pump inhibitors (PPIs) in pregnancy: a meta-analysis. Am J Gastroenterol 2009; 104:1541–1545. [Meta-analysis]

59. Pasternak B, Hviid A. The use of proton-pump inhibitors in early pregnancy and the risk of birth defects. N Engl J Med 2010; 363:2114–2123. [II-2]

60. Matok I, Gorodischer R, Karen G, et al. The safety of metoclopramide use in the first trimester of pregnancy. N Engl J Med 2009; 360:2528–2535. [II-2, n = 3458]

61. Berkovitch M, Mazzota P, Greenberg R, et al. Metoclopramide for nausea and vomiting of pregnancy: a prospective multicenter international study. Am J Perinatol 2002; 19:311–316. [II-2, n = 175 neonates exposed in 1st trimester to metoclopramide]

62. Bsat F, Hoffman DE, Seubert DE. Comparison of three outpatient regimens in the management of nausea and vomiting in pregnancy. J Perinatol 2003; 23:531–535. [RCT, n = 169]

63. Tan PC, Khine PP, Vallikkannu N, et al. Promethazine compared with metoclopramide for hyperemesis gravidarum: a randomized control trial. Obstet Gynecol 2010; 115:975–981. [RCT, n = 149]

64. Lombardi DG, Istwan NB, Rhea DJ, et al. Measuring outpatient outcomes of emesis and nausea management in pregnant women. Manag Care 2004; 13(11):48–51. [II-3]

65. Bartfai Z, Kocsis J, Puno EH, et al. A population based case-control teratologic study of promethazine use during pregnancy. Reprod Toxicol 2008; 25:276–285. [II-3]

66. Ziaei S, Hosseiney FS, Faghihzadeh S. The efficacy of low dose prednisolone in the treatment of hyperemesis gravidarum. Acta Obstet Gynecol Scand 2004; 83:272–275. [RCT, n = 80]

67. Einarson A, Maltepe C, Navioz Y, et al. The safety of ondansetron for nausea and vomiting of pregnancy: a prospective comparative study. BJOG 2004; 111:940–943. [II-2, n = 176 women with ondansetron exposure]

68. Sullivan CA, Johnson CA, Roach H, et al. A pilot study of intravenous ondansetron for hyperemesis gravidarum. Am J Obstet Gynecol 1996; 174:1565–1568. [RCT, n = 30; ondansetron 10-mg IV versus promethazine 50-mg IV, both q8h]

69. Ylikorkala O, Kauppila A, Ollanketo ML. Intramuscular ACTH or placebo in the treatment of hyperemesis gravidarum. Acta Obstet Gynecol Scand 1979; 58(5):453–455. [RCT, n = 32]

70. Yost NP, McIntire DD, Wians FH, et al. A randomized, placebo-controlled trial of corticosteroids for hyperemesis due to pregnancy. Obstet Gynecol 2003; 102:1250–1254. [RCT, n = 126]

71. Safari HR, Fassett MJ, Souter IC, et al. The efficacy of methyl-prednisolone in the treatment of hyperemesis gravidarum: a randomized, double-blind, controlled study. Am J Obstet Gynecol 1998; 179:921–924. [RCT, n = 40]

72. Nelson-Piercy C, Fayers P, de Swiet M. Randomised, double-blind, placebo-controlled trial of corticosteroids for the treatment of hyperemesis gravidarum. BJOG 2001; 108(1):9–15. [RCT, n = 24]

73. Bondok RS, El Sharnouby NM, Eid HE, et al. Pulsed steroid therapy is an effective treatment for intractable hyperemesis gravidarum. Crit Care Med 2006; 34:2781–2783. [RCT, n = 40]

74. Chiossi G, Neri I, Cavazzuti M, et al. Hyperemesis gravidarum complicated by Wernicke encephalopathy: background, case report, and review of the literature. Obstet Gynecol Surv 2006; 61(4):255–268. [III; case report and review of literature]

75. Heazell A, Thornaycroft J, Walton V, et al. Acupressure for the inpatient treatment of nausea and vomiting in early pregnancy: a randomized controlled trial. Am J Obstet Gynecol 2006; 194:815–820. [RCT, n = 80]

76. Hsu JJ, Clark-Glena R, Nelson DK, et al. Nasogastric enteral feeding in the management of hyperemesis gravidarum. Obstet Gynecol 1996; 88:343–346. [II-3]

77. Russo-Stieglitz KE, Levine AB, Wagner BA, et al. Pregnancy outcome in patients requiring parenteral nutrition. J Matern Fetal Med 1999; 8:164–167. [II-2]

78. Folk JJ, Leslie-Brown HF, Nosovitch JT, et al. Hyperemesis gravidarum: outcomes and complications with and without total parenteral nutrition. J Reprod Med 2004; 49:497–502. [II-2, n = 166]

79. Holmgren C, Aagaard-Tillery KM, Silver RM, et al. Hyperemesis in pregnancy: an evaluation of treatment strategies with maternal and neonatal outcomes. Am J Obstet Gynecol 2008; 198(1):56. [II-2]

80. Nuthalapaty FS, Beck MM, Mabie WC. Complications of central venous catheters during pregnancy and postpartum: a case series. Am J Obstet Gynecol 2009; 201:311.e1–311.e5. [II-3]

81. Trogstad LI, Stoltenberg C, Magnus P, et al. Recurrence risk in hyperemesis gravidarum. BJOG 2005; 112(12):1641–1645. [II-3]

10

Intrahepatic cholestasis of pregnancy

Aisha Nnoli and Steven K. Herrine

KEY POINTS

- The diagnosis of intrahepatic cholestasis of pregnancy (ICP) is **first onset of pruritus in the second or third trimester, elevated serum bile acids >10 µmol/L, and spontaneous relief of signs and symptoms within four weeks after delivery.**
- **ICP is diagnosed once all other forms of liver disease and cholestasis have been excluded.**
- A total bile acid level of ≥40 µmol/L represents severe disease.
- **Complications of untreated, usually severe ICP,** include spontaneous preterm birth, meconium, nonreassuring fetal heart tracing, fetal death, neonatal death, and postpartum hemorrhage. Fetal deaths occur mostly ≥37 weeks, and no increased perinatal deaths have occurred in recent series with ursodeoxycholic acid (UDCA) treatment and delivery by 37 to 38 weeks.
- **UDCA is the current treatment of choice for maternal pruritis and improvement of bile acids and transaminases. Once UDCA therapy is maximized, addition of S-adenosylmethionine is associated with further improvement.** There is insufficient evidence supporting improved neonatal outcomes.
- **Vitamin K** 10 mg once a day at onset of ICP or 34 weeks has been suggested for prevention of postpartum hemorrhage, but there is insufficient evidence for a strong recommendation.
- There are several reports of sudden fetal death within 24 hours of a reactive nonstress test (NST), and insufficient evidence for a recommended fetal testing protocol.
- Especially in severe cases, **delivery should occur by 37 to 38 weeks.**

HISTORIC NOTES

Old names such as "benign jaundice of pregnancy" or "idiopathic jaundice of pregnancy" should not be used anymore.

DIAGNOSIS/DEFINITION

Pruritus (100% of patients) **and elevated serum bile acids** >10 µmol/L (≥14 µmol/L in >90%), in the absence of other liver disease, which resolves after pregnancy (1). If normal bile acids, some accept the diagnosis with just pruritus plus abnormal transaminases (2). Other accepted names are gestational cholestasis or obstetric cholestasis. Differential diagnoses, although rare, may include pregnancy-related pruritic symptoms, cholestasis viral hepatitis, primary sclerosing cholangitis, and acute fatty liver of pregnancy (Fig. 10.1, Table 10.1) (3–5).

SYMPTOMS

Pruritus usually involves the whole body, but is most severe in palms and soles, with nocturnal predominance (6). It may also present with mild jaundice, subclinical steatorrhea, gallstone formation, cholecystitis, and vitamin K deficiency. Mild jaundice, if present, typically develops one to four weeks after onset of pruritis with serum levels of conjugated bilirubin mildly elevated.

INCIDENCE/EPIDEMIOLOGY

Incidence varies geographically, with 0.01% to 0.5% in the United States; 0.1% to 0.2% in Europe; 5% Hispanics; and 9.2% to 15.6% in South America (7).

It commonly occurs in late second and third trimester, rapidly resolves within four weeks after delivery, and is associated with adverse pregnancy outcomes (1,7).

GENETICS

Of the ICP cases, 15% to 30% have a family history of intrahepatic cholestasis (IC), but most cases are not related to known mutations of familial IC. Genetic predisposition is shown in high-prevalence regions such as Chile and Scandinavia. Data suggest mutations in phospholipid transporter ATP-cassette transporter B4 and/or multidrug-resistant protein-3 may lead to altered biliary canalicular transport and excretion of phosphatidylcholine. These genes are more frequent in women who developed severe IC (6,7).

ETIOLOGY/BASIC PATHOPHYSIOLOGY

The metabolic demands of pregnancy stress the liver and exceed the capacity for cholesterol metabolism in susceptible individuals. Bile acids such as **glycocholic and taurocholic acid** increase in serum and cause symptom of itching (6). Pathogenesis is poorly understood. Bile acids have been shown to induce contraction of chorionic veins of the placenta, and increased fetal myometrial sensitivity to oxytocin is seen after incubation with cholic acid (1).

CLASSIFICATION

A bile acid level of ≥40 mmol represents severe disease. Severe disease represents about 20% of cases of ICP. Complications happen mainly with severe ICP (8,9).

RISK FACTORS/ASSOCIATIONS

Associated family history of ICP, gestational hyperestrogenemia, abnormal progesterone metabolism, multiple pregnancies, winter season, and selenium deficiency (7,10).

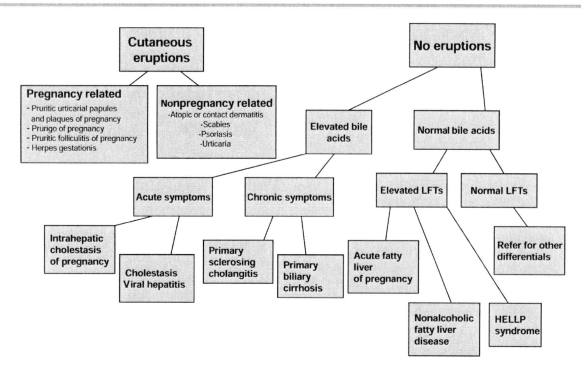

Figure 10.1 Pruritus during pregnancy. *Abbreviations*: LFT, liver function tests; HELLP, Hemolytic anemia, Elevated Liver enzymes, and Low Platelet count.

COMPLICATIONS (WITHOUT TREATMENT)

Spontaneous preterm birth (SPTB) 15%, meconium 45%, non-reassuring fetal heart testing (NRFHT) 5% to 15%, fetal death 2% to 10%, neonatal death 1% to 2%, and postpartum hemorrhage 20% to 22%. SPTB occurs mostly at 32 to 36 weeks, as for other SPTB. Fetal deaths occur mostly ≥37 weeks (3). Etiology of fetal deaths is unclear, but taurocholate is toxic to cardiomyocytes (11). Complications occur almost only in severe cases. **No increase in perinatal deaths has occurred in recent series with treatment and delivery by 37 to 38 weeks** (2,12). Subclinical steatorrhea may occur along with fat malabsorption, and this may lead to vitamin K deficiency, resulting in a prolonged prothrombin time and postpartum hemorrhage (7).

PREGNANCY CONSIDERATIONS

Up to 50% of women recall pruritus during pregnancy, but few have elevated bile acids. Bile acids may be normal at first, and increase later (usually increase an average of 3 weeks after symptoms of pruritus). Of ICP diagnoses, 80% to 86% are made after 30 weeks.

PREGNANCY MANAGEMENT/EVALUATION
Principles

Severe ICP is associated with perinatal complications, so that the largest series has proposed no intervention for milder cases (i.e., bile acids <40 mmol) (9).

Workup

Bile acids (repeat serially if initially negative and high clinical suspicion); and **Transaminases** such as AST and ALT (elevated 60% of times). GGT is not necessary, but elevated 30% of

times. **Hepatitis C antibody** can be checked, as ICP is more common in these women. One might consider a right upper quadrant ultrasound (10% have cholelithiasis) and evaluation of other differentials in uncertain cases (Fig. 10.1, Table 10.1) (3–5).

MANAGEMENT (FIG. 10.2)
Prevention

No preventive measures have been proposed.

Therapy

Ursodeoxycholic Acid (Ursodiol)

> *Mechanism of action*: Hydrophilic bile acid, which inhibits intestinal absorption of other bile acids, enhances excretory hepatocyte function and choleretic activity, stabilizing the hepatocyte cell membrane and diluting the more toxic bile acids in the enterohepatic circulation (12). It may also allow for transport of bile acids out of fetal compartment.
> *Safety*: FDA class B.
> *Dose*: 10 to 25 mg/kg divided in two doses daily. Usually start at 300 to 500 twice a day.
> *Side effects*: Diarrhea.
> *Effectiveness*: Compared to placebo, **UDCA is associated with decreased pruritus, a significantly greater reduction of bile acids and transaminases, lower incidences of preterm birth** (13–16). When compared to other interventions, UDCA has been shown in larger trials to have a **significant beneficial effect in decreasing pruritus, bile acids, and liver function tests** (17–19). The outcome of fetal death is generally uncommon, but indirect

Table 10.1 Selected Differential Diagnoses of Pregnant Women with Pruritus

	Intrahepatic cholestasis of pregnancy	Viral hepatitis	Primary sclerosing cholangitis	Primary biliary cirrhosis	Acute fatty liver of pregnancy
Common trimester presentation	Third	Any	Any	Any	Second, third
Clinical features	Severe pruritis, jaundice	Nausea, vomiting, jaundice, prolonged abdominal pain and fluctuating jaundice and pruritis	Insidious and intermittent jaundice, fatigue, pruritis, abdominal pain	Fatigue, intermittent pruritis, RUQ pain, anorexia, and jaundice	Nausea, vomiting, abdominal pain, jaundice mental status changes, +/− preeclampsia, +/− HTN
Laboratory findings	Alkpho nl or elevated Trans elevated, sometimes to 1000 U/L Bilirubin: mildly elevated	Alkpho nl Trans 1000 to 2000 U/L; ALT >AST Bilirubin: nl or mildly elevated	Alkpho 3–5 × nl Trans 4–5× nl Bilirubin: nl or mildly elevated	Alkpho 3–4 × nl Trans <3× nl Bilirubin: early stage: nl, then increases slowly, may exceed >20 mg/dL	Alkpho nl Trans nl or moderately elevated Bilirubin: elevated
Pathology	Mutation in multidrug resistance-3 gene; environmental factors Bx: Bland changes typical of cholestasis of liver biopsy	Viral infection; sequalae from acute hepatitis can lead to cholestasis Bx: Marked inflammation	Idiopathic, associated with IBS; cholangiographic findings of multifocal structuring an ectasia of biliary tree Bx: thickened, fibrotic duct wall	Autoimmune inflammatory destruction of intralobular bile ducts. Bx: Ductopenia: absence of interlobular bile ducts >50% portal tracts	Often idiopathic, some patients with inherited LCHAD deficiency; most common in primiparous and multiple gestations Bx: Microvesicular fatty liver disease
Treatments with reported benefit on symptoms	Ursodeoxycholic acid (first-line therapy); SAMe	Supportive measures	Ursodeoxycholic acid, treat underlying, liver transplant	Ursodeoxycholic acid, steroids	Delivery

Abbreviations: Alkpho, alkaline phosphatase; Bx, biopsy; HTN, hypertension; LCHAD, Long-chain 3-hydroxyacyl CoA dehydrogenase; nl, normal; RUQ, right upper quadrant; SAMe, *S*-adenosylmethionine; Trans, transaminases. *Source:* Adapted from Refs. 27–29.

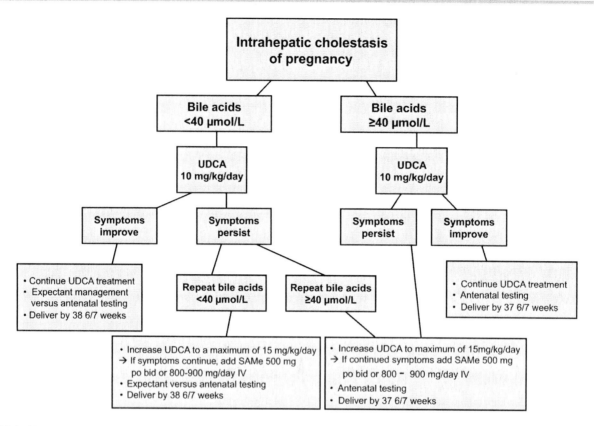

Figure 10.2 Treatment algorithm. *Abbreviations*: UDCA, ursodeoxycholic acid; SAMe, *S*-adenosylmethionine. *Source*: Adapted from Refs. 1,3,4,7.

evidence correlates lower bile acids with less fetal deaths and other complications.

S-Adenosylmethionine
S-adenosylmethionine (SAMe) has similar mechanism of action and side effects as UDCA. Dose should be 500 mg orally twice a day, or 800 to 900 mg IV infusion once a day. Compared to placebo, one trial showed significantly **greater improvements in pruritus, bile salts, and liver enzymes** with SAMe (15,16,19–22). Compared to UDCA, SAMe is less effective at improving pruritus, bile acids, transaminases, and bilirubin (15,23–25). SAMe is not commonly used by itself given the superiority of UDCA.

UDCA and SAMe
Compared to placebo or UDCA alone, **UDCA and SAMe resulted in greater improvements in pruritus, bile salts, and selected liver function assays**; UDCA and SAMe versus SAMe resulted in greater improvements in bile salts (15,16,24).

Other Therapies
Dexamethasone. Compared to dexamethasone, UDCA is associated with a greater reduction in bile acids and liver enzymes, with improved pruritus only in women with severe ICP (17).
Cholestyramine. Cholestyramine is an anion exchange resin that binds to bile acids and decreases their absorption in the ileum. Cholestyramine should not be taken with other medications because of potential effects on their absorption. Safety: FDA class C; dose: 8 g orally once a day. Significant

side effects include a decrease in intestinal absorption of fat-soluble vitamins A, D, E, and K. No studies support the use of vitamin K supplementation to decrease risks associated with deficiency. Compared with UDCA, no significant differences were observed in pruritis, bile salts, or fetal/neonatal outcomes (18).
Guar gum. Guar gum is a type of dietary fiber that decreases the bile acid pool by binding to bile acids in the intestinal lumen (6) Safety: FDA class B. Compared to placebo, there are no differences in pruritus, bile salts, or fetal/neonatal outcomes observed in a very small RCT (26).
Activated charcoal. Activated charcoal is a porous substance shown to adsorb bile salts, decrease bilirubin levels and inhibit bile acid absorption (5) Safety: FDA class C. Compared to no treatment, the reduction in bile salts was greater with charcoal, but there was no difference in pruritus relief, or fetal/neonatal outcomes in a very small RCT (27).
Hydroxyzine. Hydroxyzine antagonizes central and peripheral histamine-1 receptors. Safety: FDA class C; dose: 25 to 100 mg as needed every six hours orally. Hydroxyzine might improve tolerance to persistent itching, but this is not based on RCT data (7).
Vitamin K. Vitamin K (FDA class C) 10 mg once a day at onset of ICP or 34 weeks has been suggested for prevention of postpartum hemorrhage, but there is insufficient evidence for a strong recommendation (5).

Conclusion
Given the above results, and the greater experience with UDCA, **UDCA is the current treatment of choice for**

cholestasis of pregnancy. Once UDCA therapy is maximized, addition of SAMe is associated with further improvement. Given the low effect that UDCA and/or SAMe may have on itching, other antipruritic therapy may be required. No treatments were found to be unsafe. No study had enough data to properly assess effect on fetal/neonatal outcomes.

ANTEPARTUM TESTING
No RCT specifically addresses fetal surveillance and its frequency in ICP. Kick counts daily, and nonstress tests (NSTs) once per week starting at diagnosis (usually on or after 32 weeks) have been proposed, but there are several reports of fetal death after reactive NST (28,29).

DELIVERY
The majority of unexplained fetal deaths occurs after 37 weeks (6). Especially in severe cases (bile acid level of ≥40 mmol), consider delivery by 37 to 38 weeks (6,12,16). The pregnancy can be delivered earlier if amniocentesis is positive for fetal lung maturity or meconium. Women with mild (<40 µmol/L) ICP can probably be managed expectantly (6,9).

REFERENCES
1. Pusl T, Beuers U. Intrahepatic cholestasis of pregnancy. Orphanet J Rare Dis 2007; 2:26. [II-3]
2. Kenyon AP, Percy CN, Girling J, et al. Obstetric cholestasis, outcome with active management: a series of 70 cases. BJOG 2002; 109(3):282–288. [II-3]
3. Cappell M. Hepatic disorders severely affected by pregnancy: medical and obstetric management. Med Clin North Am 2008; 92 (4):739–760. [II-2]
4. Cappell M. Hepatic disorders mildly to moderately affected by pregnancy: medical and obstetric management. Med Clin North Am 2008; 92(4):717–737. [II-2]
5. Feldman M, Friedman L, Brandt L. Gastrointestinal and Liver Disease. 9th ed. Philadelphia, PA: Saunders, 2010. [Review]
6. Pathak B, Sheibani L, Lee R. Cholestasis of pregnancy. Obstet Gynecol Clin North Am 2010; 37(2):269–282. [II-3]
7. Saleh M, Abdo K. Intrahepatic cholestasis of pregnancy: review of the literature and evaluation of current evidence. J Womens Health 2007; 16(6):833–841. [II-3]
8. Sentilhes L, Bacq Y. The intrahepatic cholestasis of pregnancy. J Obstet Gynecol Reprod Biol 2008; 37(2):118–126. [II-3]
9. Trauner M, Meier PJ, Boyer JL. Molecular pathogenesis of cholestasis. N Engl J Med 1998; 339(17):1217–1227. [Review; nonpregnant]
10. Glantz A, Marschall HU, Mattsson LA. Intrahepatic cholestasis of pregnancy: relationships between bile acid levels and fetal complication rates. Hepatology 2004; 40(2):467–474. [II-3; n = 693, largest series]
11. Williamson C, Hems LM, Goulis DG, et al. Clinical outcome in a series of cases of obstetric cholestasis identified via a patient support group. BJOG 2004; 111(7):676–681. [II-3; n = 352]
12. Gorelik J, Shevchuk A, de Swiet M, et al. Comparison of the arrhythmogenic effects of tauro- and glycoconjugates of cholic acid in an in vitro study of rat cardiomyocytes. BJOG 2004; 111 (8):867–870. [II-2]
13. Roncaglia N, Locatelli A, Arreghini A, et al. A randomized controlled trial of ursodeoxycholic acid and S-adenosyl-L-methionine in the treatment of gestational cholestasis. BJOG 2004; 111:17–21. [RCT, n = 46]
14. Diaferia A, Nicastri PL, Tartagni M, et al. Ursodeoxycholic acid therapy in pregnant women with cholestasis. Int J Gynaecol Obstet 1996; 52(2):133–140. [RCT, n = 16]
15. Palma J, Reyes H, Ribalta J, et al. Ursodeoxycholic acid in the treatment of cholestasis of pregnancy: a randomized, double-blind study controlled with placebo. J Hepatol 2000; 27(6):1022–1028. [RCT, n = 15]
16. Nicastri PL, Diaferia A, Tartagni M, et al. A randomised placebo-controlled trial of ursodeoxycholic acid and S-adenosylmethionine in the treatment of intrahepatic cholestasis of pregnancy. BJOG 1998; 105(11):1205–1207. [RCT; UDCA = 8; SAMe = 8; both = 8; placebo = 8]
17. Burrows RF, Clavisi O, Burrows E. Interventions for treating cholestasis in pregnancy. Cochrane Database of Syst Rev 2001; (4):CD000493. [Meta-analysis; 9 RCTs, n = 227. UDCA vs. placebo: 3 RCTs, n = 56. UDCA vs. SAMe: 3 RCTs, n = 82. SAMe vs. placebo: 4 RCTs, n = 82. Guar gum: 1 RCT, n = 48. Activated charcoal: 1 RCT, n = 20. UDCA + SAMe versus placebo, UDCA or SAMe: 1 RCT, n = 32 (8/group). Sample sizes of individual studies were small, the largest study included 48 women and five of the nine studies included 20 women or fewer.]
18. Glantz A, Marschall HU, Lammert F, et al. Intrahepatic cholestasis of pregnancy: a randomized controlled trial comparing dexamethasone and ursodeoxycholic acid. Hepatology 2005; 2(6):1399–1405. [RCT, n = 130]
19. Binder T, Salaj P, Zima T, et al. Randomized prospective comparative study of ursodeoxycholic acid and S-adenosyl-L-methionine in the treatment of intrahepatic cholestasis of pregnancy. J Perinat Med 2006; 34(5):383–391. [RCT, n = 78]
20. Kondrackiene J, Beuers U, Kupcinskas L. Efficacy and safety of ursodeoxycholic acid versus cholestyramine in intrahepatic cholestasis of pregnancy. Gastroenterology 2005; 129:894–901. [RCT, n = 84]
21. Frezza M, Pozzato G, Chiesa L, et al. Reversal of intrahepatic cholestasis of pregnancy in women after high dose S-adenosyl-L-methionine administration. Hepatology 1984; 4(2):274–278. [RCT, n = 18]
22. Frezza M, Centini G, Cammareri G, et al. S-Adenosylmethionine for the treatment of intrahepatic cholestasis of pregnancy. Results of a controlled clinical trial. Hepatogastroenterology 1990; 37 (suppl 2):122–125. [RCT, n = 30]
23. Ribalta J, Reyes H, Gonzalez MC, et al. S-Adenosyl-L-methionine in the treatment of patients with intrahepatic cholestasis of pregnancy: a randomized, double-blind, placebo-controlled study with negative results. Hepatology 1991; 13(6):1084–1089. [RCT, n = 18]
24. Floreani A, Paternoster D, Melis A, et al. S-Adenosylmethionine versus ursodeoxycholic acid in the treatment of intrahepatic cholestasis of pregnancy: preliminary results of a controlled trial. Eur J Obstet Gynecol Reprod Biol 1996; 67(2):109–113. [RCT, n = 20]
25. Roncaglia N, Locatelli A, Arreghini A, et al. A randomized controlled trial of ursodeoxycholic acid and S-adenosyl-L-methionine in the treatment of gestational cholestasis. BJOG 2004; 111:17–21. [RCT, n = 66]
26. Riikonen S, Savonius H, Gylling H, et al. Oral guar gum, a gel-forming dietary fiber relieves pruritus in intrahepatic cholestasis of pregnancy. Acta Obstet Gynecol Scand 2000; 79(4):260–264. [RCT, n = 39]
27. Kaaja RJ, Kontula KK, Raiha A, et al. Treatment of cholestasis of pregnancy with peroral activated charcoal. A preliminary study. Scand J Gastroenterol 1994; 29(2):178–181. [RCT, n = 19]
28. Heinonen S, Kirkinen P. Pregnancy outcome with intrahepatic cholestasis. Obstet Gynecol 1999; 94:189–193. [II-2]
29. Alsulyman O, Ouzounian J, Ames-Castro M. Intrahepatic cholestasis of pregnancy: perinatal outcome associated with expectant management. Am J Obstet Gynecol 1996; 175:957–960. [II-2]

11

Inflammatory bowel disease

Priyadarshini Koduri and Cuckoo Choudhary

KEY POINTS

- Inflammatory bowel disease (IBD) refers to Crohn's disease (CD) and ulcerative colitis (UC).
- Pathogenesis of IBD is not well known, although both environmental and genetic factors play a role.
- If one parent has UC, the risk of the offspring developing UC is 1.6%; if one parent has CD, risk goes up to as high as 5.2%. With both parents having IBD, the offspring's risk goes up to 35%.
- Complications from IBD can be from intestinal or extraintestinal manifestations.
- **Women with IBD should be encouraged to plan conception when the disease is in remission, and when their nutritional status is optimized.**
- **Smoking cessation** is an extremely important factor in keeping women with CD quiescent.
- CD has been associated with first-trimester miscarriage, preterm birth <37 weeks, and low birth weight. Association with small for gestational age is controversial.
- UC is associated with preterm birth <37 weeks. It may be associated with an increased risk of congenital anomalies.
- Even if disease is well controlled, women with IBD remain at risk for adverse pregnancy outcomes.
- **The risk of a flare of IBD during pregnancy (33%) is similar to when they are not pregnant.**
- **Multiple medications are available for management of IBD. Most are considered safe for use in pregnancy and breast-feeding except for methotrexate and thalidomide. Aminosalicylates such as sulfasalazine or mesalamine are usually considered first-line therapies.**
- Surgical management for UC during pregnancy is only indicated in cases of massive hemorrhage, fulminant colitis unresponsive to medical management, perforation, or strongly suspected/known carcinoma. Colectomy in pregnancy is historically associated with high perinatal mortality.
- Ileal pouch–anal anastomosis does not confer additional maternal or fetal morbidity. Long-term pouch function is not affected by pregnancy or mode of delivery.
- **Mode of delivery in CD remains controversial with no randomized controlled trials available to provide guidance. Limited evidence suggests that in women with CD, vaginal delivery is appropriate in quiescent or absent perianal disease (abscess/fistula). A cesarean delivery may be performed for women with active perianal disease such as perianal abscess or fistula.**
- Thromboprophylaxis postpartum may be considered, particularly postcesarean section.
- Pregnancy and breast-feeding may have a mitigating effect on the course of IBD in the years following delivery.

BACKGROUND

Inflammatory bowel disease (IBD) refers to Crohn's disease (CD) and ulcerative colitis (UC). Both are chronic diseases that affect women of reproductive age. They have a protracted relapsing and remitting course that extends over years. Although they share several common features, there are distinct differences between the two conditions summarized in Table 11.1. Differentiating between UC and CD, however, may be impossible in 15% of patients (1).

CROHN'S DISEASE
Definition
CD is a chronic, transmural, granulomatous inflammation of the gastrointestinal system, which can involve any part of the GI tract. Although it commonly involves the colon and terminal ileum, the rectum may be involved in up to 50% of patients (1).

Diagnosis
Diagnosis is based on history and a combination of endoscopic, radiographic, and pathologic findings documenting the focal, asymmetric, and transmural features of the disease (Table 11.1). A diagnosis of CD is rarely made for the first time during pregnancy (2).

Signs/Symptoms
Manifestations of CD in pregnancy are similar to those in the nonpregnant state. Typical symptoms include chronic or intermittent diarrhea, abdominal pain, weight loss, fever and rectal bleeding. Acute ileitis may mimic appendicitis. Additional clinical features include pallor, anorexia, palpable abdominal mass/tenderness, perianal fissures, fistula, or abscess. **Perianal manifestations are unique to CD.**

Extraintestinal symptoms are not uncommon and may involve a variety of organ systems (Table 11.2). Many of these manifestations are also seen in UC.

Epidemiology/Incidence
The incidence of CD varies by geographical region, but has been rising over the past decade. The incidence of CD in developed Western countries, including the United States, is estimated at 7 per 100,000 population (3). Disease frequency is two to four times higher in Jewish populations. The peak age of onset is in the second and third decades of life. Smoking is associated with a twofold increased risk of CD (1).

Etiology/Basic Pathophysiology
Etiology remains unclear. The current hypothesis is that IBD results from a response to environmental triggers (infection,

Table 11.1 Comparison of Ulcerative Colitis and Crohn's Disease

Feature	Ulcerative colitis	Crohn's disease
Extent of inflammation	Limited to mucosa	Involves all layers (transmural)
Intestine involved	Colon only	All segments of the gastrointestinal tract; terminal ileum most common
Rectal involvement	Always	Sometimes
Pattern of spread	Contiguous	Patchy, skip lesions
Granulomas	No	Yes (sometimes)
Fistula	No	Yes
Strictures	No	Yes
Abscess	No	Yes
Perianal disease	No	Yes
Bloody diarrhea	Yes	Maybe
Ileal disease on computed tomography	No	Yes
Increased colon cancer risk	Yes	Maybe (if colonic involvement)
Cure with surgery	Yes	No
Percent of patients who will need surgery	20%	70%

Table 11.2 Extraintestinal Manifestations of IBD

Dermatologic	Erythema nodosum
	Pyoderma gangrenosum
	Aphthous stomatitis
	Pyostomatitis vegetans
	Sweet's syndrome
	Anal skin tags
Musculoskeletal	Osteopenia/osteoporosis
	Osteomalacia
	Increased risk of fractures in hips, wrist, spine and ribs
	Peripheral arthritis
	Axial arthropathies
Ocular	Conjunctivitis
	Uveitis
	Scleritis/episcleritis
Genitourinary	Nephrolithiasis
	Ureteral obstruction
	Fistulas
Hepatobiliary/pancreatic	Primary sclerosing cholangitis
	Cholelithiasis
	Pancreatitis
Thromboembolic	Increased risk of venous and arterial thromboses
	Hyperhomocysteinemia
Hematologic	Anemia
Pulmonary/cardiovascular	Chronic bronchitis
	Bronchiectasis
	Endocarditis/myocarditis
	Pleuropericarditis
	Reactive amyloidosis

Abbreviation: IBD, inflammatory bowel disease.

smoking, drugs, or other agents) in genetically susceptible individuals, resulting in a chronic dysregulation of mucosal immune function (4).

Complications

Maternal
Complications from CD may include serosal adhesions, partial and complete small bowel obstruction, fistula formation, perforation with resulting peritonitis, abscess formation, malabsorption, and perianal disease. Also, complications may arise from any extraintestinal manifestations (Table 11.2).

Fetal
The evidence related to fetal and neonatal outcomes is conflicting and limited to observational studies. Retrospective studies suggest there may be an increased risk of first-trimester miscarriage in women with CD when compared to controls (5). Several population-based studies and a recent meta-analysis have shown an increased risk of preterm birth <37 weeks and low-birth-weight infants in women with CD (6–10). There is no increased risk of stillbirths or congenital anomalies (6). The data regarding the risk of small for gestational age (SGA) infants are conflicting, but a recent meta-analysis suggests there is no increased risk (6,11).

Pregnancy Considerations
Effect of Pregnancy on CD
Pregnant women with CD are no more likely to flare compared to nonpregnant women with CD (12). Pregnancy may in fact have positive effects on disease activity as lower rates of relapse are observed in the three years following pregnancy (13,14). Lower rates of stenosis and/or resection have also been noted in women with CD who have been pregnant during their disease course (15).

Effect of CD on Pregnancy
Regardless of disease activity, women with CD are at similar risks for adverse pregnancy outcomes that have been previously outlined (16). Women with CD are at increased risk of cesarean delivery (6).

Management
Principles
Treatment of CD during pregnancy is similar to therapy in a nonpregnant patient. A multidisciplinary approach by an obstetrician/perinatologist and gastroenterologist is recommended. Most medications used in the management of CD are considered safe for use in pregnancy, and have not been shown to be teratogenic. Women maintained in remission should continue their prepregnancy medications throughout their pregnancy, unless they are on clearly teratogenic agents. Termination of pregnancy is not a therapeutic option for CD as there is no evidence that termination results in improved disease activity (17).

Workup
When a woman presents with symptomatic colitis and relapse is suspected, it is important to rule out infectious causes including *Clostridium difficile* colitis. *C. difficile* may have a more fulminant course in patients with IBD (18). Although imaging and colonoscopy/sigmoidoscopy may be indicated in the initial diagnosis of CD, they are often not necessary for workup of a relapse. Colonoscopy and/or flexible sigmoidoscopy may be performed safely during pregnancy.

Differential Diagnosis
Infectious colitis (bacterial, fungal, viral or protozoan), diverticulitis, ischemic colitis, solitary rectal ulcer syndrome, nonsteroidal anti-inflammatory drug (NSAID)-related colitis.

Table 11.3   Medications Used in IBD

Type of medication	Drug	Pregnancy category	Recommendations for pregnancy	Breast-feeding
5-Amniosalicylic acid drugs	Sulfasalazine	B	First-line therapy; low risk; women should take 2-mg folic acid daily	Likely safe
	Mesalazine	B	Low risk	Likely safe
	Olsalazine	C	Low risk	Likely safe
	Balsalazide	B	Limited information	Limited information
Immunosuppressive agents	Azathioprine/ 6-mercaptopurine	D	Continue in pregnancy if efficacious; low risk	Likely safe
	Cyclosporine	C	Moderate risk	Not recommended
	Methotrexate	X	Contraindicated; teratogenic	Contraindicated, teratogenic
Anti-TNF-alpha agents	Infliximab	B	Low risk	Likely safe
	Adalimumab	B	Limited data; low risk	Safety unknown
	Certolizumab	B	Safety unknown	Safety unknown
Corticosteroids	Prednisone	C	Low risk; possible risk of cleft palate. PPROM and GDM	Likely safe
Antibiotics	Metronidazole	B	Low risk	Likely safe
	Quinolones	C	Low risk; possible cartilage damage with first-trimester exposure	Likely safe
Miscellaneous	Thalidomide	X	Contraindicated; teratogenic	Contraindicated; teratogenic

Abbreviations: IBD, inflammatory bowel disease; TNF, tumor necrosis factor; PPROM, premature preterm rupture of membranes; GDM, gestational diabetes mellitus.

Preconception Counseling
- A woman with CD should have a detailed discussion with her primary care provider, gastroenterologist, and obstetrician about her illness. Since the clinical course of CD during pregnancy depends on CD activity at the time of conception, it is important to make sure that the disease is in remission before pregnancy is planned. **Quiescent disease at the time of conception (either spontaneous or on therapy) typically remains quiescent in two-third of patients during pregnancy while active disease remains active in up to 70% of patients.** Improvement during pregnancy is only noted in 30% (19).
- **Women are therefore encouraged to enter pregnancy while the disease is in remission and their nutritional status has been optimized.**
- Women on methotrexate (MTX) should be counseled to be off the medication at least three to six months before conceiving. Additionally, women on sulfasalazine should be on folic acid at least one month prior to conception (20).
- Counsel women on **avoidance of exacerbating factors including smoking and NSAID use** (3).
- The likelihood of a child developing CD should be discussed with parents, although pregnancy should never be discouraged due to this reason. **The risk is estimated at 5.2% if one parent has CD** and 36% if both have IBD (11,21).
- The risk of infertility in patients with CD who have not had surgery seems to be the same as that of the general population.
- Review of vaccination history is important. Women on immunosuppressants should be immunized against influenza and pneumococcal infections. Under appropriate circumstances they should also receive tetanus and meningococcal vaccines (18).

Prenatal Care
Comanagement with a gastroenterologist is recommended to ensure medication safety. Early evaluation and treatment of anemia, if applicable, is useful. To ensure appropriate weight gain during pregnancy, a nutrition consult may also be helpful. A third-trimester growth ultrasound may be helpful due to conflicting reports regarding SGA risk.

Therapy
Treatment of CD is based on disease location, severity, and extraintestinal complications. Pharmacologic therapy is the mainstay of treatment. Table 11.3 summarizes the pregnancy recommendations for commonly used drugs in the therapy of IBD.

Aminosalicylates. **Sulfasalazine, mesalamine**, balsalazide, and olsalazine are in this category. These are usually considered the first-line therapies, both in nonpregnant and pregnant women. Drugs in this category have limited placental transfer and are generally considered safe for use in pregnancy and in breast-feeding. They have not been shown to be teratogenic (22–26). They have not been shown to be associated with stillbirth, spontaneous abortion, preterm delivery, and low birth weight (22).

Because of the possible antifolate effects of sulfasalazine, women on sulfasalazine are recommended to take 2-mg folic acid/day in the prenatal period and throughout the pregnancy (11).

Corticosteroids
Prednisone is generally safe in pregnancy and breast-feeding (17). Although it does not cross the human placenta, animal studies report an increased risk of cleft palate in the offspring. Women on high doses should avoid breast-feeding within four hours of taking their dose to minimize possible neonatal effects. High-dose prednisone confers risk of diabetes (early glucola is warranted) and PPROM. A steroid taper is recommended when used for more than one week. Stress dose steroids are indicated only in special circumstances (see chap. 25, page 199).

Antibiotics
Metronidazole and quinolones have been used in the management of IBD. Metronidazole is considered safe for use in pregnancy and breast-feeding. Quinolones have a high affinity for bone tissue and cartilage. Animal studies show cartilage damage in weight-bearing joints after quinolone exposure.

Although risk with exposure is minimal, alternative therapies should be used in pregnancy when available (11). Augmentin, another antibiotic used commonly in the management of both perianal and luminal CD, can be used safely during pregnancy. Rifamixin is a relatively new antibiotic, pregnancy category C, used in management of CD.

Immunomodulators/Immunosuppressants

Azathioprine/6-mercaptopurine. Mercaptopurine and azathioprine are often used to maintain remission in steroid-dependent patients with IBD (27,28). Multiple case series and cohort studies have not demonstrated an increased risk of congenital anomalies, suggesting that these drugs are safe for use in pregnancy (28–35). **Women who conceive on these medications should be allowed to remain on them through the pregnancy.** They should be counseled not to stop 6-mercaptopurine before conceiving as that may actually increase the risk of fetal loss (36). Several series suggest that breast-feeding on azathioprine/6-mercaptopurine may be safe (37–39).

Methotrexate. MTX is clearly teratogenic and use is **contraindicated in pregnancy** and in women considering pregnancy. Use in pregnancy or during organogenesis (six to eight weeks after conception) is associated with methotrexate embryopathy. Exposure later in pregnancy may be associated with fetal toxicity and/or mortality. Women considering pregnancy should discontinue MTX three to six months before attempting conception (11). MTX is contraindicated in breast-feeding.

Cyclosporine. This drug is typically used in patients with UC who are refractory to steroids. Cyclosporine has not been found to be teratogenic in humans (40–42). Hypertension and seizures have been reported with cyclosporine use. It should preferably not be initiated during pregnancy (30,31). Breast-feeding is not recommended because of potential neonatal nephrotoxicity and immunosuppression (43,44).

Infliximab. Infliximab is a tumor necrosis factor (TNF)-alpha inhibitor used in patients with IBD (45–47). Several studies have documented the safety of infliximab in pregnancy and have shown no increased risk of congenital anomalies (48–51). Nonetheless, concerns regarding increased drug transfer across the placenta in the third trimester have been raised (52,53). As such, current recommendations suggest that pregnant women should avoid treatment after 30 weeks' gestation and if necessary the mother can be bridged with steroids to control the disease activity until delivery (53–55). The safety of infliximab in breast-feeding remains unknown although case reports of women on infliximab suggest it is safe (50,56).

Adalimumab. Adalimumab is an anti-TNF-alpha agent used in the management of CD. Human data on adalimumab use during pregnancy in IBD patients are limited. Case reports do not suggest teratogenicity (57,58). Adalimumab safety in breast-feeding remains unknown.

Certolizumab. Certolizumab has been used in the management of CD, but is a relatively new drug. Although it has decreased placental transfer compared to infliximab and adalimumab, and has not been detected in breast milk, data regarding safety of use in pregnancy or breast-feeding are limited.

Miscellaneous Agents

Natalizumab. This is a humanized IgG4 monoclonal antibody that is approved for treatment of CD. In 143 pregnant patients that were exposed to this drug, no birth defects were noted. It does cross the placenta during the third trimester of pregnancy. It is a pregnancy category C drug.

Thalidomide. Thalidomide has been successfully used in the treatment of some patients with CD (59). Use in pregnancy and while breast-feeding is unequivocally contraindicated because of its well-known teratogenic effects.

Antepartum Testing

There is no literature to support the use of routine antenatal testing in patients with CD.

Delivery

No randomized controlled trials exist to determine the best form of delivery for women with CD. By current practice, **the method of delivery should be dictated by obstetric indication.** Vaginal delivery is acceptable for women with quiescent or absent perianal disease while **cesarean delivery should be performed in those women with active perianal disease defined as perianal abscess or fistula** (60). Episiotomy should be avoided as it places women with CD at risk for perineal disease peri-delivery (61).

Women with IBD are considered "intermediate" risk for venous thromboembolism. Thromboprophylaxis (e.g., with low-molecular-weight heparin) should be considered for women postpartum (e.g., up to seven days), particularly for those women undergoing a cesarean delivery (62). The first dose should be administered no sooner than 4 hours postoperatively and no later than 24 hours postoperatively.

Postpartum/Breast-feeding

Breast-feeding is not associated with an increased risk of disease flare and may even be protective against a flare in the year following delivery (63,64).

ULCERATIVE COLITIS
Definition

UC is a chronic disease characterized by mucosal inflammation that usually involves the rectum and extends proximally to involve all or part of the colon. Disease is limited to the rectum and rectosigmoid in 40% to 50% of patients while 30% to 40% have disease extending beyond the sigmoid but not involving the whole colon. In 20% of patients the entire colon is involved (1).

Diagnosis

A diagnosis of UC is typically suspected on clinical grounds. It can be confirmed by proctosigmoidoscopy or colonoscopy, histology of biopsy specimens, and by a negative stool exam ruling out infectious causes including *C. difficile* (18).

Signs/Symptoms

The manifestations of UC are similar in pregnant and non-pregnant women. Typical symptoms include diarrhea (often nocturnal), rectal bleeding, tenesmus, passage of mucus, and crampy abdominal pain. In severe disease, liquid stool with blood, pus, and fecal matter may be experienced. Generalized symptoms may include anorexia, nausea, vomiting, fever, and weight loss. On physical examination, a tender anal canal and blood in the rectum may suggest proctitis. Severe pain and bleeding suggests toxic colitis while tympany on abdominal exam suggests megacolon. Signs of peritonitis may suggest perforation (1). Similar to CD, extraintestinal manifestations are not uncommon (Table 11.2).

Epidemiology/Incidence

The incidence of UC varies by geographical location. It is most common in Western nations and incidence in the United States is estimated at 8 to 12/100,000 population per year (18). Unlike CD, the incidence of UC has remained stable over the past several decades (18). Smoking and even a history of smoking increases the risk of UC. Former smokers have a 1.7-fold increased risk of developing UC compared to nonsmokers (1).

Etiology/Basic Pathophysiology

The etiology of UC remains unknown. The pathogenesis is currently thought to be similar to CD (see section "Etiology/ Basic Pathophysiology" described earlier for CD).

Complications

Maternal

Massive hemorrhage typically from erosions in the colon (1%), toxic megacolon (5%), perforation (rare, but fatal in 15% of cases), and strictures (5–10%) (1). The risk of colon cancer is related to the duration and extent of the disease. After 10 years, the colon cancer risk is estimated at 0.5% to 1% per year, necessitating annual or biannual colonoscopic surveillance (18). Complications may also arise from any existing extra-intestinal manifestations (Table 11.2).

In women with an ileal pouch–anal anastomosis (IPAA), pregnancy is considered safe and is not associated with an increased frequency of maternal morbidity or pouch compli-cations (65). Pouch complications reported in pregnancy include small bowel obstruction (2.8% antenatally, 6.8% post-partum), pouchitis (1.8%), and perianal abscess (0.4%) (66).

Fetal

On the basis of a large population-based study and a meta-analysis, UC is associated with preterm birth <37 weeks (6,67). Several studies suggest that UC is not associated with low birth weight, intrauterine growth restriction, SGA infants, or stillbirth (6,68–70). Although the data are conflicting, some population-based studies and a meta-analysis suggest that UC may be associated with congenital anomalies, specifically limb deficiencies, obstructive urinary abnormalities, and multiple anomalies (6,68,71). However, these findings have not been replicated in other studies (69). The presence of an IPAA does not confer additional fetal morbidity or mortality (65).

Pregnancy Considerations

Effect of Pregnancy on UC

Pregnant women with UC are just as likely to flare as non-pregnant women (72). Pregnancy may result in fewer relapses in the years following delivery in women with UC (14,15).

In women with an IPAA, there may be transient worsen-ing of pouch function during the pregnancy, but long-term function is preserved regardless of mode of delivery. Addi-tionally, long-term pouch function in women who have had a vaginal delivery is similar to women who did not have a delivery following IPAA (65,73).

Effect of UC on Pregnancy

See section "Complications: Fetal."

Management

General Principles

Management of a pregnant woman with UC is best done in partnership with a gastroenterologist. The general principles

for management of pregnant patients with UC are similar to management principles in women with CD.

Workup

See section "Workup" described earlier for CD.

Differential Diagnosis

Infectious diarrhea (bacterial, fungal, viral or protozoan), diverticulitis, ischemic colitis, solitary rectal ulcer syndrome, NSAID-related colitis.

Preconception Counseling

- Women should be encouraged to optimize the medical management before conception and optimize nutritional status (see section "Crohn's Disease").
- Discontinue known teratogenic drugs. Women on metho-trexate should wait three to six months after discontinua-tion before attempting pregnancy. Women on sulfasalazine should take 2-mg folic acid daily at least one month prior to conceiving and through the pregnancy.
- If a woman has had UC for more than eight years, it is prudent to ensure her colonoscopic surveillance is up to date before conception.
- Counsel on the risk of inheritance of UC. The risk is estimated at 1.6% if the mother has UC and 36% if both have IBD (11).
- Review of vaccination history is important. Women on immunosuppressants should be immunized against influ-enza and pneumococcal infections. Under appropriate circumstances, they should also receive tetanus and meningococcal vaccines (18).

Prenatal Care

The pregnancy should be managed in partnership with a gastroenterologist. Although the data are conflicting regarding the increased risk of congenital anomalies, a careful anatomical survey is recommended. There is no literature to support serial growth ultrasounds or antenatal surveillance.

Therapy

Pharmacological therapy. Many of the medications used to maintain remission or treat acute relapses are similar to the medications used in CD. See section "Therapy" (under CD) and Table 11.3.

Surgery. Despite medical management, some women may develop fulminant disease, necessitating operative inter-vention. Currently, total abdominal colectomy with a Brooke ileostomy is the most commonly performed procedure for patients who require urgent colectomy for fulminant or toxic UC (74). This procedure does not preclude a future IPAA.

Even when a surgical intervention for UC is performed in the third trimester, cesarean section should be reserved for obstetric indications (74).

Colectomy. Absolute indications for surgery are exsan-guinating hemorrhage, perforation, and documented/strongly suspected carcinoma (4,18). Other indications include severe colitis with or without toxic megacolon unresponsive to max-imal medical therapy (18). There are no prospective random-ized trials comparing medical with surgical treatment efficacy for any indication in UC.

Historically, colectomy in pregnancy for fulminant UC has been associated with a high fetal mortality rate (49%) and concerning maternal mortality rate (22%) (74). However, a more recent case series of women with fulminant UC undergoing total colectomy demonstrated no maternal or fetal mortality, which is consistent with other series published after 1987 (74).

Ileal Pouch–Anal Anastomosis
This is the most commonly performed procedure for UC. It involves resection of the large intestine and creation of an ileal J-pouch, which is attached to a rectal muscle cuff. It helps patient maintain their quality of life after colectomy because it maintains intestinal continuity and the function of defecation. IPAA is considered curative for UC.

However, recent data suggest that the risk of infertility in women with UC increases threefold after IPAA.

Antepartum Testing
There is no literature to base a recommendation for antenatal testing. However, in the absence of an increased risk of stillbirth, antenatal testing is not recommended.

Delivery
Similar to CD, mode of delivery should be dictated by obstetric indication. A vaginal delivery is considered safe for women with an IPAA (65,75). As in the case of a woman with CD, thromboprophylaxis (e.g., with low-molecular-weight heparin) should be considered in women with UC.

Postpartum/Breast-feeding
Breast-feeding may have a protective effect on the disease course of UC (64).

REFERENCES
1. Friedman S, Blumberg RS. Inflammatory Bowel Disease. In: Fauci AS, Braunwald E, Kasper DL, et al. Harrison's Principles of Internal Medicine. 17th ed. Available at: http://www.accessmedicine.com/content.aspx?aID=2883197. [Review]
2. Hill J, Clark A, Scott NA. Surgical treatment of acute manifestations of Crohn's disease during pregnancy. J R Soc Med 1997; 90:64–66. [II-3]
3. Lichtenstein GR, Hanauer SB, Sandborn MD, and the Practice Parameters Committee of the American College of Gastroenterology. Management of Crohn's disease in adults. Am J Gastroenterol 2009; 104(2):465–483. [III]
4. Carter MJ, Lobo AJ, Travis SPL, on behalf of the IBS Section of the British Society of Gastroenterology. Guidelines for the management of inflammatory bowel disease in adults. Gut 2004; 53(suppl V):v1–v16. Doi 10.1136/gut.2004.043372. [III]
5. Mayberry JF, Weterman IT. European survey of fertility and pregnancy in women with Crohn's disease: a case control study by European Collaborative Group. Gut 1986; 27:821–825. [II-2]
6. Cornish J, Tan E, Teare J, et al. A meta-analysis on the influence of inflammatory bowel disease on pregnancy. Gut 2007; 56:830–837. Doi: 10.1136/gut.2006.108324. [I]
7. Fonager K, Sorenson HT, Olsen J, et al. Pregnancy outcome for women with Crohn's disease: a follow-up study based on linkage between national registries. Am J Gastroenterol 1998; 93(12):2426–2430. [II-2]
8. Kornfeld D, Cnattingius S, Ekbom A. Pregnancy outcomes in women with inflammatory bowel disease—a population-based cohort study. Am J Obstet Gynecol 1997; 177(4):942–946. [II-2]
9. Baird DD, Narendranathan M, Sandler RS. Increased risk of preterm birth for women with inflammatory bowel disease. Gastroenterology 1990; 99:987–994. [II-2]
10. Reddy D, Murphy SJ, Kane SV, et al. Relapses of inflammatory bowel disease during pregnancy: in hospital management and birth outcomes. Am J Gastroenterol 2008; 103:1203–1209. [II-2]
11. Mahadevan U. Pregnancy and inflammatory bowel disease. Med Clin North Am 2010; 94:53–73. [III]
12. Nielsen OH, Andreasson B, Bondesen S, et al. Pregnancy in Crohn's disease. Scand J Gastroenterol 1984; 19(6):724–732. [II-2]
13. Agret F, Cosnes J, Hassani Z, et al. Impact of pregnancy on the clinical activity of Crohn's disease. Aliment Pharmacol Ther 2005; 21(5):509–513. [II-3]
14. Castiglione F, Pignata S, Morace F, et al. Effect of pregnancy on the clinical course of a cohort of women with inflammatory bowel disease. Ital J Gastroenterol 1996; 28(4):199–204. [II-2]
15. Riis L, Vind I, Politi P, et al. Does pregnancy change the disease course? A study in a European cohort of patients with inflammatory bowel disease. Am J Gastroenterol 2006; 101(7):1539–1545. [II-2]
16. Dubinsky M, Abraham B, Mahadevan U. Management of the pregnant IBD patient. Inflamm Bowel Dis 2008; 14(12):1736–1750. [III]
17. Mottet C, Juillerat, Gonvers J, et al. Pregnancy and Crohn's disease. Digestion 2005; 71:54–61. [III]
18. Kornbluth A, Sachar DB, and The Practice Parameters Committee of the American College of Gastroenterology. Ulcerative colitis practice guidelines in adults: American College of Gastroenterology, Practice Parameters Committee. Am J Gastroenterol 2010; 105(3):501–523. Doi: 10.1038/ajg.2009.727; published online January 12, 2010. [III]
19. Rogers RG, Katz VL. Course of Crohn's disease during pregnancy and its effect on pregnancy outcome: a retrospective review. Am J Perinatol 1995; 12:262–264. [II-3]
20. Faculty of Sexual and Reproductive Healthcare Clinical Guidance. Sexual and reproductive health for individuals with inflammatory bowel disease: clinical effectiveness unit, June 2009. [III]
21. National Association for Colitis and Crohn's Disease. Pregnancy and IBD (NACC Information Sheet). 2008. Available at: http://nacc.org.uk/downloads/factsheets/Pregnancy.pdf. Accessed March 2, 2009. [III]
22. Rahimi R, Nikfar S, Rezaie A, et al. Pregnancy outcome in women with inflammatory bowel disease following exposure to 5-aminosalicylic acid drugs: a meta-analysis. Reprod Toxicol 2008; 25:271–275. [II-1]
23. Mogadam M, Dobbin WO III, Korelitz BI, et al. Pregnancy in inflammatory bowel disease: effect of sulfasalazine and corticosteroids on fetal outcome. Gastroenterology 1981; 80(1):72–76. [II-3]
24. Norgard B, Czeizel AE, Rockenbauer M, et al. Population-based case control study of the safety of sulfasalazine use during pregnancy. Aliment Pharmacol Ther 2001; 15(4):483–486. [II-2]
25. Diav-Citrin O, Park YH, Veerasuntharam G, et al. The safety of mesalamine in human pregnancy: a prospective controlled cohort study. Gastroenterology 1998; 114:23–28. [II-2]
26. Martineau P, Tennenbaum R, Elefant E, et al. Foetal outcome in women with inflammatory bowel disease treated during pregnancy with oral mesalamine microgranules. Aliment Pharmacol Ther 1998; 12(11):1101–1108. [II-3]
27. Pearson DC, May GR, Fick G, et al. Azathioprine for maintaining remission of Crohn's disease. Cochrane Database Syst Rev 2000: CD000067. [I]
28. Gisbert JP, Linares PM, McNicholl AG, et al. Meta-analysis: the efficacy of azathioprine and mercaptopurine in ulcerative colitis. Aliment Pharmcol Ther 2009; 30:126–137. [II-1]
29. Present DH, Meltzer SJ, Krumholz MP, et al. 6-Mercaptopurine in the management of inflammatory bowel disease: short- and long-term toxicity. Ann Intern Med 1989; 111:641–649. [II-3]
30. Alstead EM. Fertility and pregnancy in inflammatory bowel syndrome. World J Gastroenterol 2001; 7:455–459. [III]
31. Alstead EM. Inflammatory bowel disease in pregnancy. Postgrad Med J 2002; 78:23–26. [III]
32. Francella A, Dyan A, Dosian C, et al. The safety of 6-mercaptopurine for childbearing patients with inflammatory bowel disease: a retrospective cohort study. Gastroenterology 2003; 124:9–17. [II-2]
33. Moskovitz DN, Bodian C, Chapman ML, et al. The effect on the fetus of medications used to treat inflammatory bowel disease patients. Am J Gastroenterol 2004; 99:656–661. [II-3]

34. Polifka JE, Friedman JM. Teratogen update: azathioprine and 6-mercaptopurine. Teratology 2002; 65:240–261. [III]
35. Langagergaard V, Pedersen L, Gislum M, et al. Birth outcome in women treated with azathioprine or mercaptopurine during pregnancy: a Danish nationwide cohort study. Aliment Pharmacol Ther 2007; 25:73–81. [II-2]
36. Zlatanic J, Korelitz BI, Rajapakse R, et al. Complications of pregnancy and child development after cessation of treatment with 6-mercaptopurinefor inflammatory bowel disease. J Clin Gastroenterol 2003; 36(4):303–309. [II-3]
37. Moretti ME, Verjee Z, Ito S, et al. Breast feeding during maternal use of azathioprine. Ann Pharmcother 2006; 40:2269–2272. [II-3]
38. Sau A, Clarke S, Bass J, et al. Azathioprine and breastfeeding: is it safe? BJOG 2007; 114:498–501. [II-3]
39. Christensen LA, Dahlerup JF, Nielsen MJ, et al. Azathioprine treatment during lactation. Aliment Pharmacol Ther 2008; 28:1209–1213. [II-3]
40. Armenti VT, Ahlswede KM, Ahlswede BA, et al. National Transplant Pregnancy Registry—outcomes of 154 pregnancies in cyclosporine-treated female kidney transplant recipients. Transplantation 1994; 57:502–506. [II-3]
41. Armenti VT, Radomski JS, Moritz MJ, et al. Report from the National Transplantation Pregnancy Registry (NTPR): outcomes of pregnancy after transplantation. Clin Transpl 2005; 69–83. [II-3]
42. Bar Oz B, Hackman R, Einarson T, et al. Pregnancy outcome after cyclosporine therapy during pregnancy: a meta-analysis. Transplantation 2001; 71:1051–1055. [II-1]
43. American Academy of Pediatrics Committee on Drugs. Transfer of drugs and other chemicals into human milk. Pediatrics 2001; 108:776–789. [III]
44. Sifontis NM, Coscia LA, Constantinescu S, et al. Pregnancy outcomes in solid organ transplant recipients with exposure to mycophenolate mofetil or sirolimus. Transplantation 2006; 82:1698–1702. [II-3]
45. Hanauer SB, Feagan BG, Lichtenstein GR, et al. Maintenance infliximab for Crohn's disease: the ACCENT I randomized trial. Lancet 2002; 359:1541–1549. [I]
46. Rutgeerts P, Sandborn WJ, Feagan BG, et al. Infliximab for induction and maintenance therapy for ulcerative colitis. N Engl J Med 2005; 353:2462–2476. [II-1]
47. Gisbert JP, Gonzalez-Lama J, Mate J. Infliximab therapy in ulcerative colitis: systematic review and meta-analysis. Ailment Pharmacol Ther 2007; 25:19–37. [II-1]
48. O'Donnell S, O'Morain C. Review article: use of antitumour necrosis factor therapy in inflammatory bowel disease during pregnancy and conception. Aliment Pharmacol Ther 2008; 27:885–894. [III]
49. Lichtenstein GR, Feagan BG, Cohen RD, et al. Serious infections and mortality in association with therapies for Crohn's disease: TREAT registry. Clin Gastroenterol Hepatol 2006; 4:621–630. [II-3]
50. Mahadevan U, Kane SV, Sandborn WJ, et al. Intentional infliximab use during pregnancy for induction or maintenance of remission in Crohn's disease. Aliment Pharmacol Ther 2005; 21:733–738. [II-3]
51. Katz JA, Antoni C, Keenan GF, et al. Outcome of pregnancy in women receiving infliximab for the treatment of Crohn's disease and rheumatoid arthritis. Am J Gastroenterol 2004; 99:2385–2392. [II-2]
52. Zelinkova Z, de Haar C, de Ridder L, et al. High intra-uterine exposure to infliximab following maternal anti-TNF treatment during pregnancy. Aliment Pharmacol Ther 2011; 33(9):1053–1058. [II-3]
53. Vasiliauskas ED, Church JA, Silverman N, et al. Case report: evidence for transplacental transfer of maternally administered infliximab to the newborn. Clin Gastroenterol Hepatol 2006; 4(10):1255–1258. [II-3]
54. Friedman S, Regueiro MD. Pregnancy and nursing in inflammatory bowel disease. Gastroenterol Clin North Am 2002; 31(1):265–273, xii. [III]
55. Hou JK, Mahadevan U. A 24 year-old woman with inflammatory bowel disease. Clin Gastroenterol Herpatol 2009; 7:944–947. [II-3]
56. Mahadevan U. Fertility and pregnancy in the patient with inflammatory bowel disease. Gut 2006; 55:1198–1206. [III]
57. Vesga L, Terdiman JP, Mahadevan U. Adalimumab use in pregnancy. Gut 2005; 54:890. [II-3]
58. Mishkin DS, Van Deinse W, Becker JM, et al. Successful use of adalimumab (Humira) for Crohn's disease in pregnancy. Inflamm Bowel Dis 2006; 12(8):827–828. [II-3]
59. Ehrenpreis ED, Kane SV, Cohen LB, et al. Thalidomide therapy for patients with refractory Crohn's disease: an open label trial. Gastroenterology 1999; 117(6):1271–1277. [II-3]
60. Ilnyckyji A, Blanchard JF, Rawsthrone P, et al. Perianal Crohn's disease and pregnancy: role of mode of delivery. Am J Gastroenterol 1999; 94(11):3274–3278. [II-2]
61. Brandt LJ, Estabrook SG, Reinus JF. Results of a survey to evaluate whether vaginal delivery and episiotomy lead to perineal involvement in women with Crohn's disease. Am J Gastroenterol 1995; 90:1918–1922. [II-3]
62. Royal College of Obstetricians and Gynaecologists. Reducing the risk of thrombosis and embolism during pregnancy and the puerperium. Green-top Guideline No. 37, 2009. [III]
63. Moffatt DC, Ilnyckyj A, Bernstein CN. A population-based study of breastfeeding in inflammatory bowel disease: initiation, duration, and effect on disease in the postpartum period. Am J Gastroenterol 2009; 104(10):2517–2523. [II-2]
64. Klement E, Cohen RV, Boxman J, et al. Breastfeeding and risk of inflammatory bowel disease: a systematic review with meta-analysis. Am J Clin Nutr 2004; 80:1342–1352. [I]
65. McLeod RS. Ileal pouch anal anastomosis: pregnancy—before, during and after. J Gastrointest Surg 2008; 12(12):2150–2152. [III]
66. Seligman N, Sbar W, Berghella V. Pouch function and gastrointestinal complications during pregnancy after ileal pouch–anal anastomosis. J Matern Fetal Neonatal Med 2011; 24(3):525–530. [II-3]
67. Norgard B, Fonager K, Sorenson HT, et al. Birth outcomes of women with ulcerative colitis: a nationwide Danish cohort study. Am J Gastroenterol 2000; 95(11):3165–3170. [II-3]
68. Dominitz JA, Young JC, Boyko EJ. Outcomes of infants born to mothers with inflammatory bowel disease: a population-based cohort study. Am J Gastroenterol 2002; 97(3):641–648. [II-2]
69. Mahadevan U, Sandborn WJ, Li DK, et al. Pregnancy outcomes in women with inflammatory bowel disease: a large community-based study from Northern California. Gastroenterology 2007; 133(4):1106–1112. [II-2]
70. Molnar T, Farkas K, Nagy F, et al. Pregnancy outcome in patients with inflammatory bowel disease according to the activity of the disease and the medical treatment: a case–control study. Scand J Gastroenterol 2010; 45(11):1302–1306. [II-2]
71. Norgard B, Puho E, Pedersen L, et al. Risk of congenital abnormalities in children born to women with ulcerative colitis: a population-based, case–control study. Am J Gastroenterol 2003; 98(9):2006–2010. [II-2]
72. Nielson OH, Andreasson B, Bondeson S, et al. Pregnancy in ulcerative colitis. Scand J Gastroentol 1983; 18(6):735–742. [II-3]
73. Ravid A, Richard CS, Spencer LM, et al. Pregnancy, delivery and pouch function after ileal pouch–anal anastomosis for ulcerative colitis. Dis Colon Rectum 2002; 45:1283–1288. [II-3]
74. Dozois EJ, Wolff BG, Tremaine WJ, et al. Maternal and fetal outcome after colectomy for fulminant ulcerative colitis during pregnancy: case series and literature review. Dis Colon Rectum 2005; 49:64–73. [II-3]
75. Illnyckyj A. Surgical treatment of inflammatory bowel diseases and pregnancy. Best Pract Res Clin Gastroenterol 2007; 21(5):819–834. [III]

12

Gallbladder disease

Priyadarshini Koduri and Cuckoo Choudhary

KEY POINTS
- Symptomatic gallstones are common in pregnant women, but acute cholecystitis is uncommon.
- Pregnancy and the postpartum period increase the risk of gallstones and acute cholecystitis.
- Biliary colic is the most common symptom associated with gallstones.
- Acute cholecystitis can be differentiated from biliary colic based on constant right upper quadrant or epigastric pain, Murphy's sign and evidence of inflammation with systemic signs.
- Diagnosis of cholelithiasis or acute cholecystitis is based on characteristic signs, symptoms, and ultrasonographic findings.
- Acute cholecystitis is associated with significant maternal and fetal risks.
- Conservative management should be initially attempted in cases of biliary colic and acute cholecystitis to avoid surgery.
- Of women with acute cholecystitis, 27% fail conservative management and require a cholecystectomy.
- Cholecystectomy is unequivocally recommended in women with sepsis, ileus, or perforation.
- Endoscopic retrograde cholangiopancreatography (ERCP) and magnetic resonance cholangiopancreatography (MRCP) are considered safe in pregnancy.
- Maternal and fetal outcomes are similar regardless of surgical approach to cholecystectomy. However, the laparoscopic approach has inherent surgical advantages. Surgery is best performed in the second trimester to minimize fetal risks.

CHOLELITHIASIS
Diagnosis/Definition
Presence of gallstones in the gallbladder. A diagnosis of cholelithiasis may be incidental or may be suspected on the basis of classic symptoms with confirmation on ultrasound.

Symptoms
Up to 50% of pregnant women with cholelithiasis are asymptomatic (1). The most common symptom reported is biliary colic—**recurrent pain in the right upper quadrant or epigastrium** that is sudden in onset and may radiate to the interscapular area or right scapula. Biliary colic results from obstruction of the cystic or common bile duct. The resulting increased intraluminal pressure is unrelieved by repeated gallbladder contractions. While nausea and vomiting often accompany biliary colic, the common triad of bloating, nausea, and heartburn are only weakly associated with the presence of gallstones (2).

Epidemiology/Incidence
Gallstones are fairly common and are found in up to 20% of women under age 40 in autopsy series (3). Gallstones have been reported in 7% of nulliparous women and 20% of multiparous women (4). Biliary sludge, which is a precursor to gallstones, is seen in up to 30% of pregnant women (2).

Etiology/Pathophysiology
Gallstones form by concretion or accretion of normal or abnormal bile constituents. Increased biliary secretion of cholesterol and gallbladder hypomotility contributes to gallstone formation. There are three major types of gallstones: cholesterol, pigment, and mixed. Cholesterol and mixed stones constitute the majority of gallstones seen (80%) while pigment stones constitute the rest (3).

Risk Factors/Associations
Common risk factors for cholelithiasis are listed in **Table 12.1**. **Pregnancy is associated with an increased risk of cholelithiasis** likely due to decreased gallbladder motility and increased lithogenicity of bile (1,5). Increased risk for cholelithiasis may remain up to five years postpartum (6). While the incidence of gallstones or sludge may increase with advancing gestation, regression in the postpartum period is not uncommon (7–11).

Differential Diagnosis
Acute cholecystitis (should be suspected if fever, chills, tachycardia, or other systemic signs accompany persistent right upper quadrant/epigastric pain), appendicitis, pancreatitis, peptic ulcer disease, pyelonephritis, HELLP syndrome, acute fatty liver disease, or hepatitis.

Complications
Maternal
> Cholecystitis, cholangitis, choledocholithiasis, pancreatitis, or ileus.

Fetal
> No reports suggest an increased fetal risk associated with biliary colic or the presence of gallstones.

Management
Principles
Conservative management may be an option at least initially in an attempt to avoid surgery. However, more recent evidence suggests having a lower threshold for surgical intervention given the safety of the laparoscopic approach and potentially improved fetal outcomes particularly in the second trimester (4,12,13).

Workup
> *Laboratory investigations.* Blood count, transaminases, total bilirubin, alkaline phosphatase, serum amylase and lipase.

Table 12.1 Risk Factors for Cholelithiasis

Cholesterol and mixed gallstones
    Race/Ethnicity: North American Indians, Hispanics
    Obesity
    Rapid weight loss (e.g., post gastric bypass)
    Female sex hormones (e.g., oral contraceptive pills)
    Ileal resection
    Advancing age
    Gallbladder hypomotility
    Diet: High calorie, high fat
Pigment stones
    Ethnicity: Asian
    Chronic hemolysis
    Alcoholic cirrhosis
    Chronic biliary tract infection, parasitic infection

Imaging. **Ultrasound is the most useful and sensitive test** for detecting sludge and gallstones even as small as 2 mm (3,14). Classic sonographic findings suggestive of gallstones include acoustic shadowing of opacities in the gallbladder lumen that change with the patient's position. The false-negative and false-positive rates for ultrasound in gallstone patients are estimated at 2% to 4% (3).

Therapy

All pregnant women with symptomatic cholelithiasis should be admitted to the hospital for observation. Although it is generally accepted that women without systemic symptoms should be conservatively managed initially in an effort to avoid surgery, this view was challenged in a recent retrospective review of 58 pregnant women with gallbladder disease, excluding those with acute cholecystitis (15). **Compared to women surgically managed, women who were conservatively managed had twice the rate of obstetric complications.** However, this difference was not statistically significant and the obstetric complications were not directly linked to gallbladder disease.

Conservative management should be attempted initially for about 24 hours. This typically includes bowel rest with NPO, intravenous hydration, and use of opioid analgesics. Surgical consultation should be obtained. **Indications for surgical management in symptomatic women without acute** cholecystitis include worsening of symptoms, inability to tolerate oral intake, increasing abdominal tenderness, and patient preference.

Pregnancy Considerations

Biliary colic alone does not appear to increase the risk of adverse obstetric outcome.

Labor and Delivery Issues

Mode of delivery is not impacted by the presence of gallstones. Cesarean section should be performed for obstetric indications.

ACUTE CHOLECYSTITIS
Diagnosis/Definition

Acute cholecystitis is inflammation of the gallbladder. A diagnosis of acute cholecystitis should be made on the basis of characteristic history and physical examination (Fig. 12.1). Murphy's sign is a physical examination finding of increased abdominal rigidity on inspiration and right upper quadrant tenderness. This sign is pathognomonic for acute cholecystitis, but may not always be present on exam, depending on gestational age and body habitus.

Symptoms

Symptoms suggestive of acute cholecystitis are similar in the pregnant and nonpregnant state. **Common signs and symptoms include constant right upper quadrant pain, fever, tachycardia, leukocytosis, anorexia, nausea, vomiting, and inability to tolerate oral intake.** Jaundice and signs consistent with peritonitis may also be present. In women with superimposed bacterial infection, sepsis may also be apparent.

Epidemiology/Incidence

Although cholelithiasis is fairly common in pregnancy, acute cholecystitis is relatively uncommon. It is estimated to complicate 0.1% of all pregnancies (16).

Risk Factors/Associations

See section "Cholelithiasis."

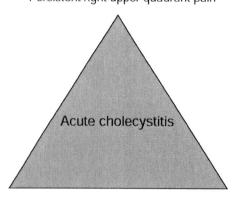

Persistent right upper quadrant pain

Right upper quadrant tenderness (with or without Murphy's sign)

Inflammatory response (indicated by symptoms and labs)

Figure 12.1 Diagnosing acute cholecystitis.

Complications

Maternal

Sepsis, cholangitis, pancreatitis, empyema of the gallbladder, gangrene and perforation, fistula formation, gallstone ileus, porcelain gallbladder with associated increased risk of gallbladder cancer.

Fetal

Fetal death (7% in women treated conservatively vs. 2% in women treated with laparoscopic cholecystectomy) (12), preterm delivery (3.5% in women treated conservatively vs. 6% in women treated surgically) (17), first-trimester miscarriage.

Etiology/Pathogenesis

The majority of cases of acute cholecystitis result from obstruction of the cystic duct by gallstones (2,18). Inflammation of the gallbladder results from three factors: mechanical inflammation from increased intraluminal pressure, resulting in ischemia of the gallbladder wall and mucosa, chemical inflammation from release of tissue factors, and bacterial inflammation. Bacterial inflammation may play a role in 20% of all patients with acute cholecystitis (18). Characteristic bacteria involved include *Escherichia coli*, *Klebsiella*, *Streptococcus faecalis*, *Staphylococcus*, and *Clostridium* (3,18).

Pregnancy Considerations

Principles

The appropriate and optimal management of pregnant women with acute cholecystitis remains controversial. Risks of conservative management include risk to the fetus from recurrent relapses, malnutrition, and other complications that may result from complicated gallbladder disease. However, surgery is not without maternal or fetal risk either. Management decisions for the pregnant woman with acute cholecystitis should be made in conjunction with a general surgeon to ensure optimal management for both mother and fetus.

Workup

> *Laboratory investigations.* Complete blood count, transaminases, total bilirubin, alkaline phosphatase, serum amylase and lipase.

> *Imaging.* **Ultrasound is the image modality of choice in pregnancy for diagnosing cholecystitis.** Classic sonographic findings suggestive of acute cholecystitis are similar in pregnant and nonpregnant women. They include a thickened gallbladder wall (>3–5 mm), pericholecystic fluid, gallstones, and a sonographic Murphy's sign (2).

> However, ultrasound is insensitive in diagnosing choledocholithiasis (presence of an obstructing gallstone in the common bile duct). If choledocholithiasis is suspected on the basis of a dilated biliary tree, abnormal liver tests or pancreatitis, further diagnostic modalities should be employed, namely MRCP or ERCP.

> MRCP Considering the safety of MRI in pregnancy, **MRCP is likely safe in pregnancy**. Nonetheless, there are no clear guidelines for use of MRCP in pregnancy. In doses several times the human dose, paramagnetic contrast agents have been associated with fetal abnormalities and increased risk of miscarriage in animals (19,20). Safety of these contrast agents during breast-feeding remains unknown.

> ERCP ERCP followed by sphincterotomy and stone extraction is now the most common treatment modality for symptomatic choledocholithiasis. In cases of acute cholecystitis, a cholecystectomy may be performed after an ERCP to prevent recurrence of obstruction. **The safety of ERCP in pregnancy is now well accepted** (21,22). Reported complication rates post-ERCP range from 7% to 16%. Possible complications include post-ERCP pancreatitis, preterm labor, and postsphincterotomy bleeding (23–27).

> ERCP is best performed in the second trimester to minimize obstetric risks (22). Fetal radiation exposure during an ERCP can vary depending on procedure time and fluoroscopy time. Although there is a correlation between fluoroscopy time and fetal radiation exposure, this relationship is not entirely linear (27). In a series of 17 patients undergoing ERCP, fetal radiation doses were <200 mrad when fluoroscopy time was limited to less than one minute (27). **Effort should be made to minimize fluoroscopy time, using shielding under the pelvis and over the lower part of the abdomen**. ERCP without use of fluoroscopy have been reported, but this may not be practical in most circumstances (28,29). Perioperative fetal monitoring is recommended.

Management

All women with suspected acute cholecystitis should be hospitalized and a surgical consultation should be obtained. If acute cholecystitis is confirmed, conservative management is a reasonable initial option to avoid surgery. **Conservative therapy typically includes NPO and bowel rest, intravenous hydration, and opioid analgesia**. Broad-spectrum antibiotics should be considered in women with systemic symptoms who do not improve in 12 to 24 hours (2).

The safety and possible efficacy of a short course of indomethacin in the second trimester to attempt to reverse the gallbladder inflammation has been reported (16). Indomethacin use should be avoided after 32 weeks to avoid premature close of the ductus arteriosus and oligohydramnios. While ursodeoxycholic acid is used in nonpregnant women to dissolve gallstones, efficacy for use in pregnancy is uncertain (30).

A **majority of patients (40–70%) who are treated conservatively relapse during the pregnancy** (4,12). Approximately 27% of women will fail conservative management and require cholecystectomy (17). **Definitive surgical therapy is required in pregnant women with sepsis, ileus, or perforation** (2).

Laparoscopic Vs. Open Cholecystectomy

A recent systematic review did not find any difference in maternal or fetal outcome when the open laparoscopic approach was compared to the open approach (17). The **laparoscopic approach has inherent advantages and is preferred when possible**. Ideally, surgery in pregnancy should be performed in the second trimester to minimize fetal risk. However, **laparoscopic cholecystectomy has been safely performed even in the third trimester** (31–34).

Regardless of mode of surgery, the pregnant patient should be placed in the left lateral position to avoid aortocaval compression. Perioperative monitoring should be performed. When the laparoscopic approach is used, care should be taken to avoid high intraperitoneal pressures, using the open technique for umbilical port insertion and using electrocautery away from the uterus. Steroids for fetal lung maturity should be considered between 23 and 33 6/7 weeks.

Labor and Delivery Considerations

Acute cholecystitis or history of cholecystectomy during the pregnancy should not impact mode of delivery. Cesarean section should be reserved for obstetric indications.

REFERENCES

1. Ramin KD, Ramsey PS. Disease of the gallbladder and pancreas in pregnancy. Obstet Gynecol Clin North Am 2001; 28:571–580. [III]
2. Gilo NB, Amini D, Landy HJ. Appendicitis and cholecystitis in pregnancy. Clin Obstet Gynecol 2009; 52(4):586–596. [III]
3. Norton J. Greenberger and Gustav Paumgartner. Diseases of the gallbladder and bile ducts. In: Fauci AS, Braunwald E, Kasper DL, et al. eds. Harrison's Principles of Internal Medicine. 15th ed. New York: McGraw-Hill, 2001. [Review]
4. Swisher SG, Schmit PJ, Hunt KK, et al. Biliary disease during pregnancy. Am J Surg 1994; 168:576–579. [II-3]
5. Everson GT. Gastrointestinal motility in pregnancy. Gastroenterol Clin North Am 1992; 21:751–776. [III]
6. Thijs C, Knipschild P, Leffers P. Pregnancy and gallstone disease: an empiric demonstration of the importance of specification of risk periods. Am J Epidemiol 1991; 134:186–195. [II-2]
7. Maringhini A, Marceno MP, Lanzarone F, et al. Sludge and stones in gallbladder after pregnancy. Prevalence and risk factors. J Hepatol 1987; 5(2):218–223. [II-3]
8. Tsimoyiannis EC, Antoniou NC, Tsaboulas C, et al. Cholelithiasis during pregnancy and lactation. Prospective study. Eur J Surg 1994; 160(11):627–631. [II-3]
9. Ko CW, Beresford SA, Schulte SJ, et al. Incidence, natural history and risk factors for biliary sludge and stones during pregnancy. Hepatology 2005; 41:359–365. [II-3]
10. Basso L, McCollum PT, Darling MR, et al. A study of cholelithiasis during pregnancy and its relationship with age, parity, menarche, breastfeeding, dysmenorrhea, oral contraception and a maternal history of cholelithiasis. Surg Gynecol Obstet 1992; 175:41–46. [II-2]
11. Valdivieso V, Covarrubias C, Siegel F, et al. Pregnancy and cholelithiasis: pathogenesis and natural course of gallstones diagnosed in early puerperium. Hepatology 1993; 17:1–4. [II-3]
12. Jelin EB, Smink DS, Vernon AH, et al. Management of biliary tract disease during pregnancy: a decision analysis. Surg Endosc 2008; 22:54–60. [II-3]
13. Barone JE, Bears S, Chen S, et al. Outcome study of cholecystectomy during pregnancy. Am J Surg 1999; 177(3):232–236. [II-3]
14. Shea JA, Berlin JA, Escarce JJ, et al. Revised estimates of diagnostic test sensitivity and specificity in suspected biliary tract disease. Arch Intern Med 1994; 154:2573–2581. [II-2]
15. Dhupar R, Smaldone GM, Hamad GG. Is there a benefit to delaying cholecystectomy for symptomatic gallbladder disease during pregnancy? Surg Endosc 2010; 24(1):108–112. [II-3]
16. Dietrich CS, Hill CC, Hueman M. Surgical disease presenting in pregnancy. Surg Clin North Am 2008; 88:408–419. [III]
17. Date RS, Kaushal M, Ramesh A. A review of the management of gallstone disease and its complications in pregnancy. Am J Surg 2008; 196(4):599–608. [III]
18. Indar AA, Beckingham IJ. Acute cholecystitis. BMJ 2002; 325:639–643. [III]
19. American College of Obstetricians and Gynecologists. Guidelines for diagnostic imaging during pregnancy. ACOG Committee Opinion No. 299. Obstet Gynecol 2004; 104(3):647–651. [III]
20. Kanal E, Borgstede JP, Barkovich AJ, et al. American College of Radiology White Paper on MR safety: 2004 update and revisions. AJR Am J Roentgenol 2004; 182(5):1111–1114. [III]
21. Chong VH, Jalihal A. Endoscopic management of biliary disorders during pregnancy. Hepatobiliary Pancreat Dis Int 2010; 9(2):180–185. [II-3]
22. Al-Hashem H, Muralisharan V, Cohen H, et al. Biliary disease in pregnancy with an emphasis on the role of ERCP. J Clin Gastroenterol 2009; 43(1):58–62. [III]
23. Gupta R, Tandan M, Lakhtakia S, et al. Safety of therapeutic ERCP in pregnancy—an Indian experience. Indian J Gastroenterol 2005; 24:161–163. [II-3]
24. Jamidar PA, Beck GJ, Hoffman BJ, et al. Endoscopic retrograde cholangiopancreatography in pregnancy. Am J Gastroenterol 1995; 90:1263–1267. [II-3]
25. Tham TC, Vandervoort J, Wong RC, et al. Safety of ERCP during pregnancy. Am J Gastroenterol 2003; 98:308–311. [II-3]
26. Tang SJ, Mayo MJ, Rodriguez-Frias E, et al. Safety and utility of ERCP during pregnancy. Gastrointest Endosc 2009; 69:453–461. [II-3]
27. Kahaleh M, Hartwell GD, Arseneau KO, et al. Safety and efficacy of ERCP in pregnancy. Gastrointest Endosc 2004; 60:287–292. [II-3]
28. Uomo G, Manes G, Picciotto FP, et al. Endoscopic treatment of acute biliary pancreatitis in pregnancy. J Clin Gastroenterol 1994; 18:250–252. [II-3]
29. Simmons SC, Tarnasky PR, Rivera-Alsira ME, et al. Endoscopic retrograde cholangiopancreatography (ERCP) in pregnancy without the use of radiation. Am J Obstet Gynecol 2004; 190:1467–1469. [II-3]
30. Ward A, Brogden R, Heel R, et al. Ursodeoxycholic acid: a review of its pharmacologic properties and therapeutic efficacy. Drugs 1984; 27:95–131. [III]
31. Coelho JC, Vianna RM, da Costa MA, et al. Laparoscopic cholecystectomy in the third trimester of pregnancy. Arq Gastroenterol 1999; 36:90–93. [II-3]
32. Eichenberg BJ, Vanderlinden J, Miguel C, et al. Laparoscopic cholecystectomy in the third trimester of pregnancy. Am Surg 1996; 62:874–877. [II-3]
33. Sen G, Nagabhushan JS, Joypaul V. Laparoscopic cholecystectomy in the third trimester of pregnancy. J Obstet Gynaecol 2002; 22:556–557. [II-3]
34. Pucci RO, Seed RW. Case report of laparoscopic cholecystetomy in the third trimester of pregnancy. Am J Obstet Gynecol 1991; 165:401–402. [II-3]

13

Pregnancy after transplantation

Vincent T. Armenti, Carlo B. Ramirez, Cataldo Doria, and Michael J. Moritz

KEY POINTS
- The best outcomes in pregnancy after liver transplant occur in patients with:
  - Good general health ≥1 year since transplant
  - Minimal or no proteinuria (<1 g/24 hr)
  - Creatinine <1.5 mg/dL
  - Well-controlled or no hypertension
  - No evidence of recent graft rejection
  - **Stable immunosuppressive regimen** and liver function.
- Potential maternal and fetal complications include **preterm birth, preeclampsia, fetal growth restriction, and low birth weight.**
- Pregnancy in and of itself does not affect previously stable hepatic allograft function.
- The effect of **comorbid conditions (i.e., diabetes, hypertension)** should be considered and their **management optimized.**
- **Transplant recipients should have their baseline kidney function** (creatinine, 24-hour urine collection for total protein) **assessed.**
- Maintenance of current immunosuppression in pregnancy is usually recommended, except for **mycophenolic acid products (MPA), for which fetal risks should be discussed, and alternatives sought if possible.**
- Summary of **management options on p. 101.**

RENAL TRANSPLANT
Please see chapter 17, "Renal Disease."

LIVER TRANSPLANT
Historic Notes
The first human liver transplant was performed in 1963 by Thomas Starzl (University of Colorado) (1). Through the years, great improvements have been made in the field because of a better understanding of the tissue compatibility and organ storage, the immune system, earlier detection and treatment of rejection, and better prevention and management of infections. As a result, among liver transplant recipients, a higher survival rate and a return to a good quality of life have been achieved. The first known posttransplantation pregnancy in a liver transplant recipient was reported in 1978 (2).

In 1991, the National Transplantation Pregnancy Registry (NTPR) was established at Thomas Jefferson University in Philadelphia, Pennsylvania, to analyze pregnancy outcomes in solid-organ transplant recipients (3) (Table 13.1).

Diagnosis/Definition
Orthotopic liver transplantation (OLTx) is the treatment of choice for all nonneoplastic end-stage liver diseases and for selected patients with nonresectable hepatic malignancies.

End-stage liver disease (ESLD) is any hepatic disease that jeopardizes the survival or that seriously modifies the quality of life of the patient, and for which the transplant is the only therapy, since no other medical or surgical treatment exists that is able to provide a reasonable chance of recovery.

Symptoms
Before undergoing OLTx, some patients remain in quite good clinical condition. There may be individual variations in terms of hospital care requirements. As the liver disease progresses, symptoms such as encephalopathy, weakness, and lethargy become more frequent. Intractable ascites, peripheral edema, anorexia, jaundice, pruritus and cholestasis, peritonitis, and pneumonia may also develop. Often the patient is severely malnourished.

Indications
The main indications for OLTx are listed in Table 13.2. Although chronic hepatitis C infection (HCV) represents the leading indication for OLTx in the United States, autoimmune hepatitis is probably the most frequent reason for transplantation among young female recipients who may become pregnant after transplant (4,5).

Epidemiology/Incidence
Approximately one-third of all patients who have undergone OLTx are women, and about 75% of female recipients are of reproductive age (4).

Pathophysiology
Patients with end-organ failure experience hypothalamic-pituitary-gonadal dysfunction and decreased ovulation or sperm maturation (5,6). Amenorrhea or menstrual abnormalities with decreased fertility occur in up to 50% of women with chronic liver disease (5,7). A successful transplant almost uniformly leads to a prompt return to normal menstrual cycles and to reproductive functions because of the recovery of the gonadotrophic function (8–10). This is an important component of the restoration of normality of life for patients of childbearing age, and it is evidenced by the increasing number of posttransplantation pregnancies reported worldwide (11–20).

Preconception Counseling
It is universally recognized that, although pregnancy in graft recipients seems to be well tolerated and associated with a

Table 13.1 NTPR: Pregnancies in Female Transplant Recipients

Organ	Recipients	Pregnancies	Outcomes[a]
Kidney	886	1422	1466
Liver	166	292	298
Liver-Kidney	4	6	7
Small-Bowel	1	1	1
Pancreas-Kidney	43	77	79
Pancreas alone	1	4	5
Heart	58	103	107
Heart-Lung	5	5	5
Lung	21	30	32
Totals	**1185**	**1940**	**2000**

[a]Includes twins, triplets, quadruplets. As of December 2010.

Table 13.2 Main Indications for Liver Transplant

Acute liver failure
Postinflammatory cirrhosis
Postalcoholic cirrhosis
Primary biliary cirrhosis
Secondary biliary cirrhosis
Primary sclerosing cholangitis
Autoimmune cirrhosis
Cirrhosis of unknown etiology
Inborn errors of metabolism
Biliary atresia
Congenital hepatic fibrosis
Cystic fibrosis
Budd–Chiari syndrome
Hepatic cysts
Hepatic trauma
Benign tumors
Primary malignant tumors

good outcome, it must be considered high risk, requiring close surveillance by a coordinated team (20). Therefore, since **a return to fertility is the rule after OLTx**, obstetricians/gynecologists and the transplant team should extensively counsel reproductive-age transplant patients, before and after transplantation, and **appropriate contraceptive plans** should be recommended. For patients wishing to avoid pregnancy, there are limited data on appropriate contraception following transplantation. Barrier methods are preferred. Oral contraceptives are relatively contraindicated because of many theoretical complications such as the risk of thromboembolism, cholestasis, exacerbated hypertension, and interference in cyclosporine metabolism. While intrauterine devices may initially increase the risks of infection especially in immunocompromised women, their use may be considered and is probably safe (6).

Ideally, patients should be vaccinated prior to transplantation against influenza, pneumococcus, hepatitis B, and tetanus. Alternatively, they should be vaccinated prepregnancy (see chap. 38).

Timing of Pregnancy

The shortest interval from OLTx to conception reported in the literature is three weeks (21). Several authors recommend **waiting for at least one to two years after OLTx**, based on rejection risks, and to allow stabilization of allograft function and of immunosuppressive regimen (6–8,20). The advice to wait for two years after a successful transplant may be too restrictive, because newer immunosuppressive regimens have decreased rejection rates in the first posttransplant year.

When choosing the timing of pregnancy after OLTx, several individual factors should be considered:

a. Good general health ≥1 year since transplant
   • Risk of acute graft rejection
   • Risk of acute infection that might impact the fetus (cytomegalovirus [CMV] acute infection is most common within 6–12 months posttransplant)
b. Proteinuria and creatinine level
   • None or minimal proteinuria (<1 g/24 hr)
   • Serum creatinine <1.5 mg/dL
c. Rejection and immunosuppression
   • No evidence of recent graft rejection (in the past year)
   • Stable immunosuppression regimen (stable dosing)
d. Stable liver function
   • Patients with stable liver function generally have a low risk for opportunistic infections
e. Maternal age
f. Medical noncompliance

Comorbidity/Risk Factors

In the presence of stable allograft and renal function, pregnancies following OLTx are generally well tolerated with a good maternal and neonatal outcome. However, several comorbid factors may influence pregnancy outcomes.

Etiology of Original Disease

Recurrent liver disease, especially viral hepatitis, appears to be one of the most serious risks for both mother and child. Vertical transmission occurs in 10% to 20% of HBsAg-positive (HBeAg-negative) nontransplant mothers without immunoprophylaxis. For prevention of vertical transmission, all newborns, born to women with hepatitis B surface antigen (HBsAg) positive, should receive immunoprophylaxis (HBIg) and HB vaccine within 12 hours of birth. This combination prevents >90% of neonatal hepatitis B virus (HBV) infection (22). Therefore, the incidence of vertical transmission to the child of HBV carriers who underwent OLTx presumptively could be quite similar.

Also, the rate of maternal-fetal HCV transmission in OLTx recipients is unclear, requiring additional analysis. The vertical infection rate in pregnant HCV RNA–positive subjects is around 3% to 5% (in absence of other viral coinfections) (23). A well-documented risk factor for HCV vertical transmission is maternal high viral load. Therefore, special attention should be given to patients with high viral load posttransplant (see chaps. 30 and 31).

Hypertension

Often in the posttransplantation population there is an increased incidence of hypertension and renal insufficiency caused by calcineurin inhibitors, that is, cyclosporine and tacrolimus. Both immunosuppressive regimens can induce endothelial cell dysfunction and decrease endogenous nitric oxide production, causing renal dysfunction and hypertension. This may contribute to the increased incidence of preeclampsia among pregnant women after OLTx (5,20).

Mild renal insufficiency or hypertension can be well controlled with the same treatment (calcium channel blockers) used in the nontransplant population (24).

Diabetes

New-onset diabetes mellitus (NODM) develops in approximately 15% of liver transplant recipients and a similar proportion of patients have diabetes prior to transplantation (25).

Preexisting diabetes and probably NODM are associated with increased mortality and risk of infection. Controversial data exist concerning the impact of immunosuppressive therapy on the development of posttransplantation diabetes mellitus. Corticosteroid exposure should be limited as much as possible. Reduction of calcineurin inhibitor dose is advised. The management of NODM is essentially similar to that of diabetes in the nontransplant population. Numerous studies have established a direct relationship between maternal glycemic control and neonatal outcomes for all types of diabetes. Evidence indicates that intrauterine exposure to diabetes increases the risk of obesity, insulin resistance, insulin secretory defect, and subsequent development of type 2 diabetes in the offspring. Early diagnosis, patient education, proper follow-up, and postpartum testing will certainly decrease poor perinatal outcomes, also enabling a secondary prevention of type 2 diabetes in the long term. Modern treatment protocols during pregnancy emphasize strict glycemic control by a combination of diet and medication. Traditionally, insulin therapy has been considered the gold standard for management of diabetes, because of its efficacy in achieving better glucose control and the fact that it does not cross the placenta (26) (see chap. 4).

CMV Acute Infection

CMV acute infection is the most common type of infection within 6 to 12 months posttransplant. It is particularly dangerous in early pregnancy. CMV infection is a causative agent of congenital malformation (microcephaly, cerebral palsy, sensorineural deafness) or congenital liver disease. Such abnormalities are seen in approximately 10% to 15% of infected pregnancies. Screen all transplant recipients with CMV IgG and IgM. If IgM positive, perform avidity testing (see chap. 46). The use of antiviral agents in the management of CMV infection during pregnancy remains controversial (7) (see chap. 46).

Rejection

Most cases of graft rejection are reported during the earlier phases of pregnancy. If the transplanted organ is functioning well before the recipient becomes pregnant, there does not seem to be a greater risk of rejection during pregnancy. It is universally recognized that immunosuppression therapy should be maintained during pregnancy by serum levels, as a reduction or discontinuation may lead to rejection of the transplanted organ. The reported incidence of biopsy-proven acute rejection ranges between 2% and 8% (3,7,20). When acute rejection is suspected, percutaneous liver biopsy is not contraindicated in pregnant patients, although ultrasound visualization is recommended to reduce the risk of complications. Evaluation of rejection includes liver Doppler ultrasound to exclude anatomic source of graft dysfunction. Although rejection is a concern, it can be successfully managed with adjustment of immunosuppressive medications. For more serious cases the use of steroids as antirejection therapy is safe. On the other hand, safety of antilymphocyte globulins and rituximab is still unknown. There have been some reports of lower birth weights and premature births in mothers who had experienced rejection during pregnancy.

Infrarenal Aortic Graft

Particular attention should be reserved for patients with infra-aortic grafts for hepatic arterial flow. One death as a result of clotting of the aortic graft by external compression from the gravid uterus has been reported (24). Therefore, patients with infra-aortic graft should be monitored with color Doppler ultrasonography during pregnancy.

Pregnancy Complications

Pregnancy does not seem to deteriorate allograft function in OLTx recipients. Although pregnancies after liver transplant are generally associated with successful outcomes, they are considered high risk because of the higher incidence of complications, requiring close surveillance by transplant clinicians, gynecologists, and obstetricians.

Pregnancy complications may include (Table 13.3) the following:

Preterm Birth and Low Birth Weight

Children born to female transplant recipients are more likely to be premature and/or small for gestational age. The risk of prematurity is up to 50% and the mean gestational age ranges between 36 and 37 weeks (3–5,20). The consequences of decreased gestational age at delivery, particularly under 34 weeks gestation, may include neonatal morbidity, mortality, and long-term morbidities.

Intrauterine Growth Restriction

The risk of intrauterine growth restriction (IUGR) is estimated to be at about 20%. The IUGR is associated with perinatal morbidity and mortality with long-term health implications. The management of IUGR is to achieve the delivery of the newborn in the best possible condition, balancing the risks of prematurity against those of continued intrauterine confinement (see chap. 44).

Preeclampsia

Hypertension and occurrence of preeclampsia are more common in OLTx recipients, with an incidence of 20%. These complications may be more common in patients taking cyclosporine, probably because of the related endothelial cell dysfunction, and less common with tacrolimus (3–5,20,24). The management of preeclampsia is the same as in the nontransplant population (see chap. 1).

Abnormal Blood Chemistry Tests and Liver Function

Pruritus and cholestasis occur frequently. Elevated alkaline phosphatase levels are found in approximately 35% of normal pregnancies after OLTx. Graft rejection needs to be considered in all cases and differentiated from other conditions. Hemolysis, low platelets syndrome, and anemia have been reported (5).

Immunosuppressive Agents Commonly Used and Their Potential Side Effects

While there are potential risks of the exposure of infants to immunosuppressive medications, data to date have been encouraging with most standard regimens (Tables 13.4 and 13.5).

Recent studies have reported an association between administration of **mycophenolic acid products (MPA) [mycophenolate mofetil (MMF) and enteric-coated mycophenolate sodium (EC-MPS)] to transplant recipients and an increased risk of adverse outcomes in pregnancy and of a specific pattern of birth defects** (27,28). In 2007, the package inserts of MMF and EC-MPS included a change from pregnancy

Table 13.3 NTPR: Pregnancy Outcomes Among Solid-Organ Transplant Recipients

	Kidney[a]	Pancreas-kidney	Liver	Heart	Lung
Maternal factors (n = pregnancies)	(987)	(75)	(287)	(103)	(30)
Mean transplant-to-conception interval (yr)	3.6–6.1	3.0–5.5	5.7 ± 4.9	6.0 ± 4.7	3.6 ± 3.3
Hypertension during pregnancy	56–65%	28–95%	32%	39%	53%
Diabetes during pregnancy	4–12%	0–5%	7%	2%	23%
Infection during pregnancy	19–23%	23–62%	26%	13%	21%
Preeclampsia	**30–32%**	**27–32%**	**22%**	**18%**	**17%**
Rejection episode during pregnancy	**1–2%**	**0–14%**	**7%**	**11%**	**6%**
Graft loss within 2 yr of delivery	8–10%	18–19%	7%	4%	14%
Outcomes (n)[b]	(1017)	(77)	(293)	(106)	(32)[c]
Therapeutic abortions	0.8–8.4%	4–5%	4%	5%	16%
Spontaneous abortions	12–26%	9–28%	18%	30%	28%
Ectopic	0.4–1%	0–3%	0.3%	2%	0
Stillborn	2–3%	0	1.7%	1%	0
Live births	**70.8–76%**	**69–86%**	**76%**	**62%**	**56%**
Live births (n)	(762)	(58)	(221)	(66)	(18)
Mean gestational age (wk)	35–35.8	34.2–34.8	36.4 ± 3.5	36.8 ± 2.6	33.9 ± 5.2
Preterm birth (<37 wk)	**52–53%**	**65–83%**	**42%**	**38%**	**61%**
Mean birth weight (g)	2470–2547	1934–2263	2674 ± 796	2600 ± 568	2206 ± 936
Low birth weight (<2500 g)	42–46%	50–68%	34%	39%	61%
Cesarean section	43–58%	61–69%	41%	40%	31%
Neonatal deaths % (n) (within 30 days of birth)	1–2%	(1)	(1)	0	(2)[b]

[a]Range of incidence because of different immunosuppressants.
[b]Includes twins, triplets, quadruplets.
[c]Includes one triplet pregnancy: one spontaneous abortion at 14 wk and two born at 22 wk and died within 24 hr of birth.

Table 13.4 Immunosuppressive Agents and Their Side Effects

Immunosuppressant	Side effect
Prednisone[a]	Glucose intolerance
Azathioprine[a]	Leukopenia
Cyclosporine[a,b]	Hypertension, nephrotoxicity
Tacrolimus[a,b]	Hypertension, nephrotoxicity, neurotoxicity, glucose intolerance, myocardial hypertrophy
Mycophenolate Mofetil	GI disturbance
Sirolimus[a,b]	Leukopenia, thrombocytopenia, hyperlipidemia

[a]There have been no known teratogenic effects.
[b]Follow with blood levels.

category C to category D (29,30). The warning states that females of childbearing potential must use contraception while taking MPA since use during pregnancy is associated with increased rates of pregnancy loss and congenital malformations. In addition to the NTPR data, postmarketing data collected by Roche Laboratories Inc. between 1995 and 2007 revealed that among the 77 women exposed to systemic MMF during pregnancy, 25 had spontaneous abortions and 14 had a malformed infant or fetus (29). Six of these 14 had ear abnormalities. Reported to the NTPR are 9 liver recipients with 14 pregnancies with exposure to MMF. Pregnancy outcomes included seven spontaneous abortions and seven live births. Three had malformations: two infants had multiple malformations and died, the other had repair of total pulmonary venous return.

Pregnancy outcomes with exposure to sirolimus remain limited. Reported to the NTPR are three liver recipients with three pregnancies (two live births, one spontaneous abortion) (3).

Workup and Management

Close surveillance by the maternal-fetal medicine and the transplant team is recommended (Table 13.6).

Table 13.5 FDA Pregnancy Categories for Commonly Used Immunosuppressive Drugs in Transplantation

Drug	Animal reproductive data	Pregnancy category[a]
Corticosteroids (prednisone, methylprednisolone, others)	Y	B
Azathioprine (Imuran[R])	Y	D
Cyclosporine (Sandimmune[R], Neoral[R], others)	Y	C
Tacrolimus, FK506 (Prograf[R], others)	Y	C
Antithymocyte globulin (Atgam[R], ATG, Thymoglobulin[R])	N	C
Orthoclone (OKT[R]3)	N	C
Mycophenolate mofetil (CellCept[R], others)	Y	D
Enteric-coated mycophenolate sodium (Myfortic[R])	Y	D
Basiliximab (Simulect[R])	Y	B
Daclizumab (Zenapax[R])	N	C
Sirolimus (Rapamune[R])	Y	C

[a]FDA categories briefly defined: B = no fetal risk, no controlled studies; C = fetal risk cannot be ruled out; D = evidence of fetal risk.

- Baseline laboratory tests should include the following:
  a. Bilirubin, creatinine
  b. Liver function test
  c. Cyclosporine level/tacrolimus level
  d. 24-hour urinary protein and creatinine clearance
  e. Urine analysis and urine culture
  f. CMV, HSV, and Toxo IgM and IgG; HBsAg, HBsAb, HepCAb

Repeat lab testing (a→e) should occur at a minimum of once every trimester until 32 weeks. After 32 weeks, obtain labs (a→d) every other week or as needed.

Table 13.6 Pregnancy after Transplantation Management Options

Prepregnancy

Patients should defer conception for at least 1 yr after transplantation, with adequate contraception

Assessment of graft function (organ specific):
- Recent biopsy
- Proteinuria (24-hr collection for total protein)
- Hepatitis B and C status (HBsAg; Hep. C Antibody)
- CMV, toxoplasmosis, herpes simplex status (IgG, IgM)

Maintenance immunosuppression options:
- Azathioprine
- Cyclosporine
- Tacrolimus
- Corticosteroids
- Mycophenolate mofetil (avoid as feasible)
- Enteric-coated mycophenolate sodium (avoid as feasible)
- Sirolimus

The effect of comorbid conditions, (i.e., diabetes, hypertension) should be considered and their management optimized

Vaccinations should be given if needed (i.e., rubella, etc.) (see chap. 38)

Explore etiology of original disease; discuss genetic issues, if relevant

Discuss the effect of pregnancy on renal allograft function

Discuss the risks of intrauterine growth restriction, preterm birth, low birth weight, etc. (Table 13.3)

Prenatal

Accurate early diagnosis and dating of pregnancy

Clinical and laboratory monitoring of functional status of transplanted organ and immunosuppressive drug levels: Consider:
- Every 4–8 wk until 36 wk
- Every 2–4 wk until delivery

Monthly urine culture

Surveillance for rejection with biopsy if it is suspected

Surveillance for bacterial or viral presence, i.e., CMV, toxoplasmosis, hepatitis

Fetal surveillance

Monitor for hypertension and nephropathy

Careful surveillance for preeclampsia

Early screening for gestational diabetes

Labor and delivery

Vaginal delivery is optimal; cesarean delivery for obstetric reasons

For heart/heart-lung/lung recipients:
- Vigilance for poor or absent cough reflex, the need for airway protection
- Unpredictable response to vasoactive medications
- Judicious use of intravenous fluids

Postnatal

Monitor immunosuppressive drug levels for at least 1 mo postpartum, especially if dosages increased during pregnancy

Surveillance for rejection with biopsy if it is suspected

Breast-feeding discussion

Contraception counseling

Source: From Ref. 3.

Elevations of liver function tests and/or bilirubin could be indicative of rejection (<10% incidence in pregnancy). Evaluation of rejection includes liver ultrasound with Doppler to exclude anatomic sources of graft dysfunction. Liver biopsy to diagnose rejection is not contraindicated in pregnancy.

Because of an increased risk of carbohydrate intolerance caused by the administration of prednisone or tacrolimus, patients should be screened with glucose tolerance tests in the first trimester, followed by routine screening between 24 and 28 weeks. There are several drugs that interact with cyclosporine.

Antepartum Testing

A dating **ultrasound** should be performed in the first trimester. A detailed anatomy ultrasound should be performed in the second trimester. During the third trimester, assessment of fetal growth should be accomplished with serial (as needed) ultrasound examinations.

Weekly nonstress tests can begin at 32 weeks, unless medical or obstetric complications indicate earlier testing.

Labor and Delivery Issues

Patients who have received extended therapy with steroids during the antepartum period should receive "stress dose" steroids (i.e., hydrocortisone 100 mg IV every 8 hours × 24 hours).

Cesarean delivery should be performed only for obstetric indications.

Breast-feeding

There are reports to the NTPR of mothers who have breast-fed their infants without reported problems. However, any immunosuppressive drug exposure to the infant could potentially exceed the threshold for safety. The relatively small amount of drug transferred and the lack of reported adverse effects together with the documented benefits of breast-feeding may outweigh the theoretical risks of this exposure. Continued study in this area is warranted, especially of infant drug exposure and immunological development (3,16,31).

THORACIC TRANSPLANT

Table 13.3 shows pregnancy outcomes in liver, heart, and lung recipients for comparison (3). Female heart transplant recipients are able to maintain pregnancy with the majority resulting in a live birth. Not all rejections are treated as some are low grade. Maternal survival, independent of pregnancy-related events, should be considered as part of prepregnancy planning.

By comparison, lung recipients have a higher incidence of more significant rejection as well as graft loss in the peripartum period with smaller newborns. Successful pregnancy is possible post–lung transplantation. Analyses of a larger number of cases may help to identify other trends in pregnancy after lung transplantation. Whether long-term maternal survival is impacted by pregnancy warrants further study.

REFERENCES

1. Starzl TE, Marchioro TL, Von Kaulla KN, et al. Homotransplantation of the liver in humans. Surg Gynecol Obstet 1963; 117:659–676. [II-3]
2. Walcott WO, Derick DE, Jolley JJ, et al. Successful pregnancy in a liver transplant patient. Am J Obstet Gynecol 1978; 132(3):340–341. [II-3]
3. Coscia LA, Constantinescu S, MoritzMJ, et al. Report from the National Transplantation Pregnancy Registry (NTPR): outcomes of pregnancy after transplantation. In: Cecka JM, Terasaki PI, eds. Clinical Transplants 2010. Los Angeles, CA: UCLA Terasaki Foundation Laboratory. 2011:65–85. [II-2]
4. Jabiry-Zieniewicz Z, Cyganek A, Luterek K, et al. Pregnancy and delivery after liver transplantation. Transplant Proc 2005; 37 (2):1197–1200. [II-2]
5. Nagy S, Bush MC, Berkowitz R, et al. Pregnancy outcome in liver transplant recipients. Obstet Gynecol 2003; 102(1):121–128. [II-2]
6. McKay DB, Josephson MA, Armenti VT, et al. Reproduction and transplantation: report on the AST Consensus Conference on

Reproductive Issues and Transplantation. Am J Transplant 2005; 5(7):1592–1599. [Review]

7. Armenti VT, Herrine SK, Radomski JS, et al. Pregnancy after liver transplantation. Liver Transpl 2000; 6(6):671–685. [II-2]

8. Bonanno C, Dove L. Pregnancy after liver transplantation. Semin Perinatol 2007; 31:348–353. [Review]

9. Cundy TF, O'Grady JG, Williams R. Recovery of menstruation and pregnancy after liver transplantation. Gut 1990; 31(3): 337–338. [II-3]

10. Parolin MB, Rabinovitch I, Urbanetz AA, et al. Impact of successful liver transplantation on reproductive function and sexuality in women with advanced liver disease. Transplant Proc 2004; 36(4):943–944. [II-3]

11. Christopher V, Al-Chalabi T, Richardson PD, et al. Pregnancy outcome after liver transplantation: a single-center experience of 71 pregnancies in 45 recipients. Liver Transpl 2006; 12:1138–1143. [II-2]

12. Dei Malatesta MF, Rossi M, Rocca B, et al. Pregnancy after liver transplantation: report of 8 new cases and review of the literature. Transpl Immunol 2006; 15(4):297–302. [II-3]

13. Pan GD, Yan LN, Li B, et al. A successful pregnancy following liver transplantation. Hepatobiliary Pancreat Dis Int 2007; 6(1):98–100. [Case report, III]

14. Jankovic Z, Stamenkovic D, Duncan B, et al. Successful outcome after technically challenging liver transplant during pregnancy. Transplant Proc 2007; 39:1704–1706. [Case report, III]

15. Jabiry-Zieniewicz Z, Bobrowska K, Pietrzak B. Mode of delivery in women after liver transplantation. Transplant Proc 2007; 39:2796–2799. [II-2]

16. Heneghan MA, Selzner M, Yoshida EM, et al. Pregnancy and sexual function in liver transplantation. J Hepatol 2008; 49(4):507–519. [Review]

17. Surti B, Tan J, Saab S. Pregnancy and liver transplantation. Liver Int 2008; 28(9):1200–1206. [Review]

18. Coffin CS, Shaheen AA, Burak KW, et al. Pregnancy outcomes among liver transplant recipients in the United States: a nationwide case-control analysis. Liver Transpl 2010; 16(1):56–63. [II-2]

19. Cash WJ, Knisely AS, Waterhouse C, et al. Successful pregnancy after liver transplantation in progressive familial intrahepatic cholestasis, type 1. Pediatr Transplant 2010; [Epub ahead of print]. [Case report, III]

20. Armenti VT, Constantinescu S, Moritz MJ, et al. Pregnancy after transplantation. Transplant Rev 2008; 22:223–240. [Review]

21. Laifer SA, Darby MJ, Scantlebury VP, et al. Pregnancy and liver transplantation. Obstet Gynecol 1990; 76(6):1083–1088. [II-2]

22. Lai CL, Ratziu V, Yuen MF, et al. Viral hepatitis B. Lancet 2003; 362:2089–2094. [Review]

23. Ferrero S, Lungaro P, Bruzzone BM, et al. Prospective study of mother-to-infant transmission of hepatitis C virus: a 10-year survey (1990–2000). Acta Obstet Gynecol Scand 2003; 82(3):229–234. [II-2]

24. Jain AB, Reyes J, Marcos A, et al. Pregnancy after liver transplantation with tacrolimus immunosuppression: a single center's experience update at 13 years. Transplantation 2003; 76(5): 827–832. [II-2]

25. Marchetti P. New-onset diabetes after liver transplantation: from pathogenesis to management. Liver Transpl 2005; 11(6):612–620. [Review]

26. Homko CJ, Sivan E, Reece AE. Is there a role for oral antihyperglycemics in gestational diabetes and type 2 diabetes during pregnancy? Treat Endocrinol 2004; 3(3):133–139. [Review]

27. Anderka MT, Lin AE, Abuelo DN, et al. Reviewing the evidence for mycophenolate mofetil as a new teratogen: case report and review of the literature. Am J Med Genet A 2009; 149A(6):1241–1248. [II-2]

28. Sifontis NM, Coscia LA, Constantinescu S, et al. Pregnancy outcomes in solid organ transplant recipients with exposure to mycophenolate mofetil or sirolimus. Transplantation 2006; 82(12):1698–1702. [II-2]

29. Roche Laboratories. Mycophenolate Mofetil Package Insert. Nutley, NJ: Roche Laboratories, 2009. [III]

30. Novartis Pharmaceuticals Corp. Mycophenolic acid package insert. East Hanover, NJ: Novartis Pharmaceuticals, 2009. [III]

31. Mastrobattista JM, Gomez-Lobo V, for the Society for Maternal-Fetal Medicine. Pregnancy after solid organ transplantation. Obstet Gynecol 2008; 112(4):919–932. [Review]

14

Maternal anemia

M. Kathryn Menard and Robert A. Strauss

KEY POINTS

- Anemia in pregnancy is defined as a **hemoglobin (Hgb) <11 g/dL in the first or third trimesters and < 10.5 g/dL in the second trimester (1).**
- The most **common cause** is **iron deficiency.**
- **All pregnant women** should have **Hgb** and mean corpuscular volume (**MCV**) evaluated.
- **All** individuals of **African ancestry** should have a **hemoglobin electrophoresis**.
- **Workup** of anemia in pregnancy is described in Tables 14.1–14.4 and Figures 14.1–14.4. **MCV**, serum **ferritin** level, and **hemoglobin electrophoresis** are key laboratory tests.
- **Iron-deficiency anemia**
  - **Universal iron supplementation during pregnancy, with or without folate, is associated with a reduced risk of anemia and iron deficiency at term.** Significant reduction in perinatal morbidity has not been demonstrated, although there are **insufficient data on this and other clinically important outcomes.**
  - **Therapy** of iron-deficiency anemia with oral iron treatment in pregnancy is associated with a **reduction in the number of women with hemoglobin <11 g/dL and a greater mean hemoglobin level**, but again there are **insufficient data on other clinically relevant outcomes.**
  - **Parenteral iron** may be considered in patients with severe iron-deficiency anemia who cannot tolerate or will not take oral iron.

For sickle cell disease, see chapter 15; for von Willebrand disease, see chapter 16; for care of Jehovah's Witness pregnant women, see chapter 9 in *Obstetric Evidence Based Guidelines*.

DEFINITION

Hemoglobin (Hgb) <11 g/dL in the first or third trimesters and <10.5 g/dL in the second trimester (1).

SYMPTOMS

Usually asymptomatic, unless hemoglobin <6 to 7 g/dL.

INCIDENCE

Iron-deficiency anemia occurs in >20% to 30% of women even in developed countries if iron supplementation is not provided.

GENETICS

See Table 14.1 for types of hemoglobinopathies. Figure 14.1 describes the embryonic developmental sequence of hemoglobin chains. Tables 14.2 and 14.3 describe the types of α- and β-thalassemias. *Cis*-α-thalassemia is more common in South-east Asian ancestry; β-thalassemia is more common in women of Mediterranean, Asian, Middle Eastern, Hispanic, and West Indian ancestry. Ethnicity is not a good predictor of risk, as ethnic background is often mixed and many marry outside their ethnic group (2).

ETIOLOGY/PATHOPHYSIOLOGY

Most common cause is iron deficiency. Some degree of anemia (i.e., Hgb 11–12 g/dL) is physiologic in pregnancy: The red blood cell (RBC) mass and plasma both increase, but the plasma increase (40–60%) is proportionally greater than the RBC increase (15–30%), resulting in a lowering of the Hgb concentration. The differential diagnosis for true anemia in pregnancy is reviewed in Tables 14.1 to 14.3 and Figure 14.2. Iron-deficiency anemia is highly prevalent during pregnancy because of the nutrient demands required for the fetus and for maternal red blood cell mass expansion.

RISK FACTORS

Short interpregnancy interval, multiple gestations, low socioeconomic status, malnutrition, pica, history of heavy menses, and gastrointestinal disease affecting absorption are risk factors for iron-deficiency anemia. Though iron-deficiency anemia from ongoing blood loss from the gastrointestinal system is less common in women of reproductive age, when iron deficiency is recognized during pregnancy, all possible causes should be considered.

COMPLICATIONS

Iron-deficiency anemia: **low birth weight, preterm birth, maternal cardiovascular compromise, or possible need for transfusion.** Maternal anemia may also be associated with postpartum depression and poor mental and psychomotor performance testing in offspring (3).

MANAGEMENT
Workup (Tables 14.1–14.4 and Figs. 14.2–14.4)

- Initial evaluation: complete blood count (CBC) with indices (**Hgb** and **mean corpuscular volume, MCV**). These two indices should be **checked in all pregnant women.**
  - Hgb <11 g/dL and **MCV** < 80 um^3 represent a microcytic anemia (Fig. 14.2). Obtain Hgb electrophoresis to assess for a hemaglobinopathy and serum ferritin to assess iron stores. Follow algorithm.
  - If Hgb < 11 g/dL and **MCV** ≥80 um^3, check reticulocyte count to determine if anemia is secondary to underproduction or hemolysis, and obtain a history to identify any evidence of active bleeding, medication exposure, chronic disease, glucose-6-phosphate dehydrogenase (G6PD) deficiency, or a family history of RBC disorders.

Table 14.1   Types of Hemoglobins

Hgb A$_1$	2 α-chains	2 β-chains	Major adult hemoglobin
Hgb A$_2$	2 α-chains	2 δ-chains	Minor adult hemoglobin
Hgb F	2 α-chains	2 γ-chains	Fetal hemoglobin
Hgb H	—	4 β-chains	α-Thalassemia major ($-/-\alpha$)
Hgb Barts	—	4 γ-chains	Hydrops fetalis ($-/-$)
Hgb Gower	2 ε-chains	2 ς-chains	Embryonic hemoglobin

Table 14.2   Types of α-Thalassemia

α-Thalassemia silent carrier (asymptomatic)	α α/α – (heterozygous α^+-thalassemia)
α-Thalassemia trait (mild anemia)	α $-/\alpha$ – (trans) (homozygous α^+-thalassemia)
	Or
	$-/\alpha$ α (cis) (heterozygous α^0-thalassemia)
α-Thalassemia major (Hgb H Disease)	α $-/-$ –
(mostly Hgb H hemolytic anemia)	(α^+-thalassemia/α^0-thalassemia)
Hydrops fetalis (80% Hgb Bart's/ 20% Hgb H)	$-$ $-/-$ – (homozygous α^0-thalassemia)

Because there are two α-chains on each chromosome 16, the possibility exists for four different disease states (unlike β-thalassemias, where only two disease states are found).

Table 14.3   Types of β-Thalassemia

β-Thalassemia trait: one β-chain affected	β/β^0
Cooley anemia: both β-chains affected	β^0/β^0

β^0 absence of β-chain production → causes more severe anemia.
β^+ decrease in β-chain production → causes milder anemia.

Table 14.4   Laboratory Ranges

Laboratory reference ranges
   Ferritin 20–150 ng/mL
   Folate 3–18 ng/mL
   B12 (cobalamin) 250–1200 pg/mL
   MCV 80–100 μm^3
Normal hemoglobin electrophoresis
   Hgb A$_1$ > 95%
   Hgb A$_2$ < 3.5%
   Hgb F < 1%

Abbreviation: MCV, mean corpuscular volume.

○ If high reticulocyte counts ($\geq$3), then anemia may be secondary to hemolysis or blood loss. Consider (*i*) peripheral blood smear and haptoglobin (decreased), (*ii*) direct coombs (suggests autoimmune hemolytic anemia), (*iii*) Hgb electrophoresis to rule out SS or SC disease, and (*iv*) hemoccult or other tests if other sources of blood loss are suggested by history.
○ If low reticulocyte count (<3), then anemia is secondary to underproduction and should be evaluated according to the algorithm.

Table 14.5   Iron Supplements

Preparation	Elemental iron content
Ferrous fumarate	106 mg per 325 mg tablet
Ferrous sulfate	65 mg per 325 mg tablet
Ferrous gluconate	34 mg per 300 mg tablet
Iron dextran	50 mg/mL, IM or IV
Ferric gluconate	12.5 mg/mL IV
Iron sucrose	20 mg/mL IV

- All individuals of **African ancestry** should have a **hemoglobin electrophoresis**. Solubility testing is inadequate for screening since they fail to identify other important hemoglobinopathies (2). If documented results from a prior hemoglobin electrophoresis can be obtained, this test should not be repeated.
- Anemia of chronic disease is usually associated with normocytic anemia (about 20% are associated with microcytic anemia). Causes include chronic liver disease, thyroid disease, uremia, chronic infections, and malignancies. A reasonable workup may include liver function tests (LFTs), blood urea nitrogen (BUN) and creatinine, thyroid-stimulating hormone (TSH), and any tests for malignancy or chronic infection indicated by patient history and risk factors. Also check serum iron, serum B12, and RBC folate to rule out combined deficiencies.
- A nutrition consult should be obtained for patients with B12, folate, and iron deficiencies.
- A **genetic consult** should be obtained for all patients with inherited disorders. Attempt to obtain a blood sample for hemoglobin electrophoresis from the father of the baby prior to the genetic consult. DNA testing for α-globin abnormalities is available.

Prevention

Iron supplementation is associated with prevention of low hemoglobin at term and at six weeks postpartum (6–8). There is no evidence, however, of significant reduction in significant perinatal outcomes such as low birth weight, preterm birth, or infection. Most of the RCTs provided very limited information about the clinical outcomes for women or their babies (6). Except in women with hemochromatosis or other genetic disorder, there is little evidence of morbidity associated with iron supplementation. **The recommended daily allowance of ferrous iron during pregnancy is 27 mg**, as present in most prenatal vitamins (1). Table 14.5 lists elemental iron content of available iron supplements.

Folate supplementation is associated with increased or maintained serum folate levels and red cell folate levels compared to placebo or no supplementation. Folate supplementation is associated with a reduction in the proportion of women with low hemoglobin level in late pregnancy and megaloblastic erythropoiesis. Compared to placebo, folate supplementation is associated with similar incidences of preeclampsia, PTB, perinatal mortality, and a possible reduction in the incidence of low birth weight. Because of limited data, there is **insufficient evidence** to assess whether folate supplementation has any substantial effect on maternal or neonatal outcomes (9).

Therapy

There is a paucity of quality trials assessing the maternal and neonatal benefits of treatment of iron-deficiency anemia in pregnancy. Compared to placebo, **oral iron treatment** in

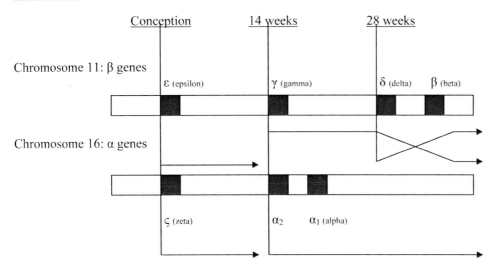

Figure 14.1 Developmental sequence of hemoglobin chains.

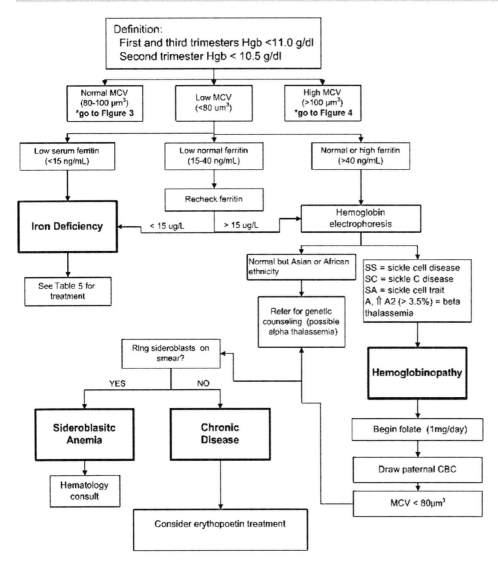

Figure 14.2 Evaluation of anemia in pregnancy.

Normocytic Anemia (Hgb < 11.0)

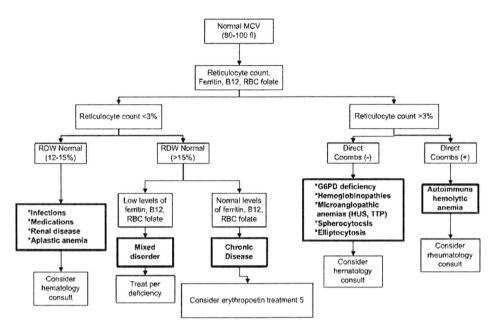

Figure 14.3 Normocytic anemia (Hgb < 11.0).

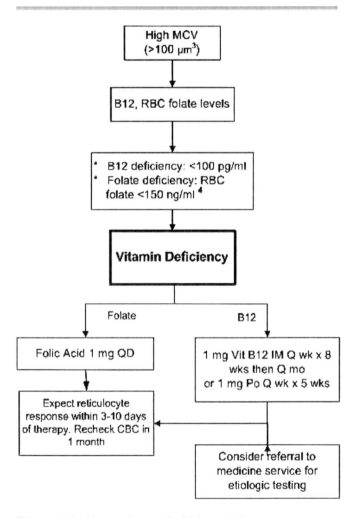

Figure 14.4 Macrocytic anemia (Hgb < 11.0).

pregnancy is associated with a reduction in the number of women with hemoglobin <11 g/dL and a greater mean hemoglobin level (9,10). Gastrointestinal side effects (e.g., constipation, nausea, and abdominal cramps) are common with oral iron treatments. Compared with standard oral preparations, **controlled release iron preparations** are associated with a diminished frequency of constipation.

The **intravenous (IV) or intramuscular (IM) routes** of administration are associated with better hematologic indices in women than the oral route, but there are insufficient data to compare potential adverse effects such as venous thrombosis and severe allergic reaction (10–12). Trials have reported that IV iron sucrose [calculated as: weight before pregnancy (kg) × (110g/L – actual hemoglobin (g/L) × 0.24 + 500 mg)] treated iron-deficiency anemia and restored iron stores faster and more effectively than oral iron polymaltose complex (300-mg elemental iron) daily or oral iron sulfate 240 mg daily without serious side effects, but again with insufficient data on important maternal or perinatal outcomes (8).

There are insufficient data to assess the effects of other forms of prevention or therapy, including self-donation during pregnancy.

Antepartum testing
Consider growth ultrasound in the third trimester.

Delivery and anethesia
Prepare team regarding increased risk in the event of hemorrhage. Consider having blood available for possible transfusion in cases of severe anemia, for example, Hgb <8 g/dL.

Postpartum/breast-feeding
There is **limited evidence** to assess different therapies for postpartum anemia. Outcome data on clinically relevant criteria are lacking. There was no apparent effect on need for blood

transfusions, although the RCTs may have been of insufficient size to rule out important clinical differences. Hematological indices (hemoglobin and hemocrit) show some increases when erythropoietin was compared to iron only, or iron and folate, but not when compared with placebo. When compared with iron therapy only, **erythropoietin** increases the likelihood of lactation at discharge from hospital in a very small trial (13). An iron-rich diet has not been studied as an intervention. **Most clinical outcomes have not been studied**.

Given that postpartum anemia is associated with several complications, including less ability to fully engage in child-care, household tasks, and exercise, as well as altered cognition, mood and productivity, preventive measures for iron-deficiency postpartum anemia are recommended.

REFERENCES

1. Recommendations to prevent and control iron deficiency in the United States. Center for Disease Control and Prevention. MMWR Recomm Rep 1998; 47(RR-3):1–29. [Level III, review]
2. American College of Obstetricians and Gynecologists. Hemoglobinopathies in pregnancy. ACOG Practice Bulletin No. 78. Obstet Gynecol 2007; 109(1):229–237. [Review]
3. American College of Obstetricians and Gynecologists. Anemia in Pregnancy. ACOG Practice Bulletin No. 95. Obstet Gynecol 2008; 112(1):210–207 reaffirmed 2010. [Review]
4. Braunwald E, Fauci AS, Isselbacher KJ, et al. eds. Ch 107: Megaloblastic anemia. In: Harrison's Online. The McGraw Hill Publishers, 2001–2004. Available at: http://harrisons.accessmedicine.com/. [Review]
5. Campbell BA. Megaloblastic anemia in pregnancy. Clin Obstet Gynecol 1995; 38(3):455–462. [Review]
6. Pena-Rosas JP, Viteri FE. Effects and safety of preventive oral iron or iron+folic acid supplementation for women during pregnancy. Cochrane Database Syst Rev 2009; (4):CD004736. [Meta-analysis; 49 trials, n = 23,200]
7. Hemminki E, Rimpela U. A randomized comparison of routine vs selective iron supplementation during pregnancy. J Am Coll Nutr 1991; 10:3–10. [RCT, n = 2694]
8. Hemminki E, Merilainen J. Long term follow-up of mothers and their infants in a randomized trial on iron prophylaxis during pregnancy. Am J Obstet Gynecol 1995; 173(1):205–209. [RCT, n = 2694]
9. Mahomed K. Folate supplementation in pregnancy. Cochrane Database Syst Rev 2007; (3):CD000183. [Meta-analysis; 21 RCTs, n = >3100]
10. Reveiz L, Gyte GML, Cuervo LG. Cochrane Database Syst Rev 2007; (2):CD003094. [Meta-analysis; 17 trials, n = 2578]
11. Baymumeu F, Subiran-Buisset C, Nour-Eddine B, et al. Iron therapy in iron deficiency anemia in pregnancy: intravenous route versus oral route. Am J Obstet Gynecol 2002; 186:518–522. [RCT]
12. Al RA, Unlubilgin E, Kandemir O, et al. Intravenous versus oral iron for treatment of anemia in pregnancy: a randomized trial. Obstet Gynecol 2005; 106(6):1335–1340. [RCT, n = 90]
13. Dodd JM, Dare MR, Middleston P. Treatment for women with postpartum iron deficiency anaemia. Cochrane Database Syst Rev 2004; (4):CD004222. [Meta-analysis; 6 trials, n = 411]

15

Sickle cell disease

Britta Panda and Jeffrey Ecker

KEY POINTS

- **Sickle cell disease** is an **autosomal recessive** disease resulting from an alteration in the structure of hemoglobin producing hemoglobin S (HbS). It is characterized by chronic hemolytic anemia and vaso-occlusive events.
- **Diagnosis is made by hemoglobin electrophoresis.**
- Severe complications during pregnancy and adverse pregnancy outcomes are most commonly experienced by women with HbSS and HbSβ^0 genotypes.
- Complications may include pregnancy loss, fetal growth restriction, preterm birth, preeclampsia, placental abnormalities, anemia, painful crises, UTI and other infections, thromboembolic events, acute chest syndrome (ACS), alloimmunization, postpartum infections, and maternal mortality.
- Pneumococcal and influenza vaccines are important prevention interventions.
- Painful crises are managed with **narcotic** (preferably morphine) therapy and **IV fluids**. Antibiotics should be added if the woman is febrile, has an infection, or has ACS; **oxygen should be added if the woman has low oxygen saturation**.
- **Prophylactic blood transfusions are not beneficial.** Blood transfusions are indicated for symptomatic or orthostatic anemia, hemoglobin <6 g/dL or hematocrit <25%, acute stroke, ACS, or multiple organ failure.
- In the 10% of patients with sickle cell disease who develop ACS, a chest X-ray is necessary. Antibiotics (usually cephalosporin and erythromycin) aimed at infectious pathogen(s) in pulmonary tree, and bronchodilators are the mainstay of therapy.

HISTORIC NOTES

Sickle cell disease was first described in 1910 by Herrick. In 1949, Linus Pauling described the molecular structure of sickle cell hemoglobin by protein electrophoresis. In 1956, Ingram and Hunt discovered the single amino acid change in sickle cell hemoglobin (1). In the 1960s, median survival age in the United States for those with sickle cell disease was estimated to be 42 years for men and 48 years for women (2). During the past two decades, improvements in medical care and earlier detection (especially through newborn screening) have led to better survival rates, improved quality of life, and better pregnancy outcomes in women with sickle cell disease (3,4).

DEFINITION

Sickle cell disease is an inherited disorder resulting from an **alteration in the structure of hemoglobin producing HbS**. It is characterized by **hemolysis and vaso-occlusive** events. Sickle cell disease is associated with a mild to moderate chronic anemia. The term sickle cell disease includes **sickle cell anemia (HbSS), hemoglobin S combined with hemoglobin C (HbSC), hemoglobin S combined with β-thalassemia (HbSβ^+ or HbSβ^0),** and other double heterozygous conditions causing sickling and thus, clinical disease (e.g., hereditary persistence of fetal hemoglobin (HgS/HPHP), and hemoglobin E (HbS/HbE) (5). The clinical manifestations vary among these genotypes, with HbSβ^0 usually with similar severe phenotype as HbSS; HbSC associated with intermediate disease; and very mild or symptom free for HbSβ^+, HbSHPHP, and HbSE (1,6).

DIAGNOSIS

The diagnosis is made by **hemoglobin electrophoresis**, according to the definition above. In all 50 U.S. states, newborns are screened for sickle cell disease at birth.

EPIDEMIOLOGY/INCIDENCE

Sickle cell disease occurs in about 1 and 600 African-Americans. Sickle cell trait occurs in 1 and 12 African-Americans, resulting in the birth of approximately 1100 infants with sickle cell disease annually in the United States. HbSS accounts for 60% to 70% of sickle cell disease in the United States. The prevalence of sickle cell disease and patients with sickle cell trait is highest in West Africa (25% of the population have one mutation), Mediterranean, Saudi Arabia, India, South and Central America, and Southeast Asia (1,6).

GENETICS/INHERITANCE

Sickle cell disease is an **autosomal recessive** disorder characterized by a mutation of a single nucleotide of the β-globin gene on chromosome 11p, changing the sixth amino acid in the β-globin chain from glutamic acid to valine. As noted above, other forms of sickle cell disease result from co-inheritance of HbS with other abnormal β-globin chain variants, the most common forms being sickle hemoglobin C disease (HbSC) and two types of sickle β-thalassemia (HbSβ^+ thalassemia and HbSβ^0 thalassemia). Inheriting one HbS gene results in sickle cell trait. Inheriting two HbS genes results in sickle cell disease. Concordant with an autosomal recessive pattern of inheritance, if both parents carry one HbS gene, the fetus has a 25% chance of having sickle cell disease, 50% chance of having sickle cell trait, and 25% chance of being unaffected (6).

PATHOPHYSIOLOGY

In most individuals without hemoglobinopathy, 96% to 97% of hemoglobin in humans is Hemoglobin A (which consists of two α- and two β-chains), with small portions of Hemoglobin A2 (two α- and two δ-chains), and at times Hemoglobin F (two α- and two γ-chains). Hemoglobin provides the oxygen carrying capacity of erythrocytes. HbS occurs because of a point mutation in which valine, a hydrophilic amino acid, is substituted for glutamic acid, a hydrophobic amino acid in the β-globin gene. This allows the sickle hemoglobin to polymerize when it is deoxygenated, triggering a cascade of repeated injury to the red-cell membrane. As a consequence, these cells become very rigid, assume a characteristic sickle shape, hemolyse, and are unable to pass through small capillaries, leading to vessel occlusion and ischemia. This tissue ischemia leads to acute and chronic pain as well as to end-organ damage. As vaso-occlusion can occur in any vessel, this is a systemic disease that can affect any organ. The life span of a sickle cell is about 10 to 20 days compared to the 120 days life span of a normal red blood cell. This chronic hemolysis contributes to the anemia (1,6,7). Dehydration, infection, decrease in oxygen tension, and acidosis, are common triggers of cell sickling and sickle cell crisis. Sickle cell crisis describes several independent acute conditions occurring in patients with sickle cell disease (vaso-occlusive crisis, aplastic crisis, hemolytic crisis).

SYMPTOMS

1. **Chronic hemolytic anemia**
   - Fatigue, pallor, shortness of breath
   - Aplastic crisis presents with severe anemia and reticulocytopenia. It is the most common hematologic crisis during pregnancy
2. **Acute vaso-occlusive episodes**
   - Pain involving the chest, lower back, abdomen, head, and bones/extremities
   - Dactylitis (inflammation of fingers and/or toes) often the first symptom of sickle cell disease
   - Exacerbated by cold, infection, stress, dehydration, alcohol, and fatigue
3. **Infections**
   - Urinary tract infections, pneumonia, osteomyelitis, endometritis
   - Organisms include *Streptococcus pneumoniae*, *Hemophilus influenza*, *Staphylococcus*, gram-negative organisms, *Salmonella*, and mycoplasma
4. **Cardiac**
   - Systolic murmur, cardiomegaly, high output failure

5. **Pulmonary**
   - ACS presents with chest pain, dyspnea, tachypnea, fever, cough, leukocytosis, and pulmonary infiltrates. It is usually a result of infection, vaso-occlusion, or bone marrow embolization
6. **Gastrointestinal**
   - Right upper quadrant syndrome presents with abdominal pain, fever, hepatomegaly, hyperbilirubinemia, and increased liver function tests. Splenomegaly is common
7. **Renal**
   - Hematuria, papillary necrosis, nephrotic syndrome, renal infarction, pyelonephritis, hyposthenuria, and renal medullary carcinoma
8. **Neurologic**
   - Transient ischemic attacks, cerebrovascular accidents, seizures, coma, hemiparesis, hemianesthesia, visual field changes, and cranial nerve palsy
   - Moyamoya disease is a progressive occlusive process of the cerebral vasculature that results in the formation of collateral vessels with the appearance of "puffs of smoke" (Moyamoya in Japanese) on angiography
9. **Skeletal**
   - Avascular necrosis most often occurs in the humeral and femoral heads and is characterized by pain

COMPLICATIONS

Pregnancy in women with sickle cell disease is complicated not only by the maternal condition characterized by years of chronic organ damage but also by the physiologic changes and adaptations of pregnancy that can often compound or exacerbate underlying organ damage. However, the majority of these women can achieve a successful pregnancy: the majority tends to deliver beyond 28 weeks' gestation with a >80% live birth rate, although 50% will require transfusion or medically indicated hospitalization and 75% will have a pain crisis during the pregnancy (8).

Several complications have been reported: effects of sickle cell disease on pregnancy—Table 15.1 (8–12); effects of pregnancy on sickle cell disease—Table 15.2 (8,11,12).

Table 15.1 Complications: Effects of Sickle Cell Disease on Pregnancy

Complication	HBSS	HBSC	HBSβ^0
Pregnancy loss (mostly first trimester)	7–36% (8–10)	9% (10)	
Fetal death	No increase (8,9)	No increase (8,9)	
Fetal growth restriction (FGR)	45% (9)	21% (9)	
Small for gestational age (SGA)[a]	21% (11)		
Acute anemia	4% (11)		15% (11)
Painful crises[b]	20–50%. (8,9,11)	19–26% (9,11)	
Urinary tract infections	15% (8)		
Preterm birth	45% (9,11)[c]	22% (9)	
Preeclampsia	10% (9,12)	3%	
Alloimmunization[d]			
Antepartum admissions[e]	62% (9)	26% 2.8(9)	
Postpartum infections[f]	1.4 (12)		

% is reported if available in the source study.
[a]Preeclampsia and acute anemia episodes are risk factors for SGA. High hemoglobin F levels are protective for fetal growth (11).
[b]There is no difference in the rate of painful episodes before, during and after pregnancies (11).
[c]The mean gestational age at delivery is 34 to 37 weeks (9,11).
[d]Any woman with sickle cell disease is at increased risk for Rh and other antibodies if she has had blood transfusions in the past.
[e]Because of all the above complications, in particular painful crises, and increased incidences of infections in general, women with sickle cell disease in pregnancy are at increased risk for hospitalization.
[f]More likely to have postpartum infections secondary to endometritis or pyelonephritis. The effect is listed as Odds Ratio compared to the African-American population. No increase risk for postpartum hemorrhage (8,9).

Table 15.2 Complications: Effects of Pregnancy on Sickle Cell Disease

Complication	HBSS
Maternal mortality	0.5–2.1% (8,11,12)
Acute chest syndrome	7–20% (8,11)
Thromboembolic events	2.5 (12)
Cerebral vein thrombosis	4.9 (12)
Pyelonephritis	1.3 (12)
Pneumonia	9.8 (12)
Sepsis	6.8 (12)
SIRS	12.6 (12)
Pulmonary hypertension	6.3 (12)
No. of blood transfusions	22.5 (12)
Postpartum infection	1.4 (12)

% is reported if available in the source study. Otherwise, the effect is listed as Odds Ratios or Relative Risks.

PREGNANCY MANAGEMENT
Principles
Multidisciplinary team approach, involving hematologist, blood bank, primary care, obstetrician, and any other involved health care workers (e.g., pulmonologist, cardiologist, pain and drug dependency services, and social services).

Workup
For diagnosis: Hemoglobin electrophoresis
For a crisis: Hemoglobin, hemoglobin electrophoresis, urine culture, and culture of any other possible infectious source; blood gas if hypoxia is present

Preventive Care
Pneumococcal and influenza vaccines; avoid triggers (especially infections), optimize hemoglobin status by educating on good nutrition and prescribe vitamins/folic acid/iron as needed, establish plan for home medication regimen, and educate on analgesia safety in pregnancy.

Preconception
Patients are no longer counseled to avoid pregnancy. Counseling should consist of a review of the effects of sickle cell disease on pregnancy, highlighting an increased risk for hospital admissions, pain crises, infections, severe anemia, maternal mortality, and others (Tables 15.1 and 15.2) (8–12). The discussion should also entail the effects of sickle cell disease on the fetus, which are early pregnancy loss, growth restriction, and perinatal mortality, as well as a risk for inherited hemoglobinopathies. Preventive care should be emphasized. Try to optimize hemoglobin status by prescribing up to **4-mg folic acid** and a prenatal vitamin (4,13). Discuss medication use during pregnancy and change/stop teratogenic medications (ACE inhibitors, iron chelators, and possibly hydroxyurea) and vaccinate as needed.

Prenatal Care
1. Initial visit: medical (assess for chronic organ damage, especially pulmonary hypertension, renal disease, and congestive heart failure), obstetrical, transfusion, and social history; nutritional assessment; discuss precipitating factors for painful crises and prior successful pain management. Counseling regarding risks (Tables 15.1 and 15.2). Advice on the need for adequate hydration and fluid intake. Preventive care.
2. Initial laboratory studies: CBC, reticulocyte count, Hb electrophoresis, serum iron studies, bilirubin, liver function tests, hepatitis A, B, and C, HIV, BUN, creatinine, antibody screen, rubella antibody titer, VDRL, tuberculosis skin test, Pap smear as appropriate, chlamydia and gonorrhea cultures.
3. Test the father of the baby (CBC, hemoglobin electrophoresis). Offer genetic counseling if father is positive for HbS. If father is positive for HbS, direct DNA analysis is available by polymerase chain reaction via chorionic villous sampling or amniocentesis. Interestingly, the vast majority of women at risk of an affected fetus decline prenatal diagnosis.
4. Serial urine cultures every four to eight weeks.
5. CBC every trimester.
6. **Folate supplementation up to 4 mg daily** plus prenatal vitamin (4,13). Ferrous sulfate 325 mg only if iron deficient (avoid iron overload).
7. Pneumococcal and influenza vaccines.
8. Consider first-trimester ultrasound for exact dating, which might be helpful in the evaluation of suspected growth restriction later during pregnancy. Ultrasound at 18 to 20 weeks for a detailed anatomy scan, and then growth scans starting at 28 to 32 weeks as clinically indicated.
9. For patients with multiple red cell alloantibodies and an anticipated need for a blood transfusion, consider to have phenotypically matched units of PRBC identified.
10. Rescreen for red cell alloantibodies in third trimester (14).

THERAPY
1. **Painful crisis** (diagnosis made by history, often no physical or laboratory finding).
   - **Narcotics:** Morphine is the preferred agent. Consider using a patient-controlled analgesia (PCA) system for severe pain. Oral controlled-release morphine is as effective as intravenous morphine in nonpregnant adults. Ask women regarding which narcotic or pain management works best for them, and implement as appropriate. After 28 to 32 weeks, avoid NSAIDs, which are safe and effective earlier in pregnancy. Prescribe stool softeners with narcotic use (15).
   - **Intravenous fluids:** Effective in nonpregnant adults. Adequate fluid intake is 60 mL/kg/24 hr in adults (15). Consider 150 cc/hr. Monitor fluid balance.
   - **Antibiotics:** Broad-spectrum antibiotics should be used if patient is febrile ($T > 38°C$), or if there is evidence of infection. Add a macrolide (e.g., erythromycin) if chest symptoms are present (15).
   - **Oxygen:** Use only for ACS or if O_2 saturation is less than patient's known state or <95% (4) (such treatment is ineffective in nonpregnant patients and may be so in pregnant women as well) (15).
   - **Labor and delivery:** There is no need to alter general recommendations for labor and delivery in women in sickle cell crisis. A crisis is not an indication for cesarean delivery or other special intervention. Close monitoring of mother and fetus for adequate oxygenation is paramount. Pain during labor can be managed with narcotics, regional anesthesia, or local anesthesia via pudendal block (19). Pediatricians should be aware of any chronic narcotic use in pregnancy, as such is a risk for neonatal withdrawal.

2. **Anemia**
   - **Transfusions:** There is limited evidence to assess the efficacy of prophylactic blood transfusions for pregnant women with sickle cell disease. Compared to transfusion only for Hb <6 g/dL, transfusion (or exchange transfusion) with two units of red cells every week for three weeks, or until hemoglobin level is 10 to 11 g/dL or HbS <35%, is associated with no significant difference in perinatal outcome (16). Prophylactic transfusions decreased the number of painful crisis (14% vs. 50%). Disadvantages of prophylactic transfusion include increase in costs, number of hospitalizations, and risk of alloimmunization (16). Therefore, prophylactic blood transfusions are not indicated universally for pregnant women with sickle cell disease.

     Indications for transfusions are: any woman who is symptomatic or orthostatic from anemia, and/or with a hemoglobin of <6 g/dL or hematocrit <25%, or with acute stroke or chest syndrome or multiple organ failure.

     Sickle cell crisis is not an absolute indication to transfusion. Persistent crises are an indication to transfusion to avoid recurrence. If blood transfusion is indicated, it should always be leukodepleted and matched for Rh and Kell antigens.

     Goal of transfusion are usually: hematocrit >35%, HbA$_1$ >40%, and HbS <35%.

     There is insufficient evidence to compare exchange versus regular blood transfusions for sickle cell disease in pregnancy. For a hematocrit <15%, a direct transfusion is always preferable. For a hematocrit >15%, an exchange transfusion can be considered.
   - **Iron, folic acid, and multivitamins**: Only prescribe iron if patient is deficient (avoid iron overload).
   - **Hydroxyurea** (hydroxycarbamide): Decreases number and severity of painful crisis and improves survival in nonpregnant adults and children (17). However, there are insufficient clinical data and trials to make a firm recommendation on its use, efficacy, and teratogenicity during pregnancy (18).

ALLOIMMUNIZATION

If the antibody screen is positive, follow recommendations in chapter 52. The antigen status of the father of the pregnancy should be tested, as he often does not carry the offending antigen, with the maternal antibody usually acquired by prior transfusions. Bilirubin level (Delta OD450) in amniotic fluid of women with sickle cell disease is unreliable for detecting fetal anemia, as maternal hemolysis and hyperbilirubinemia increase fetal and AF bilirubin levels. Fetal anemia may be assessed by middle cerebral artery Doppler (see chap. 52).

ANTENATAL TESTING

There are no prospective studies on the use of antepartum testing in sickle cell disease women (10). Fetal monitoring can be started at 32 weeks with weekly non-stress test/amniotic fluid indexes, especially if fetus is growth restricted (6).

DELIVERY

It is safe for patients to deliver vaginally. Inductions and cesarean sections should be reserved for obstetrical indications (4).

There is one case report of a sickle cell crisis triggered by induction of labor with a prostaglandin (19). Some recommend prophylactic transfusion before a cesarean delivery to avoid precipitating a crisis because of blood loss in patients with hemoglobin 7 to 8 g/dL or less (20).

ANESTHESIA

There are no contraindications to anesthesia (IV, regional, or general) (4).

POSTPARTUM

During the postpartum period, early ambulation and adequate hydration is encouraged. Compression boots and incentive spirometry should be used during bedrest. Anemia should be assessed and transfusion only if indicated (see above). Breast-feeding is encouraged. Low-dose oral contraceptives, Depoprovera injections, and intrauterine devices are all safe in pregnancy (21).

ACUTE CHEST SYNDROME
Definition

New pulmonary infiltrate of at least one complete lung segment with alveolar consolidation and excluding atelectasis; and presence of chest pain, temp T >38.5°C, tachypnea, wheezing, or cough. Hypoxia, decreasing hemoglobin levels, and progressive pneumonia are frequent. Mostly associated with pulmonary fat embolism and pulmonary infection, with 3% to 10% chance of death, related to pulmonary embolism and pneumonia.

Incidence

Acute chest syndrome develops in about 10% of women with sickle cell disease.

Pathophysiology

Cause of ACS remains mainly unknown. Infection leading to sickle crisis, anemia, hypoxia, and vaso-occlusion with ischemic damage are the most common associations.

Symptoms

Chest pain, pain in arms and legs, dypnea, fever, etc.

Complications

ACS is one of the most common causes of death (3–10%) among those with sickle cell disease. Neurologic complications, probably secondary to CNS hypoxia, occur in about 20% of patients. Pulmonary emboli and infarction can also occur.

Work up

For ACS, chest X-ray; sputum culture, nasopharyngeal sample and/or bronchoscopy washings culture (*Chlamydia pneumoniae* and *Mycoplasma pneumoniae* are most common pathogens).

Therapy

Antibiotics (usually cephalosporin and erythromycin) aimed at infectious pathogen(s) in pulmonary tree, and bronchodilators (even if no evidence of reactive airway disease). Blood transfusions (especially in hypoxic and/or anemic women), oxygen (15% need mechanical ventilation), and pain control as needed (22).

SICKLE CELL TRAIT

Pregnant women with sickle cell trait should be screened with a hemoglobin electrophoresis if this has not been done before, and testing of the father and genetic counseling should be offered.

They are at increased risk of **urinary tract infections**, and therefore should have a urine culture at first prenatal visit and in every trimester, with asymptomatic bacteriuria adequately treated.

HbSC DISEASE

HbC is due to a single nucleotide substitution (A for G) in the 6th codon of the β-globin gene (making it a Hb C gene) in chromosome 11, leading to substitution of lysine for glutamic acid on the β-globin chain, resulting in β^c globin. Of African-Americans, 1% are carriers (trait). Diagnosis is by electrophoresis. No disease with trait only.

HbSC occurs in about 1/833 African-Americans. About 40% to 60% have same clinical course as HbSS disease, while others have milder disease. Preventive and prenatal management should be as for HbSS.

HbS-βTHAL

Diagnosis by hemoglobin electrophoresis: HbS > HbA; elevated HbA$_2$, elevated HbF. Prognosis and management are as for HbSS.

HEMOGLOBIN E

Prevalent in Southeast Asia. No increase in morbidity and mortality, except possible slight decrease in birth weight and increase in abruption.

REFERENCES

1. Rust OA. Pregnancy complicated by sickle hemoglobinopathy. Clin Obstet Gynecol 1995; 38(3):472–484. [Review]
2. Serjeant GR, Higgs DR, Hambleton IR. Elderly survivors with homozygous sickle cell disease. N Engl J Med 2007; 356:642–643. [III]
3. World Health Organization. Sickle Cell Anaemia: Report by the Secretariat. 59th World Health Assembly; 2006. [III]
4. ACOG Committee on Obstetrics. Hemoglobinopathies in pregnancy. ACOG Practice Bulletin No. 78. Obstet Gynecol 2007; 109:229–237. [III]
5. Serjeant GR. The emerging understanding of sickle cell disease. Br J Haematol 2001; 112:3–18. [Review]
6. Rappaport VJ. Hemaglobinopathies in pregnancy. Obstet Gynecol Clin 2004; 31(2):25. [Review]
7. Stuart MJ, Nagel RL. Sickle-cell disease. Lancet 2004; 364:1343–1360. [Review; nonpregnant]
8. Serjeant GR, Loy LL, Crowther M, et al. Outcome of pregnancy in homozygous SSD. Obstet Gynecol 2004; 103(6):1278–1285. [II-2]
9. Sun PM. Sickle cell disease in pregnancy: twenty years of experience at Grady Memorial Hospital, Atlanta, Georgia. Am J Obstet Gynecol 2001; 184(6):1127. [II-2]
10. Milner PF, Jones BR, Dobler J. Outcome of pregnancy in sickle cell anemia and sickle cell-hemoglobin C disease. An analysis of 181 pregnancies in 98 patients, and a review of the literature. Am J Obstet Gynecol 1986; 138(3):239–245. [II-3]
11. Smith JA. Pregnancy in sickle cell disease: experience of the Cooperative Study of Sickle Cell Disease. Obstet Gynecol 1996; 87(2):199–204. [II-2]
12. Villers MS, Jamison MG, De Castro LM, et al. Morbidity associated with sickle cell disease in pregnancy. Am J Obstet Gynecol 2008; 199(2):125.e1–125.e5. [III]
13. Pregnancy, contraception and fertility. In: Bennett L, Chapman C, Davis B, et al. Standards for the Clinical Care of Adults with Sickle Cell Disease in the UK. London: Sickle Cell Society 2008:59. [III]
14. Mohomed K. Prophylactic versus selective blood transfusion for sickle cell anaemia during pregnancy. Cochrane Database Syst Rev 1996; (2):CD000040. [I]
15. ReesDC, Olujohungbe AD, Parker NE, et al.; British Committee for Standards in Haematology General Haematology Task Force by the Sickle Cell Working Party. Guidelines for the management of the acute painful crisis in sickle cell disease. Br J Hematol 2003; 120:744–752. [Guideline]
16. Koshy M. Prophylactic red-cell transfusions in pregnant patients with sickle cell disease. A randomized cooperative study. N Engl J Med 1988; 319(22):1447–1452. [RCT, $n = 72$]
17. Rees D, Williams TN, Gladwin MT. Sickle cell disease. Lancet 2010; 376:2018–2031. [Review]
18. National Institutes of Health Consensus Development Conference Proceedings. Hydroxyurea: treatment for sickle cell disease. Maryland: National Institutes of Health February 25–27, 2008. [III]
19. Faron G, Corbisier C, Tecco L, et al. First sickle cell crisis triggered by induction of labor in a primigravida. Eur J Obstet Gynecol Repro Biol 2001; 94(20):304–306. [II-3]
20. Firth PG, Alvin C. Sickle cell disease and anesthesia. J Am Anesthesiol 2004; 101(3):766–785. [Review]
21. Freie HM. Sickle cell disease and hormonal contraception. Acta Obstet Gynecol Scand 1983; 62(3):211–217. [II-3]
22. Vichinsky EP, Neumayr LD, Earles AN, et al. Causes and outcomes of the acute chest syndrome in sickle cell disease. N Engl J Med 2000; 342(25):1855–1865. [II-3]

von Willebrand disease

Dawnette Lewis

KEY POINTS

- **Ensure correct diagnosis of von Willebrand disease (vWD), which must be done while not pregnant. The diagnostic work usually includes factor VIII, vWF:Ag, and ristocetin cofactor activity.** Be aware of **physiologic increase of factor VIII and vWF levels in pregnancy.**
- Key labs: **factor VIII, vWF:Ag, and ristocetin cofactor activity.** Check factor VIII levels at least every trimester.
- **Test DDAVP responsiveness** preferably preconception, or in second or third trimester.
- **Prophylactic therapy for most common type (I) of vWD, if factor VIII is** <50% of normal, **is DDAVP.**
- **Prophylactic therapies for other types of vWD are according to type, and include DDAVP, vWF concentrates (Humate-P, Alphanate SD/HT), and/or adjuvant therapy [antifibrinolytic amino acids (amniocaproic acid and tranexamic acid), used in conjunction with desmopressin and plasma concentrates].**
- If possible, avoid pudendal blocks, operative vaginal deliveries, as well as scalp lead, scalp pH, given the 50% chance of the fetus being affected.

HISTORIC NOTES

First described in 1926 by a Finnish pediatrician, Erik von Willebrand. He also described that the condition was inherited in an autosomal dominant fashion and improved with blood transfusions.

DIAGNOSIS/DEFINITION

Diagnosis of vWD is complex (Table 16.1). For type I, the three most important laboratory tests are as follows:

- **Factor VIII** (decreased)
- **vWF:Ag** (von Willebrand factor antigen—an immunoreactive protein) (decreased)
- **Ristocetin cofactor activity** (binding of vWF:Ag to the platelet membrane glycoprotein Iba, mediated by the antibiotic ristocetin) (decreased).

vWD is usually associated with prolonged bleeding time, with thromboplastin time and partial thromboplastin time frequently normal.

In pregnancy, many of the values for diagnosis are normal, and diagnosis cannot be made reliably. For distinguishing types (Table 16.1), also send multimeric analysis, and factor VIII binding assay. Factor VIII levels are best (but not that good) at predicting surgical/soft-tissue bleeding.

SYMPTOMS

Ask detailed personal and family history. Symptoms include epistaxis, bleeding at dental surgery, bleeding from gums, ecchymoses, prolonged bleeding after minor cuts, menorrhagia, postpartum hemorrhage, delayed postpartum hemorrhage, and postoperative bleeding.

EPIDEMIOLOGY/INCIDENCE

Incidence about 1% to 2% in the general population; most common congenital hemorrhagic disease.

GENETICS

Usually autosomal dominant (Table 16.2). vWF is a large multimeric glycoprotein encoded on chromosome 12 and is synthesized and released from endothelium and megakaryocytes. There are over 250 mutations of all types known.

ETIOLOGY/BASIC PATHOPHYSIOLOGY

Decrease (quantitative: types I and III) in vWF (also known as factor VIII cofactor) or its function (qualitative: type II) (Table 16.2). This cofactor is critical for normal platelet adhesion at site of vascular injury (Fig. 16.1) (1).

TYPES (TABLE 16.2)

I. **Autosomal dominant (60–85%).** Partial quantitative decrease in vWF. **Mild-moderate decrease in vWF.** Also **decreased factor VIII** 5–30 (normal range 50–150 IU/dL); **decreased vWF:Ag; decreased** vWF:Ac (tinty), which are measured by **ristocetin**-induced **cofactor** assay.

II. Autosomal dominant (10–30%). Qualitative defect of vWF. **Normal vWF but dysfunction:**
    A. decreased vWF function;
    B. decreased vWF function causing increased binding of platelets and so **decreased platelets** by platelet agglutination.
    M and N types are uncommon.

III. Autosomal recessive (1–5%). Quantitative decrease of vWF. **No vWF** and very low factor VIII. Severe symptoms, **do not respond to DDAVP.**

Acquired: during certain disease states.

COMPLICATIONS

Intra- and postpartum hemorrhage. Postpartum hemorrhage occurs in 16% to 29% of women within 24 hours, and delayed (after 24 hours, usually within 2 weeks) in 20% to 29% of women. It does not impair fertility or increase pregnancy loss.

PREGNANCY CONSIDERATIONS

Factor VIII and vWF levels rise in pregnancy, so they might be, and in fact usually are, normal in women with vWD.

Table 16.1 Common laboratory findings in von Willebrand disease

Subtype[a]	von Willebrand factor antigen	von Willebrand factor ristocetin cofactor activity	von Willebrand factor ristocetin cofactor activity/von Willebrand factor antigen (ratio)	Factor VIII	Low-dose ristocetin-induced platelet aggregation	Multimer assay
Type 1	Low	Low	>0.5–0.7	Low or normal	No reaction	Normal
Type 2A	Low	Low	<0.5–0.7	Low or normal	No reaction	Decrease in large multimers
Type 2B	Low	Low	<0.5–0.7	Low or normal	Positive	Decrease in large multimers
Type 2M	Low	Low	<0.5–0.7	Low or normal	No reaction	Normal
Type 2N	Normal to low	Normal to low	>0.5–0.7	Low	No reaction	Normal
Type 3	Absent	Absent		Low	No reaction	Absent

Source: Adapted from Ref. 4.

Table 16.2 Mechanism, Inheritance, and Treatment for the Different Types of von Willebrand Disease

Type	Mechanism	Inheritance	Treatment	Second-line therapy
1	Quantitative (partial) decrease vWF	Autosomal dominant	DDAVP	Factor VIII/vWF concentrates
2	Qualitative/functional defect vWF	Autosomal dominant		
A	Platelet-dependent vWF— absence of large or intermediate size multimers	Autosomal dominant	Factor VIII/vWF concentrates	DDAVP
B	Large multimers absent (increase in binding with platelets and vWF)	Autosomal dominant	None	
M		Autosomal dominant	Factor VIII/vWF concentrates	DDAVP
N	Defect in binding of vWF with platelets	Autosomal dominant	Factor VIIII/vWF concentrates	DDAVP
3	Severe or absent vWF and factor VIII deficiency	Autosomal recessive	Factor VIII/vWF concentrates (without alloantibodies). Recombinant factor VIII (with alloantibodies)	
Acquired	Occurs in disease states such as cancer, valvular heart disease (aortic stenosis), thrombocythemia, autoimmune diseases	Increased clearance of vWF from plasma	Treatment of underlying condition	Desmopressin, plasma concentrates, immunoglobulin

PREGNANCY MANAGEMENT
Principles
Treat as you would in nonpregnant adult.

Workup (Labs)
See section "Diagnosis" (Tables 16.1 and 16.2).

Preconception Counseling
Obtain history, type of vWD, records, etc.; for hematology and genetic counseling, consult as necessary; baseline laboratory tests (see section "Workup"); hepatitis B vaccine. If vWD type I with factor VIII levels <50 IU/dL, type II or III, or history of severe bleeding, consider care in a high-risk center, with close collaboration with hematologist.

Prenatal Care
First trimester: See section "Preconception Counseling," if not done yet. Prenatal diagnosis, including chorionic villous sampling, is possible (give DDAVP or other prophylaxis as appropriate per type—see below).

Second/third trimester: Anesthesia consult; test response to DAVVP.

Third trimester: Monitor laboratory tests; birth plan (anesthesia, DDAVP, etc.). Aim to achieve factor VIII levels of ≥50 IU/dL, associated with very low risk of any bleeding complications (2).

Therapy (Table 16.2, Fig. 16.2)
Type I
DDAVP (desmopressin, i.e., 1-deamino-8-D-arginine vasopressin; synthetic vasopressin analog—antidiuretic hormone)

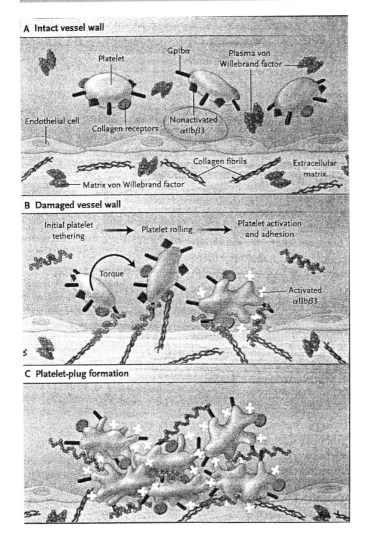

Figure 16.1 Normal platelet adhesion at site of vascular injury. (A) Intact vessel wall. (B) Damaged vessel wall. (C) Platelet-plug formation. Reprinted with permission, from[1].

0.3 µg/kg IV over 30 minutes (maximum dose: 25–30 µg). Works within one hour (peak occurs in 30–90 minutes after the infusion). Also available SQ (0.3 µg/kg) or nasal inhalation (300 µg in adults). Mechanism of action is promoting release of vWF and factor VIII from endothelial cells, so it increases ristocetin cofactor activity, and increases three times the vWF:Ag level and factor VIII procoagulant level (FVIII:C). One can give test dose, and then **check factor VIII** and ristocetin cofactor activity at peak (one hour) and clearance (four hours). It lasts up to 10 hours, so repeat q12h, usually for a maximum of two to four doses. **DDAVP is the first-line therapy for type I**.

Safe in pregnancy for mother and fetus (does not cross placenta; FDA category B) (2), and during breast-feeding.

If not responsive to DDAVP: **Alphanate** (factor VIII and vWF mixed). This is better than cryoprecipitate because there are no infectious disease issues. Otherwise, use **Humate-P** (purified factor VIII). Usual loading dose for these two vWF concentrates is 40 to 60 IU/kg.

Alternatives, especially more for treatment of hemorrhage more than prophylaxis, are **cryoprecipitate** (fibrinogen and vWF), or **FFP** (watch volume overload). Applies to all above.

Safety: limited data, but probably safe. Counsel regarding blood product precautions.

Type IIa
Preferred therapy is factor VIII/vWF concentrates (as Alphanate, Humate-P, etc.)

Type IIb
No specific treatment is available, but can treat as per Figure 16.2.

Type III
Without alloantibodies: factor VIII/vWF concentrates; with alloantibodies: recombinant factor VIII.

Antepartum Testing

Not indicated unless other complications present (no known direct fetal risks).

Delivery (Figure 16.2)

Types I and II: measure (*i*) **factor VIII**, (*ii*) vWFAg, (*iii*) ristocetin cofactor activity. **If factor VIII levels are >30% to 40% of normal (or ≥50 mU/dL), there is very low risk of bleeding with vaginal or cesarean delivery. If lower, prophylactically administer DDAVP (if DDAVP responder) or concentrates/blood products** (see above, according to type) *at time of delivery (if possible 1 hour before)*, **and 12 hours thereafter** (then as needed).

Type III: do not measure factor VIII, as always low. Treat daily as above starting before delivery.

Oxytocin dose should be carefully monitored, since fluid retention can be a side effect of both oxytocin and DDAVP, and lead to life threatening hyponatremia.

As fetus has a 50% chance of having von Willebrand disease, scalp lead, scalp pH, and operative vaginal delivery should be avoided.

Anesthesia

Regional anesthesia is safe if normal PTT, factor VIII levels of ≥50 mU/dL, and normal ristocetin cofactor activity.

Postpartum/Breast-feeding

Measure factor VIII one to two weeks postpartum, since increased level during pregnancy will again physiologically decrease in vWD disease. Risk of postpartum bleeding in fact continues for about two to four weeks, so that additional doses of DDAVP and close monitoring are required. Consider oral contraception.

As the neonate has a 50% chance of having von Willebrand disease, circumcision may need to be delayed until after testing.

FUTURE

vWF produced by recombinant DNA techniques, gene therapy.

RARE/RELATED

Glanzman disease (congenital thromboasthenia): congenital bleeding disorder defined by defective or quantitatively abnormal glycoprotein (GP) IIb/IIIa receptors (Fig. 16.1). Diagnosis: bleeding and abnormal platelet aggregation in response to

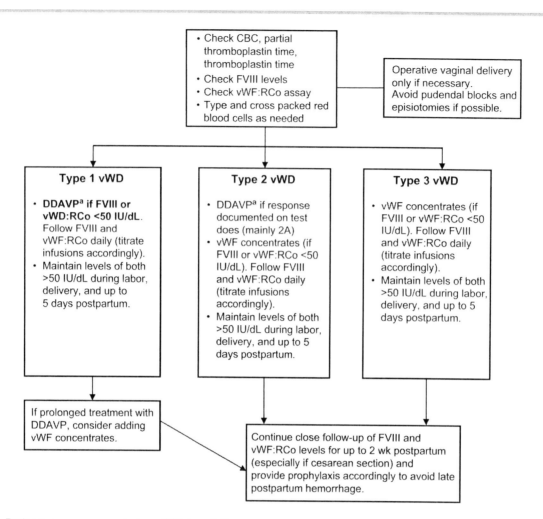

Figure 16.2 Peripartum management of von Willebrand disease.

[a]Avoid hypotonic solutions at time of delivery if using DDAVP in order to prevent hyponatremia. *Source*: Adapted from Ref. 4.

stimuli, prolonged bleeding times, and normal platelet counts (3). Four pregnancies in the world's literature up to 1978, very few after.

REFERENCES

1. Mannucci P. Treatment of von Willebrand disease. N Engl J Med 2004; 351:683–694. [Review]
2. James AH. von Willebrand disease. Obstet Gynecol Surv 2006; 61:136–145. [Review]
3. Newman PJ, Seligsohn U, Lyman S, et al. The molecular genetic basis of Glanzmann thrombasthenia in the Iraqi–Jewish and Arab populations in Israel. Proc Natl Acad Sci U S A 1991; 88(8):3160–3164. [II-3]
4. Pacheco LD, Constantine MM, Saade GR, et al. Von Willebrand disease and pregnancy: a practical approach for the diagnosis and treatment. Am J Obstet Gynecol 2010; 203:194–200. [III]

17

Renal disease

Sara Nicholas

KEY POINTS

- The frequency of complications in pregnancies with maternal renal disease is directly proportional to the initial creatinine level.
- Complications include **preterm birth, preeclampsia, fetal growth restriction, low birth weight**, and **perinatal mortality**. In women with **creatinine ≥1.4 mg/dL,** about **10%** will have progressive **renal deterioration. Creatinine >2.3 mg/dL may be regarded as a contraindication to pregnancy.**
- **Workup** includes serum **creatinine, blood urea nitrogen, and electrolytes** as well as **24-hour urine collection for protein and creatinine clearance.**
- Hypertension is commonly associated with renal disease and should be treated to **keep diastolic <90 mmHg.**
- Women with end-stage renal disease (ESRD) on **dialysis** should be counseled **preconception** that they **should receive a renal transplant** and **then wait one to two years** before attempting pregnancy. Women on dialysis or with a recently transplanted kidney should be maintained on **effective contraception.** If pregnant, counseling should include review of the very **high rates** of the above **complications.**
- There is an overall **success** of pregnancy (live births) in women after **renal transplantation** of **>90%.**
- In women with **moderate to severe** renal insufficiency, **low-dose aspirin** may reduce the incidence of **preeclampsia.**
- **Pelvic floor exercises** during and after pregnancy **decrease the incidence of urinary incontinence in the third trimester and postpartum.**

HISTORIC NOTES

"Children of women with renal disease used to be born dangerously or not at all—not at all if their doctors had their way" (1).

DIAGNOSES/DEFINITIONS

Chronic renal insufficiency (CRI): The early stage of renal failure when the kidneys no longer function properly but do not yet require dialysis. CRI can be difficult to diagnose as symptoms are not usually apparent until kidney disease has progressed significantly.

Chronic renal failure (CRF): Irreversible, progressive impaired kidney function. CRF generally progresses from CRI to ESRD.

End-stage renal disease (ESRD): Patients with ESRD no longer have kidney function adequate to sustain life and **require dialysis or kidney transplantation.** Without proper treatment, ESRD is fatal.

Nephrotic syndrome (NS): Defined by >3.5 g of proteinuria in 24 hours in nonpregnant adults. A condition caused by any disease that damages the kidneys' filtering system, the glomeruli. Nephrotic syndrome is associated with hypoalbuminemia, edema, and hypercholesterolemia.

SYMPTOMS

Include a frequent need to urinate and edema, as well as possible anemia, fatigue, weakness, headaches, and loss of appetite. As renal disease progresses, other symptoms such as nausea, vomiting, bad breath, and pruritus may develop as toxic metabolites, normally filtered out of the blood by the kidneys, build up to harmful levels.

EPIDEMIOLOGY/INCIDENCE

The overall incidence of renal disease in the general obstetric population is **0.03% to 0.2%** (2–4).

PHYSIOLOGIC RENAL CHANGES IN PREGNANCY

Pregnancy is marked by vasodilation, occurring soon after conception. This results in a drop in blood pressure, an increase in cardiac output, and an increase in renal blood flow and glomerular filtration rate (GFR). These changes persist until late gestation. Likely causes include increased progesterone, nitric oxide, relaxin, and estrogen. Functionally, there is increased renal plasma flow (peaks 60–80% in second trimester, then falls to 50–60% during third trimester). GFR increases 30% during the first trimester and peaks at 50% above prepregnancy values in the second trimester. Creatinine and urea production remains unchanged, resulting in a drop in serum creatinine and urea levels to mean values of 0.6 and 9 mg/dL, respectively. Near term, a 15% to 20% decrease in GFR occurs (5) (chap. 3, *Obstetric Evidence Based Guidelines*). Ideally, evaluation of renal function in pregnancy should be based on GFR, with creatinine clearance probably the closest way to measure GFR. There is an increase in the size of the kidneys and urinary collecting system. Kidney length increases approximately 1 cm and volume increases 30%. The entire collecting system is dilated, which may be confused with an obstructive uropathy.

CLASSIFICATION

See Table 17.1 (6,7).

Table 17.1 Classification of Renal Insufficiency

Category	Serum creatinine[a] (μmol/L [mg/dL])
Preserved	<100 (<1.1)
Mildly impaired renal function	100–124 (1.1–1.3)
Moderate renal insufficiency	125–250 (1.4–2.8)
Severe renal insufficiency	>250 (>2.8)

[a]In early pregnancy. *Source*: Adapted from Refs. 6,7.

RISK FACTORS/PRECONCEPTION COUNSELING

As functional loss progresses, the risks to mother and fetus increase substantially (6). The goal is to optimize prepregnancy health.

Specific Diseases

Vasculopathy: Patients with vasculopathy from sclero-derma and polyarteritis nodosa should be discouraged from pregnancy, because of high maternal and fetal morbidity and mortality (6,8,9).

Lupus nephritis: Patients with lupus nephritis do well when the disease is in remission for six months prior to conception, with a live birth rate up to 95% (10,11). Rates of preterm delivery and preeclampsia are based on degree of renal insufficiency. Total live birth rate for all lupus patients is 58% to 95% (10,12). Low complement levels at conception are predictive of adverse pregnancy outcomes (RR 19), while use of low-dose aspirin during pregnancy is associated with a decrease in adverse outcomes (RR 0.11) (11). In addition, the risk of flare is increased in patients with >1 g of proteinuria or GFR <60 mL/min (11) (see chap. 25).

Mild renal insufficiency: Typically successful pregnancy outcomes with no adverse affect on the course of their disease (13).

Moderate and severe renal insufficiency: Prognosis is more guarded. Deterioration in renal function is seen in 43%, of which 10% do not improve postpartum (14).

CHRONIC RENAL INSUFFICIENCY
Complications

Prognosis is directly related to the degree of renal insufficiency (Table 17.2) (9,15,16,38,47). The best outcomes are in women with preconception serum creatinine levels below 2 mg/dL and diastolic blood pressure of 90 mmHg or less (3,6). Creatinine clearance below 70 mL/min prior to conception is associated with poor outcomes even when serum creatinine levels are in the minimal dysfunction category (17). Poor prognosis is also associated with the need for more than one antihypertensive medication, with a significant decrease in live birth rate (13). Proteinuria (>1 g/24 hr) and reduced GFR (<40 mL/min) in combination are risk factors for progression of renal disease to end stage, and also predict a shorter time to dialysis therapy and lower birth weight (18).

Infertility: Conception with GFR <25 mL/min is rare secondary to alterations in hypothalamic-pituitary-adrenal (HPA) axis (19).

Hypertension: Incidence of hypertension increases from 28% at baseline to approximately 50% by the third trimester (14).

Proteinuria: Urinary protein excretion >3 g in 24 hours increases from approximately 25% to 41% during pregnancy (14).

Preeclampsia: Increased incidence. Diagnosis is difficult because of the high frequency of baseline hypertension and proteinuria.

Preterm labor: Incidence as high as 85% (20).

Low birth weight: 66% (20).

Perinatal mortality: 10% to 20% (13,14).

Cost: Women with chronic renal disease have increased median cost of pregnancy (2).

Pregnancy Considerations

Pregnancy does not appear to adversely affect the natural history of renal disease in women with mild dysfunction. Instead, 10% with moderate to severe disease will suffer irreversible deterioration during pregnancy (3,14,21).

Workup

Serum creatinine, BUN, and electrolytes as well as **24-hour urine collection for protein and creatinine clearance**. A 24-hour urine >300-mg protein is considered abnormal and correlates roughly to 1+ proteinuria on a urine dipstick. Urine dipstick should not be the only testing for women with suspected renal disease, as this can miss up to 1 in 11 hypertensive pregnant women with actual proteinuria (22). Total protein/creatinine ratio has been shown to be effective in ruling out proteinuria if it is <250 mg. Because of decreased ability to discriminate between 250 and 400 mg of proteinuria, a **24-hour urine collection is still considered the gold standard**, especially if the results are equivocal (23). Renal biopsy should be reserved to those whose diagnosis is in question.

Prevention

Aim to preserve whatever renal function remains.

Management

Patients with moderate or severe renal insufficiency should be managed with a **multidisciplinary approach**, in conjunction with a perinatologist, nephrologist, and neonatologist.

Table 17.2 Rate of Complications According to Degree of Renal Insufficiency (%)

Creatinine	PTB	Preeclampsia	HTN	FGR	Perinatal mortality	Live birth	Decline in renal function
<1.4	20	11	25	24	9	>90	16
1.4–2.8	36–60	42	56	31–37	7	>90	50
>2.8	73–86	86	56	43–57	36	N/A	40
Dialysis	48–84	20	100	50–80	60	40–50	N/A
Renal transplant	52–75	23–37	47–63	20–66	7	74–80	14

Source: From Refs. 9,15,16,38,47. *Abbreviations*: PTB, preterm birth; HTN, hypertension; FGR, fetal growth restriction; N/A, not available.

Prenatal Care

Prenatal Visits

Women may be seen every two to four weeks until 32 weeks gestation, after which they may need to be seen weekly because of the markedly increased risk for severe preeclampsia. Careful monitoring of blood pressure and proteinuria for early detection of hypertension and superimposed preeclampsia should be performed at every visit.

Laboratory Tests

Evaluation of renal function by **24-hour creatinine clearance and protein excretion** at least at the first visit in early pregnancy, and, depending on severity of renal insufficiency, each trimester. Frequent **urine culture** should be done for early detection of asymptomatic bacteriuria or confirmation of urinary tract infection. Maternal anemia should be corrected with iron supplementation or erythropoietin if severe.

Antenatal Testing

- Frequent (e.g., monthly) ultrasound for fetal growth
- Biophysical assessment (e.g., nonstress tests, biophysical profile, Doppler of umbilical artery) of fetal well-being weekly after ≥32 weeks

Patient Education

The symptoms of preterm labor and preeclampsia should be reviewed with women who have chronic renal disease.

Therapy

Hypertension

Should be treated aggressively in obstetric patients with underlying renal dysfunction to preserve kidney function. The goal is to **keep diastolic blood pressure <90 mmHg.** Use of antihypertensive medication in pregnancy is discussed in chapter 1.

Preeclampsia

Magnesium is not contraindicated, but should be **used with extreme caution**, begun at 1 to 2 g/hr, possibly without a bolus, or just given as boluses as needed. Evaluation for side effects of magnesium should occur at least hourly and magnesium levels should be checked often (e.g., every two to four hours) in labor to adjust the dose. Calcium gluconate should be available. An alternative is to use phenytoin 15 to 20 mg/kg IV. **Low-dose aspirin** should be started in the first trimester in women with moderate to severe CRI and in women with a history of lupus nephritis to reduce the incidence of preeclampsia and fetal growth restriction (FGR) (11,24).

Preterm Labor

Magnesium and indomethacin should be used with caution as they are renally excreted.

Asymptomatic Bacteriuria

Bacteriuria should be treated for one to two weeks, and suppression should be given for the remainder of the pregnancy (25).

Delivery

Delivery should be performed at a tertiary care center. Mode of delivery should be for standard obstetric indications. Deliberate preterm birth may be necessary in the face of worsening maternal renal function, severe preeclampsia, or worsening fetal status.

Postpartum/Breast-feeding

Little is known about the quantities of immunosuppressive agents in breast milk. While small series have shown little toxicity, caution should be used when recommending breast-feeding to patients taking these agents (26).

Long-Term Renal Prognosis

When kidney dysfunction is mild, pregnancy does not appear to adversely alter the natural history with the possible exception of a few disorders (13). **In women with moderate to severe renal insufficiency (maternal serum creatinine ≥ 1.4 mg/dL), 10% of patients will have progressive renal deterioration at 12 months postpartum** (14).

NEPHROTIC SYNDROME
General

Nephrotic syndrome is defined by >3.5 g of proteinuria in 24 hours in nonpregnant adults (27). The most common causes of adult nephrotic syndrome outside of pregnancy are focal glomerulosclerosis, membranous nephropathy, and minimal-change disease (28). The decrease in oncotic pressure in pregnant women with nephrotic syndrome may lead to increased edema, intravascular volume depletion, and hypoalbuminemia.

Epidemiology/Incidence

Nephrotic syndrome occurs in 0.012% to 0.025% of all pregnancies (27).

Workup

Newly diagnosed nephrotic syndrome in early pregnancy has been associated with hydatidiform molar pregnancies; therefore, this should be evaluated (27–29). If the diagnosis is made prior to pregnancy, histologic diagnosis can help direct treatment. In most cases of stable disease, renal biopsy can be deferred until postpartum if histologic diagnosis is not already made. Renal biopsy in pregnancy is considered a safe option, especially if the results are expected to potentially change management (30,31). The presence of proteinuria >1 g in combination with GFR <40 mL/min is predictive of worse prognosis in pregnancy (18). For this reason, **patients with newly diagnosed proteinuria during their prenatal care should have a 24-hour urine collection for both protein and creatinine clearance, in order to estimate GFR.**

Complications

Nephrotic syndrome rarely causes complications in pregnancy in the absence of hypertension and abnormal renal function. Most of the literature on nephrotic syndrome in pregnancy is based on case reports; therefore, the incidence of specific complications is unknown.

Specific Diseases

Membranous nephropathy is associated with increased fetal demise, preterm delivery (43%), hypertension, and a decline in maternal renal function (32).

Prenatal Care, Fetal Monitoring, and Labor Management

Should follow the recommendations for CRI. Patients should be managed with a **multidisciplinary** approach, in conjunction with a perinatologist, nephrologist, and neonatologist.

Management

It may be necessary to treat the nephrotic syndrome with steroids, which requires early and repeat screening for gestational diabetes (GDM).

Long-Term Prognosis

Relates to the specific diagnosis. Most evidence suggests that pregnancy does not worsen or accelerate the overall disease process in women with primary glomerular disease, at least at five-year follow-up (33). The exception to this appears to be women with membranous glomerulonephritis, who do worse after experiencing a pregnancy.

DIALYSIS
Principles/Counseling

Women with ESRD on dialysis have impaired fertility secondary to suppression of HPA axis function, leading to anovulation and amenorrhea. Fertility rates are improving with advances in dialysis, overall decreased serum creatinine levels, and improvement of azotemia. Published rates of fertility range from 1% to 7%. Dialysis-dependent patients with ESRD should be **offered contraception** (34).

Women on dialysis should be counseled preconception that they should receive a renal transplant and then wait for one to two years before attempting pregnancy. For successful outcomes in pregnant women on dialysis, the key is **coordination of multidisciplinary care** to maintain blood pressure control, fluid balance, and adequate nutrition. There is an overall >50% to 70% likelihood of fetal survival (35). Live births in women on dialysis during pregnancy has improved from 23% (36) to about 50% in 1994 (14), to 79% in 1998 (35), and to 92% in 2002 (34).

Complications

Stillbirth (8–50%), **neonatal death** (9–25%), **preterm delivery** (48–84%), **severe preeclampsia** (11%) (20,37), **polyhydramnios** (40%) (38), **FGR** (50–80%), **hypertension** (100%), **anemia** (100%), and even **maternal death** despite recent improved overall outcomes (34). Most of the neonatal morbidity occurs secondary to prematurity. The risk of congenital anomalies does not appear to be increased. Preeclampsia is a poor prognostic factor in these patients, associated with increased rates of stillbirth, low birth weight, and prematurity (38).

Pregnancy Management

- Counseling regarding complications should be reviewed. Because of the high incidence of complications, termination may be discussed, as well as the opportunity for possibly a better outcome after renal transplant (34).
- Intensive hemodialysis (HD) for patients with ESRD **six to seven times a week** is recommended. There appears to be a trend toward better infant survival in women who received dialysis ≥20 hr/wk (20).
- Plasma urea level appears to be the most important factor influencing pregnancy outcome in dialysis patients. A predialysis urea of 30 to 50 mg/dL (5–8 mmol/L) is associated with improved outcomes (39).
- Prepregnancy dialysis regimen should be increased by approximately 50%.
- HD may be superior to peritoneal dialysis (PD), but this has not been studied in any trial in pregnancy. Older reports have demonstrated more successful pregnancies in women undergoing HD (79%) compared to PD (33%) (35). Newer small series demonstrate comparable out-

comes between HD and PD (40,41) but no clear benefit of PD over HD. For this reason, PD is not recommended in the general pregnant patient population. If patients are already established on PD, there is no compelling evidence to change to HD (20,37).

- Aggressively use HD to decrease azotemia for improving pregnancy outcomes. As a goal, predialysis urea level should be ≤100 mg/dL and BUN should be low (7–10 mg/dL), so that there is not osmotic diuresis in the fetus.
- Avoid maternal hypotension during HD. Keep BP 130–150/80–90.
- Avoid excessive fluid shifts. Ensure minimal fluctuations and limit volume changes.
- Alter heparin regimen near delivery if possible.
- Use maternal dry weight to base HD volume.
- No studies of fetal surveillance during HD.
- Altering HD rates to achieve maximal volume control may decrease incidence of polyhydramnios.
- Nutritional consult (25).
- Other metabolic changes:
  ○ Keep bicarbonate 22 to 26.
  ○ Keep hemoglobin 11 to 12 mg/dL with erythropoietin (can be given in pregnancy, does not cross the placenta). Because of resistance to erythropoietin in pregnancy, the dose must be increased by as much as 50% to maintain the target hemoglobin (39). Anemia is associated with worse neonatal outcomes (38).
  ○ Replace calcium (≥2 g/day), phosphorus.
  ○ Dialysate: may need more potassium, less calcium.
- Adequate calorie and protein supply needs to be assured.
- Ensure good blood pressure control.
- Maintain attention toward signs and symptoms of preterm labor.
- Maternal serum screening for aneuploidy is unreliable in this group of patients (34,42).
- Indocin may worsen kidney function. Magnesium should be avoided if possible or used cautiously with frequent levels.
- Close antepartum fetal surveillance is warranted because of risk of FGR and NRFHT.
- Consider delivery at 34 to 36 weeks.
- There are insufficient data to assess the effects of antenatal steroids and the risk of GDM in HD patients.
- Neonatologists should be available to assess the neonate. Neonates are born with BUN and creatinine levels equal to the mother's and often experience osmotic diuresis, resulting in volume contraction and electrolyte abnormalities. Intrauterine hypercalcemia may result in postnatal hypocalcemia and tetany (43).

Antepartum care should otherwise be similar to those patients with chronic renal disease.

Postpartum

Most women return to prepregnancy dialysis regimens and have uncomplicated postpartum recoveries. Postpartum care must address contraception. Future pregnancies should follow renal transplant.

RENAL TRANSPLANTATION
Principles

Management should be at a center with a **transplant nephrologist**, and requires attention toward **serial assessment of renal function, diagnosis and treatment of rejection, blood** pressure control and control of anemia. There is an overall success of pregnancy (live births) in women after renal transplantation of >**90%** (44). Fertility can normalize soon after transplantation, so patients should be maintained on contraception until ready to attempt a pregnancy. If graft function is adequate and stable, pregnancy does not cause accelerated graft demise (45). However, one case-control study suggested that graft function is adversely affected by pregnancy (46). At 10-year follow-up, graft survival was 69% in pregnant patients and 100% in nonpregnant controls.

Complications
Slightly increased incidences of fetal growth restriction, premature rupture of membranes, preterm delivery, and preeclampsia.

Preconception Counseling
Ideal candidate for pregnancy is a woman with:

1. Good general health for at least one year posttransplant before attempting conception
2. Minimal (ideally <300 mg or at least <1000 mg/24 hr) proteinuria
3. Absence (ideal) or at least good control of hypertension
4. No evidence of graft rejection
5. Absence of pelvicaliceal distention on intravenous pyelogram
6. Stable renal function (maternal serum creatinine <1.4 mg/dL or ideally <1.1 mg/dL). Fetal survival improves from 75% with creatinine >1.4% to 95% with normal creatinine. **Creatinine >2.3 mg/dL may be regarded as a contraindication to pregnancy** as all transplant patients with a creatinine >2.3 mg/dL experienced progression of renal failure requiring retransplant or dialysis within two years of pregnancy (47)
7. Stable immunosuppressive regimen
8. If possible, drug therapy should be reduced to maintenance levels: prednisone <15 mg/day, azathioprine <2 mg/kg/day, cyclosporine <5 mg/kg/day (25)

Prenatal Care
Attempt to obtain operative records from transplant surgery to identify location of kidney. Be aware of side effects of immunosuppressive agents (Table 17.3). A common immunosuppressive drug is currently tacrolimus (Prograf). It crosses the placenta but has not been associated with an increase in congenital anomalies. Avoid nephrotoxic drugs. Be aware of significant drug interactions with cyclosporine (Table 17.4).

> *Antenatal visits*: should be every 2 to 4 weeks up to 32 weeks and weekly thereafter.
> *Lab work*: includes monthly assessment of: **CBC, BUN, serum creatinine, electrolytes, serum urate, 24-hour creatinine clearance and protein** levels, and urine specimen for **culture**. Initial labs should also include serum serologies for **cytomegalovirus, toxoplasmosis,** and **herpes simplex** virus (IgM and IgG for each) and **LFTs. Levels of immunosuppressive agent** (tacrolimus, cyclosporine, etc.) should be obtained at least every trimester. If the patient is on prednisone or tacrolimus, obtain a fasting and two-hour postprandial

Table 17.3 Immunosuppressive Agents Commonly Used and Their Side Effects

Agent→Side effect
- Prednisone[a]→glucose intolerance
- Azathioprine[a]→leukopenia
- Cyclosporine[a,b]→hypertension, nephrotoxicity (watch for drug interactions—see Table 17.4)
- Tacrolimus[a,b]→hypertension, nephrotoxicity, neurotoxicity, glucose intolerance, myocardial hypertrophy
- Sirolimus[b]→GI disturbance, weakness; animal studies raise concern regarding potential for human fetotoxicity, although no teratogenesis is evident.
- Mycophenolate mofetil→GI disturbance; animal studies raise concern regarding potential for human teratogenicity. At least 12 cases of human deformity associated with mycophenolate mofetil, including microtia (11), auditory canal atresia (8), cleft lip and palate (6), and micrognathia (4) (48).

[a]These have no known teratogenic effects.
[b]Follow with blood levels.

Table 17.4 Drug Interactions with Cyclosporine

Drugs that exhibit nephrotoxic synergy

Gentamicin	Cimetidine
Tobramycin	Ranitidine
Vancomycin	Diclofenac
Amphotericin B	Trimethoprim with sulfamethoxazole
Ketoconazole	Azapropazon
Melphalan	

Careful monitoring of renal function should be practiced when Sandimmun[R] (cyclosporine) is used with nephrotoxic drugs.

Drugs that alter cyclosporine levels

Cyclosporine is extensively metabolized by the liver. Therefore, circulating cyclosporine levels may be influenced by drugs that affect hepatic microsomal enzymes, particularly the cytochrome P-450 system. Substances known to inhibit these enzymes will decrease hepatic metabolism and increase cyclosporine levels. Substances that are inducers of cytochrome P-450 activity will increase hepatic metabolism and decrease cyclosporine levels. Monitoring of circulating cyclosporine levels and appropriate Sandimmun (cyclosporine) dosage adjustment are essential when these drugs are used concomitantly.

*Drugs that **increase** cyclosporine levels*

Diltiazem	Danazol
Nicardipine	Bromocriptine
Verapamil	Metoclopramide
Ketoconazole	Erythromycin
Fluconazole	Methylprednisone
Intracondazole	

*Drugs that **decrease** cyclosporine levels*

Rifampin	Phenobarbital
Phenytoin	Carbamazepine

Other drug interactions

Reduced clearance of prednisolone, digoxin, and lovastatin has been observed when these drugs are administered with Sandimmun (cyclosporine). In addition, a decrease in the apparent volume of distribution of digoxin has been reported after Sandimmun (cyclosporine) administration. Severe digitalis toxicity has been seen within days of starting cyclosporine in several patients taking digoxin. Sandimmun (cyclosporine) should not be used with potassium-sparing diuretics because hyperkalemia can occur. During treatment with Sandimmun (cyclosporine), vaccination may be less effective: and the use of live vaccines should be avoided. Myositis has occurred with concomitant lovastatin, frequent gingival hyperplasia with nifedipine, and convulsions with high dose methylprednisolone. Further information on drugs that have been reported to interact with Sandimmun (cyclosporine) is available from Sandoz Pharmaceuticals Corporation (New Jersey, U.S.).

Source: From Ref. 49.

blood sugar upon presentation. If these values are normal, perform a glucose challenge test at 24 weeks. Renal transplant patients are at considerable risk for urinary tract infections (up to 40%) and should be screened regularly (47).

Fetal surveillance: should follow the recommendations for chronic renal disease.

Labor Management

Should include careful monitoring of maternal fluid balance, cardiovascular status, and temperature. Cesarean delivery should be for obstetric indications only. Women who have received steroids for long periods during the antepartum period should receive "stress dose" steroids. Notification of the use of immunosuppressants to the pediatrician is important for proper follow-up of the neonate.

Renal Graft Rejection

Occurs in 4% to 9% pregnant allograft recipients and is difficult to diagnose. Factors that increase risk include increased number of episodes of rejection during the year prior to conception, maternal serum creatinine >2 mg/dL, proteinuria >500 mg/dL, and graft dysfunction during pregnancy (45). Clinical hallmarks include fever, oliguria, deteriorating renal function, renal enlargement, and tenderness. **Renal ultrasound** and **biopsy** for diagnosis is necessary before aggressive anti-rejection therapy is begun.

Postpartum/Breast-feeding

In general, not enough data are available to make a formal recommendation. However, breast-feeding is contraindicated in patients on cyclosporine.

Resources

USA National Transplant Pregnancy Registry. Available at: http://www.jefferson.edu/ntpr/1-877-955-6877.

URINARY TRACT INFECTIONS
Screening

All pregnant women should be screened at the first prenatal visit for asymptomatic bacteriuria. The prevalence of asymptomatic bacteriuria in pregnancy is comparable to nonpregnant patients, between 2% and 10%. If asymptomatic bacteriuria goes untreated in pregnancy, 25% to 40% of patients will develop pyelonephritis, compared to 3% of women who are treated (50,51). Women with risk factors for urinary tract infections (UTIs) (DM, GDM, neurogenic bladder, prior frequent UTIs, sickle cell disease) should be screened every trimester. Patients with sickle cell trait are at increased risk for pyelonephritis, but it has not been demonstrated that frequent screening reduces that risk (51).

Complications

Pregnant women with asymptomatic bacteriuria are at increased risk for symptomatic infection and **pyelonephritis**. There is also as a positive relationship between untreated bacteriuria, **low birth weight**, and **preterm birth**. Other complications of UTIs or pyelonephritis include fetal mortality, possibly long-term mental retardation, and developmental delay (52), preeclampsia, anemia, and pulmonary and renal insufficiency. Treatment of asymptomatic bacteriuria helps prevent these complications (see chapters 2 and 16, *Obstetric Evidence Based Guidelines*).

Prevention

Daily intake of 10 to 16 oz of **cranberry juice** decreases the incidence of recurrent *Escherichia coli* UTIs. *Lactobacillus GG* drink does not have any benefit (53).

Diagnosis

A threshold of ≥**100,000** colony-forming units (**CFUs**) is the indication for treatment. Group B *Streptococcus* should be appropriately treated at any concentration (see chapter 16, *Obstetric Evidence Based Guidelines*). It is important to avoid contamination by cleansing the perineum and then collecting "mid-stream" urine.

Treatment

Check allergies and sensitivities. If appropriate, **nitrofurantoin** 100 mg orally twice per day can be used for seven days. If not effective, oral alternatives are cephalexin 250 mg every six hours, amoxicillin 250 mg every eight hours, or trimethoprim-sulfamethoxazole 160/800 mg orally every 12 hours for 7days.

Follow-up

A **test of cure** is necessary. If positive, repeat antibiotic regimen (consider different, sensitive regimen), and assess compliance. Intramuscular treatment can be given if compliance remains an issue. Suppressive therapy (once a day of nitrofurantoin 50 mg, amoxicillin 250 mg, or cephalexin 250 mg) is indicated after two UTIs or one episode of pyelonephritis.

PYELONEPHRITIS
Incidence

1% to 2% (54).

Diagnosis

Urinary tract infection with costovertebral angle tenderness, usually accompanied by systemic symptoms such as fever and chills. Positive urine culture is necessary for diagnosis.

Management

- **Urine culture sensitivity is crucial to assure adequate antibiotic coverage**.
- Workup should include CBC, electrolytes, creatinine, and liver function tests. Intravenous fluids.
- Usually inpatient treatment. Outpatient therapy can be considered for uncomplicated compliant women with pyelonephritis after IV ceftriaxone (55,56).
- **Intravenous antibiotics** for 24 to 48 hours or at least >24 hours afebrile:
  - Drug of choice:
    - **Ceftriaxone 1 to 2 g every 24 hours** (57,58)
  - Alternatives:
    - Ancef 1 to 2 g every six hours
    - Ampicillin 1 to 2 g every six hours, with gentamicin 1.5 mg/kg every eight hours
    - Trimethoprim-sulfamethoxazole 160/800 mg every 12 hours.

- If not afebrile within 48 hours with appropriate regimen, or if recurrent pyelonephritis, consider renal ultrasound to rule out renal abscess.
- Once IV therapy completed, oral therapy for 10 to 14 days, followed by suppression and frequent urine cultures (see above) (59,60).

URINARY NEPHROLITHIASIS
Incidence
At least 1/1500, but may occur more commonly (61,62). Up to 12% of the general population has a urinary stone during their lifetime, with recurrence rates approaching 50% (61). Nephrolithiasis is also called renal calculi or stones. Given the low incidence, it is unclear if the occurrence of nephrolithiasis is or is not increased in pregnancy, with some authors reporting an incidence as high as 1/200.

Risk Factors
More common in Caucasians, second and third trimester, right side (63), recurrent UTIs, gout, prior renal stones or renal disease, family history.

Complications
Possibly increased preterm birth and pyelonephritis (64).

Diagnosis
A typical presentation for renal colic includes nausea, vomiting, hematuria, and flank or abdominal pain. Urinalysis may reveal hematuria, as well as pyuria in up to 42% of patients (65,66). The best imaging technique in the nonpregnant adult is unenhanced helical **CT scan** of the abdomen and pelvis, which has 96% sensitivity and 100% specificity (61). If CT is unavailable, **plain abdominal X ray** should be performed, since 75% to 90% of urinary stones are radiopaque. **Ultrasonography** has a sensitivity of only 11% to 24% with >90% specificity in nonpregnant adults, but because of a **sensitivity of about 67% in pregnancy**, it is currently the first-line screening test in pregnancy. Doppler ultrasound has been shown to be somewhat useful in distinguishing ureteral obstruction from physiologic hydronephrosis. A difference of >0.04 in the resistive indices of the obstructed and normal kidneys can be used to predict obstruction. In addition, comparison of bilateral ureteral jets on ultrasound can be helpful (67). If initially the ultrasound is negative, an MRU (magnetic resonance urography) (68) should be considered or, if unavailable, probably X ray second and CT third. Renal stones are poorly visualized by MRI alone. It is important to know that mild to moderate hydronephrosis is physiologic in pregnancy and is usually worse on the right kidney.

Management
Composition, location, and size of stone should be assessed. Up to 64% to 70% of women can pass stones spontaneously during pregnancy and an additional 50% of the remaining pass the stones in the postpartum period (66). Most patients with stones will not require intervention; therefore, hydration and pain control is the typical first-line management. Urgent intervention is indicated with obstruction, infected upper urinary tract, impending renal deterioration, intractable pain or vomiting, anuria, or high-grade obstruction of a solitary or transplanted kidney.

Pain Control
There are no trials in pregnancy or even in nonpregnant adults. Ketorolac and diclofenac appear to be as effective as narcotics. All can be used acutely intravenously.

Usually **increases in fluids and movement** are used as initial interventions in pregnancy as well as nonpregnant adults. Over 70% of stones in pregnancy resolve with conservative management. A urinary stone seen by ultrasound (or CT) but not X ray is probably a uric acid stone; 20 mmol of potassium citrate orally two to three times daily (aim to alkalinize urine to pH 6.5–7.0) can be effective medical therapy for dissolution of this type of stone.

If conservative therapy fails, insertion of **stents** is a safe intervention in pregnancy. Percutaneous nephrostomy is needed only rarely, but is safe in pregnancy. Ureteroscopy has also been shown to be safe and effective in pregnancy, with complication rates similar to the nonpregnant patient (61,62). Shock wave lithotripsy is considered first-line therapy for proximal ureteral stones <1 cm in nonpregnant adults, but is usually avoided in pregnancy. Inadvertent lithotripsy in pregnancy is not a cause for concern (66,69).

PREVENTION OF URINARY INCONTINENCE
Incidence
Urinary incontinence has been reported to occur in 5% to 40% of pregnant and postpartum women.

Prevention
Pelvic floor exercises *during pregnancy* decrease the incidence of urinary incontinence in the third trimester and postpartum, up to six months after birth (70–72). Pelvic floor muscle strength is also significantly higher. Group training with a physiotherapist for 60 minutes once per week and twice daily at home 8 to 12 times for a period of 12 weeks between 20 and 36 weeks holding the pelvic floor muscle contraction six to eight seconds each time with rest periods of six seconds is one accepted and effective intervention (72).

Pelvic floor muscle training *after childbirth* is **effective in prevention and treatment of urinary incontinence** (73–77).

POSTPARTUM URINARY RETENTION
Definition
Absence of spontaneous micturition six hours post vaginal delivery or six hours after catheter removal (after cesarean delivery). A residual <50 mL is normal and one >200 mL is abnormal (78).

Incidence
0.2% to 3% (79).

Risk Factors
Nulliparity, prolonged stages of labor, epidural anesthesia, operative or cesarean delivery.

Management
There are no trials to assess any intervention. Oral analgesia, standing and walking, warm bath, immersing hands in cold water may help. If bladder volume by ultrasound <400 mL, wait; if >400 mL, **intermittent catheterization every four to six hours until the woman is able to void and then the first residual volume is <150 mL** is usually recommended and

preferable to indwelling catheterization. Pharmacologic treatment should be avoided. If the woman has still retention upon discharge and/or after 48 hours, self-catheterization should be taught. Prophylactic antibiotics are indicated in women who require catheterization. There are no clear long-term sequelae of postpartum urinary retention. Complete resolution of voiding dysfunction is expected within 28 days with no increased risk for long-term voiding abnormalities. Higher postvoid residual volumes at 72 hours after delivery are predictive of a longer time to full recovery (79).

REFERENCES

1. Anonymous. Pregnancy and renal disease. Lancet 1975; 2(7939):801–802. [Review]
2. Fink JC, Schwartz SM, Benedetti TJ, et al. Increased risk of adverse maternal and infant outcomes among women with renal disease. Paediatr Perinat Epidemiol 1998; 12(3):277–287. [II-2]
3. Bar J, Ben-Rafael Z, Padoa A, et al. Prediction of pregnancy outcome in subgroups of women with renal disease. Clin Nephrol 2000; 53(6):437–444. [II-2]
4. Fischer MJ, Lehnerz SD, Hebert JR, et al. Kidney disease is an independent risk factor for adverse fetal and maternal outcomes in pregnancy. Am J Kidney Dis 2004; 43(3):415–423. [II-3]
5. Milne JE, Lindheimer MD, Davison JM. Glomerular heteroporous membrane modeling in third trimester and postpartum before and during amino acid infusion. Am J Physiol Renal Physiol 2002; 282(1):F170–F175. [II-2]
6. Lindheimer MD, Davison JM, Katz AI. The kidney and hypertension in pregnancy: twenty exciting years. Semin Nephrol 2001; 21(2):173–189. [Review]
7. Modena A, Hoffman M, Tolosa JE. Chronic renal disease in pregnancy: a modern approach to predicting outcome. Am J Obstet Gynecol 2005; 193:s86. [II-2]
8. Jungers P, Houillier P, Forget D, et al. Specific controversies concerning the natural history of renal disease in pregnancy. Am J Kidney Dis 1991; 17(2):116–122. [III]
9. Jones DC. Pregnancy complicated by chronic renal disease. Clin Perinatol 1997; 24(2):483–496. [III]
10. Huong DL, Wechsler B, Vauthier-Brouzes D, et al. Pregnancy in past or present lupus nephritis: a study of 32 pregnancies from a single centre. Ann Rheum Dis 2001; 60(6):599–604. [II-2]
11. Imbasciati E, Tincani A, Gregorini G, et al. Pregnancy in women with pre-existing lupus nephritis: predictors of fetal and maternal outcome. Nephrol Dial Transplant 2009; 24(2):519–525. [II-3]
12. Hayslett, JP. The effect of systemic lupus erythematosus on pregnancy and pregnancy outcome. Am J Reprod Immunol 1992; 28(3–4):33:199–204. [II-2]
13. Jungers P, Chauveau D, Choukroun G, et al. Pregnancy in women with impaired renal function. Clin Nephrol 1997; 47(5):281–288. [II-2]
14. Jones DC, Hayslett JP. Outcome of pregnancy in women with moderate or severe renal insufficiency. N Engl J Med 1996; 335:226–232. [II-2]
15. Hou SH. Frequency and outcome of pregnancy in women on dialysis. Am J Kid Dis 1994; 23:60–63. [II-3]
16. Armenti VT, Radomski JS, Moritz MJ, et al. Report from the national transplantation pregnancy registry (NTPR): outcomes of pregnancy after transplantation. Clin Transpl 2001:97–105. [II-2]
17. Abe S. An overview of pregnancy in women with underlying renal disorders. Am J Kidney Dis 1991; 17(2):112–115. [II-3]
18. Imbasciati E, Gregorini G, Cabiddu G, et al. Pregnancy in CKD stages 3 to 5: fetal and maternal outcomes. Am J Kidney Dis 2007; 49:753–762. [II-3]
19. Holley JL, Bernardini J, Quadri KM, et al. Pregnancy outcomes in a prospective matched control study of pregnancy and renal disease. Clin Nephrol 1996; 45(2):77–82. [II-2]
20. Okundaye I, Abrinko P, Hou S. Registry of pregnancy in dialysis patients. Am J Kidney Dis 1998; 31(5):766–773. [II-2]
21. Cunningham FG, Cox SM, Harstad TW, et al. Chronic renal disease and pregnancy outcome. Am J Obstet Gynecol 1990; 163:352–359. [II-3]
22. Phelan LK, Brown MA, Davis GK, et al. A prospective study of the impact of automated dipstick urinalysis on the diagnosis of preeclampsia. Hypertens Pregnancy 2004; 23(2):135–142. [II-2]
23. Cote AM, Brown MA, Lam E, et al. Diagnostic accuracy of urinary spot protein:creatinine ratio for proteinuria in hypertensive pregnant women: systematic review. BMJ 2008; 336 (7651):1003–1006. [Review]
24. Bujold E, Roberge S, Lacasse Y, et al. Prevention of preeclampsia and intrauterine growth restriction with aspirin started in early pregnancy: a meta-analysis. Obstet Gynecol 2010; 116:402–414. [Meta-analysis of RCTs]
25. Hou S. Pregnancy in chronic renal insufficiency and end-stage renal disease. Am J Kidney Dis 1999; 33(2):235–252. [II-3]
26. Nyberg G, Haljamae U, Frisenette-Fich C, et al. Breast-feeding during treatment with cyclosporine. Transplantation 1998; 65 (2):253–255. [II-3]
27. Cohen AW, Burton HG. Nephrotic syndrome due to preeclamptic nephropathy in a hydatidiform mole and coexistent fetus. Obstet Gynecol 1979; 53:130–134. [II-3]
28. Alvarez L, Ortega E, Rocamora N, et al. An unusual case of nephrotic syndrome and hypertension in a young woman. Nephrol Dial Transplant 2002; 17(11):2026–2029. [II-3 and review]
29. Komatsuda A, Nakamoto Y, Asakura K, et al. Nephrotic syndrome associated with a total hydatidiform mole: case report. Am J Med Sci 1992; 303:309–312. [II-3]
30. Day C, Hewins P, Hildebrand S, et al. The role of renal biopsy in women with kidney disease identified in pregnancy. Nephrol Dial Transplant 2008; 23(1):201–206. [II-2]
31. Packham DK, Fairley KF. Renal biopsy: indications and complications in pregnancy. BJOG 1987; 94(10):935–939. [II-3]
32. Packham DK, North RA, Fairley KF, et al. Membranous glomerulonephritis and pregnancy. Clin Nephrol 1987; 28(2): 56–64. [II-3]
33. Barcelo P, Lopez-Lillo J, Cabero L, et al. Successful pregnancy in primary glomerular disease. Kidney Int 1986; 30:914–919. [II-3]
34. Chao A-S, Huang J-Y, Lien R, et al. Pregnancy in women who undergo long-term hemodialysis. Am J Obstet Gynecol 2002; 187 (1):152–156. [II-3]
35. Romao JE Jr., Luders C, Kahhale S, et al. Pregnancy in women on chronic dialysis. A single-center experience with 17 cases. Nephron 1998; 78(4):416–422. [II-3]
36. Registration Committee of the European Dialysis and Transplant Association. Successful pregnancies in women treated by dialysis and transplantation. BJOG 1980; 87(10):839–845. [II-3]
37. Chan WS, Okun N, Kjellstrand CM. Pregnancy in chronic dialysis: a review and analysis of the literature. Int J Artif Organs 1998; 21(5):259–268. [II-3]
38. Luders C, Castro MC, Titan SM, et al. Obstetric outcome in pregnant women on long-term dialysis: a case series. Am J Kidney Dis 2010; 56:77–85. [II-3]
39. Asamiya Y, Otsubo S, Matsuda Y, et al. The importance of low blood urea nitrogen levels in pregnant patients undergoing hemodialysis to optimize birth weight and gestational age. Kidney Int 2009; 75(11):1217–1222. [II-2]
40. Jefferys A, Wyburn K, Chow J, et al. Peritoneal dialysis in pregnancy: a case series. Nephrology 2008; 13(5):380–383. [II-3]
41. Chou CY, Ting IW, Lin TH, et al. Pregnancy in patients on chronic dialysis: a single center experience and combined analysis of reported results. Eur J Obstet Gynecol Reprod Biol 2008; 136 (2):165–170. [II-2, review]
42. Cheng PJ, Liu CM, Chang SD, et al. Elevated second-trimester maternal serum hCG in patients undergoing haemodialysis. Prenat Diagn 1999; 19(10):955–958. [II-3]
43. Blowey DL, Warady BA. Neonatal outcome in pregnancies associated with renal replacement therapy. Adv Ren Replace Ther 1998; 5:45–52. [Review]
44. Armenti VT, Radomski JS, Moritz MJ, et al. Report from the National Transplantation Pregnancy Registry (NTPR): outcomes

of pregnancy after transplantation. Clin Transpl 2002:121–130. [II-2]

45. Armenti VT, McGrory CH, Cater JR, et al. Pregnancy outcomes in female renal transplant recipients. Transplant Proc 1998; 30 (5):1732–1734. [II-2]

46. Salmela K, Kyllonen L, Homberg C, et al. Impaired renal function after pregnancy in renal transplant recipients. Transplantation 1993; 56:1372–1375. [II-2]

47. Crowe AV, Rustom R, Gradden C, et al. Pregnancy does not adversely affect renal transplant function. QJM 1999; 92:631–635. [II-3]

48. Merlob P, Stahl B, Klinger G. Tetrada of the possible mycophenolate mofetil embryopathy: a review. Reprod Toxicol 2009; 28 (1):105–108. [Review]

49. Physician's Desk Reference. 52nd ed. Montvale, NJ: Thomson PDR, 1998.

50. Gilstrap LC, Ramin SM. Urinary tract infections during pregnancy. Obstet Gynecol Clin North Am 2001; 28(3):581–591. [Review]

51. Thurman AR, Steed LL, Hulsey T, et al. Bacteriuria in pregnant women with sickle cell trait. Am J Obstet Gynecol 2006; 194:1366–1370. [II-2]

52. McDermott S, Callaghan W, Szwejbka L, et al. Urinary tract infections during pregnancy and mental retardation and developmental delay. Obstet Gynecol 2000; 96:113–119. [II-2]

53. Kontiokari T, Sundqvist K, Nuutinen M, et al. randomized trial of cranberry–lingonberry juice and *Lactobacillus GG* drink for the prevention of urinary tract infections in women. BMJ 2001; 322:1571. [RCT, *n* = 150]

54. Hill JB, Sheffield JS, McIntire DD, et al. Acute pyelonephritis in pregnancy. Obstet Gynecol 2005; 105(1):18–23. [II-3; *n* = 440 cases of pyelonephritis]

55. Millar LK, Wing DA, Paul RH, et al. Outpatient treatment of pyelonephritis in pregnancy: a randomized controlled trial. Obstet Gynecol 1995; 86(4 pt 1):560–564. [RCT, *n* = 120]

56. Wing DA, Hendershott CM, DeBuque L, et al. Outpatient treatment of acute pyelonephritis in pregnancy after 24 weeks. Obstet Gynecol 1999; 94:683–688. [RCT, *n* = 92]

57. Sharma P, Thapa L. Acute pyelonephritis in pregnancy: a retrospective study. Aust N Z J Obstet Gynecol 2007; 47(4):313–315. [II-2]

58. Sanchez-Ramos L, McAlpine KJ, Adair CD, et al. Pyelonephritis in pregnancy: once-a-day ceftriaxone versus multiple doses of cefazolin. A randomized, double-blind trial. Am J Obstet Gynecol 1995; 172(1):129–133. [RCT, *n* = 178]

59. Van Dorsten JP, Lenke RR, Schifrin BS. Pyelonephritis in pregnancy. The role of in-hospital management and nitrofurantoin suppression. J Reprod Med 1987; 32(12):895–900. [RCT]

60. Brost BC, Campbell B, Stramm S, et al. Randomized clinical trial of antibiotic therapy for antenatal pyelonephritis. Infect Dis Obstet Gynecol 1996; 4(5):294–297. [RCT, *n* = 67]

61. Teichman JMH. Acute renal colic from ureteral calculus. N Engl J Med 2004; 350:684–693. [Nonpregnant adult review]

62. Semins MJ, Trock BJ, Matlaga BR. The safety of ureteroscopy during pregnancy: a systematic review and meta-analysis. J Urol 2009; 181:139–143. [Review]

63. Lewis DF, Robichaux AG, Jaekle RK, et al. Urolithiasis in pregnancy: diagnosis, management and pregnancy outcome. J Reprod Med 2003; 48:28–32. [II-3; *n* = 86]

64. Swartz MA, Lydon-Rochelle MT, Simon D, et al. Admission for nephrolithiasis in pregnancy and risk of adverse birth outcomes. Obstet Gynecol 2007; 109(5):1099–1104. [II-2]

65. Thomas AA, Thomas AZ, Campbell SC, et al. Urologic emergencies in pregnancy. Urology 2010; 76:453–460. [Review]

66. Stothers L, Lee LM. Renal colic in pregnancy. J Urol 1992; 148:1383–1387. [II-2]

67. Shokeir AA, Mahran MR, Abdulmaaboud M. Renal colic in pregnant women: role of renal resistive index. Urology 2000; 55:344–347. [II-2]

68. Spencer JA, Chahal R, Kelly A, et al. Evaluation of painful hydronephrosis in pregnancy: magnetic resonance urographic patterns in physiological dilatation versus calculus obstruction. J Urol 2004; 171:256–260. [II-3]

69. Asgari MA, Safarinejad MR, Hosseini SY, et al. Extracorporeal shock wave lithotripsy of renal calculi during pregnancy. BJU Int 1999; 84(6):615–617. [II-3]

70. Sampselle CM, Miler JM, Mims BL, et al. Effect of pelvic muscle exercise on transient incontinence during pregnancy and after childbirth. Obstet Gynecol 1998; 91:406–412. [RCT, *n* = 46]

71. Reilly ETC, Freeman RM, Waterfield MR, et al. Prevention of postpartum stress incontinence in primigravidae with increased bladder neck mobility: a randomized controlled trial of antenatal pelvic floor exercises. BJOG 2002; 109(1):68–76. [RCT, *n* = 268]

72. Morkved S, Bo K, Schei B, et al. Pelvic floor muscle training during pregnancy to prevent urinary incontinence: a single-blind randomized controlled trial. Obstet Gynecol 2003; 191:313–319. [RCT, *n* = 301]

73. Morkved S, Bo K. The effect of postpartum pelvic floor muscle exercise in the prevention and treatment of urinary incontinence. Int Urogynecol J 1997; 8:217–264. [RCT, *n* = 198]

74. Morkved S, Bo K. Effect of postpartum pelvic floor muscle training in prevention and treatment of urinary incontinence: a one-year follow up. BJOG 2000; 107:1022–1028. [RCT follow-up]

75. Wilson PD, Herbison GP. A randomised controlled trial of pelvic floor muscle exercises to treat postnatal urinary incontinence. Int Urogynecol J Pelvic Floor Dysfunct 1998; 9(5):257–264. [RCT, *n* = 230]

76. Chiarelli P. Female Urinary Incontinence in Australia: Prevalence and Prevention in Postpartum Women [dissertation]. Callaghan, Australia: The University of Newcastle, 2001. [RCT]

77. Glazener CMA, Herbison GP, Wilson PD, et al. Conservative management of persistent postnatal urinary and faecal incontinence: randomised controlled trial. BMJ 2001; 323:593–596. [RCT, *n* = 747]

78. Yip S-K, Sahota D, Pang M-W, et al. Postpartum urinary retention. Obstet Gynecol 2005; 106:602–606. [Review]

79. Groutz A, Levin I, Gold R, et al. Protracted postpartum urinary retention: the importance of early diagnosis and timely intervention. Neurourol Urodyn 2011; 30(1):83–86. [II-2]

18

Headache

Stephen Silberstein

KEY POINTS

- **Most causes of headache in pregnancy** are not due to ominous causes but due **to migraine or tension-type headache.**
- **Migraines affect up to 18% of pregnant women; this condition frequently has been diagnosed before pregnancy.**
- **New-onset headache in pregnancy** requires a **thorough neurological evaluation** that may include **neuroradiographic studies and/or cerebrospinal fluid (CSF) analysis.**
- Some worrisome disorders that cause headache occur more commonly in pregnant women. These include subarachnoid hemorrhage, stroke, pituitary tumor or apoplexy, and cerebral venous thrombosis.
- **Education about avoiding specific food, caffeine and alcohol triggers** for migraine may reduce the need for both preventive and acute medications. Pregnant patients with headache should **avoid skipping meals, should regularize their sleep and exercise habits, and consider yoga, meditation, or biofeedback** as an adjunctive migraine preventive modality.
- **Certain acute and preventive medication can be used** with caution in pregnancy; most are not absolutely contraindicated.
- **Most** patients with migraine without aura, and many with migraine with aura, **improve during pregnancy,** particularly during the second and third trimester.
- Patients who are unknowingly pregnant and who have taken medications in the nonsteroidal anti-inflammatory class or the triptan class early in pregnancy can be reassured that drugs of these classes have not been shown to increase the incidence of teratogenicity.
- For **acute treatment** of primary headache, **acetaminophen, alone (preferably), or with codeine (for refractory headache),** should be the first choice during all trimesters. **Naproxen and ibuprofen** are safe and well tolerated in pregnancy, but should be **avoided after 28 weeks.** Severe unrelenting migraine responds well to parenteral antiemetics, such as metaclopramide and prochlorperazine. **Propranolol can be considered as a prophylactic medication** for the pregnant patient whose headache frequency requires daily preventive medication, and for whom nonpharmacologic approaches to headache prophylaxis have failed.

BACKGROUND/EPIDEMIOLOGY

The relationship between headache and pregnancy is of concern for two reasons: First, primary headache disorders (migraine or tension-type headaches) are far more common in women than men, and the impact of headache in women is directly affected by reproductive life events. One-year migraine prevalence is 18% in women in the United States. It has a peak incidence following menarche in young girls, is most prevalent in the reproductive age of 20 to 50, is commonly exacerbated by menses, influenced by hormonal contraception and replacement therapy, and is often improved following menopause. Migraine, particularly migraine without aura, generally improves with pregnancy and worsens in the postpartum period.

Pregnancy has been a common exclusion criterion for controlled clinical trials. Therefore, data on the safety of drugs used for primary headache types in pregnant women, such as migraine and tension-type headache, are scant. Yet in a survey of drug utilization by the World Health Organization, 68% of pregnant women took some form of medication.

Clinicians should be particularly vigilant regarding secondary headaches; several ominous conditions, such as stroke, pituitary tumors, and subarachnoid hemorrhage, occur more frequently in women who are pregnant than those who are not (1).

DIAGNOSIS

Diagnostic criteria as per the International headache Society are shown in the Table 18.1 (2).

Diagnostic Considerations for Headache in Pregnancy

Some secondary causes of headache (because of another, often ominous, disorder):

- Cortical venous thrombosis or cranial sinus thrombosis
- Subarachnoid hemorrhage
- Preeclampsia or eclampsia associated with elevated blood pressure [associated with reversible cerebral vasospastic syndrome (RCVS)]
- Stroke
- Idiopathic intracranial hypertension (pseudotumor cerebri)
- Pituitary tumor and pituitary apoplexy
- Headache associated with trauma to the head or neck, or to infection or disease of the meninges, sinuses, eyes, or ears

Some primary causes of headache:

- Migraine with and without aura
- Tension-type headache
- Trigeminal autonomic cephalgias (cluster headache)
- Cough headache

Red flags suggesting a secondary (ominous) headache:

- Sudden-onset (thunderclap) headache
- Secondary risk factors (HIV, systemic cancer)

Table 18.1 International Headache Society Criteria for the Diagnosis of Migraine

---

Migraine without Aura

A. At least five attacks fulfilling criteria B–D

B. Headache duration of 4–72 hr

C. Headache with at least two of the following:
   a. Unilateral location
   b. Pulsating quality
   c. Moderate or severe pain intensity
   d. Aggravation by routine physical activity

D. During headache at least one of the following:
   a. Nausea and/or vomiting
   b. Photophobia and phonophobia

E. Not attributed to another disorder

Migraine with Aura

A. Aura consisting of at least one of the following:
   a. Fully reversible visual symptoms (flickering lights or spots) or loss of vision
   b. Fully reversible sensory symptoms (paresthesia or numbness)
   c. Fully reversible speech disturbance

B. Aura develops gradually over $\geq$5 min and lasts $\leq$60 min

C. Not attributed to another disorder

Tension-type headache

A. At least 10 episodes occurring less than 1 day/mo on average and fulfilling criteria B–D

B. Headache lasting from 30 min to 7 days

C. Headache that has at least two of the following characteristics
   a. Bilateral location
   b. Pressing/tightening (nonpulsatile) quality
   c. Mild or moderate intensity
   d. Not aggravated by routine physical activity

D. Not attributed to another disorder

Source: Adapted from Ref. 2.

- Headache associated with systemic symptoms (fever, weight loss, meningeal signs, papilledema) or focal neurologic signs (confusion, impaired alertness, or incoordination)
- New, different, or progressively worsening headache
- Positional headache that occurs only in the upright posture and is relieved with recumbency (CSF leak)

EPIDEMIOLOGY/PATHOPHYSIOLOGY

In the past year, 18% of women and 6% of men had a **migraine** headache, but nearly half of these patients remain undiagnosed. It is estimated that an even greater number of women (approximately 40%) suffer from episodic or chronic tension-type headache. Migraine usually improves during pregnancy, but a first migraine can occur during pregnancy, usually in the first trimester. The elevated and sustained levels of plasma estrogens are felt to be protective during pregnancy and the fall in estrogen at the onset of menses a factor in menstrually associated migraine. Estrogens are known to increase pain thresholds in animal studies (3) and endogenous opioids also increase as pregnancy progresses. Migraine often recurs postpartum, usually within three to six days.

The meninges, proximal cerebral blood vessels, and venous sinuses are pain sensitive. Therefore it is not surprising that subarachnoid hemorrhage from a ruptured aneurysm, or vessel distension from a venous thrombosis, would produce head pain. Pus and subarachnoid blood act as irritants, setting up an inflammatory reaction and potentially interfering with CSF reabsorption, causing hydrocephalus.

The pathophysiology of migraine is complex. Even less is known about the genesis of tension-type headache. The migraine aura is probably due to cortical spreading depression (CSD). CSD is a spreading decrease in electrical activity that moves across the cerebral cortex at 2 to 3 mm/min. It is characterized by shifts in cortical steady state potential, transient increases in potassium, nitric oxide, and glutamate, and transient increases in CBF, followed by sustained decreases. Functional MRI studies of patients with migraine show that a period of hyperemia precedes the oligemia present during the migraine aura and the headache itself can begin before hyperemia, while blood flow in the cerebral cortex is still reduced. Headache probably results from activation of meningeal and blood vessel nociceptors combined with a change in central pain modulation. Headache and its associated neurovascular changes are subserved by the trigeminal system. Stimulation results in the release of substance P and calcitonin gene related peptide (CGRP) from sensory C-fiber terminals and neurogenic inflammation (4). Neurogenic inflammation sensitizes nerve fibers (peripheral sensitization), which now respond to previously innocuous stimuli, such as blood vessel pulsations, causing, in part, the pain of migraine. Central sensitization of trigeminal nucleus caudalis neurons can also occur. Central sensitization may play a key role in maintaining the headache. The migraine aura can trigger headache: CSD activates trigeminovascular afferents. This replaces the older theories of migraine pathophysiology of aura caused by vasoconstriction and headache caused by vasodilation.

GENETICS

Migraine is a group of familial disorders with a genetic component. Familial hemiplegic migraine (FHM) is a group of autosomal dominant disorders associated with attacks of migraine, with and without aura, and hemiparesis. FHM1 accounts for approximately two-thirds of cases and is due to at least 10 different missense mutations in the CACNA1A gene, which codes for the α_1-subunit of a voltage dependent P/Q Ca^{2+} channel. FHM2 results from a new mutation in the α_2-subunit of the Na/K pump. FHM3 is due to a missense mutation in gene SCN1A (Gln1489Lys), which encodes an α_1-subunit of a neuronal voltage-gated Na+ channel ($Na_v1.1$)

PREGNANCY CONSIDERATIONS
Effect of Pregnancy on the Disorder

Several retrospective studies of the course of migraine in pregnancy have been performed (5). Most women with migraine improve during pregnancy, women without aura more commonly than women with aura, generally by the second and third trimester. Women whose migraines began during the menarche and **those with menstrually associated migraine are more likely to have headaches recede during pregnancy** (6,7).

Some women have their first attack during pregnancy; others will have increased head pain during the first trimester. In these studies, the headaches of a small percentage of women with migraine developed worse headache during pregnancy. Most of these women had migraine with aura.

Migraine often recurs postpartum or can also begin for the first time in general.

Effect of the Disorder on Pregnancy

Patients with migraine were not believed to have an increased incidence of teratogenicity, toxemia, stillbirths, or miscarriage compared with controls (8). However, one study from Denmark reported that women with migraine had a higher incidence of low-birth-weight infants than women without migraine (9). A new study from Taiwan found that women with migraines were at increased risk of having low-birth-weight preterm babies, preeclampsia, and delivery by, cesarean, compared with unaffected mothers (10).

MANAGEMENT

Evaluation of Headache in Pregnancy

Headache in pregnancy should be evaluated in the same manner as any other time, with the awareness of specific disorders that are more frequent or only occur with pregnancy. The clinician should be alert to the warning signs of ominous headache. Certain conditions that cause worrisome headache are more common in pregnancy. Headache that presents in a sudden (thunderclap) fashion may indicate subarachnoid hemorrhage, particularly if associated with a change in consciousness or focal neurologic signs. Sudden headache can also accompany preeclampsia (consider RCVS) or pituitary apoplexy. Venous or sinus thrombosis, associated with the puerperium, can present with seizure, precipitous headache, vomiting or focal signs, and, if intracranial pressure is elevated, papilledema.

Whether or not to obtain a CT or an MRI as part of the evaluation of headache in pregnancy depends on the degree of suspicion for an ominous cause of headache. Generally speaking, **head CT and MRI are safe in pregnancy**, although the decision to obtain the study should be based on the risk of missing a structural or serious cause of headache without the study. **Gadolinium**, used as a contrast agent for MRI scanning, does cross the placenta (11). However, if an intracerebral bleed, mass lesion, or meningitis is suspected, the benefit of CT, MRI, or MRA far outweighs the potential risks, including the risk of gadolinium. Gadolinium was deemed **safe** by the European Society of Radiology, because after gadolinium contrast media no effect on the fetus has been reported in the literature (12). Lumbar puncture to diagnose meningitis or hemorrhage may be delayed until CT of the brain without contrast is obtained to avoid the risk of herniation if a mass, or cerebral edema, is suspected.

Acute Therapy for Headache

Acute migraine treatments in nonpregnant women include simple analgesics (acetaminophen, aspirin), nonsteroidal anti-inflammatory drugs (NSAIDs), opioids, ergot alkaloids, isometheptene caffeine-barbiturate combinations, and triptans (Fig. 18.1).

Migraine typically improves as pregnancy progresses. However, in the first trimester, when headache often worsens, concern arises as to the potential effect of acute medication on embryogenesis. The situation is particularly poignant as many women, unknowingly pregnant, will have used acute medications to treat migraine or tension-type headache in the very early days or weeks after conception.

Acetaminophen is the drug most commonly taken during pregnancy. There is no evidence of any teratogenic effect

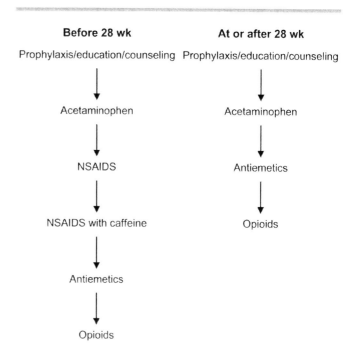

Before 28 wk
Prophylaxis/education/counseling
↓
Acetaminophen
↓
NSAIDS
↓
NSAIDS with caffeine
↓
Antiemetics
↓
Opioids

At or after 28 wk
Prophylaxis/education/counseling
↓
Acetaminophen
↓
Antiemetics
↓
Opioids

Figure 18.1 Proposed algorithm for management of primary headache in pregnancy, based on gestational age.

(FDA B). Aspirin's concerns about safety came from earlier data, when aspirin was used in therapeutic doses for analgesic or antipyretic purposes. These concerns do not appear to apply to low-dose (60–100 mg/day) aspirin (FDA C; D if third trimester). Although aspirin is labeled category C, aspirin is unique in that there are clinical trials that studied aspirin during pregnancy for conditions other than headache, for example in patients with antiphospholipid antibody syndrome (13). Recommended dosing of aspirin is high, at 500 to 1000 mg per attack (8). Other category B drugs (no evidence of risk in humans, but without controlled human studies) include, **caffeine, ibuprofen, indomethacin, and naproxen** (note **the latter three are category D at the end of the third trimester**). NSAID use has been associated with premature closure of the ductus arteriosus and pulmonary hypertension in the neonate when given late in pregnancy (14).

Meperidine and morphine are FDA category C in pregnancy, but their use should be restricted late in pregnancy (6). Prednisone and dexamethasone, which can be used to treat "status migrainosus," are both FDA category C.

Ergotamine and dihydroergotamine are category X, and should be avoided in pregnant women. Ergots are abortifacients and have been shown to cause fetal distress and birth defects.

Antiemetic medicines, such as **metaclopramide, chlorpromazine, and prochlorperazine**, are effective parenterally for the head pain itself, in addition to the nausea and vomiting that can accompany migraine, and are generally considered safe in pregnancy. Intravenous or intramuscular antiemetics, with fluid replacement, are very effective in aborting status migrainosus, or severe headache in the emergency room or urgent care center.

The triptans are 5-HT 1B/1D receptor agonists that are effective in treating migraine headache and the accompanying symptoms of photosensitivity, nausea, and vomiting. The data obtained from 12 years of prospective monitoring of pregnancies exposed to sumatriptan and naratriptan failed to show a signal for a substantial increase in the risk of all major birth defects following prenatal sumatriptan or naratriptan exposure. However, the size of the registry is currently insufficient to evaluate the risk of specific defects or to permit definitive conclusions of the risks associated with sumatriptan or naratriptan (15). The triptan class is category C, and as such is not recommended for pregnant migraineurs. However, on the basis of the pregnancy registry, if a patient has unwittingly taken **sumatriptan**, prior to knowledge of her pregnancy, **reassurance is appropriate given the lack of teratogenicity of this drug**. It is not known whether this positive outcome may also be extrapolated to other medications in the triptan class.

Headache Prophylaxis in Pregnancy

Clinicians should be encouraged to treat headaches in early pregnancy with acute medications such as acetaminophen, or low doses of codeine. **Preventive therapy should be reserved for women whose headaches continue to worsen throughout pregnancy**. There are no prospective randomized clinical trials of migraine prophylactic drugs in pregnant women.

Nonpharmacologic therapies should be initiated first. **Relaxation training and thermal biofeedback**, combined with relaxation techniques and **cognitive behavioral therapies**, have been subjected to rigorous, well-designed, randomized clinical trials and show efficacy in migraine prevention (16). In contradistinction, evidence-based therapy recommendations for acupuncture, hypnosis, and chiropractic manipulation for headache prevention are not as yet available.

Whenever a second comorbid condition exists with migraine, it is advisable to use one drug to treat both conditions. Examples include migraine and epilepsy, wherein an anticonvulsant may be effective to treat both conditions, and migraine and depression, for which a selective serotonin reuptake inhibitor (SSRI), such as fluoxetine (category B), may similarly permit monotherapy.

Propranolol is probably the safest drug to use in later pregnancy as a preventive for headache, as it is not known to have teratogenic effect (7). Verapamil (calcium channel blocker) may also be beneficial (17). Valproic acid should be avoided for headache prophylaxis because of its potential for causing neural tube defects. The use of topiramate and gabapentin should be restricted for headache prophylaxis in view of their potential association with fetal defects, although these drugs can be very effective for nonpregnant migraineurs.

Education about avoiding specific food, caffeine, and alcohol triggers for migraine may reduce reliance on both preventive and acute medications. Pregnant patients with headache should **avoid skipping meals, should regularize their sleep and exercise habits, and consider meditation or yoga**.

REFERENCES

1. Silberstein SD. Sex Hormones and Headaches. Philadelphia: Current Medicine Group, 2007. [Review]
2. International Headache Society. The international classification of headache disorders. 2nd ed. Cephalalgia 2004; 24(suppl 1):1–160. [Review]
3. Dawson-Basoa MB, Gintzler AR. 17-Beta-estradiol and progesterone modulate an intrinsic opioid analgesic system. Brain Res 1993; 601(1–2):241–245. [II-3]
4. Dimitriadou V, Buzzi MG, Theoharides TC, et al. Ultrastructural evidence for neurogenically mediated changes in blood vessels of the rat aura mater and tongue following antidromic trigeminal stimulation. Neuroscience 1992; 48:187–203. [II -2]
5. Loder E, Silberstein SD. Headaches in woman. In: Silberstein SD, Lipton RB, Dodick DW, eds. Wolff's Headache and Other Head Pain. 8th ed. New York: Oxford University Press, 2008:691–710. [Review]
6. Aube M. Migraine in pregnancy. Neurology 1999; 53(4 suppl 1): S26–S28. [Review]
7. Fox AW, Diamond ML, Spierings ELH. Migraine during pregnancy. CNS Drugs 2005; 19(6):465–481. [Review]
8. Wainscott G, Volans GN. The outcome of pregnancy in women suffering from migraine. Postgrad Med J 1978; 54:98–102. [II-2]
9. Olesen C, Steffensen FH, Sorensen HT, et al. Pregnancy outcome following prescription for sumatriptan. Headache 2000; 40(1): 20–24. [II-3]
10. Chen HM, Chen SF, Chen YH, et al. Increased risk of adverse pregnancy outcomes for woman with migraines: a nationwide population-based study. Cephalalgia 2010; 30(4):443–448. [II-2]
11. Schwartz RB. Neurodiagnostic imaging of the pregnant patient. In: Deinsky O, Feldmann E, Hainline B, eds. Neurologic Complications of Pregnancy. New York: Raven Press, 1994:243–248. [Review]
12. Webb JAW, Thomsen HS, Morcos SK. The use of iodinated and gadolinium contrast media during pregnancy and lactation. Eur Radiol 2005; 15:1234–1240. [Review]
13. Vainio M, Kujansuu E, Iso-Mustajarvi J, et al. Low dose acetylsalicylic acid in prevention of pregnancy-induced hypertension and intrauterine growth retardation in women with bilateral uterine artery notches. BJOG 2002; 109(2):161–167. [II-2]
14. Morris JL, Rosen DA, Rosen KR. Nonsteroidal anti-inflammatory agents in neonates. Paediatr Drugs 2003; 5:385–405. [Review]
15. Cunnington M, Ephross S, Churchill P. The safety of sumatriptan and naratriptan in pregnancy: what have we learned? Headache 2009; 49:1414–1422. [Review]
16. Campbell JK, Penzien DB, Wall EM, and the US Headache Consortium. Evidence-based guidelines for migraine headache: behavioral and physical treatments. In: AOA.net (online). Available at: www.aoa-net.org/MembersOnly/hcnonpharnpdf. Accessed February 25, 2003. [Review]
17. Silberstein SD, Freitag FG, Bigal ME. Migraine treatment. In: Silberstein SD, Lipton RB, Dodick DW, eds. Wolff's Headache and Other Head Pain. 8th ed. New York: Oxford University Press, 2008:177–292. [Review]

19

Seizures

Meriem Bensalem-Owen

KEY POINTS

- **Epilepsy** is a chronic neurological condition characterized by **recurrent unprovoked seizures.** The most important diagnostic tool is the **history.**
- There is **insufficient evidence to support or refute an increased risk** of a change in **seizure frequency** or **status epilepticus** during pregnancy.
- **Fetal loss, perinatal death, congenital anomalies** (4–8%, or about twice the baseline risk), **low birth weight, prematurity, induction, developmental delay,** and **childhood epilepsy** have been reported in the past to be more frequent, but more recent data do not confirm an increase in these complications.
- **Supplemental folic acid** (0.4 up to 4 mg daily) may be given to all women of childbearing age taking **antiepileptic drugs** (AEDs) prior to conception and continued during pregnancy. There is **insufficient published information** to address the **dosing of folic acid.**
- **Counsel** women with seizures or epilepsy about the risk of AED-associated teratogenicity and neurodevelopmental delay, folic acid supplementation, possible changes in seizure frequency during pregnancy, importance of medication compliance and AED level monitoring, inheritance risks for seizures, and breast-feeding.
- In general, the best choice for therapy is the AED that best controls the seizures. **Monotherapy at the lowest possible dose of the AED most efficient in controlling seizures** should be **the goal.**
- **Carbamazepine, phenobarbital, primidone, phenytoin, valproate, and topiramate** are FDA category D drugs, and should be **avoided** if possible.
- **Optimize AED therapy and complete AED changes** if possible **at least six months before planned conception.**
- **Seizure freedom for at least nine months prior to pregnancy is probably associated with a high likelihood of remaining seizure-free during pregnancy.**
- **Stopping or changing an AED during pregnancy for the sole purpose of reducing teratogenicity is not advised.**
- **Prenatal testing** should include first-trimester ultrasound, **alpha-fetoprotein (AFP) levels, anatomy and echocardiographic ultrasounds,** and if needed amniocentesis for amniotic fluid AFP and acetylcholinesterase.
- As pregnancy progresses, **both total and nonprotein bound plasma concentrations of some AEDs may decline.**
- Monitor AED levels through the eighth postpartum week.
- There is **insufficient evidence to support or refute a benefit of prenatal vitamin K supplementation for reducing the risk of hemorrhagic complications in the newborns** of women with epilepsy.
- **Encourage breast-feeding** and monitor for sedation or feeding difficulties, which can be caused by certain AEDs, usually those with low protein binding.

BACKGROUND

Recommendations and guidelines presented in this chapter are in large part based on the updated three companion Practice Parameters of the Quality Standards Subcommittee and Therapeutics and Technology Assessment Subcommittee of the American Academy of Neurology and American Epilepsy Society (1–3).

DIAGNOSES/DEFINITIONS

Seizures result from an abnormal paroxysmal discharge of a group of cerebral neurons. **Epilepsy** is a chronic neurological condition in which **recurrent seizures occur unprovoked by systemic or neurological insults.** The most important diagnostic tool is the **history.** The examination is very often normal unless the patient has a structural brain lesion. The history should include the following information:

- The presence or absence of an aura, which is a recurrent stereotypic abnormal sensation or experience. The aura is a simple partial seizure.
- Seizure description by an eye witness, including duration.
- Postictal phase, description, and duration.
- Exacerbating factors.
- Birth history, especially when the seizure onset is in the neonatal period or early childhood.
- History of febrile convulsions, central nervous system infections or head trauma with loss of consciousness.
- Family history.

Ancillary tests include **EEG**, laboratory tests as indicated by the history, and imaging of the brain. **MRI of the head** is more sensitive than CT scan for detecting subtle lesions. EEG poses no risk to the fetus, so workup for diagnosis should proceed in pregnancy just as in nonpregnant adults.

SYMPTOMS

In partial-onset seizures, some patients may experience a subjective feeling, called aura. The particular site of the brain affected determines usually the symptomatology and/or the clinical expression of the seizure.

EPIDEMIOLOGY/INCIDENCE

Epilepsy occurs in 0.5% to 0.8% of the general population, with 5% of people reporting a seizure at some time in their life. The prevalence of epilepsy in the United States indicates that approximately one half million women with epilepsy are of childbearing age (4).

ETIOLOGY/BASIC PATHOPHYSIOLOGY

Paroxysmal discharges of neurons occur when the threshold for firing of neuronal membranes is reduced. The pathophysiology of epileptic disorders is not very well understood. Structural abnormalities of neuronal transmitter receptors, channelopathies, excessive excitatory activity, cortical remodeling, and loss of inhibitory neuronal activity have all been implicated as possible mechanisms.

CLASSIFICATION

Depending on their onset, seizures are classified as either **partial** (focal) or **generalized**. The prototype for generalized seizures is the generalized tonic clonic (GTC) seizure. Partial seizures can be further subdivided into **simple partial** or **complex partial** seizures (CPS). During simple partial seizures awareness is preserved and the patient can either experience focal motor manifestations or experience a subjective feeling, called aura.

Auras can be olfactory, gustatory, sensory, auditory, visual, vertiginous sensations or psychic experiences (such as "déjà vu"). CPS are characterized by impairment of awareness; these seizures can secondarily generalize.

RISK FACTORS/ASSOCIATIONS

Risk factors for seizures are numerous, but could include malformations of cortical development, head trauma, central nervous system infections, family history, complicated febrile convulsions, and possibly history of difficult birth (anoxia or trauma) or complicated (fetal infections and/or preterm birth) pregnancy.

COMPLICATIONS

Epileptic women of childbearing age should be informed of the risks associated with antiepileptic drug (AED) use prior to conception (3), and that seizures may be harmful to mother and fetus (5).

Maternal Complications

There is insufficient evidence to support or refute an increased risk of preeclampsia, pregnancy-related hypertension, spontaneous abortion, a change in seizure frequency or an increased risk of status epilepticus in pregnant women with epilepsy. Only class IV studies could be found on this subject. On the basis of class II studies, seizure freedom for at least nine months prior to pregnancy is probably associated with a high likelihood (84–92%) of remaining seizure-free during pregnancy. Women can injure themselves during seizures, especially in the case of CPS or GTC.

Fetal Complications

GTC seizures increase the risk of hypoxia and acidosis as well as injury from blunt trauma. Generalized seizures but not partial seizures occurring during labor can affect fetal heart rate. **Fetal loss** (1.3–14%) and **perinatal death** (1.3–7.8%), **congenital malformations anomalies** (4–8%, or about twice the baseline risk), **low birth weight** (7–10%), **prematurity** (4–11%), **induction, developmental delay**, and **childhood epilepsy** can

be associated with in utero exposure to AEDs. There is insufficient evidence to determine whether the risk of neonatal hemorrhagic complications in the newborns of women with epilepsy taking AEDs is substantially increased. **Evidence is inadequate to determine whether prenatal vitamin K in women with epilepsy reduces the risk of hemorrhagic complications in the newborns.**

Most common congenital malformations, which differ for different AEDs, are cardiac, neural tube, craniofacial, fingers, and others.

Epilepsy and pregnancy registries have been operational for more than 10 years and were developed in order to better understand the risks of birth defects associated with AED treatment, and more importantly, to systematically study the range of birth defects resulting from use of each AED (6). Two class I studies, including one from the U.K. Epilepsy and Pregnancy Registry, revealed that exposure during the first trimester to valproic acid monotherapy is associated with a greater risk for major congenital malformations than carbamazepine monotherapy (7,8). Valproic acid as part of polytherapy was associated with greater risk than polytherapy without valproic acid (7).

Data from the North American Antiepileptic Drug (NAAED) Pregnancy Registry indicate that **the rate of major malformations is 10.7% with valproate** (9), **6.5% with phenobarbital, 2.7% with lamotrigine, and 2.5% with carbamazepine**. Valproic acid is associated with neural tube defects, oral clefts, hypospadias, poor cognitive outcome, and cardiac malformations. Exposure to phenytoin, carbamazepine, and lamotrigine was associated with oral clefts. Avoidance of phenobarbital may reduce the risk of cardiac malformations. A recent communication from the NAAED indicates an **increased risk of oral clefts in infants exposed to topiramate monotherapy during the first trimester of pregnancy** and an increased risk of low birth weight (<5 lb 8 oz) in babies exposed to the drug in utero.

MANAGEMENT
Principles

Effect of pregnancy on disease: Increase in hepatic cytochrome P450 enzyme activity and renal clearance causes the **concentration** of some **AEDs to fall**. Decreased protein binding results **in higher levels of unbound biologically active AEDs** and may cause toxicity (Table 19.1). On the basis of current studies, there is insufficient evidence to support or refute an increased risk of a change in seizure frequency or status epilepticus during pregnancy.

Preconception Counseling

Also include in first prenatal visit:

a. Conception should be deferred until seizures are well controlled on minimum dose of medication.
b. Monotherapy is preferable. Good compliance with AEDs is essential to avoid any seizures.
c. Inform women with epilepsy that infants exposed in utero to AED have a **4% to 8% risk of congenital malformation**, most notably neural tube defects, compared to 2% to 3% for the general population. Epilepsy pregnancy registries have been operational for more than 10 years, and collected an impressive amount of data. **Carbamazepine, phenobarbital, primidone, phenytoin, valproate and topiramate** are FDA category D drugs, and should be **avoided** if possible at least in the first trimester. Recent pregnancy databases have suggested that valproate is

Table 19.1 Pharmacokinetic Profile of the Most Commonly Used AEDs

	Mechanism	Pregnancy category	Protein binding (%)
First-generation AEDs			
Phenytoin (Dilantin)	Na	D	90
Carbamazepine (Tegretol)	Ca, GABA	D	75
Valproic acid (Depakote, Depakene)	Na, GABA	D	85–95
Ethosuximide	T-type Ca	C	0
Second- and third-generation AEDs			
Gabapentin (Neurontin)	Ca	C	0
Pregabalin (Lyrica)	Ca	C	0
Lamotrigine (Lamotrigine)	Na, Glutamate	C	55
Levetiracetam (Keppra)	SV2a	C	0
Oxcarbazepine(Oxcarbamazepine)	Na, Ca	C	40
Tiagabine (Gabatril)	GABA reuptake	C	96
Topiramate (Topiramate)	Multiple	D	10
Zonisamide (Zonegran)	Na, T-Ca	C	40–60
Lacosamide (Vimpat)	Na (slow inactivation)	C	15
Rufinamide (Banzel)	Na	C	34
Vigabatrin (Sabril)	GABA	C	0

First-generation AEDs	*Adverse effects*
Phenytoin (Dilantin)	Rash, ataxia, hirsutism, gingival hypertrophy, osteoporosis
Carbamazepine (Tegretol)	Rash, diplopia, sexual dysfunction, osteoporosis
Valproic acid (Depakote, Depakene)	Weight gain, tremor, hair loss, encephalopathy, hepatotoxicity, pancreatitis, polycystic ovaries
Ethosuximide	Nausea, vomiting, anorexia, rash
Second- and third-generation AEDs	
Gabapentin (Neurontin)	Weight gain, edema, myoclonus
Pregabalin (Lyrica)	Increased appetite, confusion, somnolence
Lamotrigine (Lamotrigine)	Rash, aseptic meningitis
Levetiracetam (Keppra)	Behavioral changes, asthenia
Oxcarbazepine (Oxcarbamazepine)	Hyponatremia, diplopia, rash
Tiagabine (Gabatril)	Encephalopathy, status epilepticus
Topiramate (Topiramate)	Renal stones, speech difficulties, paresthesias, weight loss, acidosis, closed-angle glaucoma
Zonisamide (Zonegran)	Renal stones, weight loss, paresthesias, contraindicated if history of allergy to sulfa drugs
Lacosamide (Vimpat)	Dizziness, nausea, vomiting, double vision
Rufinamide (Banzel)	Headaches, drowsiness, dizziness, vomiting
Vigabatrin (Sabril)	Visual field loss, somnolence, headaches, dizziness

Abbreviation: GABA, gamma-aminobutyric acid; AED, antiepileptic drugs.

significantly more teratogenic than carbamazepine, and the combination of valproate and lamotrigine is particularly teratogenic (10). Lamotrigine has been associated with facial clefts (11).

d. Seizure freedom for at least nine months prior to pregnancy is probably associated with a high likelihood of remaining seizure-free during pregnancy.

e. Consider neurological consultation regarding the possibility of tapering off and stopping anticonvulsant medications if the patient has been seizure-free for greater than two years and has a normal EEG. The patient should be observed for 6 to 12 months off AED before attempting conception.

f. Preconception folic acid supplementation (dose 2–4 mg) may be considered to reduce the risk of major congenital malformations.

g. Driving privileges should be suspended for several months after a seizure; the exact length varies depending on the state (12).

h. Home/work: Avoid baths, take showers instead. No manipulation of heavy machinery or working at heights (12).

i. Enzyme-inducing AEDs (Table 19.2) enhance the metabolism of oral contraceptives, therefore decreasing their efficacy. Pregnancies should be planned.

j. Emphasize that 90% of women with epilepsy have successful pregnancies and deliver healthy babies (13).

Prenatal Counseling

At the first prenatal visit and during pregnancy as necessary, counsel women with seizures or epilepsy regarding all of the above preconception issues. In addition, discuss the following:

Table 19.2 Enzyme-Inducing AEDs

Barbiturates
Primidone
Phenytoin
Carbamazepine
Oxcarbazepine
Topiramate (with doses >200 mg/day)

Abbreviation: AED, antiepileptic drugs.

- There is a possible change in seizure frequency during pregnancy.
- Although no AED is specifically indicated for use in pregnant women, the AED that renders the patient seizure-free and side effect–free should be the drug of choice during pregnancy.
- The risk-to-benefit ratio must be considered when selecting a drug.
- There is a risk of AED-associated teratogenicity and neurodevelopment delay.
- Importance of medication compliance and AED level monitoring during pregnancy. AED levels decline due to enhanced AED hepatic metabolism, changes in volume distribution, and increase in glomerular filtration rate, which leads to increased renal clearance and decreased protein binding. Therefore, levels should be measured on highly protein bound AEDs (Table 19.1).
- Breast-feeding issues (see below).
- Inheritance risks for seizures.
- Child care issues (14).

Prenatal Care

- Supplemental **folic acid** (at least 0.4 mg/day, we use 2–4 mg/day) in women with epilepsy before they become pregnant is generally recommended to reduce the risk of major congenital malformations, and although the data are insufficient to show that it is effective in women with epilepsy, there is no evidence of harm and no reason to suspect that it would not be effective in this population. The strength of this recommendation should not impact the current folic acid supplementation recommendation.
- A first-trimester ultrasound is indicated for exact dating.
- Anatomic ultrasound at 11 to 13 weeks can identify most severe defects, such as anencephaly.
- Prenatal testing for neural tube defects with **alpha-fetoprotein** levels at 15 to 18 weeks gestation (up to 21 weeks).
- If appropriate, amniocentesis for amniotic fluid alpha-fetoprotein and acetylcholinesterase levels.
- **Ultrasound at 16 to 20 weeks** gestation can assess anatomic anomalies such as orofacial clefts, heart defects, and caudal neural tube defects.
- Fetal **echocardiogram** at about 22 weeks.
- An ultrasound for growth at ≥32 weeks is not mandatory.
- Neonates should receive vitamin K, 1 mg IM at birth. The benefit of prenatal maternal vitamin K therapy is unknown, with no trial available for assessment.

THERAPY (TABLE 19.1)

- **Multidisciplinary** communication between the primary care provider, obstetrician, geneticist, and neurologist/epileptologist for counseling and management of seizures and epilepsy during pregnancy is crucial.
- **There is no trial that indicates which AED is safest during pregnancy**. The best choice is the AED that best controls the seizures. **All the AEDs are FDA category C except for the following AEDs that are category D: carbamazepine, phenobarbital, primidone, phenytoin, valproate, and topiramate** (Table 19.1). **These six AEDs should therefore be avoided if possible**, by using a different therapy beginning in the preconception period. Switching and abruptly stopping of AEDs are to be avoided.
- Regarding AED therapy, at the beginning of pregnancy it is recommended that the patient is on **monotherapy** with the AED of choice for the seizure type, achieving optimal seizure control, at the lowest effective dose.
- **Monitoring the serum levels** of **lamotrigine, carbamazepine, and phenytoin** during pregnancy should be considered and monitoring of levetiracetam and oxcarbazepine (as monohydroxy derivative) levels may be considered. Free levels (serum or saliva) are available for carbamazepine, valproic acid, phenobarbital and phenytoin. Avoid high peak levels by spreading out the total daily dose into multiple smaller doses. Studies provide some evidence supporting active monitoring of AED levels during pregnancy, particularly of lamotrigine, as changes in lamotrigine levels were associated with increased seizure frequency (15). It seems reasonable to individualize this monitoring for each patient, with the aim of maintaining a level close to preconception level, presumably the one at which the woman with epilepsy was doing well with seizure control. One study showed that during pregnancy the clearance of lamotrigine increases with a peak of 94% in the third trimester; hence, frequent adjustments of the dose are required during pregnancy (13).
- AEDs have effects on sodium, potassium, or calcium channels. They also can affect neurotransmitters enhancing the inhibitory neurotransmitter, GABA, or inhibiting the excitatory glutamate.
- AED Pregnancy Registry: Phone number 1-888-233-2334. http://www.aedpregnancyregistry.org.

DELIVERY

AED medication should be continued in labor, and in the immediate postpartum period. There is probably no substantially increased risk of cesarean delivery for women with epilepsy taking AEDs. There is possibly a substantial increased risk of premature contractions and premature labor and delivery during pregnancy for women with epilepsy who smoke (16).

POSTPARTUM/BREAST-FEEDING

Breast-feeding is not contraindicated. The greater the protein binding of AED (Table 19.1), the lower is its concentration in breast milk. Breast-feeding is not contraindicated in patients on anticonvulsant medications unless excess neonatal sedation occurs. **Monitor newborns** or infants for sedation when breast-feeding mothers with seizures take low-protein-bound AEDs. The AED concentration profiled in breast milk follows the plasma concentration curve. The total amount of drug transferred to infants via breast milk is usually much smaller than the amount transferred via the placenta during pregnancy. However, as drug elimination mechanisms are not fully developed in early infancy, repeated administration of a drug via breast milk may lead to accumulation in the infant. Extended release formulations of AEDs should be avoided.

Valproic acid, phenobarbital, phenytoin, and carbamazepine may be considered as not transferring into breast milk to as great an extent as, for example, levetiracetam, gabapentin, lamotrigine, and topiramate.

For most AEDs, the pharmacokinetics in the mother will return to prepregnancy levels within 10 to 14 days after delivery. **Monitor AED levels** through the eighth postpartum week and adjust doses accordingly to avoid toxicity. Sleep deprivation may exacerbate seizures, and should therefore be avoided. Women with epilepsy should not bathe their child while they are alone at home, should avoid stair climbing while carrying the baby; a portable changing pad placed on the floor should be used. New mothers should avoid using a carrier in front or on their back. A portable carrier with handles is a safer alternative in the event of a seizure and subsequent fall (14). Since enzyme-inducing AEDs (Table 19.1) lower estrogen concentrations by 40% to 50%, thereby compromising contraceptive effectiveness, hormonal contraceptives prescribed to women with epilepsy on these AEDs should contain ≥50 µg of ethinyl estradiol (17). Oral contraceptives induce lamotrigine metabolism requiring adjustment of its dose (18).

REFERENCES

1. Harden CL, Pennell PB, Koppel BS, et al. Practice parameter update: management issues for women with epilepsy—focus on pregnancy (an evidence-based review): III. Vitamin K, folic acid, blood levels, and breastfeeding: report of the Quality Standards Subcommittee and Therapeutics and Technology Assessment Subcommittee of the American Academy of Neurology and American Epilepsy Society. Neurology 2009; 73(2):142–149. [Guideline; III]
2. Harden CL, Hopp J, Ting TY, et al. Practice parameter update: management issues for women with epilepsy—focus on pregnancy (an evidence-based review): I. Obstetrical complications and change in seizure frequency: report of the Quality Standards Subcommittee and Therapeutics and Technology Assessment Subcommittee of the American Academy of Neurology and American Epilepsy Society. Neurology 2009; 73:126–132. [Guideline; III]
3. Harden CL, Meador KJ, Pennell PB, et al. Practice parameter update: Management issues for women with epilepsy—focus on pregnancy (an evidence-based review): II. Teratogenesis and perinatal outcomes: report of the Quality Standards Subcommittee and Therapeutics and Technology Assessment Subcommittee of the American Academy of Neurology and American Epilepsy Society. Neurology 2009; 73:133–141. [Guideline; III]
4. Hirtz D, Thurman DJ, Gwinn-Hardy K, et al. How common are the "common" neurologic disorders? Neurology 2007; 68(5):326–337. [II-3]
5. Fountain NB, Van Ness PC, Swain-Enq R, et al. Quality improvement in neurology: AAN epilepsy quality measures: report of the Quality Measurement and Reporting Subcommittee of the American Academy of Neurology. Neurology 2011; 76(1):94–99. [III]
6. Meador KJ, Pennell PB, Harden CL, et al. Pregnancy registries in epilepsy: a consensus statement on health outcomes. Neurology 2008; 71:1109–1117. [II-3]
7. Morrow J, Russell A, Guthrie E, et al. Malformations risks of antiepileptic drugs in pregnancy: a prospective study from the UK Epilepsy and Pregnancy Register. J Neurol Neurosurg Psychiatry 2006; 77(2):193–198. [II-2]
8. Wide K, Winbladh B, Kallen B. Major malformations in infants exposed to antiepileptic drugs in utero, with emphasis on carbamazepine and valproic acid: a nation-wide, population-based register study. Acta Paediatr 2004; 93(2):174–176. [II-2]
9. Wyszynski DF, Nambisan M, Surve T, et al. and for the Antiepileptic Drug Pregnancy Registry. Increased rate of major malformations in offspring exposed to valproate during pregnancy. Neurology 2005; 64(6):961–965. [II-3]
10. Tomson T, Battino D, Craig J, et al.; ILAE Commission on therapeutic strategies. Pregnancy registries: differences, similarities, and possible harmonization. Epilepsia 2010; 51(5):909–915. [III]
11. Holmes LB, Baldwin EJ, Smith CR, et al. Increased frequency of isolated cleft palate in infants exposed to lamotrigine during pregnancy. Neurology 2008; 70(22 pt 2):2152–2158. [II-2]
12. Dean P. Safety issues for women with epilepsy. In: Morrell MJ, Flynn K, eds. Women with Epilepsy. 1st ed. Cambridge: University Press, 2005:263–268. [II-3]
13. McAuley JW, Anderson GD. Treatment of epilepsy in women of reproductive age: pharmacokinetic considerations. Clin Pharmacokinet 2002; 41:559–579. [II-3]
14. Callanan M. Parenting for women with epilepsy. In: Morrell MJ, Flynn K eds. Women with Epilepsy. 1st ed. Cambridge: University Press, 2005:228–234. [III]
15. Pennell PB, Peng L, Newport DJ, et al. Lamotrigine in pregnancy: clearance, therapeutic drug monitoring, and seizure frequency. Neurology 2008; 70:2130–2136. [II-3]
16. Hvas CL, Henriksen TB, Ostergaard JR, et al. Epilepsy and pregnancy: effect of antiepileptic drugs and lifestyle on birth weight. BJOG 2000; 107:896–902. [II-3]
17. Harden CL, Leppik I. Optimizing therapy of seizures in women who use oral contraceptives. Neurology 2006; 67:S56–S58. [II-3]
18. Christensen J, Petrenaite V, Atterman J, et al. Oral contraceptives induce lamotrigine metabolism: evidence from a double-blind, placebo-controlled trial. Epilepsia 2007; 48:484–489. [RCT]

20

Spinal cord injury

Leonardo Pereira

KEY POINTS

- Spinal cord injury (SCI) in pregnant women is associated with increased risks of **urinary tract infections**, preterm birth, and anemia. **The most worrisome, potentially fatal complication is autonomic dysreflexia (ADR).**
- Antenatal management of women with preexisting SCI includes **frequent urinary cultures** *or* **antibiotic suppression (self, intermittent catheterization** is preferred); **stool softeners** and a **high-fiber diet**; routine **skin exams**, and **frequent position changes.** In women with lesions above the level of T5, baseline and serial pulmonary function tests can be used to assess vital capacity. There is insufficient data at this time to recommend universal thromboprophylaxis.
- ADR affects **up to 85% of women with lesions at or above the level of T6.** The most common sign of ADR is **systemic hypertension.** Symptoms are synchronous with uterine contractions. Prevention involves avoidance of triggers (constipation, cathetherization, exams, etc.), and **early epidural anesthesia.** Antihypertensive therapy for ADR includes: **nitroprusside amyl nitrate, trimethaphan,** and **hydralazine.**
- Several **prophylactic procedures** are necessary for **labor and delivery** in the SCI woman. Among these, **continuous hemodynamic monitoring during labor by maternal electrocardiogram, pulse oximetry, and arterial line** should be performed in patients with **baseline pulmonary insufficiency.**

DIAGNOSIS/DEFINITION

Spinal cord injury (SCI) is diagnosed neurologically. It can occur following trauma to the spinal cord, but also because of a variety of pathologies (e.g., neural tube defect, congenital, transverse myelitis, etc.).

EPIDEMIOLOGY/INCIDENCE

About 1000 new spinal cord injuries per year occur in women aged 16 to 30 in the United States. SCI diagnosed during pregnancy is rare. SCI preexisting pregnancy is relatively more common.

CLASSIFICATION

SCI is classified by its etiology, and, especially, by the level of the lesion. The higher is the functional level of the lesion, the worse are the disease and prognosis.

Complications (for women with preexisting SCI): **Asymptomatic bacteriuria, lower urinary tract infections** (up to 35% incidence) (1), and **pyelonephritis** are common. The risk of preterm birth is between 8% and 13% (1–4). Anemia can occur in 12% of women with SCI, especially with history of chronic pyelonephritis, decubitus, and/or renal failure. The most worrisome, potential fatal complication is **autonomic dysreflexia (ADR).**

PREGNANCY MANAGEMENT
Preconception Counseling

Women with preexisting SCI who are contemplating pregnancy should be referred for preconception counseling. If the spinal cord lesion is congenital or hereditary in origin then genetic counseling is warranted. Women with congenital spinal lesions such as meningomyelocele should be made aware of the increased risk of spinal cord lesions to their offspring and placed on 4 mg/day of folic acid (5). All other SCI women should take at least 400 μg of folic acid preconception.

Patients with preexisting SCI are probably at no greater risk than the general obstetric population for either congenital malformations or fetal death (6–8). In contrast to patients with SCI antecedent to pregnancy, patients who suffer traumatic SCI during pregnancy may be at risk for **spontaneous abortion, fetal malformation, abruptio placentae, or direct fetal injury** (9). A fetal malformation rate of 11% has been reported in 45 patients who suffered spinal cord injuries during pregnancy (8).

Prenatal Care
Acute SCI During Pregnancy

Acutely, SCI results in neurogenic shock or "spinal shock" because of the loss of sympathetic innervation. This typically presents with hypotension, bradycardia, and hypothermia because of parasympathetic effects. Adequate volume resuscitation and pressor support should be administered. Direct measurements of pulmonary capillary wedge pressure with a pulmonary artery catheter will assist clinical management. Internal hemorrhage should be identified and treated with the aid of a trauma surgeon if possible.

In the setting of acute SCI, initial stabilization of the neck and spinal column should occur immediately and airway patency secured. This may require a jaw thrust maneuver, nasal trumpet, or nasal intubation. Administration of methylprednisolone within eight hours of SCI may improve neurologic recovery in select cases (10). The risk of deep venous thrombosis and pulmonary embolism is greatest within eight weeks of traumatic SCI (11). Prophylactic anticoagulation should be considered during this period.

Antenatal Management of Preexisting SCI

Urinary. **Frequent urinary cultures** *or* **antibiotic suppression** (12–14). **Self, intermittent catheterization** (every four to six hours, and more frequently in third trimester) is preferred to continuous indwelling catheterization. Perineum should be cleaned before catheterization.

Gastrointestinal. **Stool softeners** and a **high-fiber diet**, to prevent constipation.

Dermatology. Routine **skin exams** for any evidence of decubitus ulcers at each visit, and **frequent position changes**. Wheelchairs may need to be resized or fitted with extra padding.

Pulmonary. In patients with high thoracic or cervical spine lesions, usually above the level of T5, baseline and serial **pulmonary function tests** to assess vital capacity (VC), and, especially if VC < 13 mL/kg, **possible need for ventilatory assistance** in labor are recommended (12,14). Supine tilted positioning is suggested for labor.

Thromboembolic. Despite a theoretical increased risk of venous thromboembolism, there are **insufficient data at this time to recommend universal thromboprophylaxis** during pregnancy. Each case should be addressed individually. Women suffering acute SCI during pregnancy should receive thromboprophylaxis for at least eight weeks post trauma on the basis of the high rate of deep venous thromboses reported in nonpregnant patients during this time period (11).

Hematology. Screen for and treat anemia aggressively.

General support. Focus on range of motion exercises in lower extremities, elevation of legs, exercises to increase upper body strength, and social support services.

Autonomic Dysreflexia. ADR is the most serious complication impacting obstetric management, affecting **up to 85% of patients with lesions at or above the level of T6** (2) (above sympathetic outflow and above the upper level of greater splanchnic flow). It is potentially fatal. It is attributed to loss of hypothalamic control over sympathetic spinal reflexes of somatic or visceral sensory impulses still active distal to the level of the lesion (15). **The most common sign of ADR is systemic hypertension** (vasoconstriction), which is often severe. Maternal clinical manifestations include hyperthermia, piloerection, diaphoresis, increased extremity spasticity, pupil dilation, nasal congestion, respiratory distress, bradycardia (most common) or tachycardia or cardiac arrhythmia, extreme fear and anxiety, headache, loss of consciousness, intracranial bleed, convulsions, and even death. **Symptoms are synchronous with uterine contractions**. BP rises with contractions, then normalizes in between.

ADR may be mistaken for preeclampsia, but several findings may help differentiate the two conditions (Table 20.1).

Triggers Afferent stimuli (usually distension) from hollow viscus (bladder, bowel, uterus) or skin (irritation or temp change) below level of the spinal cord lesion. These include uterine contractions, cervical manipulation/pelvic examinations, cold stirrups, insertion of speculum, manipulation of urinary catheters, catheter obstruction, constipation, and decubitus ulcers.

Preventive management of ADR in susceptible patients

1. Routine bladder catheterization with topical anesthetic.
2. Avoidance of constipation with bowel regimen.

3. Pelvic exams: consider pudendal block or topical anesthetic (lidocaine) prior to exams. Avoid cold stirrups or speculums if possible.
4. Prophylactic **antihypertensive therapy** (as necessary to prevent recurrent ADR) with oral nifedipine (10–20 mg), or terazosin (1–10 mg qhs) or clonidine (16).
5. **Epidural anesthesia** at the onset of labor.

Treatment of ADR

1. Remove offending stimulus. Expedite delivery if in second stage with forceps or vacuum or perform cesarean delivery (discuss this with patient prior to labor).
2. Positioning: blood pressure may be lowered by tilting head upward.
3. Antihypertensive therapy—rapid onset
   - **Nitroprusside** (0.5 μg/kg/min intravenously, titrate to BP), or sublingual sodium nitroglycerin (0.3–0.6 mL)
   - **Amyl nitrate** (one capsule crushed for inhalation)
   - Ganglionic blocking agent: **trimethaphan** (Arfonad), 1 ampule in 500 mL D5W at 3 to 4 mg/min continuous intravenously
   - α-Adrenergic blocking agent (guanethidine)
   - Direct vasodilator: **hydralazine**, 10 mg orally, or nifedipine bite and swallow tablet 10 to 20 mg
4. Anesthesia—**regional** (preferred), or general anesthesia can treat ADR.

Antepartum testing. No specific testing is recommended.

Ascertainment and preparation for (preterm or term) labor. Women with spinal cord transection above T10, especially above T6, may have **painless labor**, and are at risk for unattended delivery. Even with lower levels, if transection is complete, patients may not feel contractions. Symptoms that are related through the sympathetic nervous system may alert patients to labor. These should be reviewed with patients as they near term: abdominal or leg spasms, shortness of breath, or increased spasticity. **Uterine palpation techniques** should be reviewed with patients. Consider inpatient hospitalization, especially if patients dilated and have (>T6) high lesions (because of possible unattended delivery with ADR).

Women with SCI should have an anesthesia consult, with plan for epidural at onset of labor.

DELIVERY

Patients with spinal cord transection above the level of T10 are at risk for unattended delivery secondary to unrecognized contractions. Consider inpatient hospitalization for patients with advanced cervical dilation because of the risk of unattended delivery, or patients with spinal cord lesions above the level of T6 because of the high risk of ADR (1,14,17).

Labor is the period during which ADR is most likely to arise. Therefore, there should be a plan for delivery in a unit

Table 20.1 Differentiating ADR from Preeclampsia

Disease	Symptoms	Hematologic	Hepatic function	Urinalysis	Treatment
Preeclampsia	Independent of uterine contractions	Decreased platelets	Elevated uric acid and/or liver function tests	Proteinuria	Intravenous MgSO₄ (most commonly)
ADR	Synchronous with uterine contractions	Normal	Normal	Norepinephrine	Remove stimulus; antihypertensive therapy

Abbreviations: MgSO₄, magnesium sulfate; ADR, autonomic dysreflexia.

Table 20.2 Mode of Delivery Stratified by Level of SCI

Delivery mode	≥T6 level (%)	<T6 level (%)	All SCI (%)
NSVD	13 (29)	18 (46)	31 (37)
AVD	19[a] (42)	7 (18)	26 (31)
CD	13 (29)	14 (36)	27 (32)
Total	45 (100)	39 (100)	84 (100)

[a]Majority of assisted vaginal deliveries performed because of autonomic dysreflexia. *Abbreviations*: SCI, spinal cord injury; NSVD, normal spontaneous vaginal delivery; AVD, assisted vaginal delivery; CD, cesarean delivery.*Source*: From Refs. 1, 2, 4.

capable of invasive hemodynamic monitoring. **Appropriate antihypertensive therapy should be available at the patient's bedside during labor.** If induction is necessary, women with cervical ripening should have continuous blood pressure monitoring, and possibly an epidural. **Continuous hemodynamic monitoring during labor by maternal electrocardiogram, pulse oximetry, and arterial line** should be performed in patients with **baseline pulmonary insufficiency** (14,17). Body temperature should be closely monitored, without assuming that temperature increases are due to intra-amniotic infection (may be caused by underlying thermodisregulation). A Foley catheter may be placed during labor to avoid bladder distension or repeated catheterizations. Patients should change position and have a skin examination every two hours to prevent decubitus ulcer formation. Episiotomy should be avoided, not only because it is not beneficial in general, but also because it is a possible trigger for ADR.

The rate of spontaneous vaginal delivery and need for assisted vaginal delivery depends on the level of the spinal cord lesion. Approximately 30% of SCI patients will be delivered by cesarean (1,2,4) (Table 20.2).

ANESTHESIA
Epidural anesthesia should be administered early in labor (18,19). This is to prevent ADR, with a goal for T10 level. Prehydration is very important, as these patients tend to be hypotensive.

POSTPARTUM/BREAST-FEEDING
In the postpartum period, bladder distension and constipation should be avoided. The use of thromboprophylaxis of SCI patients during the puerperium is controversial. Breast-feeding should be encouraged. Oral contraceptive pills appear to be safe (2,20), although some authors discourage their use (21). Progesterone-only pills, transdermal patches, intramuscular medroxyprogesterone injections, condoms and spermicide, and intrauterine devices are all acceptable alternatives.

RESOURCES
SCI patients and nonmedical personnel may be referred to the following website: http://www.spinalcord.org/resources posted by the NSCIA (National Spinal Cord Injury Association) for more information.

REFERENCES
1. Wanner MB, Rageth CJ, Zach GA. Pregnancy and autonomic hyperreflexia in patients with spinal cord lesions. Paraplegia 1987; 25:482–490. [II-3]
2. Verduyn WH. Spinal cord injured women, pregnancy and delivery. Paraplegia 1986; 24:231–240. [II-3]
3. Westgren N, Hultling C, Levi R, et al. Pregnancy and delivery in women with a traumatic spinal cord injury in Sweden, 1980–1991. Obstet Gynecol 1993; 81:926–930. [II-3]
4. Hughes SJ, Short DJ, Usherwood MM, et al. Management of the pregnant woman with spinal cord injuries. BJOG 1991; 98:513–518. [II-3]
5. Centers for Disease Control: Recommendations for the use of folic acid to reduce the number of cases of spina bifida and other neural tube defects. MMWR Morb Mortal Wkly Rep 1992; 41:1–7. [Review, based on RCTs; see also chap. 2 in *Obstetric Evidence Based Guidelines*]
6. Burns AS, Jackson AB. Gynecologic and reproductive issues in women with spinal cord injury. Phys Med Rehabil Clin N Am 2001; 12:183–199. [Review]
7. McGregor JA, Meeuwsen J. Autonomic hyperreflexia: a mortal danger for spinal cord-damaged women in labor. Am J Obstet Gynecol 1985; 151:330–333. [III; one new case report of intraventricular hemorrhage because of autonomic hyperreflexia during labor]
8. Göller H, Paeslack V. Pregnancy damage and birth-complications in the children of paraplegic women. Paraplegia 1972; 10(3):213–217. [II-3]
9. Atterbury JL, Groome LJ. Pregnancy in women with spinal cord injuries. Nurs Clin North Am 1998; 33(4):603–613. [Review]
10. Gilson GJ, Miller AC, Clevenger FW, et al. Acute spinal cord injury and neurogenic shock in pregnancy. Obstet Gynecol Surv 1995; 50(7):556–560. [II-3]
11. Sugarman B. Medical complications of spinal cord injury. Q J Med 1985; 54:3–18.[II-3]
12. Obstetric management of patients with spinal cord injuries. ACOG Committee Opinion No. 275. American College of Obstetricians and Gynecologists. Obstet Gynecol 2002; 100:625–627. [Review]
13. Young BK, Katz M, Klein SA. Pregnancy after spinal cord injury: altered maternal and fetal response to labor. Obstet Gynecol 1983; 62(1):59–63. [II-3]
14. Greenspoon JS, Paul RH. Paraplegia and quadriplegia: special considerations during pregnancy and labor and delivery. Am J Obstet Gynecol 1986; 155:738–741. [III]
15. Berghella V, Spector T, Trauffer P, et al. Pregnancy in patients with preexisting transverse myelitis. Obstet Gynecol 1996; 87:809–812. [III; two new case reports of transverse myelitis]
16. Vaidyanathan S, Soni BM, Sett P, et al. Pathophysiology of autonomic dysreflexia: long-term treatment with terazosin in adult and paediatric spinal cord injury patients manifesting recurrent dysreflexic episodes. Spinal Cord 1998; 36(11):761–770. [II-2]
17. Robertson DNS. Pregnancy and labour in paraplegics. Paraplegia 1972; 10:209–212. [III]
18. Baker ER, Cardenas DD. Pregnancy in spinal cord injured women. Arch Phys Med Rehabil 1996; 77(5):501–507. [Review]
19. Pope CS, Markenson GR, Bayer-Zwirello LA, et al. Pregnancy complicated by chronic spinal cord injury and history of autonomic hyperreflexia. Obstet Gynecol 2001; 97:802–803. [III; one new case report and review]
20. Jackson AB, Wadley V. A multicenter study of women's self-reported reproductive health after spinal cord injury. Arch Phys Med Rehabil 1999; 80:1420–1428. [II-2]
21. Sipski ML. The impact of spinal cord injury on female sexuality, menstruation and pregnancy: a review of the literature. J Am Paraplegia Soc 1991; 14(3):122–126. [Review]

21

Mood disorders

Madeleine A. Becker, Tal E. Weinberger, Lex Denysenko, and Elisabeth J. S. Kunkel

KEY POINTS

- Depression is twice as common in women as in men, and rates are highest during the childbearing years.
- Depression is common in pregnancy. Up to 70% of pregnant women report symptoms of depression.
- Postpartum blues is a temporary, common condition, affecting up to 85% of new mothers.
- Postpartum depression occurs in 5% to 20% of women.
- Postpartum psychosis affects about 0.1% to 0.2% of women. There is a very high risk of postpartum psychosis in mothers with bipolar disorder.
- **Pregnant women who discontinue their antidepressant medications during pregnancy demonstrate a very high rate of relapse.**
- **Maternal depression has been associated with an increase in premature births, low birth weight, fetal growth restriction, and postnatal complications.**
- **Untreated maternal depression has been associated with an increased risk of subsequent childhood psychopathology.**
- **The Edinburgh Postnatal Depression Scale is a short and easy-to-administer screening tool to assess for postpartum depression.**
- Bipolar depression is often misdiagnosed as major depressive disorder.
- The risk of postpartum affective episodes is very high among women with bipolar disorder, with the majority of women experiencing symptoms within the first three weeks of delivery.
- The incidence of infanticide in women with untreated postpartum psychosis may be as high as 4%.
- **Patients with mood disorders should be stabilized on the minimal number of medications at the lowest effective dose before pregnancy.**
- All psychotropic medications cross the placenta and can enter breast milk.
- **Paroxetine has been associated with an increased risk in cardiac malformations and should be avoided during pregnancy if possible.**
- **Other selective serotonin reuptake inhibitors (SSRIs) have not been proven to be teratogenic.**
- **Individual decisions about medication management during pregnancy should take into account multiple factors, such as severity of maternal illness, frequency of mood episodes, efficacy of past medication trials, and strength of maternal support system.**
- In neonates exposed to lithium during the first trimester, the risk of Ebstein's anomaly is about 1:1500.
- The risk for major congenital anomalies in infants exposed to valproic acid in utero is estimated to be between 6.2% and 13.3%.
- There are still limited data regarding the safety of second-generation (atypical) antipsychotics during pregnancy.

- Sertraline and paroxetine usually produce undetectable infant levels and should be considered first-line choices postpartum in breast-feeding mothers who need to take SSRIs.

MOOD DISORDERS IN PREGNANCY AND POSTPARTUM
Definitions and Epidemiology

Major depressive disorder (MDD) is a syndrome characterized by sustained depressed mood or loss of interest in daily activities, along with "neurovegetative symptoms" of depression, which include decrease or increase in appetite, insomnia or hypersomnia, psychomotor retardation or agitation, and decreased energy. Other symptoms of MDD include feelings of worthlessness or guilt, loss of interest in usually pleasurable activities (or anhedonia), difficulty concentrating, and recurrent thoughts of death or suicidal ideation (1). Women have approximately twice the lifetime rate of depression as men (2). In women, the highest rates of major depression occur during the childbearing years, between the ages of 25 to 44. **Depression is common during pregnancy and up to 70% of pregnant women report symptoms of depression**, with 10% to 16% fulfilling the criteria for major depression (3,4).

There is a high rate of psychiatric illness in mothers after childbirth. This may be attributable to hormonal factors, but also can be associated with psychological stress and prior psychiatric illness in the mother (5,6). Syndromes causing symptoms of depression in the postpartum period include postpartum blues, postpartum depression, and postpartum psychosis.

Postpartum blues is a temporary, common condition, affecting up to 85% of new mothers. It is characterized by tearfulness, mood lability, irritability, and anxiety. Symptoms typically begin around postpartum day 2 to 4 and resolve spontaneously, usually in about two weeks. Women with postpartum blues may be at increased risk for the subsequent development of postpartum depression (7).

Postpartum depression occurs in 5% to 20% of women (8). Symptoms of postpartum depression are the same as for depression at other stages of life, and include depressed mood, insomnia, anhedonia, suicidal ideation, guilt, worthlessness, fatigue, impaired concentration, change in appetite, and change in motor activity. The *DSM-IV-TR* categorizes "postpartum onset" as a specifier of MDD, applied to the first four weeks after childbirth (ICD-10 coding permits classifications of postpartum mental disorders up to six weeks after childbirth) (1). In reality, many clinicians would consider depressive symptoms to be "postpartum depression" for a much longer period than this, generally for a year after childbirth. Proposals for revisions of such classifications include a specifier for onset within three months postpartum (9).

Postpartum psychosis is much less common than postpartum depression, affecting about 0.1% to 0.2% of all women (10). It is characterized by mood lability, agitation, confusion, thought disorganization, hallucinations, and disturbed sleep. Postpartum psychosis has been associated with an increased risk of suicide, infant neglect, and infanticide (11,12), and is considered a psychiatric emergency. Although relatively rare in the general population, the risk of postpartum psychosis is significantly increased in mothers with a history of previous inpatient psychiatric hospitalization (13,14). **There is a very high risk of postpartum psychosis in mothers with bipolar depression, reportedly as high as 46%** (3,5,6). Additionally, women who have had an episode of postpartum psychosis are at increased risk for subsequently developing bipolar affective disorder, leading many researchers to speculate that postpartum psychosis is really a subtype of bipolar disorder (15).

Risk Factors

During pregnancy, there is a high rate of relapse in patients with a history of major depression. **One study of pregnant women with a history of moderate to severe recurrent depression, who discontinued their antidepressant medication during pregnancy, demonstrated a 68% rate of relapse during pregnancy.** This was compared to a 25% relapse rate for those women who continued antidepressants throughout their pregnancies (16).

Women with a history of anxiety disorder, depression, postpartum depression, or other previous psychiatric disorders are also at an increased risk for postpartum depression (8,11,16,17). Social isolation, high parity, birth complications, and psychological distress in late pregnancy are also factors that are associated with postpartum depression (18).

Hormonal factors also have been implicated as risk factors for depression. Rapid changes in estradiol and progesterone levels have been associated with postpartum depression. Women with thyroid autoantibodies also appear to be at higher risk for postpartum depression (15).

Complications

Untreated maternal depression is associated with multiple problems, both during pregnancy and postpartum, and can negatively affect mother-child interactions. Untreated maternal depression during pregnancy may result in poor compliance with prenatal care and increased exposure risk to illicit drugs, herbal remedies, alcohol, and tobacco (3). **Maternal depression has been associated with an increase in premature births, low birth weight, fetal growth restriction, and postnatal complications** (3,19).

Infants of mothers with untreated depression have been shown to cry more, are more difficult to console, more irritable, less active, and less attentive. They also display fewer facial expressions (20,21). Mothers who are not depressed are more likely to promote childhood development by playing and talking to their baby and by following predictable routines (22,23).

Maternal depression has been associated with an increased risk of subsequent childhood psychopathology, including behavioral problems, anxiety disorders, and depression (24–28). Correspondingly, remission of maternal depression positively affects both mother and child, resulting in a significantly lower rate of childhood psychiatric symptoms and diagnoses (29).

Studies also show that mothers with depression have a poor pattern of infant health care utilization, including increased use of acute care and emergency room visits as well as decreased utilization of preventative services, including well-care visits and up-to-date vaccinations (30). Depressed mothers are less likely to continue to breast-feed (31).

Screening

The **Edinburgh Postnatal Depression Scale (EPDS)** is recommended for screening in women at risk for postpartum depression. This screening tool is short and easy to administer. It is a self-administered scale, consisting of 10 questions assessing emotional symptoms experienced by the mother over the seven days prior to evaluation. The EPDS can be completed in about five minutes (32). Scores on the EPDS range from 0 to 30 and a **score of 9 or greater should prompt further clinical evaluation**. No scale is a substitute for clinical judgment, and in any situation where there is significant clinical concern for postpartum depression, the patient should be evaluated thoroughly.

An initial validation study revealed a sensitivity of 86% and a specificity of 78% of the EPDS (32). However, a more recent review of multiple studies validating the EPDS demonstrated heterogeneity of sensitivity and specificity across different studies. This suggests that the EPDS may not be equally valid in different settings (33) (Fig. 21.1).

No laboratory findings are diagnostic of MDD. Thyroid function tests and a complete blood count are useful, however, in identifying other medical conditions that can present with symptoms of depression. Prompt psychiatric consultation should be obtained when depression is suspected, especially when symptoms are severe or when psychotic or suicidal features are present. The presence of psychosis, or suicidal or homicidal ideation or intent should be considered an emergency.

BIPOLAR DISORDER IN PREGNANCY AND POSTPARTUM
Definitions and Epidemiology

Bipolar disorder is a psychiatric illness characterized by episodes of depression alternating with sustained episodes of elevated mood and/or irritability, which are classified as either "mania" or "hypomania." Hypomania is an attenuated form of mania with no associated functional impairment. Both mania and hypomania are associated with increased energy, decreased need for sleep, rapid speech and/or thoughts, distractibility, impulsivity, mood lability, and grandiosity. "Mood swings" are not adequate for a diagnosis of bipolar disorder; rather, a patient must have a syndrome characterized by *sustained* symptoms lasting for days to weeks.

Bipolar disorder, type I (BAD I) is a severe form of bipolar disorder defined by at least one lifetime manic or mixed episode. Mixed episodes are characterized by simultaneous manic and depressive symptoms. The lifetime prevalence estimate is 1% for BAD I (34). Men and women are affected at equal rates. **Bipolar disorder, type II** (BAD II) is characterized by episodes of depression and hypomania. The lifetime prevalence estimate is 1.1% for BAD II. Women with BAD II outnumber men by a ratio of approximately 2:1 (35). The average age of onset of bipolar disorder is in the late teens to early twenties, placing affected women at high risk for mood episodes during their reproductive years. Women who have bipolar disorder spend more time in the depressed phase of the illness than men with bipolar disorder, and are more likely to have the rapid-cycling form (defined as four or more mood episodes over the course of a year) of the illness (3).

Name: _____

Address: _____

Baby's Age: _____

As you have recently had a baby, we would like to know how you are feeling. Please UNDERLINE the answer which comes closest to how you have felt IN THE PAST 7 DAYS, not just how you feel today.

1. I have been able to laugh and see the funny side of things.
   As much as I always could
   Not quite so much now
   Definitely not so much now
   Not at all

2. I have looked forward with enjoyment to things.
   As much as I ever did
   Rather less than I used to
   Definitely less than I used to
   Hardly at all

3. * I have blamed myself unnecessarily when things went wrong.
   Yes, most of the time
   Yes, some of the time
   Not very often
   No, never

4. I have been anxious or worried for no good reason.
   No, not at all
   Hardly ever
   Yes, sometimes
   Yes, very often

5. * I have felt scared or panicky for no good reason.
   Yes, quite a lot
   Yes, sometimes
   No, not much
   No, not at all

6. * Things have been getting on top of me.
   Yes, most of the time I haven't been able to cope at all
   Yes, sometimes I haven't been coping as well as usual
   No, most of the time I have coped quite well
   No, I have been coping as well as ever

7. * I have been so unhappy that I have had difficulty sleeping.
   Yes, most of the time
   Yes, sometimes
   Not very often
   No, not at all

8. * I have felt sad or miserable.
   Yes, most of the time
   Yes, quite often
   Not very often
   No, not at all

9. * I have been so unhappy that I have been crying.
   Yes, most of the time
   Yes, quite often
   Only occasionally
   No, never

10. * The thought of harming myself has occurred to me.
    Yes, quite often
    Sometimes
    Hardly ever
    Never

Response categories are scored 0, 1, 2, and 3 according to increased severity of the symptoms. Items marked with an asterisk are reverse scored (i.e., 3, 2, 1, and 0). The total score is calculated by adding together the scores for each of the ten items.

Figure 21.1 Edinburgh Postnatal Depression Scale (EPDS). *Source*: Adapted from Ref. 32.

Risk Factors

Pregnancy, once thought to be protective against affective (mood) episodes, is understood now to be a period with significant risk for recurrence (36). Women who discontinue mood stabilizer treatment shortly before or after conception have twice the risk of recurrence and a fourfold shorter latency to a new affective episode as compared to women who continue their mood stabilizers (36). Perinatal affective episodes are often depressive, rather than manic or hypomanic, and after occurring in one pregnancy, tend to recur in subsequent pregnancies (3). Maintenance of mood stability during pregnancy is crucial, as recurrence of symptoms during this time strongly predicts the onset of postpartum episodes (37).

Risk of postpartum affective episodes is extremely high in women with BAD, with a 67% risk of postpartum depression reported in one study (35). Between 25% and 50% of women with BAD will have an episode of postpartum mania; a family history of postpartum psychosis further increases the risk of a postpartum psychotic episode (35). Postpartum women have nearly seven times the risk of a psychiatric hospital admission for a first affective episode and two times the risk of a recurrent affective episode compared with pregnant and nonpregnant women (38). Onset of symptoms is often sudden. **The peak prevalence of symptom onset is between postpartum days 1 to 3, with the majority of women experiencing symptoms within three weeks after delivery** (35).

Screening

Misclassification of BAD as MDD is common in the general population. This can lead to inappropriate treatment, and consequent lack of improvement or worsening of the patient's psychiatric condition. The use of selective serotonin reuptake inhibitors (SSRIs) in bipolar disorder is controversial, but may be associated with treatment resistance or more frequent mood episodes in patients with the rapid-cycling form of the disorder (39). The administration of tricyclic antidepressants (TCAs) is known to induce mania (40). Some markers of bipolar depression (as opposed to unipolar, or major depression) include atypical symptoms (i.e., increased sleep or appetite), psychotic depression, early age of symptom onset, treatment resistance to antidepressants, and a family history of bipolar disorder (41).

Misdiagnosis of BAD as MDD in the postpartum period also may occur. Hypomania often is overlooked in the general psychiatric population, as patients often dismiss symptoms that do not disrupt (or even enhance) their functioning. Clinicians may not inquire about episodes of elevated mood. Hypomania after delivery may be misconstrued as normal joy related to the birth of a child (34).

There are no screening instruments specifically designed to detect mood episodes in patients with bipolar disorder, before or after delivery. Commonly used screening instruments, such as the EPDS, have not been validated in postpartum women with BAD (34). Of all the screening instruments for BAD used in the general population, the Mood Disorders Questionnaire has been most widely studied, both in psychiatric settings as well as primary care and community settings, with one study conducted in a perinatal population (35). No measures demonstrate high sensitivity in a community sample, making a universal screening scale difficult to recommend. Women who present with depressive symptoms during the perinatal or postpartum period should be screened clinically for BAD, given the risk of inappropriate treatment associated with misdiagnosis (35).

No screening instrument is intended to replace a thorough clinical evaluation. Any patient who has a positive screen for symptoms of mood disorder should be referred in a timely fashion for mental health evaluation. Immediate screening by a mental health professional is warranted for suspected suicidal ideation or homicidal ideation toward the baby, as well as for any concern regarding postpartum psychosis. **The incidence of infanticide in women with untreated postpartum psychosis has been estimated to be as high as 4%** (42). Emergent intervention (such as psychiatric hospitalization) may be necessary to address any immediate safety issues.

PHARMACOLOGIC MANAGEMENT OF MOOD DISORDERS

All psychotropic medications cross the placenta and can enter breast milk (3). Risks of medication exposure to the fetus need to be weighed against the risks (to both mother and fetus) of untreated maternal illness. When a mood disorder is suspected, referral to a psychiatrist is recommended. Psychotherapy should always be considered as part of the treatment plan and can be effective in many cases. Cognitive behavioral therapy and interpersonal therapy have been studied and demonstrated to be effective for some symptoms of depression in pregnancy (43). When symptoms are significant, or there is a high risk of relapse, medications can be helpful and/or necessary.

As it would be considered unethical to withhold or administer certain psychotropic medications during pregnancy, no data are available in randomized, placebo-controlled studies. As a result, most data are from nonrandomized, prospective, observational studies, or from single case reports. Mothers should be aware that the use of psychiatric medications may carry unknown adverse consequences to the unborn child, as our knowledge is based on relatively limited data.

Individual decisions about medication management during pregnancy should take into account multiple factors, such as severity of maternal illness, frequency of mood episodes, efficacy of past medication trials, and strength of maternal support system. In general, a single medication at a higher dose is preferable to multiple medications (3). Multidisciplinary collaboration regarding psychotropic medication management during pregnancy should include the obstetrician, primary care doctor, psychiatrist, pediatrician, and patient's family. The risks of discontinuing medication versus any known risks of the prenatal exposure should be fully discussed with the patient, and this discussion should be documented.

During the postpartum period, in addition to concerns about medication passage into breast milk, important considerations include the impact of sleep disruption on maternal illness. Sleep deprivation can be extremely destabilizing in women with bipolar disorder. This is particularly concerning given the fact that the postpartum period is already a time of additional vulnerability in patients with mood disorders.

Antidepressants *(Table 21.1)*

Selective serotonin reuptake inhibitors (SSRIs)

The most commonly prescribed medications for depression are the SSRIs. Compared to other classes of antidepressant medications, there are much more data available for these medications. The potential impact of maternal psychiatric depression on neonatal outcome has been difficult to evaluate independently of medication effects, resulting in some difficulty in clearly interpreting these data.

Teratogenicity

Several large reviews of the available data show **no increased rate of major malformations in women exposed to SSRIs or other antidepressants in pregnancy** (19,44). The National Birth Defects Prevention study found that there was an increased risk of omphalocele, anencephaly, and craniosynostosis, but absolute risks were small (45). These risks were found only after more than 40 statistical tests were performed, and thus, may be attributed to chance (3). In the Sloane Epidemiology Center Birth Defects Study, no increased risk of omphalocele or craniosynostosis was found to be associated with SSRI use. Both of these studies were limited by the small number of exposures for each congenital malformation (3).

There have been some reports showing that women exposed to paroxetine in the first trimester are at higher risk (1.5- to 2-fold) for *cardiac malformations* (19,46–50), but there are also reports that do not support this association (44,45,51,52). In light of these findings, the manufacturer reclassified paroxetine's pregnancy category to "D" (53). Although the data are conflicting, the majority of databases, including two recent, large, case-controlled studies, have found no significant increased rate of congenital heart defects with exposure to other SSRIs (3,19,37,44,45). In light of these findings and the FDA's warnings, paroxetine should be avoided in pregnancy. If a patient were already taking paroxetine, one should attempt to switch to another antidepressant (3), preferably before pregnancy.

Other risks concerning the use of SSRIs during pregnancy include reports of an increased risk of *persistent pulmonary hypertension of the newborn* (PPHN). PPHN involves right-to-left shunting of blood through the fetal ductus arteriosus and foramen ovale and results in neonatal hypoxia. If this is severe, it can result in right heart failure and is fatal in approximately 10% of cases. An increased risk of PPHN was found among newborns whose mothers were exposed to SSRIs later in pregnancy (after 20 weeks' gestation). PPHN was found to occur in about 3 to 6 per 1000 exposed infants. The baseline rate or occurrence of PPHN is between 0.5–2 per 1000 babies in the general population (19). Three recent studies supported an association between SSRI use and PPHN, with an adjusted odds ratio ranging from 3.44 to 6.1 (50,54,55). The mechanism may be related to high circulating levels of serotonin in the fetal lungs (54). However, there was no increased risk of PPHN in infants exposed to SSRIs found in two other large, retrospective cohort studies (56,57). Further research is needed to clarify this association.

Neonatal toxicity

SSRI exposure late in pregnancy has also been associated with transient neonatal complications. It is not clear whether the mechanism is a withdrawal syndrome or related to medication toxicity, or whether the complications may be attributable to the effects of maternal illness rather than medication exposure (58). Symptoms may include jitteriness, tachypnea, hypoglycemia, temperature instability, weak cry, poor tone, and mild respiratory distress (3). These symptoms occur in the first neonatal days and generally resolve in a period of two weeks or less (19).

Neurodevelopmental effects

Long-term neurodevolopmental effects after in utero SSRI exposure have been evaluated in a few small studies. Two studies found differences on some behavioral measures between exposed and unexposed children (59,60). However, in two studies by Nulman et al., evaluating children exposed to fluoxetine and to various TCAs, no differences were found between exposed children and controls (61,62).

Table 21.1 Antidepressants in Pregnancy and Lactation

Class	Medication	FDA risk category	Teratogenicity	Late pregnancy exposure	Neonatal toxicity	Breast-feeding
Selective serotonin reuptake inhibitors	**Citalopram** (Celexa®)	C	Most studies have not identified an increased risk of major malformations (126)	Conflicting reports regarding risk of PPHN in infants exposed to SSRIs after 20 weeks' gestation (50,54–57).	• Conflicting results regarding risk of preterm birth, low birth weight, and small for gestational age in SSRI exposed pregnancies • Late pregnancy exposure associated with neonatal adaptation problems, NICU admission, low Apgar scores • All of these findings may be attributable to maternal illness rather than medication exposure (126)	RID: <1–9% (126) Infant serum concentration low or undetectable in several studies (58) • One reported case of high infant serum levels (126)
	Fluoxetine (Prozac®, Prozac Weekly®, Sarafem®)	C	Most studies have not identified an increased risk of major malformations (126)	As above	As above	RID ≤10% Infant plasma concentration variable • Less favored because of long half-life and active metabolite • A few reports of adverse effects, but most studies with none in exposed infants (126)
	Sertraline (Zoloft®)	C	Most studies have not identified an increased risk of major malformations (126)	As above	As above	RID = 2% Infant serum concentration low to undetectable (126)
	Escitalopram (Lexapro®)	C	Very limited studies, but as escitalopram is the S-enantiomer of citalopram, it is likely comparable with this medication (126)	As above	As above	Limited data, but infant exposure thought to be similar to citalopram (126)
	Fluvoxamine (Luvox®, Luvox CR®)	C	No increased risk identified, but data are limited (126)	As above	As above	RID 1–2% Limited data; infant plasma levels variable (126)
	Paroxetine (Paxil®, Paxil CR®, Pexeva®)	D	Some data consistently supporting **increased risk of cardiac malformations** (126)	As above	As above	RID 1–3% Infant serum concentration low to undetectable (126)

Serotonin-norepinephrine reuptake inhibitors	**Venlafaxine** (Effexor®, Effexor XR®, Venlafaxine ER)	C	No increased risk identified, but data are limited (3,58)	As above	Limited data, mean infant dose is 4.7–9.2% of maternal levels; no adverse effects noted (8,94)
	Duloxetine (Cymbalta®)	C	Very limited data	As above	Very limited data available
Other	**Mirtazapine** (Remeron®, Remeron SolTab®)	C	No increased risk identified, but data very limited (3,58)	As above	Very limited data, low to undetectable infant levels; no adverse events noted (99–101)
	Bupropion (Budeprion SR, Budeprion XL, Buproban Wellbutrin®, Wellbutrin SR®, Wellbutrin XL®, Zyban®)	C	Limited data, but most studies have not identified an increased risk of major malformations (3,19, 69,70)	None reported	Limited data • One case report of a seizure in an exposed infant (97)

RID, weight adjusted relative infant dose, or % of weight adjusted maternal dose ingested by the infant.
Source: From Refs. 3,8,19,50,54–58,69,70,94,97,99–101,126.

There is limited information available on the long-term effects of antidepressant exposure. Data on this topic must be interpreted carefully, as the effects of maternal depression are also likely to have a significant impact on behavior and cognitive development (19).

Tricyclic antidepressants (TCAs)

TCAs are relatively safe and have not been shown to be associated with a higher risk of congenital malformations when taken in the first trimester (19,52,63). Perinatal complications of the newborn with tricyclic exposure later during pregnancy include tachycardia, irritability, jitteriness, hypertonia, convulsions, and anticholinergic symptoms, such as urinary retention (63).

Monoamine oxidase inhibitors (MAOIs)

Monoamine oxidase inhibitors are prescribed much less commonly because of multiple food-drug and drug-drug interactions. There are much less data available for these medications. One small study shows an increased rate of congenital malformations (64). Given the paucity of data on this class of medications, MAOIs should be avoided during pregnancy if possible (63).

Serotonin-norepinephrine reuptake inhibitors (SNRIs) and other classes

Commonly used medications in these classes include venlafaxine, duloxetine, mirtazapine, and bupropion. Overall, existing data suggest no significantly increased rate of congenital malformations with these antidepressants, but there are much less data available than for the SSRIs or TCAs (3,19,65,66). In one study, the rate of preterm delivery with the serotonin-norepinephrine reuptake inhibitors (SNRIs) or norepinephrine reuptake inhibitors (NRIs) was significantly increased and neonatal symptoms were similar to those symptoms seen in infants whose mothers were taking SSRIs during pregnancy (67). In a recent population-based case-control study, there was a small positive association with maternal bupropion use during pregnancy and left outflow tract heart defects (68). However, other studies found no increased rate of major malformations (19,69,70).

Other effects of prenatal exposure to antidepressants

There is an increased risk of *spontaneous abortion (SAB)* that is associated with the use of several classes of antidepressants in pregnancy found in some studies. Miscarriage rates were 12.4% in exposed women, versus 8.7% in women who were not exposed to medications. There were no differences found between the different classes of antidepressants. The studies were variable in controlling for confounding variables, such as health habits, smoking, and age (19,71–73). Other studies do not support this association, with incidence of SAB in women exposed to various SSRIs not exceeding the SAB rates in control groups (58).

The use of TCAs and SSRIs during pregnancy has been associated with reductions in birth weight and infants who are small for gestational age (19). Numerous studies show that SSRIs and TCAs (as well as the other antidepressants) are associated with preterm delivery (<37 weeks) (19,69). These results are not consistent and this association was not found in all studies. When effects were found, the differences in gestational age among exposed and nonexposed infants were typically modest (one week or less). As similar results were found among women using SSRIs and TCAs (which have different mechanisms of action), maternal illness rather than medication effects may explain some of these findings (50).

Expert guidelines and algorithms to guide the physician on decision-making for continuing and/or initiating medications for MDD during pregnancy have been published (see Ref. 19).

Mood Stabilizers *(Table 21.2)*

Lithium

Lithium is associated with an increased risk of Ebstein's anomaly, a cardiac defect characterized by congenital displacement of the tricuspid valve toward the apex of the right ventricle. In the general population, the risk of Ebstein's anomaly is 1:20,000. **In neonates exposed to lithium during the first trimester, the risk of Ebstein's anomaly is 1:1500** (77). Thus, while the relative risk of Ebstein's anomaly is significantly higher with prenatal lithium exposure, the absolute risk still remains small (38).

In one trial, birth weight of lithium-exposed infants was found to be significantly higher than matched controls (78). Individual cases of arrhythmia, nephrogenic diabetes insipidus, thyroid dysfunction, hypotonia, hypoglycemia, and hyperbilirubinemia have been reported. These problems are generally transient and have no long-term sequelae. Lithium-exposed infants may have poor respiratory effort and/or cyanosis at delivery. Neonatal hypotonicity, bradycardia, cyanosis, and hypoglycemia are preventable if lithium is discontinued immediately before delivery; however, given the high risk of postpartum mood episodes in these patients, lithium should be reinstated immediately afterward (79). See below for lithium in breast-feeding.

Lithium is distributed in total body fluid volume, and levels can be affected by vomiting and changes in sodium intake (38). Thyroid function should be monitored during pregnancy because of the possibility of lithium-induced thyroid toxicity. In the last trimester, renal excretion of lithium increases by 30% to 50% (79), which may necessitate a dose increase at this time. Decreasing the dose of lithium at delivery may be necessary to avoid maternal lithium toxicity associated with the dramatic decrease in vascular volume occurring at delivery. Adequate hydration should be maintained during labor (38).

Many experts recommend continuing lithium during pregnancy in women with severe symptoms who have had a good response to lithium (77). However, given the small absolute risk of Ebstein's anomaly, some patients with less frequent, less severe episodes may be able to discontinue lithium during pregnancy, or at least during the first trimester. When the decision is made to discontinue lithium, the drug should be tapered slowly (over the course of >15 days), as rapid discontinuation of lithium is associated with higher frequency of, and reduced latency to recurrence of symptoms (36). Prenatal screening, including high-resolution ultrasound and fetal echocardiography, should be conducted at 16 to 18 weeks' gestation in pregnant women with first-trimester lithium exposure (38).

Valproic acid

On the basis of data from several large antiepileptic pregnancy registries, **the risk for major congenital anomalies in infants exposed to valproic acid (VPA) in utero is estimated to be between 6.2% and 13.3%** (80). Congenital anomalies seen with VPA include neural tube defects (NTDs), cardiovascular anomalies, limb defects, and hypospadias. About 1% to 2% of exposed infants present with NTDs (80,81). Lumbosacral meningomyelocele is the most common NTD associated with VPA exposure, likely representing a drug effect on neural crest closure (38). This defect occurs 10 to 20 times more frequently in VPA-exposed infants than in the general population (81).

A specific combination of facial dysmorphic features has been described in infants exposed to VPA in utero; this same syndrome was later described in children of women using other antiepileptic drugs (AEDs) (including carbamazepine) during pregnancy. This syndrome is known as the "antiepileptic drug syndrome" and is characterized by intrauterine growth retardation, long and thin upper lip, shallow philtrum,

Table 21.2 Mood Stabilizers in Pregnancy and Lactation

Medication	FDA risk category	Teratogenicity	Neonatal toxicity	Breast-feeding	Comments
Lithium (Eskalith[R], Lithobid[R])	D	• 20–40-fold increased risk of Ebstein's anomaly but absolute risk is small (38)	Cases of transient arrythmia, nephrogenic diabetes insipidus, thyroid dysfunction, hypotonia, hypoglycemia, and hyperbilirubinemia (80). • Infants may have poor respiratory effort or cyanosis at delivery (79)	Variable infant serum levels (103,104). Risk of toxicity in the newborn. Monitor lithium levels and CBC in breast-fed exposed infants (38)	Monitor serum levels and thyroid function frequently. Fluid shifts and changes in metabolism may necessitate dose adjustment (79, 83) • High-resolution ultrasound and fetal echocardiography at 16 to 18 weeks' gestation (38)
Valproic acid (Depakene[R], Stavzor[R])/Divalproex sodium (Depakote[R], Depakote ER[R], Depakote Sprinkles[R])	D	• 6.2–13.3% risk of major anomalies: NTDs, cardiovascular anomalies, limb defects, and hypospadias • 1–2% risk of NTDs (81) • Risk of facial dysmorphic features "antiepileptic drug syndrome" (82) • Risk of cognitive deficits and ASD (81)	None noted	Considered compatible with breast-feeding (90), low infant serum levels (107)	Teratogenicity and cognitive effects likely dose dependent (1), also polytherapy associated with greater risk (81). • Supplement with high-dose folic acid (81)
Carbamazepine (Carbatrol[R], Equetro[R], Tegretol[R], Tegretol XR[R])	D	• Risk of NTD 0.5–1%; overall risk of major malformations 2.2–5.4% (80) • Risk of facial dysmorphic features "antiepileptic drug syndrome" (81)	Risk of hemorrhagic disease in the newborn because of fetal vitamin K deficiency (38)	Considered compatible with breast-feeding (90) with variable infant serum levels; few reports of infant hepatotoxicity, monitor serum levels and LFTs in exposed infants (107)	Can cause fetal vitamin K deficiency, supplementation in last month of pregnancy recommended (38) • Supplement with high-dose folic acid (38)
Oxcarbazepine (Trileptal[R])	C	Available teratogenic information is reassuring but database is too small to draw definitive conclusions (83)	None noted	Limited data	Levels may decrease during pregnancy (84)
Lamotrigine (Lamictal[R], Lamictal XR[R])	C	Conflicting results regarding risk of oral clefts (85,86,87); if elevated, absolute risk is low • May be higher risk of malformations at higher doses (80)	None noted	High infant exposure, approximately 30% of maternal levels (38) • Hypothetical risk of SJS in the newborn (113)	Changes in clearance during pregnancy and after delivery may necessitate dose adjustment (88). • Safety data are reassuring compared to other treatment options (3,80) • Periconceptional folic acid supplementation (81)

Table 21.2 Mood Stabilizers in Pregnancy and Lactation (*Continued*)

Medication	FDA risk category	Teratogenicity	Neonatal toxicity	Breast-feeding	Comments
Atypical antipsychotics **Olanzapine** (Zyprexa®, Zyprexa Zydis®) **Risperidone** (Risperdal®, Risperdal M-Tab®) **Quetiapine** (Seroquel®, Seroquel XR®) **Aripiprazole** (Abilify®, Abilify Discmelt®) **Ziprasidone** (Geodon®) **Clozapine** (Clozaril®, FazaClo®)	C: **Olanzapine, risperidone, quetiapine, aripiprazole, ziprasidone.** B: **Clozapine**	Limited data, but no evidence for increased risk with olanzapine, risperidone, clozapine, or quetiapine (37). Very limited data with aripiprazole and ziprasidone	No reports of neonatal toxicity	Limited data. Low to undetectable levels in case reports with quetiapine, risperidone, olanzapine exposure (119,120). Possibly some EPS with olanzapine exposure (119, 120). Very limited data for aripiprazole and ziprasidone. *Clozapine*: variable levels in infant serum. Hypothetical risk of agranulocytosis (8,120)	Can cause maternal weight gain and diabetes ● Some evidence of association with LGA infants (37)

Abbreviations: NTD, neural tube defects; ASD, autistic spectrum disorder; SJS, Steven's Johnson Syndrome; LGA, large for gestational age; EPS, extrapyramidal symptoms.
Source: From Refs. 3,8,37,38,79–81,83–87,88,90,103,104,107,113.

epicanthal folds, and mid-facial hypoplasia with flat nasal bridge, small upturned nose, and down-turned angles of the mouth (81). In infants exposed to VPA in utero, these features are often associated with other major anomalies and developmental delay. Cognitive deficits, attention deficit disorder, and learning difficulties have been repeatedly reported in children exposed to VPA in utero (80,81). Perinatal valproate exposure also is associated with autistic spectrum disorder (81).

Teratogenicity and cognitive effects related to prenatal VPA exposure are likely dose dependent, with doses greater than 800 to 1000 mg associated with significantly greater risk (80,82). Polytherapy with VPA and other anticonvulsants results in a higher rate of teratogenicity than monotherapy with VPA alone (81).

Valproic acid should not be used during pregnancy unless the benefits clearly outweigh the risks. Valproate is known to interfere with folic acid metabolism, so high-dose folate supplementation (4–5 mg/day) is currently recommended prior to conception and during the first trimester in women taking VPA (as well as with other anticonvulsants) during pregnancy. Folic acid supplementation decreases the incidence of NTDs, but the benefit of using high-dose folate for decreasing the rate of NTD in this population is unclear. As lamotrigine and carbamazepine interfere with folic acid absorption, supplementation is recommended in women taking these medications as well (81).

Carbamazepine and oxcarbazepine

Rates of malformations with carbamazepine exposure range from 2.2% to 5.4% in different large AED pregnancy registries. Carbamazepine is associated with a risk of NTDs of 0.5% to 1%. Recent data suggest that carbamazepine exposure may not cause cognitive impairment. Malformation rates are consistently higher with VPA than with carbamazepine (80).

Carbamazepine can cause fetal vitamin K deficiency. Vitamin K is necessary for normal mid-facial growth and for normal clotting factor function; thus, carbamazepine exposure during pregnancy may increase the risk of neonatal bleeding and mid-facial abnormalities. Many experts recommend oral vitamin K in the last month of pregnancy (38). There is currently insufficient evidence to determine whether vitamin K supplementation reduces the rate of neonatal hemorrhagic complications (82).

Data on malformation rates with oxcarbazepine exposure are still limited. A literature review on infants exposed to oxcarbazepine in utero, including data from the world wide Novartis safety database and other pregnancy registries and study centers, revealed no increased risk of malformations. However, the number of exposed pregnancies was insufficient to draw definitive conclusions regarding safety of this medication (83). Oxcarbazepine does not produce the same toxic epoxide metabolite as carbamazepine and thus, authors speculate that oxcarbazepine may be less harmful to the developing fetus (38). Plasma concentrations of oxcarbazepine may decrease during pregnancy (84), which may necessitate dose adjustment.

Lamotrigine

The reproductive safety data regarding lamotrigine seems to be reassuring compared to other treatments for BAD. The North American AED Pregnancy Registry reported a 10.4-fold increased risk of cleft lip and/or cleft palate in infants exposed to lamotrigine in utero; the absolute risk of cleft lip and/or palate in the registry was 7.3:1000 (85). Other large pregnancy registries did not substantiate this association (86,87). One pregnancy registry reported a higher risk of major malformations with lamotrigine doses greater than 200 mg/day. No effects on cognition have been found, but data remain limited (80).

Lamotrigine clearance is increased during pregnancy, which may necessitate dose increases to maintain therapeutic effect. After delivery, lamotrigine clearance returns rapidly to baseline, requiring carefully monitoring and dose adjustment to avoid toxicity (88).

Antipsychotics

There are still limited data regarding the safety of second-generation (atypical) antipsychotics during pregnancy. Current available evidence regarding olanzapine, risperidone, quetiapine, and clozapine does not reveal any increased risk for teratogenicity above that in the general population. Minimal information is available regarding ziprasidone and aripiprazole. No information is available regarding paliperidone, iloperidone, asenapine, or lurasidone. The second-generation antipsychotics are known to cause maternal weight gain and diabetes, which are independently associated with pregnancy complications. Some data indicate that second-generation antipsychotic exposure can result in a higher incidence of large-for-gestational-age infants (37).

Data regarding exposure to haloperidol, a commonly used first-generation (typical) antipsychotic, generally are reassuring. An extrapyramidal syndrome has been reported in some cases of babies exposed to first-generation antipsychotics in utero (37).

Electroconvulsive Therapy

In nonpregnant adults, electroconvulsive therapy (ECT) has well-proven efficacy in the treatment of MDD and BAD, especially when psychotic features are present or medical therapy has failed. ECT is not recommended as a first-line treatment, but may be considered in patients who have demonstrated treatment resistance. Response rates to ECT are generally higher than response rates to medication, and therapeutic effects of ECT are more rapid than those of medication. Side effects include transient memory loss, muscle soreness, and headache.

In pregnant women treated for depression, response rates to ECT were similar to response rates in nonpregnant samples (89). Risks to the mother and child are low. The most common complications of ECT in pregnant women are fetal bradyarrhythmias and induction of premature labor. Fetal bradyarrhythmias are estimated to occur at a rate of 2.7%, and likely occur as a result of hypoxia. Positioning the woman with her right hip elevated will minimize the risk of hypoxia in the fetus. Induction of labor is estimated to occur at a rate of approximately 3.5%, and may be related to postictal elevations of oxytocin. Uterine activity can be monitored during ECT administration (89).

Fetal monitoring is suggested during ECT because of the potential for fetal sedation from general anesthesia. Methohexital sodium and propofol are the anesthetic agents most commonly used for ECT in the United States; succinylcholine is generally used as a muscle relaxant. None of these agents have known teratogenicity. ECT does not generate current through the uterus. One case of fetal death after status epilepticus was reported (89). Limiting seizure duration during ECT in the general population is standard practice.

MANAGEMENT DURING LACTATION

All psychiatric medications are passed into breast milk. The American Academy of Pediatrics (AAP) has rated the compatibility of individual drugs with lactation. This rating is based on reports found in the literature and is intended to assist the physician in counseling the mother regarding breast-feeding while taking medication (90). Given the high rate of psychiatric illness during and after pregnancy, the health care practitioner should carefully evaluate the postpartum patient who is at risk for psychiatric illness to determine whether medication is necessary.

Antidepressants

The AAP Committee on Drugs rates antidepressant medications as "effects unknown, and may be of concern in breast-feeding" (90). However, a pooled analysis of antidepressant levels in lactating mothers suggests that it is probably safe to use most antidepressants during lactation (91).

Selective Serotonin Reuptake Inhibitors

The growing evidence generally is reassuring concerning safety of the use of SSRIs in breast-feeding mothers. There are few reports of adverse effects in infants exposed to these medications. The excretion of SSRIs into breast milk is relatively low to undetectable (8). Low infant plasma levels have been found with all the SSRIs, but higher concentrations have been reported for fluoxetine and citalopram (91). **Sertraline and paroxetine usually produce undetectable infant levels and should be considered first-line choices in breast-feeding mothers who need to take SSRIs** (4,91). However, if a woman has been stable on another antidepressant throughout her pregnancy, one should not always change medication as evidence suggest that most infant SSRIs levels have been found to be quite low. Fluoxetine and citalopram should not be first choices, but if needed for their effectiveness in individual women, they should be used with caution. Long-term effects of infant exposure to SSRIs through nursing have been less well studied.

Tricyclic Antidepressants

The AAP rates effects of TCAs during breast-feeding as "unknown but may be of concern." Infant plasma levels of TCAs were found to be <1% of maternal dose (92). Most reports show no adverse effects in the nursing infant (3,8,92,93). Infant respiratory depression was reported with exposure to doxepin through breast milk (3).

Monoamine Oxidase Inhibitors

No current data were found.

Venlafaxine

There are very few case reports published on the safety of venlafaxine in nursing. These show low to variable infant plasma levels in breast-fed infants. The mean infant dose or percentage of maternal intake ranged from 4.7% to 9.2% (mean of 6.4%), which is below the 10% estimated level of concern, but still relatively high compared with data published for other antidepressants (94). No adverse effects were found in exposed infants (8,94).

Duloxetine

At this time, there is an extremely limited amount of data available on effects on infants exposed to duloxetine while nursing.

Bupropion

There are no studies and only a few case reports on the safety of bupropion in breast-fed infants. Low infant serum levels were found (5,96), and no adverse effects were reported in two exposed infants (95). One study reported a seizure in a six-month-old infant, which was possibly attributable to the use of bupropion during breast-feeding (97).

Trazodone

There are very little data on trazodone. In the few cases examined, levels in breast milk have found to be low (98).

Mirtazapine

There are few published cases of infant exposure to mirtazapine. In these few cases infant levels were low to undetectable. No adverse effects were seen in the exposed infants, including sedation or weight gain, which are common side effects of this medication (99–101).

Mood Stabilizers

Lithium

The AAP Committee on Drugs considers lithium to be associated "with significant effects on some nursing infants and should be given to nursing mothers with caution." Infant levels have been reported as variable, but higher than those with many other medications, from one-half to one-third of maternal levels (102). More recent studies found considerable variability (0–30% of maternal dose) in infant serum levels of lithium, as well as levels that were generally lower than previously thought (103,104). In a few case reports, adverse infant effects have included cyanosis, hypotonia, heart murmur, EKG changes, lethargy, and hypothermia (105,106). Occasional and transient laboratory abnormalities including elevated blood urea nitrogen (BUN), creatinine, and thyroid-stimulating hormone were observed in the sample of infants studied (103). Infants may be more susceptible to both dehydration and lithium toxicity because of their immature kidney function and potential for rapid dehydration.

Valproic Acid

AAP Committee on Drugs considers valproic acid to be "compatible" with breast-feeding. Levels have found to be very low in breast milk (107). One adverse event of thrombocytopenia and anemia in an exposed infant was reported (108).

Carbamazepine

The AAP Committee on Drugs considers carbamazepine to be compatible with breast-feeding. Levels reported in infant serum were highly variable, but have not been found to penetrate breast milk in clinically significant amounts (107). In two case reports, however, carbamazepine was associated with infant hepatotoxicity (109–111). Exposed infants should be monitored by checking serum levels and liver function tests.

Lamotrigine

Effects of lamotrigine during breast-feeding are classified by the AAP as "unknown, but may be of concern." Lamotrigine is excreted in relatively high levels in breast milk. Infant serum levels were one-third (about 30%) of maternal levels, likely because of a slow, immature elimination in infants. Most of the case reports found no adverse effects in infants (107), although there were some cases of mild thrombocytosis in one study (112). There have been no reported cases of Stevens-Johnson syndrome in nursing infants to date, but since this may be a concern, infants should be closely monitored (113).

The Neurodevelopmental Effects of Antiepileptic Drugs Study is a prospective multicenter observational study examining cognitive outcomes in children at age 3 that were exposed to AEDs, both in utero and during breast-feeding. The study consisted of 199 children of mothers with epilepsy who were taking AEDs while pregnant. This study found no deleterious effects of AED therapy (valproate, carbamazepine, and lamotrigine) on cognitive outcomes of children that were exposed both in utero and while breast-feeding (114).

Although this study looked at effects on children of mothers with epilepsy rather than bipolar disorder, the effects of exposure would likely be applicable to either population.

Antipsychotics

The AAP Committee on Drugs rates the effects of haloperidol, chlorpromazine, thiothixene, mesoridazine, and trifluoperazine to be unknown and may be of concern to nursing infants. Haloperidol is excreted in relatively high amounts in breast milk, but has not been associated with adverse effects on the infant (115,116). Chlorpromazine exposure has been associated with drowsiness and lethargy in one infant (117). In one study of seven infants with exposure to chlorpromazine through breast milk, there were no adverse effects reported at 16-month and 5-year follow-up evaluations (118).

Atypical Antipsychotics

The atypical antipsychotics have not yet been rated by the AAP Committee on Drugs. There are only few case reports published. Generally, risperidone, olanzapine, and quetiapine levels have been found to be low to undetectable in samples of nursing infants and most infants showed no or few adverse effects from these medications (119,120). There was one report of an infant with cardiomegaly, jaundice, and sedation after exposure to olanzepine (119). There have also been a few cases of extrapyramidal reactions in infants exposed to olanzapine (120). The data for ziprasidone and aripiprazole are limited. In one case report, ziprasidone use in pregnancy and lactation did not result in any adverse outcomes for the infant, and in another case report, the concentration of ziprasidone in human milk was found to be low (121,122). Likewise, in one case report, aripiprazole use during pregnancy and lactation did not result in any adverse outcomes, and there were no detectable levels of aripiprazole or its metabolite in the breast milk (123).

There are very few studies published on the safety of clozapine. The AAP rates effects as "unknown and of concern" in breast-feeding. In one case report, clozapine was shown to have relatively high accumulation in breast milk (124). In an infant exposed to clozapine both prenatally and during breast-feeding, delayed speech acquisition may have been attributable to clozapine (125). Although no cases have been reported of agranulocytosis in nursing infants, it is a theoretical risk. Therefore, it is not recommended that clozapine be used during breast-feeding (8,120). With limited data available, if women decide to breast-feed while taking an antipsychotic medication, infants should be monitored for possible adverse effects.

REFERENCES

1. American Psychiatric Association. Diagnostic and Statistical Manual of Mental Disorders, 4th ed, Text Revision (DSM-IV-TR), Washington, DC: American Psychiatric Publishing, 2000. [III]
2. National Institute of Mental Health (US). The numbers count: mental disorders in America. NIH Publication No. 06-4584. Bethesda (MD): NIMH, 2006. [III]
3. ACOG Committee. Clinical Management Guidelines for Obstetrician–Gynecologists: use of psychiatric medications during pregnancy and lactation. ACOG Practice Bulletin No.92. Obstet Gynecol 2008; 111(4):1001–1020. [Review, III]
4. Gentile S. Use of contemporary antidepressants during breast-feeding: a proposal for a specific safety index. Drug Saf 2007; 30 (2):107–121. [Review, III]
5. Kendell RE, Chalmers JC, Platz C. Epidemiology of puerperal psychosis. Br J Psychiatry 1987; 150:662–673. [II-3]
6. McNeil TF. A prospective study of postpartum psychoses in a high-risk group. 1. Clinical characteristics of the current post-partum episodes. Acta Psychiatr Scand 1986; 74(2):205–216. [Prospective case-control study, II-1]
7. Newport DJ, Hostetter A, Arnold A, et al. The treatment of postpartum depression: minimizing infant exposures. J Clin Psychiatry 2002; 63(suppl 7):31–44. [Review, III]
8. Eberhard-Gran, Eskild A, Opjordsmoen S. Use of psychotropic medications in treating mood disorders during lactation: practical recommendations. CNS Drugs 2006; 20(3):187–198. [Review, III]
9. Cox J. Postnatal mental disorder: towards ICD-11. World Psychiatry 2004; 3(2):96–97. [Commentary, III]
10. Gentile S. Clinical utilization of atypical antipsychotics in pregnancy and lactation. Ann Pharmacother 2004; 38:1265–1271. [Review, III]
11. Hales RE, Yudofsky SC, eds. American Psychiatric Publishing Textbook of Clinical Psychiatry. 4th ed. Arlington, VA: American Psychiatric Publishing, 2005. [III]
12. Spinelli MG. A systematic investigation of 16 cases of neonaticide. Am J Psychiatry 2001; 158(5):811–813. [Case series, II-3]
13. Nager A, Sundquist K, Ramirez-Leon V, et al. Obstetric complications and postpartum psychosis: a follow-up study of 1.1 million first-time mothers between 1975 and 2003 in Sweden. Acta Psychiatr Scand 2008; 117(1):12–19. [Retrospective cohort, n = 1413, II-2]
14. Harlow BL, Vitonis AF, Sparen P, et al. Incidence of hospitalization for postpartum psychotic and bipolar episodes in women with and without prior prepregnancy or prenatal hospitalizations. Arch Gen Psychiatry 2007; 64(1):42–48. [Retrospective cohort, n = 2259, II-2]
15. Stewart D, Vigod S, Stotland NL. Obstetrics and gynecology. In: Levenson JL, ed. The American Psychiatric Publishing Textbook of Psychosomatic Medicine. Psychiatric Care of the Medically Ill. Washington, DC: American Psychiatric Publishing, Inc., 2010:797–826. [III]
16. Cohen LS, Altshuler LL, Harlow BL, et al. Relapse of major depression during pregnancy and in women who maintain or discontinue antidepressant treatment. JAMA 2006; 295(5):499–507. [Prospective study, n = 201, II-2]
17. Bloch M, Rotenberg N, Koren D, et al. Risk factors associated with the development of postpartum mood disorders. J Affect Disord 2005; 88(1):9–18. [Prospective study, n = 1800, II-1]
18. Nielsen Forman D, Videbech P, Hedegaard M, et al. Postpartum depression: identification of women at risk. BJOG 2000; 107 (10):1210–1217. [Prospective study, n = 5252, II-1]
19. Yonkers KA, Wisner KL, Stewart DE, et al. The management of depression during pregnancy: a report from the American Psychiatric Association and the American College of Obstetricians and Gynecologists. Gen Hosp Psychiatry 2009; 31(5):403–413. [Review, III]
20. Zuckerman B, Bauchner H, Parker S, et al. Maternal depressive symptoms during pregnancy, and newborn irritability. J Dev Behav Pediatr 1990; 11(4):190–194. [Prospective study, n = 1123, II-1]
21. Field T, Diego M, Hernandez-Reif M. Prenatal depression effects on the fetus and newborn: a review. Infant Behav Dev 2006; 29:445–455. [Review, III]
22. McLearn KT, Minkovitz CS, Strobino DM, et al. Maternal depressive symptoms at 2 to 4 months post partum and early parenting practices. Arch Pediatr Adolesc Med 2006; 160(3):279–284. [Cross-sectional cohort, n = 4874, II-3]
23. Paulson JF, Dauber S, Leiferman JA. Individual and combined effects of postpartum depression in mothers and fathers on parenting behavior. Pediatrics 2006; 118(2):659–668. [Cross-sectional cohort, n = 5089, II-3]
24. Pilowsky DJ, Wickramaratne PJ, Rush AJ, et al. Children of currently depressed mothers: a STAR*D ancillary study. J Clin Psychiatry 2006; 67(1):126–136. [Cross-sectional cohort, n = 151, II-3]
25. Biederman J, Faraone SV, Hirshfel-Becker DR, et al. Patterns of psychopathology and dysfunction in high-risk children of

parents with panic disorder and major depression. Am J Psychiatry 2001; 158(1):59–57. [Case-control, *n* = 380, II-1]

26. Brennan PA, Hammen C, Anderson MJ, et al. Chronicity, severity, and timing of maternal depressive symptoms: relationships with child outcomes at age 5. Dev Psychol 2000:36(6):759–766. [Prospective cohort, *n* = 4953, II-1]

27. Hammen C, Brennan PA. Severity, chronicity and timing of maternal depression and risk for adolescent offspring diagnosis in a community sample. Arch Gen Psychiatry 2003; 60(3):253–258. [Cross-sectional cohort, *n* = 816, II-3]

28. Gao W, Paterson J, Abbott M, et al. Maternal mental health and child behaviour problems at 2 years: findings from the Pacific Islands Families Study. Aust N Z J Psychiatry 2007; 41(11):885–895. [Prospective cohort, *n* = 1398, II-1]

29. Weissman MM, Pilowsky DJ, Wickramaratne PJ, et al. Remissions in maternal depression and child psychopathology: a STAR*D-child report. JAMA 2006; 295(12):1389–1398. [Prospective cohort, *n* = 151, II-1]

30. Minkovitz CS, Strobino D, Scharfstein D, et al. Maternal depressive symptoms and children's receipt of health care in the first 3 years of life. Pediatrics 2005; 115(2):306–314. [Prospective cohort, *n* = 5565, II-1]

31. Hatton DC, Harrison–Hohner J, Coste S, et al. Symptoms of postpartum depression and breastfeeding. J Hum Lact 2005; 21 (44):444–449. [Prospective cohort, *n* = 377, II-1]

32. Cox JL, Holden JM, Sagovsky R. Detection of postnatal depression. Development of the 10-item Edinburgh Postnatal Depression Scale. Br J Psychiatry 1987; 150:782–786. [Case-controlled validation study, II-2]

33. Gibson J, McKenzie-McHarg L, Shakespeare J, et al. A systematic review of studies validating the Edinburgh Postnatal Depression Scale in antepartum and postpartum women. Acta Psychiatr Scand 2009; 119(5):350–364. [Meta-analysis and review, III]

34. Sharma V. Management of bipolar II disorder during pregnancy and the postpartum period. Can J Clin Pharmacol 2009; 16(1):e33–e41. [Review, III]

35. Chessick CA, Dimidjian S. Screening for bipolar disorder during pregnancy and the postpartum period. Arch Womens Ment Health 2010; 13(3):233–248. [Review, III]

36. Viguera AC, Whitfield T, Baldessarini RJ, et al. Risk of recurrence in women with bipolar disorder during pregnancy: prospective study of mood stabilizer discontinuation. Am J Psychiatry 2007; 164(12):1817–1824. [Prospective cohort, *n* = 89, II-1]

37. Einarson A, Boskovic R. Use and safety of antipsychotic drugs during pregnancy. J Psychiatr Pract 2009; 15(3):183–192. [Review, III]

38. Yonkers KA, Wisner KL, Stowe Z, et al. Management of bipolar disorder during pregnancy and the postpartum period. Am J Psychiatry 2004; 161:608–620. [Review, III]

39. Ghaemi SN. Why antidepressants are not antidepressants: STEP-BD, STAR*D, and the return of neurotic depression. Bipolar Disord 2008; 10(8):957–968. [Review, III]

40. Koszewska I, Rybakowski JK. Antidepressant-induced mood conversions in bipolar disorder: a retrospective study of tricyclic versus non-tricyclic antidepressant drugs. Neuropsychobiology 2009; 59(1):12–16. [Retrospective study, *n* = 333, II-3]

41. Ghaemi SN, Ko J, Goodwin FK. The bipolar spectrum and the antidepressant view of the world. J Psychiat Pract 2001; 7(5):287–297. [Review and Editorial, III]

42. Spinelli MG. Postpartum psychosis: detection of risk and management. Am J Psychiatry 2009; 166:405–408. [Case Report and Review, III]

43. Spinelli M, Endicott J. Controlled clinical trial of interpersonal psychotherapy versus parenting education program for depressed pregnant women. Am J Psychiatry 2003; 160(3):555–562. [RCT, N = 38, I]

44. Louik C, Lin A, Werler M, et al. First-trimester use of selective serotonin-reuptake inhibitors and the risk of birth defects. N Engl J Med 2007; 356(26):2675–2683. [Retrospective observational case-controlled study, *n* = 9849, II-2]

45. Alwan S, Reefhuis J, Rasmussen SA, et al., for National Birth Defects Prevention Study. Use of selective serotonin-reuptake inhibitors in pregnancy and the risk of birth defects. N Engl J Med 2007; 356(26):2684–2692. [Cross-sectional study, *n* = 6582, II-3]

46. Wurst KE, Poole C, Ephross SA, et al. First trimester paroxetine use and the prevalence of congenital, specifically cardiac, defects: a meta-analysis of epidemiological studies. Birth Defects Res A Clin Mol Teratol 2010; 88(3):159–170. [Meta-analysis Review, III]

47. Bakker MK, Kerstjens-Frederikse WS, Buys CH, et al. First trimester use of paroxetine and congenital heart defects: a population-based case-control study. Birth Defects Res A Clin Mol Teratol 2010; 88(2):94–100. [Retrospective case-controlled study, *n* = 1293, II-2]

48. Cole JA, Ephross SA, Cosmatos IS, et al. Paroxetine in the first trimester and the prevalence of congenital malformations. Pharmacoepidemiol Drug Saf 2007; 16(10):1075–1085. [Retrospective cohort, II-3]

49. Kallen BA, Otterblad Olausson P. Maternal use of selective serontonin re-uptake inhibitors in early pregnancy and infant congenital malformations. Birth Defects Res A Clin Mol Teratol 2007; 79(4):301–308. [Retrospective cohort, II-3]

50. Reis M, Kallen B. Delivery outcome after maternal use of antidepressant drugs in pregnancy: an update using Swedish data. Psychol Med 2010; 40(10):1723–1733. [Retrospective cohort, II-3]

51. Einarson A, Pistelli A, DeSantis M, et al. Evaluation of the risk of congenital cardiovascular defects associated with the use of paroxetine during pregnancy. Am J Psychiatry 2008; 165(6):749–752. [Epidemiologic study, *n* = 3285, II-2]

52. Davis RL, Rubanowice D, McPhillips H, et al. Risk of congenital malformations and perinatal events among infants exposed to antidepressant medication during pregnancy. Pharmacoepidemiol Drug Saf 2007; 16(10):186–194. [Retrospective cohort, II-3]

53. Available at: http://www.fda.gov/Drugs/DrugSafety/PostmarketDrugSafetyInformationforPatientsandProviders/DrugSafetyInformationforHealthcareProfessionals/PublicHealthAdvisories/ucm051731.htm. [III]

54. Chambers, et al. Selective serotonin reuptake inhibitors and the risk of persistent pulmonary hypertension of the newborn. N Engl J Med 2006; 354:579–587. [Retrospective cohort-control, II-2]

55. Kallen B, Olausson PO. Maternal use of selective serotonin re-uptake inhibitors and persistent pulmonary hypertension of the newborn. Pharmacoepidemiol Drug Saf 2008; 17(8):801–806. [Retrospective cohort, II-3]

56. Andrade SE, McPhillips H, Loren D, et al. Antidepressant medication use and risk of persistent pulmonary hypertension of the newborn. Pharmacoepidemiol Drug Saf 2009; 18:246–252. [Retrospective cohort-control study, *n* = 1104 and 1104 controls, II-2]

57. Wichman CL, Moore KM, Lang TR, et al. Congenital heart disease associated with selective serotonin reuptake inhibitor use during pregnancy. Mayo Clin Proc 2009; 84:23–27. [Retrospective study, *n* = 808 and 24,406 controls, II-2]

58. Tuccori, M, et al. Safety concerns associated with the use of serotonin reuptake inhibitors and other serotonergic/noradrenergic antidepressants during pregnancy: a review. Clin Ther 2009; 31:1426–1453. [Review, III]

59. Casper RC, Fleisher BE, Lee-Ancajas JC, et al. Follow-up of children of depressed mothers exposed or not exposed to antidepressant drugs during pregnancy. J Pediatr 2003; 142:402–408. [Retrospective study, II-3]

60. Mortensen JT, Olsen J, Larsen H, et al. Psychomotor development in children exposed in utero to benzodiazepines, antidepressants, neuroleptics, and anti-epileptics. Eur J Epidemiol 2003; 18:769–771. [Retrospective study, II-3]

61. Nulman I, Rovet J, Stewart DE, et al. Neurodevelopment of children exposed in utero to antidepressant drugs. N Engl J Med 1997; 336:258–262. [Retrospective study, II-3]

62. Nulman I, Rovet J, Stewart DE, et al. Child development following exposure to tricyclic antidepressants or fluoxetine throughout fetal life: a prospective, controlled study. Am J Psychiatry 2002; 159(11):1889–1895. [II-1]

63. Altshuler LL, Cohen L, Szuba MP, et al. Pharmacologic management of psychiatric illness during pregnancy: dilemmas and guidelines. Am J Psychiatry 1996; 153-592-606. [Meta-analysis and review, III]

64. Heinonen OP, Slone D, Shapiro S. Birth Defects and Drugs in Pregnancy. Littleton, MA: Publishing Sciences Group, 1977. [III]

65. Einarson TR, Einarson A. Newer antidepressants in pregnancy and rates of major malformations: a meta-analysis of prospective comparative studies. Pharmacoepidemiol Drug Saf 2005; 14 (12):823–827. [Meta-analysis and review, III]

66. Einarson A, Choi J, Einarson TR, et al. Incidence of major malformations in infants following antidepressant exposure in pregnancy: results of a large prospective cohort study. Can J Psychiatry 2009; 54(4):242–246. [Prospective case-control, II-1]

67. Lennestal R, Kallen B. Delivery outcome in relation to maternal use of some recently introduced antidepressants. J Clin Psychopharmacol 2007; 27:607–613. [Retrospective case-control, II-2]

68. Alwan S, Reefhuis J, Botto LD, et al. Maternal use of bupropion and risk for congenital heart defects. Am J Obstet Gynecol 2010; 203(1):52.e1–52.e6. [Retrospective case-control, II-2]

69. Chun-Fai-Chan, Koren G, et al. Pregnancy outcome of women exposed to bupropion during pregnancy: a prospective comparative study. Am J Obstet Gynecol 2005; 192:932–936. [Prospective case-control, II-1]

70. Cole JA, Modell JG, Haight BR, et al. Bupropion in pregnancy and the prevalence of congenital malformations. Pharmacoepidemiol Drug Saf 2007; 16(5):474–484. [Retrospective study, II-3]

71. Einarson A, Choi J, Einarson TR, et al. Rates of spontaneous and therapeutic abortions following the use of antidepressants in pregnancy: results from a large prospective database. J Obstet Gynaecol Can 2009; 31(5):452–456. [Prospective case-control, II-1]

72. Nakhai-Pour HR, Broy P, Berard A. Use of antidepressants during pregnancy and the risk of spontaneous abortion. CMAJ 2010; 182(10):1031–1037. [Retrospective study, II-3]

73. Djulus J, Koren G, Einarson TR, et al. Exposure to mirtazapine during pregnancy: a prospective comparative study of birth outcomes. J Clin Psychiatry 2006; 67(8):1280–1284. [Prospective case-control, II-1]

74. Pastuszak A, Schick-Boschetto B, Zuber C, et al. Pregnancy outcome following first-trimester exposure to fluoxetine (Prozac). JAMA 1993; 269(17):2246–2248. [Prospective cohort control, II-1]

75. Sivojelezova A, Shuhaiber S, Sarkissian L, et al. Citalopram use in pregnancy: prospective comparative evaluation of pregnancy and fetal outcome. Am J Obstet Gynecol 2005; 193(6):2004–2009. [II-1]

76. Malm H, Klaukka T, Neuvonen P. Risks associated with selective serotonin reuptake inhibitors in pregnancy. Obstet Gynecol 2005; 106:1289–1296. [II-2]

77. Yacobi S, Ornoy A. Is lithium a real teratogen? What can we conclude from the prospective versus retrospective studies? A review. Isr J Psychiatry Relat Sci 2008; 45(2):95–106. [Review, III]

78. Jacobson SJ, Jones K, Johnson K et al. Prospective multicentre study of pregnancy outcome after lithium exposure during first trimester. Lancet 1992; 339(8792):530–533. [II-2]

79. Pinelli JM, Symington AJ, Cunningham KA, et al. Case report and review of the perinatal implications of maternal lithium use. Am J Obstet Gynecol 2002; 187:245–249. [Review, III]

80. Tomson T, Battino D. Teratogenic effects of antiepileptic medications. Neurol Clin 2009; 27:993–1002. [Review, III]

81. Ornoy A. Valproic acid in pregnancy: how much are we endangering the embryo and fetus? Reprod Toxicol 2009; 28:1–10. [Review; III]

82. Harden CL, Pennell PB, Koppel BS. Practice Parameter update: management issues for women with epilepsy—focus on pregnancy (an evidence-based review). Vitamin K, folic acid, blood levels, and breastfeeding: report of the Quality Standards Subcommittee and Therapeutics and Technology Assessment Subcommittee of the American Academy of Neurology and American Epilepsy Society. Neurology 2009; 73(142):142–149. [III]

83. Montouris G. Safety of the newer antiepileptic drug oxcarbazepine during pregnancy. Curr Med Res Opin 2005; 21(5):693–701. [III]

84. Battino D, Tomson T. Management of epilepsy during pregnancy. Drugs 2007; 67(18):2727–2746. [Review, III]

85. Holmes LB, Baldwin EJ, Smith CR, et al. Increased frequency of isolated cleft palate in infants exposed to lamotrigine during pregnancy. Neurology 2008; 70:2152–2158. [Prospective cohort, II-2]

86. Dolk H, Jentink J, Loane M, et al. Does lamotrigine use in pregnancy increase orofacial cleft risk relative to other malformations? Neurology 2008; 71:714–722. [II-2]

87. Morrow J, Russell A, Guthrie E, et al. Malformation risks of antiepileptic drugs in pregnancy: a prospective study from the UK Epilepsy and Pregnancy Register. J Neurol Neurosurg Psychiatry 2006; 77:193–198. [Prospective case-control, II-1]

88. de Haan GJ, Edelbroek P, Segers J, et al. Gestation-induced changes in lamotrigine pharmacokinetics: a monotherapy study. Neurology 2004; 63:571–573. [Case series, n = 12, II-3]

89. Anderson EL, Reti IM. ECT in pregnancy: a review of the literature from 1941 to 2007. Psychosom Med 2009; 71(2):235–242. [Review, III]

90. American Academy of Pediatrics Committee on Drugs. Transfer of drugs and other chemicals into human milk. Pediatrics 2001; 108(3):776–789. [III]

91. Weissman AM, Levy BT, Hartz AJ, et al. Pooled analysis of antidepressant levels in lactating mothers, breast milk and nursing infants. Am J Psychiatry 2004; 161(6):1066–1078. [Meta-analysis, II-2]

92. Yoshida K, Smith B, Craggs M, et al. Investigation of pharmacokinetics and possible adverse effects in infants exposed to tricyclic antidepressants in breast-milk. J Affect Disord 1997; 43 (3):225–237. [II-3]

93. Wisner KL, Perel JM, Foglia JP. Serum clomipramine and metabolite levels in four nursing mother-infant pairs. J Clin Psychiatry 1995; 56(1):17–20. [II-3]

94. Ilett KF, Kristensen JH, Hackett LP, et al. Distribution of venlafaxine and its O-desmethyl metabolite in human milk and their effects in breastfed infants. Br J Clin Pharmacol 2002; 53(1):17–22. [II-3]

95. Baab SW, Peindl KS, Piontek CM, et al. Serum bupropion levels in 2 breastfeeding mother-infant pairs. J Clin Psychiatry 2002; 63 (10):910–911. [II-3]

96. Briggs GG, Samson JH, Ambrose PJ, et al. Excretion of bupropion in breast milk. Ann Pharmacother 1993; 27(4):431–433. [II-3]

97. Chaudron LH, Schoenecker CJ. Bupropion and breastfeeding: a case of a possible infant seizure. J Clin Psychiatry 2004; 65 (6):881–882. [II-3]

98. Verbeeck RK, Ross SG, McKenna EA. Excretion of trazodone in breast milk. Br J Clin Pharmacol 1986; 22(3):367–370. [II-3]

99. Kristenen 2007, 100. Klier 2007, 101. Aichhorn 2004. Transfer of the antidepressant mirtazapine into breast milk. Br J Clin Pharmacol 2007; 63(3):322–327. [II-3]

100. Klier CM, Mossaheb N, Lee A, et al. Mirtazapine and breastfeeding: maternal and infant plasma levels. Am J Psychiatry 2007; 164(2):348–349. [II-3]

101. Aichhorn W, Whitworth AB, Weiss U, et al. Mirtazapine and breastfeeding. Am J Psychiatry 2004; 161(12):2325. [II-3]

102. Schou M, Amdison A. Lithium and pregnancy. 3. Lithium ingestion by children breast-fed by women on lithium treatment. Br Med J 1973; 2(5859):138. [II-3]

103. Viguera AC, Newport DJ, Ritchie J, et al. Lithium in breast milk and nursing infants: clinical implications. Am J Psychiatry 2007; 164(2):342–345. [II-3]

104. Moretti ME, Koren G, Verjee Z, et al. Monitoring lithium in breast milk: an individualized approach for breast-feeding mothers. Ther Drug Monit 2003; 25(3):364–366. [II-3]

105. Tunnessen WW Jr. Hertz CG. Toxic effects of lithium in newborn infants: a commentary. J Pediatr 1972; 81:804–807. [III]

106. Woody JN, London WL, Wilbanks GD Jr. Lithium toxicity in a newborn. Pediatrics 1971; 47:94–96. [Case report, III]

107. Chen L, Lui F, Yoshida S, et al. Is breastfeeding of infants advisable for epileptic mothers taking antiepileptic drugs? Psychiatry Clin Neurosci 2010; 64(5):460–468. [II-3]

108. Stahl MM, Neiderud J, Vinge E. Thrombocytopenic purpura and anemia in a breast-fed infant whose mother was treated with valproic acid. J Pediatr 1997; 130(6):1001–1003. [II-3]

109. Merlob P, Mor N, Litwin A. Transient hepatic dysfunction in an infant of an epileptic mother treated with carbamazepine during pregnancy and breastfeeding. Ann Pharmacother 1992; 26 (12):1563–1565. [II-3]

110. Frey B, Schubiger G, Musy JP. Transient cholestatic hepatitis in a neonate associated with carbamazepine exposure during pregnancy and breastfeeding. Eur J Pediatr 1990; 150(2): 136–138. [II-3]

111. Frey B, Braegger CP, Ghelfi D. Neonatal cholestatic hepatitis from carbamazepine exposure during pregnancy and breast feeding. Ann Pharmacother 2002; 36(4):644–647. [II-3]

112. Newport DJ, Pennell PB, Calamaras MR, et al. Lamotrigine in breast milk and nursing infants: determination of exposure. Pediatrics 2008; 122(1):e223–e231. [II-3]

113. Ohman I, Vitols S, Tomson T. Lamotrigine in pregnancy: pharmacokinetics during delivery, in the neonate, and during lactation. Epilepsia 2000; 41(6):709–713. [II-3]

114. Meador KJ, Baker GA, Browning N, et al. Effects of breastfeeding in children of women taking antiepileptic drugs. Neurology 2010; 75(22):1954–1960. [Prospective case-control study, II-2]

115. Whalley LJ, Blain PG, Prime JK. Haloperidol secreted in breast milk. Br Med J (Clin Res Ed) 1981; 282(6278):1746–1747. [Case report, II-3]

116. Yoshida K, Smith B, Craggs M, et al. Neuroleptic drugs in breast-milk: a study of pharmacokinetics and of possible adverse effects in breast-fed infants. Psychol Med 1998; 28 (1):81–91. [Prospective case-control study, II-2]

117. Wiles DH, Orr MW, Kolakowska T. Chlorpromazine levels in plasma and milk of nursing mothers. Br J Clin Pharmacol 1978; 5 (3):272–273. [II-3]

118. Kris EB, Carmichael DM. Chlorpromazine maintenance therapy during pregnancy and confinement. Psychiatr Q 1957; 31: 690–695. [Case series, n = 14, II-3]

119. Goldstein DJ, Corbin LA, Fung MC. Olanzapine-exposed pregnancies and lactation: early experience. J Clin Psychopharmacol 2000; 20(4):399–403. [Meta-analysis and review, III]

120. Gentile S. Infant safety with antipyschotic therapy in breastfeeding: a systematic review. J Clin Psychiatry 2008; 69(4):633–634.

121. Werremeyer A. Ziprasidone and citalopram use in pregnancy and lactation in a woman with psychotic depression. Am J Psychiatry 2009; 166(11):1298. [II-3]

122. Schlotterbeck P, Saur R, Hiemke C, et al. Low concentration of ziprasidone in human milk: a case report. Int J Neuropsychopharmacol 2009; 12(3):437–438. [II-3]

123. Lutz UC, Hiemke C, Wiatr G, et al. Aripiprazole in pregnancy and lactation: a case report. J Clin Psychopharmacol 2010; 30 (2):204–205. [II-3]

124. Barnas C, Bergant A, Hummer M, et al. Clozapine concentrations in maternal and fetal plasma, amniotic fluid and breast milk. Am J Psychiatry 1994; 151(6):945. [Case report, II-3]

125. Mendheker DN. Possible delayed speech acquisition with clozapine therapy during pregnancy and lactation. J Neuropsychiatry Clin Neurosci 2007; 19:196–197. [Case report, II-3]

126. Ellfolk, M and Malm H. Risks associated with in utero and lactation exposure to selective serotonin reuptake inhibitors (SSRIs) . Reproductive Toxicology 2010; 30: 249-260 [Review, III]

22

Smoking

Jeroen Vanderhoeven and Jorge E. Tolosa

KEY POINTS

- **Smoking** is a **preventable risk factor** associated with **low birth weight, preterm birth, perinatal death, and other maternal and perinatal complications.**
- **Smoking cessation in pregnancy reduces low birth weight, preterm birth, and perinatal death.**
- **Counseling** with behavioral and educational interventions is **associated with the highest cessation rates** (Tables 22.1–22.4).
- **Pharmacotherapies** are **either contraindicated, or their safety and efficacy is insufficiently studied in pregnancy.**
- **Nicotine replacement therapies** are safe and effective in the general population, but there is **insufficient evidence** for recommending them in pregnant smokers.
- **Nicotine replacement therapy** is associated with known **adverse fetal effects.**
- The greatest risk of **relapse** occurs in the **postpartum period.**
- There is **insufficient evidence** to recommend specific **interventions to prevent relapse in pregnant and postpartum women.**

HISTORIC NOTES

The twentieth century saw the rise of the manufactured cigarette and its popularity grew (1). People continue to smoke despite known adverse effects (1).

DIAGNOSIS/DEFINITION

Tobacco dependence is a chronic addictive condition that requires repeated intervention for cessation.

EPIDEMIOLOGY/INCIDENCE

Approximately 250 million women smoke worldwide at the beginning of the 21st century (1).

- 22% of women smoke in developed countries and 9% of women smoke in developing countries (1).
- 22.4% of American women of reproductive age smoke cigarettes (2).
- The incidence of smoking in pregnancy in the United States was 13.8% in 2005 (a significant reduction from 15.2% in 2000) (3). Estimated smoking rates during pregnancy among reproductive age women vary in different countries from 0.1% to 50% (4).
- By race, the highest prevalence of smoking occurs among those reporting multiple races and whites. The lowest prevalence occurs among Hispanics and Asian Pacific Islander women (5).
- **Women are more likely to stop smoking in pregnancy than in any other time in their lives** (6).

- Up to 46% of preconception smoking women stop smoking before their first antenatal visit or during pregnancy (7,8). Pregnancy can help motivate women to quit smoking.
- **50% to 60% of those who quit smoking in pregnancy relapse within the first four months postpartum** (3,8).
- Smokeless tobacco is an important source of nicotine exposure among pregnant women.
- Regional variations ranging from 6% (Congo) to 33.5% (Orissa, India) exist among low- and middle-income countries (9).
- Among high-income countries, both the United States and Sweden have seen increases in smokeless tobacco use that may offset decreases in cigarette consumption (10,11).

GENETICS

- Maternal genotype may affect the risk of low birth weight in cigarette smokers (12).
- The *CYP1A1*, *CYP2A6*, and *GSTT1* genes encode enzymes active in metabolism and elimination of toxic substances in cigarette smoke (12–14).
- In women who smoked, heterozygous variants of *CYP1A1* and absence of *GSTT1* genes resulted in significantly greater reductions in birth weight.

ETIOLOGY/BASIC PATHOLOGY

- Nicotine and carbon monoxide are documented fetal neurotoxins and the major compounds of tobacco smoke (15).
- Other toxic compounds include: ammonia, polycyclic aromatic hydrocarbons, hydrogen cyanide, vinyl chloride, and nitrogen oxide.
- Smoking may result in damage to fetal genetic material (16).

Nicotine

- Crosses the placenta and can be detected in the fetal circulation at levels that exceed maternal circulation by 15% (17).
- **Amniotic fluid levels** are 88% **higher than maternal plasma levels** (17).
- Causes for impaired fetal oxygen delivery: vasoconstriction and changes in capillary volume and villous membrane contribute to abnormal gas exchange within the placenta (18).
- Studies have been focused on short-term developmental fetal effects such as sympathetic activation, leading to increased fetal heart rate and reduction in fetal breathing movement. However, animal studies suggest that fetal exposure to nicotine alone impacts the incidence of late-onset diseases including type 2 diabetes, obesity, hypertension, neurobehavioral deficits, and respiratory dysfunction (19).

Table 22.1   Multiple-Choice Questionnaire Improves Initial Disclosure Rates of Smoking/Tobacco Use

(A) I have **never** smoked or I have smoked less than 100 cigarettes in my lifetime.
(B) I stopped smoking **before** I found out I was pregnant, and I am not smoking now.
(C) I stopped smoking **after** I found out I was pregnant, and I am not smoking now.
(D) I smoke some now, but I **cut down** on the number of cigarettes I smoke since I found out I was pregnant.
(E) I smoke regularly now, about the **same** as before I found out I was pregnant.
(F) Do you use any other tobacco product? (If yes, inquire about details as above)
If the patient responds to B or C, reinforce her decision to quit, congratulate her on success of quitting, and encourage her to remain smoke free.
If the patient responds to D or E, she should be classified as a smoker. Document in the chart and proceed to the other 5As of the 5A framework: Ask, Advise Assess, Assist, and Arrange.

Source: From Ref. 32.

Table 22.2   "The 5 Rs" for Smokers Who Are Unwilling to Quit Smoking

1. *Relevance:* Motivational information to a patient is more effective if it is relevant to a patient's personal circumstances (i.e., smoking can cause adverse effects in pregnancy).
2. *Risks:* Stress the acute and long-term risks of smoking. Try to associate it with the patient's current health or illnesses.
3. *Rewards:* Ask the patient to identify potential benefits of smoking.
4. *Roadblocks:* Identify barriers or impediments to quitting and note treatment options that could address the barriers.
5. *Repetition:* Repeat the motivational intervention at each visit.

Table 22.3   "The 5 As" for Patients Who Are Willing to Quit Smoking

1. *Ask*: Tobacco status is inquired and documented. A multiple-choice question method (Table 22.1) improves disclosure.
2. *Advise*: Urge all tobacco users to quit in a clear, strong, personalized manner. Review risks associated with continued smoking.
3. *Assess*: Determine the patient's willingness to quit in the next 30 days. If unwilling, the provider should ask and advise at each subsequent office visit.
4. *Assist*: Provide smoking cessation materials and provide support. Help the patient develop a plan and provide practical counseling. Pharmacotherapy may be considered for the general population of smokers, although there are insufficient data on safety and efficacy in pregnancy.
5. *Arrange*: Provide follow-up contact, either in person or by telephone soon after the quit date, and further follow-up encounters as needed. Congratulate success during each visit. Review circumstances if a relapse occurred and use it as a learning experience for the patient. Consider referral or more intensive treatment. Assess pharmacotherapy use and problems.

Table 22.4   Smoking Cessation Counseling (Skills Training and Problem Solving Techniques)

1. Identify activities that increase risk of smoking or relapse.
2. Explore coping skills and describe the time and nature of withdrawal.
3. Tell patients they may experience anxiety, frustration, depression, and intense cravings for cigarettes.
4. Withdrawal symptoms become manageable in a few weeks.
5. Make lifestyle changes to reduce stress and improve quality of life.
6. Minimize time spent in the company of smokers.
7. Provide as much information to the patient as possible: supplement discussions with pamphlets, booklets, videos, hotlines (1-800-QUIT-NOW), internet, or support groups (http://www.smokefree.gov, http://www.smokefreefamilies.org).

Carbon Monoxide

- Crosses the placenta rapidly and can be detected in the fetal circulation at **levels that exceed maternal circulation** by 15% (15,17).
- Exposure causes formation of carboxyhemoglobin. Carboxyhemoglobin is cleared slowly from the fetal circulation and diminishes tissue oxygenation via competitive inhibition with oxyhemoglobin. There is a left shift of the oxyhemoglobin dissociation curve, causing decreased availability of oxygen to the fetus (17).
- A 10% maternal carboxyhemoglobin concentration would result in a decrease of available oxygen supply to the fetus akin to a 60% reduction in blood flow.

Carcinogens

- More than 69 carcinogens have been identified.
- Levels of cyanide and at least one tobacco-specific carcinogen are higher in smokers (15,17).
- The compound is toxic to rapidly dividing cells.

RISK FACTORS

- Social disadvantage and lower education (5,20)
- Receiving Medicaid-funded maternity care
- High parity
- Low levels of support and/or being without a partner
- Exposure to domestic violence

- Having a partner that smokes or exposure to second-hand smoke at home
- Depression (20), coexisting emotional/psychiatric problems, substance abuse
- Job strain
- Poor coping skills
- Younger age
- Fear of weight gain and unsatisfied with female body image

Spontaneous quitters usually smoke less, are more likely to have stopped smoking before, are more likely to have a non-smoker partner or have more support and encouragement at home for quitting, have stronger beliefs about the dangers of smoking (6).

COMPLICATIONS (21)

Smoking is the **most modifiable risk factor associated with adverse pregnancy outcomes** (8,15,22,23). All risks are dose related. There seems to be no increase in congenital birth defects associated with smoking (24).

- *Low birth weight (LBW)*: Women who smoke are more likely to have a low-birth-weight baby (<2500 g) with relative risk (RR) of 1.3 to 10. The birth-weight **deficit is 200 to 300 g** by term (2). Up to 19% of term LBW has been attributed to smoking (25). Low birth weight causes the highest economic burden (3).
- *Preterm birth*: Women who smoke are 1.3 to 2.5 times more likely to have preterm delivery. It is estimated that up to 14% of preterm birth may be due to smoking (7).
- *Pregnancy loss*: RR of 1.2–3.4.
- *Premature rupture of membranes (PROM)*: RR of 1.9–4.2.
- *Preeclampsia*: Smoking is associated with a **reduced** incidence of preeclampsia. Quitting smoking before pregnancy precludes this decrease in preeclampsia.
- *Placental abruption*: RR of 1.4–2.5.
- *Placenta previa*: RR of 1.4–4.4.
- *Fetal death*: Large case-control and cohort studies suggest an RR of 1.2–1.4 associated with cigarette smoking.
- *Postnatal morbidities*: Increased risk of sudden infant death syndrome (SIDS), respiratory infections, reactive airway diseases, otitis media, bronchiolitis, short stature, hyperactivity, and decreased school performance. Up to 34% of cases of SIDS have been attributed to smoking (25).
- *Fetal central nervous system effects*: Abnormalities in cell proliferation and differentiation lead to decreased number of cells and eventually altered synaptic activity. Nicotine not only affects multiple transmitter pathways and influences the development of the fetal brain, but also affects eventual programming and synaptic competence (17). Resolution of any cognitive function deficit attributed to tobacco use was no longer detectable by nine years of age (26).
- *Maternal lifetime complications*: Atherosclerotic disease, lung cancer, chronic obstructive pulmonary disease, many forms of lung disease, increase risk of ectopic pregnancy, premature menopause, infertility, osteoporosis (26).
- **Second-hand** prenatal exposure to smoking has been associated with a 20% increase in **LBW** (27).

Smokeless Tobacco Complications

Adverse outcomes related to use of **smokeless tobacco** are not adequately studied. One study of the Swedish Medical Birth Registry reports an increased risk of **stillbirth** with an adjusted OR of 1.6 [CI 1.1–2.3] (28).

PREGNANCY CONSIDERATIONS

- Pregnancy is a **unique opportunity** for medical intervention and may be the only time women seek medical attention.
- Concerns over the dangers of smoking to the fetus may serve as a motivation for smoking cessation.
- Behavioral interventions such as contingency management and other support/reward programs have demonstrated efficacy in pregnancy (20,23,29).
- **The safety and efficacy of existing pharmacotherapies remain uncertain in pregnancy** (6,8).

PRINCIPLES

- Goal: Cessation of tobacco products during pregnancy.
- Tobacco dependence treatments are both clinically and cost effective relative to other medical disease prevention interventions (23).
- **Smoking cessation in pregnancy can prevent** 17% of low-birth-weight births, and 14% of preterm deliveries (7).
- Smoking in the third trimester has the greatest impact on birth weight (30).
- Women who quit smoking by the third trimester have birth weights similar to those of nonsmokers (30,31).

MANAGEMENT

- **Document smoking status at each initial prenatal visit** (32) (Table 22.1).
- The patient should also be asked about the use of any other tobacco product.
- While most pregnant women do disclose their smoking, urine cotinine testing can aid in uncovering the few who do not disclose and in managing smoking cessation (33). Biochemical verification of smoking status is an important component to the research setting and may also help to guide intervention in the clinical setting.
- Smoking cessation programs are helpful compared to no intervention at all (6).
- Most smokers make many attempts to quit before success is achieved. First-time quitters need to be aware of this trend (23).
- Explore reasons for previous failures: assess for noncompliance and improper use of cessation aides in the past (23).
- Assess for psychosocial comorbidities that may affect smoking cessation (34).
- Address second-hand tobacco exposures.
- Comprehensive tobacco control programs including **mass media campaigns** are effective in changing smoking behavior in adults (35).
- Other political and social interventions such as smoking taxation, smoking bans in public and other places, bans on tobacco advertising and promotion, increases in retail prices, antismoking advocacy, and other public policies are effective in smoking cessation (36).

THERAPY
Assessment for Intervention (23)

- Assess and document tobacco use and status at every visit. This increases the likelihood of smoking-related discussions between patients and health care providers and increase cessation rates (Table 22.1).

- The five-step assessment (the 5Rs) can be used to address the patient who is not willing to initiate smoking cessation (Table 22.2) (23).
- The five-step intervention (the 5As) is recommended in clinical practice to help pregnant women quit smoking (Table 22.3) (23). Use of the 5As is endorsed by The American College of Obstetricians and Gynecologists (8), National Cancer Institute, and the British Thoracic Society.

Counseling

- Simple advice has a small, but positive, effect on cessation rates (37).
- All health care providers should give **clear, strong, and personalized advice** to every patient to quit smoking as evidence demonstrates that a **three-minute intervention** raises abstinence rates (23).
- Disclosure rates improve 40% if a **multiple-choice format for disclosure** is used rather than a yes/no format (Table 22.1) (32).
- **Oral and written advice at each prenatal visit** regarding the risk of smoking for mother and fetus, and a plan to quit (Table 22.4) (23).
- On the basis of >56 randomized controlled trials and >21,000 women participants associated with a **23% decrease in continued smoking late in pregnancy,** support and reward techniques to help quit smoking are one of the best forms of evidence-based medicine (38,39).
- Voucher-based contingency management is a promising mode of therapy as it has been associated with increased abstinence rates and improved neonatal birth weights (20,29). Financial incentives significantly increase rates of smoking cessation (40).
- There is a strong dose-response relationship between the duration and frequency of counseling and its **effectiveness** (23). Video tapes, self-help manuals, self-help guides, telephone calls, and other interventions are other examples of effective smoking cessation interventions (8).
- Smoking cessation programs are associated with a **14% reduction in preterm birth and a 17% reduction in low birth weight** (7).
- Telephone hotlines (1-800-QUIT-NOW) and web information (http://www.smokefree.gov; http://www.smokefreefamilies.org) sites are helpful.
- Interventions to increase *smoking cessation among the partners* of pregnant women, with the additional aim of facilitating cessation by the women themselves, have been insufficiently studied (6). Nonetheless, from studies including nonpregnant women, partner smoking cessation should be performed during pregnancy.

Pharmacotherapies
Nicotine Replacement Therapy

- General
  - Nicotine replacement therapy (NRT) includes patches, gums, inhalers, lozenges, and nasal spray.
  - NRT is a part of an effective strategy to promote smoking cessation in the **general nonpregnant** population (41) (Table 22.5). All of the commercially available forms of NRT (gum, transdermal patch, nasal spray, inhaler, and sublingual tablets/lozenges) can help people who make a quit attempt to increase their chances of successfully stopping smoking. NRTs increase the rate of quitting by about 50% to 70%, regardless of setting. Quit rates are increased 43% with nicotine gum (4 mg more effective than 2 mg), and 66% with the patch. In fewer trials, nicotine inhaler, tablets/lozengers, and nasal spray are associated with 90% to 100% increase in quit rates. All these effects were largely independent of the duration of therapy, the intensity of additional support provided or the setting in which the NRT was offered (41).
  - In pregnancy, NRT may help with nicotine withdrawal, but has not yet been shown to have a significant advantage over other types of interventions (7,42).
  - In pregnancy, some studies show that NRT is associated with a trend for benefit (43–46), but safety/efficacy concerns remain (7,8,24).
  - There is a risk of adverse effects of nicotine on the fetus through alterations in the uterine, placental, or blood flow to the brain (7).
  - Animal studies suggest nicotine may be toxic to the developing central nervous systems (7).
  - The American College of Obstetricians and Gynecologists cautions that the use of NRT should only be undertaken with close supervision and after careful consideration and discussion with the patient of the known risk of continued smoking and the possible risks of NRT (8).
  - There is **insufficient evidence to assure safety or efficacy in pregnancy, with unclear ratio of risks and benefits** (6,8).
  - Biomarkers such as plasma, urine, or salivary nicotine, thiocyanate, carboxyhemoglobin, or cotinine may need to be used to monitor NRT use in pregnancy.

Table 22.5 Nicotine Replacement Therapy

Only recommended in the general nonpregnant population

Nicotine replacement	Dosing regimen	Advantages	Disadvantages
Nicotine patch: Nicoderm DQ or Nicotrol	Nicoderm DQ: 21 mg/day for 6 wk, then 14 mg/day for 2 wk, then 7 mg/day for 2 wk. Nicotrol: single dose patch for 16 hr/day for 6 wk (no tapering recommended)	Over-the-counter, easy dosing	Local skin irritation in up to 50% of users, insomnia with 24 hr dosing. 30–60 min required for maximal effect
Nicotine gum or lozenge	Start on quit date: 2 mg tab if <25 cigarettes per day or 4 mg tab if >25 cigarettes per day	Over-the-counter, satisfy oral behavior	Low nicotine levels, multiple dosing
Nicotine nasal spray	1–2 doses per hr × 3 mo. Most patients require from 7–40 sprays over 24 hr	Rapid and higher nicotine levels	Initial adverse effects may include throat and nasal irritation, discouraging use
Nicotine Inhaler	10 mg cartridges used over 20 min. 6–16 cartridges per day	Substitutes for smoking behavior	Low nicotine levels

- Nicotine gum
  - FDA class C drug with known adverse effect on fetus in animal models.
  - Nicotine gum 2 mg was associated with a nonsignificant increase in smoking cessation from 10% to 13%, and significantly increased birth weights and gestational age at birth, compared to placebo (47).
- Nicotine patch
  - Class D drugs with known human risk in pregnancies.
  - **Nicotine patches** during pregnancy have been associated with nonsignificant effects on **smoking cessation** in pregnant smokers (45,48).
  - No significant effect on birth weight or preterm birth were associated with nicotine patch use (43,45,48).
- Nicotine inhaler, tablets/lozengers, and nasal spray
  - Class D drugs with known human risk in pregnancies.
  - There is insufficient evidence to assess the safety and effectiveness of nicotine inhaler, tablets/lozengers, and nasal spray, with no RCTs of pregnant smokers.

Bupropion HCl (Zyban®, Wellbutrin®)

- Class C drug in pregnancy, with no known adverse fetal effects.
- There is an FDA black box warning relating to the risk of serious neuropsychiatric events including suicide.
- In controlled clinical trials, this antidepressant increased success for moderate to heavy smokers >15 cigarettes/day by 50% to 100% in the general population of nonpregnant smokers (6).
- **There are no published clinical trials to assess the safety and efficacy of bupropion as a smoking cessation intervention in pregnancy** (6,42).
- Dose: 300 mg/day (in two divided doses to minimize side effects). Start 2 weeks prior to anticipated quit date and continue up to 7 to 12 weeks.
- Advantages: nonnicotine, may be used in combination with patch for greater efficacy, provides therapy for comorbid depression.
- Disadvantages: contraindicated if history of seizures, head trauma, alcohol abuse, or anorexia. Multiple-drug interactions with anti-HIV medications.

Varenicline (Chantix®)

- Class C drug in pregnancy with no adequate or well-controlled studies in pregnant women.
- There is an FDA black box warning relating to the risk of serious neuropsychiatric events including suicide.
- Varenicline is a partial nicotine agonist sharing structural similarity with nicotine and competitively binds nicotine acetylcholine receptors.
- In nonpregnant populations, a meta-analysis of nine randomized trials shows that varenicline increased abstinence over placebo at six months or longer [RR 2.33 (CI 1.95–2.80)], over bupropion at one year [RR 1.52 (CI 1.22–1.88)], and over NRT at one year [RR 1.31 (CI 1.01–1.71)] (49).
- **There are no published clinical trials to assess the safety and efficacy of varenicline as a smoking cessation intervention in pregnancy** (42).
- As varenicline shares close structural similarity to nicotine and occupies identical receptor sites, it is not advisable to use nicotine or varenicline during gestation and lactation.
- Dose: titrate to 1 mg twice daily over one week. Start 0.5 mg once daily (days 1–3). Increase to 0.5 mg twice daily (days 4–7).

- Start 1 week prior to anticipated quit date and continue up to 12 weeks.
- Advantages: nonnicotine, reduced cravings, may be more economical than NRT under some insurance plans.
- Disadvantages: risk of serious neuropsychiatric events; risk of angioedema and serious skin reactions; twofold increase in adverse effects of nausea, vomiting, vivid dreams, and constipation compared to placebo.

Combination Therapies

More studies are needed to determine whether combination therapy of NRT or other pharmaceutical in combination with behavioral modification, such as contingency management, increases efficacy or safety (46,50–52).

NOT Recommended

- *Clonidine*: Limited efficacy. Superior to placebo, but not statistically significant. Side effects include drowsiness, fatigue, and dry mouth (53)
- *Nortriptyline (a tricyclic agent)*: Some benefit but not FDA approved. Class C drug. Unsafe in pregnancy (54,55)
- *Maclobemide (a monoamine oxidase inhibitor)*: Some benefit but not FDA approved. Class C drug. Uncertain safety in pregnancy (54)
- *Serotonin reuptake inhibitors*: Not effective (55)
- *Opioids*: Naloxone and naltrexone. Not effective (56)

Alternative Treatments

- *Acupuncture:* There is no clear evidence that acupuncture, acupressure, laser therapy, or electrostimulation are effective at smoking cessation more than placebo effect (57).
- Hypnosis and meditation have been insufficiently studied in pregnant smokers to make a recommendation (8).
- *Stages of change* or *feedback* do not show benefit (6).

BREAST-FEEDING

- Abstinence increases breast-feeding initiation and duration (58).
- Breast-fed infants of smoking mothers have urinary cotinine levels 50 times higher than breast-fed infants of nonsmoking mothers and 10 times higher in bottle-fed infants of women who smoke (22). Mothers unable to quit smoking in the postpartum period should still be encouraged to breast-feed. Mothers should be counseled to avoid smoking at home (59).
- Incentive-based programs for tobacco cessation may increase duration of breast-feeding (58).

POSTPARTUM

- **50% to 60% of those who quit smoking relapse in first four months after delivery** (3,8), likely due to period of great stress and emotional fluctuations.
- Risk factors include depression, family members who smoke, prepregnancy tobacco use, and low weight gain in pregnancy (60).
- Effective strategies for preventing relapse have not yet been identified (61), but smoking cessation interventions should be continued, in collaborations with primary physicians and other health care personnel (Table 22.5).

PREVENTION
Relapse Prevention

- Insufficient evidence to support use of any specific interventions for helping smokers who have successfully quit for a short time and prevent relapse (58).
- It may be more efficient to focus efforts on initial cessation attempts (6,61).
- Biochemical markers may be used to monitor abstinence once cessation has occurred: carbon monoxide and urinary cotinine (22). More research is needed to validate this method (6).

Reduce Initiation of Smoking

Prevent sale of tobacco to young people, prohibit smoking in public places, increase tobacco taxation, workplace smoking cessation programs, ban on tobacco sponsorship of sporting and cultural events (6,35,36,62).

FUTURE

- Development of clinical trials needed to determine safety and efficacy of pharmacologic therapies such as nicotine replacement, bupropion, and varenicline (6–8,42).
- Clinical trials of alternative interventions such as contingency management to reduce tobacco use, and of use of biochemical markers of exposure to tobacco in pregnancy and the postpartum period.
- Existing tobacco surveillance practices should be modified to include use of presentations of smokeless tobacco.
- Current investigations should include an antinicotine vaccine and new pharmaceutical approaches.

REFERENCES

1. Shafey O, Eriksen M, Ross H, et al. The Tobacco Atlas. 3rd ed. Atlanta, GA: American Cancer Society, 2009. [Epidemiologic data]
2. Center for Disease Control and Prevention (CDC). Smoking prevalence among women of reproductive age—United States, 2006. MMWR Morb Mortal Wkly Rep 2008; 57(31):849–852. [Epidemiologic data]
3. Tong VT, Jones JR, Dietz PM, et al. Trends in smoking before, during, and after pregnancy—Pregnancy Risk Assessment Monitoring System (PRAMS), United States, 31 sites, 2000–2005. MMWR Surveill Summ 2009; 58(4):1–29. [II-2]
4. WHO Report on the Global Tobacco Epidemic, 2009: Implementing smoke-free environments, World Health Organization, 2009. [III]
5. Center for Disease Control and Prevention (CDC). Cigarette smoking among adults and trends in smoking cessation—United States, 2009. MMWR Morb Mortal Wkly Rep 2010; 59(35):1135–1140. [Epidemiologic data]
6. U.S. Department of Health and Human Services. Women and Smoking: A Report of the Surgeon General. Rockville: U.S. Department of Health and Human Services, Public Health Service, Office of the Surgeon General, 2001. [Epidemiologic data]
7. Lumley J, Chamberlain C, Dowswell T, et al. Interventions for promoting smoking cessation during pregnancy. Cochrane Database Syst Rev 2009; (3):CD001055. [72 trials, n ≥25,000]

   Update of previous Cochrane Review on this topic. Seven new RCTs included and four cluster RCTs. Smoking cessation interventions significantly reduced low birth weight (RR 0.83; 0.73–0.95) and preterm birth (RR 0.86: 0.74–0.98), as well as smoking in pregnancy (RR 0.94: 0.93–0.96). Eight trials of smoking relapse prevention (n > 1000) showed no significant reduction in relapse rates.

8. ACOG. Smoking cessation during pregnancy. ACOG Committee Opinion No. 471. Obstet Gynecol 2010; 116(5):1241–1244. [Guideline]
9. England LJ, Kim YS, Tomar SL, et al. Non-cigarette tobacco use among women and adverse pregnancy outcomes. Acta Obstet Gynecol 2010; 89:454–464. [Review]
10. Swedish National Board of Health and Welfare. Available at: http://www.socialstyrelsen.se/publikationer2008/2008-125-18. Accessed 2/16/2011. [II-2]

    Observational study spanning 2000–2006 of Swedish cigarette and other tobacco product use in pregnancy using national database.

11. Connolly GN, Alpert HR. Trends in the use of cigarettes and other tobacco products, 2000–2007. JAMA 2008; 299:2629–2630. [II-3]
12. Wang X, Zuckerman B, Pearson C, et al. Maternal cigarette smoking, metabolic gene polymorphism, and infant birth weight. JAMA 2002; 287:195–202. [II-2, n = 741]

    Case-control study. Mothers of singleton live births were evaluated by PTB, LBW, and maternal smoking status in pregnancy. The maternal genotype of CYP1A1 and GSTT1 genotypes for each variable was assessed. The greatest reduction for birth weight was found in smoking mothers with CYP1A1 Aa/aa genotypes with absent GSTT1 (−1285 g, p < 0.001). LBW infants and PTB were also significantly more prevalent in pregnant smokers with CYP1A1 Aa/aa genotypes with absent GSTT1.

13. Tyndale RF. Genetics of alcohol and tobacco use in humans. Ann Med 2003; 35:94–121. [Review]
14. Aagaard-Tillery K, Spong KY, Thom E, et al. Pharmacogenomics of maternal tobacco use: metabolic gene polymorphisms and risk of adverse pregnancy outcomes. Obstet Gynecol 2010; 115: 568–577. [II-2, n = 1004]

    Case-control study of 502 smokers with matched controls were evaluated for adverse pregnancy outcome on the basis of GSTT1 (del), CYP1A1, and CYP2A6 gene polymorphisms in mother and fetus. Fetal GSTT1(del) was significantly and specifically associated with low birth weight in pregnant smokers. Other adverse pregnancy outcomes were not associated with the gene polymorphisms studied.

15. Dempsey DA, Benowitz NL. Risks and benefits of nicotine to aid smoking cessation in pregnancy. Drug Safety 2001; 24:277–322. [Review]
16. Chica RA, Ribas I, Giraldo J, et al. Chromosomal instability in amniocytes from fetuses of mothers who smoke. JAMA 2005; 293:1212–1222. [II-1]
17. Andres RL, Day MC. Perinatal complications associated with maternal tobacco use. Semin Neonatol 2000; 5:231–241. [II-2]
18. Burton GJ, Palmer ME, Dalton KJ. Morphometric differences between the placental vasculature of non-smokers, smokers, and ex-smokers. BJOG 1989; 96(8):907–915. [II-3]
19. Bruin JE, Hertzel CG, Holloway AC. Long-term consequences of fetal and neonatal nicotine exposure: a critical review. Toxicol Sci 2010; 116:364–374. [Review]

    Landmark toxicology review with focus on long-term effects of developmental nicotine exposure using existing data from animal models.
    "The evidence provided in this review overwhelmingly indicates that nicotine should no longer be considered the 'safe' component of cigarette smoke. In fact, many of the adverse postnatal health outcomes associated with maternal smoking during pregnancy may be attributable, at least in part, to nicotine alone."

20. Heil SH, Scott TL, Higgins ST. An overview of principles of effective treatment of substance use disorders and their potential application to pregnant cigarette smokers. Drug Alcohol Depend 2009; 104(suppl 1):S106–S114. [Review]

Novel interventions for tobacco cessation in pregnancy can be found from interventions for other substance use disorders. Promising modalities include contingency management using alternative reinforcers that accommodate deficits in D2 dopamine receptor density (voucher-based CM); medications modafinil and deprnyl; cotreatment of depression.
"Certainly, pharmacotherapies offer a potentially important treatment strategy for improving outcomes with pregnant smokers." "The evidence that cessation medications increase abstinence rates in pregnant smokers in inconclusive."

21. Castles A, Adams EK, Melvin CL, et al. Effects of smoking during pregnancy: five meta-analyses. Am J Prev Med 1999; 16(3): 208–215. [Meta-analyses, 34 articles]

    Meta-analyses of 34 articles culled from 124 evaluating relative risk and odd's ratio for PPROM, preeclampsia, abruption, placenta previa, and ectopic pregnancy among smokers in pregnancy.

22. UpToDate: Smoking and Pregnancy, 2011. Available at: http://www.uptodate.com. [Review]
23. Fiore MC, Jaen CR, Baker TB, et al. Treating Tobacco Use and Dependence: 2008 Update. Clinical Practice Guideline. Rockville, MD: U.S. Department of Health and Human Services, Public Health Service, 2008. [Guideline]
24. Morales-Suarez MM, Bille C, Christensen K, et al. Smoking habits, nicotine use, and congenital malformations. Obstet Gynecol 2006; 107:51–57. [II-2]
25. Dietz PM, England LJ, Shapiro-Mendoza CK, et al. Infant morbidity and mortality attributable to prenatal smoking in the U.S. Am J Prev Med 2010; 39(1):45–52. [II-2]
26. MacArthur C, Knox EG, Lancashire RJ. Effects at age nine of maternal smoking in pregnancy: experimental and observational findings. BJOG 2001; 108(1):67–73. [II-2]
27. Heggard HK, Kjaergaad H, Moller LF, et al. The effect of environmental tobacco smoke during pregnancy on birth weight. Acta Obstet Gynecol Scand 2006; 85(6):675–681. [II-2]
28. Wikstrom AK, Cnattingius S, Stephansson O. Maternal use of Swedish snuff (snus) and risk of stillbirth. Epidemiology 2010; 21 (6):772–778. [II-2]

    Population-based cohort study of Swedish Medical Birth Register involving 7629 snuff users, 41,488 smokers of 1 to 10 daily cigarettes, and 17,014 smokers of greater than 10 cigarettes. Stillbirth rate was significantly elevated for snuff users [aOR 1.6 (1.1–2.3)], "light" smokers [aOR 1.4 (1.2–1.7)], and heavy smokers [aOR 2.4 (2.0–3.0)] when compared to 504,531 nonsmoking controls.

29. Heil SH, Higgins ST, Bernstein IM. Effects of voucher-based incentives on abstinence from cigarette smoking and fetal growth among pregnant women. Addiction 2008; 103(6):1009–1018. [I, n = 82 pregnant tobacco users]

    Participants were randomized to contingent or noncontingent voucher conditions. Vouchers could be exchanged for retail items during pregnancy and up to 12 weeks postpartum. Contingent vouchers were earned for biochemically verified abstinence. Participants in the contingent voucher system had significantly increased abstinence at delivery (41% vs. 10%; p = 0.003) and 12-week postpartum (24% vs. 3%; p = 0.006). Birth weight was significantly increased (3355 g vs. 3102 g, p = 0.06). Trend toward lower %LBW and %PTB was observed but not significant. Cost of incentive was $334 per participant.

30. Lieberman E, Gremy I, Lang JM, et al. Low birthweight at term and timing of fetal exposure to maternal smoking. Am J Public Health 1994; 84(7):1127–1131. [II-2]
31. McCowan LM, Dekker GA, Chan E, et al. Spontaneous preterm birth and small for gestational age infants in women who stop smoking early in pregnancy: prospective cohort study. BMJ 2009; 338:b1081. [II-2, n = 2504]

    Prospective cohort study. No differences noted in rate of PTB or SGA between nonsmokers and cessation in early pregnancy. Tobacco users screening positive at 14 to 16 wga had higher rates of spontaneous PTB (10% vs. 4%, p = 0.006) and SGA (17% vs. 10%, p = 0.03) than those who accomplished cessation in early pregnancy. Rates of adverse effects may be mitigated with cessation prior to 14 wga.

32. Mullen PD, Carbonari JP, Tabak ER, et al. Improving disclosure of smoking by pregnant women. Am J Obstet Gynecol 1991; 165 (2):409–413. [II-3]
33. Swamy GK, Reddick KL, Brouwer RJ, et al. Smoking prevalence in early pregnancy: comparison of self-report and anonymous urine cotinine testing. J Matern Fetal Neonatal Med 2011; 24 (1):86–90. [II-3]
34. Kleber HD, Weiss RD, Anton RF Jr, et al. Treatment of patients with substance use disorders, second edition. American Psychiatric Association. Am J Psychiatry 2007; 164(4 suppl):5–123. [Guideline]
35. Bala M, Strzeszynski L, Cahill K. Mass media interventions for smoking cessation in adults. Cochrane Database Syst Rev 2008; (1):CD004704. [Meta-analysis; 11 "campaigns"]
36. Ali MK, Koplan JP. Promoting health through tobacco taxation. JAMA 2010; 303(4):357–358. [Review III]
37. Lancaster T, Bergson G, Stead LF. Physician advice for smoking cessation. Cochrane Database Syst Rev 2008; (4):CD000165. [Meta-analysis; 41 trials, n = 31,000 nonpregnant participants]

    Brief advice versus no advice detected a significant increase in quitting (RR 1.66; 1.42–1.94, 17 trials). More intensive intervention increased estimated effect (RR 1.84; 1.60–2.13, 11 trials). A small benefit of more intensive intervention over brief advice was noted. Assuming an unassisted quit rate of 2% to 3%, quit rates may increase further 1% to 3%.

38. Sexton M, Hebel JR. A clinical trial of change in maternal smoking and its effect on birth weight. JAMA 1984; 251(7):911–915. [RCT]
39. Donatelle RJ, Prows SL, Champeau D, et al. Randomised controlled trial using social support and financial incentives for high risk pregnant smokers: Significant Other Supporter (SOS) program. Tob Control 2000; 9(suppl 3):iii67–iii69. [RCT]
40. Volpp KG, Troxel AB, Pauly MV, et al. A randomized, controlled trial of financial incentives for smoking cessation. N Engl J Med 2009; 360:699–709. [RCT, n = 878 nonpregnant adults]
41. Stead LF, Perera R, Bullen C, et al. Nicotine replacement therapy for smoking cessation. Cochrane Database Syst Rev 2008; (1):CD000146. [Meta-analysis; 111 trials, N > 40,000 nonpregnant adults]

    NRT of any type resulted in abstinence compared to control (RR 1.58; 1.50–1.66): Nicotine gum (RR 1.43; 1.33–1.53), nicotine patch (RR 1.66; 1.53–1.81), nicotine inhaler (RR 1.90; 1.36–2.67), lozenge (RR 1.2.00; 1.63–2.45), and nasal spray (RR 2.02; 1.49–3.73). 4 mg gum was associated with significant benefit when compared to 2 mg gum in heavy smokers. Quit rates were increased by 50% to 70% with the addition of an NRT.

42. Oncken CA, Kranzler HR. What do we know about the role of pharmacotherapy for smoking cessation before or during pregnancy? Nicotine Tob Res 2009; 11:1265–1273. [Review]

    NRT has not been demonstrated to have an advantage over placebo treatment. Studies are limited to small sample size and/ or poor medication compliance. NRT use is associated with increased birth weight. Psychosocial interventions should be first treatment option for pregnant smokers.

43. Pollack KJ, Oncken CA, Lipkus IM, et al. Nicotine replacement and behavioral therapy for smoking cessation in pregnancy. Am J Prev Med 2007; 33:297–305. [RCT, n = 181]

Women were randomized to a self-selected NRT arm (patch, gum, lozenge, or no therapy arm) (N = 122) versus behavioral modification (N = 59). This trial was stopped by DSMB after an a priori criterion of a near-twofold increase in adverse pregnancy outcomes in the NRT arm (30% vs. 17%). Further analysis revealed that this effect was no longer present when controlling for history of preterm birth (32% vs. 12% respectively).

44. Wisborg K, Henriksen TB, Secher NJ. A prospective intervention study of stopping smoking in pregnancy in a routine antenatal care setting. BJOG 1998; 105(11):1171–1176. [RCT, *n* = 250]
45. Kapur B, Hackman R, Selby P, et al. Randomized, double blind, placebo-controlled trial of nicotine replacement therapy in pregnancy. Curr Ther Res 2001; 62(4):274. [RCT, *n* = 30]
46. Hegaard H, Hjaergaard H, Moller L, et al. Multimodel intervention raises smoking cessation rate during pregnancy. Acta Obstet Gynecol Scand 2003; 82:813–819. [RCT]
47. Oncken C, Dornelas E, Greene J, et al. Nicotine gum for pregnant smokers: a randomized controlled trial. Obstet Gynecol 2008; 112:859–867. [RCT, *n* = 194]

RCT women randomized to 2 mg nicotine gum (N = 100) versus placebo (N = 94) for six weeks. NRT group was associated with higher birth weight, decreased LBW, and lower risk of delivery prior to 37 weeks' gestation. The mean gestational age at delivery was clinically significant (38.9 vs. 38 weeks, P < 0.014). The cessation rate was low (13% NRT vs. 9.6% on placebo) at six weeks. This trial remained underpowered and was suspended by the DSMB for poor cessation.

48. Wisborg K, Henriksen TB, Jespersen LB, et al. Nicotine patches for pregnant smokers: a randomized controlled study. Obstet Gynecol 2000; 96:967–971. [RCT, *n* = 250]

Behavior modification therapy combined with either 15-mg NRT patch for eight weeks followed by 10-mg NRT patch for three weeks (N = 120) or placebo (N = 122). No differences in birth weight, LBW, preterm birth with adequate power. Only 11% of those in the treatment group completed a full course of therapy.

49. Cahill K, Stead LF, Lancaster T. Nicotine receptor partial agonists for smoking cessation. Cochrane Database Syst Rev 2008; (3): CD006103. [Meta-analysis; nine RCTs, *n* = 7627]

Meta-analysis of nine randomized trials of varenicline increased abstinence over placebo at six months or longer (RR 2.33; 1.95–2.80) and over bupropion at one year (RR 1.52; 1.22–1.88) and over NRT at one year (RR 1.31; 1.01–1.71). There is a need for independent community-based trials of varenicline, to test its efficacy and safety in smokers with varying comorbidities and risk patterns. There is a need for further trials of the efficacy of treatment extended beyond 12 weeks.

50. Simon JA, Duncan C, Carmody TP, et al. Bupropion for smoking cessation: a randomized trial. Arch Intern Med 2004; 164 (16):1797–1803. [RCT]
51. Jorenby DE, Leischow SJ, Nides MA, et al. A controlled trial of sustained-release bupropion, a nicotine patch, or both for smoking cessation. N Engl J Med 1999; 340(9):685–691. [RCT]
52. Oncken CA, Dietz PM, Tong VT, et al. Prenatal tobacco prevention and cessation interventions for women in low- and middle-income countries. Acta Obstet Gynecol Scand 2010; 89(4):442–453. [Review]

Tobacco prevention and intervention strategies for decreasing tobacco exposure and use in LMIC countries are reviewed. Recommendations of a working group of tobacco control and perinatal experts are reviewed. Key research priorities are identified including evaluating the impact of tobacco control policy on tobacco use and SHS exposure among pregnant and reproductive age women, development of culturally adapted interventions, exploring use of

concurrent population level and clinical interventions for cessation among pregnant and reproductive age women.

53. Gourlay SG, Stead LF, Benowitz NL. Clonidine for smoking cessation. Cochrane Database Syst Rev 2004; (3):CD000058. [Meta-analysis]
54. UpToDate. Overview of Smoking Cessation. 2011. Available at: http://www.uptodate.com. [Review]
55. Hughes JR, Stead LF, Lancaster T. Antidepressants for smoking cessation. Cochrane Database Syst Rev 2007; (1):CD000031. [Meta-analysis; 66 trials]

Meta-analysis of 66 trials using antidepressants for smoking cessation. Bupropion (36 trials, n = 11140, RR 1.69; 1.53–1.85), nortryptilene (6 trials, n = 975, RR 2.03; 1.48–2.78); both increased long-term cessation. Insufficient evidence to demonstrate any additional benefit with the addition of NRT to these medications. There is no significant effect of SSRIs, MAOi, or venlafaxine.

56. David S, Lancaster T, Stead LF. Opioid antagonists for smoking cessation. Cochrane Database Syst Rev 2001; (3):CD003086. [Meta-analysis; four trials]

No significant differences in long-term (6 months) abstinence rates.

57. White AR, Rampes H, Campbell JL. Acupuncture and related interventions for smoking cessation. Cochrane Database Syst Rev 2006; (1):CD000009. [Meta-analysis; 24 studies]

No significant differences in short- or long-term abstinence rates.

58. Higgins TM, Higgins ST, Heil SH, et al. Effects of cigarette smoking cessation on breastfeeding duration. Nicotine Tob Res 2010; 12(5):483–488. [II-1, *n* = 158]

RCT where first 32 participants were assigned (not randomized) to their treatment or control group for pilot study purposes. Participants received incentive-based intervention or routine administration of comparable vouchers (control). Women receiving incentive-based treatment have significantly higher breastfeeding duration 35% versus 17% at 12 weeks postpartum (p = 0.002) as well as abstinence 25% versus 3% (p < 0.01).

59. Gartner L, Morton J, Lawrence RA, et al. American academy of pediatrics policy statement: breastfeeding and the use of human milk. Pediatrics 2005; 115(2):496–506. [Guideline]
60. Soloman LJ, Higgins ST, Heil SH, et al. Predictors of postpartum relapse to smoking. Drug Alcohol Depend 2007; 90(2–3):224–227. [II-3, *n* = 87]

Multivariate analyses of predictors of postpartum relapse of women who quit smoking in pregnancy. Relapse rate of 48% within 6 months postpartum. Friends/family members who smoke, heavy prepregnancy smoking, higher depression scores, and lower weight gain concerns were associated with increased risk of relapse. Interventions at targeting postpartum relapse include reducing postpartum depression.

61. Hajek P, Stead LF, West R. Relapse prevention interventions for smoking cessation. Cochrane Database Syst Rev 2009; (1): CD003999 [Meta-analysis, 36 RCTs]

There is insufficient evidence to support the use of any specific behavioral or pharmacologic intervention for helping smokers who have successfully quit for a short time and avoid relapse.

62. Cahill K, Moher M, Lancaster T. Workplace interventions for smoking cessation 2008. Cochrane Database Syst Rev 2008; (4): CD003440. [51 studies]

23

Drug abuse

Neil S. Seligman

KEY POINTS

- Estimates of the incidence of drug abuse during pregnancy, based on patient interview and toxicologic testing, vary from 0.4% to 27%.
- All pregnant women should be screened for illicit drug using tools such as the **CAGE-AID questionnaire**.
- Treatment of substance-abusing pregnant women requires a multidisciplinary team.
- Promoting **preconception behavioral change**, or ideally education and counseling to prevent substance abuse, is preferred over drug abuse treatment during pregnancy.
- Polysubstance abuse (including tobacco and alcohol) is common.

Opiods

- Infections (including hepatitis, HIV, and others) account for the majority of complications related to parenteral opioid use.
- **Neonatal withdrawal from opioids occurs in 60% to 70% of exposed neonates**.
- **Oral replacement therapy is the standard treatment for opioid addiction**. Replacement therapy diminishes the risks of perinatal transmission of hepatitis C and HIV, and increases utilization of prenatal care, among other benefits. Higher recidivism rates and an increased rate of complications are seen with detoxification. **Methadone (preferred) and buprenorphine are the most common options for replacement therapy**. Methadone is titrated to the lowest effective dose that prevents withdrawal symptoms.
- Opioids decrease baseline fetal heart rate and variability. Optimal timing of a nonstress test or biophysical profile is at least four to six hours following the last dose of medication.

Cocaine

- Systemic effects of cocaine include hypertension, tachycardia, and mydriasis. Pregnancy is associated with increased sensitivity of the cardiovascular system to the harmful effects of cocaine such as arrhythmias and myocardial infarction.
- Fetal and neonatal effects of cocaine include higher rates of congenital malformations, intrauterine growth restriction, low birth weight (<2500 g), small for gestational age, preterm premature rupture of membranes, preterm birth, abruption, stillbirth, and emergent delivery. Cocaine exposure also results in shorter gestation, smaller head circumference, decreased length, and withdrawal symptoms.

- Interventions for cocaine dependence primarily involve **psychosocial therapies**; currently, there are no Food and Drug Administration (FDA)-approved pharmacotherapies for treatment of cocaine dependence during pregnancy.

Others

- The incidence of amphetamine use during pregnancy varies from 0.1% to 1.0% whereas methamphetamine use may be up to 5.2% in some high prevalence areas. Ecstasy use among pregnant women varies from 0.6% to 8.8%.
- Amphetamine and methamphetamine use during pregnancy has been associated with an increased risk of malformations (cardiac and cleft lip), preterm birth, alterations in fetal and neonatal size, neonatal withdrawal, and long-term developmental consequences. The complications of ecstasy use during pregnancy are not well characterized.
- Benzodiazepine exposure is associated with preterm birth (aOR, 1.48), delivery by cesarean section (aOR, 1.53), low birth weight (aOR, 1.30–1.89), low Apgar score (aOR, 2.02), and neonatal sedation and withdrawal.
- Marijuana is the most commonly used drug during pregnancy; approximately 1 in 20 pregnant women use marijuana.
- The effects of marijuana exposure are mild, limited to decreased length of gestation (0.8 weeks) and birth weight (131 g), and are likely the result of alterations in hemodynamics. Marijuana use during pregnancy may increase the risk of sudden infant death syndrome.
- Phencyclidine does not appear to cause congenital malformations but is associated with a higher incidence of prematurity (20–22%), intrauterine growth restriction (32%), low birth weight (30%), and small for gestational age infants (17%). Developmental effects, including neurological effects, behavioral problems, and sleep disturbances, have been noted.
- An increased risk of limb reduction defects, central nervous system anomalies, and neural tube defects has been reported in association with lysergic acid diethylamide (LSD) use.

BACKGROUND

Drug use can be categorized into different patterns (Table 23.1). However, there is no safe pattern of illicit substance use.

INCIDENCE

Patient interviews and urine toxicologic testing at the initial prenatal visit and at delivery suggest that substance use

Table 23.1 Patterns of Drug Use

Use: sporadic consumption of drugs without adverse consequences

Abuse: variable consumption resulting in adverse consequences including (one or more in 12 months): (*i*) social or interpersonal consequences, (*ii*) failure to fulfill obligations at work, school, or home, (*iii*) physically hazardous situations, (*iv*) legal consequences

Substance dependence: a maladaptive pattern of substance use leading to impairment or distress as manifest by (any three in 12 months): (*i*) tolerance, (*ii*) withdrawal, (*iii*) substance is taken in larger amounts and for longer than was expected, (*iv*) persistent desire or unsuccessful efforts to cut down, (*v*) excessive time is spent in obtaining or using the substance, (*vi*) substance use interferes with work, recreation, or social life, (*vi*) substance use is continued despite knowledge of the adverse consequences

Addiction: a primary chronic disease characterized by impaired control over behavior, drug craving, inability to consistently abstain from drug use, and diminished recognition of significant problems with behaviors and interpersonal relationships

Table 23.2 Common Signs and Symptoms That Should Indicate a High Risk of Drug Use

Late or no prenatal care
Multiple missed prenatal care appointments
Impaired school or work performance
History of unexplained adverse obstetrical or neonatal outcomes (e.g., abruption)
Children with neurodevelopmental problems
Children not currently living in the home or involvement by child protective services
Medical history of other substance abuse or drug abuse related problems
Family history of drug abuse
Frequent encounters with law enforcement
Partners who have a history of substance abuse
Sudden behavioral changes
Stigmata of drug use (track marks, related infections)
History of physical or sexual abuse
Signs or symptoms of intoxication

Table 23.3 CAGE-AID

1. Have you felt you ought to cut down on your drinking or drug use?
2. Have people annoyed you by criticizing your drinking or drug use?
3. Have you felt bad or guilty about your drinking or drug use?
4. Have you ever had a drink or used drugs first thing in the morning to steady your nerves or to get rid of a hangover (eye-opener)?

during pregnancy ranges from **0.4% to 27%**, depending on the population surveyed (1). According to the 2009 National Survey on Drug Use and Health, there were 21.8 million Americans (8.7%) aged 12 and older who admitted to drug use in the past month and 3.9 million were diagnosed with substance dependence or abuse (2).

The most commonly used illicit drugs are marijuana, nonmedical use of psychotherapeutics (narcotics, tranquilizers, stimulants, sedatives), cocaine, and hallucinogens (2). The rate of substance abuse is lower in females (6.6%) than in males (10.8%) (2). Substance use by reproductive age females represents possible exposures. Among pregnant women 15 to 44 years old, the rate of current illicit drug use was 4.5% (2). Estimates based on surveys may underestimate the rate of substance abuse by as much as 50% or more. In a study of universal screening for substance abuse in an inner city population, 19% of women screened positive for one or more substances at the time of admission to labor and delivery, of which, only 32.6% gave a history of drug use (3).

RISK FACTORS

Attributes common among pregnant substance-abusing women include a history of sexual assault, poor self-esteem, and difficulty with relationships. Addiction and needle use increases the risk of sexually transmitted infections, including hepatitis C and HIV, endocarditis, and tuberculosis (4) through needle sharing, risky sexual behaviors (e.g., unprotected intercourse, sex with multiple partners, and trading drugs for sex, prostitution), and incarceration (resulting from the purchase and sale of illicit drugs, prostitution, or theft). Consistent with general recommendations for prenatal care, all pregnant women with a history of drug abuse should be offered HIV counseling and testing. Drug-dependent women have higher rates of psychopathology, which may impede optimal management.

Factors that may heighten the suspicion of drug abuse are shown in Table 23.2.

WORKUP

Options for the evaluation of illicit substance use include interview, questionnaires, and chemical tests. Use of open-ended

questions and motivational interviewing techniques may be helpful (5). There are no validated questionnaires for substance abuse screening in pregnant women; however, the **CAGE-AID questionnaire** is frequently used (Table 23.3). The Drug Abuse Screening Test (DAST) is another available option.

Chemical tests using samples of maternal blood, hair, saliva, sweat, or urine, or fetal/neonatal specimens (amniotic fluid, cord blood, meconium, blood, hair, or urine) are available for most illicit substances. Verbal consent should be obtained before obtaining these tests. Urinalysis is the most commonly used laboratory screening for substance use. False-negative test results can occur when drug ingestion occurred too recently for the substance to appear in the urine, when sufficient time has passed to allow complete drug clearance, or with dilute urine (Table 23.4). Likewise, the physician should also be aware of the limitations of neonatal testing. Drugs may be present in meconium for months, making it difficult to differentiate between the occasional user, continued substance use, and women on

Table 23.4 Length of Time Drugs Are Present in Urine

Opioids	
Codeine	2 days
Morphine	2 days
Heroin	1 day
Methadone	3 days
Cocaine	1–3 days
Amphetamines	2 days
Benzodiazepines	
Single use	3 days
Chronic use	6 wk
Marijuana	
Single use	3 days
Chronic use	30 days

treatment (e.g., methadone maintenance therapy) with no recent substance use. When maternal history and/or laboratory tests are positive for illicit drug use, a complete drug history should be obtained for each substance. The acronym "DRUG" may be useful to remember the components of the drug history.

> **D**rug name
> **R**oute (e.g., intravenous, oral)
> **U**sed how much, how often
> **G**otten how (e.g., prostitution, theft)

The initial evaluation of substance-abusing pregnant women presenting to the labor and delivery unit for any reason should include a urine drug screen, ideally with consent.

MANAGEMENT

In general, pregnant women are highly motivated to decrease or stop using illicit substances to avoid potential negative consequences for the fetus. Women who acknowledge their use of illicit substances should be counseled and offered treatment as necessary (6,7). Treatment of substance-abusing pregnant women requires a **multidisciplinary team**. Providers must be aware of the specific needs of the pregnant substance abuser. Management options include **psychosocial treatments** (1) **such as motivational interviewing** (5), **cognitive behavioral therapies, 12-step approaches, community/social network approaches, and contingency management, pharmacologic therapies, and inpatient treatment. Contingency management strategies (rewards for good behavior) are effective in improving retention of pregnant women in illicit drug treatment programs** (8).

PREVENTION

The prevention of drug abuse is paramount to drug abuse treatment. Prevention strategies are focused on **increasing public awareness of the harmful effects of drug use through advertising campaigns, school programs, and encouraging parents to educate their children. Physicians** should take an active role in drug abuse prevention by **routinely counseling their patients about the negative consequences of drug abuse**.

PRECONCEPTION COUNSELING

Substance use is an important component of the history in women seeking preconception counseling because fetal drug exposure is preventable. Women with a positive history and/or laboratory testing for substance abuse should be counseled about the reproductive effects of the specific substances along with the risks and benefits of pharmacological and nonpharmacologic treatment. Women should be encouraged to postpone conception until after completing drug treatment. Because of the reproductive risks of certain pharmacological treatments, reliable methods of contraception should be encouraged. Anovulatory cycles and infertility are more common in substance-abusing women, especially with opioid use; however, it should be stressed that pregnancy can definitely occur without adequate contraception. There is some evidence that **prepregnancy health promotion is associated with a positive effect on maternal behavior change (specifically binge drinking)** but more research is needed (9) (see chap. 1, *Obstetric Evidence Based Guidelines*).

Table 23.5 Elements of the Initial Evaluation

History of drug sequelae (thrombophlebitis, bacterial endocarditis, hepatitis)
Psychosocial history (abuse, domestic violence, depression/anxiety/bipolar, inpatient psych admission)
Thorough drug history (what, how much, how often, how obtained, taken how)
Physical exam (sequelae of drug use: track marks, abscess scars, dentition)
Dating ultrasound
Laboratory evaluation: CBC with differential, basic metabolic panel, liver function tests, hepatitis B and C antibody, RPR, blood type and antibody screen, HIV (with counseling), urinalysis and culture, TB skin test

PRENATAL CARE

All pregnant women should be screened for the use of illicit substances (10). In fact, all patients over 12 years old should be screened (11). Obtaining a history of drug abuse may be facilitated by creating a private, safe, nonjudgmental atmosphere (see earlier section "Workup"). Maternal history alone may not be sufficient when there is a high suspicion of substance abuse. Reluctance to admit substance use may stem from fear of legal repercussions and involvement of child protective services. Some states consider substance abuse during pregnancy a form of child endangerment and have laws requiring mandatory reporting of substance abuse during pregnancy. Components of the history and physical exam and the recommended laboratory evaluation are shown in Table 23.5.

OPIOIDS: HEROIN, PRESCRIPTION NARCOTICS
Historic Notes

Opioids are among the world's oldest known drugs. Opium is the dried "latex" of the opium poppy, which is grown mainly in southeast Asia. Use of opium for its therapeutic benefits predates recorded history. Opium has incited a great deal of social, political, and economic strife. Opium contains morphine, codeine, and thebaine (converted chemically into oxycodone, oxymorphone, nalbuphine, naloxone, naltrexone, and buprenorphine). Opium can also be converted into heroin for illicit use, although its origin dates to 1874 when it was first introduced as a cure for morphine addiction (12).

Diagnosis/Definition

Opioids are chemicals that bind to the opioid receptor. The term "opiate" is used to refer to naturally occurring alkaloids found in opium. Street names for heroin in the United States include "big H," "black tar," "chiva," hell dust," "horse," "negra," and "smack." Opioids can be taken orally, sniffed, smoked, absorbed through the skin, or injected (most common route of administration for heroin). Heroin may be "cut" with adulterants such as quinine, cornstarch, and baby formula powder.

Symptoms

Acute intoxication causes euphoria, altered pain sensation, and sedation; however, opioids can affect multiple organ systems (e.g., hypotension because of decreased vascular tone). **Withdrawal** presents as restlessness, insomnia, mydriasis, tachycardia, tachypnea, hypertension, lacrimation, rinorrhea, yawning, and piloerection. Opioid overdose, the most serious complication, presents with decreased respiratory rate, miotic pupils, pulmonary edema, obtundation, and/or coma. Overdose because of opioids is usually managed by securing an airway, supporting respiration, and administration of naloxone (Narcan).

Epidemiology/Incidence

1/1000 pregnant women reported heroin use during pregnancy, and an additional 12/1000 pregnant women reported using prescription narcotic analgesics (13). However, estimates range from <1% to as high as 21% depending on the population (14). Oxycodone and hydrocodone are the most commonly abused prescription narcotic analgesics (15).

Risk Factors/Associations

Many opioid-addicted pregnant women are unmarried (18%), poorly educated (20% finished high school), and prostitute themselves (22%) (12). The percentage women who do not receive prenatal care is as high as 80% (12).

Complications

Maternal medical complications because of chronic parenteral opiate abuse account for much of the obstetrical issues in these women. Of greatest concern are infections, especially **hepatitis B, hepatitis C, and HIV**. However, other sequelae include, but are not limited to, **bacteremia/sepsis, cellulitis, endocarditis, tuberculosis/pneumonia, and sexually transmitted infections** (16). Recent literature on obstetrical complications pertains mainly to women on methadone maintenance. For the purpose of this section, studies of methadone-maintained women were largely excluded. Few studies have independently evaluated nonsupervised or "street" methadone or nonprescription use of narcotic analgesics. Complications related to illicit opioid (e.g., heroin) use and prescribed opioid use may not be comparable.

- *Congenital anomalies*: There is no established increased risk of congenital anomalies or pattern of malformations related to fetal opioid exposure; however, a recent case-control study demonstrated an association between opioid analgesic treatment and certain birth defects—conoventricular septal defects (OR, 2.7; 95% CI, 1.1–6.3), atrioventricular septal defects (OR, 2.0; 95% CI, 1.2–3.6), hypoplastic left heart syndrome (OR, 2.4; 95% CI, 1.4–4.1), spina bifida (OR, 2.0; 95% CI, 1.3–3.2), or gastroschisis (OR, 1.8; 95% CI, 1.1–2.9) (17). Most prescription opioid analgesics are FDA pregnancy category B and C.
- *Obstetrical complications*: *Heroin* abuse during the first half of pregnancy has been associated with **miscarriage**, but not occasional use of *prescription opioids* (18). The rate of prematurity has not been estimated from controlled studies; however, the average of four observational studies gives a **28% rate of preterm birth (PTB)** [range 17–45% (19)] among women addicted to heroin (12). The incidence of meconium staining ranges from 21% to 46% compared to 12% to 13.8% in drug-free controls (12); however some studies have reported no difference. Additionally, the rates of malpresentation (breech), low Apgar score at five minutes, stillbirth, preterm premature rupture of membranes (PPROM), abruption, and preeclampsia are increased in some studies while others report no increase (12). A retrospective cohort study examining the effect of the type of narcotic used demonstrated rates of "fetal distress" between 47% and 52% for women abusing unsupervised methadone, heroin, and polydrug abuse

(20). Respiratory distress may be less common because of fetal stress from repeated episodes of withdrawal.
- *Fetal/neonatal morphometrics*: Opioids cross the placenta binding to opioid receptors in the fetus. Heroin may affect birth weight by lowering fetal plasma leptin levels. Heroin use is associated with **decreased birth weight**. In a retrospective study, mean birth weight of infants exposed to heroin during pregnancy was lower than controls (2490 g vs. 3176 g) (21). Combining the results of four controlled studies yielded similar results (mean 2553 g; −691 g compared to controls) (12). It is **not entirely clear whether the decrease in birth weight is entirely due to heroin or is secondary to other aspects related to heroin addiction (e.g., malnutrition and smoking)**. Likewise, low birth weight (LBW) is more common among heroin-exposed neonates. The results averaged from controlled studies give a 41% rate of low birth weight (vs. 26% in methadone, $p \leq 0.01$ and 19% in drug-free controls, $p \leq 0.0025$) (12), much of which is due to a higher incidence of intrauterine growth restriction (20% vs. 4%) (22), and small for gestational age (SGA) infants (18% vs. 12% in methadone and 5% in drug-free controls) (12).
- *Neonatal withdrawal*: The **incidence of withdrawal** is approximately 60–70% among opioid-exposed neonates. Neonatal withdrawal, also called neonatal abstinence syndrome (NAS), is characterized by central nervous system hyperirritability, gastrointestinal dysfunction, respiratory distress, and autonomic symptoms (16,23). The most serious, life-threatening sequela of NAS is seizures. Up to 30% of opioid-exposed neonates will demonstrate abnormalities on electroencephalogram and 2% to 11% will have overt seizures (24). There are several scoring systems to measure the severity of NAS, the most common of which was proposed by Finnegan (25). Neonates with high NAS scores (e.g., a cumulative Finnegan score of ≥ 24) may be candidates for replacement therapy (usually neonatal opium solution, morphine, clonidine, or phenobarbital, but buprenorphine has also been recently studied with promising results) (26).
- *Long-term neonatal outcome*: With the exception of methadone, data on long-term outcome of infants exposed to opioids are limited. In a study using video-taped interactions between drug-dependent women and their infants at four months, global ratings of interaction quality were lower compared to non–drug-exposed dyads (23). Greater body tension and poorer coordination was also observed in the drug-exposed infants. Neurological impairment was also more common at 18 months and 3 years of age (27).

Therapy

The incidence of obstetrical complications is lower among women undergoing treatment (16). **Oral replacement therapy is the standard treatment for opioid addiction**. Randomized controlled trials demonstrate an approximate threefold reduction in heroin use and a threefold increase in retention in treatment relative to nonpharmacologic treatment (28,29). In pregnancy, the **maternal and fetal benefits** are extensive and, among others, include **diminished risks of acquiring and vertically transmitting hepatitis C and HIV and increased utilization of prenatal care**. Two approaches to pharmacological treatment are maintenance and detoxification.

The goal of **maintenance therapy** is to substitute heroin with another licit drug in quantities sufficient to prevent symptoms of withdrawal and drug craving. **Detoxification**, however, aims to replace heroin with progressively lower doses of a licit substance until treatment is no longer required. **High rates of return to illicit opioid use has been observed with detoxification in pregnant women** (30,31) and nonpregnant individuals (28,32,33); however, these two approaches to therapy have not been compared in randomized controlled trials or pregnant women. Additionally, the safety of detoxification during pregnancy is not well studied. **Detoxification has been associated with miscarriage, stillbirth, and alterations in fetal adrenal hormone levels** (34,35), but larger, more recent studies have not confirmed these findings (36,37).

Methadone
Methadone (FDA category C), a long-acting synthetic μ receptor agonist, is the **preferred treatment for opioid addiction during pregnancy**. Four randomized controlled trials have shown that **methadone maintenance decreases illicit opioid use, criminal activity, and mortality rates in heroin-addicted nonpregnant adults** (38). Initial stabilization with methadone should be done under supervision in an inpatient setting because of possible dangerous interactions between methadone and other substances. Typical initial stabilization doses range from 10 to 30 mg with the dose increased in 5 to 10 mg increments thereafter. The most appropriate methadone dose is controversial. Doses of at least 60 mg are more effective than lower doses (28,39). We **recommend titrating the daily methadone dose to achieve the lowest effective dose that prevents symptoms of withdrawal and drug cravings**. In our experience the average maintenance dose of methadone is approximately 120 mg/day. As a result of the physiologic changes that occur during pregnancy (decreased plasma levels and increased clearance) dose increases are often needed in the later part of pregnancy to prevent withdrawal. A methadone trough level may be useful in guiding dose adjustments as symptomatic women have significantly lower mean methadone levels than asymptomatic women (0.18 mg/L vs. 0.24 mg/L) (40). Likewise, trough levels >0.3 mg/L should be correlated to urine drug screen results because of possibility of withdrawal from other illicit substances. Caution should be taken when prescribing other medications to women on methadone because of the potential for drug-drug interactions. For example, both methadone and the commonly prescribed antibiotic metronidazole increase the QTc interval, which can lead to potentially fatal ventricular arrhythmias.

Methadone maintenance is associated with improved obstetrical and neonatal outcome compared to illicit opioid abuse (more adequate prenatal care, longer gestation, increased birth weight and head circumference, etc.) but not to the level of drug-free controls. However, the rate of continued illicit substance abuse is as high as 88% in some studies and this continued substance abuse may attenuate some of the beneficial effects of drug treatment programs (19,41).

The most common neonatal sequela of opioid exposure is **neonatal withdrawal**, also referred to as **NAS**. Rates of NAS reported in the literature range from 31% to 80% (40,42). However, **maternal methadone has not been shown conclusively to be associated with either the incidence of NAS or the length of neonatal treatment for NAS** (43–45). Methadone has also been associated with decreased birth weight and head circumference (46), jaundice, and thrombocytosis. Less commonly recognized is the effect of methadone on the developing visual system. In a group of 20 exposed infants and children, ophthalmic abnormalities included decreased visual acuity (95%), nystagmus (70%), delayed visual maturation (50%), strabismus (30%), refractive errors (30%), and cerebral visual impairments (25%) (47). Neither the long-term effects nor the independent effect of other illicit substances are clear.

Buprenorphine
Buprenorphine (Subutex, FDA category C) is a partial μ receptor agonist and κ receptor antagonist. Randomized trials demonstrate that buprenorphine increases treatment retention (RR 1.21–1.52) and decreases heroin use (28,29) in nonpregnant adults compared to methadone. The main advantages of buprenorphine are that it does not require supervised daily administration and can be prescribed by any physician with appropriate training (48). **The benefits of buprenorphine compared to methadone in pregnancy are still insufficiently studied.** In a Cochrane systematic review of maintenance agonist treatments for opiate-dependent pregnant women, which included two randomized trials of methadone versus buprenorphine, there was no difference in dropout [RR 1.00 (0.41–2.44)], continued illicit heroin use [RR 2.50 (0.11–54.87)], rate of neonatal treatment for NAS [RR 1.28 (0.58–2.85)], and length of neonatal treatment for NAS [RR 0.50 (−1.84, 2.84)] (49). A recent randomized, placebo-controlled trial comparing methadone and buprenorphine for treatment of maternal opioid dependency found that buprenorphine was associated with significantly lower doses of morphine for treatment of NAS (mean total amount 1.1 vs. 10.4 mg), shorter duration of treatment for NAS (4.1 vs. 9.9 days), and shorter neonatal hospital stay (10.0 versus 17.5 days) but no difference in continued illicit substance use (15% vs. 9%, p = 0.27) or the rate of neonatal treatment for NAS (57% vs. 47%, p = 0.26) (50). This trial has yet to be included in the Cochrane systematic review. A limitation of the trial was a markedly higher attrition rate from the buprenorphine treatment arm than from the methadone arm (18% versus 33%, p = 0.02). **Suboxone** is a combination of buprenorphine and naltrexone. The addition of naltrexone is meant to deter parenteral use of buprenorphine. In general, women taking Suboxone should be switched to an equivalent dose of buprenorphine (Subutex).

Other Treatments
Other treatments for opioid-addicted pregnant women include oral slow-release morphine, heroin-assisted treatment, L-A-acetylmethadol (LAAM), and clonidine. In a small randomized controlled trial, oral slow-release morphine was superior to methadone in abstinence from heroin, but there was no statistically significant difference in birth weight or duration of NAS (49,51). There are two case reports of "heroin-assisted" treatment in a total of five pregnant women. Heroin-assisted treatment combines methadone and injectable heroin. The selection criteria for this program are a history of addiction for more than two years, failure of at least two alternative treatments, and risk of further physical or social decline. The authors observed a higher birth weight compared to women treated with methadone alone (52). LAAM is a μ receptor agonist with a longer half-life than methadone. LAAM was taken off of the market in 2003 because it prolongs the QT interval, leading to potentially life-threatening ventricular arrhythmias. Clonidine, an α-agonist antihypertensive medication, has been used alone or in addition to other medications for mild withdrawal. The blood pressure lowering effect of clonidine is due to its α_2-agonist properties. Likewise, clonidine prevents withdrawal symptoms through the same mechanism. In summary, treatments other than methadone or buprenorphine have limited evidence for safety and efficacy and therefore should be avoided.

Antepartum Testing

Reports of an increased risk of intrauterine fetal demise associated with intravenous opiate abuse (16) have led some authors to suggest weekly fetal monitoring beginning at 32 weeks. However, **for women in a treatment program who have repetitively negative urine drug screens, antepartum testing should be reserved for standard obstetrical indications** (e.g., intrauterine growth restriction (IUGR)). Opiates are associated with decreases in baseline and variability. Ideally, to avoid misinterpretation, women on methadone or other prescribed narcotics should have nonstress test or biophysical profile scheduled before or at least four to six hours after a dose of methadone.

Delivery

As per common obstetric practices.

Anesthesia

Peripheral intravenous access can be difficult in chronic intravenous drug abusers. Dosing of other opioid analgesics for pain control during labor and postpartum can be challenging because of tolerance as a result of chronic receptor stimulation (53). In a retrospective study, methadone-maintained women required 70% more oxycodone equivalents after cesarean section than controls (54). Opioid antagonists or agonist-antagonists can precipitate acute withdrawal (54). Examples of these drugs are Nubain®, Talwin®, Stadol®, and Narcan®. If any of these drugs are accidentally given, withdrawal can also be reversed with any opioid (54). Regional anesthesia is safe. However, hypotension may occur more frequently because of concomitant malnutrition and/or liver disease. After delivery, fluid shifts may increase opiate levels. However, we have not observed any cases of over sedation or other complications postpartum.

Postpartum/Breast-feeding

The American Academy of Pediatrics (AAP) Committee on Drugs strongly advises that women should not use heroin while breast-feeding as it may be hazardous to the infant and nursing mother. Tremors, restlessness, vomiting, and poor feeding have been reported in breast-fed infants of women using heroin (55). Breast-feeding is not contraindicated in women taking opioids for acute (e.g., Percocet for postoperative pain) or chronic pain.

Women taking methadone should be **encouraged to breast-feed**; some of the benefits include improved maternal-infant bonding and favorable effects on NAS (56–59). It is not clear whether the favorable effects of breast-feeding on NAS are related to methadone in breast milk or the act of breast-feeding itself (60). The AAP lists methadone as compatible with breast-feeding at any dose (55).

The use of buprenorphine is acceptable while breast-feeding (61).

COCAINE
Historic Notes

Cocaine was purified from the coca plant in 1862 by Albert Neiman. Sigmund Freud first introduced cocaine into modern medicine in 1884 with his treatise "On Coca," but its use as a topical anesthetic (cocaine-saturated saliva) dates back thousands of years. Cocaine is still used in some ophthalmologic procedures. Coca-Cola® contained cocaine until 1903; today the soft drink still contains a non-narcotic extract prepared from the coca plant.

Diagnosis/Definition

Cocaine is prepared from the leaves of the *Erythroxylon coca* plant. As a hydrochloride, cocaine (also known as "snow") is sold in the form of a powder, or as granules or crystals. Crack, also known as crack cocaine, rock, or freebase, is cocaine returned to its alkalinized form by heating it with baking soda and water. Cocaine can be injected, snorted, or smoked (in cigarettes or with marijuana). Inhalation is the preferred route of administration by crack users (62).

Symptoms

Cocaine produces a brief euphoria by interfering with presynaptic neurotransmitter uptake, thereby increasing sympathomimetic neurotransmitters (63). Systemic effects include **hypertension, tachycardia, and dilated pupils.**

Pregnancy is associated with increased sensitivity of the cardiovascular system to cocaine (64,65). Plasma cholinesterase activity, the enzyme responsible for metabolizing cocaine, is decreased during pregnancy, which prolongs the adverse effects of cocaine (66). Additionally, other physiologic changes during pregnancy (increased oxygen demand and limited or decreased supply because of increases in heart rate blood pressure and left ventricular contractility) (63) increase the cardiopulmonary toxicity of cocaine (66,67).

Serious complications of acute cocaine use include **arrhythmias, myocardial infarction, crack cocaine–induced pulmonary edema, alveolar rupture, spontaneous pneumothorax, stroke, seizures, gastrointestinal ischemia, hyperthermia, and death.** Cocaine use may present as the constellation hypertension, proteinuria, and edema, and therefore may be confused for preeclampsia. Withdrawal symptoms from cocaine include drug craving, fatigue, and mental depression.

Epidemiology/Incidence

Cocaine use peaked in the 1980s (8–17% in urban hospitals) (68) and has since declined. From 1993 to 1995, 9.1% of pregnant women used cocaine by self-report or positive meconium at four urban centers (3.4% history and positive meconium) (69). According to another study, in the late 1990s, the prevalence of cocaine use by pregnant women was approximately **0.28% (1/10th of overall drug use during pregnancy)** (70). More recently, between 2000 and 2001, at a public hospital in São Paulo, Brazil, the rate of cocaine use by pregnant teens 11 to 19 years in the third trimester was 1.7% using hair analysis.

Etiology/Basic Pathophysiology

Cocaine readily crosses the placenta and can be detected in fetal blood and tissues (68). The maternal and fetal sequelae of cocaine may be related to the effects of cocaine on the cardiovascular system (67,71). Uterine artery vasospasm and vasoconstriction in response to cocaine results in decreased uteroplacental blood flow and uteroplacental insufficiency, which can lead to fetal acidosis, hypoxia, and distress. Additionally, cocaine has β-agonist properties that stimulate uterine contractions (70), an effect that has been reproduced in vitro (72). Uterine contractions and acute vasoconstriction of vessels in the placental bed are thought to be the mechanisms of abruption related to cocaine use (66,73). Cocaine has the ability to potentiate the effects of or be potentiated by other drugs. The combination of cocaine and ethanol produces cocaethylene, a biologically active substance with unknown reproductive effects (67).

Risk Factors/Associations

As with other substances, women who use cocaine are more likely to use other illicit substances, tobacco, and/or alcohol. Cocaine use during pregnancy is more common among black women compared with the racial distribution of other substances. Pregnant women who use cocaine also tend to be older, have less than a high school education, higher gravidity, and are more likely to have had a prior abortion (74).

Complications

* *Congenital anomalies*: Cocaine use alone (RR 1.7, 95% CI 1.12–2.60) or cocaine in addition to other drugs (RR 2.10, 95% CI 1.42–3.09) during pregnancy is associated with a **higher rate of congenital malformations** (genitourinary, cardiac, and limb reduction defects) (68,75). Neonates exposed to cocaine are at risk for structural and functional (arrhythmias, conduction abnormalities, etc.) congenital heart disease (76). Exposure to cocaine has been suggested in the etiology of hydranencephaly (67).

* *Obstetrical complications*: **IUGR, shorter gestation** (−1.47 weeks 95% CI −1.97 to −0.98), **PTB** (OR, 3.38; 95% CI 2.72–4.21), **PPROM** (RR 1.85, 95% CI 1.35–2.52 cocaine alone; RR 3.18, 95% CI 1.61–6.29 cocaine with other drugs), **abruption** (RR 4.55, 95% CI 3.19–6.50 cocaine alone; RR 4.95, 95% CI 2.08–11.81 cocaine with other drugs), and **stillbirth** (as a consequence of abruption) are the most frequently cited obstetrical complications of cocaine use (67,68,75,77,78,79). Women presenting with PPROM in association with cocaine exhibit more advanced cervical dilation (80,81). Body packing, the ingestion of multiple packets of cocaine for the purpose of smuggling, can cause serious complications if a packet ruptures and at least one case of perimortem cesarean section has been reported in this situation (82). Women who use cocaine during pregnancy are four times more likely to require **emergent delivery**.

* *Fetal/neonatal morphometrics*: Cocaine use during pregnancy is associated with **lower birth weight** (−492 g, 95% CI −562– to −421), **LBW** (OR, 3.66; 95% CI 2.90–4.63), SGA **infants** (OR, 3.23; 95% CI 2.43–4.30), **decreased head circumference** (−1.21 to −1.72 cm), **and decreased length** (−2.17 to −2.57 cm) (75,77). Bowel perforation and necrotizing enterocolitis associated with cocaine exposure have been reported (67).

* *Neonatal withdrawal*: Abrupt discontinuation of cocaine at birth results in a constellation of withdrawal symptoms, best described as "neonatal toxicity." These symptoms include **jitteriness/tremulousness** (OR, 2.17; 95% CI 1.44–3.29), **irritability** (OR, 1.81; 95% CI 1.18–2.80), **excessive suck** (OR, 3.58; 95% CI 1.63–7.88), **hyperalertness** (OR, 7.78; 95% CI 1.72–35.06), and **autonomic instability** (OR, 2.64; 95% CI 1.17–5.95) (69).

* *Long-term neonatal outcome*: Initial studies reported adverse neurological consequences of antenatal cocaine exposure (so-called crack babies); however, more recent studies have found that much of the effect is related to co-occurring exposures. Nonetheless, cocaine is not without consequence. Cocaine exposure was related to **lower scores on tests of short-term memory, more behavioral problems, and changes in temperament** at three years of age compared to nonexposed children (83). Cocaine also has **effects on the visual system**. Strabismus and refractive errors are more likely among children prenatally exposed to cocaine. Cases of permanent eyelid edema have also been reported. Cocaine use more than three times per week was associated with higher rates of **childhood obesity** (84). The mechanism that has been postulated to explain this finding is poor maternal nutrition and LBW, which has been linked to later obesity.

Therapy

There are currently no FDA-approved pharmacologic therapies available for detoxification or maintenance of cocaine dependence. Interventions for cocaine dependence primarily involve **psychosocial therapies** (e.g., cognitive behavioral therapy, motivational interviewing). Very few interventions have been specifically studied in pregnancy. Treatment programs for cocaine have a favorable impact on pregnancy outcome; rates of PTB and LBW were decreased by 67% and 84% (71). Motivational enhancement therapy was compared to "usual" counseling for pregnant women abusing cocaine in a randomized trial that found no difference in treatment utilization. The use of motivational incentives, also known as **voucher-based contingency management**, was studied in a small, randomized trial of pregnant women abusing cocaine. Treatment retention and abstinence from cocaine was high in both groups and there was a trend toward increased attendance at prenatal care visits (*p* = 0.077) (85). In a separate study, **motivational interviewing** was associated with a significant reduction in neonatal intensive care unit admission and length of stay and cost savings amounted to $5000 per mother/infant pair above the cost of the program (86).

Withdrawal from cocaine is usually mild, if present, and not life threatening for the mother or fetus. Benzodiazepines can be given to relieve symptoms (70). Rarely, psychotic symptoms during withdrawal may require treatment with antipsychotic medications.

Antepartum Testing

The role of antepartum testing (ultrasound and nonstress tests or biophysical profiles) for cocaine use is insufficiently studied to make recommendations. Serial ultrasounds have been used to assess fetal growth (70).

Anesthesia

Regional anesthesia should be used with caution because of combative behavior, altered perception of pain, cocaine-induced thrombocytopenia, and ephedrine-resistant hypotension (usually responds to phenylephrine). Women may perceive pain despite adequate spinal/epidural anesthesia levels (76). Hydralazine is the drug of choice for management of cocaine-induced hypertension, but treatment with labetalol plus nitroglycerin may be a reasonable alternative (79). Propranolol should be avoided because of the potential for unopposed α-adrenergic stimulation.

Postpartum/Breast-feeding

The AAP Committee on Drugs strongly advises that women should not use cocaine while breast-feeding as it may be hazardous to the infant and nursing mother. Cocaine intoxication has been reported in breast-fed infants of women using cocaine (55).

AMPHETAMINES: AMPHETAMINE, METHAMPHETAMINE, 3,4-METHYLENEDIOXYMETHAMPHETAMINE (ECSTASY)
Historic Notes
Amphetamines were first synthesized in 1887 (87). Amphetamine is FDA approved (schedule II) for the treatment of attention-deficit hyperactivity disorder (ADHD) and narcolepsy. Methamphetamine (schedule II) is FDA approved for the treatment of ADHD and obesity. Methamphetamine is easily made from over-the-counter cold medications and addiction can occur after as little as one use (88). Ecstasy was patented in 1912 (89). In the 1970s, psychotherapists used ecstasy to enhance "openness" with their patients (89). Ecstasy was classified as a schedule I drug in 1985 (89).

Diagnosis/Definition
Amphetamines are structurally similar to norepinephrine (90) and act primarily by increasing levels of norepinephrine and other biogenic amines (87,90). Street names for amphetamines include dexies, bennies, ice (methamphetamine), and crystal (methamphetamine). Amphetamines can be taken orally, injected, or smoked (78.3% for methamphetamines) (91). Gamma-hydroxybutyrate (GHB) is sometimes referred to as "liquid ecstasy" but is chemically and pharmacologically unrelated to 3,4-methylenedioxymethamphetamine.

Symptoms
Symptoms of amphetamine use include alertness, decreased fatigue, sleeplessness, euphoria, exhilaration, emotional openness, reduction of negativity, and decreased inhibition (92). Systemic effects include hypertension, dilated pupils, tremor, and hyperactivity (90). Release of serotonin is responsible for some of the hallucinogenic effects of amphetamines (90). Rarely, at high doses, toxicity mimicking cocaine toxicity can be seen, including hypertension, retinal damage, cardiac arrhythmia, hyperthermia, seizure, shock, stroke, and death (90). Methamphetamine abuse can cause toxic hepatitis, which presents similarly to acute viral hepatitis.

Epidemiology/Incidence
Amphetamines are the most abused prescription medication (93). Use of methamphetamine, the most commonly abused amphetamine, is an escalating problem in the United States and other parts of the world (89,94,95). The reported incidence of methamphetamine use during pregnancy is between **0.1% and 1.0%** (96). Methamphetamine use during pregnancy is significantly more common (5.2%) in cities where methamphetamine use is prevalent (97) and more common in the West, Midwest, and Southeast United States (91). Methamphetamines may account for nearly a quarter of drug treatment admissions during pregnancy in some areas (91). The rate of ecstasy exposure during pregnancy is less clear. Ecstasy is one of the most widely used illicit drugs in the United Kingdom where the rate of self-reported use ranged from 0.6% to 8.8% in 2004 (89). In the United States, ecstasy use peaked in 2001 and has since declined.

Etiology/Basic Pathophysiology
Methamphetamine crosses the placenta and is detectable in fetal tissues. Studies of methamphetamine in pregnant sheep suggest that vasoconstriction may be the mechanism that leads to obstetrical and neonatal complications (98).

Risk Factors/Associations
Women who use ecstasy during pregnancy are more likely to be younger (mean 23.2 years vs. 31.2 years, $p < 0.0001$), report that the pregnancy was unplanned (84% vs. 54%, $p < 0.05$), use alcohol (66% vs. 31%, $p < 0.0001$), smoke cigarettes (54% vs. 20%, $p < 0.0001$), and use other illicit drugs during pregnancy compared to nonusers (94,99). Similar patterns of polysubstance abuse are observed among women who abuse amphetamine and methamphetamine (91,94,100).

Complications
Given that amphetamines and cocaine have similar effects on the central nervous system, both agents produce similar effects during pregnancy and are often combined in studies.

- *Congenital anomalies*: There is insufficient information on which to make a definitive conclusion about the developmental toxicity of *amphetamine and methamphetamine*. However, an increased risk of **cardiac malformations and cleft lip** has been reported. Data from the United Kingdom National Teratology Information Service demonstrated a 15% rate of congenital anomalies after prenatal *ecstasy* exposure (expected 2–3%). Among these malformations, talipes equinovarus occurred more frequently than expected [all three female, 38/1000 (95% CI 8.0–109.0) vs. expected 3:1 male predominance, 1/1000] (101). There was also a trend toward higher-than-expected rates of congenital heart disease [26/1000 (95% CI 3.0–90.0) vs. expected 5–10/1000].

- *Obstetrical and neonatal complications*: Several case series of *amphetamine*-addicted women have demonstrated higher-than-expected rates of **abruption, PTB, IUGR, and LBW** (102,103). In another retrospective study evaluating the effects of methamphetamine use, complications that occurred significantly more frequently included PTB (52% vs. 17%, $p < 0.001$), low five-minute Apgar score (6% vs. 1%, $p < 0.001$), and neonatal mortality (4% vs. 1%, $p < 0.001$) (95). *Methamphetamine* exposure has also been associated with an increased OR of SGA (2.05–3.5), and decreased birth weight and head circumference (98,100,104). The obstetrical and neonatal complications of ecstasy use are insufficiently studied.

- *Neonatal withdrawal*: Neonatal withdrawal from *amphetamine and methamphetamine* is characterized by abnormal sleep, poor feeding, tremors, and hypertonia.

- *Long-term neurodevelopmental outcome*: In a 14-year follow-up study of Swedish children exposed to *amphetamine* prenatally, the children demonstrated **deficits in school performance** including language, mathematics, and physical training at age 14 years (105). Earlier follow-up of these children showed increased **sleepiness, characteristics of autism, speech abnormalities, and stranger anxiety** by 1 year old, **lower IQ** at 4 years old, and **aggressive behavior and difficulty with peers** at 8 years old (106). *Methamphetamine*-exposed neonates have been found to have higher physiological **stress** (difficulty maintaining normal, regular respiration) (106). Magnetic resonance imaging–based studies of children up to 16 years old suggest that *methamphetamine* exposure may cause damage to brain structures involved in **executive functioning (e.g., attention deficit) and verbal memory** (107–109). No long-term studies of prenatal *ecstasy* exposure are available (89).

Therapy
There is currently no FDA-approved medications available for detoxification or maintenance of amphetamine dependence.

Antepartum Testing
The role of antepartum surveillance for exposure to amphetamines is insufficiently studied to make recommendations.

Anesthesia
Sympathectomy caused by regional anesthesia can result in profound hypotension in women using amphetamines, and vasopressors should be used with caution (53). Dosing of general anesthetics may be altered by acute and chronic amphetamine use (53).

Postpartum/Breast-feeding
The AAP Committee on Drugs strongly advises that women should not ingest amphetamines while breast-feeding. Amphetamine, in particular, is concentrated in human milk and adverse effects on the neonate have been reported (irritability and poor sleep) (55).

BENZODIAZEPINES
Historic Notes
Benzodiazepines have been studied as potential treatments for threatened abortion, preterm labor, preeclampsia, and as adjuncts for pain management in labor.

Diagnosis/Definition
Benzodiazepines are a group of compounds formed through the fusion of a benzene and a diazepine ring. They are categorized by half-life as short, medium, and long acting. Street names for benzodiazepines include "benzos," "downers," "nerve pills," and "tranks." Benzodiazepines are usually taken orally.

Symptoms
Benzodiazepines are sedative drugs, used mainly for the treatment of anxiety, and have the potential for addiction.

Epidemiology/Incidence
Benzodiazepines were the most commonly prescribed drugs in pregnancy (110). In the 1970s and 1980s, 1.6% to 2.2% of pregnant women in the United States and Europe used benzodiazepines during pregnancy; however, the exact incidence of benzodiazepine exposure is unclear with rates varying from <1% to 40% (111).

Etiology/Basic Pathophysiology
Benzodiazepines cross the placenta; fetal and neonatal concentration vary between benzodiazepines. Whereas diazepam levels in the neonate are one- to threefold higher than those of the mother, neonatal levels of midazolam are lower than those of the mother (110).

Risk Factors/Associations
Benzodiazepine exposure in Swedish women is associated with older age, higher incidence of smoking, less education, and use of other psychoactive drugs (111).

Complications
A clear understanding of the effects benzodiazepines is limited by significant heterogeneity between studies: benzodiazepines studied as a class versus individual agents; effect of the underlying medical condition (e.g., epilepsy) or obstetrical complication (e.g., preeclampsia); licit versus illicit use; concomitant use of other psychoactive drugs, illicit substances, tobacco, or alcohol.

- *Congenital anomalies*: Several studies, including approximately 350 women exposed to benzodiazepines, do not indicate an increased risk of facial clefts or other congenital malformations but only a portion of the women were exposed in the first trimester (110). A meta-analysis showed an **increased risk of major malformations** (OR, 3.01; 95% CI 1.32–6.84), using data pooled from seven case-control studies, but the pooled risk calculated from four cohort studies was not significant (OR, 0.90; 95% CI 0.61–1.35) (112). Similarly, there was an increased risk of oral clefts associated with benzodiazepine exposure (OR, 1.79; 95% CI 1.13–2.82), when data from six case-control studies were combined but not from the combination of three cohort studies (OR, 1.19; 95% CI 0.34–4.15) (112); but studies including induced abortions were excluded (113). Among 1979 neonates with benzodiazepine exposure in Sweden between 1994 and 2005, the rate of congenital malformations was 5.3% compared to a background rate of 4.7% during the same time period; however, pyloric stenosis and alimentary tract atresia occurred more often than expected (RR 4.9, 95% CI 1.3–12.5) (114). An increased risk of gastrointestinal anomalies was also observed in a study of 262 benzodiazepine-exposed neonates where the OR for anal atresia was 6.19 (95% CI 2.44–15.74) following exposure to lorazepam (115). According to an American College of Obstetrics and Gynecology Practice Bulletin, benzodiazepines do not carry a significant risk of teratogenesis (116). The absolute risk of oral cleft from prenatal benzodiazepine exposure was increased by 0.01%, from 6 in 10,000 to 7 in 10,000 in one meta-analysis (117). In a recent case-control study, an association with congenital anomalies, including oral clefts with exposure to five different benzodiazepines, was not found (118).
- *Obstetrical and neonatal complications*: **PTB and LBW** (aOR, 1.48; 95% CI 1.26–1.75), **cesarean section** (aOR, 1.53; 95% CI 1.37–1.70), **low birth weight** (early exposure: aOR, 1.30; 95% CI 1.06–1.59; late exposure: aOR, 1.89; 95% CI 1.89–2.76), **low Apgar scores** <7 at five minutes (late exposure: aOR, 2.02; 95% CI 1.13–3.65), all have been associated with benzodiazepine exposure (111). After exclusion of women with reported use of antidepressants, there was no significant increased risk of PTB or low APGAR score <7 at five minutes. Benzodiazepine use immediately prior to delivery may result in delivery of a **sedated neonate** (119,120).
- *Neonatal withdrawal*: Neonatal withdrawal from benzodiazepines is characterized by **hypoventilation, irritability, hypertonicity, and "floppy infant syndrome" (hypotonia, lethargy, poor respiratory effort, and feeding difficulties)**. Other withdrawal symptoms include

restlessness, hypertonia, hyperreflexia, tremulousness, and gastrointestinal symptoms (diarrhea and vomiting) (116). Symptoms of withdrawal may be delayed, not occurring until day 12 to 21, and may last for several months (116,121). We recommend, if clinically feasible, avoiding administration of benzodiazepines to pregnant women, especially those on methadone maintenance therapy. Benzodiazepine use by women on methadone maintenance therapy is associated with more severe neonatal opiate withdrawal (i.e., NAS) (24,38,45,122). In a multivariate analysis, the mean length of treatment was two weeks longer among neonates exposed to methadone and benzodiazepines versus methadone alone (45).

- *Long-term neonatal outcome*: Behavioral effects of benzodiazepines have not been definitively proven (110,116); 17 children of women treated with benzodiazepines were followed to 18 months. Compared to children of women without psychiatric disorders, the benzodiazepine (mainly diazepam)-exposed children showed impaired fine motor skills and abnormal tone and patterns of movement (e.g., walking) (123). However, in a study of children with prenatal exposure to chlordiazepoxide, there was no evidence of abnormal neurodevelopment (IQ or motor status) at 8 months ($n = 501$ children) or 4 years ($n = 435$ children) (124).

Therapy

Abrupt discontinuation of benzodiazepines may cause serious maternal withdrawal symptoms. Benzodiazepine withdrawal is less likely if a woman has not taken therapeutic doses (i.e., three to four times per day) for ≥4 weeks. These women should be reassessed for benzodiazepine withdrawal if they have changes in vital signs (systolic blood pressure ≥150 mmHg, diastolic blood pressure ≥100 mmHg, pulse >110 beats/min, temperature >101°F, or SpO_2 <96%) or symptoms of anxiety or agitation.

   Psychiatry consultation is suggested for women who are dependent on benzodiazepines (i.e., use of benzodiazepine at therapeutic doses for ≥4 weeks). **Typically, a longer-acting benzodiazepine (e.g., Klonopin) is substituted to reduce the risk of benzodiazepine withdrawal seizure.** There are currently no FDA-approved medications available for detoxification or maintenance of benzodiazepine dependence.

Antepartum Testing

The role of antepartum surveillance for benzodiazepine exposure is insufficiently studied to make a recommendation.

Postpartum/Breast-feeding

Most benzodiazepines are "moderately safe" (lactation risk category L3) during breast-feeding. Approximately 0.1% to 11% of the weight adjusted maternal dose is transferred to the breast milk and is drug specific (110). No significant adverse neonatal reactions have been reported (55,110).

CANNABIS (MARIJUANA)
Historic Notes

Cannabis has been used for medicinal purposes for thousands of years and is among the earliest non–food-bearing plants cultivated by humans (125).

Diagnosis/Definition

More than 400 chemicals are found in *Cannabis sativa*. The primary active ingredient in marijuana is **tetrahydrocannabinol (THC)**. Marinol (dronabinol), a synthetic preparation of Δ^9-THC, is indicated for treatment of anorexia and weight loss in patients with AIDS and of nausea and vomiting associated with chemotherapy. Dried cannabis leaves contain 2% to 4% THC. Some common street names for marijuana include pot, grass, herb, weed, Mary Jane, reefer, skunk, boom, gangster, kif, chronic, and ganja. Marijuana is most commonly smoked but can also be taken orally.

Symptoms

The symptoms of marijuana intoxication include euphoria, tachycardia, conjunctival congestion, and anxiety (126).

Epidemiology/Incidence

Marijuana is the **most commonly used illicit drug**. In the United States, among women who use illicit drugs during pregnancy, 75% to 80% use marijuana (127). The incidence of marijuana use during pregnancy is approximately **5%** (127–129), but has been reported to be as high as 27% (53). More than 40% of reproductive age women have tried marijuana at least once (130).

Etiology/Basic Pathophysiology

Marijuana crosses the placenta and can be detected in fetal tissues for several weeks after use (131). Chronic marijuana use alters uterine artery blood flow (132) and may **decrease uteroplacental perfusion** (133). When taken in combination, marijuana can potentiate the effects of other illicit drugs.

Risk Factors/Associations

Marijuana use during pregnancy is most highly associated with not only cigarette smoking and alcohol consumption, but also lower socioeconomic status and less education (129,134).

Complications

Although it is difficult to separate the effects of marijuana from its contextual associations of use, subtle effects could have a large impact because exposure is so frequent (135). The risk of obstetrical and/or neonatal complications increases in relation to the amount of marijuana use and is greatest among frequent users (≥4–6 times per week) (136). Infrequent use appears to pose limited risk.

- *Congenital anomalies*: There is no obvious pattern of malformations associated with first trimester marijuana use. Congenital anomalies are slightly more common among marijuana users but the difference was not statistically significant (133,136).
- *Obstetrical complications*: Frequent marijuana use ≥6 times per week is associated with a 0.8-week **reduction in length of gestation** (137). Marijuana does not appear to contribute to excess PTB (129,138), stillbirth, perinatal mortality, or neonatal intensive care unit admission (150,158).
- *Fetal/neonatal morphometrics*: Marijuana **use ≥4 times per week** was associated with a 131 g (95% CI 209–52) **reduction in mean birth weight** in a meta-analysis of five studies (138). Less frequent use was not associated with significant alterations in birth weight (139). Additionally,

there is no association with low birth weight (139). The effect, if any, on length and head circumference is small (approximately 0.5 cm) (127,130,140). Only one study reported an increased incidence of SGA (OR, 3.8; 95% CI 1.2–14).

- *Neonatal withdrawal*: Examination of **neonates** of moderate to heavy marijuana smokers using the Brazelton Neonatal Assessment Scale demonstrated **altered responses to visual stimuli, increased tremulousness, and a high-pitched cry** (134). These findings were no longer present by one month of age.
- *Long-term neonatal outcome*: Frequent, more than weekly, maternal marijuana use may be a risk factor for sudden infant death syndrome (141). Studies including children up to 12 years old, who were prenatally exposed to marijuana, demonstrate normal language and intelligence; however, there are conflicting findings with regard to behavior, namely hyperactivity and attention (131).

Therapy
Currently, there is no approved pharmacotherapy for marijuana abuse.

Antepartum Testing
The role of antepartum surveillance for marijuana exposure is insufficiently studied to make recommendations.

Anesthesia
Drugs affecting maternal heart rate and blood pressure should be used with caution. Adverse interactions have been reported between marijuana and drugs such as propranolol (53). Likewise, during cesarean section under general anesthesia, the combination of marijuana and certain inhaled anesthetics can result in pronounced myocardial depression (53). If general anesthesia is planned, the airway effects of chronic smoke inhalation should be considered (53). Cross-tolerance to opioids and benzodiazepines may make dosing difficult (53).

Postpartum/Breast-feeding
THC levels in breast milk are up to eight times higher than in maternal serum (131,142). The AAP Committee on Drugs strongly advises that women should not use marijuana while breast-feeding as it may be hazardous to the infant and nursing mother (55).

PHENCYCLIDINE
Historic Notes
Phencyclidine (PCP) was developed as an anesthetic agent and produced effective anesthesia and analgesia with minimal respiratory and cardiovascular depression but was removed from the market because of a high incidence of delirium, agitation, and violence (143). The dissociative anesthetic ketamine is a derivative of PCP (143).

Diagnosis/Definition
The chemical name of PCP is 1-(1-phenylcyclohexyl) piperidine. Street names for PCP include angel dust, hog, ozone, rocket fuel, shermans, wack, crystal, and embalming fluid. PCP is most commonly smoked (73%) or snorted (13%), but can also be swallowed (12%) or injected (2%) (144,145).

Symptoms
Most women who abuse PCP do so only occasionally and a typical dose is 5 mg. Chronic use may lead to habituation and the need for doses as high as 100 mg to achieve the same feeling (146). Common symptoms of intoxication are nystagmus, hypertension, altered consciousness (e.g., depressed), mental status changes (e.g., disorientation and hallucinations), and bizarre behavior (e.g., agitation and violence) (143). Although rare, acute psychosis and death have been reported (147).

Epidemiology/Incidence
Although popular in the 1970s, PCP abuse declined in the late 1980s and 1990s but has recently reemerged as a drug of abuse (148). In the early 1980s, PCP use by pregnant women in Cleveland ranged from 5.8% (by testing) to 6.4% (by history) (145,149). A more recent estimate is unavailable.

Etiology/Basic Pathophysiology
The exact mechanism of action of PCP is unclear. PCP is an *N*-methyl D-aspartate (NMDA) receptor antagonist (150). PCP crosses the placenta and can be detected in amniotic fluid, umbilical cord blood (151–153), and neonatal urine (154). Concentrations in the fetus may exceed maternal levels (12,90,95).

Risk Factors/Associations
The rate of concomitant tobacco use ranges from 43% to 84% (146,155–157). The majority of pregnant women that use PCP during pregnancy also abuse other illicit drugs (e.g., cocaine) and alcohol.

Pregnancy Complications
There is a **high rate of polysubstance abuse by women using PCP**, which limits the ability to tease out the obstetrical and neonatal effects PCP abuse. The use of matched, non–drug-exposed controls was infrequent.

- *Congenital anomalies*: Although there were early case reports of infants exposed antenatally to PCP born with dysmorphic facial features (149,158) and a report of an infant with a cerebellar malformation, **no increased rate of congenital malformations** have been reported in a literature review totaling 206 neonates with prenatal PCP exposure (159).
- *Obstetrical complications*: The rate of **PTB** among PCP-exposed neonates was 20% to 22% (155,158).
- *Fetal/neonatal morphometrics*: Prenatal exposure to PCP has not been consistently shown to affect birth weight, length, or head circumference (145,156,157). However, higher-than-expected rates of **IUGR** (32%) (155), **LBW** (30%) (158), and **SGA** (17%) (158) have been reported.
- *Neonatal withdrawal*: Neonatal withdrawal from PCP is characterized by neurological (e.g., tremor, abnormal tone, and hypertonic reflexes) and gastrointestinal (e.g., emesis and diarrhea) symptoms, irritability, exaggerated responses to auditory and tactile stimuli, and rapid shifts in consciousness (145,146,154,157,158,160). Symptoms of withdrawal were reported in 55% of 22 infants with exposure to PCP alone (158). Symptoms of withdrawal can be managed conservatively (e.g., swaddling), by acidification of the urine, or when medications are indicated, with phenobarbital, diazepam, or paregoric.

- *Long-term neonatal outcome*: Studies of long-term neuro-developmental outcome are limited by small size and dropout rates of over 50%. At 12 to 18 months of age, exposed infants demonstrated **impaired fine motor skills** (160). Caretakers reported **behavioral problems (e.g., temper tantrums and oppositional behaviors), inconsolability, and sleep disturbances** (158,160).

Therapy

Mild symptoms can be managed with isolation and by "talking-down." Additional symptoms and their treatments are as follows: convulsions are treated with diazepam, hypertension with antihypertensives (e.g., hydralazine), fever with antipyretics, and severe rigidity and rhabdomyolysis with dantrolene (12,161). There are currently no FDA-approved medications available for detoxification or maintenance of PCP dependence.

Antepartum Testing

The role of antepartum surveillance is insufficiently studied to make recommendations. However, hypertension in response to moderate to high doses of PCP may be an indication for non-stress testing and/or ultrasound to estimate fetal weight (12).

Postpartum/Breast-feeding

PCP is present in breast milk (151,152). The AAP Committee on Drugs strongly advises that women should not use PCP while breast-feeding as it may be hazardous to the infant and nursing mother (55).

HALLUCINOGENS: LYSERGIC ACID DIETHYLAMIDE, PSILOCYBIN (MAGIC MUSHROOMS), PEYOTE (MESCALINE)
Historic Notes

Naturally occurring hallucinogens have been used for centuries as part of religious and cultural activities. LSD, the prototypical synthetic hallucinogen, was synthesized in 1938 by the chemist Albert Hofmann who recognized its hallucinogenic capabilities when he was accidentally exposed.

Diagnosis/Definition

The active ingredients in psilocybin and peyote are psilocin (*N*, *N*-dimethyl-4-phosphoryloxytryptamine) and 3,4,5-trimethoxy-pheneylamine. LSD is an ergot (rye fungus) derivative. Street names are as follows:

- LSD: acid, trips, microdots, dots, blotters (or named by the design on the blotting paper), mellow or tabs
- Psilocybin: magic mushrooms, shrooms, magics, blue meanies, liberty caps, golden tops, mushies
- Peyote: buttons, cactus, mesc

LSD can be taken orally as a tablet, capsule or liquid applied to blotter paper, sniffed, injected, or smoked. Psilocybin and peyote are usually taken orally; peyote can also be smoked.

Symptoms

Hallucinogens principally alter sensory perceptions, mood, and thought patterns. Vital sign abnormalities are uncommon, but may include increased blood pressure and heart rate. Rare complications include hyperthermia and serotonin syndrome.

Epidemiology/Incidence

According to the National Household Survey on Drug Abuse, 0.2% of reproductive age women aged 15 to 44 years reported hallucinogen use in the past month. Among pregnant women screened for inclusion in a study of prenatal methamphetamine exposure, <0.5% used hallucinogens.

Etiology/Basic Pathophysiology

Evidence that LSD causes DNA damage in vitro raises concerns about its potential as a teratogen (162).

Complications

The effects of hallucinogen exposure on obstetrical neonatal outcome are not well studied.

- *Congenital anomalies*: In a literature review including 162 pregnancies with parental LSD use before or during pregnancy, there were 7 anomalies (4.3%) not attributable to other causes. **Limb reduction defects** accounted for 5 of the 7 anomalies; a higher-than-expected incidence (1.78/1000) (163). Another series of 148 pregnancies, including specimens from spontaneous and induced abortions, with parental LSD use showed a 9.6% rate of major anomalies that were mainly **central nervous system** (hydrocephalus and arteriovenous malformations) and **neural tube defects**. Because of lack of appropriate controls and confounding by use of other illicit substances, tobacco, and alcohol, a cause-and-effect relationship cannot be established (163,164). There are no reports of human teratogenesis because of psilocybin or peyote (162).
- *Obstetrical and neonatal complications*: There is no evidence that LSD, or other hallucinogens, increased the risk of PTB or have an effect on birth weight.
- *Long-term neonatal outcome*: Follow-up of children, whose parents used LSD, to 2.5 years old showed no growth or developmental abnormalities (164).

Therapy

In most cases, supportive care is all that is necessary. Benzodiazepines are the first-line treatment for acute agitation. Rarely, severe hyperthermia may require paralysis. There are currently no FDA-approved medications available for detoxification or maintenance of hallucinogen dependence.

Antepartum Testing

The role of antepartum surveillance is insufficiently studied to make recommendations. However, hyperthermia and serotonin syndrome may be an indication for fetal monitoring.

REFERENCES

1. Rayburn WF, Bogenschutz MP. Pharmacotherapy for pregnant women with addictions. Am J Obstet Gynecol 2004; 191(6):1885–1897. [Review; III]
2. National Survey on Drug Use & Health. Available at: http://www.oas.samhsa.gov/nhsda.htm. Last accessed February 13, 2011. [Survey; level III]
3. Azadi A, Dildy GA 3rd. Universal screening for substance abuse at the time of parturition. Am J Obstet Gynecol 2008; 198(5):e30–e32. [II-3]
4. Martin J, Payte JT, Zweben JE. Methadone maintenance treatment: a primer for physicians. J Psychoactive Drugs 1991; 23 (2):165–176. [Review; III]

5. ACOG. Motivational interviewing: a tool for behavioral change. ACOG Committee Opinion No. 423. Obstet Gynecol 2009; 113 (1):243–246. [III]

6. Kuczkowski KM. The effects of drug abuse on pregnancy. Curr Opin Obstet Gynecol 2007; 19(6):578–585. [Review; III]

7. ACOG. Cocaine in pregnancy. ACOG Committee Opinion No. 114. Int J Gynaecol Obstet 1993; 41(1):102–105. [III]

8. Terplan M, Lui S. Psychosocial interventions for pregnant women in outpatient illicit drug treatment programs compared to other interventions. Cochrane Database Syst Rev 2007; 17(4): CD006037. [Systematic Review; I]

9. Whitworth M, Dowswell T. Routine pre-pregnancy health promotion for improving pregnancy outcomes. Cochrane Database Syst Rev 2009; 7(4):CD007536. [Systematic Review; I]

10. ACOG. Substance abuse in pregnancy. ACOG Technical Bulletin No. 195. Int J Gynaecol Obstet 1994; 47(1):73–80. [III]

11. National Institute on Drug. Abuse screening for drug use in general medical settings. Available at: http://www.nida.nih. gov/nidamed/resguide/resourceguide.pdf. Last accessed May 6, 2011. [III]

12. Glantz CJ, Woods JR Jr. Cocaine, heroin, and phencyclidine: obstetric perspective. Clin Obstet Gynecol 1993; 36(2):279–301. [Review; III]

13. Wilbourne P, Wallerstedt C, Dorato V, et al. Clinical management of methadone dependence during pregnancy. J Perinat Neonatal Nurs 2001; 14(4):26–45.[Review; III]

14. Brown HL, Britton KA, Mahaffey D, et al. Methadone maintenance in pregnancy: a reappraisal. Am J Obstet Gynecol 1998; 179(2):459–463. [Review; III]

15. U.S. Drug Enforcement Administration. Heroin. Available at: http://www.justice.gov/dea/concern/heroin.html. Last accessed May 6, 2011.

16. Kaltenbach K, Berghella V, Finnegan L. Opioid dependence during pregnancy: effects and management. Obstet Gynecol Clin North Am 1998; 25(1):139–151. [Review; III]

17. Broussard CS, Rasmussen SA, Reefhuis J, et al. for the National Birth Defects Prevention Study. Maternal treatment with opioid analgesics and risk for birth defects. Am J Obstet Gynecol 2011; 204(4):314.e1–e11. [II-2]

18. Organization for Teratology Information Specialists. Prescription Opioids and Pregnancy. Available at: http://www.otis-pregnancy.org/files/rxopioids.pdf. Last accessed May 6, 2011.[III]

19. Almario CV, Seligman NS, Dysart KC, et al. Risk factors for preterm birth among opiate-addicted gravid women in a methadone treatment program. Am J Obstet Gynecol 2009; 201(3):326. e1–326.e6. [II-2]

20. Stimmel B, Goldberg J, Reisman A, et al. Fetal outcome in narcotic-dependent women: the importance of the type of maternal narcotic used. Am J Drug Alcohol Abuse 1982; 9(4):383–395. [II-2]

21. Kandall SR, Albin S, Lowinson J, et al. Differential effects of maternal heroin and methadone use on birthweight. Pediatrics 1976; 58(5):681–685. [II-2]

22. Doberczak TM, Thronton JC, Bernstein J, et al. Impact of maternal drug dependency on birth weight and head circumference of offspring. Am J Dis Child 1987; 141(11):1163–1167. [II-2]

23. Kaltenbach K, Silverman N, Wapner RJ. Methadone maintenance during pregnancy. In: Parrino MW, ed. State Methadone Treatment Guidelines. Rockville, MD: U.S. Department of Health and Human Services, Center for Substance Abuse Treatment, 1992:85–93. [Review III]

24. Oei J, Lui K. Management of the newborn affected by maternal opiates and other drugs of dependency. J Paediatr Child Health 2007; 43(1–2):9–18. [Review; III]

25. Finnegan LP, Connaughton JF Jr., Kron RE, et al. Neonatal abstinence syndrome: assessment and management. Addict Dis 1975; 2(1–2):141–158. [II-3]

26. Kraft WK, Gibson E, Dysart K, et al. Sublingual buprenorphine for treatment of neonatal abstinence syndrome: a randomized trial. Pediatrics 2008; 122(3):e601–e607. [RCT, n = 26; I]

27. Hunt RW, Tzioumi D, Collins E, et al. Adverse neurodevelopmental outcome of infants exposed to opiates in-utero. Early Hum Dev 2008; 84(1):29–35. [Review; III]

28. Rayburn W, Bogenschutz M. Pharmacotherapy for pregnant women with addictions. Am J Obstet Gynecol 2004; 191 (6):1885–1897. [Review III]

29. Mattick RP, Breen C, Kimber J, et al. Buprenorphine maintenance versus placebo or methadone maintenance for opioid dependence. Cochrane Database Syst Rev 2008; 16(2):CD002207. [Systematic Review; I]

30. Dashe JS, Sheffield JS, Olscher DA, et al. Relationship between maternal methadone dosage and neonatal withdrawal. Obstet Gynecol 2002; 100(6):1244–1249. [II-2]

31. Maas U, Kattner E, Weingart-Jesse B, et al. Infrequent neonatal opiate withdrawal following maternal methadone detoxification during pregnancy. J Perinat Med 1990; 18(2):111–118. [II-2]

32. Amato L, Davoli M, Minozzi S, et al. Methadone at tapered doses for the management of opioid withdrawal. Cochrane Database Syst Rev 2005; 20(3):CD003409. [Systematic Review; I]

33. Maura S, Resemble A. Leaving methadone treatment: lessons learned, lessons forgotten, lessons ignored. Mt Sinai J Med 2001; 68:62–74. [Review; III]

34. Rementeriá JL, Nunag NN. Narcotic withdrawal in pregnancy: stillbirth incidence with a case report. Am J Obstet Gynecol 1973; 116(8):1152–1155. [II-3]

35. Zuspan FP, Gumpel JA, Mejia-Zelaya A, et al. Fetal stress from methadone withdrawal. Am J Obstet Gynecol 1975; 122(1):43–46.

36. Dashe JS, Jackson GL, Olscher DA, et al. Opioid detoxification in pregnancy. Obstet Gynecol 1998; 92(5):854–858. [II-3]

37. Blinick G, Wallach RC, Jerez E. Pregnancy in narcotics addicts treated by medical withdrawal. The methadone detoxification program. Am J Obstet Gynecol 1969; 105(7):997–1003.

38. Berghella V, Lim PJ, Hill MK, et al. Maternal methadone dose and neonatal withdrawal. Am J Obstet Gynecol 2003; 189(2): 312–317. [II-2]

39. Seligman NS, Weiner SM, Berghella V. Methadone maintenance therapy during pregnancy. In: Basow DS, ed. UpToDate. Waltham: UpToDate, 2011.[Review; III]

40. Drozdick JD, Berghella V, Hill MK, et al. Methadone trough levels in pregnancy. Am J Obstet Gynecol 2002; 187(5):1184–1188. [II-2]

41. Edelin KC, Gurganious L, Golar K, et al. Methadone maintenance in pregnancy: consequences to care and outcome. Obstet Gynecol 1988; 71(3 pt 1):399–404. [II-2]

42. Strauss ME, Andresko M, Stryker JC, et al. Relationship of neonatal withdrawal to maternal methadone dose. Am J Drug Alcohol Abuse 1976; 3(2):339–345. [II-2]

43. Cleary BJ, Donnelly J, Strawbridge J, et al. Methadone dose and neonatal abstinence syndrome-systematic review and meta-analysis. Addiction 2010; 105(12):2071–2084.[Meta-analysis]

44. Seligman NS, Almario CV, Hayes EJ, et al. Relationship between maternal methadone dose at delivery and neonatal abstinence syndrome. J Pediatr 2010; 57(3):428–433, 433.e1. [II-2]

45. Seligman NS, Salva N, Hayes EJ, et al. Predicting length of treatment for neonatal abstinence syndrome in methadone-exposed neonates. Am J Obstet Gynecol 2008; 199(4):396.e1–396.e7. [II-2]

46. Hayes E, Seligman N, Horowitz K, et al. 252: Dose-response relationship between maternal methadone dose and decreased neonatal head circumference. Am J Obstet Gynecol 2007; 197(6 suppl):s81. [II-2]

47. Hamilton R, McGlone L, MacKinnon JR, et al. Ophthalmic, clinical, and visual electrophysiological findings in children born to mothers prescribed substitute methadone in pregnancy. Br J Ophthalmol 2010; 94(6):696–700. [II-3]

48. Physician Buprenorphine Training Events. Available at: http:// buprenorphine.samhsa.gov/pls/bwns/training. Last accessed May 6, 2011. [III]

49. Minozzi S, Amato L, Vecchi S, et al. Maintenance agonist treatments for opiate dependent pregnant women. Cochrane Database Syst Rev 2008; 16(2):CD006318. [Systematic Review; I]

50. Jones H, Kaltenbach K, Heil SH, et al. Neonatal abstinence syndrome after methadone or buprenorphine exposure. N Engl J Med 2010; 363(24):2320–2331. [RCT]

51. Fischer G, Jagsch R, Eder H, et al. Comparison of methadone and slow- release morphine maintenance in pregnant addicts. Addiction 1999; 94(2):231–239. [RCT, n = 48; I]

52. Kashiwagi M, Arlettaz R, Lauper U, et al. Methadone maintenance program in a Swiss perinatal center: (I): management and outcome of 89 pregnancies. Acta Obstet Gynecol Scand 2005; 84 (2):140–144. [II-3]

53. Kuczkowski KM. Anesthetic implications of drug abuse in pregnancy. J Clin Anesth 2003; 15(5):382–394. [Review; III]

54. Meyer M, Wagner K, Benvenuto A, et al. Intrapartum and post-partum analgesia for women maintained on methadone during pregnancy. Obstet Gynecol 2007; 110(2, pt 1):261–266. [II-2]

55. American Academy of Pediatrics Committee on Drugs. Transfer of drugs and other chemicals into human milk. Pediatrics 2001; 108(3):776–789. [III]

56. Lim S, Prasad MR, Samuels P, et al. High-dose methadone in pregnant women and its effect on duration of neonatal absti-nence syndrome. Am J Obstet Gynecol 2009; 200(1):70.e1–70.e5. [II-2]

57. Abdel-Latif ME, Pinner J, Clews S, et al. Effects of breast milk on the severity and outcome of neonatal abstinence syndrome among infants of drug-dependent mothers. Pediatrics 2006; 117(6):e1163–e1169. [II-2]

58. Jansson LM, Choo R, Velez ML, et al. Methadone maintenance and breastfeeding in the neonatal period. Pediatrics 2008; 121 (1):106–114. [II-2]

59. Ballard JL. Treatment of neonatal abstinence syndrome with breast milk containing methadone. J Perinat Neonatal Nurs 2002; 15(4):76–85. [III]

60. Liu AJ, Nanan R. Letter to the Editor: methadone maintenance and breastfeeding in the neonatal period. Pediatrics 2008; 121 (4):869. [III]

61. Drug and Lactation Database: Buprenorphine. Available at: http://toxnet.nlm.nih.gov/cgi-bin/sis/htmlgen?LACT, CAS#52485-79-7. [III]

62. Drugs and Chemical of Concern: Cocaine. Available at: http://www.deadiversion.usdoj.gov/drugs_concern/cocaine/cocaine. htm. Last accessed February 7, 2011. [III]

63. Hernandez M, Birnbach DJ, Van Zundert AJ. Anesthetic man-agement of the illicit-substance-using patient. Curr Opin Anaes-thesiol 2005; 18(3):3115–3124. [Review; III]

64. Woods JR Jr. Pregnancy increases cardiovascular toxicity to cocaine. Am J Obstet Gynecol 1990; 162(2):529–533. [II-2]

65. Plessinger MA, Woods JR Jr. Maternal, placental, and fetal pathophysiology of cocaine exposure during pregnancy. Clin Obstet Gynecol 1993; 36(2):267–278. [Review; III]

66. Gaither K. Cocaine abuse in pregnancy: an evolution from panacea to pandemonium. South Med J 2008; 101(8):783–784. [Editorial]

67. Plessinger MA, Woods JR Jr. Cocaine in pregnancy: recent data on maternal and fetal risks. Obstet Gynecol Clin North Am 1998; 25(1):99–118. [Review; III]

68. Richardson GA, Day NL, McGauhey PJ. Impact of prenatal marijuana and cocaine use on the infant and child. Clin Obstet Gynecol 1993; 36(2):302–318. [Review; III]

69. Bauer CR, Langer JC, Shankaran S, et al. Acute neonatal effects of cocaine exposure during pregnancy. Arch Pediatr Adolesc Med 2005; 159(9):824–834. [II-2]

70. Bhuvaneswar CG, Chnag G, Epstein LA, et al. Cocaine and opioid use during pregnancy: prevalence and management. Prim Care Companion J Clin Psychiatry 2008; 10(1):59–65. [Review III]

71. Hull L, May J, Farrell-Moore D, et al. Treatment of cocaine abuse during pregnancy: translating research to clinical practice. Curr Psychiatry Rep 2010; 12(5):454–461. [Review III]

72. Monga M, Weisbrodt NW, Andres RL, et al. The acute effect of cocaine exposure on pregnant human myometrial contractile activity. Am J Obstet Gynecol 1993; 169(4):782–785. [II-3]

73. Oyelese Y, Ananth CV. Placental abruption. Obstet Gynecol 2006; 108(4):1005–1016. [Review III]

74. Day NL, Cottreau CM, Richardson GA. The epidemiology of alcohol, marijuana, and cocaine use among women of child-bearing age and pregnant women. Clin Obstet Gynecol 1993; 36 (2):232–245. [Review III]

75. Addis A, Moretti ME, Syed FA, et al. Fetal effects of cocaine: an updated meta-analysis. Reprod Toxicol 2001; 15:341–369. [Meta-analysis]

76. Meyer KD, Zhang L. Short- and long-term adverse effects of cocaine abuse during pregnancy on the heart development. Ther Adv Cardiovasc Dis 2009; 3(1):7–16. [Review III]

77. Gouin K, Murphy K, Shah PS, and the Knowledge Synthesis Group on Determinants of Low Birth Weight and Preterm Births. Effects of cocaine use during pregnancy on low birth-weight and preterm birth: systematic review and metaanaly-ses. Am J Obstet Gynecol 2011; 204:304.e1–304.e12. [Meta-analysis]

78. Bingol N, Fuchs M, Diaz V, et al. Teratogenicity of cocaine in humans. J Pediatr 1987; 110(1):93–96. [II-2]

79. Kuczkowski KM. The cocaine abusing parturient: a review of anesthetic considerations. Can J Anesth 2004; 51(2):145–154. [Review III]

80. DeLaney DB, Larrabee KD, Monga M. Preterm premature rup-ture of the membranes associated with recent cocaine use. Am J Perinatol 1997; 14(5):285–288. [II-2]

81. Dinsmoor MJ, Iron SJ, Christmas JT. Preterm premature rupture of the membranes associated with recent cocaine use. Am J Obstet Gynecol 1994; 171(2):305–308. [II-2]

82. Cordero DR, Medina C, Helfgott A. Cocaine body packing in pregnancy. Ann Emerg Med 2006; 48(3):323–325. [II-3]

83. Richardson GA, Goldschmidt L, Willford J. Continued effects of prenatal cocaine use: preschool development. Neurotoxicol Ter-atol 2009; 31(6):325–333. [II-2]

84. Shankaran S, Banh CM, Bauer CR, et al. Prenatal cocaine expo-sure and BMI and blood pressure at 9 years of age. J Hypertens 2010; 28(6):1166–1175. [II-2]

85. Elk R, Mangus L, Rhoades H, et al. Cessation of cocaine use during pregnancy: effects of contingency management interven-tions on maintaining abstinence and complying with prenatal care. Addict Behav 1998; 23(1):57–64. [RCT, n = 12; I]

86. Svikis DS, Golden AS, Huggins GR, et al. Cost-effectiveness of treatment for drug-abusing pregnant women. Drug Alcohol Depend 1997; 45(1–2):105–113. [III]

87. Berman S, O'Neill J, Fears S, et al. Abuse of amphetamines and structural abnormalities in brain. Ann N Y Acad Sci 2008; 1141:195–220. [Review; III]

88. Anglin MD, Burke C, Perrochet B, et al. History of the meth-amphetamine problem. J Psychoactive Drugs 2000; 32(2):137–141. [Review; III]

89. Skelton MR, Williams MT, Vorhees CV. Developmental effects of 3,4-methylenedioxymethamphetamine: a review. Behav Phar-macol 2008; 19(2):91–111. [Review; III]

90. Plessinger MA. Prenatal exposure to amphetamines. Risks and adverse outcomes in pregnancy. Obstet Gynecol Clin North Am 1998; 25(1):119–138. [Review III]

91. Terplan M, Smith EJ, Kozloski MJ, et al. Methamphetamine use among pregnant women. Obstet Gynecol 2009; 113(6):1285–1291. [II-3]

92. Green AR, Mechan AO, Elliott JM, et al. The pharmacology and clinical pharmacology of 3,4-methylenedioxymethamphetamine (MDMA, "ecstasy"). Pharmacol Rev 2003; 55(3):463–508. [Review; III]

93. Johnston LD, O'Malley PM, Bachman JG, et al. Monitoring the Future national survey results on drug use, 1975–2006. Volume I: secondary school students (NIH Publication No. 07-6202). Bethesda, MD: National Institute on Drug Abuse, 2007. [II-3]

94. Ho E, Karimi-Tabesh L, Gideon K. Characteristics of pregnant women who use Ecstasy (3, 4-methylenedioxymethamphet-amine. Neurotoxicol Teratol 2001; 23(6):561–567. [II-2]

95. Good MM, Solt I, Acuna JG, et al. Methamphetamine use during pregnancy: maternal and neonatal implications. Obstet Gynecol 2010; 116(2 pt 1):330–334. [II-2, $n = 276$]

96. Della Grotta S, LaGrasse LL, Arria AM, et al. Patterns of methamphetamine use during pregnancy: results from the Infant Development, Environment, and Lifestyle (IDEAL) study. Matern Child Health J 2010; 14(4):519–527. [II-2]

97. Arria AM, Derauf C, Lagasse LL, et al. Methamphetamine and other substance use during pregnancy: preliminary estimates from the Infant Development, Environment, and Lifestyle (IDEAL) study. Matern Child Health J 2006; 10(3):293–302. [II-3]

98. Nguyen D, Smith LM, LaGrasse LL, et al. Intrauterine growth of infants exposed to prenatal methamphetamine: results from the infant development, environment, and lifestyle study. J Pediatr 2010; 157(2):337–339. [II-2]

99. Derauf C, LaGrasse LL, Smith LM, et al. Demographic and psychosocial characteristics of mothers using methamphetamine during pregnancy: preliminary results of the Infant Development, Environment, and Lifestyle Study (IDEAL). Am J Drug Alcohol Abuse 2007; 33(2):281–289. [II-2]

100. Smith LM, LaGrasse LL, Derauf C, et al. The Infant Development, Environment, and Lifestyle Study (IDEAL): effects of prenatal methamphetamine exposure, polydrug exposure, and poverty on intrauterine growth. Pediatrics 2006; 118(3): 1149–1156. [II-2]

101. McElhatton PR, Bateman DN, Evans C, et al. Congenital anomalies after prenatal ecstasy exposure. Lancet 1999; 354:1441–1442. [II-3]

102. Eriksson M, Larsson G, Windbladh B, et al. The influence of amphetamine addiction on pregnancy and the newborn. Acta Paediatr Scand 1978; 67(1):95–99. [II-3]

103. Eriksson M, Larsson G, Zetterström R. Amphetamine addiction and pregnancy. II. Pregnancy, delivery and the neonatal period. Socio-medical aspects. Acta Obstet Gynecol Scand 1981; 60 (3):253–259. [II-2]

104. Oro AS, Dixon SD. Perinatal cocaine and methamphetamine exposure: maternal and neonatal correlates. J Pediatr 1987; 111 (4):571–578. [II-2]

105. Cernerud L, Eriksson M, Jonsson B, et al. Amphetamine addiction during pregnancy: 14-year follow-up of growth and school performance. Acta Paediatr 1996; 85(2):204–208. [II-2]

106. Smith LM, LaGasse LL, Derauf C, et al. Prenatal methamphetamine use and neonatal neurobehavioral outcome. Neurotoxical Teratol 2008; 30(1):20–28. [II-2]

107. Smith LM, Chang L, Yonekura ML, et al. Brain proton magnetic resonance spectroscopy in children exposed to methamphetamine in utero. Neurology 2001; 57(2):255–260. [II-2]

108. Chang L, Smith LM, LoPresti C, et al. Smaller subcortical volumes and cognitive deficits in children with prenatal methamphetamine exposure. Psychiatry Res 2004; 132(2):95–106. [II-2]

109. Lu LH, Johnson A, O'Hare ED, et al. Effects of prenatal methamphetamine exposure on verbal memory revealed with fMRI. J Dev Behav Pediatr 2009; 30(3):185–192. [II-2]

110. McElhatton PR. The effects of benzodiazepine use during pregnancy and lactation. Reprod Toxicol 1994; 8(6):461–475. [Review; III]

111. Wikner BN, Stiller CO, Bergman U, et al. Use of benzodiazepines and benzodiazepine receptor agonists during pregnancy: neonatal outcome and congenital malformations. Pharmacoepidemiol Drug Saf 2007; 16(11):1203–1210. [II-2]

112. Dolovich LR, Addis A, Vaillancourt JM, et al. Benzodiazepine use in pregnancy and major malformations or oral cleft: meta-analysis of cohort and case-control studies. BMJ 1998; 317 (7162):839–843. [Meta-analysis]

113. Garne E, Bergman U. Benzodiazepine use in pregnancy and major malformations or oral clefts: Induced abortions should be included. BMJ 1999; 319(7214):918. [III]

114. Wikner BN, Stiller CO, Källén B, et al. Use of benzodiazepines and benzodiazepine receptor agonists during pregnancy: maternal characteristics. Pharmacoepidemiol Drug Saf 2007; 16 (9):988–994. [II-2]

115. Bonnot O, Vollset SE, Godet PF, et al. Maternal exposure to lorazepam and anal atresia in newborns: results from a hypothesis-generating study of benzodiazepines and malformations. J Clin Psychopharmacol 2001; 21(4):456–458. [II-2]

116. ACOG. Use of psychiatric medication during pregnancy and lactation. ACOG Practice Bulletin No. 92. Obstet Gynecol 2008; 111(4):1001–1020. [III]

117. Altshuler LL, Cohen L, Szuba MP, et al. Pharmacologic management of psychiatric illness during pregnancy: dilemmas and guidelines. Am J Psychiatry 1996; 153(5):592–606. [III]

118. Eros E, Czeizel AE, Rockenbauer M, et al. A population-based case-control teratologic study of nitrazepam, medazepam, tofisopam, alprazolum and clonazepam treatment during pregnancy. Eur J Obstet Gynecol Reprod Biol 2002; 101(2):147–154. [II-2]

119. Cree JE, Meyer J, Hailey DM. Diazepam in labour: its metabolism and effect on the clinical condition and thermogenesis of the newborn. Br Med J 1973; 4(5887):251–255. [II-3]

120. Whitelaw AGL, Cummings AJ, McFadyen IR. Effects of maternal lorazepam on the neonate. Br Med J 1981; 282(6270): 1106–1108. [II-3]

121. American Academy of Pediatrics Committee on Drugs. Neonatal drug withdrawal. Pediatrics 1998; 101(6):1079–1088. [III]

122. Sutton LR, Hinderliter SA. Diazepam abuse in pregnant women on methadone maintenance. Implications for the neonate. Clin Pediatr 1990; 29(2):108–111. [II-3]

123. Lagreid L, Hagberg G, Lundberg A. Neurodevelopment in late infancy after prenatal exposure to benzodiazepines—a prospective study. Neuropediatrics 1992; 23(2):60–67. [II-2]

124. Hartz SC, Heinonen OP, Shapiro S, et al. Antenatal exposure to meprobamate and chlordiazepoxide in relation to malformations, mental development, and childhood mortality. N Engl J Med 1975; 292(14):726–728. [II-2]

125. Childers SR, Breivogel CS. Cannabis and endogenous cannabinoid systems. Drug Alcohol Depend 1998; 51(1–2):173–187. [Review; III]

126. Kuczkowski KM. Marijuana in pregnancy. Ann Acad Med Singapore 2004; 33(3):336–339. [III]

127. de Moraes Barros MC, Guinsburg R, de Arújo Peres C, et al. Exposure to marijuana during pregnancy alters neurobehavior in the early neonatal period. J Pediatr 2006; 149(6):781–787. [Review; III]

128. Fergusson DM, Horwood LJ, Northstone K, ALSPAC Study Team. Maternal use of cannabis and pregnancy outcome. BJOG 2002; 109(1):21–27. [II-2]

129. Witter FR, Niebyl JR. Marijuana use in pregnancy and pregnancy outcome. Am J Perinatol 1990; 7(1):36–38. [II-2]

130. Bada HS, Reynolds EW, Hansen WF. Marijuana use, adolescent pregnancy, and alteration in newborn behavior: how complex can it get? J Pediatr 2006; 149(6):742–745. [Comment]

131. Kozer E, Koren G. Effects of prenatal exposure to marijuana. Can Fam Physician 2001; 47:264–264. [III]

132. El Marroun H, Tiemeier H, Steegers EA, et al. A prospective study on intrauterine cannabis exposure and fetal blood flow. Early Hum Dev 2010; 86(4):231–236. [II-2]

133. Cornelius MD, Taylor PM, Geva D, et al. Prenatal tobacco and marijuana use among adolescents: effects on offspring gestational age, growth, and morphology. Pediatrics 1995; 95(5): 738–743. [II-2]

134. Fried PA. Prenatal exposure to tobacco and marijuana: effect during pregnancy, infancy, and early childhood. Clin Obstet Gynecol 1993; 36(2):319–337. [Review III]

135. Jobe AH. Marijuana effects on neurobehavior of newborns. J Pediatr 2006; 149(6):a1. [III]

136. Linn S, Schoenbaum SC, Monson RR, et al. The association of marijuana use with outcome of pregnancy. Am J Public Health 1983; 73(10):1161–1164. [II-2]

137. Fried PA, Watkinson B, Willan A. Marijuana use during pregnancy and decreased length of gestation. Am J Obstet Gynecol 1984; 150(1):23–27. [II-2]

138. English DR, Hulse GK, Milne E, et al. Maternal cannabis use and birth weight: a meta-analysis. Addiction 1997; 92(11):1553–1560. [Meta-analysis]

139. Zuckerman B, Frank DA, Hingson R, et al. Effects of maternal marijuana and cocaine use on fetal growth. N Engl J Med 1989; 320(12):762–768. [II-2]

140. Hatch EE, Bracken MB. Effect of Marijuana use in pregnancy on fetal growth. Am J Epidemiol 1986; 124(6):986–993. [II-2]

141. Scragg RK, Mitchell EA, Ford RP, et al. Maternal cannabis use in the sudden death syndrome. Acta Paediatr 2001; 90(1):57–60. [II-2]

142. Perez-Reyes M, Wall ME. Presence of delta9-tetrahydrocannabinol in human milk. N Engl J Med 1982; 307(13):819–820. [II-3]

143. Baldridge EB, Bessen HA. Phencycldine. Emerg Med Clin North Am 1990; 8(3):541–550. [Review III]

144. McCarron MM, Schulze BW, Thompson GA, et al. Acute phencyclidine intoxication: incidence of clinical findings in 1000 cases. Ann Emerg Med 1981; 10:237. [II-3]

145. Golden NL, Kuhnert BR, Sokol RJ, et al. Neonatal manifestation of maternal phencyclidine exposure. J Perinat Med 1987; 15 (2):185–191. [II-2]

146. Golden NL, Kuhnert BR, Sokol RJ, et al. Phencyclidine use during pregnancy. Am J Obstet Gynecol 1984; 148(3):254–259. [II-2]

147. Petrucha RA, Kaufman K, Pitts FN. Phencyclidine in pregnancy: a case report. J Reprod Med 1982; 27(5):301–303. [II-3]

148. Drugs and Chemical of Concern: Phencycldine. Available at: http://www.deadiversion.usdoj.gov/drugs_concern/pcp.htm. Last accessed February 4, 2010. [III]

149. Golden NL, Sokol RJ, Rubin IL. Angel dust: possible effects on the fetus. Pediatrics 1980; 65(1):18–20. [II-3]

150. Deutsch SI, Mastropaolo, Rosse RB. Neurodevelopmental consequences of early exposure to phencyclidine and related drugs. Clin Neuropharmacol 1998; 21(6):320–332. [Review; III]

151. Nicholas JM, Lipshitz J, Schreiber EC. Phencyclidine: its transfer across the placenta as well as into breast milk. Am J Obstet Gynecol 1982; 18:143–146. [II-3]

152. Kaufman KR, Petrucha RA, Pitts FN, et al. PCP in amniotic fluid and breast milk: case report. J Clin Psychiatry 1983; 44(7):269–270. [II-3]

153. Kaufman KR, Petrucha RA, Pitts FN Jr., et al. Phencyclidine in umbilical cord blood: preliminary data. Am J Psychiatry 1983; 140(4):40–452. [II-3]

154. Strauss AA, Mondanlou HD, Bosu SK. Neonatal manifestations of maternal phencyclidine (PCP) abuse. Pediatrics 1981; 68 (4):550–552. [II-3]

155. Tabor BL, Smith Wallace T, Yonekura ML. Perinatal outcome associated with PCP versus cocaine use. Am J Drug Alcohol Abuse 1990; 16(3–4):337–348. [II-2]

156. Mvula MM, Miller JM, Ragan FA. Relationship of phencyclidine and pregnancy outcome. J Reprod Med 1999; 44(12):1021–1024. [II-2]

157. Chasnoff IJ, Burns WJ, Hatcher RP, et al. Phencyclidine: effects on the fetus and neonate. Dev Pharmacol Ther 1983; 6(6):404–408. [II-2]

158. Wachsman L, Schuetz S, Chan LS, et al. What happens to babies exposed to phencyclidine (PCP) in utero? Am J Drug Alcohol Abuse 1989; 15(1):31–39. [II-3]

159. Fico TA, VanderWende C. Phencyclidine during pregnancy: behavioral and neurochemical effects in the offspring. Ann N Y Acad Sci 1989; 562:319–326. [II-3]

160. Howard J, Kropenske V, Tyler R. The long-term effects on neurodevelopment in infants exposed prenatally to PCP. NIDA Res Monogr 1986; 64:237–251. [II-3]

161. McCarron MM. Phencyclidine intoxication. NIDA Res Monogr 1986; 64:209–217. [II-3]

162. Illinois Teratogen Information Service. ITIS Newsletters: the effects of hallucinogen use during pregnancy. 2000; 8(2). Available at: http://www.fetal-exposure.org/resources/index.php/2000/10/01/the-effects-of-hallucinogen-use-during-pregnancy. Last accessed February 7, 2011. [II-3]

163. Long SY. Does LSD induce chromosomal damage and malformations? A review of the literature. Teratology 1972; 6(1):75–90. [Review; III]

164. Jacobson CB, Berlin CM. Possible reproductive detriment of LSD users. JAMA 1972; 222(11):1367–1373. [II-2]

24

Respiratory diseases: asthma, pneumonia, influenza, and tuberculosis

Lauren A. Plante and Laura A. Hart

ASTHMA
Key Points

- Asthma is characterized by airway obstruction, inflammation, and increased responsiveness to stimuli. To be certain of diagnosis, once abnormal forced expiratory volume in one second (FEV_1) is found in a patient with historic and physical exams findings consistent with asthma, other differential diagnoses must be excluded.
- Asthma is classified as **mild intermittent, mild persistent, moderate persistent, and severe persistent** by symptoms and peak expiratory flow rate (PEFR) or spirometry.
- Asthma has historically been associated with small increased risks of preterm birth, low birth weight, perinatal mortality, and preeclampsia, but these risks are probably associated just with undertreatment of asthma; **if asthma is adequately treated, it is not associated with a significant increase in adverse perinatal outcomes**.
- Pregnancy has a variable effect on asthma severity, with about two-thirds getting better and one-third worse.
- The **management** of asthma in pregnant women should follow the **same guidelines as for other nonpregnant patients**.
- Management is based on objective measurements of pulmonary function (PEFR) (Table 24.1). The management plan should include use of environmental control measures, adequate pharmacotherapy, and patient education regarding symptoms, management, and compliance.
- **Inhalation therapy is preferred to systemic treatments**, with **inhaled corticosteroids, NOT inhaled β-agonist, the mainstay of therapy**.
- Prostaglandin F2α should be avoided.

Diagnosis
Asthma is characterized by episodic symptoms of airway obstruction, which is at least in part reversible; alternative explanations must be excluded. Airway inflammation with edema and remodeling, rather than simply bronchospasm, is the key. Increased airway responsiveness to stimuli is characteristic. Indicators that suggest a diagnosis of asthma include wheezing, history of recurrent cough, chest tightness or difficulty in breathing; worsening of symptoms with exercise, viral infection, exposure to animal fur or feathers, mold, pollen, house dust mites, tobacco or wood smoke, changes in weather, airborne chemicals or dusts; or worsening of symptoms at night. Physical examination is not always reliable, and may include thoracic hyperexpansion or chest deformity, hunching of shoulders or use of accessory muscles, audible wheezing or a prolonged expiratory phase, increased nasal discharge or nasal polyps, or any manifestation of an allergic skin condition. The more indicators present, the more likely the diagnosis; however, the absence of wheezing does not equal the absence of asthma. If a diagnosis of asthma is being considered, the next step is spirometry to determine whether airflow obstruction is present, and, if so, whether it is reversible. Forced vital capacity (FVC), FEV_1, and FEV_1/FVC ratio are measured before and after administration of a short-acting bronchodilator. Reduced FEV_1 or FEV_1/FVC shows airflow limitation, and a 12% or greater improvement in FEV_1 after the administration of inhaled albuterol confirms reversibility. (1)

To be certain of an asthma diagnosis, **once abnormal FEV_1 is found in a patient with history and physical exam findings consistent with asthma, other differential diagnoses must be excluded**, such as chronic obstructive pulmonary disease, congestive heart failure, pulmonary embolus, laryngeal or vocal cord dysfunction, and mechanical airway obstruction.

Symptoms
Wheezing, shortness of breath, coughing, chest tightness, difficulty in breathing, dyspnea.

Incidence
Asthma affects approximately 8% of pregnant women (2). Among U.S. women aged 18 to 44, 5% reported an asthma attack within the preceding 12 months. However, 12% to 14% had received a diagnosis of asthma at some point during their lifetimes (2). Thus, this is a common disease among women of reproductive age.

Etiology and Basic Pathophysiology
Airway obstruction and inflammation, usually because of excessive response to stimuli, as described above.

Classification
Asthma severity, that is, the intrinsic intensity of the disease, is classified into four stages (Table 24.1) (1). Severity is most easily measured in a patient who is not receiving long-term control therapy. Severity can also be measured, once asthma control is achieved, by the amount of medication required to maintain control (Tables 24.2–24.4).

National Heart, Lung, and Blood Institute (NHLBI) classification is as follows.

Mild Intermittent Asthma

Fewer than two episodes per week AND fewer than two nocturnal episodes per month, plus
PEFR better than 80% of personal best (or FEV_1 > 80% of predicted), plus
Less than 20% variation in PEFR in the course of a day.

Table 24.1 Classification of Asthma Severity

	Mild intermittent	Mild persistent	Moderate persistent	Severe persistent
Symptoms	$\leq$2 times a week	>2 times a week but <1 time a day	Daily	Continuous
	Asymptomatic between exacerbations		Exacerbations occur $\geq$2 times a week	Frequent exacerbations
Pulmonary function	Normal PEFR between exacerbations		FEV_1 or PEFR 60% to 80% of predicted	FEV_1 or PEFR <60% of predicted
FEV_1 or PEFR in relation to predicted	$\geq$ 80%	>80%		
PEFR variability	PEFR variability <20%	PEFR variability 20% to 30%	PEFR variability >30%	PEFR variability >30%
Nocturnal awakening	$\leq$2 times a month	>2 times a month	>1 time a week	Nightly awakenings
Interference with daily activities	None	Mild	Some interference with normal activities but rare severe exacerbation	Limitations of physical activity
Treatment	Step 1	Step 2	Step 3 or Step 4	Step 5

Abbreviations: NAEPP, National Asthma Education and Prevention Program; PEFR, peak expiratory flow rate; FEV_1, forced expiratory volume in one second. *Source*: Adapted from Ref. 1.

Mild Persistent Asthma

Symptoms more than twice a week (but not daily), or nocturnal symptoms more than twice per month, plus
Peak expiratory flow (PEF) better than 80% of personal best (or FEV_1 > 80% of predicted), plus
No more than 20% to 30% variation in PEFR in the course of a day.

Moderate Persistent Asthma

Daily symptoms, or nocturnal symptoms more than once per week, or
PEF between 60% and 80% of personal best (FEV_1 60–80% of predicted), or
PEF variation > 30%.

Severe Persistent Asthma

Continuous daytime symptoms, or
Frequent nocturnal symptoms, or
PEF <60% of personal best (FEV_1 < 60% of predicted).
PEF variation is typically > 30%.

Pregnancy Complications

Asthma has historically been associated with small increased risks of preterm birth, low birth weight, perinatal mortality, congenital malformations, and preeclampsia (3,4). These risks are probably associated just with undertreatment of asthma: **if asthma is adequately controlled, it is not associated with a significant increase in adverse perinatal outcomes** (5,6). A relationship has been reported between decreased FEV_1 during pregnancy and increased risk of low birth weight and prematurity (7). In addition, women who required hospitalization for asthma during pregnancy, or who reported their asthma control to be poor during pregnancy, were at higher risk for preterm birth, though not for growth restriction (6). Large studies indicate that therapy tailored according to asthma severity can result in excellent infant and maternal outcomes (5,8). There are no randomized prospective trials comparing pregnancy outcomes in treated and untreated asthmatics. Women who decrease their asthma medication during pregnancy deliver infants of lower birth weight and slightly shorter gestational age than those who either increase their medication or make no change (9).

Pregnancy Considerations

Pregnant women are less likely than others to receive appropriate asthma care (10). Pregnant women are equally likely to be admitted for an asthma attack, but are less likely to receive corticosteroids in the emergency department (ED), and those who are sent home are less likely to be prescribed outpatient steroids. Pregnant women are far more likely than nonpregnant counterparts to report ongoing symptoms two weeks after an ED visit, perhaps because of the difference in steroid use (10). Adherence to treatment with inhaled corticosteroids has been reported to be poor in many studies. For example, women reported to decrease their use of inhaled corticosteroids during early pregnancy, as compared with their use of these agents in the 20 weeks before their last menstrual period; this may be due to their reported concern regarding the safety of inhaled corticosteroids during pregnancy (3).

Pregnancy has a variable effect on asthma severity, which may improve, worsen, or remain unchanged. In general, **about two-thirds get better, and one-third get worse** (2). **Most exacerbations occur between 24 and 36 weeks**, while the fewest symptoms occur at term. Of patients with mild disease, 2% were hospitalized during pregnancy, 13% were noted to have an exacerbation, and 13% had symptoms at time of delivery (7). For patients with moderate asthma, 7% were hospitalized and 26% had an exacerbation during pregnancy, with 21% symptomatic at delivery. Among severe asthmatics, 27% were hospitalized and 52% had an exacerbation during pregnancy, and 46% of severe asthmatics were symptomatic at delivery (7). A number of factors have been proposed as predictors of disease worsening during pregnancy (smoking, carrying a female fetus, worsening of rhinitis) but studies are inconsistent (11–13).

Table 24.2 Usual Drugs & Dosages for Long-Term Control Medication During Pregnancy

Medication	Dosage		
	Low dose	Medium dose	High dose
Inhaled corticosteroid			
Beclomethasone CFC 42 or 84 μg/puff	168–504 μg TDD	504–840 μg TDD	>840 μg TDD
Beclomethasone HFA 40 or 80 μg/puff	80–240 μg TDD	240–480 μg TDD	>480 μg TDD
Budesonide dry powder 200 μg/inhalation	200–600 μg TDD	600–1200 μg TDD	>1200 μg TDD
Flunisolide 250 μg/puff	500–1000 μg TDD	1000–2000 μg TDD	>2000 μg TDD
Fluticasone			
Metered dose inhaler: 44, 88, 220 μg/puff	MDI: 88–264 μg TDD	MDI: 264–660 μg TDD	MDI: >660 μg TDD
Dry powder inhaler: 50, 100, 250 μg/inhalation	DPI: 100–300 μg TDD	DPI: 300–750 μg TDD	DPI: >750 μg TDD
Triamcinolone acetonide 100 μg/puff	400–1000 μg TDD	1000–2000 μg TDD	>2000 μg TDD
Systemic corticosteroid	**How supplied**	**Daily dose** (all three drugs are dosed the same)	**Short burst to achieve control** (all dosed the same)
Methylprednisolone	Tablets: 2,4,8,16,32 mg	7.5–60 mg daily	40–60 mg/day
Prednisolone	Tablets: 5 mg Syrup: 5 mg/5 mL, 15 mg/5 mL	As a single dose in AM	As a single dose, or as two divided doses
Prednisone	Tablets: 1,2.5,5,10,20,50 mg Oral solution: 5 mg/mL	Every other day as needed for control	For 3–10 days
Long-acting β-agonist (LABA): Not for symptom relief, and not used alone; use with inhaled corticosteroids			
Salmeterol	MDI: 21 μg/puff DPI: 50 μg/blister	MDI: 2 puffs q12h DPI: 1 blister q12h	
Formoterol	DPI: 12 μg per single-use capsule	1 capsule q12h	
Combination: LABA plus inhaled corticosteroid			
Fluticasone/salmeterol	DPI: fluticasone dose varies 100,250 or 500 μg /puff; Salmeterol always 50 μg/puff	One inhalation twice daily	Fluticasone dose depends on asthma severity
Cromolyn	MDI: 1 mg/puff Nebulizer 20 mg/amp	MDI: 2–4 puffs, 3–4 × daily Or 1 ampule nebulized 3–4 × daily	
Leukotriene receptor antagonists			
Montelukast	10 mg tablet	10 mg qhs	
Zafirlukast	Tablet, 10 or 20 mg	40 mg daily	
Theophylline	Liquids; sustained-release tablets; capsules	Starting dose 10 mg/kg/day	Maximum dose 800 mg/day; serum drug monitoring, 5–12 μg/mL is therapeutic

Abbreviations: TDD, total daily dose; NAEPP, National Asthma Education and Prevention Program; PEFR, peak expiratory flow rate; FEV_1, forced expiratory volume in one second; CFC, chlorofluorocarbons; HFA, hydrofluoroalkane; MOI, metered-dose inhaler; DPI, dry powder inhaler.
Source: From Ref. 1.

Management

Principles

The management of asthma in pregnant women should follow the same guidelines as for other patients. The goal is to maintain asthma control during pregnancy. In 2004, the National Asthma Education and Prevention Program (NAEPP) stated, "it is safer for pregnant women with asthma to be treated with asthma medications than it is for them to have asthma symptoms and exacerbations" (14). Recent recommendations for asthma management and control are available from the 2007 NAEPP Guidelines (1), the NAEPP update on managing asthma in pregnancy (14), and from the American College of Obstetricians and Gynecologists (15). However, the latter two publications acknowledge that evidence quality is often limited to consensus or expert opinion.

Table 24.3 Quick-Relief Short-Acting β-Agonists

Medication	How provided	Dose (all same)
Albuterol CFC	90 μg/puff (200 puffs/canister)	Two puffs 5 min before anticipated exercise
Albuterol HFA	90 μg/puff (200 puffs/canister)	OR
Pirbuterol CFC	200 μg/puff (400 puffs/canister)	Two puffs q4–6h, as needed
Levalbuterol HFA	45 μg/puff (200 puffs/canister)	

Abbreviations: CFC, chlorofluorocarbons; HFA, hydrofluoroalkane.
Source: Adapted From Ref. 1.

Table 24.5 Environmental Control Measures for Asthma Management

Reduce or eliminate allergens
    Cockroaches
    Pollen
    Mold
    Animal dander
    House dust mites
    Encase mattresses and pillows in allergen-impermeable covers
    Remove carpets from bedroom
    Reduce indoor humidity
Eliminate or reduce exposure to tobacco smoke
Reduce exposure to indoor and outdoor pollutants
    Wood-burning stoves, fireplaces
    Unvented stoves or heaters
    Irritants such as perfumes and cleaning products

Table 24.4 Medications for Asthma Exacerbations During Pregnancy

Medication	Dose	Comment
Short-acting inhaled β-agonist		
Albuterol		
Nebulizer solutions 5 mg/mL, or 2.5 mg/3 mL, 1.25 mg/mL	Nebulizer: 2.5–5 mg q 20 min × 3 doses; follow with 2.5–10 mg q1–4h as needed or 10–15 mg/hr continuously	Dilute to minimum of 3 mL, use gas flow 6–8 L/min
MDI: 90 μg/puff	MDI: 4–8 puffs q20 min up to 4 hr; then q1–4h as needed	MDI is as effective as nebulizer if patient is able to coordinate
Levalbuterol	1.25–2.5 mg q 20 min × 3 doses, then	
Nebulizer solutions 1.25 mg/3 mL, 0.63 mg/3 mL	1.25–5 mg q1–4h as needed, or 5–7.5 mg/hr continuously	
Bitolterol, pirbuterol		Has not been studied in severe exacerbations
Injected β-agonists		
Epinephrine 1:1000 (1 mg/mL)	0.3–0.5 mg sq q20 min × 3 doses	No proven advantage of injection over aerosol
Terbutaline 1 mg/mL	0.25 mg sq q20 min × 3 doses	No proven advantage of injection over aerosol
Anticholinergics		
Ipratroprium bromide		Not as first-line monotherapy
Nebulizer solution 0.25 mg/mL	Nebulizer: 0.5 mg q30 min × 3 doses, then q2–4h as needed	May mix in nebulizer with albuterol
Ipratroprium plus albuterol		
Nebulizer solution: each 3-mL vial contains 0.5-mg ipratroprium bromide + 2.5-mg albuterol	Nebulizer: 3 mL q30 min × 3 doses, then q2–4h as needed	
MDI: each puff contains 18-μg ipratroprium bromide + 90-μg albuterol	4–8 puffs as needed	
Systemic corticosteroids	(dose all three the same)	
Prednisone	120—180 mg/day, in three or four divided doses, × 48 hr	
Methylprednisolone	60–80 mg/day until	
Prednisolone	PEFR reaches 70% of predicted or 70% of personal best	

Prevention
Eliminate or mitigate asthma triggers. Environmental control measures are shown in Table 24.5.

Preconception Care
Multidisciplinary care is recommended for preparation of pregnancy and during pregnancy. Education regarding prognosis, complications, and management of asthma therapy should be reviewed, with emphasis on the fact that asthma therapy should not change in pregnancy compared to the nonpregnant state, but should still aim for maximal relief of symptoms and best pulmonary function, through attentive patient compliance with suggested management.

Prenatal Care
Achieving and maintaining asthma control requires four components of care:

1. Use of *objective* measures of lung function such as PEFR, both to ascertain severity, assess asthma control, and to monitor therapy, rather than relying on symptoms.

2. Control of environmental factors and comorbid conditions to eliminate or mitigate asthma triggers.
3. Pharmacotherapy designed to prevent or reverse airway inflammation typical of asthma, as well as drug treatment for exacerbations.
4. Patient education regarding symptoms, management, and compliance.

Workup of Asthma Control

Asthma control should be assessed on a regular basis (at least at each prenatal visit) by review of symptoms, medications used, and quality of life over the preceding weeks. The **PEF can be measured by peak flow meters**, which are portable, inexpensive, and disposable. Both FEV_1 and PEF remain unchanged in pregnancy in the normal state. **Predicted PEF values are based on age, gender, and height. For women, they range from 380 to 550 L/min. Each pregnant woman should establish her personal best during quiescent asthma. PEF > 80% of personal best are normal; values between 50% and 80% are intermediate; values <50% are associated with severe asthma exacerbation.** Daily peak flow monitoring using an inexpensive home meter is advisable in cases of moderate or severe asthma, in order to identify presymptomatic airflow obstruction, which may require escalation of therapy. Outcomes have not been proven to be different when symptom-based monitoring is used rather than PEF monitoring (1), but objective measures are particularly valuable for patients with a history of exacerbations, when evaluating a change in therapy, or for those patients whose perception of airflow is poor. PEF results should be recorded in a log and brought to each prenatal visit.

Therapy

General

Inhalation therapy is preferred to systemic treatments, because of direct delivery to airway and fewer side effects. Spacer devices can increase delivery to the lungs and minimize oral absorption. For all except the mild intermittent type of asthma, **inhaled corticosteroids, NOT inhaled β-agonists, are the mainstay of therapy.**

Use of one or more canister of β-agonist per month indicates inadequate asthma control. Gain control as quickly as possible; a short course of oral steroids may be helpful. Review symptoms monthly. Other indicators of a need for stepped-up therapy are symptoms more than twice per week; three or more nighttime awakenings related to asthma symptoms; and limitation or interference with normal activity. Step-down therapy may be attempted only if symptoms are well controlled.

An individualized action plan should be generated for an asthmatic patient. This incorporates frequent self-assessment, a daily self-management plan, long-term self-management plan, and an asthma action plan based on symptoms, peak flow, and medications used. The action plan allows patients to step-up therapy at home with exacerbations, and provides criteria for contacting the physician or seeking care in an ED. Sample action plans can be found online at http://www.nhlbi.nih.gov/health/public/lung/asthma/asthma_act-plan.pdf and http://www.nhlbi.nih.gov/health/public/lung/asthma/actionplan_text.htm.

If symptoms are not adequately controlled, review compliance, inhalation technique, and environmental control. If no room for improvement in these areas, step up to the next level of therapy. At step 3 or 4 (moderate or severe persistent disease), or if patient required >2 bursts of oral systemic corticosteroids in one year, or has an exacerbation requiring hospitalization, refer to a specialist in asthma (if one is not already involved).

Goals

- No limitations at school or work
- Normal or near-normal pulmonary function assessed by PEF (or FEV_1)
- Prevent hypoxemia
- Minimal-to-none exacerbations, chronic symptoms, use of short-term β-agonists, or medication side effects

Suggested Medications

A stepwise approach to manage asthma is recommended to gain and maintain control (Fig. 24.1). Usual drug doses are shown in Table 24.2. Medications for exacerbation are shown in Table 24.3 and 24.4 (all tables are adapted from the NAEPP) (1). Algorithms for home and hospital management of exacerbation can be found in the NAEPP guidelines (Figs. 24.2 and 24.3) (1). Number and frequency of medications increase with increasing asthma severity. On the basis of clinical trials, medications are considered to be "preferred" or "alternative" at each step of therapy. For patients who are not already taking long-term control medications, assess asthma severity and initiate therapy according to level of severity. For patients who are already taking long-term control medications, assess asthma control and step-up therapy if the patient's asthma is not well controlled on current therapy. In general, **using short-acting β-agonists (SABA) >2 days a week indicates the need for starting or increasing long-term control medications.**

Mild intermittent asthma. These patients require **no daily medication** (step 1). Quick relief can be provided in the form of two to four puffs of a SABA bronchodilator as needed. In the event of exacerbation, PEFR 50 to 80% of predicted should be treated with an inhaled short-acting β-mimetic immediately. Values <50% require the same therapy plus immediate visit to emergency room. However, the need to use rescue twice a week or more means a step-up in therapy and a reclassification of severity. These patients can have severe exacerbations interrupting long periods of normal lung function, in which case systemic steroids should be offered.

Mild persistent asthma. Treat with a **daily inhaled corticosteroid** (low dose). Alternative therapies include inhaled cromolyn, leukotriene receptor antagonist (LTRA), or sustained-release theophylline adjusted to serum level of 5 to 12 µg/mL (step 2).

Moderate persistent asthma. Treat with either a **medium-dose inhaled corticosteroid or a low-dose inhaled corticosteroid plus a long-acting inhaled β-agonist** (step 3). If necessary, give the long-acting β-agonist (LABA) with a medium-dose corticosteroid (step 4).

Alternative therapies include low-dose or medium-dose inhaled corticosteroid in combination with either theophylline or a LTRA.

Severe persistent asthma. These patients require **both a high-dose inhaled corticosteroid and a long-acting inhaled β-agonist** (step 5) and may also require **oral corticosteroids** (step 6); when feasible, the oral corticosteroids should be discontinued and control maintained with inhaled agents.

An alternative therapy would be high-dose inhaled corticosteroid plus sustained-release theophylline titrated to therapeutic serum levels, as above.

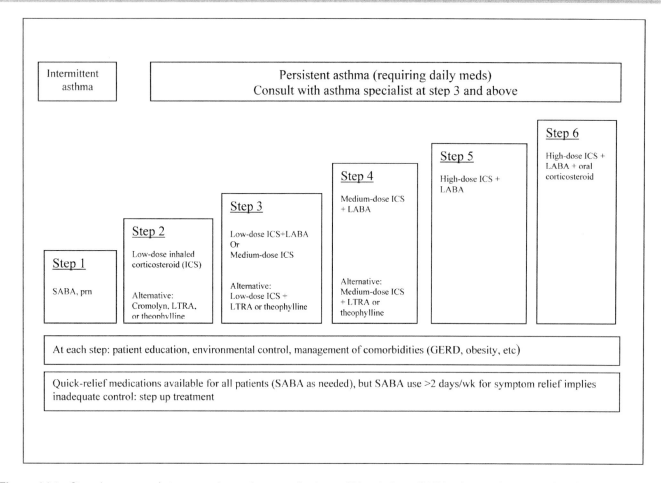

Figure 24.1 Stepwise approach to managing asthma medications. *Abbreviations*: SABA, short-acting β-agonists; LTRA, leukotriene receptor antagonist; LABA, long-acting β-agonist; GERD, gastroesophageal reflux disease. *Source*: Adapted from Ref. 1.

Inhaled Steroids
Anti-inflammatory agents decrease edema and secretions in the bronchioles. Indications are shown in Figure 24.1. They are used not for acute relief, but for long-term management (four weeks for maximal benefit). **Inhaled corticosteroids are the most consistently effective long-term control medication at all steps of care for persistent asthma. If β-agonist (e.g., albuterol) is used two times a week, inhaled steroid therapy should be started.** Most of the data on inhaled steroids in human pregnancy come from budesonide (Pulmacort) (12). Inhaled beclomethasone is associated with improved FEV$_1$ and fewer side effects compared to oral theophylline in the only trial comparing them in pregnancy (16). In a large, double-blind, randomized trial, treatment with low-dose budesonide had no adverse effects on the outcome of pregnancy (17). There is no evidence of increased rates of congenital malformations with the use of inhaled corticosteroids in pregnancy (4,14). Nor is there an effect on fetal growth, preterm birth, rates of gestational hypertension, preeclampsia, and perinatal mortality (6,7,18–20) A meta-analysis concludes that they are safe in pregnancy (21).

β-Agonists
β-Agonists relax bronchiolar smooth muscle. There is no consistent evidence of increased rates of congenital malformations with the use of β-agonists in pregnancy (14) despite a recent

case-control study suggesting an increased risk of gastroschisis when bronchodilators were used during the periconception period (22). Without having adjusted for severity of maternal asthma, it would be premature to conclude that β-agonists correlate with gastroschisis. Use of inhaled β-agonists does not appear to increase perinatal risks in pregnant asthmatic patients (including gestational hypertension, preterm birth, low birth weight, fetal growth, and small for gestational age) (6,7).

Short-acting β-agonists. These are the treatment of choice for relief of acute symptoms. Regularly scheduled, daily, chronic use of SABA is **not** recommended. The onset of action is <5 minutes, with a duration of only four to six hours.

Long-acting β-agonists. Produce bronchodilation for at least 12 hours after a single dose. They are not to be used as monotherapy for long-term control of asthma. Instead, they are used in combination with inhaled corticosteroids for long-term control and prevention of symptoms in moderate or severe persistent asthma. Long-acting β-agonists have been shown to be more effective than LTRA or theophylline as add-on therapy to inhaled corticosteroids (1).

Combination of Inhaled Corticosteroids and Long-Acting β-Agonists (Fixed-Drug Combination)
Fluticasone and salmeterol (Advair) combination is more effective than either drug alone in nonpregnant trials.

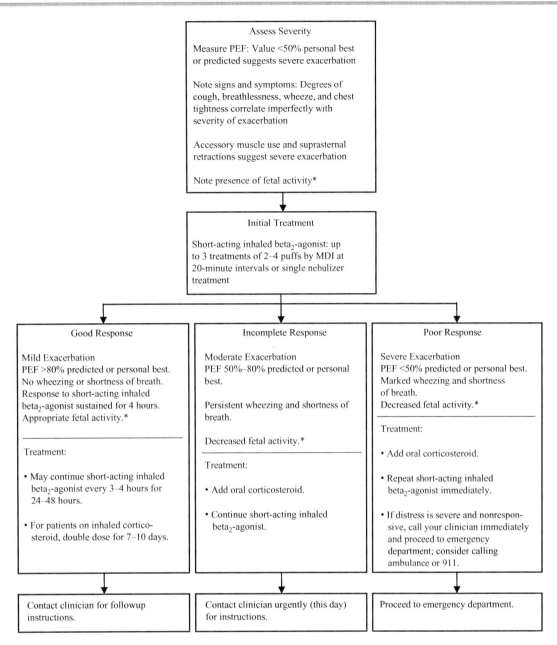

Figure 24.2 Management of asthma exacerbations during pregnancy and lactation: home treatment. *Source*: From Ref. 14.

Cromolyn
Cromolyn sodium is a nonsteroidal anti-inflammatory agent used for chronic management of asthma, not acute exacerbations (four weeks for maximal benefit). There is **no evidence of increased rates of congenital malformations** with the use of cromolyn in pregnancy (14); this is a safe drug in pregnancy, as is nedocromil.

Theophylline
Theophylline has a long record of use in pregnancy and no teratogenic effects are known; however, the narrow therapeutic window and potential for maternal and fetal toxicity mandates close monitoring of serum levels. Low-dose theo-

phylline is an alternative to a LABA when inhaled corticosteroids do not suffice to control symptoms, but this is not a preferred therapy (1). Recommendations for target serum theophylline levels have been changed to 5 to 12 µg/mL.

Leukotriene Receptor Antagonists
Limited human data are available on the use of LTRA during pregnancy. Several small studies have not shown an increase in the rate of major malformations in offspring of women who took LTRA during pregnancy (23,24). Mean birth weight was lower and risk of low birth weight and fetal distress was higher in the montelukast-exposed group, a difference that may have been related to asthma severity rather than drug effect. In nonpregnant individuals, these drugs are less

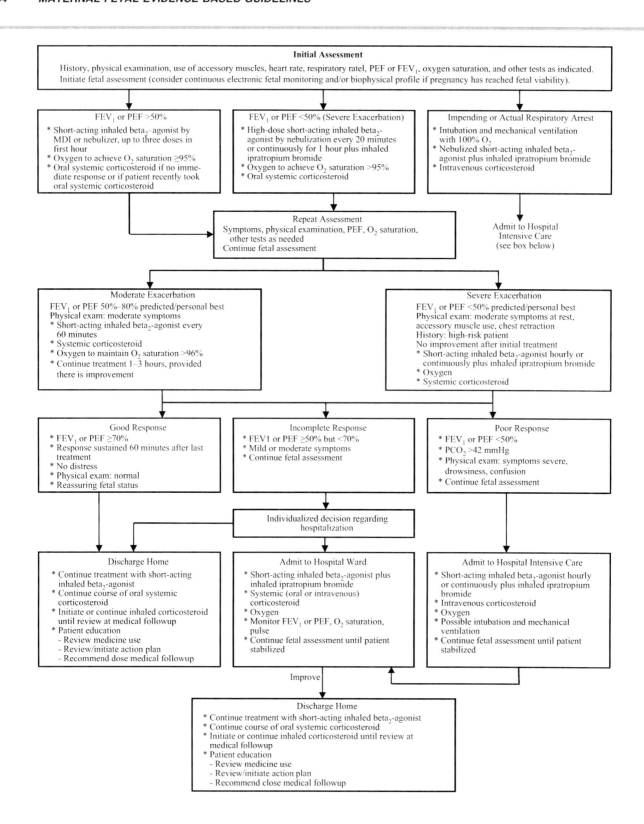

FEV₁, forced expiratory volume in 1 second: MDI, metered-dose inhaler: PCO₂, carbon dicodde partial pressure; PEF, peak expiratory flow.

Figure 24.3 Management of asthma exacerbations during pregnancy and lactation: emergency department and hospital based care. *Source*: From Ref. 14.

effective than inhaled corticosteroids, and do not add much benefit to women already on inhaled steroids. They do not reduce the risk of exacerbation requiring systemic steroids, and are associated with modest improvement in PEF, with very modest decrease in use of rescue short-acting β-2 agonists (25). These drugs may be considered during pregnancy for women who had a good response to them prior to pregnancy, but they are not a preferred option when initiating therapy. Montelukast and zafirlukast are safe in pregnancy. Zileuton, a 5-lipoxygenase inhibitor, has been advised against in pregnancy based on animal data: human data are lacking (14).

Anticholinergics

Anticholinergics inhibit muscarinic cholinergic receptors and reduce intrinsic vagal tone of the airway. Ipratropium bromide provides additive benefit to SABA in moderate or severe exacerbations in the emergency care setting, not the hospital setting.

Oral Corticosteroids

Oral corticosteroids are **indicated when combinations of inhaled steroids, β-agonists, and cromolyn do not control asthma**. Oral steroid use in the first trimester is associated with a possible increased risk of cleft lip (with or without cleft palate) from the background rate of 0.1% to 0.3%, a small excess risk. The use of oral corticosteroids during pregnancy is associated with an increase in incidence of gestational diabetes, preeclampsia, preterm delivery, and low birth weight. These outcomes may be attributed to either the drug or the severity of the disease process. Available data do not allow for the distinction (7).

Intravenous corticosteroids may be indicated in severe asthma exacerbation.

Status Asthmaticus

Recommendations for management are either anecdotal or extrapolated from management of status asthmaticus outside of pregnancy (26,27).

Antepartum Testing

No specific indication.

Delivery

Asthma medications should be continued in labor. Although asthma is typically quiescent during labor and delivery, PEF should be measured upon admission, and again every 12 hours in labor.

The idea of giving stress doses of steroids in labor or perioperatively is poorly supported by research (See chapter 25, page 199). Individuals receiving long-term corticosteroids have not, in randomized studies, proven incapable of endogenous steroid production perioperatively. A recent systematic review concludes that there is no need to add stress-dose steroids in the perioperative period, as long as patients continue to get their usual daily dose of steroids; this would not, however, be true for patients with primary adrenal failure or other primary dysfunction of the hypothalamic-pituitary axis, who would still require additional glucocorticoid coverage. Thus, extrapolating from work done on surgical patients, one would not expect adrenal crisis, and it would seem satisfactory to continue their regular daily steroid dosing during labor for women who are on prednisone, without adding additional "stress doses." Blood pressure should, of course, be carefully monitored (28).

Prostaglandin E1 and E2 are safe. **Prostaglandin F2α should be avoided**, as it can cause bronchospasm.

Anesthesia

No specific changes; as a rule, regional anesthetics are preferred to general.

Postpartum/Breast-feeding

The NAEPP found that the use of prednisone, theophylline, antihistamines, inhaled corticosteroids, β2-agonists, and cromolyn is not contraindicated for breast-feeding (14). Breast-feeding does not protect against asthma in offspring (29).

PNEUMONIA
Key Points

- The presence of an **infiltrate on chest X ray** confirms the diagnosis of pneumonia.
- Complications of community-acquired pneumonia (CAP) include mechanical ventilation, maternal mortality, low-birth-weight infant, and perinatal mortality.
- **Prompt administration** of antibiotics without delay **and appropriate antibiotic therapy** are the most important principles for effective management.
- Hospitalization is indicated when a pregnant woman with CAP has coexisting medical conditions such as malignancy, renal failure, immunosuppression, cerebrovascular disease, diabetes, or valvular heart disease, RR $\geq$30, diastolic BP $\leq$60, systolic BP $\leq$90, HR $\geq$125, altered mental status, PaCO$_2$ < 60 on room air, presence of a pleural effusion, hematocrit <30, arterial pH<7.35, or multilobe involvement.
- **Most cases of low-risk CAP in pregnancy can be treated with a macrolide, while the more high-risk ones can be treated with a macrolide and a β-lactam.**
- Antibiotic therapy should not be changed within the first 72 hours unless clinical deterioration is overt or organism sensitivities become available.

Diagnosis

Pneumonia is an infectious process of the lower respiratory tract, which should be suspected if a patient presents with new respiratory symptoms of cough, dyspnea, or sputum production, particularly if fever and abnormal breath sounds are also present. The presence of an infiltrate on chest X ray confirms the diagnosis.

Etiology/Basic Pathophysiology

Etiology is usually bacterial, viral, or fungal infection of the lungs. *Streptococcus pneumoniae* (5–30%) and *Mycoplasma pneumoniae* (5–30%) are the most common pathogens, but dozens of different organisms can cause pneumonia (Table 24.6) (30,31). In CAP, the causative agent is identified in only 40% to 60% of the cases (32).

Classification

The distinction between CAP and hospital-acquired pneumonia is made in practice. In the majority of cases, clinical signs and symptoms do not distinguish one pathogen from another. **The vast majority of cases of pneumonia in pregnant women in clinical practice and in the literature are cases of CAP.**

Table 24.6   Pathogens Isolated in Patients with Community-Acquired Pneumonia

Bacterial
- Common: *Streptococcus pneumoniae, Mycoplasma pneumoniae, Haemophilus influenza, Staphylococcus aureus, Chlamydophila pneumoniae,* and psittaci
- Less common: *Pseudomonas aeruginosa, Legionella* spp., *Klebsiella* spp., *Moraxella catarrhalis, Bordetella pertussis, Escherichia coli, Enterobacter* spp., *Serratia* spp.

Viral
- Common: influenza A and B and varicella-zoster virus
- Less common: adenovirus species, enteroviruses (echovirus, coxsackievirus, poliovirus), Epstein–Barr virus, cytomegalovirus, respiratory syncytial virus (common in children), parainfluenza virus, human metapneumovirus, herpes simplex virus, coronaviruses, measles virus, hantavirus

Fungal
- Uncommon: *Histoplasma capsulatum, Coccidioides immitis, Cryptococcus neoformans, Blastomyces hominis, Aspergillus* spp., *Candida* spp., Mucormycotic fungi

Other Causes
- Uncommon: *Mycobacterium tuberculosis, Pneumocystis jirovecii, Toxoplasma gondii, Ascaris lumbricoides, Strongyloides stercoralis, Coxiella burnetii, Rickettsia rickettsii*

Source: Adapted from Ref. 31.

The Infectious Diseases Society of America (IDSA) and The American Thoracic Society (ATS) use the Pneumonia Severity Index (PSI) to stratify CAP by comorbidity and mortality rates (33). Most pregnant patients with CAP will fall into subset I; this is a group that, if nonpregnant, would be appropriately treated as outpatients. There are, however, no reliable data as to inpatient versus outpatient therapy in pregnancy.

Symptoms
Respiratory symptoms: cough, dyspnea, or sputum production; usually fever.

Epidemiology
The attack rate for CAP is no different among pregnant women than among women of reproductive age who are not pregnant, approximately 1.5 per 1000 (34). Pregnant women hospitalized with CAP have lower severity scores than their nonpregnant counterparts; this may reflect either a tendency for the disease process to be less severe or a lower threshold for hospitalization during pregnancy. Pneumonia incidence is evenly distributed throughout pregnancy; that is, there is no specific period of vulnerability.

Risk Factors
Smoking; asthma.

Complications
Approximately **2% of pregnant women with pneumonia require intubation and mechanical ventilation** (35). The risk of **maternal mortality with CAP was 2.9% from reports in the 1990s** (36). Among women hospitalized for pneumonia during pregnancy, the risk of delivering a small-for-gestational-age infant is increased relative to controls, although this may be confounded by different health behaviors in the two groups. Rates of preterm birth and perinatal mortality are increased after pregnancy complicated by pneumonia, though not to statistical significance. Term and preterm premature rupture of membranes have been shown to be increased in women with viral and bacterial pneumonia (37).

Pregnancy Considerations
Women hospitalized for CAP during pregnancy appear to be less ill than their nonpregnant counterparts, measured by either severity score or length of stay, but this probably reflects a tendency to hospitalize for less severe disease because of the pregnancy. The rate of preterm delivery is higher among women with a diagnosis of pneumonia than among those with upper-tract respiratory infection or with no respiratory infection (38). In addition, the risk of placental abruption is twice as high among pregnant women hospitalized for pneumonia compared to a control group without respiratory disease (39) although in this large dataset obtained from the National Hospital Discharge Survey, the highest risk of abruption followed not pneumonia but chronic bronchitis.

Management
Principles
Prompt administration of antibiotics without delay and appropriate antibiotic therapy are the most important principles for effective management.

Prevention
Pneumococcal vaccine prevents 71% of cases of CAP and 32% of related mortality in nonpregnant adults (30). For details on recommended pneumococcal and influenza vaccines, see chapter 38.

Workup
Assess severity of illness by physical findings (blood pressure, respiratory rate, mental status, state of hydration) and by radiographic findings (e.g., multilobar involvement and pleural effusion). Laboratory testing for a specific cause is controversial and frequently nonrevealing. The Infectious Disease Society of America and the American Thoracic Society have recommended that diagnostic testing be initiated to determine the cause of CAP if the results would change treatment decisions, for example antimicrobial regimens. This would be most useful in areas of high antibiotic resistance or if unusual pathogens are suspected. A list of clinical indications for more extensive diagnostic testing can be found in the IDSA/ATS Consensus Guidelines (33). Routine diagnostic tests to identify an etiologic diagnosis are optional for the mildly ill, but patients with severe CAP should have the following diagnostic tests: blood cultures, urinary antigen assays for *Legionella* spp. and *S. pneumoniae*, and expectorated sputum samples/endotracheal aspirates.

Blood culture is positive in 5% to 11% of cases; positive blood cultures are more common in those with severe CAP (40). Blood cultures should be obtained before antibiotic administration.

Treatment

Hospitalization

The initial management decision after diagnosis is to determine the site of care, that is, outpatient, hospital ward, or ICU. There are no trials addressing benefits of outpatient versus inpatient care for the pregnant woman with pneumonia. Keeping this in mind, physicians may still begin treatment decisions by using a prediction tool for increased mortality, such as the PSI, combined with clinical judgment (33). The PSI was developed to assist physicians in identifying patients at a higher risk of complications and who are more likely to benefit from hospitalization, that is, those with comorbidities, hypoxemia, alteration in vital signs, etc. It has not been validated in pregnancy. Direct admission to ICU is required for patients with septic shock requiring vasopressors, or with acute respiratory failure requiring intubation and mechanical ventilation.

The majority of obstetrical patients will fail to qualify as high risk by these criteria. Retrospectively applying American Thoracic Society guidelines in place at the time of the study (similar to above), only 25% of pregnant patients with a diagnosis of CAP could have been assigned to outpatient care (35). A 23-hour observation period might be useful in deciding whether inpatient treatment is warranted in the pregnant patient.

Antibiotics

There are no trials to determine which antibiotic regimen is most beneficial for the pregnant woman with pneumonia. No published treatment guidelines alter therapy for pneumonia because of pregnancy. Antibiotic selection should take into account the common causes of CAP, local antibiotic resistance patterns, clinical presentation, comorbid conditions, and recent antibiotic use. The fluoroquinolones are generally avoided in pregnancy because of concerns about interference with cartilage formation in the fetus, and the tetracyclines because of concerns about dentition. However, depending on drug allergies and microbiologic sensitivities, it may be necessary to alter these preferences. Initial choice of antimicrobial treatment is empirical. The ATS and IDSA recommend antibiotic regimens for adults with CAP (40); they are adapted here to exclude, where possible, quinolones and tetracyclines.

- Previously healthy patient, no recent antibiotic therapy, no risk factors for drug-resistant *S. pneumoniae*:
  - Erythromycin, azithromycin, or clarithromycin: only 1% of pregnant women with CAP remained febrile with erythromycin 500 mg every six hours (35).
- Previously healthy, but antibiotics within the past three months for any reason; or comorbidities (chronic heart/lung/liver/kidney disease, or diabetes, or asplenia); or immunocompromise, including immunosuppressant drugs:
  - *β*-**lactam plus macrolide**; high-dose amoxicillin (1 g po tid) or high-dose amoxicillin-clavulanate (2 g po bid) are preferred; alternatives include ceftriaxone, cefpodoxime, or cefuroxime (500 mg po bid).
- Inpatient, not in ICU:
  - *β*-lactam (cefotaxime, ceftriaxone, or ampicillin) **plus** a macrolide.

- Inpatient, ICU:
  - *β*-lactam **plus** azithromycin.
- For *Pseudomonas*:
  - Piperacillin-tazobactam, cefepime, imipenem, or meropenem **plus** ciprofloxacin or levofloxacin,
    Or
  - Piperacillin-tazobactam, cefepime, imipenem, or meropenem **plus** aminoglycoside **plus** azithromycin.
- For community-acquired methicillin-resistant *Staphylococcus aureus*:
  - Add vancomycin or linezolid

In summary, **most cases of low-risk CAP in pregnancy can be treated with a macrolide, while the more high-risk ones can be treated with a macrolide and a *β*-lactam.** Uncommon pathogens do exist, and should be considered if response to therapy is inadequate or incomplete.

Typical responses to therapy include defervescence in two to four days, with resolution of leukocytosis in the same time period. The chest X ray may take longer to clear, as may the auscultatory findings. **Antibiotic therapy should not be changed within the first 72 hours unless clinical deterioration is overt or organism sensitivities become available.** There is no evidence in nonpregnant adults that intravenous and oral therapy differ in efficacy. Patients should be switched from intravenous to oral therapy when hemodynamically stable and improving clinically, able to ingest medications and have a normally functioning GI tract. If the pathogen and sensitivities are known, the narrowest spectrum agent should be chosen for oral therapy, but in most cases this will not be possible, and oral agents should duplicate the spectrum of the parenteral agents used. The American Thoracic Society and the Infectious Diseases Society of America recommend **discharge to home the same day that clinical stability is achieved (afebrile, no tachypnea nor tachycardia, normotensive, normoxemic, normal mental status, and able to tolerate oral intake) and the switch to oral agents is made.** Inpatient observation while receiving oral therapy is not necessary. A follow-up inpatient chest X ray is not indicated.

There are inadequate data to determine the best duration of antimicrobial treatment for CAP. With older agents, a **duration of 10 to 14 days is commonly prescribed**, but newer agents have longer half-lives and therefore may be curative over shorter courses of therapy, for example, five to seven days; trials are under way. Regardless of the total duration, it is recommended that patients with CAP be treated for a minimum of five days, should be afebrile for 48 to 72 hours, and should be clinically stable before discontinuation of therapy (40).

Oxygen support should be provided as needed.

Antepartum Testing

No specific indication.

Delivery

No specific changes.

Anesthesia

No specific changes.

Postpartum/Breast-feeding

No specific changes.

INFLUENZA
Key Points

- Trivalent inactivated influenza vaccine is recommended for all pregnant and postpartum patients.
- **In addition to the protective effect of vaccination on women themselves, infants born to vaccinated mothers have fewer episodes of influenza, fever, and respiratory illness in their first six months of life.**
- Influenza antiviral medications should be started **as soon as possible after** symptom onset, ideally within 48 hours of symptom onset. **Treatment should not wait for laboratory confirmation of influenza.**
- Risk of severe illness and mortality because of influenza appear to be higher among pregnant women.

Epidemiology/Incidence

Annual epidemics of influenza typically occur during the late fall through early spring. In addition to seasonal flu, epidemics or pandemics arise unpredictably. The pattern of emergence is usually in the Southern Hemisphere first, during the austral winter.

Etiology/Basic Pathophysiology

Influenza illnesses are caused by infection with one of the three types of circulating RNA viruses: A, B, or C (41). While B and C are almost exclusive to humans, A is avian in origin, although capable of infecting a range of warm-blooded animals. Both A and B types cause epidemic human disease. Influenza A viruses are subtyped by their surface antigens hemagglutinin (H) and neuraminidase (N).

High mutation rates and the potential for cross-species genetic reassortment are characteristic of influenza A (41). New influenza A subtypes have the potential to cause a pandemic, as demonstrated most recently in the 2009 H1N1 pandemic. The 2009 pandemic influenza A (H1N) virus contains a combination of gene segments that had not been reported previously in animals or humans.

Influenza spread is by aerosolized droplets. The incubation period for influenza is one to four days; patients are likely infectious one day before symptom onset.

Symptoms

Infection with influenza virus can range from asymptomatic infection to uncomplicated upper respiratory tract disease to serious complicated illness such as secondary bacterial pneumonia, sepsis, and organ failure. Symptoms include fever, cough, sore throat, nasal congestion or rhinorrhea, headache, myalgia, and malaise.

Diagnosis

A variety of laboratory tests are available (Table 24.7). Testing should occur if the result would influence clinical management. For screening during influenza season, antigen-based rapid testing is appropriate, but positive predictive value is poor when influenza prevalence is low.

Complications

Largely maternal. In influenza pandemics, the maternal mortality case–fatality ratio is higher than that of the general population. In the most recent pandemic (2009), pregnant women, who represented approximately 1% of the U.S. population, accounted for 5% of deaths from 2009 influenza A (H1N1) (42,43). In a case series from the 2009 H1N1 pandemic, 7% of deaths occurred in the first trimester, 27% in the second, and 64% in the third trimester (43). This study is consistent with previous pandemics and seasonal influenza studies, which usually suggest that the risk of influenza complications is higher in the second and third trimester of pregnancy than in the first trimester (44,45).

Transplacental passage of influenza virus appears to be rare (46). Infants born to women with laboratory-confirmed seasonal influenza during pregnancy do not have higher rates of low birth weight or lower Apgar scores (46,47). The effect of influenza on perinatal outcomes is inconsistent. In most studies, there are no significant differences in mode of delivery, duration of delivery admission, episodes of preterm labor, and adverse perinatal outcomes between the influenza and non-influenza groups (48,49), although a large U.S. study of 2009 pandemic H1N1 influenza demonstrated a 30% risk of preterm birth among affected women (43). Severe maternal illness, of course, such as overt respiratory failure, is associated with significantly worse perinatal outcome than in most seasonal or even pandemic influenza (50–52).

Pregnancy Considerations

Changes in the immune, respiratory, and cardiovascular systems result in pregnant women being more severely affected. Pregnant women are at higher risk for severe complications

Table 24.7 Influenza Testing Methods

Test	Method	Time	Comment
PCR	Gel-based reverse transcriptase PCR	≥2 hr	High sensitivity Very high specificity
Immunofluorescence	Direct or indirect fluorescent antibody stain	2–4 hr	Moderate-to-high sensitivity High specificity
Rapid tests	Antigen detection; enzyme immunoassay	10–30 min	Low to moderate sensitivity High specificity Limitations: may not distinguish influenza A and B Positive predictive value poor outside of influenza season
Viral culture	Shell vial culture or cell culture	2–10 days	Moderate-to-high sensitivity, highest specificity; useful for public health surveillance, not for clinician
Serology	Acute paired & convalescent samples: ELISA, complement fixation, hemagglutination, or neutralization	Weeks to months	Reference laboratories only; useful for public health surveillance, no help in clinical management

Source: From Ref. 61.

and death from influenza, both H1N1 influenza and seasonal influenza.

During periods of seasonal flu, pregnant women account for excess health care visits related to respiratory complaints and excess hospitalizations (above what would be expected outside of pregnancy); this is true for both healthy women and those with chronic conditions. The rate of hospitalization for seasonal (not pandemic) influenza among healthy nonpregnant women in Canada has been reported as 17/100,000, but 156/100,000 among healthy women who were pregnant. The 10-fold difference in influenza hospitalization persisted among women with comorbidities, but as expected the absolute rates are higher (53). Pregnant women are at increased risk for hospitalization during influenza season, and those hospitalized for respiratory illness stay longer (43,53,54). During the 2009 H1N1 influenza pandemic, pregnant and postpartum women with H1N1 influenza had a seven times higher risk of admission to ICU than nonpregnant women in the same age group, and after 20 weeks of pregnancy the relative risk of ICU admission was 13 times higher (52). The severity of disease is demonstrated by utilization of extracorporeal membrane oxygenation (ECMO): in 2009 in Australia and New Zealand, 16% of all ECMO interventions for respiratory failure in H1N1 were performed on pregnant or postpartum patients (55); these are patients whom conventional mechanical ventilation could not adequately oxygenate.

Management
Prevention
Annual influenza vaccination is the most effective method for preventing influenza infection and its complications (56). The vaccine is reformulated yearly to cover the strains predicted to be in circulation. The trivalent inactivated vaccine (TIV) for individuals is recommended for women who are pregnant, postpartum, or breast-feeding during the influenza season. TIV contains noninfectious killed viruses and cannot cause influenza. It can be given in any trimester of pregnancy. Safety is not a concern: there is no suggestion of fetal harm after TIV administration to pregnant women (57) and no difference in rate of preterm birth and cesarean delivery (58). The live attenuated influenza vaccine (given intranasally), like other live-virus vaccines, should not be given during pregnancy (see also chapter 38).

In addition to the protective effect of vaccination on women themselves, infants born to vaccinated mothers have fewer episodes of influenza, fever, and respiratory illness in their first six months of life (59), which may represent antibody transfer (60). Each season, influenza vaccines are reformulated. Vaccination providers may check updated information at the Centers for Disease Control and Prevention (http://www.cdc.gov/flu), Food and Drug Administration (http://www.fda.gov/BiologicsBloodVaccines/SafetyAvailability/vaccinesafety/default.htm), or World Health Organization (WHO) (http://www.who.int/csr/disease/influenza/vaccinerecommendations/en/index.html). However, national health authorities approve the specific composition and formulation of yearly vaccines for individual countries.

Prophylaxis After Suspected Exposure
Chemoprophylaxis after exposure to influenza is recommended for individuals at high risk of complications from influenza, which would include pregnant and postpartum women (61). For household exposures, this means a 10-day course of either oseltamivir 75 mg once daily, or zanamivir as two 5-mg inhalations once daily. There are no RCTs of postexposure influenza prophylaxis among pregnant women.

Therapy
There are four licensed antiviral agents in the United States. The M2 ion channel inhibitors (amantadine and rimantadine) are effective only for prophylaxis and treatment of influenza A, and resistance is not uncommon. The neuraminidase inhibitors, oseltamivir and zanamivir, are effective against both influenza A (including H1N1) and influenza B. Although the manufacturer has conducted no studies to assess safety of these medications for pregnant women, available risk-benefit data clearly indicate that **pregnant women with suspected or confirmed influenza should receive prompt antiviral therapy.**

The standard dose for oseltamivir is 75 mg po bid for five days (62). The standard dose for zanamivir is two inhalations twice daily for five days; this drug should be avoided in case of chronic respiratory disease, including asthma. If oseltamivir resistance is suspected, use zanamivir.

Treatment should be started as soon as possible, preferably within the first 48 hours. Delayed treatment of antiviral therapy has been associated with more severe illness and death in both seasonal influenza and 2009 influenza A (H1N1), whereas early initiation of treatment has been associated with reduced duration of illness, severity, mortality, and incidence of complications (43,50,63–66). **Laboratory confirmation of influenza virus infection is not necessary for the initiation of treatment.** For uncomplicated influenza infection, a five-day course of antiviral medication is prescribed (62).

Several recent systematic reviews of neuraminidase inhibitors in nonpregnant adults (65–67) confirm a statistically significant advantage for oseltamivir compared to placebo in reduction of symptoms (HR = 1.20; 95% CI, 1.06, 1.35), with a reduction in duration of illness of about one day. The major advantage appears to be in decreasing the risk of severe respiratory complications. However, among pregnant women specifically, those who received no antiviral treatment had a fourfold higher risk of ICU admission and a fivefold higher risk of mechanical ventilation (43). Delayed or inadequate treatment was associated with up to a 50-fold higher risk of death.

There is limited evidence regarding the safety of oseltamivir use in pregnancy. A single-cotyledon perfused placental model showed that oseltamivir is extensively metabolized by the placenta (68) with minimal accumulation of the metabolite on the fetal side. In a population of 90 Japanese women who received oseltamivir during pregnancy, the incidence of malformation (1.1%) was similar to the incidence of major malformations in the general population (69). A retrospective cohort study of 239 pregnant women in Texas demonstrated no association of antepartum exposure to amantadine, rimantadine, or oseltamivir with adverse fetal outcomes (70). The limited (albeit reassuring) information on fetal effects is trumped by the importance of antiviral therapy for pregnant women.

Antepartum Testing
No evidence for recommendations.

Delivery
No evidence for recommendations.

Postpartum/Breast-feeding

Whether influenza viruses are passed into human milk is not known; however, respiratory droplets are believed to be the main mode of viral transmission. Because of the anti-infective benefits of human milk for infants, continuation of breast-feeding is recommended while the mother is receiving treatment for influenza infection. The concentration of oseltamivir found in breast milk equates to much lower doses than the therapeutic dose given to infants (71).

TUBERCULOSIS
Key Points

- Definite diagnosis of **active infection** is based on culture (of suspected site: sputum for pulmonary TB) for *Mycobacterium tuberculosis*. Sputum culture is also important for drug sensitivity testing.
- Diagnosis of **latent tuberculosis infection** is based on a positive tuberculin test (or interferon gamma-release assay, IGRA) and the absence of signs, symptoms, or proof of active disease.
- Pregnancy does not influence the progression from latent to active disease.
- The treatment for latent tuberculosis infection in pregnancy is isoniazid 300 mg daily for six to nine months.
- Treatment of active tuberculosis consists of an initial two-month phase of therapy, including isoniazid, rifampin, pyrazinamide, and ethambutol. Directly observed therapy is usually recommended. For the following four months, continue isoniazid and rifampin. **Treatment for active tuberculosis is not altered by pregnancy**.

Epidemiology/Incidence

Although still rare in the developed world, there were nine million new TB cases in 2009 worldwide, and 1.5 million deaths; TB is one of the top three causes of death for women of reproductive age (72). HIV coinfection (about 12% worldwide) accounts for a significant portion of the tuberculosis burden. Even resource-rich countries have seen a resurgence of TB over the past few years, as a result of an increase in immigrant populations. The national incidence of TB in pregnancy in the UK in 2008 was estimated at 4 per 100,000 maternities (73). All but one of the TB patients in this study were non-Western immigrants, and half had extrapulmonary disease. Few had undergone tuberculin skin testing, despite recommendations to the contrary.

Symptoms (of active disease)

Cough, lethargy, dyspnea, malaise, fever, sweating, weight loss. Hemoptysis is a late finding.

Etiology/Basic Pathophysiology

The pathogenesis of tuberculosis infection and disease in pregnant women is similar to that in nonpregnant women. Spread (by airborne droplets) is facilitated by the ability of these small particles to remain airborne for hours after being emitted from an infected respiratory tract. Once the *Mycobacterium* is taken up by alveolar macrophages, the infection may either be contained by granuloma formation or may progress to active disease (74). Most patients develop cell-mediated immunity, which is demonstrated by conversion of the tuberculin skin test, and which constitutes latent tuberculosis infection. In some patients, the replication of *M. tuberculosis* cannot be contained, and active disease occurs. Latent tuberculosis infection can develop into active tuberculosis, especially in individuals with risk factors. Pulmonary disease is the most common but not the only form of active tuberculosis, which can manifest in 20% of cases (extrapulmonary tuberculosis) as meningitis, osteitis, genitourinary involvement, or disseminated disease.

Risk Factors/Associations

HIV is the most important risk factor. Poorly controlled diabetes, renal failure, malignancy, steroids, malnutrition, and vitamin A or D deficiency are other risk factors for acquiring active *M. tuberculosis* infection (74).

Diagnosis

Definitive diagnosis of **active** infection is still made by **culture** (of suspected site, e.g., sputum) **for *M. tuberculosis***. Smear demonstrating acid-fast bacilli is a technique for rapid diagnosis (74). Diagnosis of **latent tuberculosis** requires a newly positive tuberculin test in the absence of disease (thus no symptoms, X-ray findings, bacilli on smear, or positive culture).

The most widely used method to detect respiratory TB in most disease-endemic countries is the sputum smear microscopy test developed in the 19th century, drawbacks of which include low sensitivity (especially in children and in HIV-positive individuals), inability to determine drug susceptibility, and variable performance depending on operator training and skill. In December 2010, the WHO endorsed a novel rapid test for tuberculosis, a fully automated molecular test for TB case detection plus rifampicin resistance testing. Other than adding sputum and reagent to the cartridge, there is little for the technician to do (75). In a multinational study of about 1500 nonpregnant adults, this assay identified 98% of patients with smear-positive and culture-positive tuberculosis (including more than 70% of patients with smear-negative and culture-positive disease) and correctly identified 98% of bacteria that were resistant to rifampin (75). The effect of pregnancy on this test has not been studied, but it is counterintuitive to assume pregnancy would affect it.

Pregnancy Considerations

Tuberculosis attack rates appear to be comparable in the pregnant and nonpregnant states. Presentation is similar among both pregnant and nonpregnant patients, but diagnosis may be delayed in pregnancy because of the ubiquity of constitutional complaints during early pregnancy. **Pregnancy is not known to influence the progression from latent to active disease,** nor has it been shown to affect the response to treatment. Pregnancy is not associated with higher (or lower) prevalence of anergy compared to other HIV-negative adults.

There are conflicting data on the effect of TB on maternal and neonatal outcomes. In a recent population-based study in Taiwan, women known to have TB during pregnancy—all of whom were treated—demonstrated an absolute increase of 2–3% in the rate of low-birth-weight babies, with no difference in preterm births, compared to controls (76). An earlier case-control study from India suggested higher rates of both preterm birth and small for gestational age newborns among women undergoing treatment for pulmonary TB, compared to matched controls (77), but a later Indian case-control study found no difference in perinatal outcome (78).

Congenital TB, which is very rare, is associated with maternal HIV infection, tuberculous endometritis, and miliary tuberculosis (79). It can occur hematogenously via the placenta and umbilical vein or by fetal aspiration or ingestion of infected amniotic fluid. Neonatal TB develops following exposure of an infant to the mother's aerosolized respiratory sections. This is more common than congenital TB, and diagnosis of neonatal TB can lead to diagnosis of previously unrecognized TB in the mother (80).

Pregnancy Management

Principles

Management of *M. tuberculosis* infection in pregnancy should be multidisciplinary, with involvement of obstetrician, maternal-fetal medicine, and infectious diseases specialists.

Screening

Tuberculin Skin Testing

Tuberculin skin testing (TST) is the method historically used to detect both latent and active disease. TST can be performed safely in pregnant women, and pregnancy does not alter the response to the TST (81). Using standardized **purified protein derivative (PPD)**, 0.1 mL (5 tuberculin units) is administered intradermally in the volar surface of the forearm. The reaction is read 48 to 72 hours after the injection, although reading is accurate up to a week after challenge. Targeted (not universal) tuberculin testing is recommended so as to identify individuals who are at increased risk for developing *M. tuberculosis* infection and who would benefit by treatment of latent tuberculosis infection. **Testing is discouraged among persons without these risk factors.** Persons at increased risk for development of active disease are those who were recently infected (i.e., converted from a positive to a negative skin test within the preceding two years), as well as those who have latent infection plus an increased risk of progression to overt disease. Table 24.8 shows some of **indications for testing in pregnancy**: it is not an exhaustive list but is limited to those conditions that may be found in pregnancy. **Interpretation of PPD results** is shown in Table 24.9 (82).

A decision to test is a decision to treat. Therefore, do not test unless prepared to treat. With a positive skin test, **chest X ray** (and perhaps additional testing) is indicated to differenti-

Table 24.8 Indications for Tuberculin Skin Testing in Pregnancy (Factors Which Predispose to Progression from Latent to Active Disease)

Recent conversion
Household contacts of persons with infectious pulmonary TB
Recent immigration from parts of the world with high rates of TB
Homelessness
HIV infection
Living or working in institutional setting in which TB is common (hospital, jail, homeless shelter)
Injection drug use
Renal failure on hemodialysis
Diabetes
Solid organ transplantation
Certain cancers; certain surgeries such as gastrectomy or jejunal bypass
High-dose corticosteroids for prolonged periods (lower limit not known)
Significantly underweight/poor nutrition

Table 24.9 Interpretation of Tuberculin Skin Testing

Size of reaction	Persons in whom reaction is considered positive
≥5 mm	HIV-infected persons
	Close contacts of persons with infectious tuberculosis
	Persons with an abnormal chest radiograph consistent with previous tuberculosis
	Immunosuppressed patients receiving the equivalent of ≥15 mg of prednisone per day for ≥1 mo
≥10 mm	Foreign-born persons recently arrived (<5 yr earlier) from country with high prevalence of tuberculosis
	Persons with a medical condition that increases the risk of tuberculosis[a]
	Injection-drug users
	Members of medically underserved, low-income populations (e.g., homeless persons)
	Residents and staff members of long-term care facilities (e.g., nursing homes, correctional institutions, and homeless shelters)
	Health care workers
	Children <4 yr of age
	Persons with conversion on a tuberculin skin test (increase in duration of ≥10 mm within a 2-yr period)
≥15 mm	All others

[a]Medical conditions that increase the risk of tuberculosis: silicosis, end-stage renal disease, malnutrition, diabetes mellitus, carcinoma of the head and neck or lung, immunosuppressive therapy, lymphoma, leukemia, loss of >10% of ideal body weight, gastrectomy, and jejunoileal bypass. *Source*: From Ref. 81.

ate latent from active infection, as the therapy is different. The screening algorithm is shown in Figure 24.4.

Selective immunological testing (IGRA) for tuberculosis antigens, performed on whole blood, has become available. This appears to correlate better with recent TB exposure than does TST, is less likely to be affected by prior BCG vaccination, and is less likely to produce a false-positive result (83). Data in pregnancy are limited at this time, although a single trial in Kenya of cryopreserved specimens obtained from HIV-positive pregnant women suggested that positive IGRA testing correlated strongly with the development of active TB postpartum (84). IGRA may, in future, replace TST as the standard screen for TB exposure, latent infection, or disease. At this time it may be used to screen adults in any situation in which TST would be considered (85), including women with prior BCG vaccine.

Workup

Women with a cough lasting for > 2 weeks or with symptoms as described above, especially with risk factors or from high-prevalence areas, should be worked up for tuberculosis. **Radiographic** findings suggesting tuberculosis include upper lobe infiltrate, cavitary lesions, and hilar adenopathy. Sputum smear can be negative even in active disease (15–20% of cases). Sputum culture is required both for definite diagnosis and for drug sensitivity testing (74), although both false-positive and false-negative results have been reported. Growth generally occurs in 7 to 21 days, but may take 6 weeks or longer.

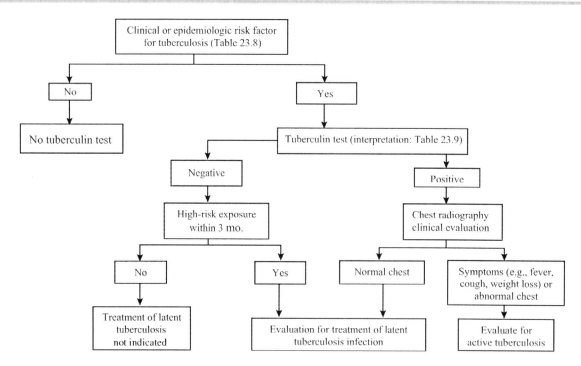

Figure 24.4 Tuberculosis screening algorithm. *Source*: From Ref. 81.

Management

Prevention

BCG (bacille Calmette–Guerin) vaccine has >70% efficacy in preventing *M. tuberculosis* infection in children, but not great efficacy in adults. TST cannot distinguish between induration induced by BCG or *M. tuberculosis* infection. A history of BCG vaccination is ignored when administering and interpreting a tuberculin skin test. BCG should not be administered during pregnancy for the prevention of tuberculosis, since it is a live vaccine. IGRA testing is useful in evaluating for TB in women with prior BCG vaccine.

Therapy

Latent Tuberculosis Infection

The treatment for latent tuberculosis infection in pregnancy is **isoniazid 300 mg daily for six to nine months** (81). Alternative rifampin-based regimens have not been evaluated in pregnancy. Because isoniazid can interfere with pyridoxine metabolism and thereby precipitate peripheral neuropathy, **coadministration of pyridoxine 25 mg/day is advisable**. Isoniazid is 60% to 90% effective in reducing the risk of progression from tuberculosis latent infection to active disease. The most important but rare (1/1000) side effect of isoniazid is hepatitis; the concern that this may be more common among pregnant women (which prompted a consideration of routinely deferring treatment to the puerperium) is based on a single investigation in which five cases of isoniazid hepatitis were identified among nearly 4000 pregnant women (86): statistical significance was absent. Age > 35 years is no longer considered a contraindication to isoniazid use (82). **Pregnant and postpartum women should have pretreatment liver transaminases and bilirubin function tests**, and if these are normal, isoniazid can be started. Liver function tests should be obtained monthly. Isoniazid should be discontinued in a symptomatic or jaundiced patient if alanine aminotransferase (ALT) is more than three times the upper limit of normal, and in an asymptomatic patient if ALT is more than five times the upper limit of normal (87).

Advantages of beginning treatment during pregnancy include better compliance and less loss to follow-up. A decision analysis suggests that antepartum treatment of latent tuberculosis infection is more efficient at preventing additional cases of TB within the population (88). Recent infection with tuberculosis (i.e., a recent conversion of TST) or HIV coinfection increases the risk for transplacental spread of tubercle bacilli, and thus for congenital tuberculosis, which implies that treatment for latent infection in these cases should be especially expeditious and compliant.

Active Tuberculosis Infection

Single-drug therapy is not acceptable for active TB. Multiple drugs for six months or more can cure > 95% of patients (Tables 24.10 and 24.11) (88). The treatment regimen is two-part, with an initial period of intensive therapy to kill actively growing bacilli, shortening the time the individual is infectious to others, followed by a second phase in which microbiologic cure is the goal. **The usual treatment for new patients with TB is an initial two-month phase of isoniazid, rifampin,**

Table 24.10 Recommended Daily Doses of First-Line Anti-Tuberculosis Drugs (Adults)

Isoniazid	4–6 mg/kg	Maximum 300 mg
Rifampicin	8–12 mg/kg	Maximum 600 mg
Pyrazinamide	20–30 mg/kg	
Ethambutol	12–18 mg/kg	

Daily dosing is optimal. Dosing three times a week instead of daily is an alternative for HIV-negative patients, assuming that therapy is directly observed. In the case of three times weekly treatment, doses of isoniazid, pyrazinamide, and ethambutol are higher than listed here. *Source*: Adapted from Ref. 89.

Table 24.11 WHO-Recommended Treatment Regimens

Treatment category	Patients	Tuberculosis treatment[a]	
		Initial phase	Continuation
I	New cases of smear-positive pulmonary TB; or severe extrapulmonary TB; or severe smear-negative pulmonary TB; or severe concomitant HIV disease	2 mo $H_3R_3Z_3E_3$ or 2 mo $H_3R_3Z_3S_3$	4 mo H_3R_3
II	Previously treated smear-positive pulmonary TB; relapse; treatment failure; treatment after default	2 mo HRZE or 2 mo HRZS 2 mo $H_3R_3Z_3E_3S_3$/1 mo $H_3R_3Z_3E_3$	4 mo HR 5 mo $H_3R_3E_3$
III	New cases of smear-negative pulmonary TB, or with less severe forms of extrapulmonary TB	2 mo HRZES/1 mo HRZE 2 mo $H_3R_3Z_3E_3$	5 mo HRE 4 mo H_3R_3 4 mo HR

[a]Subscript refers to the number of doses per week; for daily dosing, no subscript. H, isoniazid; R, rifampicin; Z, pyrazinamide; S, streptomycin; E, ethambutol. *Source*: Adapted from Ref. 89.

pyrazinamide, and ethambutol. Drugs may be given as fixed-dose combinations. Strict adherence to the regimen is important in minimizing drug resistance; for this reason directly observed therapy is usually recommended. **For the following four months, isoniazid and rifampin are continued**. In settings where isoniazid resistance is high and the patient's strain of TB has not been tested for isoniazid resistance, the four-month continuation phase should also include ethambutol.

Treatment regimens and alternatives are available from the Centers for Disease Control and Prevention, the American Thoracic Society, the National Institute for Clinical Excellence, and the WHO. Those interested in these topics may bookmark the CDC's *Find TB Resources* Web site at http://www.findtbresources.org/scripts/index.cfm, which contains links to these sites.

In the case of multidrug-resistant (MDR) or extensively drug-resistant (XDR) tuberculosis, treatment becomes considerably more complex. Retreatment is beyond the scope of this chapter.

Tuberculosis treatment is not altered by pregnancy. Isoniazid, rifampin, pyrazinamide, and ethambutol are not teratogenic, and the WHO recommends their use in pregnant women (89). Streptomycin exposure in utero has been associated with infant hearing loss, and so it is contraindicated in pregnancy. There are no adequate well-controlled reliable studies in human pregnancy. Although there has been some discussion in the literature about deferring treatment of latent tuberculosis infection to the postpartum period (see above), **there is no defensible argument for deferring treatment of active disease during pregnancy**. Pregnant women who are untreated pose an infection risk to the population at large as well as to their own infants.

Drug Resistance
MDR-TB—resistant to isoniazid and rifampin—accounts for about 1% of isolates in the United States. (90) Worldwide, MDR-TB accounts for about 4% of cases (91), although in some areas of the Russian Federation this rate is as high as 25%. Approximately 5% to 10% of MDR-TB strains are believed to be XDR, that is, also resistant to second-line anti-TB drugs. Pregnant women with MDR tuberculosis should be treated despite the limited safety data, because of the grave public health implications. Tuberculosis strains that are known to be resistant to one or more of the first-line drugs are treated with alternative agents, for example, capreomycin, cycloserine, fluoroquinolones, para-aminosalicylate, thiacetazone, amoxacillin-clavulanic acid, clofazimine, or clarithromycin. Kanamycin,

streptomycin, and amikacin, which are ototoxic, have been associated with hearing loss in newborns whose mothers were treated during pregnancy. Ethionamide not only worsens nausea associated with pregnancy but has also been associated with congenital anomalies in animal studies: the WHO recommends against its use in pregnancy, if possible (92). For all the second-line drugs, well-designed controlled studies in pregnant women are unavailable. The literature on treatment of drug-resistant TB during pregnancy is limited to case reports or case series (93–96). Therapy of MDR tuberculosis during pregnancy should be driven by microbiologic susceptibility patterns (obtained by direct culture or known to be prevalent in the area), modified where possible by fetal concerns. For example, the WHO suggests that therapy of drug-resistant TB may be delayed until the second trimester after a discussion with the patient of the risks and benefits (90). The individual practitioner is unlikely to make solo decisions about the treatment of MDR-TB, as this is a role commonly filled by the health authority. The WHO maintains a tuberculosis gateway that provides links to epidemiology and to treatment of tuberculosis: http://www.who.int/tb/en/.

Coinfection with TB and HIV During Pregnancy
This is a large and growing public health problem, directly affecting global maternal mortality (97), which is nevertheless beyond the scope of this chapter. The interested reader is referred to a recent review of the topic (98) and to online resources at CDC and WHO.

Infection Control Issues
Women with active pulmonary tuberculosis are infectious, but if the organism is sensitive, two weeks of multidrug therapy renders them noninfectious, so special precautions are not necessary thereafter. If the duration of therapy is shorter, or if MDR tuberculosis is present or suspected, the mother must be isolated in a negative pressure room for labor, and personal protective equipment should be worn by staff. Measures for the infant may include prophylactic isoniazid, BCG vaccination, or—in cases of MDR or XDR tuberculosis—separation from the mother.

Antepartum Testing
No specific indications.

Delivery
Cord blood and placenta should be tested for acid-fast bacilli.

Postpartum/Breast-feeding

Maternal tuberculosis treatment is not altered by breast-feeding. Pyridoxine should be administered to the breast-feeding infant even if the infant is not receiving isoniazid therapy (79,81). Neonate should undergo TST, chest X ray, lumbar puncture, and *M. tuberculosis* smear and culture if mother had TB during pregnancy. If tuberculosis is suspected in the child, the child should be adequately treated.

REFERENCES

1. National Asthma Education and Prevention Program. Expert Panel Report 3: guidelines for the diagnosis and management of asthma: full report 2007. Available at: http://www.nhlbi.nih.gov/guidelines/asthma/asthgdln.pdf. [Guideline]
2. Kwon HL, Triche EW, Belanger K, et al. The epidemiology of asthma during pregnancy: prevalence, diagnosis, and symptoms. Immunol Allergy Clin North Am 2006; 26:29–62. [III]
3. Enriquez R, Wu P, Griffin MR, et al. Cessation of asthma medication in early pregnancy. Am J Obstet Gynecol 2006; 195:149–153. [II-2]
4. Blais L, Kettani FZ, Elftough N, et al. Effect of maternal asthma on the risk of specific congenital malformations: a population-based cohort study. Birth Defects Res A Clin Mol Teratol 2010; 88:216–222. [II-2]
5. Dombrowski MP, Schatz M, Wise R, et al., for the National Institute of Child Health and Human Development Maternal-Fetal Medicine Units Network and the National Heart, Lung and Blood Institute. Asthma during pregnancy. Obstet Gynecol 2004; 103:5–12. [II-2]
6. Bakhireva LN, Schatz M, Jones KL, et al. Asthma control during pregnancy and the risk of preterm delivery or impaired fetal growth. Ann Allergy Asthma Immunol 2008; 101:137–143. [II-3]
7. Schatz M, Dombrowski MP, Wise R, et al. Spirometry is related to perinatal outcomes in pregnant women with asthma. Am J Obstet Gynecol 2006; 194:120–126. [II-3]
8. Bracken MB, Triche EW, Belanger K, et al. Asthma symptoms, severity, and drug therapy; a prospective study of effects on 2205 pregnancies. Obstet Gynecol 2003; 102:739–752. [II-2]
9. Olesen C, Thrane N, Nielsen GL, et al. A population-based prescription study of asthma drugs during pregnancy: changing the intensity of asthma therapy and perinatal outcomes. Respiration 2001; 68:256–261. [II-2]
10. Cydulka RK, Emerman CL, Schreiber D, et al. Acute asthma among pregnant women presenting to the emergency department. Am J Respir Crit Care Med 1999; 160:887–892. [II-3]
11. Kircher S, Schatz M, Long B. Variables affecting asthma course during pregnancy. Ann Allergy Asthma Immunol 2002; 89:463–466. [II-3]
12. Gluck JC, Gluck PA. The effect of pregnancy on the course of asthma. Immunol Allergy Clin North Am 2000; 20:729–743. [II-3]
13. Beecroft N, Cochrane GM, Milburn HF. Effect of sex of fetus on asthma during pregnancy: blind prospective study. BMJ 1998; 317(7162):856–857. [II-3]
14. National Asthma Education and Prevention Program. NAEPP Working Group Report on managing asthma during pregnancy: recommendations for pharmacologic treatment—update 2004. NIH Publication 05-3279. Available at: http://www.nhlbi.nih.gov/health/prof/lung/asthma/astpreg/astpreg_full.pdf. Accessed November 15, 2010. [Guideline]
15. Dombrowski MP, Schatz M, ACOG Committee on Practice Bulletins-Obstetrics. Asthma in pregnancy. ACOG Practice Bulletin No. 90. Obstet Gynecol. 2008; 111(2 pt 1):457–464. [III]
16. Dombrowski MP, Schatz M, Wise R, et al. Randomized trial of inhaled beclomethasone dipropionate versus theophylline for moderate asthma during pregnancy. Am J Obstet Gynecol 2004; 190:737–744. [I, *n* = 385]
17. Silverman M, Sheffer A, Diaz, P, et al. Outcome of pregnancy in a randomized controlled study of patients with asthma exposed to budesonide. Ann Allergy Asthma Immunol 2005; 95:566–570. [I, *n* = 313]
18. Namazy J, Schatz M, Long L, et al. Use of inhaled steroids by pregnant asthmatic women does not reduce intrauterine growth. J Allergy Clin Immunol 2004; 113:427–432. [II-2]
19. Martel M-J, Rey E, Beauchesne M-F, et al. Use of inhaled corticosteroids during pregnancy and risk of pregnancy-induced hypertension: nested case-control study. BMJ 2005; 330:230–236. [II-2]
20. Breton MC, Beauchesne MF, Lemiere C, et al. Risk of perinatal mortality associated with inhaled corticosteroid use for the treatment of asthma during pregnancy. J Allergy Clin Immunol 2010; 126:772–777. [II-2]
21. Rahimi R, Nikfar S, Abdollahi M. Meta-analysis finds use of inhaled corticosteroids during pregnancy safe: a systematic meta-analysis review. Hum Exp Toxicol 2006; 25(8):447–452. [I]
22. Lin S, Munsie JPW, Herdt-Losavio ML, et al. Maternal asthma medication use and the risk of gastroschisis. Am J Epidemiol 2008; 168:73–79. [II-2]
23. Bakhireva LN, Jones KL, Schatz M, et al. Safety of leukotriene receptor antagonists in pregnancy. J Allergy Clin Immunol 2007; 119:618–625. [II-2]
24. Sarkar M, Koren G, Kalra S, et al. Montelukast use during pregnancy: a multicentre, prospective, comparative study of infant outcomes. Eur J Pharmacol 2009; 65:1259–1264. [II-2]
25. Ducharme FM. Addition of anti-leukotriene agents to inhaled corticosteroids for chronic asthma. Cochrane Database of Systematic Reviews 2004(1). Art. No.: CD003133. DOI: 10/1002/14651858.CD003133.pub2. [Meta-analysis]
26. Siddiqi AK, Gouda H, Multz AS, et al. Ventilator strategy for status asthmaticus in pregnancy: a case-based review. J Asthma 2005; 42:159–162. [II-3]
27. Elsavegh D, Shapiro JM. Management of the obstetric patient with status asthmaticus. J Intensive Care Med 2008; 23:396–402. [II-3]
28. Marik PE, Varon J. Requirement of perioperative stress doses of corticosteroids: a systematic review of the literature. Arch Surg 2008; 143:1222–1226. [Review]
29. Rust GS, Thompson CJ, Minor P, et al. Does breastfeeding protect children from asthma? Analysis of NHANES III survey data. J Natl Med Assoc 2001; 93:139–148. [II-3]
30. File TM. Community-acquired pneumonia. Lancet 2003; 362:1991–2001. [review]
31. Sheffield JS, Cunningham FG. Community-acquired pneumonia in pregnancy. Obstet Gynecol 2009; 114(4):915–922. [Review]
32. Goodnight WH, Soper DE. Pneumonia in pregnancy. Crit Care Med 2005; 33(suppl):S390–S397. [Review]
33. Fine MJ, Auble TE, Yealy DM, et al. A prediction rule to identify low-risk patients with community-acquired pneumonia. N Engl J Med 1997; 336:243–250. [II-3]
34. Jin Y, Carriere KC, Marrie TJ, et al. The effects of community-acquired pneumonia during pregnancy ending with a live birth. Am J Obstet Gynecol 2003; 18:800–806. [II-3]
35. Yost NP, Bloom SL, Richey SD, et al. An appraisal of treatment guidelines for community-acquired pneumonia. Am J Obstet Gynecol 2000; 183:131–135. [II-3]
36. Bloom SL, Ramin S, Cunningham FG. A prediction rule for community-acquired pneumonia. N Engl J Med 1997; 336:1913–1914. [Meta-analysis in letter to the editor]
37. Getahun D, Ananth CV, Oyelese Y, et al. Acute and chronic respiratory diseases in pregnancy: associations with spontaneous premature rupture of membranes. J Matern Fetal Neonatal Med 2007; 20:669–675. [II-2]
38. Banhidy F, Acs N, Puho EH, et al. Maternal acute respiratory infectious diseases during pregnancy and birth outcomes. Eur J Epidemiol 2008; 23:29–35. [II-2]
39. Getahun D, Ananth CV, Peltier MR, et al. Acute and chronic respiratory diseases in pregnancy: associations with placental abruption. Am J Obstet Gynecol 2006; 195:1180–1184. [II-2]
40. Mandell LA, Wunderink RG, Anzueto A, et al. Infectious Diseases Society of America/American Thoracic Society Consensus Guidelines on the management of community-acquired pneumonia in adults. Clin Infect Dis 2007; 44(suppl):S27–S72. [Guideline]
41. Taubenberger JK, Morens DM. Influenza: the once and future pandemic. Public Health Rep 2010; 125(suppl 3):16–26. [Review]

42. Jamieson DJ, Honein MA, Rasmussen SA, et al. H1N1 2009 influenza virus infection during pregnancy in the USA. Lancet 2009; 374:451–458. [II-3]

43. Siston AM, Rasmussen SA, Honein MA, et al. Pandemic 2009 influenza A (H1N1) virus illness among pregnant women in the United States. JAMA 2010; 303:1517–1525. [II-3]

44. Dodds L, McNeil SA, Fell DB, et al. Impact of influenza exposure on rates of hospital admissions and physician visits because of respiratory illness among pregnant women. CMAJ 2007; 176: 463–468. [II-2]

45. Tamma PD Steinhoff MC, Omer SB. Influenza infection and vaccination in pregnant women. Expert Rev Respir Med 2010; 4:321–328. [Review]

46. Irving WL, James DK, Stephenson T, et al. Influenza virus infection in the second and third trimesters of pregnancy: a clinical and seroepidemiological study. BJOG 2000; 107:1282–1289. [II-2]

47. Griffiths PD, Ronalds CJ, Heath RB. A prospective study of influenza infections during pregnancy. J Epidemiol Community Health 1980; 34:124–128. [II-2]

48. Hartert TV, Neuzil KM, Shintani AK, et al. Maternal morbidity and perinatal outcomes among pregnant women with respiratory hospitalizations during influenza season. Am J Obstet Gynecol 2003; 189:1705–1712. [II-2]

49. Acs N, Banhidy F, Puho E, et al. Pregnancy complications and delivery outcomes of pregnant women with influenza. J Matern Fetal Neonat Med 2006; 19:135–140. [II-2]

50. Louie KJ, Acosta M, Jamieson DJ, et al. for the California Pandemic Working Group. Severe H1N1 influenza in pregnant and postpartum women in California. N Engl J Med 2010; 362:27–35. [II-3]

51. ANZIC Influenza Investigators and Australasian Maternity Outcomes Surveillance System. Critical illness due to 2009 A/H1N1 influenza in pregnant and postpartum women: population based cohort study. BMJ 2010; 340:c1279. [II-2]

52. Oluyomi-Obi T, Avery L, Schneider C, et al. Perinatal and maternal outcomes in critically ill obstetrics patients with pandemic H1N1 influenza A. J Obstet Gynaecol Can 2010; 32:443–447. [II-3]

53. Schanzer DL, Langley JM, Tam TWS. Influenza-attributed hospitalization rates among pregnant women in Canada 1994–2000. J Obstet Gynecol Can 2007; 29:622–629. [II-2]

54. Cox S, Posner SF, McPheeters M, et al. Hospitalizations with respiratory illness among pregnant women during influenza season. Obstet Gynecol 2006; 107:1315–1322. [III]

55. Davies AR, Jones D, Bailey M, et al., for the Australia and New Zealand Extracorporeal Membrane Oxygenation (ANZ ECMO) Influenza Investigators. Extracorporeal membrane oxygenation for 2009 influenza A(H1N1) acute respiratory distress syndrome. JAMA 2009; 302(17):1888–1895. [II-3]

56. Cox NJ, Subbarao K. Influenza. Lancet 1999; 354:1277–1282. [III]

57. Mak TK, Mangtani P, Leese J, et al. Influenza vaccination in pregnancy: current evidence and selected national policies. Lancet Infect Dis 2008; 8:44–52. [III]

58. Munoz FM, Greisinger AJ, Wehmanen OA, et al. Safety of influenza vaccination during pregnancy. Am J Obstet Gynecol 2005; 192:1098–1106. [II-2]

59. Zaman K, Roy E, Arifeen SE, et al. Effectiveness of maternal influenza immunization in mothers and infants. N Engl J Med 2008; 359:1555–1564. [RCT, n = 340]

60. Steinhoff MC, Omer SB, Roy E, et al. Influenza immunization in pregnancy—antibody responses in mothers and infants. N Engl J Med 2010; 362:1644–1646. [III]

61. Harper SA, Bradley JS, Englund JA, et al. Seasonal influenza in adults and children: diagnosis, treatment, chemoprophylaxis, and institutional outbreak management: clinical practice guidelines of the Infectious Diseases Society of America. Clin Infect Dis 2009; 48:1003–1032. [Guideline]

62. World Health Organization. WHO guidelines for pharmacological management of pandemic (H1N1) 2009 influenza and other influenza viruses. Available at: http://www.who.int/csr/resources/publications/swineflu/h1n1_use_antivirals_20090820/en/index.html. Accessed December 20, 2010. [Guideline]

63. Aoki FY, Macleod MD, Paggiaro P, et al. IMPACT Study Group. Early administration of oral oseltamivir increases the benefits of influenza treatment. J Antimicrob Chemother 2003; 51:123–129. [II-2]

64. Kaiser L, Wat C, Mills T, et al. Impact of oseltamivir treatment on influenza-related lower respiratory tract complications and hospitalizations. Arch Intern Med. 2003; 163(14):1667–1672. [I]

65. Nicholson KG, Aoki FY, Osterhaus AD, et al. Efficacy and safety of oseltamivir in treatment of acute influenza: a randomised controlled trial. Neuraminidase Inhibitor Flu Treatment Investigator Group. Lancet 2000; 355(9218):1845–1850. [I]

66. Treanor JJ, Hayden FG, Vrooman PS, et al. Efficacy and safety of the oral neuraminidase inhibitor oseltamivir in treating acute influenza: a randomized controlled trial. U.S. Oral Neuraminidase Study Group. JAMA 2000; 283:1016–1024. [I]

67. Jefferson T, Jones M, Doshi P, et al. Neuraminidase inhibitors for preventing and treating influenza in healthy adults: systematic review and meta-analysis. BMJ 2009; 339:b5106. [Review]

68. Worley KC, Roberts SW, Bawdon RE. The metabolism and transplacental transfer of oseltamivir in the ex vivo human model. Infect Dis Obstet Gynecol 2008; 2008:927574. [II-3]

69. Tanaka T, Nakajima K, Murashima A, et al. Safety of neuraminidase inhibitors against novel influenza A (H1N1) in pregnant and breastfeeding women. CMAJ 2009; 181(1–2):55–58. [Review]

70. Greer, LG, Sheffield JS, Rogers VL, et al. Maternal and neonatal outcomes after anterpartum treatment of influenza with antiviral medications. Obstet Gynecol 2010; 115:711–716. [II-2]

71. Wentges-van Holthe N, van Eijkeren M, van der Laan JW. Oseltamivir and breastfeeding. Int J Infect Dis 2008; 12:451. [III]

72. World Health Organization. Global tuberculosis control 2010. Available at: http://whqlibdoc.who.int/publications/2010/9789241564069_eng.pdf. Accessed December 31, 2010. [III]

73. Knight M, Kurinczuk J, Nelson-Piercy C, et al., on behalf of the United Kingdom Obstetric Surveillance System (UKOSS). Tuberculosis in pregnancy in the UK. BJOG 2009; 116:584–588. [III]

74. Frieden TR, Sterling TR, Munsiff SS, et al. Tuberculosis. Lancet 2003; 362:887–892. [Review]

75. Boehme CC, Nabeta P, Hillemann D, et al. Rapid molecular detection of tuberculosis and rifampin resistance. N Engl J Med 2010; 363:1005–1015. [II-2]

76. Lin HC, Lin HC, Chen SF. Increased risk of low birthweight and small for gestational age infants among women with tuberculosis. BJOG 2010; 117:585–590. [II-2]

77. Jana N, Vasishta K, Jindal SK, et al. Perinatal outcome in pregnancies complicated by pulmonary tuberculosis. Int J Gynecol Obstet 1994; 44:119–124. [II-2]

78. Tripathy S. Tuberculosis and pregnancy. Int J Gynaecol Obstet 2003; 80:247–253. [II-1]

79. American Thoracic Society, CDC, and Infectious Diseases Society of America. Treatment of tuberculosis. MMWR Recomm Rep 2003; 52(RR-11):1–77. [Review]

80. Laibl V, Sheffield J. Tuberculosis in pregnancy. Clin Perinatol 2005; 32:739. [Review]

81. American Thoracic Society. Targeted tuberculin testing and treatment of latent tuberculosis infection. Am J Respir Crit Care Med 2000; 161:S221–S247. [Review]

82. Jasmer RM, Nahid P, Hopewell PC. Latent tuberculosis infection. N Engl J Med 2002; 347:1860–1866. [Review]

83. Royal College of Physicians, for the National Collaborating Centre for Chronic Conditions. Tuberculosis: clinical diagnosis and management of tuberculosis, and measures for its prevention and control. National Institute for Clinical Excellence 2006. Available at http://www.nice.org.uk/nicemedia/live/10980/30020/30020.pdf. Accessed December 28, 2010. [Guideline]

84. Jonnalagadda S, Payne BL, Brown E, et al. Latent tuberculosis detection by interferon γ release assay during pregnancy predicts active tuberculosis and mortality in human immunodeficiency virus type 1-infected women and their children. J Infect Dis 2010; 202:1826–1835. [III]

85. Mazurek GH, Jereb J, Vernon A, et al. IGRA Expert Committee, Centers for Disease Control and Prevention (CDC). Updated

guidelines for using Interferon Gamma Release Assays to detect *Mycobacterium tuberculosis* infection—United States, 2010. MMWR Recomm Rep 2010; 59(RR–5):1–25. [Guideline]

86. Franks AL, Binkin NJ, Snider DE, et al. Isoniazid hepatitis among pregnant and postpartum Hispanic patients. Public Health Rep 1989; 104:151–155. [II-3]

87. Saukkonen J, Cohn D, Jasmer R, et al. An official ATS statement: hepatotoxicity of antituberculosis therapy. Am J Respir Crit Care Med 2006; 174:935–952. [III]

88. Boggess KA, Myers ER, Hamilton CD. Antepartum or postpartum isoniazid treatment of latent tuberculosis infection. Obstet Gynecol 2000; 96:757–762. [II-2]

89. World Health Organization. Treatment of Tuberculosis: Guidelines for National Programmes. 4th ed, 2010. Available at: http://www.who.int/tb/publications/tb_treatmentguidelines/en/index.html. Accessed December 26, 2010. [Guideline]

90. Centers for Disease Control and Prevention. Reported Tuberculosis in the United States, 2009. Atlanta, GA: U.S. Department of Health and Human Services, CDC, 2010. Available at: http://www.cdc.gov/tb/statistics/reports/2009/pdf/report2009.pdf. Accessed December 31, 2010. [Review]

91. World Health Organization. Multidrug and extensively drug-resistant TB (M/XDR-TB). 2010 Global Report on Surveillance and Response. Available at: http://whqlibdoc.who.int/publications/2010/9789241599191_eng.pdf. Accessed December 31, 2010. [Review]

92. World Health Organization. Guidelines for the programmatic management of drug-resistant tuberculosis. Emergency update 2008. Available at: http://whqlibdoc.who.int/publications/2008/9789241547581_eng.pdf. Accessed December 30, 2010. [Guideline]

93. Lessnau K, Qarah S. Multidrug-resistant tuberculosis in pregnancy: case report and review of the literature. Chest 2003; 123:953–956. [III]

94. Shin S, Guerra D, Rich M, et al. Treatment of multidrug-resistant tuberculosis during pregnancy: a report of 7 cases. Clin Infect Dis 2003; 36:996–1003. [II-3]

95. Drobac P, delCastillo H, Sweetland A, et al. Treatment of multi-drug-resistant tuberculosis during pregnancy: long-term follow-up of 6 children with intrauterine exposure to second-line agents. Clin Infect Dis 2005; 40:1689–1692. [II-3]

96. Palacios E, Dallman R, Munoz M, et al. Drug-resistant tuberculosis and pregnancy: treatment outcomes of 38 cases in Lima, Peru. Clin Infect Dis 2009; 48:1413–1419. [II-2]

97. Grange J, Adhikari M, Ahmed Y, et al. Tuberculosis in association with HIV/AIDS emerges as a major nonobstetric cause of maternal mortality in Sub-Saharan Africa. Int J Gynaecol Obstet 2010; 108(3):181–183. [III]

98. Adhikari M. Tuberculosis and tuberculosis/HIV co-infection in pregnancy. Semin Fetal Neonatal Med 2009; 234–240. [Review]

25

Systemic lupus erythematosus

Maria A. Giraldo-Isaza

KEY POINTS

- **Diagnosis:** ≥4/11 American Rheumatologic Association criteria.
- **Preconception counseling:** Feto-neonatal and maternal **complications** are primarily seen in systemic lupus erythematosus (SLE) patients **with active disease periconception or patients with hypertension, renal, heart, lungs or brain disease, or antiphospholipid, or SSA/SSB antibodies.** Therefore, it is recommended to screen for all above, and to start pregnancy with SLE in remission. Optimize medical therapy preconception.
- **Laboratories:** CBC with platelets, transaminases, creatinine, BUN, anti-Ro (SSA) and anti-La (SSB), anticardiolipin antibodies (ACA), lupus anticoagulant (LA) or dilute Russell's viper venom time (DRVVT), anti beta-2 glycoprotein-I, antinuclear antibodies (ANA), anti–ds DNA, C3, C4, urine sediment, 24-hour urine for total protein and creatinine clearance.
- **If stable with no recent flares on azathioprine and/or hydroxychloroquine (Plaquenil), it is recommended to continue them in pregnancy and postpartum.** Keep at lowest possible efficacious dose of medications, including steroids.
- Low-dose aspirin (50–150 mg daily), if indicated, should be ideally initiated prior to 16 weeks for prevention of preeclampsia, fetal growth restriction (FGR), and preterm birth.
- **For women with APS, see chapter 26.**
- Women with **SSA/SSB antibodies** have a **2% to 5% risk of congenital heart block (CHB);** preventive screening and therapy for CHB are not evidence based. Women with fetuses with CHB should be managed and delivered at a tertiary care center with the availability of immediate neonatal pacing.

HISTORIC NOTES

In the 1950s, SLE 5-year survival: 50%; in 1990s, 10-year survival: 95%.

DIAGNOSIS

American Rheumatologic Association (**ARA**) **criteria:** need ≥4 out of the following 11 criteria to make diagnosis of SLE—either serially or simultaneously (1).

1. Malar rash
2. Discoid rash
3. Photosensitivity
4. Oral ulcers—painless
5. Arthritis (nonerosive, involving two or more peripheral joints)
6. Serositis: pleuritis or pericarditis, conjunctivitis
7. Renal disorder: persistent proteinuria >0.5 g/day, or cellular casts
8. Neurologic disorder: seizure or psychosis
9. Hematologic disorder: hemolytic anemia with reticulocytosis, or leukopenia <4000/mm^3, or lymphopenia <1500/mm^3, or thrombocytopenia <100,000/mm^3
10. Immunologic disorder: positive lupus erythematosus cell preparation, or anti–double-stranded (ds) DNA, or anti-Smith (SM) antibody, or false-positive serologic test for syphilis
11. Antinuclear antibodies (ANA) in abnormal titers

SYMPTOMS

See the 11 diagnostic criteria. Also general (fatigue, fever, malaise, weight loss); GI (anorexia, ascites, vasculitis); thrombosis, Raynaud's phenomenon, among others.

EPIDEMIOLOGY/INCIDENCE

1:700 to 2000 general population (1:200 in African Americans). 90% in women. 1/500 in childbearing age. Table 25.1 has a list of incidence of abnormal laboratory tests. 25% of SLE patients meet criteria for antiphospholipid syndrome (APS) (see chap. 26).

ETIOLOGY/BASIC PATHOPHYSIOLOGY

Autoantibody (Ab) to fixed tissue antigen (Ag) in vessel wall, nucleus, cytoplasmic membranes, etc.; Ag-Ab complexes in serum.

COMPLICATIONS
Maternal

Hypertension (4–20%), preeclampsia (8–20%), eclampsia (0.5–1%), preterm birth (20–50%) [spontaneous—preterm premature repture of membranes (PPROM) and preterm labor (PTL)—and indicated], cesarean section (30–40%), lupus flare (20–30%), nephritis (10–20%); hematologic complications including thrombocytopenia (4%), anemia (13%), antepartum bleeding (2%), blood transfusion (3%) (2-4). There is also increased risk (1–2%) for infections, thrombosis, and maternal death when compared with non-SLE pregnant women (4). Increased risk of diabetes is associated to treatment with steroids during pregnancy.

Fetal/Neonatal

Increased incidence of first-trimester spontaneous pregnancy loss (10–20%), fetal death (1–5%), FGR (5–20%), CHB (see below), neonatal lupus (see below) (2–4). Independent risk factors for pregnancy loss in SLE women are proteinuria (≥ 500 mg in 24 hours), APS, thrombocytopenia (≤150,000/mm^3), and hypertension (≥140/90 mmHg) (5).

These adverse outcomes are primarily seen in SLE patients with active disease periconceptionally, or in patients

Table 25.1 Selected Laboratory Tests for SLE

Test	Prevalence in SLE patients	Associations/comments
ANA	95%	Not specific or pathognomonic
Anti–double-stranded (ds) DNA	70%	Clinical activity and flares; renal
Anti-Ro (SSA)	30%	Congenital heart block (CHB), neonatal lupus, Sjogren's syndrome
Anti-La (SSB)	15%	CHB, neonatal lupus, Sjogren's syndrome
Anticardiolipin antibodies (ACA)	50%	APS (see chap. 26), thrombosis
Lupus anticoagulant (LA)	26%	FGR, fetal death, preeclampsia
Anti-SM	20%	Specific for SLE
Anti-RNP	40%	Neonatal lupus, mixed connective tissue (CT) disorder
Anticentromere		90% in CREST variant of scleroderma

Abbreviations: SLE, systemic lupus erythematosus; ANA, antinuclear antibodies.

with hypertension, renal, cardiac, pulmonary or neurologic disease, or antiphospholipid antibodies. APS is associated with most fetal deaths in SLE. Renal disease is present in 50% of SLE patients. Lupus nephritis and APS are associated with higher incidence of PTL and hypertensive disorders. Above complications may also be seen more frequently in multiple pregnancies with SLE.

PREGNANCY CONSIDERATIONS
Effect of Pregnancy on SLE
Pregnancy usually does not affect long-term prognosis of SLE. Incidence of flares varies widely, depending on the definition of flare, patient selection, and clinical status at conception. About 50% of patients will have measurable lupus activity during pregnancy. Flares can occur in any trimester, but are most common in late pregnancy and post-partum. Most flares in pregnancy are mild (90%), musculoskeletal, and hematologic. Prednisone $\geq$20 mg only is usually required for severe flares.

Effect of SLE on Pregnancy
Increased incidence of complications (see above). If renal SLE, 50% have hypertension, 10% to 30% worsening but usually reversible renal disease. If creatinine $\geq$1.3 mg/dL, and/or creatinine clearance <50 mL/min, and/or proteinuria >3 g in 24 hour preconceptionally, there is small risk of irreversible renal deterioration. Patients with SLE that undergo kidney transplant have a pregnancy outcome similar to those patients that have kidney transplants for other indications (6) (see chaps. 13 and 17).

MANAGEMENT
Principles
Over 90% of women without end-organ disease or antiphospholipid antibodies (APAs) do well, and take home babies. Goal: pregnancy with SLE in remission. **Start pregnancy with SLE in remission.** To achieve this, usually **need to optimize medical therapy preconceptionally.** Most drugs are safe (see below), and should be continued throughout pregnancy.

Workup
Baseline prenatal laboratory tests should include the following (Table 25.1): **CBC with platelets, transaminases, creatinine, blood urea nitrogen (BUN), anti-Ro (SSA), anti-La (SSB), ACA, LA, anti-beta 2-glycoprotein-I, ANA, anti–ds DNA, C3, C4, urine sediment, 24-hour urine for total protein and creatinine clearance.**

Differential diagnosis to distinguish SLE flare from preeclampsia includes the following: C3, C4 ($\downarrow$ in SLE), and anti–ds DNA ($\uparrow$ in SLE), urine sediment (red and white cells and cellular casts seen in SLE). Gestational age (GA) at onset of symptoms is also helpful, with preeclampsia usually only after 24 weeks.

Preconception Counseling
Review all of above with patient and family, especially diagnosis, risks and complications, and management. Evaluate by history, physical exam, and laboratory tests. Obtain records. Discuss current medications. To insure pregnancy is conceived with SLE quiescent, encourage patient to wait at least six months without flares/active disease before attempting conception. Discuss contraception. **If stable with no recent flares on azathioprine and/or hydroxychloroquine, it is recommended to continue them in pregnancy and postpartum. Keep at lowest possible efficacious dose of steroids.** Substitute teratogenic medications (e.g., mycophenolate mofetil) with safe medications prior to conception. Consider multidisciplinary management with rheumatologist/nephrologist if lupus nephritis.

Prenatal Care
For women with positive antiphospholipid antibody, see chapter 26. Treatment decisions are based on the past obstetric history and any history of prior thromboembolic events. Identify and manage risk factors for early pregnancy loss. The use of medications to treat or suppress SLE flares will need to be evaluated on an individual basis. If patients have been maintained on medication(s) throughout the pregnancy, these should be continued through the postpartum period. Counsel regarding avoiding excessive sun exposure or fatigue.

Therapy
NSAIDs (Nonsteroidal Anti-inflammatory Drugs)
Safe up to 28 to 30 weeks. Side effects: fetal ductal closure and oligohydramnios, especially after 30 weeks. Low-dose aspirin (50–150 mg daily) should ideally be initiated prior to 16 weeks for prevention of preeclampsia, FGR, and preterm birth (7).

Corticosteroids
Mechanism of action: $\downarrow$ antibody levels. Prednisone: 5 to 80 mg usual daily dose. Try to keep maintenance doses $\leq$20 mg/day. For treatment of flares, usually need $\geq$60 mg/day for three weeks. Safe in pregnancy (metabolized by placenta, does not cross it). Animal studies report facial clefts. Safe for breastfeeding. High doses: risk of diabetes (perform early glucola), PPROM, hypertension, and FGR. Taper if used more than seven days. Side effects: increased bone loss, especially together with heparin (give calcium). Fluorinated corticosteroids (dexamethasone and betamethasone) cross the placenta and should not be used to treat lupus activity.

In general, there is no need for stress steroids peripartum. The usual oral daily dose should be given peripartum. **Stress dose of steroids are indicated only if prednisone ≥20 mg daily or equivalent dose of a different steroid given for >3 weeks** (8,9). This is to prevent Addisonian collapse, manifested as general malaise, nausea/vomiting, and skin changes, which is extremely rare. If used, stress dose of steroids can be given as hydrocortisone 100 mg IV when patient is in active labor or prior to induction of anesthesia if cesarean delivery, followed by hydrocortisone 50 mg IV q8h for 24 hours. Usual oral dose should be restarted postpartum.

Azathioprine (Azasan, Imuran)
Daily 50 to 100 mg orally or divided bid. Increase after six to eight weeks. Safe in pregnancy. FGR association is probably due to SLE, not azathioprine. It induces chromosomal breaks, which disappear as infant grows.

Hydroxychloroquine Sulfate (Plaquenil)
Antimalarian drug. 400 to 600 mg orally daily, then ↓ 200 to 400 mg daily. **Safe in pregnancy** (10). No increased risk of miscarriage, stillbirth, pregnancy loss, and congenital anomalies in exposed pregnancies when compared to nonexposed group (11). If stopped, 2.5 times risk of flare compared to placebo (12). **Important not to stop drug periconception (11,13). In fact, if stable with no recent flares on hydroxychloroquine, it is recommended to continue it in pregnancy and postpartum.** No long-term effects. Safe in breast-feeding.

Bromocriptine
Inhibitor of prolactin secretion. Pilot study shows potential benefit if given in second and third trimester in a dose of 2.5 mg daily. It decreases lupus activity, PPROM, preterm birth, and low birth weight. No risk of congenital anomalies or spontaneous abortion (14). If given for two weeks postpartum, 2.5 mg bid starting 12 hours after delivery in nonnursing mothers, it can also decrease SLE flares (15). Insufficient data for recommendation, further studies are needed.

Immunoglobulin
Used as 0.5 g/kg initiated after positive pregnancy test until 33 weeks of gestation. It has been associated in a nonrandomized study with decrease in the rate of miscarriage in patients with history of recurrent pregnancy loss (25% pregnancy loss in nontreated group vs. 0% in treated group) with or without associated APS, decrease in doses of concomitant medications including prednisolone, decrease in lupus activity, and improvement in laboratory values (anti-ds DNA, anti-Ro, and anti-LA antibodies) (16). Insufficient data for recommendation; further studies are needed.

Other Agents
Acethaminophen or paracetamol: safe throughout pregnancy. Usually not as effective as other therapies. Cyclophosphamide, methotrexate, penicillamine, and mycophenolate mofetil: avoid; not safe in pregnancy. Plasmapheresis: last resort, consult rheumatology.

ANTEPARTUM TESTING
Accurate gestational age assessment is important; therefore, a first-trimester ultrasound examination is indicated.

Fetal growth can be evaluated throughout the pregnancy with q4–6weeks ultrasound examinations. For women with SSA/SSB, see section "Congenital Heart Block." A fetal echo-

cardiogram is indicated if CHB, arrhythmia or hydropic signs are detected.

Patients in whom disease activity is quiescent, and there is no evidence of hypertension, renal disease, FGR, or preeclampsia, can begin weekly fetal testing at 34 to 36 weeks' gestation. Patients with active disease, antiphospholipid antibodies, renal disease, hypertension, or FGR can begin antepartum testing earlier, for example, 30 to 32 weeks.

DELIVERY
Stress dose steroids are indicated only if prednisone ≥20 mg daily or equivalent dose of a different steroid is given for >3 weeks. See section "Corticosteroids."

POSTPARTUM/BREAST-FEEDING
Flares are more common. Continue and consider increasing SLE therapies. Breast-feeding usually safe depending on medications.

CONGENITAL HEART BLOCK
Incidence
The incidence of CHB is about 2% to 5% of SSA/SSB positive women.

Etiology
SSA/SSB antibodies cause myocarditis and fibrosis in the AV node and bundle of HIS regions. Maternal antibodies are necessary to cause CHB, but evidence suggests that there are other factors involved in the development of CHB.

Counseling
Usually permanent, with pacemaker needed in two-third of surviving affected children before adulthood. One-third of untreated CHB infants die within three years (sudden death). 10% to 15% of affected offspring will have a life-threatening cardiomyopathy. There is about a 19% recurrence in future siblings. Complications: congestive heart failure (hydrops).

Management
Prevention
If positive for SSA/SSB, consider following with weekly fetal pulse Doppler echocardiography or fetal kinetocardiogram/tissue Doppler echocardiography (FKCG) from 16 to 26 weeks and every other week from 26 to 34 weeks to look for prolonged PR (AV) interval and any dysrrhythmia, especially looking for incomplete (first or second) degree block. This screening may not be cost-effective given CHB is uncommon in prospective series even with positive SSA/SSB, and is not evidenced-based (17). The fetal mechanical PR interval is measured from simultaneous mitral and aortic Doppler waveforms (17). FKCG, a tissue velocity–based measurement of AV conduction, appears to be superior to the pulse Doppler echocardiography (18). Data from prospective series revealed that the FKCG can detect first-degree AV block in ~8.5% of these high risk fetuses and that Doppler can detect PR prolongation in only ~3% of these fetuses and did not precede the occurrence of third-degree block (19,21). Treatment with dexamethasone (4 mg/day) upon detection has been reported as possibly associated with normalization of AV conduction (19). Recent studies (nonrandomized) suggest dexamethasone 4 mg daily is likely beneficial in treating fetuses with first-degree AV block, possibly beneficial in treating second-degree block, and not beneficial and possibly harmful for third-degree block (20–22). Risks-benefits of prolonged

steroid treatment should be discussed with the patient. Even it remains unclear if cardiac injury is progressive and could be prevented if diagnosed and treated early, prolongation of the PR interval>150 ms, moderate or severe tricuspide regurgitation, and/or atrial echodensity appear to be potential early biomarkers of reversible cardiac injury. Intravenous immunoglobulin (IVIg) at a dose of 400 mg/kg every three weeks is not effective in reducing recurrent CHB in high-risk patients (23–25).

Prenatal Care

Fetal echocardiography should be performed (see also section "Prevention"). Of CHB cases, 10% to 20% have CHD and not SSA/SSB, but 95% of CHB without CHD have SSA/SSB. For fetuses with hydrops, see also chapter 53.

Therapy

Once complete (third degree) CHB, this is considered to be irreversible. No randomized trials have demonstrated the effectiveness of steroid, (20,25–28) beta-mimetic, (29,30) digoxin, IVIg and other therapies to normalize conduction or improve outcome. **Women with fetuses with CHB should be managed and delivered at a tertiary care center with the availability of immediate neonatal pacing.**

Delivery

While trial of labor (TOL) by repeated scalp sampling to assure fetal well-being can be attempted, TOL is often difficult to manage clinically.

NEONATAL LUPUS

Transient neonatal SLE, because of maternal IgG through placenta. Usually IgG and association with SSA-SSB occurs in 10% of SSA/SSB pregnancies. So prophylaxis not indicated. F:M 14:1. Not always mother has diagnosis of SLE. Characterized by photosensitive annular erythematous rash, elevated liver enzymes, cholestasis, fulminant liver disease, thrombocytopenia or pancytopenia, heart block, and cardiomyopathy. Most cases are cutaneous (transient rash) and have thrombocytopenia. Can last for 14 to 16 weeks. Neonatal death rate is 1% to 2%.

REFERENCES

1. Tan EM, Cohan AS, Aries JF, et al. The 1982 revised criteria for the classification of systemic lupus erythematosus. Arthritis Rheum 1982; 25:1271. [III]
2. Smyth A, Oliveira GH, Lahr BD, et al. A systematic review and meta-analysis of pregnancy outcomes in patients with systemic lupus erythematosus and lupus nephritis. Clin J Am Soc Nephrol 2010; 5(11):2060–2068. [II-2]
3. Chakravarty EF, Nelson L, Krishnan E. Obstetric hospitalizations in the United States for women with systemic lupus erythematosus and rheumatoid arthritis. Arthritis Rheum 2006; 54(3):899–907. [II-2]
4. Clowse ME, Jamison M, Myers E, et al. A national study of the complications of lupus in pregnancy. Am J Obstet Gynecol 2008; 199(2):127.e1–127.e6. [II-2]
5. Clowse ME, Magder LS, Witter F, et al. Early risk factors for pregnancy loss in lupus. Obstet Gynecol 2006; 107(2 pt 1):293–299. [II-2]
6. McGrory CH, McCloskey LJ, DeHoratius RJ, et al. Pregnancy outcomes in female renal recipients: a comparison of systemic lupus erythematosus with other diagnoses. Am J Transplant 2003; 3(1):35–42. [II-2]
7. Bujold E, Roberge S, Lacasse Y, et al. Prevention of preeclampsia and intrauterine growth restriction with aspirin started in early pregnancy: a meta-analysis. Obstet Gynecol 2010; 116(2 pt 1):402–414. [I]
8. Marik PE, Varon J. Requirement of perioperative stress doses of corticosteroids: a systematic review of the literature. Arch Surg 2008; 143(12):1222–1226. [II-2]
9. The American College of Obstetricians and Gynecologists. Steroid use in pregnancy. PROLOG Obstetrics, 6th ed., 46–47. [III]
10. Costedoat-Chalumeau N, Amoura Z, Duhaut P, et al. Safety of hydroxychloroquine in pregnant patients with connective tissue diseases: a study of one-hundred thirty-three cases compared to a control group. Arthritis Rheum 2003; 48:3207–3211. [II-1]
11. Clowse ME, Magder L, Witter F, et al. Hydroxychloroquine in lupus pregnancy. Arthritis Rheum 2006; 54(11):3640–3647. [II-2]
12. The Canadian Hydroxychloroquine Study Group. A randomized study of the effect of withdrawing hydroxychloroquine sulfate in systemic lupus erythematosus. N Engl J Med 1991; 324:150–154. [RCT]
13. Levy RA, Vilela VS, Cataldo MJ, et al. Hydroxychloroquine in lupus pregnancy: double-blind and placebo-controlled study. Lupus 2001; 10:401–404. [RCT, $n = 20$]
14. Jara LJ, Cruz-Cruz P, Saavedra MA, et al. Bromocriptine during pregnancy in systemic lupus erythematosus: a pilot clinical trial. Ann N Y Acad Sci 2007; 1110:297–304. [II-1]
15. Yang XY, Liang LQ, Xu HS, et al. Efficacy of oral bromocriptine in protecting the postpartum systemic lupus erythematosus patients from disease relapse. Zhonghua Nei Ke Za Zhi 2003; 42(9):621–624. [II-1]
16. Perricone R, De Carolis C, Kröegler B, et al. Intravenous immunoglobulin therapy in pregnant patients affected with systemic lupus erythematosus and recurrent spontaneous abortion. Rheumatology (Oxford) 2008; 47(5):646–651. [II-2]
17. Van Bergen AH, Cuneo BF, Davis N. Prospective echocardiographic evaluation of atrioventricular conduction in fetuses with maternal Sjogren's antibodies. Am J Obstet Gynecol 2004; 191:1014–1018. [II-3]
18. Nii M, Hamilton RM, Fenwick L, et al. Assessment of fetal atrioventricular time intervals by tissue Doppler and pulse Doppler echocardiography: normal values and correlation with fetal electrocardiography. Heart 2006; 92(12):1831–1837. [II-2]
19. Rein AJ, Mevorach D, Perles Z, et al. Early diagnosis and treatment of atrioventricular block in the fetus exposed to maternal anti-SSA/Ro-SSB/La antibodies: a prospective, observational, fetal kinetocardiogram-based study. Circulation 2009; 119(14):1867–1872. [II-1]
20. Copel JA, Buyon JP, Kleinman CS. Successful in-utero therapy of fetal heart block. Am J Obstet Gynecol 1995; 173:1384–1390. [II-3]
21. Friedman DM, Kim MY, Copel JA, et al. PRIDE Investigators Utility of cardiac monitoring in fetuses at risk for congenital heart block: the PR Interval and Dexamethasone Evaluation (PRIDE) prospective study. Circulation 2008; 117(4):485–493. [II-1]
22. Friedman DM, Kim MY, Copel JA, et al. Prospective evaluation of fetuses with autoimmune-associated congenital heart block followed in the PR Interval and Dexamethasone Evaluation (PRIDE) Study. Am J Cardiol 2009; 103(8):1102–1106. [II-1]
23. Friedman DM, Llanos C, Izmirly PM, et al. Evaluation of fetuses in a study of intravenous immunoglobulin as preventive therapy for congenital heart block: results of a multicenter, prospective, open-label clinical trial. Arthritis Rheum 2010; 62(4):1138–1146. [II-1]
24. Pisoni CN, Brucato A, Ruffatti A, et al. Failure of intravenous immunoglobulin to prevent congenital heart block: findings of a multicenter, prospective, observational study. Arthritis Rheum 2010; 62(4):1147–1152. [II-2]
25. Buyon JP, Waltuck J, Kleinman C, et al. In-utero identification and therapy of congenital heart block. Lupus 1995; 4:116–121. [II-3]

26. Saleeb S, Copel J, Friedman D, et al. Comparison of treatment with fluorinated glucocorticoids to the natural history of auto-antibody-associated congenital heart block. Arthritis Rheum 1999; 42:2335–2345. [II-3]

27. Shinohara K, Miyagawa S, Fujita T, et al. Neonatal lupus erythematosus: results of maternal corticosteroid therapy. Obstet Gynecol 1999; 93:952–957. [II-3]

28. Narne S, Berghella V, Weiner S, et al. Outcome in fetuses with auto-antibody associated congenital heart block treated with dexamethasone. Obstet Gynecol 2004; 103:106s. [II-3]

29. Novi JM, Mulvihill BHK. Use of subcutaneous B-sympathomimetic pump for the treatment of fetal congenital complete heart block. J Repro Med 2003; 48:893–895. [II-3]

30. Eronen M, Heikkila P, Teramo K. Congenital complete heart block in the fetus: hemodynamic features, antenatal treatment, and outcome in six cases. Pediatr Cardiol 2001; 5:385–392. [II-3]

26

Antiphospholipid syndrome

James A. Airoldi

KEY POINTS

- The **diagnosis** of antiphospholipid syndrome (APS) requires the presence of at least **one clinical and one laboratory** criteria (Tables 26.1 and 26.2).
- **APS is associated with venous thromboembolism (VTE), early onset preeclampsia, early pregnancy loss, fetal growth restriction (FGR), fetal death, preterm birth, and other complications**.
- Therapy should be as follows:
  - For APS with ≥3 **unexplained consecutive pregnancy losses at <10 weeks: low-dose ASA** and **prophylactic heparin** (either unfractionated or low molecular weight).
  - For APS with VTE during the current pregnancy: **therapeutic anticoagulation.**
  - For APS with **VTE prior to pregnancy: prophylactic heparin.**
  - There are no trials to assess therapy for APS with a history of preeclampsia and/or FGR prior to 34 weeks' gestation.
- If on low-molecular-weight heparin, regional anesthesia may need to be delayed until ≥24 hours after the last dose.

HISTORIC NOTES

Lupus anticoagulant (LA) was first described in early 1950s as prolonging certain clotting assays. A few years later, LA was found to be associated with the false-positive test for syphilis and, paradoxically, thrombosis.

DIAGNOSIS

The diagnosis of APS requires the presence of **at least one clinical** (Table 26.1) **and one laboratory** (Table 26.2) criteria (1,2). Abnormal laboratory tests must occur in **more than two occasions, ≥12 weeks apart.** The two tests must occur within a five-year time frame. There are no time limits on the interval between the clinical and laboratory events. Once the diagnosis is established by the criteria above, subsequent negative results decrease but do not eliminate the risks of complications.

ANTIPHOSPHOLIPID ANTIBODY TESTING

Antiphospholipid antibodies (APAs) are directed against phospholipids, and include anticardiolipin antibodies (ACAs), LA, and anti–beta-2 glycoprotein-I (B2GP-I) (Table 26.2). LA is a double misnomer. LA is seen in many patients without systemic lupus erythematosus (SLE), and is associated with thrombosis, not anticoagulation (see chap. 25). Possible testing for LA is shown in Figure 26.1. ACAs strongly correlate with LA and thrombosis. ACAs require the presence of plasma phospholipids–binding protein B2 glycoprotein I to bind to cardiolipin. In contrast, ACAs from patients with syphilis or other infections are B2 glycoprotein I independent. Approximately 80% of patients with LA have ACAs, while 20% of patients with ACAs are found positive for LA (2). Substantial **interlaboratory variation** when testing the same sera remains a **serious problem**.

SYMPTOMS

Clinical manifestations of APS may include any organ system, including vascular (arterial or venous), cardiac, cutaneous, endocrine/reproductive, gastrointestinal, hematologic, neurologic, obstetrical, ophthalmologic, pulmonary, renal, and others.

EPIDEMIOLOGY/INCIDENCE

APAs are found in up to 5% of healthy controls. The prospective risks in this are unknown. Of SLE patients, 25% to 35% have APS (see chap. 25). ACAs are present in 15% women with recurrent miscarriage; LA is found in 8% of patients with recurrent miscarriage. In women with mid-trimester fetal loss, LA is seen in up to 30%. Of definite APS patients, 70% have both ACAs and LA.

ETIOLOGY/BASIC PATHOPHYSIOLOGY

APAs may cause pregnancy loss by thrombosis of placental vessels, interference with coagulation factors (reduce levels of annexin V), inhibition of proliferation of trophoblasts, complement activation, or other yet unknown mechanisms.

CLASSIFICATION

Primary APS refers to patients with APS but no other autoimmune disorders. *Secondary* APS refers to patients with other autoimmune disorders (e.g., SLE) (2).

COMPLICATIONS
Maternal

- **Venous, and arterial, thromboembolism:** Risk is 5% to 12% in pregnancy; there are no adequate cohort or case-control studies to validate these estimates of VTE with APS pregnant women (3). 0.5% to 2% of asymptomatic nonpregnant people incidentally found to have APAs have thromboses each year. Most thrombotic events are venous (65–70%). Arterial thromboses can occur in atypical sites such as the retina, the subclavian artery, or the middle cerebral artery (the most common vessel involved when a stroke occurs in these patients).
- **Preeclampsia:** There is a statistically significant association especially between preeclampsia and ACA (3)

Table 26.1 Clinical Criteria for Diagnosis of Antiphospholipid Syndrome

1. *Vascular thrombosis*

   One or more clinical episodes of arterial, venous, or small vessel thrombosis, in any tissue or organ. Thrombosis must be confirmed by objective criteria (e.g., imaging or Doppler studies or histopathology).

   And/or

2. *Pregnancy morbidity*

   (A). **One or more unexplained deaths** of a morphologically normal fetus **at or beyond the 10th week** of gestation, with normal fetal morphology documented by ultrasound or by direct examination of the fetus.

   And/or

   (B). **One or more premature births** of a morphologically normal neonate **before the 34th week** of gestation **because of: eclampsia or severe preeclampsia, or features consistent with placental insufficiency** (e.g., abnormal Doppler flow, abnormal fetal testing, AFI < 5, SGA).

   And/or

   (C). **Three or more unexplained consecutive spontaneous abortions before the 10th week** of pregnancy, with maternal anatomic or hormonal abnormalities and paternal and maternal chromosomal causes excluded.

Abbreviations: AFI, amniotic fluid index; SGA, small for gestational age. *Source*: Modified from Refs. 1,2.

Incidence of preeclampsia is about 18% to 48% of women with APS.

- **Autoimmune thrombocytopenia:** Risk is 40% to 50%. Heparin-induced thrombocytopenia [less with low-molecular-weight heparin (LMWH)] can also occur, as well as lupus flare in patients with coexisting SLE.

Fetal

- **Pregnancy loss and fetal death:** These complications can occur in any trimester, and be recurrent. About 5% to 20% of women with recurrent pregnancy losses have APAs (2). While all APAs are associated with pregnancy loss and fetal death, early pregnancy loss has been associated in a review with both ACA and LA; recurrent first trimester

Table 26.2 Laboratory Criteria for the Diagnosis of Antiphospholipid Syndrome

1. **Lupus anticoagulant** present in plasma, on two or more occasions **at least 12 wk apart**. Examples are lupus anticoagulant, DRVVT, or aPTT test (Fig. 26.1).

And/or

2. **Anticardiolipin antibody** of IgG and/or IgM isotype in serum or plasma, present as >**40 GPL or MPL**, or > 99th percentile, on two or more occasions, **at least 12 wks apart.**

And/or

3. **Anti-B2 glycoprotein-I of IgG and/or IgM** isotype in serum or plasma (in titer >**99**th **percentile** for a normal population as defined by the laboratory performing the test), present on two or more occasions, **at least 12 wks apart.**

Abbreviations: DRVVT, dilute Russell's viper venom time; aPTT, activated partial thromboplastin time. *Source*: Modified from Refs. 1,2.

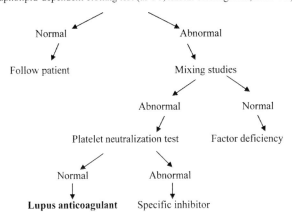

Figure 26.1 Algorithm for interpretation of lupus anticoagulant test. *Abbreviations*: aPTT, activated partial thromboplastin time; DRVVT, dilute Russell's viper venom time. *Source*: From Refs. 1,2.

with ACA; second trimester with LA; third trimester with ACA (3).

- **FGR** (in particular with ACA) (3).
- **Preterm birth** (33%, secondary to gestational hypertension or placental insufficiency, either spontaneous or iatrogenic).
- **Placental abruption** (not associated with ACA or LA in a review) (3).

PREGNANCY CONSIDERATIONS

Complications are less if pregnancy starts when APS is "quiescent" without symptoms and with negative levels of APAs, while complications are more frequent and severe if APS is active with high levels of APAs. As other autoimmune disorders, APS can exacerbate postpartum: fever, pulmonary infiltrates, pleural effusion, occasionally renal, pulmonary complications, VTE; rarely DIC and mortality.

MANAGEMENT
Principles

Multidisciplinary management with rheumatologist or internal medicine specialist is recommended.

Screening

Women with the following risk factors should be screened for ACA, LA, and B2GP-I:

- Three or more spontaneous unexplained first-trimester losses <10 weeks
- One or more unexplained fetal loss/death ≥ 10 weeks
- Early onset (<34 weeks) preeclampsia or FGR, leading to indicated PTB
- SLE
- History of vascular thrombosis (VTEs such as deep-vein thrombosis, pulmonary embolus, and stroke)

Workup

Laboratory tests include ACA, LA, and B2GP-I tests (Table 26.2). Testing for APAs other than LA, ACA, and B2GP-I is not clinically useful in the evaluation of recurrent pregnancy loss and should not be performed.

Prevention

There is no preventive strategy available.

Therapy

Evidence

- Compared to placebo or usual care, low-dose aspirin *alone* is not associated with any difference in outcome in pregnant women with APS (4–6). The summary relative risk for recurrent pregnancy loss is 1.05, 95% CI 0.66, 1.68 (7).
- Compared to low-dose aspirin alone, the **combination of unfractionated heparin (UFH) and low-dose aspirin** in APS patients **with recurrent first-trimester losses** is associated with significant **reduction in early pregnancy loss** (OR 0.26, 95% CI 0.14–0.48; number needed to treat 4) (7–10). **Low molecular weight heparin** (LMWH) did not show a benefit when combined with aspirin (OR 0.70, 95% CI 0.34–1.45) (11,12). This could be attributed to the lower efficacy of LMWH or to several other parameters such as the paucity of studies on LMWH and small study samples, low cutoff threshold for APAs positivity, coexistence of other thrombophilic disorders within the same study, or late entry into the studies that may preclude many early losses, non-acceptance of randomization, and the crossover from assigned treatments (11,12). These five studies have recently been reviewed and published as a systematic review (13).
- Two small RCTs have directly compared LMWH to UFH, and despite the small number of patients recruited, **effectiveness of LMWH appears comparable with that of UFH** (14,15).
- Compared to low-dose aspirin alone, the combination of low-dose aspirin and either UFH or LMWH in patients with a late pregnancy loss showed no benefit in reducing the risk of late pregnancy loss (OR 1.07, 95% CI 0.36–3.16) (8–12).
- Compared to low-dose aspirin alone or placebo, prednisone and low-dose aspirin are not associated with a significant difference in pregnancy loss (RR 0.85, 95% CI 0.53, 1.36) (16,17). However, there were significant higher rates of preterm birth in the prednisone groups in both trials and higher NICU admissions in one study (17). There were also lower birth weights in the prednisone group in one of the studies (16).
- Compared to heparin and low-dose aspirin, prednisone and low-dose aspirin are associated with no difference in pregnancy loss rates, but again the prednisone group had a significantly higher rate of preterm birth (18).
- In women already on heparin and aspirin, the addition of IVIG does not affect pregnancy loss rates in a very small trial, but is associated with a significantly higher preterm birth rate (19). This therapy is very expensive, and the only treatment shown to lower anticardiolipin levels.

Actual Therapy (Table 26.3)

- **APS with early (usually <10 weeks) recurrent pregnancy loss: low-dose aspirin (ASA)** and **prophylactic heparin (either** UFH or LMWH) (20,21).

    Therapy is usually begun once fetal viability is established, but **there is insufficient evidence regarding best time of initiation of therapy**. Low-dose aspirin dose is usually about 75 to 100 mg daily (and some experts recommend starting it even preconception in severe cases) (20). Dose for prophylactic UFH is usually: 5000 to 7500 U first trimester, 7500 to 10000 U second trimester, 10,000 U third trimester SQ q12h. Dose for prophylactic LMWH is usually: enoxaparin (Lovenox) 30 to 40 mg SQ q12h or dalteparin (Fragmin) 5000 U SQ q12h. One may adjust prophylaxis in high-risk cases to a heparin (anti-Xa) level range of 0.2 to 0.4. Anti-Xa level is usually drawn four hours after injection. Anti-Xa levels have not been adequately evaluated prospectively to show a reduction in the incidence of complications.

- **APS with VTE during the current pregnancy: therapeutic anticoagulation** (20,21).

    Therapeutic intravenous UFH doses need to be adjusted to keep activated partial thromboplastin time (aPTT) two to three times normal. Therapeutic LMWH is usually enoxaparin 1 mg/kg q12h SQ, or dalteparin 200 U/kg q12h SQ. Therapeutic LMWH must be adjusted to heparin (anti-Xa) level 0.5 to 1.2. After initial therapy, subcutaneous therapeutic LMWH or UFH should be continued for a minimum total duration of six months.

Table 26.3 Suggested Prophylaxis for APS and Selected Pregnancy Complications

Antiphospholipid syndrome without previous thrombosis, and recurrent early (usually <10 wk) miscarriage	Low-dose aspirin with either • UFH 5000–7500 U first trimester; 7500–10,000 U second trimester; 10,000 U third trimester SQ q12h, or • LMWH, e.g., enoxaparin (Lovenox) 30–40 mg SQ q12h or dalteparin (Fragmin) 5000 U SQ q12h
Antiphospholipid syndrome with previous VTE	Low-dose aspirin with either • UFH 5000–7500 U first trimester; 7500–10,000 U second trimester; 10,000 U third trimester SQ q12h, or • LMWH, e.g., enoxaparin (Lovenox) 30–40 mg SQ q12h or dalteparin (Fragmin) 5000 U SQ q12h

Abbreviations: APS, antiphospholipid syndrome; UFH, unfractionated heparin; LMWH, low-molecular-weight heparin; SQ, subcutaneous.

Anticoagulation should also be used for six weeks postpartum. Postpartum anticoagulation could be at therapeutic doses if the VTE occurred late in pregnancy, or it could be at prophylactic doses if the VTE occurred early in pregnancy.

- **APS with VTE in a prior pregnancy: prophylactic heparin (either UFH or LMWH) both in the antepartun and postpartum period (six weeks)** (20,21).

  Therapy is usually begun once fetal viability is established, but there is insufficient evidence regarding best time of initiation of therapy. Low-dose aspirin dose is usually about 75 to 100 mg daily. Prophylactic UFH dose is usually 5000 to 7500 U first trimester, 7500 to 10,000 U second trimester, 10,000 U third trimester SQ q12h. Prophylactic LMWH dose are usually enoxaparin (Lovenox) 30 to 40 mg SQ q12h, or dalteparin (Fragmin) 5000 U SQ q12h. One may adjust prophylaxis in high-risk cases to a heparin (anti-Xa) level range of 0.2 to 0.4. Anti-Xa level is usually drawn four hours after injection. Anti-Xa levels have not been adequately evaluated prospectively to show a reduction in the incidence of complications.

- **APS with late fetal death:** Treatment trials have not shown a significant benefit at this time. The two trials that addressed this issue had some weaknesses, and thus no recommendations can be made at this time (11,12).

- **APS with a medically indicated preterm birth secondary to early onset intrauterine growth restriction (IUGR) or severe preeclampsia:** There are no treatment trials to assess any therapy, and no recommendations can be made at this time. Some experts have suggested prophylaxis similar to that shown in Table 26.3 (21).

Other Issues with Therapy

Heparin is associated with a 5% decrease in bone mass density and, therefore, osteoporosis. Supplemental calcium (calcium gluconate/carbonate 1500 mg daily) and vitamin D, as well as resistance exercise, should be encouraged. Idiosyncratic thrombocytopenia known as **heparin-induced thrombocytopenia (HIT)** occurs in <5% of women on heparin therapy, is usually mild, and starts usually 3 to 15 days after initiation of therapy. HIT is less common with LMWH. If on heparin (either type), consider checking an anti-Xa level at least once in three weeks after initiating heparin. **Check platelet counts initially and then weekly in the first three weeks to assure that there is no evidence of HIT.** There is no evidence to assess warfarin therapy for women with extreme thrombotic histories, including recurrent thromboses or cerebral thrombosis (see also chap. 28).

ANTEPARTUM TESTING

- Early ultrasound is essential for accurate dating.
- Detailed ultrasound at about 18 to 20 weeks and follow-up ultrasounds about every 4 to 6 weeks for growth, fluid volume, and (if necessary) Doppler evaluation of the fetus.
- Fetal surveillance testing (e.g., NSTs and/or BPPs) starting at 32 weeks.
- Daily fetal kick counts.

PREPARATIONS FOR DELIVERY

- Consider delivery by EDC.
- If on LMWH, consider switching to UFH at 36 weeks to allow regional anesthesia.

DELIVERY

Consider sending the placenta to pathology, to check for decreased placental weight, ischemic-hypoxic changes—infarctions, decidual and fetal thrombi, chronic villitis.

ANESTHESIA

If on UFH, regional anesthesia can be administered usually six to eight hours after the dose, or at least when the aPTT is within normal limits. **If on LMWH, regional anesthesia should be delayed until ≥24 hours after the last dose,** since there is a risk of spinal hematoma if regional anesthesia is performed within 24 hours. That is why a woman on LMWH might be switched off LMWH on to UFH weeks before any chance of labor or delivery (usually around 36 weeks if no other risk of preterm birth).

POSTPARTUM/BREAST-FEEDING

- In women with APS based on recurrent embryonic loss <10 weeks, the use of anticoagulation in the postpartum period has never been shown to be helpful.
- In women with APS based on fetal loss ≥ 10 weeks and no thrombotic events, anticoagulation for six weeks is usually recommended in the United States (2) (only three to five days in the United Kingdom).
- Women with APS based on prior thrombotic events should be switched to warfarin therapy. Warfarin therapy is safe in breast-feeding women. An INR of 3.0 is desirable.

Estrogen-containing oral contraceptives should be avoided, as they further increase the VTE risk.

It is imperative that women with APS be followed closely by a medical or hematological specialist after pregnancy. About 50% of women with APS develop thromboses in the 3 to 10 years after delivery, and about 10% develop SLE (2).

REFERENCES

1. Miyakis S, Lockshin MD, Atsumi T, et al. International consensus statement on an update of the classification criteria for definite antiphospholipid syndrome (APS). J Thromb Haemost 2006; 4:295–306. [Review]
2. American College of Obstetricians and Gynecologists. Antiphospholipid syndrome. ACOG Practice Bulletin No. 118. Obstet Gynecol 2011; 117:192–199. [Review]
3. Robertson L, Wu O, Langhorne S, et al. Thrombphilia in pregnancy: a systematic review. Br J Haematol 2006; 132:171–196. [Review]
4. Pattison NS, Chamley LW, Birdsall M, et al. Does aspirin have a role in improving pregnancy outcome for women with the antiphospholipid syndrome? A randomized controlled trial. Am J Obstet Gynecol 2000; 183:1008–1012. [RCT, *n* = 50]
5. Cowchock S, Reece EA. Do low-risk pregnant women with antiphospholipid antibodies need to be treated? Am J Obstet Gynecol 1997; 176:1099–1100. [RCT, *n* = 19]
6. Tulppala M, Marttunen M, Soderstrom-Anttila V, et al. Low-dose aspirin prevention of miscarriage in women with unexplained or autoimmune related recurrent miscarriage: effect on prostacyclin and thromboxane A2 production. Hum Reprod 1997; 12:1567–1572. [RCT, *n* = 66]
7. Empson M, Lassere M, Craig JC, et al. Recurrent pregnancy loss with antiphospholipid antibody: a systematic review of therapeutic trials. Obstet Gynecol 2002; 99:135–144. [Meta-analysis; 10 RCTs; includes Refs. 2,3,4,6,8,9,10,11,12; *n* = 627]

8. Rai R, Cohen H, Dave M, et al. Randomised controlled trial of aspirin and aspirin plus heparin in pregnant women with recurrent miscarriage associated with phospholipids antibodies. BMJ 1997; 314:253–257. [RCT, *n* = 90]

9. Kutteh WH. Antiphospholipid antibody-associated recurrent pregnancy loss: treatment with heparin and low dose aspirin is superior to low-dose aspirin alone. Am J Obstet Gynecol 1996; 174:1584–1589. [RCT, *n* = 50]

10. Goel N, Tuli A, Choudhry R. The role of aspirin versus aspirin and heparin in cases of recurrent abortions with raised anticardiolipin antibodies. Med Sci Monit 2006; 12:CR132–CR136. [RCT, *n* = 72]

11. Farquharson RG, Quenby S, Greaves M. Antiphospholipid syndrome in pregnancy: a randomized controlled trial of treatment. Lupus 2002; 100:408–413. [RCT, *n* = 98]

12. Laskin CA, Spitzer KA, Clark CA, et al. Low molecular weight heparin and aspirin for recurrent pregnancy loss: results from the randomized, controlled HepASA Trial. J Rheumatol 2009; 36:279–287. [RCT, *n* = 88]

13. Ziakas P, Pavlou M, Voulgarelis M. Heparin treatment in antiphospholipid syndrome with recurrent pregnancy loss. Obstet Gynecol 2010; 115:1256–1262. [Review]

14. Noble LS, Kutteh WH, Lashey N, et al. Antiphospholipid antibodies associated with recurrent pregnancy loss: prospective, multicenter, controlled pilot study comparing treatment with low-molecular-weight heparin versus unfractionated heparin. Fertil Steril 2005; 83:684–690. [RCT, *n* = 50]

15. Stephenson MD, Ballem PJ, Tsang P, et al. Treatment of antiphospholipid antibody syndrome (APS) in pregnancy: a randomized pilot trial comparing low molecular weight heparin to unfractionated heparin. J Obstet Gynaecol Can 2004; 26:729–734. [RCT, *n* = 26]

16. Silver RK, MacGregor SN, Sholl JS, et al. Comparative trial of prednisone plus aspirin vs. aspirin alone in the treatment of anticardiolipin antibody positive obstetric patients. Am J Obstet Gynecol 1993; 169:1411–1417. [RCT, *n* = 39]

17. Laskin CA, Bombardier C, Hannah ME, et al. Prednisone and aspirin in women with autoantibodies and unexplained recurrent fetal loss. N Engl J Med 1997; 337:148–153. [RCT, *n* = 202]

18. Cowchock FS, Reece EA, Balaban D, et al. Repeated fetal losses associated with antiphospholipid antibodies: a collaborative randomized trial comparing prednisone with low-dose heparin treatment. Am J Obstet Gynecol 1992; 166:1318–1323. [RCT, *n* = 45]

19. Branch DW, Peaceman AM, Druzin M, et al. A multicenter placebo-controlled pilot study of intravenous immune globulin treatment of antiphospholipid syndrome during pregnancy. The Pregnancy Loss Study Group. Am J Obstet Gynecol 2000; 182:122–127. [RCT, *n* = 16]

20. Bates S, Greer I, Pabinger I, et al. Venous thromboembolism, thrombophilia antithrombotic therapy and pregnancy. Chest 2008; 133:844–886. [Review]

21. Ruiz-Irastorza G, Crowther M, Branch W, et al. Antiphospholipid syndrome. Lancet 2010; 376:1498–1509. [Review; III]

27

Inherited thrombophilia

James A. Airoldi

KEY POINTS

- Inherited thrombophilias are genetic conditions that increase the risk of thromboembolic disease.
- The risk of thrombotic events is affected by numerous factors including thrombophilia, personal history of deep vein thrombosis (DVT), family history of DVT, surgery, age over 35 years, high parity, high body mass index, smoking, and immobilization.
- The prevalence and thrombogenic potential of the inherited thrombophilias are shown in Tables 27.1 and 27.2.
- There are statistically significant associations in retrospective cohort with venous thromboembolism (VTE) and factor V Leiden (FVL), prothrombin 20210A gene mutation (PGM), antithrombin III (ATIII) deficiency, decreased protein C (PC) and protein S (PS). Two prospective cohort studies showed an association of VTE and FVL, and one did not.
- The presence of inherited thrombophilias has not been associated with adverse pregnancy outcomes when the best studies (prospective, large, etc.) are evaluated. Prior adverse pregnancy outcomes include intrauterine growth restriction (IUGR), preeclampsia, intrauterine fetal demise (IUFD), abruptio placentae, and early pregnancy loss.
- Fetal carriage of inherited thrombophilia mutations may also have adverse clinical consequences, but the evidence is insufficient for clinical recommendation.
- Screening for inherited thrombophilias:
  - Universal screening for inherited thrombophilias is not recommended.
  - It is reasonable to screen any pregnant woman with a prior personal history of VTE, as this could affect anticoagulation recommendations. Screening can include at least FVL, PGM, and ATIII, and also PS and PC if the etiology was nonrecurrent (e.g., broken bone).
  - In a woman with VTE in the current pregnancy, screening can be performed for at least FVL, PGM, and ATIII.
  - In an otherwise healthy pregnant woman with no personal history of VTE or adverse pregnancy outcomes, but whose first-degree relative has a genetic thrombophilia, there is insufficient evidence to recommend any type of screening.
  - In an otherwise healthy pregnant woman with a prior adverse pregnancy outcome but no major risk factors for VTE, there is insufficient evidence to support screening.
- Treatment for inherited thrombophilias and related conditions:
  - If PC, PS, heterozygous FVL, or PGM are detected in a woman with prior VTE, prophylactic anticoagulation is reasonable.
  - If homozygous FVL or PGM or an ATIII deficiency or a compound heterozygote is detected in a woman with a prior VTE, full therapeutic anticoagulation is indicated.
  - In a woman with a prior personal history of a VTE and a recurring etiology, prophylactic anticoagulation is recommended.
  - Among women with a nonrecurring cause for the prior VTE and no thrombophilia, the risk of recurrent antepartum VTE is low; therefore, routine antepartum prophylaxis with heparin may not be warranted. Anticoagulation could still be given postpartum.
  - In women with one unexplained pregnancy loss at ≥10th week and either heterozygous FVL mutation, prothrombin G20210A mutation, or PS deficiency, LMWH enoxaparin 40 mg starting at eight weeks is associated with a higher (86% vs. 29%) incidence of a healthy live birth compared to low-dose aspirin in one trial.

See also chapters 25, 26, and 28.

HISTORIC NOTES

Antithrombin deficiency and dysfibrinogenemia, the first inherited thrombophilias to be described (1965), were found in studies of families in which several members were affected by venous thrombosis (1,2). Later, heterozygous deficiencies of protein C (PC) (3) and protein S (PS) (4) were identified as causes of inherited thrombophilia. In 1993, resistance to activated PC, the most common cause of inherited thrombophilia, was discovered (5,6). In most cases, it results from a mutation of the factor V gene (G1691A), resulting in a protein called factor V Leiden (FVL) (7). In 1996, the 20210 mutation of the prothrombin gene was found to be another cause of thrombophilia (8).

DEFINITION

Inherited thrombophilias are genetic conditions that increase the risk of VTE and possibly some pregnancy complications (9).

EPIDEMIOLOGY/INCIDENCE

VTE is the leading cause of pregnancy-related maternal morbidity and mortality in the developed world (10). Estimates for the incidence of thrombotic events occurring during pregnancy and the puerperium vary from 0.2 to 2 per 1000 births (10,11). During pregnancy, women have a fivefold increased risk of VTE compared with nonpregnant women (11), and cesarean delivery carries a fivefold higher risk of thrombosis relative to vaginal delivery (12,13). The frequency of thrombotic events is equal in the antepartum and postpartum periods. Antepartum risk is equally divided for each trimester

Table 27.1   Prevalence of Different Thrombophilias in the General and At-Risk Population

	Prevalence in general population (%)	Prevalence in patients with history of thrombosis (%)
Factor V Leiden (heterozygous)	1–15	10–50
Prothrombin gene (heterozygous)	2–5	6–18
ATIII deficiency	0.02	1–3
Protein S deficiency	0.1–1.3	1–5
Protein C deficiency	0.2–0.4	3–5
Hyperhomocysteinemia	5	10
MTHFR (C677T heterozygous)	5–14	–

Source: From Refs. 15, 16.

Table 27.2   Risk of VTE with Different Thrombophilias

	VTE potential (RR of VTE)	VTE risk per pregnancy		% of all VTE
		No history (%)	*Prior VTE* (%)	
Factor V Leiden heterozygote	5–7	0.25	10	40
Factor V Leiden homozygote	25	1.5	17	2
Prothrombin gene heterozygote	3–9	0.5	>10	17
Prothrombin gene homozygote	25	2–3	>17	0.5
FVL/prothrombin compound heterozygote	84	4.5–5	>20	1–3
Antithrombin III activity <60%	50–100	0.4–7	40	1
Protein C activity <50%	10–13	0.1–0.8	4–17	14
Protein S free antigen <55%	2–10	0.1	0–22	3
Hyperhomocysteinemia (>16 μM)	3–6	0.2	NA	<5%

Abbreviation: VTE, venous thromboembolism; RR, risk ratio. *Source*: From Refs. 15, 16, 44.

(11). Therefore, if anticoagulation is warranted, it should begin very early in pregnancy as coagulation factors increase early in pregnancy. Pulmonary embolism is more common postpartum (11).

Up to 50% of women who have thrombotic events during pregnancy possess an underlying **congenital or acquired thrombophilia** (14). The frequency of the major inherited thrombophilias varies substantially within healthy populations and among patients with previous venous thrombosis (Table 27.1) (15,16). The most common inherited thrombophilias are heterozygosity for the FVL gene mutation, the prothrombin G20210A gene mutation (PGM), and the thermolabile variant of methylenetetrahydrofolate reductase (C677T MTHFR), the most common cause of hyperhomocysteinemia. Less common thrombophilias include autosomal-dominant deficiencies of antithrombin, PC, and PS. Factor V Leiden and the G20210A mutation in the prothrombin gene are common among Caucasians but are extremely rare among Asians and Africans (17). The population prevalence of FVL mutation shows racial differences. In a recent prospective cohort study, the carrier rate was 6.1% in Caucasians, 0.8% in African-Americans, 1.7% in Hispanics, and 1.9% in others (18) (Table 27.1).

ETIOLOGY/BASIC PATHOPHYSIOLOGY

Changes in the coagulation system, an increase in venous stasis, and vascular injury at delivery substantially increase the risk of developing VTE in pregnancy compared with the nonpregnant state (10). Coagulation system changes include increases in fibrinogen and factors II, VII, VIII, IX, X, and XII, an increase in the activity of the fibrinolytic inhibitors as evidenced by increases in plasminogen-activator inhibitor 1 (PAI-1) and 2 (PAI-2), a decrease in PS activity (because of estrogen-induced decreases in total PS and increases in the complement 4b binding protein, which binds PS), and an

increase in resistance to activated PC in the second and third trimesters (19,20) (see chapter 3, *Obstetric Evidence Based Guidelines*). In approximately 50% of patients with a hereditary thrombophilia, the initial thrombotic event occurs in the presence of an additional risk factor such as pregnancy, personal or family history, high body mass index, smoking, oral contraceptive use, orthopedic trauma, immobilization, or surgery (21,22). Histologic examination of uteroplacental vessels and intervillous architecture from pathologic pregnancies typically display increased fibrin deposition, thrombosis, and hypoxia-associated endothelial and trophoblast changes (23). Another placental pathology study of women with and without thrombophilia who had severe preeclampsia, intrauterine growth retardation, severe abruptio placentae, or stillbirth showed lower placental weight, and higher number of villous infarcts and fibrinoid necrosis in the thrombophilic women but no higher rate of thrombosis in the placenta. This study questions whether thrombosis of the placental vessels is the main cause of the outcomes (24). Antiphospholipid antibodies inhibit extravillous trophoblastic differentiation, and heparin and aspirin attenuate trophoblastic apoptosis (25,26). Altered regulation of complement may play a significant role in this pathologic process, and heparin inhibits activation of complement (27).

GENETICS/CLASSIFICATION OF EACH INHERITED THROMBOPHILIA (TABLES 27.1 AND 27.2)
Factor V Leiden

The FVL mutation arises from a (G → A) mutation in nucleotide 1691 of the factor V gene's 10th exon, resulting in a substitution of a glutamine for an arginine at position 506 in the factor V polypeptide (factor V Q506). The resultant amino acid substitution impairs the activated PC and PS complex inactivation of factor Va. This defect is termed the FVL mutation and is primarily inherited in an **autosomal-dominant** fashion. It is the most common cause of activated PC resistance. Its prevalence is about 5% to 10% in Europeans, 3% in Afro-Americans, and rare in Asian and African populations (Table 27.1). Homozygosity for the mutation, although rare, confers a far higher risk of thromboembolism. Compound heterozygotes should be treated similar to homozygous women (17).

Prothrombin G20210A

Heterozygosity for a mutation in the promoter of the prothrombin gene (G20210A) leads to increased (150–200%) circulating levels of prothrombin and an increased risk of thromboembolism. Homozygosity for the prothrombin mutation confers a risk of thrombosis equivalent to that of FVL homozygosity. It is inherited in an **autosomal-dominant** fashion (17).

Antithrombin III

Antithrombin III (ATIII) deficiency is the **most thrombogenic** of the inherited thrombophilias with a 70% to 90% lifetime risk of thromboembolism. Deficiencies in AT result from numerous point mutations, deletions, and insertions, and are usually inherited in an **autosomal-dominant** fashion. Because the prevalence of AT deficiency is low, 1/1000 to 1/5000, it is only present in 1% of patients with thromboembolism (17). The appropriate **cutoff of abnormal activity is <60%.**

Protein C

PC is a vitamin K–dependent polypeptide synthesized primarily in the liver. Activated PC combines with free PS to inhibit factors V and VIII (see Fig. 28.1). PC levels can be decreased by warfarin. Its deficiency can result from numerous mutations. Different mutations have highly variable procoagulant sequelae, making it extremely difficult to predict which patients with PC or PS deficiencies will develop thromboembolism (17). The inheritance is **autosomal dominant.** PC deficiency is best diagnosed by a **functional assay activity cutoff of <50%,** which is present in only 0.3% of the populations.

Protein S

PS is a vitamin K–dependent polypeptide synthesized primarily in the liver. PS is present in plasma in its free (40%) and bound (60%) forms, but it is the free form that is functional. PS specifically functions as a cofactor with PC (see Fig. 28.1). Its deficiency presents with one of three phenotypes: (*i*) type I, marked by reduced total and free immunoreactive forms; (*ii*) type II, characterized by normal free immunoreactive levels but reduced activated protein C (APC) cofactor activity; and (*iii*) type III, in which there are normal total immunoreactive but reduced free immunoreactive levels. The inheritance is **autosomal dominant. Protein S decreases normally** by about 40% **during pregnancy,** and thus screening during pregnancy is not recommended. The decrease in pregnancy is due to estrogen-induced decreases in total PS and increases in the complement 4b binding protein, which binds PS. A **free PS antigen <55%** in nonpregnant women should be detected at least twice to detect true deficiency, and best correlate with genetic deficiency. If screening in pregnancy is necessary, cutoff values in the second and third trimesters have been identified at <30% and <24%, respectively (28).

MTHFR/Homocysteinemia

The most common form of genetic hyperhomocysteinemia results from the production of a thermolabile variant of **methylenetetrahydrofolate reductase (MTHFR)** with reduced enzymatic activity (T mutation) (29). The gene encoding for this variant contains an alanine-to-valine substitution at amino acid 677 (C677T) (30). The responsible gene is common, with a population frequency estimated between 5% and 14% (31,32). A MTHFR polymorphism at A1298C is less common. Homozygosity for the thermolabile variant of MTHFR (TT genotype) is a relatively common cause of mildly elevated plasma homocysteine levels in the general population, often occurring in association with low serum folate levels (33,34). Increased blood levels of homocysteine may reflect deficiency of folate, vitamin B6, and/or vitamin B12 (35–38). Plasma folate and B12 levels, in particular, are strong determinants of the homocysteine concentration. Homocysteine levels are inversely related to folate consumption, reaching a stable baseline level when folate intake exceeds 400 μg/day (39,40). Vitamin B6 is a weaker determinant (40). Isolated MTHFR mutations are not associated with increased risk of VTE, and therefore, should not be categorized as thrombophilias (11,41).

RISK FACTORS/ASSOCIATIONS

The risk of thrombotic events is affected by numerous factors including **thrombophilia, personal history of DVT, family history of DVT, surgery, age over 35 years, high parity, high body mass index, smoking, and immobilization** (42,43).

COMPLICATIONS
VTE

The thrombogenic potential of the inherited thrombophilias and the probability of thrombosis per pregnancy in affected individuals are shown in Table 27.2 (15,16,44,45). If the woman is a heterozygote for both FVL and PGM, the probability of thrombosis per pregnancy is 4.6% (44). Data from older case-control studies show significant associations between thrombophilias and VTE in women with no personal history (14). The largest nested case-control study showed no association between FVL and VTE in women with no personal history (18). Data from older case-control studies show significant associations between thrombophilias (FVL and prothrombin) and VTE in women with prior VTE (45).

Adverse Pregnancy Outcome (Table 27.3)

To assess the true association between thrombophilias and pregnancy complications, prospective cohort studies are preferred over retrospective cohort and case-control studies. Meta-analyses of retrospective cohort and case-control studies show many significant associations between various thrombophilias and adverse pregnancy outcomes (46–53). Confounders were assessed and included ethnicity, genetic testing only, and severity of illness (54).

Two large case-control studies assessed this relationship. In one study, FVL mutation showed no relationship with pregnancy loss (any trimester), placental abruption, preeclampsia, or fetal growth restriction (18). In another large case-control study, there was no significant association between preeclampsia and four different thrombophilias (FVL, prothrombin gene mutation, MTHFR C677T mutation, or homocysteine) (55).

Table 27.3 Associations Between Inherited Thrombophilias and Adverse Pregnancy Outcomes

	Factor V	PT 20210	MTHFR (C677T)
First trimester loss	No (18,58,60) Yes (59)	No (56)	No (59)
Second or third trimester loss	No (18,58,60) Yes (57)	No (56,57)	No (57) Yes (61)
IUGR	No (18,57–60)	No (56,57)	No (57,59)
Preeclampsia	No (18,55,57–60)	No (55–57)	No (55,57,59) Yes (61)
Placental abruption	No (18)	No (56) Yes (57)	No (57)

Based on six prospective cohort studies and two large case-control studies. *Abbreviations*: PT, prothrombin; MTHFR (C677T), methylenetetrahydrofolate reductase. *Source*: From Refs. 18,55–61.

Six prospective cohort studies are noted in the most current literature. **All were performed in low-risk women, which is probably not the targeted population.**

In the first study, there was no association between the prothrombin G20210A mutation and pregnancy loss, preeclampsia, abruption, or SGA neonates in a low-risk, prospective cohort (56).

In the second study, some statistically significant findings were noted (57):

- Women who carried the prothrombin gene mutation had an odds ratio (OR) of 3.58 [95% confidence interval (CI) 1.20–10.61, $P = 0.02$] for the development of the composite primary outcome (abruption, stillbirth, or neonatal death).
- Homozygous carriers of the MTHFR 1298 polymorphism had an odds ratio of 0.26 (95% CI 0.08–0.86, $P = 0.03$) for the composite outcome, denoting a protective effect.
- None of the other polymorphisms studied showed a significant association with the composite outcome.
- Placental abruption was significantly associated with prothrombin gene mutation (OR 12.15, 95% CI 2.45–60.39, $P = 0.002$).
- FVL conferred an increased risk of stillbirth (OR 8.85, 95% CI 1.60–48.92, $P = 0.01$).

In the third study, there was no significant association between FVL and preeclampsia, intrauterine growth restriction, or pregnancy loss. FVL was associated with birth weights >90th percentile (OR 1.81; 95% CI 1.04–3.31) and neonatal death (OR 14.79; 95% CI 2.71–80.74) (58).

In the fourth study, the frequency of FVL and MTHFR was no higher in those who subsequently developed preeclampsia or intrauterine growth retardation, and none of the screened population developed thrombosis (59).

In the fifth study, the APC-resistant subgroup did not differ significantly from the non–APC-resistant subgroup in terms of pregnancy complications, but was characterized by an eightfold higher risk of VTE (3/270 vs. 3/2210), a lower rate of profuse intrapartum hemorrhage (3.7% vs. 7.9%) ($P = 0.02$), and less intrapartum blood loss (340 mL vs. 361 mL) ($P = 0.04$) (60).

In the sixth study, women with hyperhomocysteinemia had severe preeclampsia (2/35 vs. 5/714, $P < 0.01$) and stillbirth (2/35 vs. 10/714, $P < 0.05$) more frequently than normohomocysteinemia (61).

In summary, there are no consistent results from these six prospective cohort studies, and therefore the conclusion at this time is that **the presence of inherited thrombophilias has not been consistently associated with adverse pregnancy outcomes.**

FETAL THROMBOPHILIAS

Fetal carriage of thrombophilic mutations may also have adverse clinical consequences. A case-control study evaluated abortuses for the presence of FVL (62). The mutation was present more frequently among abortuses than in unselected pregnancies. If the placenta showed >10% infarction, the fetus was 10 times more likely to have the mutation than when the placenta was normal. Carriers of multiple or homozygous thrombophilic defects were at increased risk of having a birth weight in the lowest quartile or lowest decile in a retrospective study (63). In a prospective study (18), there was no statistical significance between fetal thrombophilia and any adverse pregnancy outcome. However, fetal FVL mutation carriage was associated with more frequent preeclampsia among African-American women and Hispanic women compared to Caucasian women.

DOSE DEPENDENCY OF THROMBOPHILIA

A case-control study nested in the European Prospective Cohort on Thrombophilia (EPCOT) compared 571 women with thrombophilia, with 395 control patients, and reported an increased risk of fetal loss (miscarriage and stillbirth) among the former patients (29.4% vs. 23.5%; $P = 0.04$) (64). The risk of loss was greater after 28 weeks than at or before 28 weeks (OR 3.6; 95% CI 1.4–9.4 vs. OR 1.27; 95% CI 0.94–1.71). **The highest risk for stillbirth was observed in women with combined thrombophilic defects and antithrombin and PC deficiencies.** This suggests that often single genetic defects, such as FVL, may not lead to thrombosis, but rather it is the presence of multiple defects that causes a problem.

In another study (65), the FVL homozygous genotype increased the risk of late fetal loss. However, the overall likelihood of a positive outcome was high in women who were homozygous for factor V.

MANAGEMENT
Screening (Table 27.4)

The decision to perform screening should clearly be influenced by the following:

- The prevalence of the risk factor in the studied population
- Whether the information gathered would impact on clinical management

There is **insufficient evidence to support universal screening,** given the overall low prevalence of thrombophilias in the general population, and the low prevalence of VTE and adverse pregnancy outcomes.

It would be reasonable to screen with a full panel any pregnant women with a **prior personal history of VTE,** especially when due to a **nonrecurring etiology** (e.g., immobilization after an accident). Among women with a history of VTE, older case-control studies have demonstrated that recurrent VTE occurs frequently during pregnancy in thrombophilic women (45). In a prospective study (30), the frequency of FVL in women with a history of thrombosis was higher than expected, (15% vs. 2%), but not for MTHFR (about 505 in cases

Table 27.4 Who to Screen (or Not to Screen) for Inherited Thrombophilias

	Screen for
Prior VTE with nonrecurrent etiology	Factor V, PT 20210; ATIII; PC; PS
Prior VTE with recurrent etiology	Factor V; PT 20210; ATIII
VTE in current pregnancy	Factor V; PT 20210; ATIII
General population	No screening
Relative with inherited thrombophilia but no personal history of VTE	No screening
Prior adverse pregnancy outcome	No screening

Abbreviations: VTE, venous thromboembolism; PT, prothrombin; PC, protein C; PS, protein S; ATIII, antithrombin III.

and controls). In another prospective study (66), pregnant women with a single previous episode of VTE without antepartum anticoagulation had a 2.4% antepartum recurrence of VTE. There were **no recurrences in the 44 women who had no evidence of thrombophilia and who also had a previous episode of thrombosis that was associated with a nonrecurring risk factor.** Among the 51 women with abnormal laboratory results or a previous episode of idiopathic thrombosis, or both, 5.9% had an antepartum recurrence of VTE. Among **women with a nonrecurring cause for the prior VTE and no thrombophilia,** the risk of recurrent antepartum VTE is low; therefore, **routine antepartum prophylaxis with heparin may not be warranted.** Anticoagulation should still be given postpartum. **If PC, PS, heterozygous FVL, or PGM are detected in this group of women, prophylactic anticoagulation would seem reasonable. If homozygous FVL or PGM or an ATIII deficiency or a compound heterozygote are detected, full therapeutic anticoagulation would be indicated.** An elevated homocysteine and a low folate, B6, or B12 level should prompt replacement. Screening for MTHFR is not recommended.

In a woman with a **prior personal history of a VTE** and a **recurring etiology** (i.e., oral contraceptives), **prophylactic anticoagulation** is usually recommended. Being positive for PC or PS would not change clinical management, thus screening should be avoided. **Screening would be indicated for FVL, PGM, and ATIII,** as homozygous FVL, homozygous PGM, compound heterozygote, or an ATIII deficiency would prompt therapeutic anticoagulation. An elevated homocysteine and a low folate, B6, or B12 level should prompt replacement. Screening for MTHFR is not recommended.

In a woman with a **VTE in the current pregnancy,** screening should only be performed for **FVL, PGM, and ATIII.** A homozygous FVL, a homozygous PGM, a compound heterozygote, a double heterozygote, or an ATIII deficiency might extend the duration of therapeutic anticoagulation, and once switched over to prophylactic doses, again may extend the duration of treatment. Screening for PC or PS and obtaining a positive result would not change the clinical recommendations for anticoagulation greatly (nor would heterozygous FVL or PGM change recommendations); therefore, screening is not recommended in pregnancy. An elevated homocysteine and a low folate, B6, or B12 level should prompt replacement. Screening for MTHFR is not recommended.

In pregnant women with **multiple risk factors for VTE** (67) (e.g., AMA, obese, and first-degree relative positive for thrombophilia) who is now postpartum (especially if delivered via cesarean section), it may be reasonable to screen for thrombophilias (full panel) at that time (postpartum), as a positive result may influence the decision to use prophylactic anticoagulation for six weeks postpartum.

In an otherwise **healthy pregnant woman** with no personal history of VTE or adverse pregnancy outcomes, but whose **first-degree relative has a genetic thrombophilia,** there is **insufficient evidence** to recommend any type of screening. Postpartum screening may be reasonable if delivered via cesarean section. If such information has already been screened for and is positive, therapeutic anticoagulation should be offered for homozygous FVL, homozygous PGM, compound heterozygote, or ATIII deficiency. However, there is insufficient evidence that prophylactic anticoagulation for PC, PS or heterozygous FVL, or heterozygous PGM will support a healthy outcome. An elevated homocysteine and a low folate, B6, or B12 level should prompt replacement. Screening for MTHFR is not recommended.

In an otherwise **healthy pregnant woman** with a **prior adverse pregnancy outcome** but no major risk factors for VTE, there is **insufficient evidence** to support screening either antepartum or postpartum. If such information has already been screened for and is positive, therapeutic anticoagulation should be offered for homozygous FVL, homozygous PGM, compound heterozygote, or ATIII deficiency. However, there is no convincing evidence that prophylactic anticoagulation for PC, PS or heterozygous FVL or heterozygous PGM will support a healthy outcome. An elevated homocysteine and a low folate, B6, or B12 level should prompt replacement.

Diagnosis

Table 27.5 describes testing of thrombophilias. The following are the potential causes of false-positive results when testing for thrombophilias (68):

- *Hyperhomocysteinemia:* deficiencies of folic acid, vitamin B12, or vitamin B6; older age, renal failure, smoking

Table 27.5 Testing Characteristics for Different Thrombophilias

	Testing method	Can patients be tested during pregnancy?	Is the test reliable during acute thrombosis?	Is the test reliable while on anticoagulation?
Factor V Leiden	APC resistance assay	No	Yes	Yes
	DNA analysis	Yes	Yes	Yes
Prothrombin gene mutation G20210A	DNA analysis	Yes	Yes	Yes
Protein C deficiency	Protein C activity (<50%)	Yes	No	No
Protein S deficiency	Free protein S antigen (<55%)	No[a]	No	No
ATIII deficiency	ATIII activity (<60%)	Yes	No	No
Hyperhomocysteinemia	Fasting plasma homocysteine	Yes	Unclear	Yes

[a]Protein S cutoffs that can be used in pregnancy (but testing should be repeated more than six weeks postpartum): <30% in second and <24% in third trimesters (30). *Abbreviation*: ATIII, antithrombin III. *Source*: From Ref. 68.

- *Protein C activity:* liver disease, childhood, use of oral anticoagulants, vitamin K deficiency, disseminated intravascular coagulation (DIC), the presence of antibodies against PC
- *Protein S total and free antigen:* pregnancy, liver disease, childhood, use of oral anticoagulants, vitamin K deficiency, DIC, use of oral contraceptives, nephrotic syndrome, the presence of antibodies to PS
- *Antithrombin III activity:* liver disease, use of heparin therapy, nephrotic syndrome, DIC

Therapy (See Table 28.5)

There is only one RCT on congenital thrombophilias and pregnancy complications; therefore, there is **insufficient evidence** to make any recommendation in this area. In the first treatment trial, a prospective randomized, nonblinded non–placebo-controlled randomized trial evaluated the effect of thromboprophylaxis in women with **one unexplained pregnancy loss** at ≥ 10th week of amenorrhea and either heterozygous **FVL mutation**, **prothrombin G20210A** mutation, or **PS deficiency** (free antigen <55%) (69). Women were given 5-mg folic acid daily before conception, to be continued during pregnancy, and either **low-dose aspirin** 100 mg daily **or LMWH** enoxaparin 40 mg starting at eight weeks. LMWH was associated with a higher (86% vs. 29%) incidence of a **healthy live birth,** and lower incidence of low birth weight (10% vs. 30%). No significant side effects of the treatments could be evidenced in patients or newborns. This was not a blinded trial. As there is no argument to prove that low-dose aspirin may have been deleterious, these results support enoxaparin use during such at-risk pregnancies.

A cohort study showed that in women with a **thrombophilia** (heterozygous factor V, activated PC resistance, MTHFR 677 TT genotype, PS deficiency, heterozygous prothrombin 20210, antithrombin II deficiency, hyperhomocysteinemia, and/or PC deficiency) and a **history of ≥3 first trimester losses, ≥2 second trimester losses, or a fetal death in the third trimester,** enoxaparin 40 mg/day was associated with an approximate 80% rate of live births, similar to enoxaparin 80 mg/day (70).

Hyperhomocysteinemia

There are no trials to assess interventions for the pregnant woman with hyperhomocysteinemia. It might be reasonable to suggest safe therapy aimed to normalize the homocysteine level, with folic acid 4 mg once a day, in addition to vitamin B6 25 mg three to four times a day and vitamin B12 100 mg once a day, but counseling should emphasize that this therapy has not been tested in trials in pregnant women. This therapy has been tested in the nonpregnant population. The Vitamins and Thrombosis (VITRO) study investigated the effect of homocysteine lowering by daily supplementation of B vitamins on the risk reduction of DVT and pulmonary embolism (PE) (71). The results did not show that homocysteine lowering by vitamin B supplementation prevents recurrent venous thrombosis, even though homocysteine levels were lowered back to the normal range with therapy.

For **antepartum testing, delivery, anesthesia,** and **postpartum/breast-feeding,** see chapter 28.

REFERENCES

1. Egeberg O. Inherited antithrombin III deficiency causing thrombophilia. Thromb Diath Haemorrh 1965; 13:516–530. [II-3]
2. Beck EA, Charache P, Jackson DP. A new inherited coagulation disorder caused by an abnormal fibrinogen ("fibrinogen Baltimore"). Nature 1965; 208:143–145. [II-3]
3. Griffin JH, Evatt B, Zimmerman TS, et al. Deficiency of protein C in congenital thrombotic disease. J Clin Invest 1981; 68:1370–1373. [II-3]
4. Comp PC, Esmon CT. Recurrent venous thromboembolism in patients with a partial deficiency of protein S. N Engl J Med 1984; 311:1525–1528. [II-2]
5. Koeleman BP, Reitsma PH, Bertina RM. Familial thrombophilia: a complex genetic disorder. Semin Hematol 1997; 34:256–264. [II-2]
6. Dahlback B, Carlsson M, Svensson PJ. Familial thrombophilia due to a previously unrecognized mechanism characterized by poor anticoagulant response to activated protein C: prediction of a cofactor to activated protein C. Proc Natl Acad Sci U S A 1993; 90:1004–1008. [II-3]
7. Bertina RM, Koeleman BP, Koster T, et al. Mutation in blood coagulation factor V associated with resistance to activated protein C. Nature 1994; 369:64–67. [II-2]
8. Poort SR, Rosendaal FR, Reitsma PH, et al. A common genetic variation in the 3′-untranslated region of the prothrombin gene is associated with elevated plasma prothrombin levels and an increase in venous thrombosis. Blood 1996; 88:3698–3703. [II-2]
9. Lockwood CJ. Inherited thrombophilias in pregnant patients. Prenat Neonat Med 2001; 6:3–14. [Review]
10. Greer IA. Thrombosis in pregnancy: maternal and fetal issues. Lancet 1999; 353:1258–1265. [Review]
11. Inherited thrombophilias in pregnancy. Practice bulletin No. 113. American College of Obstetricians and Gynecologists. Obstet Gynecol 2010; 116:212–222. [Review]
12. Lindqvist P, Dahlback B, Marsal K. Thrombotic risk during pregnancy: a population study. Obstet Gynecol 1999; 94:595–599. [II-2]
13. Macklon NS, Greer IA. Venous thromboembolic disease in obstetrics and gynaecology: the Scottish experience. Scott Med J 1996; 41:83–86. [II-2]
14. Grandone E, Margaglione M, Colaizzo D, et al. Genetic susceptibility to pregnancy-related venous thromboembolism: roles of factor V Leiden, prothrombin G20210A, and methylenetetrahydrofolate reductase C677T mutations. Am J Obstet Gynecol 1998; 179:1324–1328. [II-2]
15. Franco RF, Reitsma PH. Genetic risk factors of venous thrombosis. Hum Genet 2001; 109:369–384. [II-2]
16. Haverkate F, Samama M. Familial dysfibrinogenaemia and thrombophilia. Report on a study of the SSC Subcommittee on fibrinogen. Thromb Haemost 1995; 73:151–161. [II-2]
17. Lockwood C. Inherited thrombophilias in pregnant patients: detection and treatment paradigm. Obstet Gynecol 2002; 99:333–341. [Review]
18. Dizon-Townsend D, Miller C, Sibai B, et al. The relationship of the factor V Leiden mutation and pregnancy outcomes for mother and fetus. Obstet Gynecol 2005; 106:517–524. [II-2]
19. Lockwood CJ. Heritable coagulopathies in pregnancy. Obstet Gynecol Surv 1999; 54:754. [Review]
20. Walker MC, Garner PR, Keely EJ, et al. Changes in activated protein C resistance during normal pregnancy. Am J Obstet Gynecol 1997; 77:162. [II-3]
21. De Stefano V, Leone G, Mastrangelo S, et al. Clinical manifestations and management of inherited thrombophilia: retrospective analysis and follow-up after diagnosis of 238 patients with congenital deficiency of antithrombin III, protein C, protein S. Thromb Haemost 1994; 72:352–358. [II-3]
22. Middledorp S, Henkens CM, Koopman MM, et al. The incidence of venous thromboembolism in family members of patients with factor V Leiden mutation and venous thrombosis. Ann Intern Med 1998; 128:15–20. [II-2]
23. Kingdom JC, Kaufmann P. Oxygen and placental villous development: origins of fetal hypoxia. Placenta 1997; 18:613–621. [II-3]
24. Many A, Schreiber L, Rosner S, et al. Pathologic features of the placenta in women with severe pregnancy complications and thrombophilia. Obstet Gynecol 2001; 98(6):1041–1044.[II-3]

25. Quenby S, Mountfield S, Cartwright J, et al. Antiphospholipid antibodies prevent extravillous trophoblast differentiation. Fertil Steril 2005; 83:691–698.[II-2]

26. Bose P, Black S, Kadyrov M, et al. Heparin and aspirin attenuate placental apoptosis in vitro: Implications for early pregnancy failure Am J Obstet Gynecol 2005; 192:23–30.[II-2]

27. Salmon JE, Girardi G. Antiphospholipid antibodies and pregnancy loss: a disorder of inflammation. J Reprod Immunol 2008; 77:51–56.[Review]

28. Paidas MJ, Ku DH, Lee MJ, et al. Protein Z, protec S levels are lower in patients with thrombophilia and subsequent pregnancy complications. J Thromb Haemost 2005; 3:497–501. [II-2]

29. Kang SS, Wong PWK, Susmano A, et al. Thermolabile methylenetetrahydrofolate reductase: an inherited risk factor for coronary artery disease. Am J Hum Genet 1991; 48:536. [II-3]

30. Frosst P, Blom HJ, Milos R, et al. A candidate genetic risk factor for vascular disease: a common mutation in methylenetetrahydrofolate reductase. Nat Genet 1995; 10:111. [II-3]

31. Gallagher PM, Meleady R, Shields DC, et al. Homocysteine and risk of premature coronary heart disease: evidence for a common gene mutation. Circulation 1996; 94:2154. [II-3]

32. Guttormsen AB, Ueland PM, Nesthus I, et al. Determinants and vitamin responsiveness of intermediate hyperhomocysteinemia (40 μmol/L). J Clin Invest 1996; 98:2174. [II-3]

33. Harmon DL, Woodside JV, Yarnell JW, et al. The common "thermolabile" variant of methylenetetrahydrofolate reductase is a major determinant of mild hyperhomocysteinemia. QJM 1996; 89:571. [II-3]

34. Kluijtmans LA, Young IS, Boreham CA, et al. Genetic and nutritional factors contributing to hyperhomocysteinemia in young adults. Blood 2003; 101:2483. [II-3]

35. Robinson K, Arheart K, Refsum H, et al. for the European COMCAC Group. Low circulating folate and vitamin B6 concentrations. Risk factors for stroke, peripheral vascular disease, and coronary artery disease. Circulation 1998; 97:437. [II-2]

36. Rimm EB, Willett WC, Hu FB, et al. Folate and vitamin B6 from diet and supplements in relation to risk of coronary heart disease among women. JAMA 1998; 279:359. [II-2]

37. Voutilainen S, Rissanen TH, Virtanen J, et al. Low dietary folate intake is associated with an excess incidence of acute coronary events: The Kuopio Ischemic Heart Disease Risk Factor Study. Circulation 2001; 103:2674. [II-1]

38. Vermeulen EG, Stehouwer CD, Twisk JW, et al. Effect of homocysteine-lowering treatment with folic acid plus vitamin B6 on progression of subclinical atherosclerosis: a randomised, placebo- controlled trial. Lancet 2000; 355:517. [RCT *n* = 158]

39. Selhub J, Jacques PF, Wilson PW, et al. Vitamin status and intake as primary determinants of homocysteinemia in an elderly population. JAMA 1993; 270:2693. [II-1]

40. Ubbink JR, Vermaak WJ, van der Merwe A, et al. Vitamin B-12, vitamin B-6, and folate nutritional status in men with hyperhomocysteinemia. Am J Clin Nutr 1993; 57:47. [II-2]

41. McColl MD, Ellison J, Reid F, et al. Prothrombin 20210, MTHFR C677T mutations in women with venous thromboembolism associated with pregnancy. BJOG 2000; 107:565–569. [III]]

42. Zotz RB, Gerhardt A, Scharf RE. Inherited thrombophilia and gestational venous thromboembolism. Best Pract Res Clin Haematol 2003; 16:243. [Review]

43. British Society of Hematology. Investigation and management of heritable thrombophilia. Br J Haematol 2001; 114:512. [Review]

44. Gerhardt A, Scharf RE, Beckmann MW, et al. Prothrombin and factor V mutations in women with a history of thrombosis during pregnancy and the puerperium. N Engl J Med 2000; 342:374–380. [II-2]

45. Simioni P, Tormene D, Prandoni P, et al. Pregnancy related recurrent events in thrombophilic women with previous venous thromboembolism. Thromb Haemost 2001; 86:929. [II-2]

46. Robertson L, Wu O, Langhorne S, et al. Thrombophilia in pregnancy: a systematic review. Br J Haematol 2006; 132:171–196. [Review]

47. Rey E, Kahn SR, David M, et al. Thrombophilic disorders and fetal loss: a meta-analysis. Lancet 2003; 361:901. [II-2]

48. Howley HE, Walker M, Rodger MA. A systematic review of the association between factor V Leiden or prothrombin gene variant and intrauterine growth restriction. Am J Obstet Gynecol 2005; 192:694. [II-2]

49. Lin J, August P Genetic Thrombophilias and preeclampsia: a meta-analysis. Obstet Gynecol 2005; 105:182–192. [II-2]

50. Roque H, Paidas MJ, Funai EF, et al. Maternal thrombophilias are not associated with early pregnancy loss. Thromb Haemost 2004; 91:290. [II-2]

51. Infante-Rivard C, Rivard GE, Yotov WV, et al. Absence of association of thrombophilia polymorphisms with intrauterine growth restriction. N Engl J Med 2002; 347:1. [II-2]

52. Prochazka M, Happach C, Marsal K, et al. Factor V Leiden in pregnancies complicated by placental abruption. BJOG 2003; 110:462–466. [II-2]

53. Facco F, You W, Grobman W. Genetic thrombophilias and intrauterine growth restriction. A meta-analysis. Obstet Gynecol 2009; 113:1206–1216.[Review]

54. Kist W, Janssen, N, Kalk, J et al. Thrombophilias and adverse pregnancy outcome – a confounded problem. Thromb Haemost 2008; 99:77–85.[II-3]

55. Kahn S, Platt R, McNamara H, et al. Inherited thrombophilia and preeclampsia within a multicenter cohort: the Montreal Preeclampsia study. Am J Obstet Gynecol 2009; 200:151–159.[II-3]

56. Silver R, Zhao Y, Spong Y, et al. Prothrombin gene G20210A mutation and obstetric complications. Obstet Gynecol 2010; 115:14–20.[II-2]

57. Said JM, Higgins J, Moses E, et al. Inherited thrombophilia polymorphisms and pregnancy outcomes in nulliparous women. Obstet Gynecol 2010; 115:5–13.[II-2]

58. Clark P, Walker I, Govan L, et al. The GOAL study: a prospective examination of the impact of factor V Leiden and ABO(H) blood groups on haemorrhagic and thrombotic pregnancy outcomes. Br J Haematol 2008; 140:236–240.[II-2]

59. Murphy RP, Donoghue R, Nallen R. Prospective evaluation of the risk conferred by factor V Leiden and thermolabile methylenetetrahydrofolate reductase polymorphisms in pregnancy. Arterioscler Thromb Vasc Biol 2000; 20:266–270. [II-2]

60. Lindqvist PG, Svensson PJ, Marsal K, et al. Activated protein c resistance (FVQ506) and pregnancy. Thromb Haemost 1999; 81:532–537. [II-2]

61. Murakamis S, Matsubara N, Miyakaw S, et al. The relation between homocysteine concentration and methylenetetrahydrofolate reductase genetic polymorphism in pregnant women. J Obstet Gynaecol Res 2001; 27:349–352. [II-2]

62. Dizon-Townson DS, Meline L, Nelson LM, et al. Fetal carriers of the factor V Leiden mutation are prone to miscarriage and placental infarction. Am J Obstet Gynecol 1997; 177:402. [II-2]

63. von Kries R, Junker R, Oberle D, et al. Foetal growth restriction in children with prothrombotic risk factors. Thromb Haemost 2001; 86:1012. [II-2]

64. Preston FE, Rosendaal FR, Walker ID, et al. Increased fetal loss in women with heritable thrombophilia. Lancet 1996; 348:913–916. [II-2]

65. Biron-Andréani C, Bauters A, Le Cam-Duchez V, et al. Factor V Leiden homozygous genotype and pregnancy outcomes. Obstet Gynecol 2009; 114:1249–1253.[II-2]

66. Brill-Edwards P, Ginsberg JS, Gent M, et al. Safety of withholding heparin in pregnant women with a history of venous thromboembolism. N Engl J Med 2000; 343:1439–1444. [II-1, *n* = 125]

67. Lindqvist PG, Olofsson P, Dahlback B. Use of selective factor V Leiden screening in pregnancy to identify candidates for anticoagulation. Obstet Gynecol 2002; 100:332. [II-3]

68. Seligsohn U, Lubetsky A. Medical progress: genetic susceptibility to venous thrombosis. N Engl J Med 2001; 344:1222–1231. [Review]

69. Gris JC, Mercier E, Quere I, et al. Low molecular weight heparin verses low-dose aspirin in women with one fetal loss and a constitutional thrombophilic disorder. Blood 2004; 103:3695. [RCT, $n = 160$]

70. Brenner B, Hoffman R, Carp H, et al. Efficacy and safety of two doses of enoxaparin in women with thrombophilia and recurrent pregnancy loss: the LIVE-ENOX study. J Thromb Haemost 2005; 3:227–229. [II-2]

71. den Heijer M, Willems H, Blom H, et al. Homocysteine lowering by B vitamins and the secondary prevention of deep vein thrombosis and pulmonary embolism: a randomized, placebo-controlled, double-blind. Blood 2007; 109:139–144.[RCT, $n = 325$]

28

Venous thromboembolism and anticoagulation

James A. Airoldi

KEY POINTS

- Venous thromboembolism (VTE) is the **leading cause of pregnancy-related maternal morbidity and mortality in the developed world.**
- Risk factors for VTE are listed in Table 28.1, and include pregnancy, **prior thromboembolism, age of 35 years or more, increased parity, increased maternal weight, instrument-assisted deliveries or cesarean section, prolonged immobilization, smoking, and the presence of an acquired or inherited thrombophilia.**
- **Compressive ultrasonography** is the **primary modality for the diagnosis** of deep vein thrombosis (DVT) in pregnancy.
- The **ventilation/perfusion (V/Q) scan** or a **computerized tomography pulmonary angiography (CTPA)** are fairly equivalent first-line imaging tests for the diagnosis of **pulmonary embolism** in pregnant patients although some experts favor V/Q scans.
- The three anticoagulant typically used are **unfractionated heparin (UFH), low-molecular-weight heparin (LMWH),** and **warfarin**.
- **Platelet counts** should be checked five days after initiation of UFH, and periodically for the first three weeks of **heparin therapy**.
- **LMWH is at least as effective and safe as UFH** for the treatment of patients with acute DVT, and for the prevention of DVT. **LMWH and UFH do not cross the placenta,** and are safe for the fetus. The incidences of bleeding, osteopenia, and heparin-induced thrombocytopenia with LMWH are probably decreased compared to UFH in pregnant patients. Pregnant women may require higher doses and these risks could be dose related. **The dosing of LMWH in pregnancy remains controversial.**
- Warfarin derivatives **cross the placenta** and have the potential to cause both **bleeding in the fetus and teratogenicity.** Warfarin use is believed to be safe in the first six weeks of gestation, but has been **associated with warfarin embryopathy in 4% to 5% of fetuses when maternal exposure occurs between six and nine weeks' gestation.**
- In the pregnant patient with **acute VTE, either therapeutic LMWH throughout pregnancy or intravenous UFH** for at least five days, followed by therapeutic UFH or LMWH for a minimum of six months, is the recommended approach. Anticoagulants should be administered for at least six weeks postpartum.
- There are **three general approaches** to the antepartum management of pregnant patients with **previous VTE: UFH, LMWH, or close surveillance.**
  - ○ Among women with a **nonrecurring cause for the prior VTE and no thrombophilia,** the risk of recurrent antepartum VTE is low, and therefore **routine antepartum prophylaxis with heparin is not warranted.**

However, postpartum low-dose prophylaxis is still recommended.
  - ■ If there is a potential recurring cause, prophylactic anticoagulation is recommended.
  - ○ In pregnant women with a **prior VTE with** history of a **low-risk thrombophilia (heterozygous factor V or prothrombin gene, protein C or S), prophylactic anticoagulation is recommended.**
  - ○ **Therapeutic anticoagulation** is recommended for prior VTE and **high-risk thrombophilia (ATIII deficiency, homozygous factor V or prothrombin gene, or compound heterozygote).**
  - ○ **Therapeutic anticoagulation** should be used in pregnant women if the woman has had **recurrent VTE episodes, life-threatening thrombosis, or thrombosis while receiving chronic anticoagulation.** Filters in the inferior vena cava should be considered in this situation as well.
- It is recommended that pregnant patients with recurrent early pregnancy losses and **antiphospholipid syndrome (APS)** who do not have a history of venous thrombosis receive a prophylactic regimen of heparin (and low-dose aspirin), and that those with previous thrombosis and APS receive a similar prophylactic dose regimen of heparin (see chap. 26).
- The antepartum management of pregnant women with **known thrombophilia** and **no prior VTE** remains controversial because of our limited knowledge of the natural histories of various thrombophilias and a lack of trials of VTE prophylaxis. Currently, there is **no evidence to suggest prophylactic anticoagulation** (see chap. 27).
- In pregnant women with **mechanical heart valves,** it appears reasonable to use one of the following four regimens: (*i*) therapeutic LMWH or UFH between 6 and 12 weeks and close to term only, and vitamin K antagonists (VKAs) at other times; (*ii*) careful therapeutic UFH throughout pregnancy; (*iii*) careful therapeutic LMWH throughout pregnancy; or (*iv*) VKAs throughout pregnancy.

DEFINITION

Venous thromboembolism (VTE) includes any thromboembolic event in a vein, including deep vein thrombosis (DVT) and pulmonary embolism (PE), which are the most common, and others [cerebrovascular event (CVA or stroke), etc.].

SYMPTOMS

DVT can present with leg swelling, erythema, pain and calor, with about 25% of patients with these symptoms having DVT. PE is not detected clinically in 70% to 80% of patients in whom it is detected postmortem. Most patients who die of PE do so within 30 minutes of the event, reinforcing the need for rapid and accurate diagnosis (1).

EPIDEMIOLOGY/INCIDENCE

VTE is the **leading cause of pregnancy-related maternal morbidity and mortality in the developed world** (2). Fatal PE remains the leading cause of maternal mortality, accounting for 19.6 % of all maternal deaths. Interestingly, hemorrhage is the second leading cause of maternal deaths (about 17%), thus signifying the delicate balance between coagulation and anticoagulation in pregnancy. The incidence of all thromboembolic events averages about **1.3** (range 0.5–3) **per 1000 pregnancies** (3), and about an equal number are identified antepartum and in the puerperium (4). There is an equal frequency in all three trimesters. Pulmonary emboli are more frequent postpartum (4). During pregnancy and postpartum, women in general have a **fivefold increased risk of VTE compared with nonpregnant women** (4). The risk is increased approximately twofold during the antepartun period, and 14-fold in the postpartum period, especially after cesarean delivery. DVT is more common in the left than the right leg. PE occurs in 15% of untreated DVTs, with a mortality rate of 15%. PE occurs in 4.5% of treated DVTs, with a mortality rate of 1% (5). Death from PE occurs about every 1.1 to 1.5 per 100,000 pregnancies (6).

GENETICS

About 50% of patients with thrombosis have an identifiable underlying genetic disorder (7). Moreover, approximately 50% to 60% of patients with a hereditary basis for thrombosis, or a thrombophilia, do not experience a thrombotic event until one other risk factor is present (4) (see chap. 27).

ETIOLOGY/BASIC PATHOPHYSIOLOGY

The coagulation cascade is briefly and schematically shown in Figure 28.1. Pregnancy is associated with marked alterations in the proteins of the coagulation and fibrinolytic systems (8,9) (see chap. 3, *Obstetric Evidence Based Guidelines*). A tendency for excessive clotting seems to be an adaptive mechanism to prevent excessive bleeding at delivery. At delivery, about 120 spiral arteries are denuded while carrying about 12% of the woman's cardiac output every minute. Much of the prevention in bleeding is due to myometrial contraction, but there are also marked increased clotting capacity, impaired fibrinolysis, and decreased natural anticoagulant activity in pregnancy. Three main factors, those in Virchow's triad, contribute to the increased risk of VTE in pregnancy:

- *Hypercoagulable blood*: The levels of coagulation factors II, V, VII, VIII, IX, X, and XII increase substantially by the middle of pregnancy. The generation of fibrin also increases markedly. Levels of the anticoagulant protein S appear to decrease about 40% throughout pregnancy, although levels of protein C remain normal. The fibrinolytic system is also inhibited, most substantially in the third trimester. These clotting factor changes occur very early in pregnancy, and thus anticoagulation should be started early in pregnancy if it is going to be started.
- *Stasis*: compression of iliac veins; hormonally mediated vein dilation; immobilization.
- *Vascular damage*: vascular compression at delivery; assisted or operative delivery.

RISK FACTORS/ASSOCIATIONS

Venous thromboembolism is a multifactorial disease process. Risk factors are shown in Table 28.1, with those most common in pregnancy including **prior thromboembolism, age of 35 years or more, increased parity, increased maternal weight, multiple pregnancy, instrument-assisted deliveries or cesarean section, prolonged immobilization, smoking, and the presence of an acquired or inherited thrombophilia** (see chaps. 26 and 27) (10–12). About 50% of cases of VTE in pregnancy are associated with an inherited or acquired thrombophilia (6).

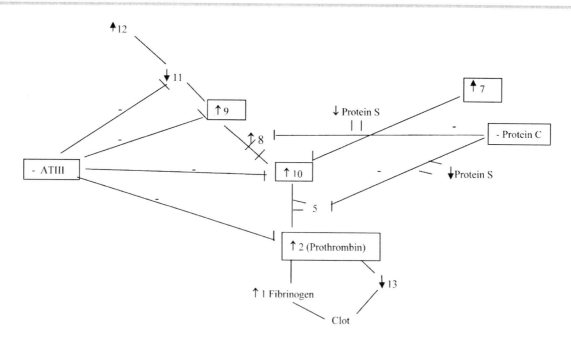

Figure 28.1 Coagulations cascade and some pregnancy changes. *Abbreviations*: ↑↓, change in pregnancy; □; , vitamin K dependent; −, negative feedback.

Table 28.1 Conditions Associated with Increased Risk for VTE (Pregnant and Nonpregnant Women)

Advancing age
Obesity
Previous venous thromboembolism
Surgery
Trauma
Active cancer
Acute medical illnesses—e.g., acute myocardial infarction, heart
   failure, respiratory failure, infection
Inflammatory bowel disease
Antiphospholipid syndrome
Dyslipoproteinemia
Nephrotic syndrome
Paroxysmal nocturnal hemoglobinuria
Myeloproliferative diseases
Behcet's syndrome
Varicose veins
Superficial vein thrombosis
Congenital venous malformation
Long-distance travel
Prolonged bed rest
Immobilization
Limb paresis
Chronic care facility stay
Pregnancy/puerperium
Oral contraceptives
Hormone replacement therapy
Heparin-induced thrombocytopenia
Other drugs
   Chemotherapy
   Tamoxifen
   Thalidomide
   Antipsychotics
Central venous catheter
Vena cava filter
Intravenous drug abuse

Abbreviation: VTE, venous thromboembolism. *Source*: From Ref. 11.

Table 28.2 Radiation Exposures of Diagnostic Tests for VTE

Test	Radiation exposure (in rads)
Chest X ray	0.001
Perfusion scan	0.018
Ventilation scan	0.019
Helical CT	0.005
Limited venography	0.050
Pulmonary angiography	0.221
Compression U/S	none
MRI	none

Abbreviation: VTE, venous thromboembolism.

COMPLICATIONS

VTE in general: risk of recurrence is about 7% to 12%
DVT: risk of PE, postthrombotic syndrome
PE: risk of death, pulmonary hypertension

MANAGEMENT
Principles
Given the paucity of data regarding diagnosis and treatment in pregnancy, most data are derived from the nonpregnant general population.

Diagnosis
To diagnose VTE, clinical suspicion must remain high. Clinical evaluation alone cannot confirm or refute a diagnosis of VTE in the nonpregnant state, and diagnosing VTE in pregnancy is even more challenging. Epidemiologic studies have shown that exposure to radiation of less than a total cumulative dose of 5 rads has not been associated with significant risk for fetal injury (13). The diagnostic tests shown in Table 28.2 are all below the safe limit, and most combinations of these tests are also below the 5 rads limit, although they may increase the risks for childhood cancers (14,15).

Deep Vein Thrombosis (Fig. 28.2) (12)
During pregnancy, thrombosis most frequently begins in the veins of the calf or in the iliofemoral segment of the deep

venous system and has a striking predilection for the **left leg** (16–18) (85–90%), possibly because of the compressive effects on the left iliac vein by the right iliac artery where they cross (19). Only about 25% of symptomatic patients have a thrombus, and thus the physical exam has low predictability.

    Compressive ultrasonography is now the **primary modality** for the diagnosis of DVT in pregnancy. It has a sensitivity of 97% and a specificity of 94% for the diagnosis of proximal DVT in the nonpregnant population (15,20). It is less accurate for symptomatic calf DVTs (21). It is inadequate for iliac vein thrombosis for which only magnetic resonance imaging (MRI) has shown a high degree of sensitivity and specificity (20).

    Venography was widely held to be the standard for establishing a diagnosis of DVT (22). However, exposure to radiation and the invasive nature of the test has led to its replacement by compressive ultrasound.

    D-dimer testing has been noted to have a role in diagnosing VTE in nonpregnant patients and may be useful during pregnancy. D-dimer is a measurement of the degradation products of cross-linked fibrin. Pregnancy itself may increase D-dimer levels, increasing with gestational age. Preterm labor, preeclampsia, and placental abruption also can elevate levels significantly (23). Sensitivities vary widely with different assays, ranging from 80% to 100% (24), but the main use is derived from a high negative predictive value. The approach using D-dimer is not validated in pregnancy.

    Patients who, on clinical evidence, are likely to have thrombosis but whose initial test results are negative, should undergo either venography or serial noninvasive testing. Diagnosis of pelvic vein and internal iliac thrombosis is difficult, and may require MRI.

Pulmonary Embolism (Fig. 28.3) (25)
The **ventilation/perfusion (V/Q) scan** is one of the two **primary tools** for the diagnosis of PE in pregnant patients. If a perfusion defect is seen in a patient with symptoms of PE, this finding can be considered diagnostic. The ventilation portion of the test is useful to distinguish matched defects from unmatched defects if a perfusion defect is not clearly caused by a PE. About 40% to 60% of V/Q scans are diagnostic (either high probability or normal). For nondiagnostic tests, further studies are necessary (26). Given lower radiation exposure, high proportion of normal or near-normal perfusion scans, and uncertainty regarding finding of subsegmental PE on computerized tomography pulmonary angiography (CTPA), V/Q scan is often preferred by experts as the first-line radiologic diagnostic study (27).

    CTPA has provided an additional first-line imaging test and has become the most widespread imaging test in non-pregnant adults (25). The sensitivity varies from 57% to 100%

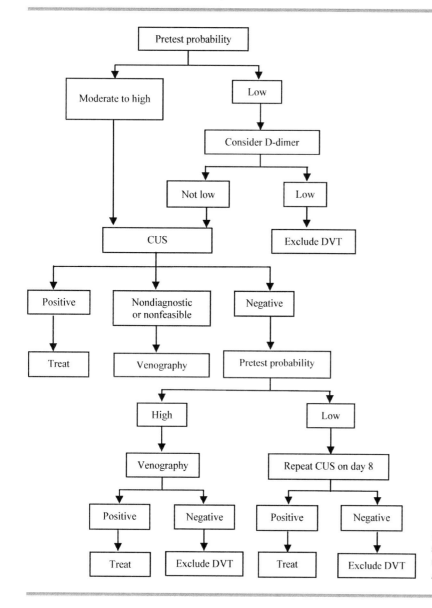

Figure 28.2 Suggested management in patient with symptoms of DVT. *Abbreviations*: CUS, compression ultrasound; DVT, deep vein thrombosis. *Source*: Adapted from Ref. 12

and the specificity varies between 64% and 100% (20,24,28). The location of the embolus affects the sensitivity and specificity of CTPA. CTPA scanning is more sensitive for detecting emboli in the central arteries and is less sensitive for detecting subsegmental emboli (29). With CTPA, the thrombus is directly visualized, and both mediastinal and parenchymal structures are evaluated, which may provide important alternative or additional diagnoses. CTPA is associated with a higher risk of maternal breast cancer than V/Q scanning.

Pulmonary angiography remains the gold standard for ruling out PE. The test requires expertise for performance and interpretation and is invasive. Thus, this test is held in reserve for patients in whom the diagnosis cannot be made or excluded on the basis of less invasive testing.

Therapy

Agents

Given the paucity of data regarding the efficacy of **anticoagulants** during pregnancy, recommendations about their use during pregnancy are based largely on data from nonpregnant patients. The three anticoagulant typically used are unfractio-

nated heparin (UFH), low-molecular-weight heparin (LMWH), and warfarin. **Heparin** (UFH or LMWH) is the anticoagulant most often used given its safety and efficacy during pregnancy (30–43). Warfarin is also an alternative anticoagulant in certain situations. All three choices are safe during breast-feeding. These anticoagulants can be used either as a low-dose **prophylactic** dose (Table 28.3) or as a (sometimes weight-adjusted) **therapeutic** dose (usually with monitoring, Table 28.4).

Unfractionated heparin. The word heparin derives from the Greek "hepar," liver, the organ where it was first isolated from. UFH exerts its anticoagulation action by two mechanisms of action: (*i*) stimulation of antithrombin III (ATIII) activity, which is an inhibitor of factors 2, 9, 10 (especially), and 11; (*ii*) direct factor 10 inhibition (Fig. 28.1). UFH half-life is about 1.5 hours.

Approximately 3% of nonpregnant patients receiving UFH acquire immune-mediated (IgG) **thrombocytopenia** (heparin-induced thrombocytopenia, **HIT**), which is frequently complicated by extension of preexisting VTE or new arterial thrombosis (44). HIT is diagnosed by antibodies

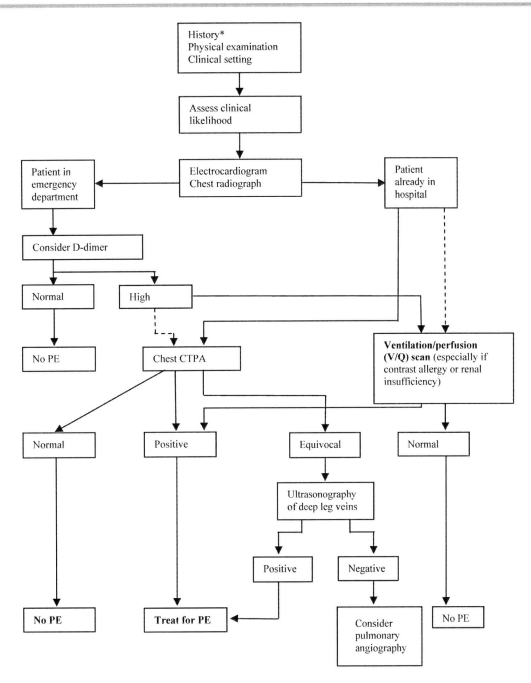

*If leg symptoms, perform CUS.

Figure 28.3 Diagnostic algorithm for suspected pulmonary embolism. *Abbreviations*: PE, pulmonary embolism; CTPA, computerized tomography pulmonary angiography; CUS, compression ultrasound. *Source*: Adapted from Ref. 25.

Table 28.3 Examples of Prophylaxic (Low-Dose) Anticoagulation Subcutaneous Regimens During Pregnancy (e.g., for Prior VTE)

- **Unfractionated heparin, 5000–7500 U every 12 hr during the first trimester; 7500–10,000 U every 12 hr during the second trimester; 10,000 U every 12 hr during the third trimester**, unless the aPTT is elevated
- Unfractionated heparin, 5000–10,000 U every 12 hr throughout pregnancy
- Unfractionated heparin dosed twice daily to target anti–factor Xa activity 0.2–0.4 U/mL
- **Enoxaparin, 40 mg once or twice daily**
- Dalteparin, 5000 U once or twice daily

Abbreviations: VTE, venous thromboembolism; aPTT, activated partial thromboplastin time.

Table 28.4 Examples of Therapeutic (Sometimes Adjusted Dose) Anticoagulation Subcutaneous Regimens (e.g., for Acute VTE in Pregnancy)

- Unfractionated heparin, (usually ≥10,000 U) given 2–3 times per day to achieve aPTT prolongation of 1.5 to 2.5
- Enoxaparin, 30–80 mg (or more) every 12 hr
- Dalteparin, 5000–10,000 U every 12 hr
- **Weight-adjusted doses of enoxaparin (1 mg/kg every 12 hr)** or dalteparin (200 U/kg every 24 hr)
- Weight-adjusted low-molecular-weight heparin with dose sufficient enough to achieve a peak anti–factor Xa level of 0.5–1.2 U/mL

Abbreviations: VTE, venous thromboembolism; aPTT, activated partial thromboplastin time.

to heparin, fall in platelet count >50%, skin lesions at the injection site, and systemic reactions after IV injection (45). HIT encompasses a range of presentations, from asymptomatic antibodies without thrombocytopenia, to thrombocytopenia, to thrombocytopenia with thrombosis. The mortality rate from untreated HIT and new thrombotic complications is 20% to 30% (46). This should be differentiated from an early, benign, transient thrombocytopenia that can occur with initiation of UFH due primarily to platelet clumping. It should be suspected when the platelet count falls to <100 × 10⁹/L or <50% of the baseline value **5 to 15 days** after commencing heparin, or sooner with recent heparin exposure (44). **Platelet counts should be checked about five days after initiation of UFH, and periodically for the first two weeks of UFH therapy**. In pregnant women who acquire HIT and require ongoing anticoagulant therapy, use of the heparinoid **danaparoid sodium** is recommended because it is an effective antithrombotic agent (40), does not cross the placenta, has much less cross-reactivity with UFH, and therefore, has less potential to produce recurrent HIT than LMWH (47). Alternatives may include fondaparinox or lepirudin (45). LMWH treatment for VTE has in general been associated with decrease in the incidence of HIT (44,47), but not in all studies (38).

Heparin therapy has been associated with **osteopenia** in pregnant women. Long-term prophylactic UFH therapy during pregnancy is associated with a 2.2% incidence of vertebral fracture (49). The mean bone loss is about 5%, with unclear reversibility. **LMWHs have a lower risk of osteopenia than UFH**. UFH and dalteparin for thromboprophylaxis in pregnancy are associated with similar bone mineral density in the lumbar spine for up to three years after delivery between healthy control subjects and the dalteparin group (50). Bone mineral density was significantly lower in the UFH group when compared to both control subjects and dalteparin-treated women in this trial. Multiple logistic regressions found that the type of heparin therapy was the only independent factor associated with reduced bone mass. Cohort studies (51) have also reported no association with osteopenia and LMWH therapy.

Given that UFH **does not cross the placenta,** there is no risk of teratogenicity. The rate of **major maternal bleeding** in pregnant patients treated with UFH therapy is about **2%,** which is consistent with the reported rates of bleeding associated with heparin therapy in nonpregnant patients (52) and with warfarin therapy (53) when used for the treatment of DVT. There is insufficient evidence to assess whether UFH is associated with different incidence of bleeding complications compared to LMWH in RCTs (54). Bleeding at the uteroplacental junction is still possible. The short half-life makes UFH the optimal anticoagulation around the time of delivery or surgery. The anticoagulant effect lasts for about 8 to 12 hours. Protamine sulfate can be used to reverse the effects of UFH. Recent UFH administration is not a contraindication to

regional anesthesia as long as the partial thromboplastin time (PTT) is not prolonged.

Low-molecular-weight heparin. LMWH exerts its anticoagulation action by stimulation of ATIII activity, inhibiting in particular factor 10 (not factor 2). There is accumulating experience with the use of LMWHs, both in pregnant and nonpregnant patients, for the prevention and treatment of VTE (36–41). On the basis of the results of large clinical trials in nonpregnant patients, **LMWH is at least as effective and safe as UFH** for the treatment of patients with acute proximal DVT (38,40), and for the prevention of DVT in patients who undergo surgery (41).

LMWH does not cross the placenta, and LMWH is safe for the fetus (37,51). The half-life is usually about four to seven hours (e.g., enoxaparin).

Bleeding complications appear to be very uncommon with LMWH. LMWH might have fewer associated risks for bleeding, HIT, and osteoporotic fractures than UFH (44,48), but the incidence of these complications have not been well established for LMWH use in pregnant patients. Pregnant women may require higher doses and these risks could be dose related.

The dosing of LMWH remains controversial. The anticoagulant effect of LMWH lasts for 18 to 24 hours. Pregnant women may require increases in dalteparin dose of 10% to 20% compared with doses of nonpregnant women to reach the target anti-Xa levels (55–57). Anticoagulation with LMWH may need to be monitored in pregnant women and the dose adjusted to reach the target Xa level, which decreases the logistical and financial benefits of LMWH. The therapeutic anti-Xa level for adjusted-dose therapy is 0.5 to 1.2 U/mL. The target anti-Xa level for prophylactic dose therapy is 0.2 to 0.4 U/mL. To achieve these levels, **often dosing every 12 hours is necessary even for prophylaxis in pregnancy**. Twice-daily dosing of enoxaparin may be necessary to maintain anti–factor Xa activity above 0.1 IU/mL throughout a 24-hour period in pregnant women (6,56,58). Enoxaparin 40 mg every 12 hours (instead of once daily) has been suggested for prophylactic anticoagulation in women at or above 90 kg (6). It is not known whether a specific minimum level of anti–factor Xa activity is necessary throughout the day to prevent thrombosis in pregnancy or whether maintaining a specific minimum level of anti–factor Xa activity for only a portion of the day is sufficient. Anti-Xa levels may be used especially for obese and for renal disease patients (6).

Warfarin (Coumadin). Warfarin derivatives are vitamin K antagonists (VKAs). Vitamin K derives its name from the German word "koagulation." Warfarin inhibits the effects of vitamin K, and hence vitamin K–dependent factors (factors 2,7,9, and 10) (Fig. 28.1). Consequently, warfarin decreases levels of proteins C and S. Warfarin derivatives **cross the placenta** and have the potential to cause both **bleeding in the fetus and teratogenicity** (58,59). Warfarin use is believed to be safe in the first six weeks of gestation, but has been associated with warfarin embryopathy in 4% to 5% of fetuses when maternal exposure occurs between six and nine weeks gestation. First-trimester warfarin embryopathy includes skeletal, (involving stippled epiphyses), nasal, and limb (hypoplasia) involvement. Bleeding in the fetus can occur during any trimester. Some recommend the use of warfarin during pregnancy anyway for specific patients, such as women with mechanical heart valves, those who have a recurrence while receiving heparin, and those with contraindications to heparin therapy. If warfarin is used during pregnancy, patients must be fully informed about the potential adverse effects on the fetus. Warfarin does not induce an anticoagulant effect in the breastfed infant when the drug is given to a nursing mother (60,61). Therefore, the use of warfarin in breast-feeding women who require postpartum anticoagulant therapy is safe.

Aspirin. Potential complications of aspirin use during the first trimester of pregnancy include birth defects (e.g., gastroschisis) and bleeding in the neonate and in the mother. **Low-dose** (60 to 150 mg/day) aspirin therapy administered during the second and third trimesters of pregnancy in women at risk for hypertensive complications and/or FGR is **safe** for the mother and fetus (62,63). The safety of higher doses of aspirin and/or aspirin ingestion during the first trimester remains uncertain.

Treatment of Acute VTE in Pregnancy (Table 28.5)
There are no RCTs for treatment of DVT specific to pregnant women (64). There are now many well-designed randomized trials and meta-analyses comparing IV UFH and SC LMWH for the treatment of acute DVT and PE in nonpregnant patients (38). They show that LMWH is at least as safe and effective as UFH. However, there are **no trials** comparing UFH to LMWH for the treatment of acute VTE in pregnancy. Therefore, in the pregnant patient with acute VTE, either (**weight-adjusted)**

therapeutic doses of SC **LMWH, or** IV **UFH** [80 IU/kg bolus followed by a continuous infusion (at least 1300/hour) to maintain the aPTT in the therapeutic range] for at least five days, followed by adjusted-dose UFH or LMWH for the remainder of the pregnancy, is the suggested approach (Table 28.4). The therapeutic dose regimen of subcutaneous UFH was shown to have equal efficacy in preventing recurrent VTE as compared to warfarin in the first three months after an acute VTE (52). Interestingly, three patients had recurrent VTE during therapy, but all were associated with interruption of anticoagulation (52). Anticoagulants should be administered **for about six months in adjusted dose** (12), and at least six weeks postpartum as well. There is insufficient evidence to assess if continuing adjusted-dose anticoagulation until six weeks postpartum is associated with any benefit or detriment. Women with antithrombin deficiency, antiphospholipid antibodies, homozygous or combined thrombophilias, or previous VTE may benefit from indefinite anticoagulation, but this should be decided by an internist after pregnancy (12). Long-term, low-intensity warfarin therapy is associated with an about 50% prevention of recurrent VTE, major hemorrhage, or death in patients with a prior idiopathic VTE (65).

Filters in the inferior vena cava have been used safely and effectively in pregnant women (66,67). Suprarenal placement is recommended. No important maternal or fetal morbidity associated with the filters has been reported. **The indications for their use are the same as in nonpregnant patients**: any contraindication to anticoagulant therapy; serious complication of anticoagulation, such as HIT; and the recurrence of PE in patients with adequate anticoagulant therapy.

The **use of thrombolytic agents** during pregnancy has been limited to life-threatening situations because of the risk of substantial maternal bleeding, especially at the time of

Table 28.5 Suggested Pregnancy Management Based on VTE (Current or Prior) and Thrombophilia

Clinical scenario	Antepartum management
VTE develops during pregnancy	**Therapeutic[a] (adjusted dose) LMWH (or intravenous UFH for 5–7 days followed by subcutaneous adjusted-dose UFH or LMWH) for 6 months (or the remainder of the pregnancy)**
Prior VTE related to a recurring factor (pregnancy or OC use) and no known thrombophilia	**Prophylactic anticoagulation[b]**
Prior VTE associated with a nonrecurring (transient) risk factor and no known thrombophilia	**Surveillance only or Prophylactic anticoagulation (if workup incomplete)**
"Low-risk" thrombophilia (heterozygous FVL or PGM, protein C, protein S) AND	
No prior VTE	**Surveillance only or Prophylactic anticoagulation if risk factors[c]**
Prior VTE	**Prophylactic anticoagulation**
"High-risk" thrombophilia (ATIII def, homozygous FVL or PGM, or double heterozygote)	
No prior VTE	**Prophylactic anticoagulation**
Prior VTE	**Therapeutic anticoagulation**
History of recurrent thrombosis, or receiving chronic therapeutic anticoagulation	**Therapeutic anticoagulation Consider IVC filter in certain cases**
Antiphospholipid syndrome and prior VTE	**Prophylactic anticoagulation (see chap. 26)**
Pregnant women with mechanical heart valves	**Warfarin throughout pregnancy except during gestational weeks 6–12 where aggressive adjusted dose UFH or LMWH should be used. Alternatively warfarin could be used during entire pregnancy after appropriate counseling**

[a]Therapeutic anticoagulation: see Table 28.4.
[b]Prophylactic anticoagulation: see Table 28.3.
[c]Risk factors: first-degree relative with VTE before age 50, or obesity, prolonged immobility, etc.
Abbreviations: VTE, Venous thromboembolism; LMWH, low-molecular-weight heparin; UFH, unfractionated heparin; FVL, factor V Leiden; PGM, prothrombin gene mutation; ATIII, antithrombin III; IVC, inferior vena cava.

delivery and immediately postpartum (68). The risk of placental abruption and fetal death because of these drugs is currently unknown.

Embolectomy, another treatment option when conservative treatment fails, is indicated to prevent death in patients who are hemodynamically unstable despite anticoagulation and treatment with vasopressors (69). Embolectomy has been associated with a 20% to 40% incidence of fetal loss (70), so this treatment must be restricted to cases in which the woman's life is endangered.

Prevention of VTE in Pregnancy (Table 28.5)
Avoidance of risk factors shown in Table 28.1 can provide important prevention of VTE and its complications. **Preconception counseling** should review these preventive measures, as well as review in detail any prior history of VTE and risk factors (see Table 27.2).

Women with a history of VTE (with or without thrombophilia) are believed to have a higher **risk of recurrence** in subsequent pregnancies. Estimates of the rate of recurrent venous thrombosis during pregnancy in women with a history of VTE have varied **between 1% and 10%** (71–74). The higher of these estimates has prompted recommendation for anticoagulant prophylaxis during pregnancy and the postpartum period in women with a history of VTE. However, the risk is likely to be lower than has been suggested by some of these studies because they were retrospective, with the possibility of significant bias. The risk is dramatically influenced by risk factors, in particular the presence of thrombophilias (see Table 27.2).

There are very few trials for the prevention of VTE in pregnancy (both antepartum and postpartum). The sample sizes of all trials are small and cannot be combined. There is **insufficient evidence** on which to base recommendations for thromboprophylaxis during pregnancy and the early postnatal period, because of limited data, especially regarding rare outcomes such as death and thromboembolic disease and osteoporosis. In general, care must be individualized according to risk factors (Table 28.5).

Antenatal prophylactic anticoagulation (usually for prior VTE) (Table 28.5). Compared to UFH, LMWH is associated with a 72% decrease in bleeding episodes; however, all other outcome variables showed no significant differences (75,76).

Compared to aspirin alone, in pregnant women with recurrent miscarriage associated with antiphospholipid antibodies, **aspirin plus heparin** appears to be associated with a 70% lower risk of fetal loss (77).

Compared to UFH only postpartum, UFH antepartum and postpartum is associated with similar results in one very small (*n* = 40) trial, which could not possibly detect significant differences given the sample size (78).

In summary, there is **insufficient evidence** on which to base recommendations for VTE prophylaxis during pregnancy and the early postnatal period (79). In general, in pregnant women with a **prior history of VTE, prophylactic anticoagulation** can be used. This may be modified on the basis of the cause of the first VTE and the presence of a thrombophilia. **If the prior VTE was related to a nonrecurrent cause** (i.e., broken bone and immobilization) **and the thrombophilia workup is negative**, the risk of recurrence is very low, and **prophylaxis may be avoided**, especially in women without other risk factors except pregnancy. In fact, the risk of recurrence was 0% in such 44 women followed without antepartum anticoagulation (80). Postpartum prophylaxis is suggested in all women with prior VTE. Both antepartum and postpartum

prophylaxis may be suggested to the woman with prior VTE and thrombophilia, prior unexplained VTE, or a current major risk factor. There are two general therapies for management of pregnant patients with previous VTE who require prophylaxis: UFH or LMWH. For low-dose prophylaxis of VTE during pregnancy, see Table 28.3.

Approximately 50% to 80% of gestational VTEs are associated with **heritable thrombophilia** (see chap. 27). Given that the background rate of VTE during pregnancy is approximately 1:1000, the absolute risk of VTE remains modest for majority of these thrombophilias, except antithrombin deficiency, homozygosity for factor V Leiden mutation and for prothrombin mutation, and combined defects. The absolute risk of pregnancy-associated VTE has been reported to range from 9% to 16% in homozygotes for the factor V Leiden mutation (81–84). Double heterozygosity for the factor V Leiden and prothrombin gene mutations has been reported to have an absolute risk of pregnancy-associated VTE of 4.0% (95% CI, 1.4–16.9%) (79). These data suggest that women with antithrombin deficiency, homozygosity for factor V Leiden mutation or the prothrombin mutation as well as double heterozygotes should be managed more aggressively than those with other low-risk inherited thrombophilias; thus, **adjusted-dose therapeutic anticoagulation is recommended for prior DVT and a high-risk thrombophilia** (ATIII deficiency, homozygous factor V or prothrombin gene mutation, or double heterozygote). Therapeutic anticoagulation may also be used in pregnant women if the woman has had recurrent VTE episodes, life-threatening thrombosis, or thrombosis while receiving chronic anticoagulation. Filters in the inferior vena cava should be considered in this situation as well. In pregnant women with **prior VTE with a history of low-risk thrombophilia** (heterozygous factor V or prothrombin gene, protein C or S), **prophylactic anticoagulation is recommended**. Persistent antiphospholipid antibodies are associated with an increased risk of VTE during pregnancy and the puerperium (48). It has been suggested that pregnant patients with the antiphospholipid syndrome who do not have a history of venous thrombosis receive a low-dose prophylactic regimen of heparin, as well as those with previous thrombosis (48) (see also chap. 26). The antepartum management of pregnant women with known thrombophilia and no prior VTE remains controversial because of our limited knowledge of the natural histories of various thrombophilias and a lack of trials of VTE prophylaxis. Prospective data are lacking regarding the issue of the incidence of VTE in a large group of pregnant women with known thrombophilia and no prior VTE. Currently, there is no evidence to suggest prophylactic, low-dose anticoagulation in this group. If there is a very strong family history of VTE (especially at young ages), consideration can be made for low-dose prophylactic anticoagulation. Individualized risk assessment should be performed in this situation.

Postnatal prophylaxis after cesarean delivery. Available data suggest that the risk of VTE is higher after **cesarean section** (especially emergent surgery) than after vaginal delivery (3). The presence of additional risk factors for pregnancy-associated VTE (e.g., prior VTE, thrombophilia, age > 35 years, obesity, prolonged bed rest, and concomitant acute medical illness) may exacerbate this risk. Clinical judgment should be used to decide on anticoagulation after cesarean section, taking into account all of the patients risk factors.

Evidence from small trials revealed that for post–cesarean delivery VTE prophylaxis, the following are observed: Compared to placebo, heparin (either UFH or LMWH) is associated with similar outcomes in two trials (85,86).

Compared to UFH, LMWH is associated with similar outcomes in one trial (87). Compared to UFH, hydroxyethyl starch is associated with similar outcomes in one trial (88).

It has been recommended that **graduated compression stockings** or intermittent pneumatic compression devices be used during and after cesarean section in patients considered to be at "moderate risk" of VTE and that **LMWH or UFH prophylaxis** be added in those thought to be at "high risk" (6,89). However, there are **no RCTs** on this subject (see chap. 13, *Obstetric Evidence Based Guidelines*).

Prophylaxis in women with mechanical heart valves. Women who anticipate ultimately needing valve replacement surgery should be encouraged to complete childbearing before valve replacement. The highest risk for VTE is with first-generation mechanical valves (Starr–Edwards, Bjork–Shiley) in the mitral position, followed by second-generation valves (St. Jude) in the aortic position (see also chap. 2). These women need to be **therapeutically anticoagulated throughout pregnancy and postpartum, with blood levels frequently (usually weekly) checked to ensure therapeutic levels of anticoagulation**. Pregnant women with prosthetic heart valves pose a problem because of the **lack of trials** regarding the efficacy and safety of antithrombotic therapy during pregnancy. There are insufficient data to make definitive recommendations about optimal anticoagulation in pregnant patients with mechanical heart valves.

There are in general **four regimens** that can be considered: (*i*) VKAs throughout pregnancy; (*ii*) either therapeutic LMWH or UFH between 6 and 12 weeks and close to term only, and VKAs at other times; (*iii*) careful therapeutic UFH throughout pregnancy; (*iv*) careful therapeutic LMWH throughout pregnancy. Before any of these approaches is used, it is crucial to explain the risks/benefits carefully to the patient.

In a review, **VKAs throughout pregnancy** was the **regimen associated with the lowest risk of valve thrombosis/ systemic embolism** (3.9%); using UFH only between 6 and 12 weeks gestation was associated with an increased risk of valve thrombosis (9.2%) (90). This analysis suggests that VKAs are more efficacious than UFH for thromboembolic prophylaxis of women with mechanical heart valves in pregnancy; however, coumarins increase the risk of **embryopathy**. In the first trimester, coumarin is associated with a 10% to 15% teratogenic risk (nasal hypoplasia, optic atrophy, digital anomalies, mental impairment). European experts have recommended warfarin therapy throughout pregnancy in view of the reports of poor maternal outcomes with heparin and their impression that the risk of embryopathy with coumarin derivatives has been overstated (91). If coumarin is used, the dose should be adjusted to attain a target INR of 3.0 (range, 2.5–3.5).

A common option utilizes **UFH during the first trimester to minimize teratogenesis, warfarin for the majority of pregnancy (12–36 weeks), and UFH again in the last month to prepare for delivery and allow for epidural anesthesia**. While this may be efficacious, fetal risk is not completely eliminated. **Substituting VKAs with heparin between 6 and 12 weeks** reduces the risk of fetopathic effects but possibly subjects the woman to an increased risk of thromboembolic complications. The reported high rates of thromboembolism with **UFH** might be explained by inadequate dosing and/or the use of an inappropriate target therapeutic range.

The use of **weight-adjusted therapeutic UFH** warrants careful monitoring and appropriate dose adjustment. A target aPTT ratio of at least twice the control should be attained (92). If used, SC UFH should be initiated in high doses, usually every eight hours, and adjusted to prolong a six-hour post-injection aPTT into the therapeutic range (usually 60–80 seconds); strong efforts should be made to ensure an adequate anticoagulant effect.

LMWH use in pregnant women with prosthetic heart valves (93–99) has been associated with treatment failures (96–99), and the use of LMWH for this indication has recently become controversial because of a warning from a LMWH manufacturer regarding their safety in this situation (100). If used, LMWH should be administered twice daily and dosed to achieve anti-Xa levels of 1.0 to 1.2 U/mL four to six hours (peak) after SC injection, with trough 0.6 to 0.7.

Extrapolating from data in nonpregnant patients with mechanical valves receiving warfarin therapy (101), for some high-risk women, **the addition of low-dose aspirin**, 75 to 162 mg/day, can be considered in an attempt to reduce the risk of thrombosis, recognizing that it increases the risk of bleeding.

ANTEPARTUM TESTING
No specific recommendations.

DELIVERY
In order to avoid an unwanted anticoagulant effect during delivery (and also for allowing neuroaxial anesthesia) in women receiving therapeutic UFH (9,102) or LMWH (30–39), it is suggested that heparin be discontinued about 24 hour prior to planned induction of labor or cesarean section. If spontaneous labor occurs in women receiving therapeutic LMWH or UFH, careful monitoring of the aPTT may be necessary. If it is markedly prolonged near delivery, protamine sulfate may be required to reduce the risk of bleeding. Therapeutic heparin can be restarted about 6 to 12 hours after delivery, and warfarin restarted in an overlapping fashion (to avoid paradoxical thrombosis) 24 to 36 hours after delivery (the night after delivery).

In women with **mechanical heart valves**, therapeutic anticoagulation can be continued IV (half-life: 1½ hour) until active labor, and then stopped during active labor and for delivery, with therapeutic heparin restarted about 6 to 12 hours after delivery, and warfarin restarted in an overlapping fashion (to avoid paradoxical thrombosis) 24 to 36 hours after delivery (the night after delivery). Extensive counseling on all these options and risks is required.

ANESTHESIA
UFH ≤5000 IU twice a day does not pose a risk for spinal hematoma. Low-dose prophylactic UFH and LMWH probably do not cause a risk for spinal hematoma (1). For precaution, women on low-dose prophylactic LMWH should not receive regional anesthesia sooner than 12 hours after the last dose. Women on therapeutic LMWH should not receive regional anesthesia sooner than 24 hours after the last dose (6,103).

POSTPARTUM/BREAST-FEEDING
For women necessitating low-dose prophylactic anticoagulation, UFH or LMWH can be restarted 12 to 24 hours postpartum, after removal of epidural catheter, depending on risk. For women necessitating therapeutic adjusted-dose anticoagulation, heparin can be restarted (either UFH or LMWH) 6 to 12 hours postpartum, with warfarin also started about 24 to 36 hours later, overlapping for the first five to seven days until warfarin is therapeutic (INR 2.0–3.0). In general, postpartum anticoagulation should be at levels at or higher those antepartum (Table 28.5). Graduated compression stockings should

also be used while not fully able to mobilize. Breast-feeding is safe while on anticoagulation (with UFH, LMWH, or warfarin). Estrogen-containing hormonal contraception should be avoided in women remaining at high risk for VTE, such as those with prior VTE and/or thrombophilias.

REFERENCES

1. American College of Obstetrics and Gynecology. Prevention of deep vein thrombosis and pulmonary embolism. ACOG Practice Bulletin No. 21. Washington, DC: ACOG, 2000; re-evaluated in 2008. [Review]
2. Greer IA. Thrombosis in pregnancy: maternal and fetal issues. Lancet 1999; 353:1258–1265. [Review]
3. Lindqvist P, Dahlback B, Marsal K. Thrombotic risk during pregnancy: a population study. Obstet Gynecol 1999; 94: 595–599. [II-2]
4. National Institutes of Health Consensus Development Conference. Prevention of venous thrombosis and pulmonary embolism. JAMA 1986; 256:744–749. [Review]
5. Gherman RB, Goodwin TM, Leung B, et al. Incidence, clinical characteristics and timing of objectively diagnosed venous thromboembolism during pregnancy. Obstet Gynecol 1999; 94:730–734. [II-2]
6. Marik PE, Plante LA. Venous thromboembolic disease and pregnancy. N Engl J Med 2008; 359:2025–2033. [III]
7. Grandone E, Margaglione M, Colaizzo D, et al. Genetic susceptibility to pregnancy-related venous thromboembolism: roles of factor V Leiden, prothrombin G20210A, and methylenetetrahydrofolate reductase C677T mutations. Am J Obstet Gynecol 1998; 179:1324–1328. [II-2]
8. Lockwood CJ. Heritable coagulopathies in pregnancy. Obstet Gynecol Surv 1999; 54:754. [Review]
9. Walker MC, Garner PR, Keely EJ, et al. Changes in activated protein C resistance during normal pregnancy. Am J Obstet Gynecol 1997; 77:162. [II-3]
10. Zotz RB, Gerhardt A, Scharf RE. Inherited thrombophilia and gestational venous thromboembolism. Best Pract Res Clin Haematol 2003; 16:243. [Review]
11. Investigation and management of heritable thrombophilia. Br J Haematol 2001; 114:512. [II-2]
12. Kyrle PA, Eichinger S. Deep vein thrombosis. Lancet 2005; 365:1163–1174. [Review]
13. Pabinger I, Grafenhofer H. Thrombosis during pregnancy: risk factors, diagnosis and treatment. Pathophysiol Haemost Thromb 2002; 32:322–324. [Review]
14. Ginsberg JS, Hirsh J, Rainbow AJ, et al. Risks to the fetus of radiologic procedures used in the diagnosis of maternal venous thromboembolic disease. Thromb Haemost 1989; 61:189–196. [II-2]
15. Kearon C, Julian JA, Newman TE, et al. Noninvasive diagnosis of deep vein thrombosis: McMaster diagnostic imaging practice guidelines initiative. Ann Intern Med 1998; 128:663–677. [Guideline]
16. Bergqvist D, Hedner U. Pregnancy and venous thromboembolism. Acta Obstet Gynecol Scand 1983; 62:449–453. [Review]
17. Bergqvist A, Bergqvist D, Hallbook T. Deep vein thrombosis during pregnancy: a prospective study. Acta Obstet Gynecol Scand 1983; 62:443–448. [II-1]
18. Hull RD, Raskob GE, Carter CJ. Serial impedance plethysmography in pregnant patients with clinically suspected deep-vein thrombosis: clinical validity of negative findings. Ann Intern Med 1990; 112:663–667. [II-2]
19. Cockett FB, Thomas ML, Negus D. Iliac vein compression: its relation to iliofemoral thrombosis and the post-thrombotic syndrome. BMJ 1967; 2:14–16. [II-2]
20. Chan WS, Ginsberg JS. Diagnosis of deep vein thrombosis and pulmonary embolism in pregnancy. Thromb Res 2002; 107: 85–91. [II-2]
21. Heijboer C, Beuller HR, Lensing AW, et al. A comparison of real time diagnosis of deep vein thrombosis in symptomatic outpatients. N Engl J Med 1993; 329:1365–1369. [II-2]
22. Weinmann EE, Salzman EW. Deep-vein thrombosis. N Engl J Med 1994; 331:1630–1641. [review]
23. Nolan TE, Smith RP, Devoe LD. Maternal plasma D-dimer levels in normal and complicated pregnancies. Obstet Gynecol 1993; 81:235–238. [II-2]
24. Fedullo Pf, Tapson VF. Clinical Practice: the evaluation of suspected pulmonary embolism. N Engl J Med 2003; 349: 1247–1256. [Review]
25. Goldhaber SZ. Pulmonary embolism. Lancet 2004; 363: 1295–1305. [Review]
26. The PIOPED Investigators. Value of the ventilation/perfusion scan in acute pulmonary embolism: results of the prospective investigation of pulmonary embolism diagnosis (PIOPED). JAMA 1990; 263:2753–2759. [II-2]
27. Bourjely G, paidas M, Khalil H, et al. Pulmonary embolism in pregnancy. Lancet 2010; 375:500–512. [III]
28. Rathbun SW, Raskob GE, Whitsett TL. Sensitivity and specificity of helical computed tomography in the diagnosis of pulmonary embolism: a systematic review. Ann Intern Med 2000; 132: 227–232. [Review]
29. Goodman LR, Curtin JJ, Mewissen MW et al. Detection of pulmonary embolism in patients with unresolved clinical and scintigraphic diagnosis: helical CT versus angiography. Am J Roentgenol 1995; 164:1369–1374. [II-2]
30. Hunt BJ, Doughty HA, Majumdar G, et al. Thromboprophylaxis with low molecular weight heparin (Fragmin) in high risk pregnancies. Thromb Haemost 1997; 77:39–43. [II-2]
31. Blomback M, Bremme K, Hellgren M, et al. Thromboprophylaxis with low molecular mass heparin, "Fragmin" (dalteparin), during pregnancy: longitudinal safety study. Blood Coagul Fibrinolysis 1998; 9:1–9. [II-2]
32. Blomback M, Bremme K, Hellgren M, et al. A pharmacokinetic study of dalteparin during late pregnancy. Blood Coagul Fibrinolysis 1998; 9:343–350. [II-2]
33. Brennand JE, Walker ID, Greer IA. Anti-activated factor X profiles in pregnant women receiving antenatal thromboprophylaxis with enoxaparin. Acta Haematol 1999; 101:53–55. [II-3]
34. Dulitzki M, Pauzner R, Langevitz P, et al. Low molecular weight heparin during pregnancy and delivery: preliminary experience with 41 pregnancies. Obstet Gynecol 1996; 87:380–383. [II-3]
35. Casele HL, Laifer SA, Woelkers DA, et al. Changes in the pharmacokinetics of the low molecular weight heparin enoxaparin sodium during pregnancy. Am J Obstet Gynecol 1999; 181:1113–1117. [II-3]
36. Ellison J, Walker ID, Greer IA. Anti-factor Xa profiles in pregnant women receiving antenatal thromboprophylaxis with enoxaparin for prevention and treatment of thromboembolism in pregnancy. BJOG 2000; 107:1116–1121. [II-3]
37. Lepercq J, Conard J, Borel-Derlon A, et al. Venous thromboembolism during pregnancy: a retrospective study of enoxaparin safety in 624 pregnancies. BJOG 2001; 108:1134–1140. [II-2]
38. Dolovich L, Ginsberg JS, Douketis JD, et al. A meta-analysis comparing low molecular weight heparins to unfractionated heparin in the treatment of venous thromboembolism: examining some unanswered questions regarding location of treatment, product type, and dosing frequency. Arch Intern Med 2000; 160:181–188. [Meta-analysis]
39. Gould MK, Dembitzer AD, Doyle RL, et al. Low-molecular-weight heparins compared with unfractionated heparin for treatment of acute deep venous thrombosis: a meta-analysis of randomized, controlled trials. Ann Intern Med 1999; 130:800–809. [Meta-analysis]
40. de Valek HW, Banga JD, Wester JWJ, et al. Comparing subcutaneous danaparoid with intravenous unfractionated heparin for the treatment of venous thromboembolism: a randomized controlled trial. Ann Intern Med 1995; 123:1–9. [RCT]
41. Nurmohamed MT, Rosendaal FR, Buller HR, et al. Low-molecular-weight heparin versus standard heparin in general and orthopedic surgery: a meta-analysis. Lancet 1992; 340:152–156. [Meta-analysis]

42. Weitz JI. Low-molecular-weight heparins. N Engl J Med 1997; 337:688–698. [Review]

43. Nelson-Piercy C, Letsky EA, de Swiet M. Low-molecular-weight heparin for obstetric thromboprophylaxis: experience of sixty-nine pregnancies in sixty-one women at high risk. Am J Obstet Gynecol 1997; 176:1062–1068. [II-3]

44. Warkentin TE, Levine MN, Hirsh J, et al. Heparin-induced thrombocytopenia in patients treated with low-molecular-weight heparin or unfractionated heparin. N Engl J Med 1995; 332:1330–1335. [II-2]

45. Silver RM. New anticoagulants in pregnancy. Obstet Gynecol 2008; 112:419–420. [III]

46. Pravinkumar E, Webster NR. HIT/HITT and alternative anti-coagulation: current concepts. Br J Anaesth 2003; 90:676–685. [Review]

47. Magnani HN. Heparin-induced thrombocytopenia (HIT): an overview of 230 patients treated with Orgaran (Org 10172). Thromb Haemost 1993; 70:554–561. [II-3]

48. Ginsberg JS, Hirsh J. Use of antithrombotic agents during pregnancy. Chest 1995; 108(suppl):305S–311S. [Review]

49. Dahlman TC. Osteoporotic fractures and the recurrence of thromboembolism during pregnancy and the puerperium in 184 women undergoing thromboprophylaxis with heparin. Am J Obstet Gynecol 1993; 168:1265–1270. [II-3, n = 184]

50. Pettila V, Leinonen P, Markkola A, et al. Postpartum bone mineral density in women treated for thromboprophylaxis with unfractionated heparin or LMW heparin. Thromb Haemost 2002; 87:182–186. [RCT]

51. Sanson BJ, Lensing AWA, Prins MH, et al. Safety of low-molecular-weight heparin in pregnancy: a systematic review. Thromb Haemost 1999; 81:668–672. [Review]

52. Hull RD, Delmore TJ, Carter CJ, et al. Adjusted subcutaneous heparin versus warfarin sodium in the long-term treatment of venous thrombosis. N Engl J Med 1982; 306:189–194. [RCT]

53. Hull RD, Hirsh J, Jay R, et al. Different intensities of oral anticoagulant therapy in the treatment of proximal-vein thrombosis. N Engl J Med 1982; 307:1676–1681. [RCT]

54. Tooher R, Gates S, Dowswell T, et al. Prophylaxis for venous thromboembolic disease in pregnancy and the early postnatal period. Cochrane Database Syst Rev 2010; (5):CD001689. [Meta-analysis]

55. Barbour LA, Oja JL, Schultz LK. A prospective trial that demonstrates that dalteparin requirements increase in pregnancy to maintain therapeutic levels of anticoagulation. Am J Obstet Gynecol 2004; 191:1024–1029. [II-1]

56. Casele HL, Laifer SA, Wolkers DA, et al. Changes in the pharmacokinetics of the low-molecular-weight heparin enoxaparin sodium during pregnancy. Am J Obstet Gynecol 1999; 181:1113–1117. [II-2]

57. Sephton V, Farquharson RG, Topping J, et al. A longitudinal study of maternal dose response to low molecular weight heparin in pregnancy. Obstet Gynecol 2003; 101:1307–1311. [II-2]

58. Ginsberg JS, Hirsh J, Turner CD, et al. Risks to the fetus of anticoagulant therapy during pregnancy. Thromb Haemost 1989; 61:197–203. [II-3]

59. Hall JAG, Paul RM, Wilson KM. Maternal and fetal sequelae of anticoagulation during pregnancy Am J Med 1980; 68:122–140. [II-3]

60. Orme L'E, Lewis M, de Swiet M, et al. May mothers given warfarin breast-feed their infants? BMJ 1977; 1:1564–1565. [II-3]

61. McKenna R, Cole ER, Vasan V. Is warfarin sodium contraindicated in the lactating mother? J Pediatr 1983; 103:325–327. [II-3]

62. Imperiale TF, Petrulis AS. A meta-analysis of low-dose aspirin for prevention of pregnancy-induced hypertensive disease. JAMA 1991; 266:260–264. [Meta-analysis]

63. CLASP Collaborative Group. CLASP: a randomised trial of low dose aspirin for the prevention and treatment of pre-eclampsia among 9,364 pregnant women. Lancet 1994; 343:619–629. [RCT]

64. Che Yaakob A, Dzarr AA, Ismail AA, et al. Anticoagulant therapy for deep vein thrombosis (DVT) in pregnancy. Cochrane Database Syst Rev 2010; (6):CD007801. [Meta-analysis]

65. Ridker PM, Goldhaber SZ, Danielson E, et al. Long-term, low-intensity warfarin therapy for the prevention of recurrent venous thromboembolism. N Engl J Med 2003; 348:1425–1434. [RCT]

66. Greenfield LJ, Cho KJ, Proctor MC, et al. Late results of supra-renal Greenfield vena cava filter placement. Arch Surg 1992; 127:969–967. [II-2]

67. Narayan H, Cullimore J, Krarup K, et al. Experience with the cardial inferior vena cava filter as prophylaxis against pulmonary embolism in pregnant women with extensive deep venous thrombosis. BJOG 1992; 99:637–640. [II-3]

68. Fagher B, Ahlgren M, Astedt B. Acute massive pulmonary embolism treated with streptokinase during labor and the early puerperium. Acta Obstet Gynecol Scand 1990; 69:659–661. [II-3]

69. Riedel M. Acute pulmonary embolism 2: treatment. Heart 2001; 85:351–360. [Review]

70. Ahearn GS, Hadjiliadis D, Govert JA, et al. Massive pulmonary embolism during pregnancy successfully treated with recombinant tissue plasminogen activator: a case report and review of treatment options. Arch Intern Med 2002; 162:1221–1227. [II-3]

71. De Swiet M, Floyd E, Letsky E. Low risk of recurrent thromboembolism in pregnancy. Br J Hosp Med 1987; 38:264. [Letter]

72. Howell R, Fidler J, Letsky E, et al. The risk of antenatal subcutaneous heparin prophylaxis: a controlled trial. BJOG 1983; 90:1124–1128. [RCT]

73. Badaracco MA, Vessey M. Recurrent venous thromboembolic disease and use of oral contraceptives. BMJ 1974; 1:215–217. [II-2]

74. Tengborn L. Recurrent thromboembolism in pregnancy and puerperium: is there a need for thromboprophylaxis? Am J Obstet Gynecol 1989; 160:90–94. [II-2]

75. Pettila V, Kaaja R, Leinonen P, et al. Thromboprophylaxis with low molecular weight heparin (dalteparin) in pregnancy. Thromb Res 1999; 96:275–282. [II-2]

76. Hamersley S, Landy H. Low molecular weight heparin is associated with less peripartum blood loss than unfractionated heparin [abstract]. Am J Obstet Gynecol 1998; 178 (1 pt 2):S66. [II-1]

77. Rai R, Cohen H, Dave M, et al. Randomised controlled trial of aspirin and aspirin plus heparin in pregnant women with recurrent miscarriage associated with phospholipid antibodies (or antiphospholipid antibodies). BMJ 1997; 314:253–257. [RCT]

78. Howell R, Fidler J, Letsky E, et al. The risks of antenatal subcutaneous heparin prophylaxis: a controlled trial. BJOG 1983; 90:1124–1128. [RCT]

79. Gates S, Brocklehurst P, Davis LJ. Prophylaxis for venous thromboembolic disease in pregnancy and the early postnatal period. Cochrane Database Syst Rev 4, 2005. [Meta-analysis]

80. Brill-Edwards. Safety of withholding heparin in pregnant women with a history of venous thromboembolism. N Engl J Med 2000; 343:1439–1444. [II-2]

81. Middledorp S, Van der Meer J, Hamulyak K, et al. Counseling women with factor V Leiden homozygosity: use absolute instead of relative risks. Thromb Haemost 2001; 87:360–361. [Review]

82. Middledorp S, Libourel EJ, Hamulyak K, et al. The risk of pregnancy-related venous thromboembolism in women who are homozygous for factor V Leiden. Br J Haematol 2001; 113:553–555. [II-2]

83. Martinelli I, Legnani C, Bucciarelli P, et al. Risk of pregnancy-related venous thrombosis in carriers of severe inherited thrombophilia. Thromb Haemost 2001; 86:800–803. [II-2]

84. Pabinger I, Nemes L, Rintelen C, et al. Pregnancy-associated risk for venous thromboembolism and pregnancy outcome in women homozygous for factor V Leiden. Hematol J 2000; 1:37–41. [II-2]

85. Hill NCW, Hill JG, Sargent JM, et al. Effect of low dose heparin on blood loss at caesarean section. BMJ 1988; 296:505–506. [II-3]

86. Burrows RF, Gan ET, Gallus AS, et al. A randomised, double blind placebo controlled trial of low molecular weight heparin

as prophylaxis in preventing venous thromboembolic events after caesarean section: a pilot study. BJOG 2001; 108:835–839. [RCT]

87. Gibson JL, Ekevall K, Walker I, et al. Puerperal thromboprophylaxis: comparison of the anti-Xa activity of enoxaparin and unfractionated heparin. BJOG 1998; 105:795–797. [II-1]

88. Heilman L, Heitz R, Koch FU, et al. Perioperative thrombosis prophylaxis at the time of caesarean section: results of a randomised prospective comparative study with 6% hydroxyethyl starch 0.62 and low dose heparin. [Die perioperative thromboseprophylaxe beim kaiserschnitt: ergebnisse einer randomisierten prospektiven vergleichsuntersuchung mit 6% hydroxyathylstarke 0.62 und low-dose-heparin.] Z Geburtsh Perinatol 1991; 195:10–15. [RCT]

89. Report of the RCOG Working Party on Prophylaxis Against Thromboembolism in Gynaecology and Obstetrics. London, UK: Royal College of Obstetricians and Gynaecologists, 1995. [Review]

90. Chan WS, Anand S, Ginsberg JS. Anticoagulation of pregnant women with mechanical heart valves: a systematic review of the literature. Arch Intern Med 2000; 160:191–196. [Review]

91. Sbarouni E, Oakley CM. Outcome of pregnancy in women with valve prostheses. Br Heart J 1994; 71:196–201. [II-2]

92. Brill-Edwards P, Ginsberg JS, Johnston M, et al. Establishing a therapeutic range for heparin. Ann Intern Med 1993; 119:104–109. [II-2]

93. Arnaout MS, Kazma H, Khalil A, et al. Is there a safe anticoagulation protocol for pregnant women with prosthetic valves? Clin Exp Obstet Gynecol 1998; 25:101–104. [II-2]

94. Lee LH, Liauw PC, Ng AS. Low molecular weight heparin for thromboprophylaxis during pregnancy in 2 patients with mechanical mitral valve replacement. Thromb Haemost 1996; 76:628–630. [Letter]

95. Rowan JA, McCowan LM, Raudkivi PJ, et al. Enoxaparin treatment in women with mechanical heart valves during pregnancy. Am J Obstet Gynecol 2001; 185:633–637. [II-2]

96. Roberts N, Ross D, Flint SK, et al. Thromboembolism in pregnant women with mechanical prosthetic heart valves anticoagulated with low molecular weight heparin. BJOG 2001; 108: 327–329. [II-2]

97. Leyh RG, Fischer S, Ruhparwar A, et al. Anticoagulation for prosthetic heart valves during pregnancy: is low-molecular-weight heparin an alternative? Eur J Cardiothorac Surg 2002; 21:577–579. [II-2]

98. Mahesh B, Evans S, Bryan AJ. Failure of low molecular-weight heparin in the prevention of prosthetic mitral valve thrombosis during pregnancy: case report and review of options for anticoagulation. J Heart Valve Dis 2002; 11:745–750. [II-3]

99. Lev-Ran O, Kramer A, Gurevitch J, et al. Low-molecular-weight heparin for prosthetic heart valves: treatment failure. Ann Thorac Surg 2000; 69:264–265. [II-3]

100. Lovenox Injection (package insert). Bridgewater, NJ: Aventis Pharmaceuticals, 2004. [Package insert]

101. Turpie AGG, Gent M, Laupacis A, et al. A comparison of aspirin with placebo in patients treated with warfarin after heart-valve replacement. N Engl J Med 1993; 329:524–529. [RCT]

102. Anderson DR, Ginsberg JS, Burrows R, et al. Subcutaneous heparin therapy during pregnancy: a need for concern at the time of delivery. Thromb Haemost 1991; 63:248–250. [II-2]

103. American Society of Regional Anesthesia (ASRA). Recommendations for Neuroaxial Anesthesia and Anticoagulation. Richmond, VA: ASRA, 1998. [Guideline]

29

Hepatitis A

Cassie Leonard and Neil Silverman

KEY POINTS

- The vast majority of hepatitis A virus (HAV) infections are self-limited.
- There is no perinatal transmission of HAV.
- The inactivated HAV vaccine can be safely used for prevention, including during pregnancy if a patient is at risk for HAV exposure.
- Exposed pregnant women can receive immune globulin injections, which are >85% effective in preventing HAV infection if given within two weeks of exposure.
- Therapy of acute HAV infection in pregnancy is supportive.

DIAGNOSIS

Anti–hepatitis A virus (HAV) IgM is the diagnostic criterion for acute HAV infection.

SYMPTOMS

Fever, malaise, decreased appetite, nausea, abdominal discomfort, dark urine, jaundice.

EPIDEMIOLOGY/INCIDENCE

Less than or equal to 1 per 1000 pregnancies (1). Worldwide, geographic areas can be characterized by high, intermediate, or low levels of endemicity (Fig. 29.1). Levels of endemicity are related to hygienic and sanitary conditions in the geographic areas. HAV infection is common (high or intermediate endemicity) throughout the developing world, where infections most frequently are acquired during early childhood and usually are asymptomatic or mild. In areas of high endemicity, adults are usually immune and epidemics of hepatitis A are uncommon.

There were about 17,000 cases in the United States in 1999 (down almost 50% from 1995), although rates have been shown to decline nationally even more lately as a result of implementation of vaccine protocols, particularly among children (2). In fact, national incidence of acute hepatitis A (new cases) has recently declined 92%, from 12.0 cases per 100,000 persons in 1995 to 1.0 per 100,000 persons in 2007—the lowest rate ever recorded (3). About 40% of population is HAV IgG+ (usually immune from old infection).

GENETICS

RNA piconavirus (family of enteroviruses).

ETIOLOGY/BASIC PATHOPHYSIOLOGY

Fecal/oral contact with infected person or contaminated food/water; rarely from blood transmission. Most U.S. cases are from person-to-person or sexual contacts or transmission during outbreaks. Average incubation period is 28 (15–49) days, then abrupt onset. HAV infection can be not only symptomatic (adults) but also asymptomatic (mostly children <6 years old). Symptoms last usually less than two months (up to six months in 10–15% patients). The vast majority of cases are self-limited.

RISK FACTORS/ASSOCIATIONS

Increased risk of acquiring HAV infection in: travelers to developing/high prevalence countries; men who have sex with men; intravenous drug abusers; people who work with nonhuman primates; people with chronic liver disease.

COMPLICATIONS

Mortality is <0.3%. Chronic carrier state does not exist.

PREGNANCY CONSIDERATIONS

No perinatal transmission.

PREGNANCY MANAGEMENT
Workup

HAV IgM and IgG. HAV IgM is detectable 5 to 10 days before the onset of symptoms and usually decreases to undetectable concentrations within six months after recovery (4). Consider rest of hepatitis workup (see chapters 30 and 31). Check AST/ALT, bilirubin.

Prevention/ Preconception Counseling

Avoid fecal-oral contamination by washing all foods and keeping hands clean. Be aware of frequent source (40%) being contact with children. Havrix (Smith Kline Beecham Biologicals, Belgium) and Vaqta (Merck and Co, Inc., New Jersey, U.S.) are inactived live virus vaccines. Two doses IM (Havrix 1 mL [50 U] or Vaqta 1 g [1440 U]), given 6 to 12 months apart, are needed to confer immunity. They can be safely used during pregnancy if a patient is at risk for HAV exposure. HA vaccine is also available in combination with HB vaccine. Immunity after vaccination lasts >10 years.

Prenatal Care
Therapy
   Acute infection. No anti-HAV drug is available at present. Supportive therapies can be offered as outpatient. Consider hospitalization only in rare cases of severe dehydration, encephalopathy, or coagulopathy.

   Exposed pregnant women can receive immune globulin injections (0.02 mg/kg IM), which are >85% effective in preventing HAV infection if given within two weeks of exposure (close personal or sexual contact). The HAV vaccine series should also be initiated (1).

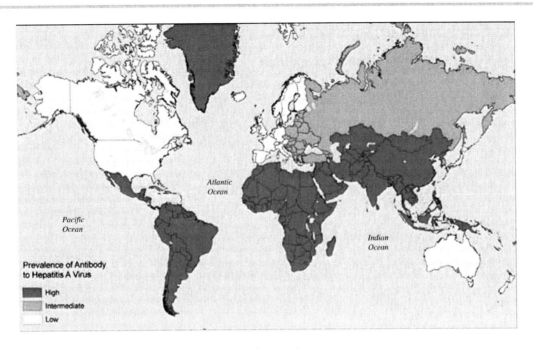

Figure 29.1   Endemicity of hepatitis A in the world. *Source*: http://www.cdc.gov.

ANTEPARTUM TESTING
Not indicated.

DELIVERY
Follow obstetrical indications.

ANESTHESIA
No particular precautions necessary.

POSTPARTUM/BREAST-FEEDING
Breast-feeding is not contraindicated.

REFERENCES
1. ACOG. Viral hepatitis in pregnancy. ACOG Practice Bulletin No. 86. Obstet Gynecol 2007; 110(4):941–956. [Review; III]
2. APGO Educational Series on Women's Health. Hepatitis B and C. In: Sexually Transmitted Infections: The Ob/Gyn's Role. Maryland: APGO, 2003. [Review; III]
3. Daniels D, Grytdal S, Wasley A. Surveillance for acute viral hepatitis—United States, 2007. MMWR Surveill Summ 2009; 58 (SS03):1–27. [Review]
4. Centers for Disease Control and Prevention. Prevention of hepatitis A through active or passive immunization: recommendations of the Advisory Committee on Immunization Practices (ACIP). MMWR Recomm Rep 2006; 55(RR-07):1–23. [Guideline; III]

30

Hepatitis B

Cassie Leonard and Neil Silverman

KEY POINTS

- Universal precautions, proper hygiene, avoidance of high-risk behavior with contact with potentially infectious body fluids (blood, semen, and saliva) must be employed by the mother (or potential mother) to avoid acquiring the infection.
- Hepatitis B virus (HBV) vaccine should be administered preconception or early in pregnancy to every reproductive age woman who is susceptible.
- All women should be screened for HBV infection during pregnancy: HBsAg is the appropriate screening test.
- Vertical transmission of HBV occurs in 90% to 95% of women with HBeAg+, and 90% of women with acute hepatitis in the third trimester.
- Vertical transmission can occur in about 20% to 30% of women who are HBsAg+ but HBeAg−.
- 90% of newborns infected with HBV develop chronic HB without intervention, with 25% of chronic HB carrier eventually dying of complications (cirrhosis, hepatocellular cancer) of HBV infection.
- All newborns born to women with HBsAg+ should receive both HBIg and HB vaccine within 12 hours of birth. This prevents 85% to 95% of neonatal HBV infection.
- Breast-feeding is not contraindicated, as long as the newborn receives appropriate immunoprophylaxis.

DIAGNOSIS/DEFINITION
Adults (Table 30.1)

Acute: HBsAg+, HBcAb+, HBcIgM+, HBsAb−
Chronic: HBsAg+ >6 months, HBsAb− (1,2)

The virus can be found by PCR in blood, urine, feces, seminal fluid, saliva, and GI tract. Serum, semen, and saliva are infectious. The initial differential diagnosis of hepatitis includes hepatic A, B, or C virus (HAV, HBV, HCV), cytomegalovirus (CMV), Epstein–Barr, varicella (VZV), coxsackie B, herpes (HSV), rubella, and autoimmune.

Infants
The diagnosis is made by detection of persistent (e.g., >9 months of age) HBsAg. Only HbsAb is attributable to newborn vaccination: HBcAb arises only as the result of actual HBV infection.

SYMPTOMS
Only 30% to 50% of patients acutely infected have symptoms such as loss of appetite, malaise, nausea, and vomiting. About 10% have jaundice. The onset is usually insidious.

EPIDEMIOLOGY/INCIDENCE
More than 400 million worldwide have chronic HBV infection. Most acquire the infection at birth or in the first one to two years of life. More than 300,000 liver cancers per year are due to HBV (>50% of 530,000 cases—118,000 cases due to HCV—so hepatitis is responsible for 82% of all liver cancer). One-third of the world's population (two billion people) have been infected with HBV: 90% have complete resolution, while about 10% overall develop chronic HBV infection; but this incidence is 90% in children <1 year old, and only 2% in persons >5 years old. About 25% of HBV chronic infection patients die of liver disease (4000/yr in the United States, >1 million/yr worldwide—0.5% mortality) (3).

The vaccine is about 95% effective against HBV. More than 90 countries implement universal vaccination: the worldwide eradication of HBV is a distinct possibility, but far away at present. More than 75% of chronic HBV infection patients are Chinese, second is sub-Saharan Africa (10–20% incidence in these countries). Incidence is 0.2% to 0.5% in North America, Europe, and Australia. The incidence of HBV infection has decreased >60% in the United States from 1985 to 1995.

GENETICS
Small partially double-stranded DNA virus.

ETIOLOGY/BASIC PATHOPHYSIOLOGY
HB virus exposure, then incubation of about 60 to 90 days (depends on the amount of viral exposure), then laboratory changes (Table 30.1).

- Antigens
  - "s" surface—infected. If present >6 months, chronic HBV infection
  - "c"—core
  - "e"—infectious
- Antibodies
  - "s"—immune
  - "c"—covers "window" period, and usually precedes HBsAb conversion

The presence of HbsAb is diagnostic for immunity, whether it results from vaccination or from natural (but cleared, or resolved) infection. HBcAb arises only as a result of natural infection, and coexists with HBsAb in individuals who have cleared their acute infection. In contrast, HBsAb and HBsAg do not coexist in standard clinical testing, since HBsAg is the clearance, or neutralizing antibody, for the antigen.

About 5% of HBV infections become chronic. This can lead to cirrhosis, hepatocellular carcinoma, and death.

CLASSIFICATION
See Table 30.1.

Table 30.1 Interpretation of the Hepatitis B Panel

Test	Results	Interpretation	Vertical transmission[a]
HbsAg Anti-HBc Anti-HBs	Negative Negative Negative	Susceptible	0%
HbsAg Anti-HBc Anti-HBs	Negative Positive Positive	Immune because of natural infection	0%
HbsAg Anti-HBc Anti-HBs	Negative Negative Positive	Immune because of hepatitis B vaccination	0%
HbsAg Anti-HBc Anti-HBc IgM Anti-HBs	Positive Positive Positive Negative	Acutely infected	First trimester: 10% Third trimester: 80–90% HBeAg−: 10–20% HBeAg+: 90%
HbsAg Anti-HBc Anti-HBc IgM Anti-HBs	Positive Positive Negative Negative	Chronically infected	HBeAg−: 2–10% HBeAg+: 80–90%
HbsAg Anti-HBc Anti-HBs	Negative Positive Negative	Four interpretations possible: 1. May be recovering from acute HBV infection 2. May be distantly immune and test is not sensitive enough to detect very low level of anti-HBs in serum 3. May be susceptible with false-positive anti-HBc 4. May be an undetectable level of HBsAg present in the serum and the person is actually a carrier	0%

[a]Assuming HIV negative, and no HB vaccine and immunoprophylaxis of neonate. *Source*: Adapted From Ref. 2.

RISK FACTORS/ASSOCIATIONS

Transmission is parenteral (percutaneous) and sexual (mucosal). The greatest source of chronic HBV infection worldwide is perinatal transmission from HBV-infected mothers. 25% of sexual contacts become positive. Intravenous drug abuse (IVDA), sexually transmitted diseases (STDs), multiple sex partners, house contacts, metal institution/prison, acupuncture are other risk factors, as is the rare HBV-infected blood transfusion. The risk of transfusion-attributable HBV infections is about 1 per 137,000 transfused units of screened blood (1). HBV-infected patients are at higher risk of HIV and HCV infections.

COMPLICATIONS

Ninety percent of patients resolve the infection (clear the s and e Ag) and develop HBsAb; 10% develop chronic HB (maintain HBsAg). Of these, most are asymptomatic with normal liver function tests (LFTs), and no HBV detectable by PCR. The other 15% to 30% of chronic HB has persistent viral replication: these patients can develop cirrhosis and hepatocellular cancer. Mortality is 0.5% to 1%.

PREGNANCY CONSIDERATIONS

Vertical transmission occurs in about **20% to 30% of children born to HbsAg+/HBeAg− mothers**, if no neonatal immunoprophylaxis is given. **If the woman is also HBeAg+, the risk for vertical transmission is about 90% to 95%, with 90% of infected neonates becoming chronic carriers as a result.** Vertical transmission is lowest (<10%) if HBeAb+. **Vertical transmission** is also **trimester dependent: first trimester 10%, third trimester 80% to 90%**, of which 90% occurs because of intrapartum exposure to blood and secretions. Only about 5% to 10% of all transmission is transplacental hematogenous or from breast-feeding. Risk of vertical transmission of HBV is not higher in HBV-infected women who undergo amniocentesis versus HBV-infected women who do not (1), but data are limited. There are insufficient data to assess the risk of in utero infection related to chorionic villus sampling in HBV-infected women (4). Pregnancy course is otherwise not altered by HBV (same incidences of pregnancy loss, congenital anomalies, etc.), except for higher preterm birth rates for acute third-trimester HBV infection.

MANAGEMENT
Principles
Main goal is prevention of vertical transmission.

Workup
HBsAg, HBsAb, HBcAb, HBcIgM, HBeAg. See Table 30.1 for interpretation of diagnosis, disease stage.

Other
- HBV DNA by quantitative PCR (to monitor risk of vertical transmission, progression of disease and effectiveness of treatment)
- Liver biopsy (consider for initial assessment of severity of disease for chronic HBV).

Prevention/Preconception Counseling (1,3)
Universal precautions, proper hygiene, avoidance of high-risk behavior with contact with potentially infected fluids (e.g., serum, semen, and saliva) must be employed by the mother (or potential mother) to avoid acquiring the infection.

HBV vaccine should be administered preconception or early in pregnancy to every reproductive age woman who is susceptible.

Universal maternal screening with HBsAg is recommended at first visit or preconception.

If HBsAg+, test for HBsAb, eAg, eAb, cAb. All HBsAg+ women should have their neonate receive HBIg and HB vaccine within 12 hours of birth. This combination prevents >90% of vertical transmission.

If HBsAg−, consider vaccine in pregnancy for all, and especially high-risk groups such as STDs, HIV+, HepC+, and IVDA.

Women who are known to be or found to be chronically HBV infected (HBsAg+) should also be screened for prior hepatitis A virus (HAV-IgG) and vaccinated if non-immune, since coinfection with other hepatitis viruses has additive morbidity.

Prenatal Care

Universal maternal screening with HBsAg at first visit or preconception. If HBsAg+, send workup as above. If HBsAg−, no further workup. Consider repeating in early third trimester in high-risk groups, such as sex with acutely or chronically HBV-infected person, sex workers, multiple/new partner, multiple STDs, HIV, IVDA, occupational contact with blood, receivers of unscreened blood, hemodialysis patients, household contacts of infected patients, persons in prisons, institutions or countries with high rates of HBV infections.

Therapy

Main intervention therapies (1–3,5,6):

HB Vaccine

Series of three IM injections in deltoid muscle over six months of recombinant DNA; 95% seroconversion (HBsAb+ and immune) rate. It is safe in pregnancy and for neonate. Two vaccines available:

1. Recombivax HB (Merck and Co, Inc., New Jersey, U.S.): adults >20 years old = 10 mg (1 mL); 11–19 years old = 5 (0.5); <11 years old = 2.5 (0.25); within 12 hours of delivery and maternal HBeAg+ = 5; within 12 hours of delivery and maternal HBeAg− = 2.5.
2. Engerix-B (Smith Kline Beecham Biologicals, Belgium): adults >20 years old—20 mg (1 mL); 11 to 19 years old—20 (1); <11 years old—10 (0.5); within 12 hours of delivery and mat. HBeAg+ = 10; within 12 hours of delivery and mat. HBeAg− = 10.

There is also one combination (HA and HB) vaccine available (Twinrix) (1).

HBIg

Immunoglobulins specific for HB (0.5 mL/kg IM for adult; 0.13 mL/kg for neonate). It is safe in pregnancy and for neonate.

Interferon-α

Immunomodulator. Safety: see chapter 31. Efficacy: 35% interferon-α vs. 15% placebo for achieving above goals.

Nucleoside/Nucleotide Analogs

Safety: generally safe. Example: Lamividune is FDA category B (7). Efficacy (Lamivudine): >95% to achieve <150,000 HBV DNA, 167% HbeAg negativity; can reverse cirrhosis of the liver. Lamivudine, given usually as 100 mg from 28 weeks to one month after birth in HBV carrier mothers, has been associated with a significant decrease in the HBV mother-to-child transmission (8). Current recommendations have not been changed on the basis of these meta-analysis data as yet,

given the high levels of HB seropositivity in controls and low quality of some of the included studies. Tenofovir, entecavir, adefovir, dipivoxil, and other newer nucleoside and nucleotide analogs have limited pregnancy data yet, but appear to be promising therapies based on reports from trials in nonpregnant adults (7). In time, third-trimester treatment of HBV-infected women with high viral titers in an attempt to lower the rates of in utero transmission may emerge as more standard therapy. However, there is an overall low rate of this occurrence (5–10%) with proper neonatal care, as well as concerns about maternal drug resistance resulting from single-agent therapy should treatment for her own health be undertaken after the pregnancy. As has evolved with HIV infection, combination maternal therapy to decrease fetal/neonatal HBV infection has biologic validity and awaits validation in future trials.

Conditions

- *Acute Hepatitis B* in pregnancy: diagnosis: document conversion from HBsAg− to HBsAg+. Check all labs as above. Outpatient supportive therapy. Consider hospitalization for severe anemia, diabetes mellitus, severe dehydration, coagulopathy, bilirubin >15. Consider interferon (see chap. 31, and below), nucleoside/nucleotide, and/or HBIg therapy. Vitamin K 10 mg IM (or po) q8h × 3 can be given to pregnant women with coagulopathy. Mortality is about 1% (1). Sexual, needle, and household contacts should be informed by the patient.

- *Exposure to HB* in pregnancy: Check all labs as above. If HBsAg− and sAb−, give HBIg and begin the HB vaccine series (preferably within 24 hours of exposure): this combination will prevent 75% of transmission. Must give HBIg within 14 days of sexual contact. Repeat HBIg within one month if blood or mucous membrane exposure.

- *Vertical transmission prevention*: **All newborns born to women with HBsAg+ should receive HBIg and HB vaccine** within 12 hours of birth, given simultaneously at different sites IM (1,2). This combination is about 95% effective in preventing neonatal HBV infection.

- *Maternal chronic hepatitis B:* While no maternal treatment aimed at interfering with disease progression and vertical transmission is commonly implemented in pregnancy, this is being reconsidered, especially as more reassuring safety and efficacy data are becoming available for interferon as well as newer nucleoside and nucleotide analogues. Therapy for nonpregnant adults is usually suggested if ALT (alanine transaminase) >1.5 upper limit of normal, **and** HBV DNA > about 150,000. Exact cutoffs for both these end points are controversial, and still being researched. Goals of therapy are sustained suppression of HBV DNA levels to very low (preferably undetectable) levels, ALT lower than half the upper limit of the normal range, and the traditional goal of undetectable HBeAg (5,6). Before therapy, liver biopsy may be considered as baseline. Consider a hepatology and/or infectious disease consult. Sexual, needle, and household contacts should be informed by the patient. Some state or local health departments require reporting.

ANTEPARTUM TESTING

Not indicated.

DELIVERY
Per obstetrical indications.

ANESTHESIA
No particular precautions necessary.

POSTPARTUM/BREAST-FEEDING
Breast-feeding is not contraindicated, as long as the mother is HBeAg− and HIV−, and the neonate receives HBIg and HB vaccine as above (1,9).

RARE/RELATED
Hepatitis D virus: incomplete RNA virus, which can super-infect 20% to 25% of chronic HBV-infected patients. HDV infection worsens chronic HBV infection, so that 25% may die from disease. If HBV is prevented, HDV infection is prevented too. HDV has no effect on pregnancy or fetus/neonate.

REFERENCES
1. American College of Obstetricians and Gynecologists. Viral hepatitis in pregnancy. ACOG Practice Bulletin No. 86. Obstet Gynecol 2007; 110(4):941–956. [Review]
2. APGO Educational Series on Women's Health. Hepatitis B and C. In: Sexually Transmitted Infections: The Ob/Gyn's Role. Maryland: APGO, 2003. [Good pregnancy review]
3. Mast EE, Weinbaum CM, Fiore AE, et al. A comprehensive immunization strategy to eliminate transmission of hepatitis B virus infection in the United States: recommendations of the advisory committee on immunization practices (ACIP) part II: immunization in adults. MMWR Recomm Rep 2006; 55(RR–16):1–33; quiz CE1–4. [Review]
4. Towers CV, Asrat T, Rumney P. The presence of hepatitis B surface antigen and deoxyribonucleic acid in amniotic fluid and cord blood. Am J Obstet Gynecol 2001; 184:1514–1520. [II-3]
5. Lai CL, Ratziu V, Yuen MF, et al. Viral hepatitis B. Lancet 2003; 362:2089–2094. [General review, nonpregnant]
6. Lai C-L, Yuen M-F. Chronic hepatitis B—new goals, new treatments. N Engl J Med 2008; 359:2488–2491. [Review, nonpregnant, III]
7. Watts DH, Covington DL, Beckerman K, et al. Assessing the risk of birth defects associated with antiretroviral exposure during pregnancy. Am J Obstet Gynecol 2004; 191:985–992. [II-2]
8. Shi Z, Yang Y, Ma L, et al. Lamivudine in late pregnancy to interrupt in utero transmission of hepatitis B. Obstet Gynecol 2010; 116:147–159. [Meta-analysis, 10 RCTs, *n* = 951 women]
9. Hill JB, Sheffield JS, Kim MJ, et al. Risk of hepatitis B transmission in breast-fed infants of chronic hepatitis B carriers. Obstet Gynecol 2002; 99:1049–1052. [II-1]

31

Hepatitis C

Cassie Leonard and Neil Silverman

KEY POINTS

- Chronic hepatitis C virus (HCV) infection is defined as HCV IgG+ with detectable HCV RNA. Chronic active HCV infection is defined as chronic HCV infection with abnormal liver function tests.
- HCV is acquired via infected blood, sexual contact, or mother-to-infant (vertical transmission).
- Complications of chronic HCV infection include cirrhosis and hepatocellular carcinoma.
- Mother-to-infant transmission is diagnosed by positive neonatal serum HCV RNA on two occasions 3 to 4 months apart after the infant is 2 months old, and/or anti-HCV detected after the infant is 18 months old. Coinfection with HIV and high maternal viral load are associated with higher risk of transmission.
- Risk factors (Table 31.2) for HCV should be avoided to prevent HCV infection, and be used for screening.
- HCV-positive pregnant women should be evaluated with HCV RNA viral load; hepatitis B surface antigen and hepatitis A antibody; liver function testing; HIV screening; gastroenterology referral; STD screening.
- Patients with HCV infection are at high risk for other viral hepatitis infections: if they are nonimmune to HAV and/or hepatitis B virus (HBV), appropriate vaccination should be given, since coinfection has additive morbidity and can be prevented with vaccination.
- Treatment for HCV chronic infection can be effective with combination antiviral therapy (pegylated alpha interferon and ribavirin) for nonpregnant adults, but cannot be used during or immediately prior to pregnancy, because of teratogenicity of ribavirin.
- In HCV-positive but HIV-negative women, cesarean delivery should be reserved for obstetrical indications.
- Breast-feeding is generally not considered to be a risk factor for vertical transmission of HCV in non-HIV infected women. Breast-feeding is instead contraindicated in women with both HCV and HIV infections.
- Therapy with ribavirin and alpha interferon (or other newer antiviral agents as they become available and are shown to be safe and effective) should be started postpartum for the same indications as in other nonpregnant adults.

DIAGNOSIS/DEFINITION

Adults (Table 31.1)

Acute HCV infection: HCV IgM+.
Chronic HCV infection: HCV IgG+ with detectable HCV DNA.
Chronic active HCV disease: HCV IgG+ with detectable HCV DNA and abnormal liver function tests (LFTs).

However, if screening is performed in a low-risk population, there will be a higher false-positive rate for HCV IgG via standard ELISA assays, and confirmatory antibody testing (such as RIBA) may be necessary. For this reason, HCV screening should be reserved for pregnant women in high-risk categories. The virus can be found by PCR in blood, urine, feces, seminal fluid, saliva, GI tract (1,2). The initial differential diagnosis of hepatitis includes hepatitis A, B, or C virus (HAV, HBV, or HCV), cytomegalovirus (CMV), Epstein–Barr, varicella (VZV), coxsackie B, herpes (HSV), rubella, autoimmune, etc.

Infants

Infection is diagnosed by positive serum HCV RNA on two occasions 3 to 4 months apart after the infant is 2 months old, or anti-HCV detected after the child is 18 months old.

SYMPTOMS

Most HCV infections (75%) are asymptomatic. Symptomatic patients present with malaise, fever, abdominal pains, and jaundice.

EPIDEMIOLOGY/INCIDENCE

In the United States, 0.6% to 4.5% of pregnant women have HCV antibodies, with considerable worldwide geographic variation. HCV is the most common chronic blood-borne infection in the United States (while HBV is worldwide), and is responsible for 20% to 40% of all cases of acute hepatitis. Worldwide, over 170 million people are chronically infected with HCV. Of noninstitutionalized U.S. citizens, 1.8% (3.9 millions) carry HCV antibodies; 74% of these (2.7 millions) have detectable viral RNA in their serum (chronic disease). The prevalence is projected to decrease from the current about 1.8% to about 1% by the year 2030. On the contrary, the prevalence of liver disease caused by HCV is on the rise. This is because of the significant lag time, often 20 years or longer, between the onset of infection and clinical manifestations of liver disease.

GENETICS

Single-stranded RNA virus; striking genetic heterogeneity, including six major genotypes, with rapid accumulation of mutations.

ETIOLOGY/BASIC PATHOPHYSIOLOGY

HCV is acquired via infected blood, sexual contact, or mother-to-infant (vertical transmission). The incubation time is usually 30 to 60 days. Chronic HCV (the presence of

Table 31.1 Definitions of Various Types of HCV Infections

HCV	HCV Ab positive
Chronic HCV	HCV Ab positive and HCV RNA positive
Chronic active HCV	HCV Ab positive, HCV RNA positive, and elevated LFTs

Abbreviations: HCV, hepatitis C virus (infection); Ab, antibody; LFTs, liver function tests.

Table 31.2 Risk Factors for HCV Infection

- History of **intravenous drug abuse**
- History of blood transfusion or exposure to blood products
- History of multiple sexually transmitted diseases
- HIV infection
- Hepatitis B viral infection
- Sexual partner who abuses intravenous drugs or has HIV, HBV, or HCV infection
- Three or more lifetime sexual partners
- Incarceration
- History of body piercing and tattooing
- Recipient of organ transplants before 1992
- Unexplained elevated transaminases
- Patient or staff members involved in chronic dialysis programs
- Participant in in vitro fertilization programs from anonymous donors

serum RNA) develops in 50% to 75% of adult and pediatric patients. The course of chronic HCV infection is usually insidious. Chronic active disease (elevation in LFTs) develops in at least 20% of chronic HCV infection.

CLASSIFICATION
Genotype 1 (subtypes 1a and 1b) is most common in United States and Western Europe, and is associated with lower response to antiviral therapy.

RISK FACTORS/ASSOCIATIONS
In the United States, the primary risk factor for HCV infection is parenteral (injected or inhaled) drug abuse (Table 31.2). The risk of HCV infection via blood transfusion is now <1/million in the United States (1). Up to 40% of HCV-infected women have no risk factors. HCV can be found in semen (2) and acquired through artificial insemination (3).

COMPLICATIONS
Complications of chronic infection include **cirrhosis** (10–20%) and **hepatocellular carcinoma** (1–5%).

PREGNANCY CONSIDERATIONS
Mother-to-Infant Transmission
Diagnostic confirmation of vertical transmission is obtained with **positive serum HCV RNA on two occasions 3 to 4 months apart after the infant is 2 months old, or anti-HCV detected after the child is 18 months old.** Table 31.3 summarizes transmission rates compiled from 77 studies and 383 cases of mother-to-infant transmission cases (1,4). **Coinfection with HIV greatly increases** vertical transmission (4). Highly active antiretroviral therapy has been shown to decrease HCV transmission in HCV-HIV coinfected women (5). Vertical transmission also correlates with **high maternal HC viral**

Table 31.3 Rate of Vertical Transmission of Hepatitis C

	Weighted rate (%)[a]
Anti-HCV only (RNA negative)	1–2
Viremic (HCV RNA positive)	4–6
HIV positive	19–40
HIV negative	3–5
Anti-HCV and injection drug use	9

[a]Weighted rate adjusts for sample size of study and variance.
Source: From Refs. 14,15.

load (6), but a specific cutoff that predicts transmission has not been identified. Vertical transmission **does not correlate with mode of delivery** in non-HIV women. HIV coinfected women delivered by cesarean section were 60% less likely to have a HCV-infected child than those delivered vaginally (7). It is controversial whether prolonged rupture of the membranes (i.e., for >6 hours) increases risk. The use of **scalp electrode is discouraged**. There is no association between gestational age and risk of transmission. Amniocentesis does not appear to significantly increase the risk (8), but very few studies have addressed this. If amniocentesis is requested, transplacental needle insertion should be avoided. There are no data regarding CVS and in utero transmission: appropriate counseling should be undertaken if an HCV-infected woman requests CVS, and the availability of amniocentesis should be discussed as a potentially less-invasive and vasodisruptive procedure.

MANAGEMENT
Prevention
There is no HCV vaccine available. **Risk factors** for HCV (Table 31.2) should be **avoided**. Prevention of complication of liver disease includes avoidance of alcohol and hepatotoxic medicines (including alternative and herbal remedies) and foods.

Principles
Effect of Pregnancy on Hepatitis C
Pregnancy does not affect the clinical course of acute or chronic hepatitis C. There is an improvement in biochemical markers of liver damage in HCV-positive women during pregnancy (9). There is a linear increase in HCV viremia throughout pregnancy (2), 50% above baseline (9).

Effect of Hepatitis C on Pregnancy
Chronic active hepatitis in the pregnant woman is associated with an increased incidence of preterm delivery, intrauterine growth restriction, small for gestational age, and NICU admission (10–12). HCV vertical transmission and its consequences can affect the neonate. Long-term complications of HCV infection for either the mother or the baby can lead to cirrhosis, cancer, and mortality.

Screening
It is neither cost effective nor appropriate to screen universally for HCV among low-risk pregnant women, given the false-positive rates for ELISA when done in a large-scale low-risk population. **Screening is recommended in women with risk factors for HCV infection** (Table 31.2). Screening is performed with anti-HCV (HCV IgG) antibody. Universal screening may become recommended when therapy for HCV in pregnancy is deemed safe and effective.

Workup

Any woman with anti-HCV (HCV IgG) antibody should have **HCV RNA viral load; hepatitis B surface antigen and hepatitis A antibody; liver function testing; HIV screening; gastroenterology referral; STD screening.** Vaccination against HAV and/or HBV should be administered if the woman is nonimmune for either or both, to avoid the comorbidities of superimposed hepatitis viral infections, which can be substantial.

Preconception/Pregnancy Counseling

Effect of pregnancy on HCV infection and vice versa should be reviewed. Counseling of the pregnant woman with HCV infection should include review of risk factors known to increase mother-to-infant transmission (HIV coinfection, HCV viremia especially with high viral loads, vaginal delivery in HIV coinfected women, scalp electrode, and breast-feeding in HIV coinfected women), and reassurance for factors known not to increase transmission (vaginal delivery in HIV-negative women, gestational age at time of infection, chorioamnionitis, and breast-feeding in HIV-negative women). Amniocentesis, especially nontransplacental, is associated with minimal risk of HCV vertical transmission. Counseling should also include other possible complications, management, and postpartum follow-up.

Therapy

Currently there is no approved treatment for HCV infection during pregnancy. Pegylated alpha interferon and ribavirin can eradicate the virus in >50% of nonpregnant patients, reduce liver fibrosis progression, and reverse cirrhosis. **Treatment with this efficacious therapy for nonpregnant adults cannot be used during or immediately prior to pregnancy, because of teratogenicity of ribavirin.** While interferon has had no teratogenic effects reported in approximately 35 cases of fetal exposure (13), these data are insufficient, and its use in pregnancy cannot be recommended at present. It would not be indicated at present for use as a single agent to treat HCV in any event. Recently, telaprevir has been associated with even higher sustained virologic response when used with both interferon and ribavirin (14), but this drug is not yet FDA approved, with insufficient pregnancy safety data. There is no HCV vaccine or immune globulin available.

ANTEPARTUM TESTING

Not indicated for HCV infection alone.

DELIVERY

In HCV-positive but HIV-negative women, mode of delivery does not affect vertical transmission, so that **cesarean delivery should be reserved for obstetrical indications.** In HCV- and HIV-positive women, mode of delivery should be cesarean delivery if the HIV viral load is ≥1000 (7).

ANESTHESIA

No particular precautions necessary.

POSTPARTUM

Patients with hepatitis C should be immunized against hepatitis A and B during pregnancy, as these vaccines are safe. If unfortunately immunization has not occurred antenatally, hepatitis A and B vaccines (or their combination) should be given postpartum, even if breast-feeding (12).

BREAST-FEEDING

Breast-feeding is generally not considered to be a risk factor for vertical transmission of HCV in non-HIV infected women (1). The safety of breast-feeding operates on the assumption that traumatized, cracked, or bleeding nipples are not present. However, with HIV coinfection, those who breast-fed were four times more likely to infect their children than those who bottle-fed (7). **Breast-feeding is therefore contraindicated in women with both HCV and HIV infections. Therapy with ribavirin and interferon should be started postpartum for the same indications as in other nonpregnant adults** (15,16).

REFERENCES

1. Viral hepatitis in pregnancy. ACOG Educational Bulletin No. 86. American College of Obstetricians and Gynecologists. Obstet Gynecol 2007; 110:941–955. [Review]
2. Leurez-Ville M, Kunstmann JM, De Almeida M, et al. Detection of hepatitis C virus in the semen of infected men. Lancet 2000; 356:42–43. [II-2]
3. Lesourd F, Izopet J, Mervan C, et al. Transmission of hepatitis C during the ancillary procedures for assisted conception: case report. Hum Reprod 2000; 15:1083–1085. [II-3]
4. Yeung LT, King SM, Roberts EA. Mother-to-infant transmission of hepatitis C virus. Hepatology 2001; 34:223–229. [II-2]
5. Zanetti AR, Tanzi E, Paccagnini S, et al. Mother-to-infant transmission of hepatitis C virus. Lombard Study Group on vertical HCV transmission. Lancet 1995; 345:289–291. [II-2]
6. Ohto H, Terazawa S, Sasaki N, et al. Transmission of hepatitis C virus from mothers to infants. N Engl J Med 1994; 330:744–750. [II-2]
7. European Paediatric Hepatitis C Virus Network. Effects of mode of delivery and infant feeding on the risk of mother-to-child transmission of hepatitis C virus. Br J Obstet Gynecol 2001; 108:371–377. [II-2]
8. Delamare C, Carbonne B, Heim N, et al. Detection of hepatitis C virus RNA (HCV RNA) in amniotic fluid: a prospective study. J Hepatol 1999; 31:416–420. [II-2]
9. Conte D, Fraquelli M, Prati D, et al. Prevalence and clinical course of chronic hepatitis C virus (HCV) infection and the rate of vertical transmission in a cohort of 15,250 women. Hepatology 2000; 31:751–755. [II-2]
10. Simms J, Duff P. Viral hepatitis in pregnancy. Semin Perinatol 1993; 17:384–393. [Review]
11. Zanetti AR, Tanzi E, Newell ML. Mother-to-infant transmission of hepatitis C virus. J Hepatol 1999; 3(suppl 1):S96–S100. [II-2]
12. Pergam S, Wang C, Gardella CM, et al. Pregnancy complications associated with Hepatitis C: data from 2003-2005 Washington state birth cohort. Am J Obstet Gynecol 2008; 199:38.e1–38.e9. [II-3]
13. Pelham J, Berghella V. Alpha interferon use in pregnancy. Obstet Gynecol 2004; 103:77s. [II-3]
14. Hoofnagle JH. A step forward in therapy for hepatitis C. N Engl J Med 2009; 360:1899–1901. [III]
15. Poynard T, Yuen M-F, Ratziu V, et al. Viral hepatitis C. Lancet 2003; 362:2095—2100. [Review]
16. Airoldi J, Berghella V. Hepatitis C and pregnancy. Obstet Gynecol Surv 2006; 61:10. [Review]

32

HIV

Amanda Cotter and William R. Short

KEY POINTS

- **Identification** of HIV infection in pregnancy is **essential for the prevention of perinatal transmission. Therefore, universal screening is recommended in the first trimester or at entry into prenatal care. An opt-out approach** has been shown to increase acceptance rates for HIV testing in pregnant women and is the recommended approach to universal prenatal screening.
- Screening should be **repeated preferably before 36 weeks in cases of high-risk behavior, high-prevalence area, or previously declined testing**.
- **Rapid testing** is recommended for previously untested women presenting in labor, or those expected to be delivered for maternal or fetal indications before results of conventional testing can be obtained. If a rapid HIV test result is positive, antiretroviral prophylaxis should be offered without waiting for the results of the confirmatory conventional tests.
- The **goal** of HIV treatment in pregnancy is to **prevent vertical transmission** primarily by reducing maternal **viral load to <1000 copies/mL or below the limit of detection of the assay**.
- **Rate of perinatal transmission** is directly **correlated to maternal viral load, but other factors also appear to play a role. Perinatal transmission can occur at any HIV RNA level, including in women with an undetectable viral load.**
- All HIV-positive women should be offered **a combination high-active antiretroviral therapy (HAART) including** azidothymidine (zidovudine) **(AZT) where feasible** regardless of clinical or immunological diagnosis to maximally suppress viral replication, reduce the risk of perinatal transmission, and minimize the risk of development of resistant virus.
- Plasma **HIV-1 RNA levels** should be **monitored serially, at least initially, and in the third trimester, to assess both effectiveness of HAART and options for best mode of delivery.**
- Women with a **viral load >1000 copies/mL** should be counseled regarding the **benefit of planned cesarean delivery at 38 weeks** to reduce the risk of transmission.
- With effective antiretroviral therapy leading to undetectable viral load, planned cesarean delivery for viral load ≥1000, and formula feeding, the risk of perinatal transmission is reduced to <2%.

HISTORICAL NOTES

The first cases of what would soon thereafter be called AIDS were reported in homosexual males on June 5, 1981. In 1994, the PACTG-076 regimen of antepartum and intrapartum AZT administered to the mother and then to the newborn for six weeks resulted in a reduction of maternal-infant transmission of HIV-1 from 25.5% to 8% (1).

DIAGNOSIS

Diagnosis is made when a screening **ELISA** is **positive** and is followed by a **confirmatory positive Western blot**. Regarding **rapid testing**, the sensitivity and specificity of each of the available rapid testing assays ranges from 95% to 100%, while the positive predictive value depends on the prevalence of disease in the population. In a population with low prevalence of disease, the positive predictive value is low while the false-positive rate is high. For example, with a prevalence of disease of ~1% in the population, the positive predictive value of the test may be as low as 60%.

EPIDEMIOLOGY

The total number of cases of HIV/AIDS in adolescents and adults worldwide is currently estimated to be 33.3 million, with approximately 50% of those cases occurring in women (2). There is great variation in distribution and prevalence from region to region as shown in Table 32.1. More than 90% of all infected persons live in the developing world. Nigeria, Ethiopia, Russia, India, and China together make up 40% of the world's population, and all have early- to middle-stage HIV epidemics. Transmission of HIV in all five of these countries is projected to increase steeply and outside of high-risk populations, such as commercial sex workers and injection drug users, to the general population through unsafe heterosexual contact and the movement of migrant or displaced populations (3). The projected increase will have significant implications for women, infants, and children in these populations. A second human immunodeficiency virus, HIV-2, is found primarily in West Africa and rarely in Angola and Mozambique. In the United States, 27% of all HIV/AIDS cases are among women, up from 7% in 1985. Black and Hispanic women have been disproportionately affected, accounting for 67% of the diagnoses of HIV infections among adult and adolescent females in 2008, by race/ethnicity, from 37 states with confidential name-based reporting. Heterosexual contact is the major mode of transmission among females accounting for 87% in Black/African-American, 84% in Hispanic/Latino, and 75% in White females in the United States (4). Worldwide, heterosexual contact is also the predominant mode of transmission in women, followed by intravenous drug use with sharing of needles.

Over 90% of pediatric HIV/AIDS cases result from perinatal transmission/breast-feeding. In developed countries, continued perinatal transmission can be attributed to a lack of awareness among pregnant women about their HIV status, the increase in HIV infection among women of childbearing age, absent or delayed prenatal care especially in women using

Table 32.1 Prevalence of HIV Infection in Various Regions of the World in 2009

Region	Number of cases	Prevalence (%)	Cases in women (%)
Sub-Saharan Africa	22.5 million	5.0	60
Caribbean	240,000	1.0	52
Eastern Europe/ Central Asia	1.4 million	0.8	44
South/Southeast Asia	4.1 million	0.3	30
Central and South America	1.4 million	0.5	35
North America	1.5 million	0.5	25
West/Central Europe	820,000	0.2	26
North Africa/Middle East	460,000	0.2	48
East Asia	770,000	0.1	22
Oceania	57,000	0.3	

Source: Adapted from Ref. 2.

illicit drugs, acute or primary infection in late pregnancy or in women who are breast-feeding, poor adherence to prescribed antiretroviral (ARV) regimens, and lack of full implementation of routine universal prenatal HIV counseling and testing. HIV status was known before the pregnancy for 68% of HIV-infected women in the United States and 3% were diagnosed during labor and delivery (4). In undeveloped countries, the lack of access to prophylactic treatment in women whom are aware of their status presents an additional risk for perinatal transmission.

PATHOPHYSIOLOGY

HIV primarily infects T lymphocytes that express the CD4 antigen, resulting in a progressive loss of these cells and impairment of cellular immunity as well as humoral immunity. When CD4 lymphocytes are sufficiently depleted there is the progression to AIDS, characterized by the development of opportunistic infections and malignancies.

CLASSIFICATION

The CDC classification is based on clinical and laboratory evaluations (Table 32.2). There are three clinical categories: (A) asymptomatic, (B) symptomatic, or (C) an AIDS-defining condition; and three ranges of CD4 count: (*i*) >500, (*ii*) 200 to 499, (*iii*) <200 cells/mm^3. Regardless of symptoms, a CD4 <200 cells/mm^3 or the presence of an AIDS-defining illness in an HIV-positive person is an AIDS diagnosis (5).

RISK FACTORS

Risk of perinatal transmission is closely related to viral load (VL) at the time of delivery (6–8). Other risk factors include low CD4+ T-lymphocyte count, lack of ARV therapy, biologic phenotype of the virus, substance abuse, prolonged duration of membrane rupture, HCV coinfection, sexually transmitted infections (STIs), preterm birth, and chorioamnionitis (9–11). Risk factors for maternal infection include unprotected sexual contact with an infected person, sharing drug needles or syringes, sexual contact with someone whose HIV status is unknown, transfusions of contaminated blood or blood components. The presence of ulcerating or nonulcerating STIs including syphilis, genital herpes, chlamydial infection, gonorrhea, or bacterial vaginosis increases susceptibility to HIV infection during sex with infected partners. There is no evidence that HIV is spread through sweat, tears, urine, feces, or by insect bites such as mosquito bites.

COMPLICATIONS
Maternal

Increased risks of chorioamnionitis, postpartum endometritis, and wound infection have been reported. The risk of peripartum infection is inversely proportional to the CD4+ count at the time of delivery.

Fetal

Possible increased risk of preterm delivery if on a protease inhibitor (PI) containing regimen, but no increased risk of FGR, stillbirth, or low Apgar scores (12–14).

PREGNANCY CONSIDERATIONS
Effect of Pregnancy on Disease

Pregnancy has no clear effect on HIV progression. A transient but clinically insignificant decrease in the CD4+ T-lymphocyte count has been described.

Effect of Disease on Pregnancy

Perinatal transmission can occur antepartum (25–40%), intrapartum (60–75%), or postpartum with breast-feeding (14%). **Perinatal transmission appears closely related to VL.** There is a strong correlation between high maternal VL at delivery and risk of transmission, but transmission has occurred at all levels of VL (15). Transmission rates are about 1.2% on HAART, 10.4% on AZT monotherapy, and 25% on no ARV (6).

PREGNANCY MANAGEMENT
Screening

Regulations and policies about HIV screening in pregnancy vary from state to state. Given the effectiveness of intervention,

Table 32.2 Classification for HIV Infection

	Clinical categories		
	A	B	C
CD4 count	Asymptomatic, acute (primary) HIV, or PGL	Symptomatic, not A or C conditions	AIDS-indicator conditions
1. ≥500/μL	A1	B1	C1
2. 200–499/μL	A2	B2	C2
3. <200/μL AIDS-indicator T-cell count	A3	B3	C3

Abbreviation: PGL, persistent generalized lymphadenopathy. *Source*: From Ref. 5.

standard serologic testing with counseling is recommended for all pregnant women at the initiation of prenatal care with a screening ELISA, which if positive is followed by a confirmatory Western blot. An opt-out approach in which the patient is informed that she will be tested for HIV along with other standard prenatal labs unless she declines has been shown in several studies to significantly increase testing rates from less than 40% to 85–98% (16–20). Screening should be repeated at 28 to 32 weeks in the case of high-risk behavior, high-prevalence area, or previously declined testing (20). Rapid testing is recommended for previously untested women presenting in labor, or those expected to be delivered for maternal or fetal indications before results of conventional testing can be obtained (20,21). If a rapid HIV test result is positive, ARV prophylaxis should be offered without waiting for the results of the confirmatory conventional tests.

Principles

The goal of HIV therapy is to achieve a HIV-1 RNA level <1000 copies/mL or below the limit of detection of the assay. The risk of perinatal transmission can be <2% with effective ARV therapy (Table 32.3), planned cesarean delivery (CD) as appropriate, and formula feeding. ARV therapy is recommended in pregnancy predominantly to decrease maternal VL and thereby decrease the risk of perinatal transmission and to improve maternal health. Combination ARV therapy is indicated in pregnancy regardless of clinical or immunological status. When combination ARV therapy is not available, or the patient chooses not to undertake this therapy, several short-course peripartum drug regimens have been shown to significantly decrease the risk of vertical transmission to ~10%.

Preconception Counseling

Many HIV-positive women enter pregnancy aware of their diagnosis, and more than half of these women enter the first trimester on ARV therapy. Preconception counseling should include the following:

- Initiate or modify ARV therapy, avoiding potentially teratogenic agents
- Opportunistic infection prophylaxis as indicated by CD4 count
- Appropriate immunizations
- Optimize maternal nutritional status, initiating folic acid supplementation
- Screen for and treat STIs
- Screen for psychological and substance abuse disorders
- Advise how to optimize the chance of conception while minimizing the risk of sexual transmission
- Prevent unwanted pregnancies

Prenatal Care

Care in pregnancy should be multidisciplinary, with close collaboration between the obstetrician, maternal-fetal medicine, and infectious disease specialists. A specialist with experience in the treatment of pregnant women with HIV-1 infection should be involved in the prenatal care.

Initial Prenatal Visit
   History.

- Complete medical and obstetric/gynecologic history at first prenatal visit.
- Document history of prior or current ARV use.

- Evaluation for symptoms of AIDS should include fever, night sweats, weight loss, a new persistent dry cough, diarrhea, refractory vaginal candidiasis, oral candidiasis, new outbreaks of herpes.
- Assess need for prophylaxis against opportunistic infections such as Pneumocystis pneumonia (PCP) or Mycobacterium avium complex (MAC).

   Physical examination. Complete physical exam at initial visit. During subsequent visits, screen for HIV disease progression. With CD4 <200 cells/mm^3, specifically evaluate for thrush, HSV, lymphadenopathy, or a rash.

   Labs. Baseline (and follow-up) laboratory investigations should include the following:

- Hepatitis B surface antigen and antibody, hepatitis B core antibody, hepatitis C antibody.
- CBC with differential, liver, and renal profile to be repeated each trimester.
- VDRL/RPR, gonorrhea, and chlamydia testing.
- PPD.
- Early diabetes screening of patients with a history of prolonged protease inhibitor (PI) exposure.
- Pap smear (all abnormal Pap smears require colposcopy).
- CD4 cell count (should be monitored at the initial visit and at least every three months in pregnancy).
- Plasma HIV RNA levels (should be monitored at the initial visit, 2 to 4 weeks after initiating or changing therapy, monthly until HIV RNA levels are undetectable, and then at about 34 to 36 weeks gestation to make a decision regarding mode of delivery. The VL should decrease by 1 to 2 logs within 4 weeks of starting therapy).
- Resistance testing should be performed prior to starting ART, in women who enter pregnancy with a HIV RNA level above the threshold for resistance testing on therapy, in women with suboptimal viral suppression after initiation of therapy, and in women with a persistently detectable plasma VL on therapy which previously suppressed the virus to below the assay level of detection. Genotyping is preferable to phenotyping because it is less expensive, it has a faster turnaround time, and a greater sensitivity for detecting mixtures of wild-type and resistant virus.
- HLA B-5701 testing if abacavir use is anticipated.

   Counseling.

- Discuss risk of transmission and factors that modify those risks.
- Discuss risk and benefits of ART for both the patient and the fetus.
- Educate on safe sex practices with condoms.

Antiretroviral Therapy (Figs. 32.1 and 32.2 and Table 32.3)

If a patient is newly diagnosed in the first trimester of pregnancy and she does not meet guidelines to start ARV therapy for herself then treatment is deferred until 14 weeks to eliminate the potential for embryopathy related to medications. Women who would not require HIV treatment outside of pregnancy are offered antiretroviral therapy for the duration of the pregnancy to prevent perinatal transmission. Antiretroviral therapy should be started by 28 weeks to achieve undetectable VL in the mother prior to delivery for optimal benefit (lowest chance of transmission). Treatment protocols must be individualized for each patient. Resistance to therapeutic agents and regimen failure are commonly related to patient

Table 32.3 Antiretroviral Therapy in Pregnancy

	NRTI		NNRTI		PI	
Recommended agents	Zidovudine (AZT) Lamivudine (3TC)	• Efficacy studies and extensive experience • AZT + 3TC is the recommended dual NRTI backbone	Nevirapine	• No evidence of teratogenicity • Increased risk of liver toxicity in women who start Nevirapine with CD4 >250 cells/mm³ • In women with CD4 <250 cells/mm³, nevirapine is acceptable • Monitor closely, especially in first 18 wk of therapy • No liver toxicity seen with single dose in labor	Lopinavir/ritonavir	• PK studies and extensive experience • Preferred PI for combination therapy
Alternate agents	Didanosine (ddI) Emtricitabine Stavudine (d4T) Abacavir	• Cases of fatal lactic acidosis have occurred with ddI + d4T. Use ONLY if no other alternative			Indinavir	• Lower drug levels in pregnancy • Unboosted indinavir NOT recommended • Requires boosting with ritonavir, but optimal dosing in pregnancy is not known • Possible elevated bilirubin in neonate
					Nelfinavir	• No evidence of human teratogenicity • Well tolerated • Lower viral response rate compared to Lopinavir/ritonavir
					Atazanavir Saquinavir	• No evidence of human teratogenicity • PK studies and moderate experience
Use in special circumstances	Tenofovir	• Limited studies in human pregnancies • Concern for bone demineralization with chronic use	Efavirenz	• Teratogenic in monkeys • Cases of CNS defects in humans • Pregnancy category D • Avoid in first trimester • Avoid in women who may become pregnant • Consider after first trimester only if no alternative	Amprenavir	• No studies in human pregnancy • Oral solution contains ethylene glycol and is contraindicated
					Atazanavir	• No studies in human pregnancy • Possible elevated bilirubin in neonate
					Fosamprenavir	• No studies in human pregnancy
Insufficient data to recommend					Darunavir Fosamprenavir Tipranavir	• No PK studies in pregnancy • No PK studies in pregnancy • No PK studies in pregnancy

Abbreviations: NRTI, nucleoside reverse transcriptase inhibitor; NNRTI, non–nucleoside reverse transcriptase inhibitor; PI, protease inhibitor.

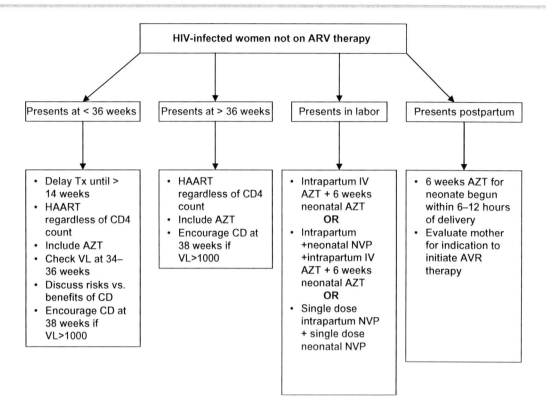

Figure 32.1 Regimens for untreated women and their infants. *Abbreviations*: Tx, therapy; ART, antiretroviral; HAART, highly active antiretroviral therapy; AZT, azidothymidine (zidovudine); NVP, nevirapine; VL, viral load; IV, intravenous; CD, cesarean delivery.

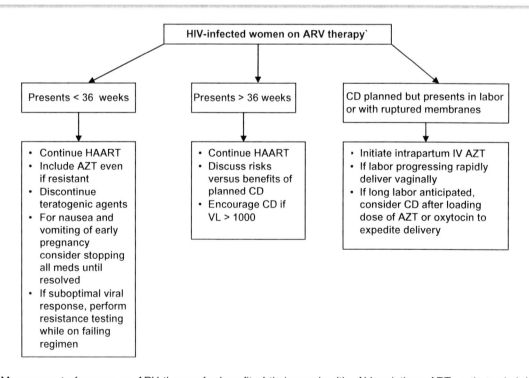

Figure 32.2 Management of women on ARV therapy for benefit of their own health. *Abbreviations*: ART, antiretroviral; HAART, highly active antiretroviral therapy; AZT, azidothymidine (zidovudine); NVP, nevirapine; VL, viral load; IV, intravenous; CD, cesarean delivery.

noncompliance. Therefore, regimens are tailored to maximize compliance (22).

Studies of zidovudine for prevention of perinatal transmission suggest that pre-exposure prophylaxis of the infant from transplacental passage is an important component of prevention. Thus, when selecting an ARV regimen for a pregnant woman, at least one nucleoside reverse transcriptase inhibitor (NRTI) with high placental transfer (zidovudine/lamivudine/stavudine/tenofovir/abacavir) should be included if possible.

AZT (1) should be part of the regimen in all pregnant women unless contraindicated: antepartum AZT orally 300 mg bid from week 14 until delivery; intrapartum infusion of AZT IV 2 mg/kg over the first hour followed by a continuous infusion of 1 mg/kg/hr until delivery. The newborn should receive AZT for at least the first four to six weeks of life (dose 2 mg/kg qid). AZT can cause anemia and neutropenia, so monitor CBC.

Regimens for Second and Third Trimester
In women who meet the criteria for ARV therapy outside of pregnancy, use optimal ARVs for the woman's health but consider the potential impact on the fetus. **Use standard ARV regimens as in nonpregnant women, but include AZT.**

Medications/Combinations to Avoid
Efavirenz, hydroxyurea, amprenavir solution, combinations of AZT with d4T or d4T with ddI.

Support decision-making by the woman after discussion of risks and benefits of ART (Table 32.1) (14,22).

Regimens for Untreated Women and Their Infants
See Figure 32.1.

Monitor for Side Effects (14,22)
Nucleoside reverse transcriptase inhibitor—AZT. Indications of toxicity that require interrupting or stopping AZT include hemoglobin <8 g/dL, absolute neutrophil count <750 cells/mm^3, AST or ALT >5 times the upper limit of normal. Potential toxicities that may affect the neonate must be considered. Animal data have noted an association between AZT use and squamous tumors in rats in later life. NRTI use has rarely been linked to mitochondrial toxicity in neonates.

Protease inhibitor—hyperglycemia. New-onset diabetes mellitus or exacerbation of existing diabetes mellitus, hyperglycemia, and diabetic ketoacidosis have been reported in patients taking PIs. There are no studies that report an increased risk of pregnancy-associated hyperglycemia in women on a PI-containing regimen. One large prospective cohort of nonpregnant women demonstrated a threefold increased risk for developing diabetes mellitus while on PI therapy (23). Pregnant women taking PIs should be screened for diabetes each trimester. Amprenavir solutions should be avoided because of potential propylene glycol toxicity.

Nucleoside analogue drugs—mitochondrial toxicity and clinical disorders. Clinical disorders include neuropathy, cardiomyopathy, myopathy, pancreatitis, hepatic steatosis, and lactic acidosis which could be confused with HELLP syndrome or acute fatty liver of pregnancy. Monitor liver enzymes and electrolytes in the third trimester. Fatalities due to lactic acidosis during pregnancy or in the early postpartum period have been reported in women on ART regimens that included the combination of d4T and ddI.

Non–nucleoside reverse transcriptase inhibitor—nevirapine—rash and hepatotoxicity. The risk is higher in women especially if CD4>250 cells/mm^3. Women entering pregnancy on an effective nevirapine (NVP)-containing regimen may continue NVP. Pregnant women on NVP should have transaminase levels monitored especially in the first 18 weeks of treatment. If the patient is symptomatic with even mildly elevated transaminase levels, or asymptomatic with severely elevated levels, NVP should be stopped and avoided in the future. **Efavirenz**—animal teratology studies demonstrated increased incidence of neural tube defects.

PROPHYLAXIS FOR OPPORTUNISTIC INFECTIONS
See Table 32.4.

IMMUNIZATIONS
Although HIV infection is primarily a disease of cell-mediated immunity, humoral immunity is also impaired in HIV-positive individuals. Serologic response to vaccination may be suboptimal, especially in advanced disease. Live virus vaccines have historically been withheld from HIV-positive individuals because of the risk of contracting the disease from the vaccine. Vaccines should be administered early in the course of HIV infection if possible to increase the likelihood of adequate responses and to minimize the risk of disseminated infection from live vaccines in immunocompromised patients.

All patients should receive **Pneumovax, hepatitis B** vaccine series, and **influenza** vaccine. Patients who are HCV positive should also be offered the **hepatitis A** vaccine series.

Tetanus and diphtheria immunization should be updated (24–26).

Inactivated polio vaccine as a primary series or booster should be administered to those at risk of exposure.

If risk of exposure to yellow fever is high and CD4 count is >200, yellow fever vaccine may be administered; however, serologic response may be as low as 35% (27).

Patients who are rubella nonimmune and have a CD4 count >200 should be offered vaccination in the postpartum period (28).

Varicella vaccine is currently being evaluated in HIV-positive adults, and as of this writing is **not** recommended in the postpartum period for varicella nonimmune women.

BCG vaccine should **not** be administered to HIV-infected women or their newborns—even if the risk of acquiring TB is high. Disseminated BCG has been reported after immunization (28,29).

ANEUPLOIDY SCREENING
There is limited evidence on the effect of HIV infection on prenatal aneuploidy screening. Currently, serum screening appears not affected sufficiently to alter its accuracy. Routine counseling should occur regarding noninvasive prenatal aneuploidy screening (30).

ANTEPARTUM TESTING
Ultrasound evaluation should be performed for the usual obstetric indications including confirmation of gestational age and assessing fetal anatomy (31). Invasive procedures such as amniocentesis, chorionic villus sampling, and cordocentesis indicated for diagnostic or therapeutic purposes may place the fetus at increased risk of transmission of the HIV virus, and appropriate counseling with review of indication for these interventions is recommended (32). Among women on HAART, no perinatal transmissions have been reported after **amniocentesis** but a small risk of transmission cannot be ruled out (32). If an amniocentesis is planned, it **should be**

Table 32.4   Prophylaxis for Opportunistic Infections

Infection	Indication	First-line Tx	Alternate Tx
Pneumocystis jiroveci pneumonia[a]	• CD4 count <200 • CD4 % <14 • History of AIDS-defining illness • History of oropharyngeal candidiasis • History of *Pneumocystis jiroveci* pneumonia (secondary prophylaxis)	Trimethoprim-sulfamethoxazole (TMP-SMZ) one DS tablet daily	TMP-SMZ one SS tablet daily OR one DS tablet 3 times/wk Dapsone 50 mg bid or 100 mg daily Atovaquone 750 mg bid or 1500 mg daily Aerosolized pentamidine 300 mg monthly
Toxoplasmic encephalitis[b]	CD4 < 100 cells/μL and Seropositive for *T. gondii* IgG	Trimethoprim-sulfamethoxazole (TMP-SMZ) one DS tablet daily	TMP-SMZ one SS tablet daily Dapsone 200 mg po + leucovorin 25 mg po weekly and pyrimethamne 75 mg weekly Atovaquone with or without pyrimethamine
Disseminated *Mycobacterium avium* complex[c]	CD4 count <50 cells/μL	Azithromycin 1200 mg po/wk	Rifabutin 300 mg po daily OR Rifabutin 300 mg po daily + azithromycin 1200 mg po weekly
Mycobacterium tuberculosis	PPD ≥ 5mm OR Prior positive PPD without adequate treatment OR Contact with person with active TB regardless of PPD status	INH sensitive: INH 300 mg po + pyridoxine 50 mg po daily for 9 mo OR INH 900 mg po + pyridoxine 100 mg po twice weekly for 9 mo INH resistant: Rifampin 600 mg po daily OR rifabutin 300 mg po daily for 4 mo	Rifampin 600 mg po daily OR rifabutin 300 mg po daily for 4 mo
Varicella zoster virus	Varicella nonimmune and exposed to chickenpox or shingles	Varicella Zoster immune globulin—5 vials (1.25 mL each) within 48–96 hours of exposure	

[a]Primary prophylaxis should be discontinued after sustained response to HAART with a CD4 count >200 cells/μL for >3 months. Secondary prophylaxis should be discontinued if CD4 count increases from <200 cells/μL to >200 cells/μL for >3 months.
[b]Discontinue primary prophylaxis after sustained response to HAART with CD4 count >200 cells/μL for >3 months. Discontinue secondary prophylaxis when initial therapy completed and asymptomatic with sustained CD4 count >200 cells/μL for >6 months.
[c]Discontinue primary prophylaxis after sustained response to HAART with CD4 count >100 cells/μL for >3 months. *Abbreviations*: HAART, highly active antiretroviral therapy; DS, double strength; SS, single strength; INH, isoniazid.

performed after initiation of an effective combination ART regimen and when the VL is nondetectable avoiding traversing the placenta.

PRETERM PREMATURE RUPTURE OF MEMBRANES

The risks of prematurity-related morbidity/mortality must be balanced against the risk of vertical transmission with prolonged rupture of membranes. If PPROM occurs prior to 32 weeks, expectant management with administration of corticosteroids for fetal lung maturity and antibiotics for latency is recommended. At a gestational age ≥32 weeks, delivery without the benefit of corticosteroids should be considered if appropriate support is immediately available to care for the premature infant. Consultation with a neonatologist should be sought if considering delivery prior to 32 weeks without the benefit of steroids as prognosis is dependent on resources available for care of the preterm infant (9,10).

DELIVERY

Maintain universal body fluid precautions for all deliveries. Inform pediatrician of mother's status. Bulb suction baby at delivery and wash off maternal secretions as soon as possible after birth.

Use the most recent VL level to counsel regarding **mode of delivery**. Risk of perinatal transmission with persistently undetectable VL on ARV therapy is <2% regardless of mode of delivery. Honor the woman's decision regarding mode of delivery. **Women with a VL >1000 copies/mL should be counseled regarding the potential benefit of scheduled CD to reduce the risk of transmission** (33). Some recommend that the absence of ARV therapy or AZT monotherapy only is indication for CD (34). Continue HAART therapy as usual and initiate **AZT infusion for three hours prior to CD** and continue until cord is clamped. Women with a low CD4 count may be at increased risk of complications after CD. All women should receive prophylactic antibiotics about 30 minutes before incision to reduce the risk of postpartum infection (35). Women with a recent VL <1000 copies/mL can be counseled that trial of labor and vaginal delivery does not significantly increase the very low (<2%) risk of perinatal transmission. It remains unclear how soon after the onset of labor or rupture of membranes the benefit of CD is lost; the delivery plan in these situations should be individualized.

INTRAPARTUM CARE

Induction of labor should be reserved for obstetric indications. Admit in early labor and augment labor to expedite delivery.

Continue the oral HAART regimen in labor; administer intravenous AZT in labor with loading and maintenance dosing continuously until the umbilical cord is clamped. Delay amniotomy; however, it is not contraindicated and may be used to augment labor later in the active phase. Avoid invasive fetal monitoring, intrauterine pressure catheter (IUPC), fetal scalp electrode (FSE), fetal blood sampling (FBS), episiotomy, forceps, or vacuum delivery (10,36).

BREAST-FEEDING

Women with HIV infection who have access to an adequate supply of infant formula or other suitable source of nutrition should not breast-feed (37). If access to an alternate nutrition source is not sufficient to completely replace breast-feeding, then exclusive breast-feeding is preferable to alternating breast-feeding/formula-feeding regimens. Any woman considering breast-feeding should be aware of her HIV status. A decision not to breast-feed may raise issues regarding confidentiality of a mothers HIV diagnosis and requires sensitivity and supportive interventions (38,39).

MATERNAL POSTPARTUM CARE

Establish ongoing primary care for HIV disease. Long-term planning is essential to ensure that the woman does not fall out of the health care system. Prevent nosocomial infection. Rubella vaccines should be administered postpartum to those women with CD4 count > 200 (28). Following delivery, considerations regarding continuation of the ARV regimen for maternal therapeutic indications are the same as for nonpregnant individuals. The pros and cons of continuing versus discontinuing therapy postpartum should be discussed with the woman so that she can make an educated decision prior to delivery regarding postpartum ART use. In general, once ART is commenced, it is continued for lifetime.

Family planning is critical to the prevention of perinatal transmission. Condom use should be strongly encouraged. Monitor for gynecological manifestations associated with disease progression. Pap smear every six months with colposcopy for any abnormal Pap smear are suggested.

FOLLOW-UP OF INFANTS

The baby should be bathed soon after delivery to remove potentially infectious maternal secretions. Baseline CBC followed by AZT prophylaxis and referral to an HIV specialist are recommended. HIV diagnostic testing to establish or rule out HIV infection as early as possible is suggested. Initiate PCP prophylaxis at six weeks (until there are two consecutive negative HIV results). Long-term follow-up of HIV and ARV exposed infants is important.

DIAGNOSIS OF HIV INFECTION IN THE INFANT

Establishing the diagnosis of HIV infection in the neonate is complicated by the presence of transplacentally acquired maternal antibodies, which makes serologic testing unreliable. The mean time to clear maternal antibodies is 10.3 months, but it can take up to 18 months (40). For this reason, a qualitative HIV-1 DNA PCR assay that detects HIV proviral DNA in peripheral blood mononuclear cells is the primary test used for the diagnosis of HIV-1 perinatally acquired infection in developed countries. HIV virologic testing should be performed at a minimum age of 14 to 21 days, 1 to 2 months, and 4 to 6 months. Some experts also test at birth especially if there is

poor control in pregnancy. HIV may be presumptively excluded with two or more negative tests with one at ≥ 14 days and another at ≥ 1 month of age. Many experts confirm HIV-negative status with an HIV antibody test at 12 to 18 months (41).

While HIV clade B is the predominant viral strain in the United States, non–clade B strains are more prevalent in other parts of the world. Some HIV DNA PCR assays may be less sensitive in detecting non–clade B. Assays for HIV-1 RNA detection are available and have comparable sensitivity and specificity for detection of neonatal infection to those of DNA-based assays; however, these assays may be less reliable in infants exposed to ART with an undetectable VL (42).

ACUTE HIV INFECTION

Primary or acute HIV infection in pregnancy is associated with an increased risk of perinatal transmission. When acute retroviral syndrome is suspected in pregnancy or during breast-feeding, a plasma HIV RNA test should be performed (which is usually >100,000 copies/mL) with an HIV antibody test to diagnose acute infection (43). Repeat HIV antibody testing is recommended in the third trimester for pregnant women with an initial negative HIV antibody test who are known to be at risk for HIV (44). All pregnant women with acute or recent HIV infection should start a combination regimen as soon as possible to prevent perinatal transmission aiming to suppress the VL to nondetectable. Resistance testing should be performed but initiation should not be delayed pending the results. Since clinically significant resistance to PIs is less common than resistance to NNRTIs in naïve patients, a ritonavir boosted PI-based regimen should be used if initiated prior to resistance testing results becoming available. If acute HIV infection occurs in pregnancy, plans for a CD at 38 weeks should be considered.

REFERENCES

1. Connor EM, Sperling RS, Gelber R, et al. Reduction of maternal-infant transmission of human immunodeficiency virus type 1 with zidovudine treatment. Pediatric AIDS clinical trials group protocol 076 study group. N Engl J Med 1994; 331(18):1173–1180. [RCT, *n* = 363]
2. UNAIDS Report on the Global AIDS Epidemic: 2010. Available at: http://www.unaids.org/globalreport/documents/20101123_GlobalReport_full_en.pdf. Accessed May 20, 2011. [Epidemiology report]
3. National Intelligence Council. The Next Wave of HIV/AIDS: Nigeria, Ethiopia, Russia, India, and China. Washington, DC: NIC, 2002. [Epidemiology report]
4. Centers for Disease Control and Prevention. Enhanced perinatal surveillance–15 areas, 2005–2008. *HIV Surveillance Supplemental Report* 2011; 16(No. 2). Available at: http://www.cdc.gov/hiv/topics/surveillance/resources/reports/. Published April 2011. Accessed May 17, 2011. [Guideline]
5. Castro KG, Ward JW, Slutsker L, et al. 1993 revised classification system for HIV infection and expanded surveillance case definition for AIDS among adolescents and adults. MMWR Recomm Rep 1992; 41(RR-17):1–19. [Guideline]
6. Cooper ER, Charurat M, Mofenson L, et al. Combination antiretroviral strategies for the treatment of pregnant HIV-1-infected women and prevention of perinatal HIV-1 transmission. J Acquir Immune Defic Syndr 2002; 29(5):484–494. [Review]
7. Garcia PM, Kalish LA, Pitt J, et al. Maternal levels of plasma human immunodeficiency virus type 1 RNA and the risk of perinatal transmission. Women and infants transmission study group. N Engl J Med 1999; 341(6):394–402. [II-2]

8. Mofenson LM, Lambert JS, Stiehm ER, et al. Risk factors for perinatal transmission of human immunodeficiency virus type 1 in women treated with zidovudine. Pediatric AIDS Clinical Trials Group Study 185 Team. N Engl J Med 1999; 341(6):385–393. [II-2]

9. Landesman SH, Kalish LA, Burns DN, et al. Obstetrical factors and the transmission of human immunodeficiency virus type 1 from mother to child. The women and infants transmission study. N Engl J Med 1996; 334(25):1617–1623. [II-2]

10. International Perinatal HIV Group. Duration of ruptured membranes and vertical transmission of HIV-1: A meta-analysis from 15 prospective cohort studies. AIDS 2001; 15(3):357–368. [Meta-analysis, 15 studies]

11. Minkoff H, Burns DN, Landesman S, et al. The relationship of the duration of ruptured membranes to vertical transmission of human immunodeficiency virus. Am J Obstet Gynecol 1995; 173 (2):585–589. [II-2]

12. European Collaborative Study, Swiss Mother and Child HIV Cohort Study. Combination antiretroviral therapy and duration of pregnancy. AIDS 2000; 14(18):2913–2920. [II-3]

13. Cotter A, Gonzalez Garcia A, Duthely L, et al. Is antiretroviral therapy associated with an increased risk of preterm delivery, low birth weight or stillbirth? J Infect Dis 2006; 193:1195–1201. [II-2]

14. Tuomala RE, Shapiro DE, Mofenson LM, et al. Antiretroviral therapy during pregnancy and the risk of an adverse outcome. N Engl J Med 2002; 346(24):1863–1870. [II-2]

15. Ioannidis JP, Abrams EJ, Ammann A, et al. Perinatal transmission of human immunodeficiency virus type 1 by pregnant women with RNA virus loads <1000 copies/ml. J Infect Dis 2001; 183 (4):539–545. [II-2]

16. Stanley B, Fraser J, Cox NH. Uptake of HIV screening in genito-urinary medicine after change to "opt-out" consent. Br Med J 2003; 326(7400):1174. [II-2]

17. Mossman CL, Ratnam S. Opt-out prenatal HIV testing in New-foundland and Labrador. Can Med Assoc J 2002; 167(6):630; author reply 630–631. [II-2]

18. Jayaraman GC, Preiksaitis JK, Larke B. Mandatory reporting of HIV infection and opt-out prenatal screening for HIV infection: effect on testing rates. Can Med Assoc J 2003; 168(6):679–682. [II-2]

19. Center For Disease Control And Prevention. HIV Testing Among Pregnant Women – United States and Canada, 1998-2001. Morbidity and Mortality Weekly Report, 2002. [Epidemiology report]

20. Prenatal and perinatal human immunodeficiency virus testing: Expanded recommendations. American College of Obstetricians and Gynecologists committee opinion number 418. Obstet Gynecol 2008; 112:739–742. [Review]

21. Bulterys M, Jamieson DJ, O'Sullivan MJ, et al. Rapid HIV-1 testing during labor: a multicenter study. J Am Med Assoc 2004; 292(2):219–223. [II-2]

22. United States Public Health Service Task Force. Perinatal HIV Guidelines Working Group Members. Public health service task force recommendations for use of antiretroviral drugs in pregnant HIV-1-infected women for maternal health and interventions to reduce perinatal HIV-1 transmission in the United States (revised May, 2010). [Guideline]

23. Justman JE, Benning L, Danoff A, et al. Protease inhibitor use and the incidence of diabetes mellitus in a large cohort of HIV-infected women. J Acquir Immune Defic Syndr 2003; 32(3):298–302. [II-2]

24. Laurence JC. Hepatitis A and B immunizations of individuals infected with human immunodeficiency virus. Am J Med 2005; 118(suppl 10A):75S–83S. [II-3]

25. McDonald P, Lighton L, Anderson R. Pneumococcal vaccine for HIV patients. Patients with HIV infection should be immunised. Br Med J 1995; 311(7001):387–388. [II-3]

26. Poland GA, Love KR, Hughes CE. Routine immunization of the HIV-positive asymptomatic patient. J Gen Intern Med 1990; 5 (2):147–152. [II-3]

27. Centers for Disease Control and Prevention. Yellow fever vaccine. Recommendations of the Advisory Committee on Immunization Practices. Morb Mortal Wkly Rep 2002; RR-17:1–11. [Guideline]

28. Center for Disease Control and Prevention, Division of Tuberculosis Elimination. Fact Sheet—BCG Vaccine. Center for Disease Control and Prevention, 2005. [Guideline]

29. Hussey G, Hawkridge T, Eley B, et al. Adverse effects of bacille calmette-guerin vaccination in HIV-positive infants. Clin Infect Dis 2004; 38(9):1333–1334; author reply 1334–1335. [II-2]

30. LaVigne KA, Seligman NS, Berghella V. Offering aneuploidy screening to HIV infected women: routine counseling. Br J Obstet Gynecol 2011; 118(7):775–778. [III]

31. ACOG Committee on Practice Bulletin 2004. ACOG Practice Bulletin No. 58. Ultrasonography in pregnancy. Obstet Gynecol 2004; 104(6):1449–1458. [Guideline]

32. Mandelbrot L, Jasseron C, Ekoukou D, et al. Amniocentesis and mother to child HIV transmission in the Agence Nationale de Recherches sur le SIDA et les Hepatites Virales French Perinatal Cohort. Am J Obstet Gynecol 2009; 200(2):160.e1–160.e9. [II-2]

33. Committee on Obstetric Practice. ACOG committee opinion. Scheduled cesarean delivery and the prevention of vertical transmission of HIV infection. Number 234, May 2000. Obstet Gynecol 2001; 73(3):279–281. [Guideline]

34. The International Perinatal HIV Group. The mode of delivery and the risk of vertical transmission of human immunodeficiency virus type 1—a meta-analysis of 15 prospective cohort studies. The International Perinatal HIV Group. N Engl J Med 1999; 340 (13):977–987. [II-2]

35. American College of Obstetricians and Gynecologists. ACOG practice bulletin number 47, October 2003: Prophylactic antibiotics in labor and delivery. Obstet Gynecol 2003; 102(4):875–882. [Review]

36. Mandelbrot L, Mayaux MJ, Bongain A, et al. Obstetric factors and mother-to-child transmission of human immunodeficiency virus type 1: the French perinatal cohorts. SEROGEST French pediatric HIV infection study group. Am J Obstet Gynecol 1996; 175(3 pt 1): 661–667. [II-2]

37. Coutsoudis A. Breastfeeding and the HIV positive mother: The debate continues. Early Hum Dev 2005; 81(1):87–93. [Review]

38. Dunn DT, Newell ML, Ades AE, et al. Risk of human immunodeficiency virus type 1 transmission through breastfeeding. Lancet 1992; 340(8819):585–588. [II-2]

39. Tess BH, Rodrigues LC, Newell ML, et al. Infant feeding and risk of mother-to-child transmission of HIV-1 in Sao Paulo State, Brazil. Sao Paulo collaborative study for vertical transmission of HIV-1. J Acquir Immune Defic Syndr Hum Retrovirol 1998; 19 (2):189–194. [II-2]

40. Louisirirotchanakul S, Kanoksinsombat C, Likanonsakul S, et al. Patterns of anti-HIV IgG3, IgA and p24Ag in perinatally HIV-1 infected infants. Asian Pac J Allergy Immunol 2002; 20(2):99–104. [II-3]

41. Centers for Disease Control and Prevention. Revised surveillance case definitions for HIV infection among adults, adolescents and children aged <18 months and for HIV infection and AIDS among children aged 18 months to <13 years, United States, 2008. MMWR 2008; 57(RR-10):1–12. [Review]

42. Nesheim S, Palumbo P, Sullivan K, et al. Quantitative RNA testing for diagnosis of HIV-infected infants. J Acquir Immune Defic Syndr 2003; 32(2):192–195. [II-3]

43. Hecht FM, Busch MP, Rawal B, et al. Use of laboratory tests and clinical symptoms for identification of primary HIV infection. AIDS 2002; 16(8):1119–1129. [II-2]

44. Nesheim S, Jamieson DJ, Danner SP, et al. Primary human immunodeficiency virus infection during pregnancy detected by repeat testing. Am J Obstet Gynecol 2007; 197(2):149 e 1–5. [II-2]

33

Gonorrhea

A. Marie O'Neill

KEY POINTS

- Gonorrhea has been associated with an increased risk of spontaneous abortion, premature labor, early rupture of fetal membranes, chorioamnionitis, and perinatal mortality, as well as neonatal conjunctivitis leading to blindness, increased HIV transmission, and postpartum infection.
- Prevention strategies shown to be effective include use of **condoms, screening high-risk populations, early diagnosis and treatment**, and **partner notification and treatment without clinical assessment.**
- There is insufficient evidence to recommend screening of low-risk pregnant women.
- Pregnant women at **high risk** for gonorrhea are those of **age <25 years, with prior sexually transmitted infection (STI), having multiple sexual partners, having a partner with a past history of any sexually transmitted disease (STD), sex work, drug use, or inconsistent condom use.** These women should be **screened** in pregnancy **for gonorrhea.**
- Definitive **diagnosis** requires isolation by **culture** *and* confirmation by **nucleic acid amplification tests.**
- First-line treatment for gonorrhea in pregnancy in the United States and most of western Europe is **ceftriaxone 125 mg IM** or **cefixime 400 mg po, each as a single dose.**
- However, in a number of Asian countries oral cephalosporins are no longer recommended because of drug resistance.
- If chlamydial infection has not been ruled out, cotreatment with azithromycin (preferred) or amoxicillin should be provided.
- Patients presenting with preterm premature rupture of membranes and having active gonorrheal infection can be managed expectantly as long as prompt treatment for gonorrhea is instituted.
- Because of the potential for concomitant infection, **testing for *Chlamydia trachomatis*, syphylis, HIV, and hepatitis B is recommended.**

EPIDEMIOLOGY/INCIDENCE

Worldwide, it is estimated that 62 million new cases of gonorrhea occur annually (1). The highest incidences of gonorrhea and its complications occur in developing countries. As a result of a national gonorrhea control program implemented in the United States in 1970s, the national rate of gonorrheal infection has decreased >75% over the last three decades. The number of cases reported in the United States continues to decrease annually. In 2009, there were 301,174 cases of gonorrhea reported to the Center for Disease Control (CDC) with approximately 40,000 of these infections occurring in pregnant women. The CDC estimated that only about half of all infections are reported (2). The incidence is substantially lower in all countries of western Europe than in the United States, but high and rising rates have been documented in eastern Europe. Gonorrhea disproportionately affects African-Americans with the reported rate of infection in this population being 19 times greater than that in whites (2,3). The median prevalence of gonorrhea in unselected populations of pregnant women has been estimated to be 10% in Africa, 5% in Latin America, and 4% in Asia (4).

ETIOLOGY

Neisseria gonorrhoeae is a gram-negative diplococcus that primarily infects nonciliated, columnar or cuboidal epithelium of the endocervix, urethra, rectum, or pharynx. Gonococci are obligate human pathogens and can survive only briefly outside of the human reservoir.

PATHOPHYSIOLOGY/TRANSMISSION

N. gonorrhoeae is easily transmitted during oral, vaginal, or anal sex. The transmission rate from male to female during vaginal intercourse is approximately 50% per contact, rising to 90% after three exposures (5). The incubation period for *N. gonorrhoeae* is on average 2 to 7 days, but may vary between 1 and 14 days. **Vertical transmission to the infant occurs in 30% to 47% cases if cervical infection is present at the time of delivery.** The eye is the most common site of neonatal infection, but disseminated gonococcal infection or gonococcal arthritis may also occur in the newborn (6,7). The vast majority of vertical transmission occurs **during vaginal delivery**; however, transmission has been reported after cesarean delivery in patients with ruptured membranes.

SYMPTOMS

The clinical manifestations of gonorrhea are unchanged in pregnant women, except that PID and perihepatitis are uncommon after the first trimester. Cervical infection is **asymptomatic in up to 80% of women** (8). When symptoms are present they include a purulent or mucopurulent cervical exudate, edema, easily induced cervical or endocervical bleeding. Urethral infection is present in 70% to 90% of women who have gonococcal cervicitis—most will present with dysuria (9). *N. gonorrhoeae* does not cause vaginitis, however coinfection with bacterial vaginosis, trichomonas, or *C. trachomatis* is common and often causes abnormal vaginal discharge. Pharyngeal infection is typically asymptomatic, but may cause exudative pharyngitis and cervical lymphadenopathy. This occurs in 10% to 20% of women with cervical gonorrhea (10,11). Rectal infection is typically asymptomatic, but may cause anal pruritus, mucopurulent discharge, and sometimes pain, tenesmus, and bleeding. This occurs in about 40% of women with cervical gonorrhea (8). Disseminated gonococcal infection occurs in 0.5% to 3% of infected individuals, and usually causes septic arthritis accompanied by a rash of hemorrhagic papules and pustules (12). There are conflicting reports as to whether pregnancy is a risk factor for disseminated infection; however, a recent publication reports an incidence of 0.04% to 0.09% in pregnancy (13).

COMPLICATIONS

- Gonorrhea has been associated with an increased risk of **spontaneous abortion, premature labor, early rupture of fetal membranes, chorioamnionitis, and perinatal mortality**. It is not clear if these complications are a direct result of gonococcal infection, or if infection is a marker for other high-risk factors (14–16).
- Vertical transmission to the infant can cause conjunctivitis, which if left untreated may result in **blindness**. Prior to routine prophylaxis of all infants at the time of birth, approximately 25% of congenital blindness in the United States was caused by gonorrheal conjunctivitis, and it remains a major cause of congenital blindness in under-developed countries (7,17).
- Epidemiologic and biologic studies provide strong evidence that gonococcal infections **facilitate the transmission of HIV infection** which has major implications for the pregnancy (18).
- Women with active cervical infection at the time of delivery are at increased risk for **postpartum infection** (19).

MANAGEMENT
Prevention

Condoms, when used correctly and consistently, provide a high degree of protection from gonorrheal infection, as well as from other STDs (20). Other important practices for prevention of gonorrhea are **screening to identify asymptomatic cases in high-risk populations, early diagnosis and treatment, and partner notification and treatment**. Several recent randomized trials reported a reduction in the rate of reinfection with an expedited approach to partner therapy whereby **partners are treated without a clinical assessment**. In this approach, the patient delivers either medication or prescriptions to their partner (21,22). The legal status of such an approach is uncertain in some states.

Screening (Table 33.1) (23–25)
There is no evidence that screening low-risk pregnant women is beneficial.

Screening pregnant women at high risk for gonorrhea may prevent other complications associated with gonococcal infection during pregnancy. **Risk factors include age <25, prior STI, multiple sexual partners, having a partner with a past history of any STD, sex work, drug use, or inconsistent condom use**. Because *N. gonorrhoeae* can cause infection at a variety of body sites, the decision of which sites to test should be guided by sexual history and physical exam findings.

Diagnosis (Table 33.1) (23–25)
Isolation of *N. gonorrhoeae* by culture is the historic mainstay of gonorrhea diagnosis. A definitive diagnosis requires isolation by culture *and* confirmation of isolates by biochemical, enzymatic, serologic, or nucleic acid testing. In most laboratories, culture has been replaced by **nucleic acid amplification tests** (NAATs), including ligase (LCR), polymerase chain reaction (PCR), transcription-mediated amplification (TMA), and strand-displacement amplification (SDA), or by unamplified DNA probe tests (non-NAATs). Clinicians who perform STD screening tests should be aware of the prevalence of STDs in the population being screened and have a conceptual understanding of positive predictive value and the impact of screening low-risk individuals with a test that has limited specificity. The positive predictive value of nucleic acid-based tests is <60% when the prevalence of infection in the population is <1%. Some assays can detect *C. trachomatis* or *N. gonorrhoeae* in a single specimen. Several of these combined assays do not

Table 33.1 Screening and Diagnostic Tests for Gonorrhea

	Sensitivity	Specificity	Advantages	Disadvantages
NAAT	96.7% compared to culture	98%	• High sensitivity • Approved for testing on voided urine • Approved for testing on liquid-based pap medium • Rapid results • Specimen less affected by handling and transport	• Most expensive option • No isolate preserved for forensics or sensitivity testing • Highest false-positive rate when persons at low risk are tested • Limited to cervical or urine specimens • Nonviable organisms or contaminants will give false-positive result
Culture	80–90%	100%	• Can obtain specimen from any potentially infected site • Preserves and isolate for antimicrobial sensitivity testing and forensics	• Organism is especially fastidious—can be difficult to grow in culture • Overgrowth of contaminating microorganisms can give a false-negative result • Organism can be rendered nonviable during transport if incorrect media used or delay in transport • 48–72 hr to complete
Gram stain	40–60% compared to culture	70–90%	• Rapid results • Negative predictive value is 99–100% • In setting of limited resources can be used for screening with follow-up testing of screen positives	• Least sensitive/specific • Higher false-negative rate results in more failure to treat
Non-NAAT	92.1% compared to culture	99%	• Inexpensive • Rapid results • Specimen less affected by handling and transport	• Nonviable organisms or contaminants will give false-positive result • Limited to cervical specimens

Source: From Refs. 23–25. *Abbreviation*: NAAT, nucleic acid amplification test.

Table 33.2 Current CDC Recommendations for Treatment of Gonorrhea Infection

Site of Infection	Recommended	Alternate
Cervix/urethra/rectum	**Ceftriaxone** 125 mg IM single dose (99.1% efficacy) **OR** **Cefixime** 400 mg po single dose (97.4% efficacy)	Spectinomycin 2 g IM single dose if allergic to cephalosporins (98.2% efficacy)
Pharynx	Ceftriaxone 125 mg IM single dose (99% efficacy) **PLUS** Azithromycin 1 g orally in a single dose	Spectinomycin 2 g IM single dose (only 50% efficacy)
Conjunctiva	Ceftriaxone 1 g IM in a single dose	

Source: From Refs. 27–29.

differentiate between the two organisms, so a positive result should be followed by tests for each organism to obtain an organism-specific result. NAAT tests are not FDA approved for use on rectal, pharyngeal, or conjunctival specimens; however, some labs have developed performance specifications for using NAATs on these specimens and results are used for clinical management (2). **Because of the continued increase in antibiotic resistant strains, suspected treatment failures must be evaluated with culture rather than a NAAT so that antibiotic sensitivity can be evaluated.**

Treatment

Antimicrobial resistance is an important consideration in the treatment of gonorrhea. The Gonococcal Isolate Surveillance Project (GISP) of the CDC has reported resistance to penicillins, tetracyclines, and fluoroquinolones. Recently, the emergence and spread of gonococcal strains resistant to oral cephalosporins has been reported and is of great concern. The majority of these resistant strains were identified in Japan, China, Hong Kong, and Taiwan (26). In the United States, Australia, and a number of western European countries an increasing number of isolates have demonstrated decreased susceptibility to ceftriaxone or cefixime but overt resistance has not yet been reported. **Current CDC recommendations for treatment are presented in** Table 33.2 (27–29), but as resistance patterns change so too may treatment recommendations. **Ceftriaxone IM or cefixime orally are currently the preferred first-line regimes for genital infection.** Updates can be found at http://www.cdc.gov/STD/treatment/. The only outcome included in the two available trials evaluating the treatment of gonorrhea in pregnancy was the incidence of "cure" assessed by bacterial culture (30). Failure to achieve "microbiological cure" was similar for each antibiotic regimen: amoxicillin plus probenecid compared with spectinomycin, amoxicillin plus probenecid compared with ceftriaxone, and ceftriaxone compared with cefixime. Side effects were uncommon for all the tested regimens. Although no differences were detected between the different antibiotic regimens, the trials were limited by their small sample size in their ability to detect important but modest differences. For women who are allergic to penicillin, treatment with ceftriaxone or spectinomycin appears to have similar effectiveness in producing microbiological cure (30).

For uncomplicated gonococcal infection treated with one of the recommended regimens, a test of cure is *not* necessary. However, if other treatment regimens are used, consider performing a test of cure four to six weeks after completing the treatment. **Of women who have endocervical gonorrhea, 35% to 50% are coinfected with *C. trachomatis*. If chlamydial infection has not been ruled out, cotreatment with erythromycin base 500 mg po qid × 7 days, or amoxicillin 500 mg po tid × 7 days should be provided.**

If a patient fails one of the recommended treatment regimens, a culture should be obtained for antimicrobial susceptibility testing. Treatment is considered to have failed if the patient reports compliance with medication regimen, simultaneous treatment of her partner, and no sexual activity without barrier protection after completing treatment. It is difficult to exclude reinfection as the cause of a positive result on repeat testing. In the United States, clinicians should contact their local or state health department or the CDC for guidance and assistance in follow-up of these patients as part of the ongoing GISP.

Patients presenting with preterm premature rupture of membranes who are found to have active gonorrheal infection can be managed expectantly as long as treatment for gonorrhea is initiated promptly (31).

Azithromycin 2 g, as a single oral dose, has demonstrated an efficacy of 99.2% for urogenital and rectal infections, and treatment efficacy of 100% for pharyngeal infection in nonpregnant adults, but has not been studied for safety or efficacy in pregnancy.

Because of the potential for concomitant infection, testing for *C. trachomatis*, syphylis, HIV, and hepatitis B is recommended.

REFERENCES

1. World Health Organization. World Health Report 1998. Geneva, Switzerland: WHO, 1998. [Epidemiologic data]
2. Centers for Disease Control and Prevention. Sexually Transmitted Disease Surveillance, 2008. Atlanta, GA: U.S. Department of Health and Human Services, 2009. [Epidemiologic data]
3. Centers for Disease Control and Prevention. STD's and Pregnancy Fact Sheet. Atlanta, GA: Department of Health and Human Services, 2007. [Review]
4. Handsfield HH, Sparling FP. *Neisseria gonorrhoeae*. In: Mandell GL, Bennett JE, Dolin R, eds. Principles and Practices of Infectious Diseases. 6th ed. Philadelphia, USA: Churchill and Livingstone, Inc., 2005:2514–2527. [Review]
5. Lin JS, Donegan SP, Heeren TC, et al. Transmission of *Chlamydia trachomatis* and *Neisseria gonorrhoeae* among men with urethritis and their female sex partners. J Infect Dis 1998; 178(6):1707–1712. [II-2]
6. Fransen L, Nsanze H, Klauss V, et al. Ophthalmia neonatorum in Nairobi, Kenya: the roles of *Neisseria gonorrhoeae* and *Chlamydia trachomatis*. J Infect Dis 1986; 153(5):862–869. [II-3]
7. Galega FP, Heymann DL, Nasah BT. Gonococcal ophthalmia neonatorum: the case for prophylaxis in tropical Africa. Bull World Health Organ 1984; 62(1):95–98. [Review]
8. McCormack WM, Stumacher RJ, Johnson K, et al. Clinical spectrum of gonococcal infection in women. Lancet 1977; 1 (8023):1182–1185. [Review]
9. Brunham RC, Paavonen J, Stevens CE, et al. Mucopurulent cervicitis—the ignored counterpart in women of urethritis in men. N Engl J Med 1984; 311(1):1–6. [II-2]
10. Wiesner PJ. Gonococcal pharyngeal infection. Clin Obstet Gynecol 1975; 18(1):121–129. [II-2]

11. Wiesner PJ, Tronca E, Bonin P, et al. Clinical spectrum of pharyngeal gonococcal infection. N Engl J Med 1973; 288(4):181–185. [II-3]

12. Holmes KK, Counts GW, Beaty HN. Disseminated gonococcal infection. Ann Intern Med 1971; 74(6):979–993. [II-3]

13. Phupong V, Sittisomwong T, Wisawasukmongchol W. Disseminated gonococcal infection during pregnancy. Arch Gynecol Obstet 2005; 273(3):185–186. [II-3]

14. Edwards LE, Barrada MI, Hamann AA, et al. Gonorrhea in pregnancy. Am J Obstet Gynecol 1978; 132(6):637–641. [II-3]

15. Schulz KF, Cates W Jr., O'Mara PR. Pregnancy loss, infant death, and suffering: legacy of syphilis and gonorrhoea in Africa. Genitourin Med 1987; 63(5):320–325. [II-3]

16. McGregor JA, French JI, Richter R, et al. Antenatal microbiologic and maternal risk factors associated with prematurity. Am J Obstet Gynecol 1990; 163(5 pt 1):1465–1473. [II-2]

17. Fox KK, Whittington WL, Levine WC, et al. Gonorrhea in the United States, 1981-1996. Demographic and geographic trends. Sex Transm Dis 1998; 25(7):386–393. [Epidemiologic data]

18. Cohen MS, Hoffman IF, Royce RA, et al. Reduction of concentration of HIV-1 in semen after treatment of urethritis: implications for prevention of sexual transmission of HIV-1. AIDSCAP Malawi Research Group. Lancet 1997; 349(9069):1868–1873. [II-2]

19. Alger LS, Lovchik JC, Hebel JR, et al. The association of *Chlamydia trachomatis*, *Neisseria gonorrhoeae*, and group B streptococci with preterm rupture of the membranes and pregnancy outcome. Am J Obstet Gynecol 1988; 159(2):397–404. [II-2]

20. Paz-Bailey G, Koumans EH, Sternberg M, et al. The effect of correct and consistent condom use on chlamydial and gonococcal infection among urban adolescents. Arch Pediatr Adolesc Med 2005; 159(6):536–542. [II-2]

21. Golden MR, Whittington WL, Handsfield HH, et al. Effect of expedited treatment of sex partners on recurrent or persistent gonorrhea or chlamydial infection. N Engl J Med 2005; 352 (7):676–685. [II-2]

22. Kissinger P, Mohammed H, Richardson-Alston G, et al. Patient-delivered partner treatment for male urethritis: a randomized, controlled trial. Clin Infect Dis 2005; 41(5):623–629. [RCT]

23. Crotchfelt KA, Welsh LE, DeBonville D, et al. Detection of *Neisseria gonorrhoeae* and *Chlamydia trachomatis* in genitourinary specimens from men and women by a coamplification PCR assay. J Clin Microbiol 1997; 35(6):1536–1540. [II-2]

24. Koumans EH, Black CM, Markowitz LE, et al. Comparison of methods for detection of *Chlamydia trachomatis* and *Neisseria gonorrhoeae* using commercially available nucleic acid amplification tests and a liquid pap smear medium. J Clin Microbiol 2003; 41(4):1507–1511. [II-2]

25. Martin DH, Cammarata C, Van Der Pol B, et al. Multicenter evaluation of AMPLICOR and automated COBAS AMPLICOR CT/NG tests for *Neisseria gonorrhoeae*. J Clin Microbiol 2000; 38(10):3544–3549. [II-2]

26. Barry PM, Klausner JD. The use of cephalosporins for gonorrhea: the impending problem of resistance. Expert Opin Pharmacol 2009; 10(4):555–577.

27. Ramus RM, Sheffield JS, Mayfield JA, et al. A randomized trial that compared oral cefixime and intramuscular ceftriaxone for the treatment of gonorrhea in pregnancy. Am J Obstet Gynecol 2001; 185(3):629–632. [RCT]

28. Centers for Disease Control and Prevention. Sexually Transmitted Diseases Treatment Guidelines 2002. MMWR, 2002. [Epidemiologic data]

29. Cavenee MR, Farris JR, Spalding TR, et al. Treatment of gonorrhea in pregnancy. Obstet Gynecol 1993; 81(1):33–38. [Review]

30. Brocklehurst P. Antibiotics for gonorrhoea in pregnancy. Cochrane Database Syst Rev 2002(2):CD000098. [Meta-analysis; 2 RCTs, $n = 346$]

31. Maxwell GL, Watson WJ. Preterm premature rupture of membranes: results of expectant management in patients with cervical cultures positive for group B streptococcus or *Neisseria gonorrhoeae*. Am J Obstet Gynecol 1992; 166(3):945–949. [II-3]

34

Chlamydia

A. Marie O'Neill

KEY POINTS

- Untreated maternal genital *Chlamydia trachomatis* has been associated with increased **preterm premature rupture of membranes, preterm birth, low birth weight, and decreased perinatal survival.**
- **Neonatal infection** is associated with neonatal **conjunctivitis** and **pneumonitis.**
- **Prevention strategies shown to be effective** include **condoms, screening to identify asymptomatic cases in high-risk populations, early diagnosis and treatment,** and **partner notification and treatment without a clinical assessment.**
- Screening and treatment of women at risk for chlamydial infection improves pregnancy outcome.
- **Pregnant women with risk factors should undergo screening: age < 25 years** (strongest risk factor), **multiple sex partners, new partner within last 3 months, single marital status, inconsistent use of barrier contraception, previous or concurrent sexually transmitted infection (STI), vaginal discharge, mucopurulent cervicitis, friable cervix, or signs of cervicitis on physical examination.**
- There is insufficient evidence to recommend for or against routine screening of asymptomatic, low-risk pregnant women aged 26 years and older for chlamydial infection.
- **A nucleic acid amplification test (NAAT) (e.g., LCR or PCR) screening test, confirmed by another NAAT test,** achieves highest predictive accuracy for the **diagnosis of maternal genital** *chlamydial* **infection.**
- **Azythromycin 1 g orally as a single dose, amoxicillin,** and **erythromycin** (in order of preference) are all accepted treatments of maternal genital *chlamydial* infection.
- A **test of cure** approximately three weeks after completion of therapy with a recommended regimen and **repeat testing in the third trimester,** as well as **testing for *N. gonorrhea*,** syphilis, HIV, and hepatitis B are recommended for those women with positive testing earlier in pregnancy.

BACKGROUND

The major sexually transmitted diseases caused by *C. trachomatis* are cervicitis, urethritis, proctitis, and lymphogranuloma venerum (LGV). *C. trachomatis* is also a significant pathogen causing conjunctivitis in both the newborn and in sexually active adolescents and adults.

EPIDEMIOLOGY/INCIDENCE

Worldwide it is estimated that over 92 million chlamydial infections occur annually, with just less than half of those in women (1). The incidence of chlamydial infections in the United States and worldwide continues to rise annually. In 2009, a total of 1,244,180 chlamydial infections were reported to the Center for Disease Control (CDC); however, the CDC estimates that there are approximately 4 million new chlamydial infections annually in the United States, and approximately 200,000 of these occur in pregnant women (2). The increase in the number of cases reported annually is known to be due in part to expansion of screening programs for at-risk women. The age-specific rate for chlamydial infection is highest in the 15- to 24-year-old age category. The rate of chlamydia in African-American females in the United States is more than 7.5 times higher than the rate among white females (2). The prevalence of chlamydia varies significantly across the world. The rates of genital *C. trachomatis* infection in pregnant women are shown in Table 34.1.

Ocular trachoma, a chronic keratoconjunctivitis caused by *C. trachomatis*, is rare in the developed world, but worldwide it is estimated that 7 to 9 million people are blind as a result of this condition (3).

LGV occurs sporadically in developed countries but is endemic in Africa, India, Southeast Asia, South America, and the Caribbean. The WHO and several partner organizations have initiated a program for global elimination of ocular trachoma as a disease of public health importance by the year 2020. Infection with *C. trachomatis* confers little protection against reinfection, and the limited protection that is conferred is short lived.

SYMPTOMS

C. trachomatis **infections** can be divided into **four clinical categories:**

- **Classic ocular trachoma**
- **Other ocular and genital diseases in adults**
- **LGV**
- **Perinatal infection—primarily conjunctivitis and pneumonia**

In pregnant women, genital infection including LGV, and conjunctivitis are the most clinically significant.

Maternal Genital Infection

The clinical manifestations of *C. trachomatis* are unchanged in pregnant women, except that pelvic inflamatory disease and perihepatitis are uncommon after the first trimester. About 70% to 90% of women with cervical or urethral *C. trachomatis* infection are asymptomatic.

Cervicitis/Urethritis

Mucopurulent cervicitis that may be perceived as vaginal discharge, cervical edema and friability, dysuria if urethritis present, and low abdominal pain if upper genital tract infection present.

Table 34.1   The Rates of Chlamydial Infection in Pregnant Women

United States	5%	India	17%
Italy	2.7%	Papua New Guinea	26%
Iceland	8%	Tanzania	6%
Brazil	2.1%	Cape Verde	13%
Thailand	5.7%		

Source: From Ref. 1.

Proctitis/Proctocolitis
Results from anal intercourse or secondary spread of secretions from the cervix.

- Serovars D through K—anal pruritus and a mucous rectal discharge that may become mucopurulent. The infection remains superficial, is limited to the rectum, and closely resembles gonococcal proctitis. Infection is often asymptomatic.
- LGV strains—rectal pain, tenesmus, rectal bleeding, and fever. The disease extends into the colon. The rectal and colonic mucosa become ulcerated, and a granulomatous inflammatory process occurs in the bowel wall, with both noncaseating granulomas and crypt abscesses. Sinus tract formation can lead to rectovaginal fistulas in women.

Chlamydial conjunctivitis is the most common cause of chronic follicular conjunctivitis. Common manifestations are a unilateral or bilateral asymmetric conjunctivitis associated with moderate hyperemia and mucopurulent discharge.

LGV
Often a difficult diagnosis to make because it is not thought of in the differential.

- The first stage is the formation of a primary lesion—a small papule or herpetiform ulcer—usually on genital mucosa or adjacent skin and causes little or no symptoms.
- The secondary stage occurs days to weeks later and is characterized by painful inguinal lymphadenopathy and systemic symptoms.
- The third stage manifests as hypertrophic chronic granulomatous enlargement with ulceration of the external genitalia. Lymphatic obstruction may also lead to elephantiasis of the genitalia.

PATHOPHYSIOLOGY/ETIOLOGY

C. trachomatis is an **obligate intracellular** pathogen that exhibits morphologic and structural similarities to gram-negative bacteria. The organism has a unique life cycle that includes an extracellular infectious form and an intracellular replicative form. The target cells of *C. trachomatis* are the squamocolumnar epithelial cells of the endocervix and upper genital tract, the conjunctiva, urethra, and rectum.

Target cells of the trachoma biovar of *C. trachomatis* are the squamocolumnar epithelial cells of the endocervix and upper genital tract, conjunctiva, urethra, and rectum. LGV biovar of *C. trachomatis* penetrates breaks in the skin or infects epithelial cells of the mucous membranes of the genital tract or rectum. It is then carried by lymphatic drainage to the regional lymph nodes, where it multiplies inside mononuclear phagocytes. *C. trachomatis* serovars D through K cause conjunctivitis in neonates as well as in adults. The incubation for *C. trachomatis* is variable depending on the type of infection, but in general is 7 to 21 days.

TRANSMISSION

- *C. trachomatis* is readily transmitted during vaginal, oral, or anal sex, and mother-to-infant transmission commonly occurs at delivery.
- The risk of acquisition of *C. trachomatis* with a single episode of sexual intercourse with an infected partner is not known. However, it appears to be substantially less than that for *Neisseria gonorrhoeae* (4).
- Between 22% and 44% of infants born to infected women develop neonatal conjunctivitis (5).
- Between 11% and 20% of infants born to infected mothers develop pneumonia caused by *C. trachomatis* (6).

COMPLICATIONS/RISKS

Untreated maternal genital *C. trachomatis* has been associated to be an independent risk factor for the statistically significant increase in **preterm premature rupture of membranes, preterm birth, low birth weight, and decreased perinatal survival** when compared to either treated women or controls without the infection (7). Successful treatment is therefore associated with prevention of premature rupture of membranes and small-for-gestational-age infants (8).

Neonatal infection acquired from an infected maternal genital tract at the time of delivery is associated with neonatal **conjunctivitis** and **pneumonitis**.

MANAGEMENT
Prevention

Condoms, when used correctly and consistently, provide a high degree of protection from chlamydia and other STIs (9). Other important practices for prevention of chlamydia are **screening to identify asymptomatic cases in high-risk populations, early diagnosis and treatment**, and **partner notification and treatment**. The rate of reinfection is reduced with an expedited approach to partner therapy whereby **partners are treated without a clinical assessment**. In this approach, the patient delivers either medication or prescriptions to their partner. The legal status of such an approach is uncertain in some states (10,11).

Screening

There is no trial to assess the efficacy of universal or risk-based screening for *chlamydial* genital infection in pregnancy. The Canadian Task Force, the CDC, the American College of Obstetricians and Gynecologists (ACOG), and the American Academy of Pediatrics (AAP) recommend that all pregnant women be screened for chlamydial infection (12–14). The U.S. Preventative Services Task Force recommends screening all pregnant women aged 24 and younger, and those over age 24 who have risk factors for infection (15). **Risk factors** for acquiring chlamydial infection (extrapolated mainly from nonpregnant studies) are **age <25 years** (strongest risk factor), **multiple sex partners, new partner within last 3 months, single marital status, inconsistent use of barrier contraception, previous or concurrent STI, vaginal discharge, mucopurulent cervicitis, friable cervix, and cervical ectopy.**

Diagnosis

A NAAT [e.g., ligase chain reaction (LCR) or polymerase chain reaction (PCR)] screening test, confirmed by another NAAT test, achieves highest predictive accuracy for the

Table 34.2 Test for Diagnosis of Maternal Genital Chlamydial Infection

	Sensitivity (%)	Specificity (%)	Advantages	Disadvantages
Culture	40–80 (29)	99.9	High specificity	• Handling requirements limit utility—temperature for storage must be 4°C and time to inoculation < 24 hr • Limited availability • Long incubation in tissue culture(48–72 hr)
DFA	50–80	99.8	Relatively quick results	• Requires a highly skilled microscopist for proper interpretation • Some assays can cross-react with other bacteria, including other species of Chlamydiae
EIA	40–60	99.5	• Not technically demanding to perform • Less expensive than nucleic acid based tests • Relatively quick results	Relatively low sensitivity
NAAT	Cervix 81–100 Urine 80–96	99.7	• Highest sensitivity and specificity comparable to culture • Can be used on voided urine specimen • Faster results than culture • Relatively quick results	Expensive
Non-NAAT	40–65	99	• Relatively easy to perform and interpret • Relatively quick results	Relatively low sensitivity

Source: From Refs. 16–21. *Abbreviations*: DFA, direct fluorescent antibody test; EIA, enzyme-linked immunosorbent assay; NAAT, nucleic acid amplification tests.

diagnosis of maternal genital *chlamydial* **infection** (16,17) (Table 34.2).

- Anti-*Chlamydia* IgM is uncommon in adults with genital tract infection. The prevalence of anti-*Chlamydia* IgG is high in sexually active adults (30–60%), even in those who do not have an active infection, and is probably due to past infection. The sensitivity, specificity, and predictive values of serologies are not high enough to make them clinically useful in the diagnosis of active disease Thus, **chlamydial serologies are not recommended for diagnosis** of active disease except in suspected cases of LGV.
- Two prospective studies compared an LCR NAAT performed on voided urine to endocervical culture in pregnant women, and found LCR to be more sensitive (18,19).
- A prospective study comparing endocervical culture with endocervical DFA, EIA, and PCR found that **nonculture tests have a higher sensitivity**, even in a population with a prevalence rate as low as 4.3% (20).
- Clinicians who perform STD screening tests should be aware of the prevalence of STDs in the population being screened and have a conceptual understanding of positive predictive value and the implications of screening low-risk individuals with a test that has limited specificity. In low-prevalence populations (<5% infected), a significant proportion of positive test results are false-positives. For example, with a prevalence of 3%, out of 1000 patients 30 are infected. A test with a sensitivity of 80% and a specificity of 99% detects 24 of the infected people but falsely identifies 10 uninfected as infected. The positive predictive value in this example is 70%.
- The Centers for Disease Control and Prevention recommended confirming positive screening tests for *C. trachomatis* when positive predictive values are <90%.
- **A positive result on a nonculture test should be considered presumptive evidence of infection in a low-prevalence population. Consideration should be given to performing an additional test after a positive screening** test and requiring that both the screening test and additional test be positive to make a diagnosis of *C. trachomatis* infection.
- Because of the greater sensitivity of NAATs, a NAAT is the only recommended additional test to verify a result from another NAAT and is, potentially, a superior additional test to verify a non-NAAT result.
- Except for using culture to obtain an isolate, a non-NAAT should not be used as an additional test after a NAAT because of the lower sensitivity of the non-NAAT.
- The majority of commercial NAATs have been cleared by the Food and Drug Administration (FDA) to detect *C. trachomatis* in endocervical swabs and urine from women.
- Other specimens (e.g., those from the vagina and eye) have been used with satisfactory performance, although these applications have not been cleared by FDA. Testing of rectal and oropharyngeal specimens with NAATs has had limited evaluation and is not recommended (21).

TREATMENT

Azithromycin, amoxicillin, and **erythromycin** (in order of preference) are all accepted treatments of maternal genital *chlamydial* infection. Compared to erythromycin, azithromycin is associated with similar efficacy (test of cure rates 93% for erythromycin and 100% for azithromycin) but higher compliance and fewer reported side effects in pregnant women (22–25). Compared to erythromycin, amoxicillin is associated with similar efficacy in achieving a negative test of cure, and is better tolerated in pregnant women (26–29). That is why azithromycin can be the first choice, despite slightly different CDC recommendations (Table 34.3). Clindamycin may be considered if azithromycin, erythromycin, and amoxycillin are contraindicated or not tolerated (30).

Doxycycline is the treatment of choice in nonpregnant women, but is not recommended in pregnancy because it may cause permanent discoloration in developing fetal teeth.

Table 34.3 Treatment of Chlamydial Infection in Pregnancy

	Recommended	Alternate
Cervicitis/urethritis/ proctitis	**Erythromycin base** 500 mg orally four times a day for 7 days **OR** **Amoxicillin** 500 mg orally three times a day for 7 days	**Azithromycin** 1 g orally single dose **OR** **Erythromycin base** 250 mg orally four times a day for 14 days **OR** **Erythromycin ethylsuccinate** 800 mg orally four times a day for 7 days **OR** **Erythromycin ethylsuccinate** 400 mg orally four times a day for 14 days
Conjunctivitis	**Azithromycin** 1 g orally single dose	**Erythromycin base** 250 mg orally four times a day for 21 days
Lymphogranuloma venerum	**Erythromycin base** 500 mg orally four times a day for 21 days	

Source: From Ref. 13.

Results of clinical trials in nonpregnant populations indicate that azithromycin and doxycycline are equally efficacious with 97% and 99% negative test of cure rates, respectively (31). In vitro studies suggest that *C. trachomatis* is not sufficiently sensitive to amoxicillin to be considered as an appropriate treatment; however, several randomized trials have demonstrated that amoxicillin does eradicate chlamydial infection in pregnancy. Treatment for LGV and conjunctivitis caused by *C. trachomatis* has not been studied in pregnancy. Recommendations are based on treatment recommendations in nonpregnant populations.

Treatment of sexual partners has been shown to decrease reinfection rates. Common partner-management options include partner notification (partners are notified and instructed to seek evaluation and treatment) and patient-delivered partner therapy (partner is treated without previous medical evaluation or prevention counseling). No single partner-management intervention has been shown to be more effective than any other in reducing reinfection rates, and some strategies are legally prohibited in some locations (2).

A follow-up test of cure is recommended in pregnant women treated for *chlamydia*. If a nucleic acid–based test is used, follow-up testing should be performed at least three weeks posttreatment because nonviable organisms may remain present for some days after successful treatment and can give a false-positive test result.

Concurrent treatment for gonorrhea is not indicated unless a positive test for this organism is obtained. **Because of the potential for concomitant infection, testing for** *N. gonorrhea*, **syphilis, HIV, and hepatitis B is recommended**.

One prospective study of cervical chlamydial infection in women presenting with preterm premature rupture of mem-branes who were conservatively managed and not treated for *Chlamydia* showed no effect on duration of latency and no increase in the incidence of chorioamnionitis or early endometritis (32).

Repeat testing in the third trimester of pregnancy is recommended for women who test positive earlier in pregnancy to reduce transmission to the neonate at birth (13).

REFERENCES

1. World Health Organization Department of HIV/AIDS. Global Prevalence and Incidence of Selected Curable Sexually Transmitted Infections. Geneva: World Health Organization, 2001. [Epidemiologic data]
2. Centers for Disease Control and Prevention. Sexually Transmitted Disease Surveillance, 2009. Atlanta, GA: U.S. Department of Health and Human Services, 2010. [Epidemiologic data]
3. Chidambaram JD, Melese M, Alemayehu W, et al. Mass antibiotic treatment and community protection in trachoma control programs. Clin Infect Dis 2004; 39(9):e95–e97. [II-2]
4. Lycke E, Lowhagen GB, Hallhagen G, et al. The risk of transmission of genital *Chlamydia trachomatis* infection is less than that of genital *Neisseria gonorrhoeae* infection. Sex Transm Dis 1980; 7 (1):6–10. [II-2]
5. Hammerschlag MR, Roblin PM, Gelling M, et al. Use of polymerase chain reaction for the detection of *Chlamydia trachomatis* in ocular and nasopharyngeal specimen from infants with conjunctivitis. Pediatr Infect Dis J 1997; 16(3):293–297. [II-2]
6. Schachter J, Grossman M, Sweet RL, et al. Prospective study of perinatal transmission of *Chlamydia trachomatis*. J Am Med Assoc 1986; 255(24):3374–3377. [II-2]
7. Ryan GM Jr., Abdella TN, McNeeley SG, et al. *Chlamydia trachomatis* infection in pregnancy and effect of treatment on outcome. Am J Obstet Gynecol 1990; 162(1):34–39. [II-2]
8. Cohen I, Veille JC, Calkins BM. Improved pregnancy outcome following successful treatment of chlamydial infection [see comment]. J Am Med Assoc 1990; 263(23):3160–3163. [1110 Chlamydia-positive women who were not treated in pregnancy, 1323 chlamydia-positive women who were treated in pregnancy, and 9111 women with negative *Chlamydia* cultures in pregnancy; II-2]
9. Paz-Bailey G, Koumans EH, Sternberg M, et al. The effect of correct and consistent condom use on chlamydial and gonococcal infection among urban adolescents. Arch Pediatr Adolesc Med 2005; 159(6):536–542. [II-2, $n = 509$]
10. Golden MR, Whittington WL, Handsfield HH, et al. Effect of expedited treatment of sex partners on recurrent or persistent gonorrhea or chlamydial infection. N Engl J Med 2005; 352 (7):676–685. [II-2]
11. Kissinger P, Mohammed H, Richardson-Alston G, et al. Patient-delivered partner treatment for male urethritis: a randomized, controlled trial. Clin Infect Dis 2005; 41(5):623–629. [RCT]
12. Davies HD, Wang EE. Periodic health examination, 1996 update: 2. Screening for chlamydial infections. Canadian task force on the periodic health examination. Can Med Assoc J 1996; 154(11):1631–1644. [Review and guideline]
13. Centers for Disease Control and Prevention. Sexually Transmitted Diseases Treatment Guidelines 2010. MMWR 2010; 59 (RR-12):8–9. [Guideline]
14. American Academy of Pediatrics and American College of Obstetricians and Gynecologists. Guidelines for Perinatal Care. 6th ed. Washington, DC: American College of Obstetricians and Gynecologists, 2007. [Guideline]
15. U.S. Preventative Services Tasks Force. Screening for chlamydial infection: U.S. Preventative Services Tasks Force Recommendation Statement. Ann Intern Med 2007; 147:128–133. [Guideline]
16. Dille BJ, Butzen CC, Birkenmeyer LG. Amplification of *Chlamydia trachomatis* DNA by ligase chain reaction. J Clin Microbiol 1993; 31(3):729–731. [II-3]
17. Ossewaarde JM, Rieffe M, Rozenberg-Arska M, et al. Development and clinical evaluation of a polymerase chain reaction test

for detection of *Chlamydia trachomatis*. J Clin Microbiol 1992; 30 (8):2122–2128. [II-3]

18. Andrews WW, Lee HH, Roden WJ, et al. Detection of genitourinary tract *Chlamydia trachomatis* infection in pregnant women by ligase chain reaction assay. Obstet Gynecol 1997; 89(4):556–560. [II-3]

19. Gaydos CA, Howell MR, Quinn TC, et al. Use of ligase chain reaction with urine versus cervical culture for detection of *Chlamydia trachomatis* in an asymptomatic military population of pregnant and nonpregnant females attending papanicolaou smear clinics. J Clin Microbiol 1998; 36(5):1300–1304. [II-2]

20. Thejls H, Gnarpe J, Gnarpe H, et al. Expanded gold standard in the diagnosis of *Chlamydia trachomatis* in a low prevalence population: diagnostic efficacy of tissue culture, direct immunofluorescence, enzyme immunoassay, PCR and serology. Genitourin Med 1994; 70(5):300–303. [II-2]

21. Mahony JB, Luinstra KE, Waner J, et al. Interlaboratory agreement study of a double set of PCR plasmid primers for detection of *Chlamydia trachomatis* in a variety of genitourinary specimens. J Clin Microbiol 1994; 32(1):87–91.

22. Adair CD, Gunter M, Stovall TG, et al. *Chlamydia* in pregnancy: a randomized trial of azithromycin and erythromycin. Obstet Gynecol 1998; 91(2):165–168. [RCT, *n* = 106]

23. Bush MR, Rosa C. Azithromycin and erythromycin in the treatment of cervical chlamydial infection during pregnancy. Obstet Gynecol 1994; 84(1):61–63. [II-2]

24. Edwards MS, Newman RB, Carter SG, et al. Randomized clinical trial of azithromycin vs erythromycin for the treatment of *Chlamydia* cervicitis in pregnancy. Infect Dis Obstet Gynecol 1996; 4:333–337. [RCT, *n* = 140]

25. Rosenn MF, Macones GA, Silverman NS. Randomized trial of erythromycin and azithromycin for treatment of chlamydial infection in pregnancy. Infect Dis Obstet Gynecol 1995; 3:241–244. [RCT, *n* = 48]

26. Alary M, Joly JR, Moutquin JM, et al. Randomised comparison of amoxycillin and erythromycin in treatment of genital chlamydial infection in pregnancy. Lancet 1994; 344(8935):1461–1465. [RCT, *n* = 210]

27. Silverman NS, Sullivan M, Hochman M, et al. A randomized, prospective trial comparing amoxicillin and erythromycin for the treatment of *Chlamydia trachomatis* in pregnancy. Am J Obstet Gynecol 1994; 170(3):829–832. [RCT, *n* = 74]

28. Magat AH, Alger LS, Nagey DA, et al. Double-blind randomized study comparing amoxicillin and erythromycin for the treatment of *Chlamydia trachomatis* in pregnancy. Obstet Gynecol 1993; 81 (5 pt 1):745–749. [RCT, *n* = 143]

29. Turrentine MA, Troyer L, Gonik B. Randomized prospective study comparing erythromycin, amoxicillin, and clindamycin for the treatment of *Chlamydia trachomatis* in pregnancy. Infect Dis Obstet Gynecol 1995; 2:205–209. [RCT, *n* = 174]

30. Brocklehurst P, Rooney G. Interventions for treating genital *Chlamydia trachomatis* infection in pregnancy. Cochrane Database of Syst Rev 2009; 4. [Meta-analysis, 11 RCT, *n* > 300]

31. Thorpe EM Jr., Stamm WE, Hook EW 3rd, et al. Chlamydial cervicitis and urethritis: single dose treatment compared with doxycycline for seven days in community based practices. Genitourin Med 1996; 72(2):93–97. [RCT, *n* =597]

32. Ismail MA, Pridjian G, Hibbard JU, et al. Significance of positive cervical cultures for *Chlamydia trachomatis* in patients with preterm premature rupture of membranes. Am J Perinatol 1992; 9(5–6):368–370. [II-3]

35

Syphilis

A. Marie O'Neill

KEY POINTS

- **Prenatal screening** and treatment of pregnant women for syphilis is **cost-effective, even in areas of low prevalence of the disease** (<0.1%).
- **All pregnant women should be screened with a serologic test for syphilis at the first prenatal visit. Women who are at high risk, live in areas of high syphilis morbidity, or are previously untested should be screened at 28 weeks and again at delivery.**
- **Penicillin** (parenteral penicillin G, 2.4 million units IM, either once or repeated weekly for three weeks depending on stage) remains the only recommended **treatment** for syphilis in pregnancy.
- Pregnant women with a **penicillin allergy** should be **desensitized** and then treated with penicillin.
- Staging of disease and penicillin dosing are not altered by pregnancy.
- Current treatment regimens are based on over 50 years of clinical experience with penicillin, expert opinion, and observational clinical studies rather than on randomized clinical trials.

DEFINITION

Treponema pallidum is the causative agent of syphilis.

INCIDENCE/EPIDEMIOLOGY

- Worldwide, it is estimated that over 10.7 million new cases of syphilis occur annually (1).
- **Each year at least half a million infants are born with congenital syphilis worldwide, and another half million stillbirths and spontaneous abortions occur as a result of maternal infection.**
- Over 90% of new cases occur in developing countries. These cases are more likely to remain untreated and result in significant morbidity and mortality. In sub-Saharan Africa, an estimated 2 million pregnant women are infected with syphilis annually, and 80% of these infections remain undiagnosed (2). Syphilis is responsible for 21% of perinatal deaths in Zimbabwe making it the leading cause of perinatal mortality (3). In Latin America, the overall prevalence of syphilis in pregnant women is 3.1%. The prevalence in pregnant women in Paraguay is 6.2%, and in Honduras 1.2% of all live births are affected with congenital syphilis (4). Since 1989, the newly independent states of the former Soviet Union have experienced a 43-fold increase in reported cases with rises proportionally larger among reproductive-aged women (5). In south and southeast Asia, over 2 million reproductive-aged women are infected with syphilis annually (1).

- The rate of primary and secondary syphilis in the United States declined by 89.7% between 1990 and 2000, but then increased annually from 2001 to 2009. In 2009, there were 13,997 cases of primary and secondary syphilis reported to the Center for Disease Control (CDC). Approximately 20% of these infections occur in reproductive-aged women (6). The number of cases of congenital syphilis increased annually from 2003 to 2007, and from 2007 to 2008 remained unchanged with 431 cases reported (6). Syphilis disproportionately affects African-Americans with the reported rate of infection in this population being 5.6 times greater than that in whites (6,7). The Syphilis Elimination Effort (SEE) is a national initiative launched by the Center for Disease Control and Prevention in 1999 to reduce or eliminate syphilis in the United States. Updates on the progress of this project can be found at http://www.cdc.gov/stopsyphilis/.

PATHOPHYSIOLOGY AND TRANSMISSION

T. pallidum is a gram-negative spirochete unable to survive outside the human host, and therefore has never been grown in culture. Unlike most other infectious diseases, it is rarely if ever diagnosed by isolation and characterization of the causative organism. *T. pallidum* can survive in the human host for several decades.

    T. pallidum is easily transmitted by sexual contact, and an overwhelming majority of cases are transmitted by **sexual intercourse**. Endemic syphilis is transmitted nonvenerally by close contact with an active lesion and occurs in communities living under poor hygiene conditions. Syphilis is rarely transmitted during transfusion of blood or blood products or through needle sharing by intravenous drug abusers. The organism generally enters the body through small breaches in epithelial surfaces of genital, anorectal, oropharyngeal, or other cutaneous sites; however; penetration of intact mucous membranes can occur. Once inside the body it rapidly disseminates. The **incubation period** for *T. pallidum* averages 3 weeks, but can range from 10 to 90 days. During the incubation period infected patients have, by definition, neither clinical nor serologic evidence of disease but are potentially infectious. The period of greatest infectivity is early in the disease when a chancre, mucous patch, or condyloma latum is present. Infectivity decreases over time, and after four years it is very unlikely that an untreated individual will spread syphilis, even by sexual contact. The risk of infection during a single sexual encounter with an infected individual is up to 60% depending on the stage of disease, and approaches 100% after five sexual encounters (8).

    Fetal syphilis occurs as a result of transplacental passage of the spirochete that enters fetal circulation causing infection. **Neonates** may acquire syphilis at the time of delivery by contact with infectious maternal secretions, blood, or genital lesions. Perinatal transmission may occur during any stage of maternal disease; however, it is most common in cases of maternal primary, secondary, or early latent syphilis with up to 83% of fetuses and newborns being affected (9).

SYMPTOMS AND CLASSIFICATION

Syphilis has been called "the great pretender" because of the **myriad of clinical manifestations** it can produce. It is a chronic, systemic infection characterized by several stages. The immune response to *T. pallidum* plays a significant role in the manifestations of all stages of syphilis. Much of the pathology observed in the disease is attributable to **vascular abnormalities caused by proliferative endarteritis** that occurs in all stages of syphilis. The pathophysiology of the endarteritis is not known, although the scarcity of treponemes and the intense inflammatory infiltrate suggest that the immune response plays a role in the development of these lesions. **Manifestations of syphilis are not altered by pregnancy.**

Incubation Period

- Asymptomatic with no serologic evidence of disease. Transmission can occur during this period.

Primary Syphilis (8,10–12)

- Symptoms develop at the site of initial treponemal invasion as a result of local replication of the organism.
- Treponemes also spread throughout the body by hematologic and lymphatic dissemination, even before the appearance of the chancre.
- Regional **adenopathy** often develops within the first week and usually consists of several discrete nontender, rubbery nodes. Inguinal adenopathy is often bilateral.
- Primary lesions are popular, but rapidly ulcerate to form a chancre.
- The classic **chancre** is a solitary, painless lesion with raised, firm, everted edges, central ulceration, and a granular base. However, up to 40% of individuals have multiple chancres.
- The most common site is the labia or cervix in females, but primary lesions may also occur on the lips, breasts, mouth, and anus.
- Without treatment, the local lesion **spontaneously resolve within three to six weeks**.
- Approximately 25% of individuals will have an adequate immune response and the infection will be spontaneously cleared.

Secondary Syphilis (8,10–12)

- If the primary infection is untreated, **secondary syphilis develops two to eight weeks later in approximately 75% of untreated individuals**.
- Secondary infection demonstrates a wide diversity in physical features involving virtually any organ and is often not thought of early in the diagnostic process.
- Generally begins with a **nonspecific constitutional illness** that commonly includes a sore throat, low-grade fever, myalgias, and generalized lymphadenopathy.
- **Skin rashes** are the classic and most commonly recognized lesions, but the appearance is highly variable, and differential diagnosis is often challenging.

- Rash is often initially macular and nonpruritic, and becomes papular by three months.
- Rash frequently involves the **palms of the hands** and **soles of the feet**, and may be accompanied by mucous patches in the mouth, pharynx, or cervix and condyloma lata in the anogenital region or axilla. **Condyloma lata** are hypertrophic lesions resembling flat warts that occur in moist areas.
- Individuals are highly contagious during this stage, especially upon contact with mucous patches or condyloma lata.
- Secondary disease **lasts for an average of 3.6 months** and spontaneously resolves. Approximately 25% of individuals experience a relapse of secondary disease during the first year of infection.

Latent Syphilis (8,10–12)

- In latent syphilis, by definition, there are **no clinical stigmata of active disease**, although disease remains detectable by **positive specific treponemal serologic tests** [FTA-ABS (fluorescent treponemal antibody absorption) or MHA-TP (microhemagglutination assay for *T. pallidum*)]. Latent syphilis is further subdivided into stages based on the duration of infection: early latent, late latent, and latent of unknown duration.

Early Latent Syphilis

- Early latency is defined as the time period within one year of initial infection.
- 90% of relapse occurs during this time period; mucocutaneous lesions are most common. Patient *is* infectious while lesions are present.
- Patients are believed to be potentially infectious in the absence of lesions.
- Vertical transmission of infection may occur.

Late Latent Syphilis

- Initial infection has occurred greater than one year previously.
- Associated with host resistance to reinfection.
- Sexual transmission is unlikely.
- Transplacental infection of the fetus can occur, but is less likely than with earlier stages of disease.
- Infection via blood transfusion is possible.

Latent Syphilis of Unknown Duration

- Date of initial infection cannot be established as having occurred within the previous year *and* patient is aged 13 to 35 years *and* has a nontreponemal titer $\geq$1:32.

Late Benign Syphilis (Tertiary Syphilis) (8,10–12)

- Without treatment at earlier stages of disease, tertiary syphilis eventually develops in 30% to 40% of infected patients.
- Usually becomes clinically manifest **after a period of 15 to 30 years** of untreated infection.
- Characteristic manifestations of tertiary disease include cardiovascular and gummatous lesions.
- **Cardiovascular** syphilis typically presents as inflammatory lesions of the cardiovascular system—especially aortitis.

- **Gummas** are granulomatous, nodular lesions that can occur in a variety of organs, most commonly skin, and bone.
- In patients with untreated syphilis, about 10% develop cardiovascular syphilis, 16% develop gummatous syphilis, and 6.5% develop symptomatic neurosyphilis (10).
- The diagnosis of late syphilis is confounded by the lack of sensitivity of the nontreponemal tests in these conditions.
- If a patient suspected of having late syphilis has a non-reactive nontreponemal test, a confirmatory treponemal test should be performed.
- Approximately one-third of patients will remain seroreactive for decades, but will *not* develop clinical manifestations of tertiary syphilis.
- Treatment of tertiary syphilis achieves a microbiologic cure, but many of the clinical manifestations will be irreversible.

Neurosyphilis (8,10–12)

- The diagnosis of neurosyphilis is made at **any** stage of disease when *both* clinical and laboratory criteria are met.
- *T. pallidum* disseminates widely after initial infection. Examination of **cerebrospinal fluid** will reveal evidence of infection [elevated lymphocytes and protein, **positive VDRL (**Venereal Disease Research Laboratory)] in approximately 15% of patients with primary syphilis, and as many as 40% of patients with secondary syphilis.
- Many patients with CSF evidence of infection will be asymptomatic in the early stages of disease.
- Persistence of CSF abnormalities for over five years in the untreated patient is highly predictive of the development of clinical neurosyphilis.
- Clinical evidence of central nervous system infection with *T. pallidum* includes the following:
  - Acute syphilitic meningitis
  - Meningovascular syphilis/seizures/stroke syndrome
  - General paresis/dementia/depression/memory loss/change in personality
  - Argyle Robertson pupils—small fixed pupils that do not react to light but do react to convergence-accommodation
  - Tabes dorsalis—paresthesias, abnormal gait, shooting pains in the extremities or trunk, diminished peripheral reflexes, loss of position and vibration senses
- Laboratory evidence of neurosyphilis includes a reactive serologic test for syphilis and a reactive VDRL in the CSF.
- The CSF-VDRL is a highly specific test, but has a **sensitivity of only about 30%**.
- Treponemal-specific **testing of CSF is helpful only when negative**—this rules out neurosyphilis. IgG antibodies cross the blood-brain barrier and can give a positive result in the absence of neurosyphilis, so **a positive treponemal-specific test is not helpful in making the diagnosis.**
- CSF examination is essential in patients with signs or symptoms of neurologic involvement at any stage of *T. pallidum* infection, and is also recommended in **all patients with untreated syphilis of unknown duration or of duration greater than one year**.
- CSF evaluation should include a cell count, protein level, and VDRL. Elevated lymphocytes and protein, positive VDRL are typical findings.
- Treatment of neurosyphilis achieves a microbiologic cure, but many of the neurologic manifestations will be irreversible.

RISK FACTORS

Risk factors for maternal infection include: multiple sexual partners, unprotected sex, sex in exchange for money or drugs, presence of other sexually transmitted infections, African-American race, spending time in a correctional facility.

The **single most significant risk factor for congenital syphilis infection is the maternal stage of disease**. With early-stage disease (primary, secondary, and early latent), up to 83% of fetuses and newborns are affected (9).

COMPLICATIONS

- Untreated syphilis can profoundly affect pregnancy outcome resulting in **spontaneous abortion, stillbirth, non-immune hydrops fetalis, preterm birth, or perinatal morbidity and mortality**. **Fetal syphilis** has similar complications and manifestations to those seen in neonatal syphilis: hepatomegaly, ascites, elevated transaminases, anemia, and thrombocytopenia are common (9).
- The longer the interval between infection and pregnancy, the more benign the outcome for the infant (13).
- In general, infection during early gestation ends in spontaneous abortion or stillbirth; infection in late gestation results in full-term delivery of an infant with congenital syphilis; while infection in the distant past often results in an unaffected infant (13).
- The greatest risk of stillbirth caused by congenital syphilis occurs at 24 to 32 weeks' gestation (14).
- Rates of **vertical transmission** in untreated women based on stage of disease (14):
  - 70% to 100% in primary syphilis
  - 40% in early latent syphilis
  - 10% in late latent disease

MANAGEMENT
Prevention

Important practices for prevention of syphilis are early diagnosis and treatment, partner notification and treatment, and screening to identify asymptomatic cases in high-risk populations.

Screening (Table 35.1) (15,16)

- Most pregnant women with syphilis are asymptomatic and can only be identified through serological screening.
- Prenatal screening and treatment programs are limited or nonexistent in many developing countries where the incidence and burden of disease is greatest.
- **Screening all pregnant women for syphilis and appropriately treating those found to be reactive effectively reduces complications associated with infection during pregnancy** (17).
- In the United States, serologic screening during pregnancy has been legislated since the 1930s; however, only 90% of states currently have statutes requiring antepartum syphilis screening (18). Of those states with mandatory screening, 76% require one prenatal test early in pregnancy, and 24% require repeat screening in the third trimester. The most cost-effective approach is to screen all pregnant women at their initial prenatal visit, and to repeat screening in the third trimester in those women with significant risk factors (17).

Table 35.1 Screening Tests for Syphilis

	Sensitivity (%)	Specificity (%)	Advantages	Disadvantages
Serology	85.5	97.1	• Relatively inexpensive • Rapid • Technically simple	• Not useful in primary disease • RPR and VDRL detect antigens NOT specific to treponemes
Dark-field microscopy	80	99–100	• Useful in evaluating lesions of primary disease • Immediate diagnosis if positive findings	• Not widely available—requires special equipment and an experienced operator
ICS	84.1–95.3	92	• Point-of-care testing • Inexpensive • Can be used in the most resource-poor settings	• Slightly lower sensitivity than other methods
PCR	95.8	95.7	• In trials PCR does differentiate syphilis from other treponematoses • May be useful in primary disease	• Expensive • Not yet available for clinical use

Abbreviations: RPR, Rapid Plasma Reagin; VDRL, Venereal Disease Research Laboratory; ICS, immunochromatographic strip; PCR, polymerase chain reaction. *Source*: From Refs. 15,16.

- **The CDC and** American College of Obstetricians and Gynecologists **(ACOG) recommend screening all pregnant women with a serologic test at the first prenatal visit. Women who are at high risk, live in areas of high syphilis morbidity, or are previously untested should be screened at 28 weeks and again at delivery** (6,19).
- The genus *Treponema* includes *T. carateum*, the causative agent of *pinta*, and *T. pallidum*. The latter species is subdivided into three subspecies: *T. pallidum* subspecies *pallidum*, which causes *syphilis*; *T. pallidum* subspecies *pertenue*, which causes *yaws*; and *T. pallidum* subspecies *endemicum*, which causes *bejel*. The subspecies causing pinta, yaws, and bejel are morphologically and serologically indistinguishable from *T. pallidum pallidum* (syphilis), so there is no test in current clinical use which can differentiate one of these treponemal infections from another. The transmission of yaws, pinta, or bejal is not via sexual contact and the clinical course of each disease is significantly different, which differentiates them from syphilis.
- **Serologic testing** remains the mainstay for screening and laboratory diagnosis of secondary, latent, and tertiary syphilis. These tests include nontreponemal and treponemal antibody detection.
- Nontreponemal tests are useful for screening. These include the Rapid Plasma Reagin (**RPR**) card test and the **VDRL**.
- Nontreponemal tests are also useful for monitoring treatment as titers drop over time, and often revert to negative; however, with repeated infection complete seroreversion may not occur.

Diagnosis

- Treponemal tests are used to confirm the diagnosis. These include the serum **FTA-ABS** and the **MHA-TP** tests.
- Treponemal tests remain reactive for many years in over 85% of persons adequately treated, and they give a false-positive result in about 1% of the general population, and should therefore not be used for screening (20).
- Serologic tests are generally not reactive until several weeks after the appearance of the primary lesion, and therefore are not useful in diagnosing primary syphilis.
- Dark-field microscopy and direct fluorescent-antibody testing for *T. pallidum* (DFA-TP) are diagnostic options for primary syphilis.

- **Dark-field microscopy** is the most specific technique for diagnosing syphilis when an active chancre or condyloma latum is present. Its sensitivity is limited by the experience of the operator performing the test, the number of live treponemes in the lesion, and the presence of nonpathologic treponemes in oral or anal lesions. Given the inherent difficulties of dark-field microscopy, negative examinations on three different days are necessary before a lesion may be considered negative for *T. pallidum* (21).
- A new screening test that consists of an immunochromatographic strip (ICS) impregnated with treponemal antigen which tests blood obtained by finger prick and offers immediate results is available (15). It has been found to be cost-effective, and has the potential to have a significant impact on the epidemiology of this disease in undeveloped, resource-poor countries.
- The complete genome of *T. pallidum* has been sequenced, and specific PCR primers have been developed; however, PCR is not yet available for routine clinical use (22,23).

Workup

- **Lumbar puncture** is indicated with
  - Neurologic/ophthalmologic signs
  - Aortitis/gummas
  - Treatment failure/treatment with agent other than penicillin
  - HIV infection
  - Titer > 1:32
- Cerebral spinal fluid with a positive VDRL is diagnostic for neurosyphilis

Treatment (Table 35.2) (24)

- The efficacy of penicillin for the treatment of syphilis was well established through clinical experience before the value of randomized controlled clinical trials was recognized. Therefore, almost all the recommendations for the treatment of syphilis are based on the opinions of persons having knowledge about STDs and are reinforced by case series, clinical trials, and more than 50 years of clinical experience.
- While erythromycin, azithromycin, and ceftriaxone are routinely used to treat syphilis in nonpregnant patients, they have not been shown to reliably cure maternal infection or prevent congenital syphilis (24).

Table 35.2   Treatment of Syphilis

Primary syphilis	**Benzathine penicillin G** 2.4 million units IM in a single dose
Secondary syphilis	**Benzathine penicillin G** 2.4 million units IM in a single dose
Early latent syphilis	**Benzathine penicillin G** 2.4 million units IM in a single dose
Late latent syphilis*	**Benzathine penicillin G** 2.4 million units IM each at 1-wk intervals × 3 wk 7.2 million units total
Tertiary syphilis	**Benzathine penicillin G** 2.4 million units IM each at 1-wk intervals × 3 wk 7.2 million units total
Neurosyphilis	**Aqueous crystalline penicillin G** 18–24 million units per day, administered as 3–4 million units IV every 4 hr or continuous infusion, for 10–14 days OR **Procaine penicillin** 2.4 million units IM once daily *PLUS* **Probenecid** 500 mg orally four times a day, both for 10–14 days

Source: From Ref. 24.
*or syphilis of unknown duration

- **Parenteral penicillin G** is the only therapy with documented efficacy for syphilis during pregnancy. The success of therapy is >98% (25).
- The highest risk of fetal treatment failure exists with maternal secondary syphilis (25).
- High VDRL titers at treatment and delivery, earlier maternal stage of syphilis, the interval from treatment to delivery, and delivery of an infant at ≤36 weeks' gestation are associated with the delivery of a congenitally infected neonate after adequate treatment for maternal syphilis (26).
- Pregnant women with syphilis in any stage who report **penicillin allergy** should be evaluated to determine the need for **desensitization, and treated with penicillin** (Table 35.3) (27).
- Women with a penicillin reaction other than anaphylaxis should undergo skin testing. Those with a history of anaphylaxis or a positive skin test to one of the penicillin determinants should be desensitized and treated with penicillin.
- Desensitization is a straightforward, relatively safe procedure that can be done orally or intravenously. Oral desensitization is regarded as safer, and is easier to perform. Patients should be desensitized in a hospital setting because serious IgE-mediated allergic reaction can rarely occur. Desensitization is typically completed in approximately four hours, after which the first treatment dose of

penicillin is administered. After desensitization, patients must be maintained on a penicillin regimen for the duration of therapy if multiple weekly doses are indicated by stage of disease.
- The **Jarisch–Herxheimer** reaction is an acute febrile reaction frequently accompanied by headache, myalgias, and other symptoms that usually occurs within the first 24 hours after any therapy for syphilis. It occurs most often in early disease—especially primary—and is thought to represent massive lysis of treponemes. The reaction begins within one to two hours of treatment, peaks at eight hours, and typically resolves within 24 to 48 hours. It **occurs in up to 45%** of pregnant women treated for syphilis. The Jarisch–Herxheimer reaction may induce labor or cause fetal distress in pregnant women; however, these concerns should **not** prevent or delay therapy.
- Ultrasonography provides a noninvasive means to evaluate the fetus for signs of syphilis. Abnormal findings indicate a risk for obstetric complications and fetal treatment failure (28).
- **Sexual contacts must be elicited, tracked, and treated** (by law in the United States).

Follow-Up After Treatment

- Nontreponemal antibody serologic titers should be checked at 1, 3, 6, 12, and 24 months following treatment (13).
- Among patients with primary and secondary syphilis, **a fourfold decline** (two dilutions) **by 6 months and an eightfold decline** (four dilutions) **by 12 months are expected**.
- Among patients with early latent syphilis a fourfold decline by 12 months is expected.
- Titers that show a fourfold rise or do not decrease appropriately suggest either treatment failure or reinfection. The treatment regimen should be repeated in these cases.
- It is important that the same testing method (RPR or VDRL) be used for all follow-up examinations since titers may vary by one to two dilutions if different tests are used.
- Patients with neurosyphilis should have repeat CSF evaluation every six months for the first two years, or until the CSF shows no evidence of disease (13).
- Treponemal tests usually stay positive for life.

NEONATAL

Neonatal congenital syphilis is characterized by macopapular rash, hepatosplenomegaly, osteochondritis/periostosis (do X ray of long bones: 95% of these infants will have osteochondritis), jaundice, ascites/hydrops, petechiae/purpura, lymphadenopathy, chorioretinitis, anemia, thrombocytopenia,

Table 35.3   Oral Desensitization Protocol for Patients with a Positive Skin Test

Penicillin V suspension dose no.	Units	Cumulative dose (Units)
1	100	100
2	200	300
3	400	700
4	800	1,500
5	1,600	3,100
6	3,200	6,300
7	6,400	12,700
8	12,000	24,700
9	24,000	48,700
10	48,000	96,700
11	80,000	176,700
12	160,000	336,700
13	320,000	656,700
14	640,000	1,296,700

Note: Observation period: 30 minutes before parenteral administration of penicillin. Interval between doses, 15 minutes; elapsed time, 3 hours and 45 minutes; cumulative dose, 1.3 million units. *Source*: Adapted from Ref. 27.

hyperbilirubinemia, elevated liver enzymes, reactive syphilis serologic tests in blood/cerebral spinal fluid. Babies can be asymptomatic. Out of the congenitally affected babies, 50% are born to mothers without prenatal care. **Infants of mothers with** untreated syphilis, relapse/reinfection, treated with erythromycin, treated <1 month before delivery, without good history of treatment, without fourfold decrease in titers, or without enough serologic follow-up **should be treated.** **Lumbar puncture** should be done on any infant suspected to have congenital syphilis.

REFERENCES

1. World Health Organization Department of HIV/AIDS. Glogal Incidence and Prevalence of four curable Curable Sexually Transmitted Infections (STI's): New estimates from WHO. Geneva: World Health Organization, 2009. [Epidemiologic data]
2. Deperthes BD, Meheus A, O'Reilly K, et al. Maternal and congenital syphilis programmes: case studies in Bolivia, Kenya, and South Africa. Gen Bull World Health Organ 2004; 82:410–416. [Epidemiologic data]
3. Aiken CG. The causes of perinatal mortality in Bulawayo, Zimbabwe. Cent Afr J Med 1992; 38:263–281. [II-3]
4. Valderrama J, Zacarias F, Mazin R. Maternal syphilis and congenital syphilis in Latin America: big problem, simple solution. Rev Panam Salud Publica 2004; 16(3):211–217. [Review]
5. Borisenko KK, Tichonova LI, Renton AM. Syphilis and other sexually transmitted infections in the Russian federation. Int J STD AIDS 1999; 10(10):665–668. [Epidemiologic data]
6. Centers for Disease Control and Prevention. Sexually Transmitted Disease Surveillance, 2008. Atlanta, GA: U.S. Department of Health and Human Services, 2009. [Review]
7. Centers for Disease Control and Prevention. STD's and Pregnancy Fact Sheet. Atlanta, GA: Department of Health and Human Services, 2004. [Review]
8. Garnett GP, Aral SO, Hoyle DV, et al. The natural history of syphilis. Implications for the transmission dynamics and control of infection. Sex Transm Dis 1997; 24(4):185–200. [Review]
9. Hollier LM, Harstad TW, Sanchez PJ, et al. Fetal syphilis: clinical and laboratory characteristics. Obstet Gynecol 2001; 97(6):947–953. [II-2]
10. Clark EG, Danbolt N. The Oslo study of the natural history of untreated syphilis; an epidemiologic investigation based on a restudy of the Boeck-Bruusgaard material; a review and appraisal. J Chronic Dis 1955; 2(3):311–344. [II-2]
11. Danbolt N, Clark EG, Gjestland T. The Oslo study of untreated syphilis; a re-study of the Boeck-Bruusgaard material concerning the fate of syphilitics who receive no specific treatment; a preliminary report. Acta Derm Venereol 1954; 34(1–2):34–38. [II-2]
12. Rockwell DH, Yobs AR, Moore MB Jr. The tuskegee study of untreated syphilis; the 30th year of observation. Arch Intern Med 1964; 114:792–798. [II-2]
13. Singh AE, Romanowski B. Syphilis: review with emphasis on clinical, epidemiologic, and some biologic features. Clin Microbiol Rev 1999; 12(2):187–209. [Review]
14. Fiumara NJ. Review of congenital syphilis. Sex Transm Dis 1984; 11(1):49–50. [Review]
15. Montoya PJ, Lukehart SA, Brentlinger PE, et al. Comparison of the diagnostic accuracy of a rapid immunochromatographic test and the rapid plasma reagin test for antenatal syphilis screening in Mozambique. Bull World Health Organ 2006; 84(2):97–104. [II-3]
16. Young H. Syphilis serology. Dermatol Clin 1998; 16(4):691–698. [II-3]
17. United States Preventive Services Task Force. Screening for syphilis infection: recommendation statement. Rockville, MD: Agency for Healthcare Research and Quality, 2004. [Guideline]
18. Hollier LM, Hill J, Sheffield JS, et al. State laws regarding prenatal syphilis screening in the United States. Am J Obstet Gynecol 2003; 189(4):1178–1183. [Review]
19. American College of Obstetricians and Gynecologists and American Academy of Pediatrics. Guidelines for Perinatal Care. 6th ed. Elk Grove Village (IL): AAP; Washington, DC: ACOG, 2007. [III]
20. Larsen SA, Steiner BM, Rudolph AH. Laboratory diagnosis and interpretation of tests for syphilis. Clin Microbiol Rev 1995; 8 (1):1–21. [II-3]
21. Cummings MC, Lukehart SA, Marra C, et al. Comparison of methods for the detection of *Treponema pallidum* in lesions of early syphilis. Sex Transm Dis 1996; 23(5):366–369. [II-1]
22. Liu H, Rodes B, Chen CY, et al. New tests for syphilis: rational design of a PCR method for detection of *Treponema pallidum* in clinical specimens using unique regions of the DNA polymerase I gene. J Clin Microbiol 2001; 39(5):1941–1946. [II-2]
23. Serwin AB, Kohl PK, Chodynicka B. The centenary of Wassermann reaction—the future of serological diagnosis of syphilis, up-to-date studies. Przegl Epidemiol 2005; 59(3):633–640. [Review]
24. Centers for Disease Control and Prevention. Sexually Transmitted Diseases Treatment Guidelines 2010. Morb Mort Week Rep 2010; 59(RR-12):35–36. [Guidelines]
25. Alexander JM, Sheffield JS, Sanchez PJ, et al. Efficacy of treatment for syphilis in pregnancy. Obstet Gynecol 1999; 93(1):5–8. [II-2]
26. Sheffield JS, Sanchez PJ, Morris G, et al. Congenital syphilis after maternal treatment for syphilis during pregnancy. Am J Obstet Gynecol 2002; 186(3):569–573. [II-2]
27. Wendel GD Jr., Stark BJ, Jamison RB, et al. Penicillin allergy and desensitization in serious infections during pregnancy. N Engl J Med 1985; 312(19):1229–1232. [II-2]
28. Wendel GD Jr., Sheffield JS, Hollier LM, et al. Treatment of syphilis in pregnancy and prevention of congenital syphilis. Clin Infect Dis 2002; 35(suppl 2):S200–S209. [II-2]

36

Trichomonas

A. Marie O'Neill

KEY POINTS

- Pregnant women colonized with *Trichomonas vaginalis* in the second trimester have a **higher risk of delivering an infant with low birth weight** *or* **delivering before term**, but unfortunately **metronidazole treatment** has been **associated with an increased risk of preterm birth**.
- *T. vaginalis* infection is a **risk factor for sexual transmission of HIV-1, with a twofold increase reported**.
- **Condoms,** when used correctly and consistently, provide a high degree of **protection from many STIs, including** *T. vaginalis*.
- There is no evidence that identifying asymptomatic *T. vaginalis* is beneficial in reducing the associated risk of preterm delivery or delivery of a low-birth-weight infant. Therefore, **there is insufficient evidence to recommend screening of asymptomatic pregnant women**, and some evidence that **treatment of these patients may in fact be harmful**.
- **Metronidazole as a single 2-g oral dose, or 500 mg twice a day for seven days**, at any gestational age is the treatment of choice for **symptomatic** *T. vaginalis* infection.
- **Concurrent treatment of sexual partners** is recommended to prevent reinfection.

EPIDEMIOLOGY/INCIDENCE

Worldwide, it is estimated that 180 million new cases of trichomoniasis occur annually (1). Developing countries account for a disproportionate number of cases. Trichomoniasis affects 2 to 3 million women and approximately 80,000 pregnant women in the United States annually. The frequency of infection in European women is similar. The WHO estimates 30 million new infections annually in Africa (2). In contrast to bacterial STIs such as *Neisseria gonorrhoeae* and *Chlamydia trachomatis*, *T. vaginalis* infection rates are as high or higher in middle-aged women when compared to adolescents. Incidence is highest among women with multiple sexual partners, and in populations with high rates of other sexually transmitted infections.

SYMPTOMS/SIGNS

The clinical manifestations of trichomoniasis are unchanged in pregnant women. Infection is **asymptomatic in up to 50% of women**. The most common symptoms include vulvovaginal pruritis (23–82%), vaginal discharge (50–75%), dysuria (30–50%), and dyspareunia (10–50%). The most common signs are copious vaginal discharge (50–75%) (yellow/green in 5–20%, frothy in 10–50%), inflammation of vaginal mucosa (40–75%), and vulvar erythema (10–20%).

PATHOPHYSIOLOGY/ETIOLOGY

Trichomoniasis is caused by the protozoan *T. vaginalis*, which had been previously thought to be a harmless commensal. *T. vaginalis* can infect the vagina and the Skene's glands of the urethra. The incubation period for *T. vaginalis* is 4 to 7 days on average, but ranges from 2 to 28 days.

TRANSMISSION

T. vaginalis is easily transmitted during **vaginal intercourse**. The organism will survive for several hours in moist environment outside the host and is rarely transmitted nonvenerally. The transmission rate from male to female during vaginal intercourse has been reported to be 66% to 100% (3). Vertical transmission to a female infant occurs in 2% to 17% if vaginal infection is present at the time of delivery (4).

COMPLICATIONS/RISKS

Pregnant women colonized with *T. vaginalis* in the second trimester had a 30% **higher risk of delivering an infant with low birth weight** *or* **delivering before term**, and a 40% higher risk of giving birth to an infant who was both preterm *and* of low birth weight (5). In pregnant women with *T. vaginalis*, unfortunately **metronidazole treatment** (two 2-g doses given 48 hours apart at 16–23 weeks) has been **associated with an 80% increase of preterm birth** compared to no treatment, with the majority of the increase in preterm delivery attributed to spontaneous preterm labor (6–8). The proposed mechanism for treatment with metronidazole causing preterm labor is that lysis of dying trichomonads elicits an inflammatory response that triggers labor (6–8) (see also chap. 16, *Obstetric Evidence Based Guidelines*).

T. vaginalis infection is a **risk factor for sexual transmission of HIV-1** in women. Studies from Africa have suggested that *T. vaginalis* infection approximately doubles the rate of HIV transmission (9). The proposed mechanism for this increased risk is twofold: local infiltration of large number of leukocytes including CD4+ lymphocytes—the primary target of HIV infection—and disruption in the integrity of the vaginal mucosa allowing access to viral particles. HIV-positive women who become infected with *T. vaginalis* have been shown to shed more HIV virus in their vaginal secretions, and therefore pose a higher risk for transmission.

Epidemiologic studies of *T. vaginalis* infection in the neonate have reported vertical transmission rates ranging from 0.1% to 4.8% (4), causing vaginal, urinary, and respiratory infection in these neonates.

MANAGEMENT
Prevention

Condoms, when used correctly and consistently, provide a high degree of protection from many STIs (10).

Table 36.1 Screening/Diagnostic Tests for *T. vaginalis*

	Sensitivity (%)	Specificity (%)	Advantages	Disadvantages
Wet mount	62–80	>99	• Rapid results • Inexpensive • High specificity	• Low sensitivity compared to culture • Sensitivity and specificity are strongly dependent on the skills and experience of the microscopist and also on the quality of the sample
Culture	95	100	• High sensitivity and specificity	• Organism can be rendered nonviable if incorrect media used or delay in transport • 3–7 days to complete • Not available in most clinical labs
PCR/NAAT	95	98	• Results available more quickly than with culture	• Most expensive option • Limited availability

Abbreviations: PCR, polymerase chain reaction; NAAT, nucleic acid amplification test. *Source*: From Refs. 15–17.

Most cases of reinfection result from sexual contact with an untreated partner. Adequate treatment of sexual partners has been shown to decrease reinfection (11).

Screening

There is no evidence that identifying asymptomatic *T. vaginalis* is beneficial in reducing the associated risk of preterm delivery or delivery of a low-birth-weight infant.

Diagnosis

Wet mount preparation of vaginal secretions suspended in normal saline with microscopic observation of motile trichomonads is the most **commonly utilized** method of diagnosing trichomoniasis in women; however, the **sensitivity** of this method is **low**.

Isolation of *T. vaginalis* by **culture is the gold standard**, but the greater cost and longer time to diagnosis make this an underutilized diagnostic option. Commonly used culture media include (12,13):

Modified Diamond's broth media	Sensitivity 95%
InPouch™ transport and test system	Sensitivity 87%
Modified Columbia agar	Sensitivity 98%

To increase the detection rate in a high-risk population without substantially increasing cost, culture could be performed on those symptomatic patients with a negative wet mount. Although nucleic acid–based tests are available, they are not yet widely used. Conventional Pap smear is not considered accurate for the identification of *T. vaginalis*. Confirmatory testing is necessary for those cases reported by Pap: sensitivity = 60% to 70%, specificity = 88%. Liquid-based Pap smear is accurate for the identification of *T. vaginalis* and warrants treatment without further testing; however, the sensitivity is low (61.4%) (14). Clinicians who perform STD screening tests should be aware of the prevalence of STDs in the population being screened and have a conceptual understanding of positive predictive value and the impact screening low-risk individuals has with a test that has limited specificity (Table 36.1) (15–17).

PCR and nucleic acid amplification tests that can be performed as rapid point of care testing are commercially available outside of the United States. To date, none of these assays are FDA approved.

Treatment

The nitroimidazoles are the only class of drugs useful for the oral or parenteral treatment of trichomoniasis. In randomized clinical trials, oral nitroimidazoles have resulted in parasitologic cure rates of 90% to 95%. Metronidazole and tinidazole are most commonly used. **Metronidazole can be given as a single 2-g oral dose, or 500 mg twice a day for seven days,** and can be given to symptomatic women **at any gestational age** (7). Multiple studies and meta-analyses have not demonstrated a definitive association between metronidazole use during pregnancy and teratogenic or mutagenic effects in infants (18,19). Tinidazole is given as a single 2-g oral dose. Its use is contraindicated in the first trimester of pregnancy. Metronidazole resistance is increasingly common. The CDC estimated that **5% of clinical isolates of *T. vaginalis* exhibit** some degree of **metronidazole resistance**. An escalated dosing regimen of metronidazole 2 g daily for three to five days has been successful in some cases of resistant infection, but in general **not more than a single 2-g dose should be given to prevent possible increase in preterm birth** (7). Tinidazole is effective in treating up to 60% of metronidazole-resistant *T. vaginalis* infections. **Concurrent treatment of sexual partners** is recommended to prevent reinfection.

REFERENCES

1. World Health Organization. World Health Report 1998. Geneva, Switzerland: WHO, 1998. [Epidemiologic data]
2. Gerbase AC, Mertens TE. Sexually transmitted diseases in Africa: time for action. Afr Health 1998; 20(3):10–12. [Review]
3. Krieger JN. Trichomoniasis in men: old issues and new data. Sex Transm Dis 1995; 22(2):83–96. [II-3]
4. Danesh IS, Stephen JM, Gorbach J. Neonatal *Trichomonas vaginalis* infection. J Emerg Med 1995; 13(1):51–54. [II-3]
5. Cotch MF, Pastorek JG II, Nugent RP, et al. *Trichomonas vaginalis* associated with low birth weight and preterm delivery. The Vaginal Infections and Prematurity Study Group. Sex Transm Dis 1997; 24(6):353–360. [II-2]
6. Klebanoff MA, Carey JC, Hauth JC, et al. Failure of metronidazole to prevent preterm delivery among pregnant women with asymptomatic *Trichomonas vaginalis* infection. N Engl J Med 2001; 345(7):487–493. [RCT; *n* = 617. 2 g metronidazole q48h × 2 doses]
7. Gulmezoglu AM. Interventions for trichomoniasis in pregnancy. Cochrane Database of Syst Rev 1, 2011. [Meta-analysis; two RCTs; *n* = 842]
8. Ross SM, Van Middelkoop A. Trichomonas infection in pregnancy: does it affect outcome? S Afr Med J 1983; 63:566–567.

[RCT; n = 225; 2 g metronidazole × 1 dose to women and their partners]

9. Laga M, Manoka A, Kivuvu M, et al. Non-ulcerative sexually transmitted diseases as risk factors for HIV-1 transmission in women: results from a cohort study. AIDS 1993; 7(1):95–102. [II-2]

10. Paz-Bailey G, Koumans EH, Sternberg M, et al. The effect of correct and consistent condom use on chlamydial and gonococcal infection among urban adolescents. Arch Pediatr Adolesc Med 2005; 159(6):536–542. [II-3]

11. Schwebke JR, Desomnd RA. A randomized controlled trial of partner notification methods for prevention of *Trichomonas* in women. Sex Transm Dis 2010; 37:392–396. [RCT, n = 484]

12. Borchardt KA, Zhang MZ, Shing H, et al. A comparison of the sensitivity of the InPouch TV, diamond's and trichosel media for detection of Trichomonas vaginalis. Genitourin Med 1997; 73 (4):297–298. [II-2]

13. Stary A, Kuchinka-Koch A, Teodorowicz L. Detection of *Trichomonas vaginalis* on modified Columbia agar in the routine laboratory. J Clin Microbiol 2002; 40(9):3277–3280. [II-2]

14. Lara-Torre E, Pinkerton JS. Accuracy of detection of *Trichomonas vaginalis* organisms on a liquid-based Papanicolaou smear. Am J Obstet Gynecol 2003; 188(2):354–356. [II-2]

15. Radonjic IV, Dzamic AM, Mitrovic SM, et al. Diagnosis of *Trichomonas vaginalis* infection: the sensitivities and specificities of microscopy, culture and PCR assay. Eur J Obstet Gynecol Reprod Biol 2006; 126: 116–20. [II-2]

16. Aslan DL, Gulbahce HE, Stelow EB, et al. The diagnosis of *Trichomonas vaginalis* in liquid-based pap tests: correlation with PCR. Diagn Cytopathol 2005; 32(6):341–344. [II-3]

17. Patel SR, Wiese W, Patel SC, et al. Systematic review of diagnostic tests for vaginal trichomoniasis. Infect Dis Obstet Gynecol 2000; 8(5–6):248–257. [Review]

18. Burtin P, Taddio A, Ariburnu O, et al. Safety of metronidazole in pregnancy: a meta-analysis. Am J Obstet Gynecol 1995; 172(2 pt 1):525–529. [Meta-analysis]

19. Sorensen HT, Larsen H, Jensen ES, et al. Safety of metronidazole during pregnancy: a cohort study of risk of congenital abnormalities, preterm delivery and low birth weight in 124 women. J Antimicrob Chemother 1999; 44(6):854–856. [II-2]

37

Group B *Streptococcus*

M. Kathryn Menard

KEY POINTS

- Asymptomatic group B streptococcus (GBS) colonization in the mother is associated with an incidence of neonatal GBS disease of ~1% to 2% without intervention. **Neonatal disease** is divided in **early onset** or **late onset**, with possible complications being **sepsis, pneumonia, meningitis,** and less frequently **focal infections** and death.
- Major **risk factors** for neonatal GBS sepsis are **prolonged rupture of membranes ($\geq$18 h), preterm delivery,** and **temperature $\geq$100.4°F ($\geq$38°C).**
- **Universal prenatal maternal screening and intrapartum antibiotic treatment** is the most efficacious of the current strategies for prevention of early-onset disease, and >50% more effective than a risk factor–based strategy. There is no known effective preventive strategy for late-onset GBS sepsis.
- **Women with GBS bacteriuria [>10,000 colony-forming units (CFU)]** in the current pregnancy or who had a **prior infant with GBS sepsis** are candidates for **intrapartum antibiotics prophylaxis,** and should be the only two groups **not screened** in the third trimester.
- **Screening** involves collecting an **anovaginal specimen at 35 to 37 weeks** (labeled penicillin-allergic if appropriate). Women who are GBS positive are treated with **penicillin in labor.** Ampicillin is a reasonable alternative. If the patient is penicillin-allergic but not at high risk for anaphylaxis, cefazolin is the agent of choice.
- For women at high risk for anaphylaxis, GBS isolate should be tested for susceptibility to clindamycin and erythromycin. **Vancomycin is recommended if isolate is resistant to either clindamycin or erythromycin.**
- **Intrapartum treatment for chorioamnionitis is recommended regardless of GBS maternal status.**

DIAGNOSIS/DEFINITION

GBS, also known as *Streptococcus agalactiae*, is a cause of morbidity and mortality primarily in pregnant or postpartum women and newborns.

SYMPTOMS

In the **mother**, GBS is usually **asymptomatic**. It can cause urinary tract infection, chorioamnionitis, endometritis, bacteremia, and stillbirth. Two forms of infection occur in **newborns**: **early onset** and **late onset**. Early-onset GBS disease usually causes illness within the first 24 hours of life. However, illness can occur up to six days after birth. Late-onset disease usually occurs at three to four weeks of age; it can occur any time from seven days to three months of age. Symptoms of neonatal GBS include breathing problems, not eating well, irritability, extreme drowsiness, unstable temperature (low or high), weakness, or listlessness (in late onset).

EPIDEMIOLOGY/INCIDENCE (FIG. 37.1)

GBS is a major cause of infectious morbidity among infants. In the United States, it is the most common cause of serious bacterial sepsis, including neonatal meningitis. The prevalence of asymptomatic GBS anovaginal colonization in pregnant women is **about 20%**, with a range of 10% to 30% (1). GBS colonization during pregnancy can be transient or persistent. A substantial portion of women who are colonized during one pregnancy will not have GBS colonization during a subsequent pregnancy. Usually 40% to 75% of neonates born to colonized mothers are colonized themselves (2). As a result of prevention efforts employing screening and antibiotic prophylaxis, the incidence of **early-onset GBS sepsis** fell in United States from 1.7 cases per 1000 live births in 1990 to **0.34 to 0.37 per 1000 live births** in 2004 through 2008 (1).

ETIOLOGY/BASIC PATHOPHYSIOLOGY

GBS is an encapsulated gram-positive coccus that colonizes the vaginal and gastrointestinal tract (reservoir) in 10% to 30% of healthy pregnant women (2–5). GBS may cause maternal urinary tract infection, amnionitis, endomyometritis, and maternal sepsis. Neonates acquire the organism as a result of **vertical transmission from the maternal genital tract** to the infant in utero or **usually at delivery**.

CLASSIFICATION

Disease in the neonate is divided into early and late disease (Table 37.1). **Early neonatal sepsis** with GBS often is observed within 24 hours of delivery. Early-onset disease presents within the first six days of life with breathing difficulty, shock, pneumonia, and occasionally meningitis (1). Nothing specific regarding the clinical presentation in early disease differentiates GBS as the etiology from other pathogens. Pneumonia with bacteremia is common and meningitis less likely. **Late-onset GBS disease** is defined as infection after one week and before three months after birth. Late disease is commonly characterized by bacteremia and meningitis. Infections in the infant can be localized, or may involve the entire body.

RISK FACTORS/ASSOCIATIONS

For early-onset GBS disease, **prolonged rupture of membranes (ROM) ($\geq$18 hours), preterm delivery (but >80% GBS neonates are term), temperature $\geq$ 100.4°F ($\geq$38°C),** maternal GBS colonization between 35 and 37 weeks, birth of a previous infant with invasive GBS disease, maternal chorioamnionitis, young maternal age, African-American race, Hispanic ethnicity, GBS bacteriuria during pregnancy. Diabetes or maternal GBS colonization in a previous pregnancy are not risk factors for early-onset GBS disease.

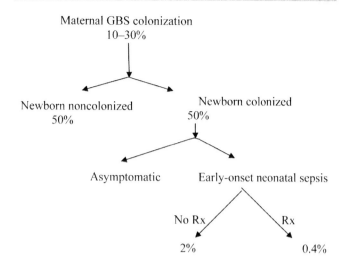

Figure 37.1 GBS infection: maternal to infant transmission. Rx, treatment.

COMPLICATIONS (TABLE 37.1)

In newborns, GBS can cause **sepsis, pneumonia, meningitis,** and less frequently **focal infections** such as osteomyelitis, septic arthritis, or cellulites. Early-onset GBS sepsis is defined as occurring within the first week of life, usually around 48 hours and within 72 hours. Neonatal death occurs in 4% to 6% of cases of early-onset disease. Mortality is higher among preterm infants, 20% to 30% if <33 weeks gestation, compared with 2% to 3% among full-term infants (1).

MANAGEMENT
Principles/Prevention

Several approaches to the prevention of **early-onset** GBS neonatal infection have been studied or devised (6). There are **no trials** to assess the effectiveness of any of these approaches, probably because they would have to include about >100,000 screened pregnancies to show a difference in early-onset GBS sepsis, given the current incidence of the disease (<0.5%). Potential strategies are outlined in the following sections.

Maternal Vaccination

Vaccination against GBS is potentially the most effective method of preventing the morbidity and mortality caused by infection. GBS vaccines have been investigated as a tool to reduce maternal colonization and prevent transmission to the neonate; however, a licensed vaccine is not yet available (1). GBS capsular polysaccharide (CPS)–based protein conjugate vaccines have been produced and tested in animals (7). The first capsular polysaccharide vaccines was poorly immunogenic, so a trial of protein conjugate vaccines followed, using tetanus toxoid as the conjugate. They were shown to be safe and well tolerated, and the antibody response was persistent for over a year in the mother and the passive protection in the neonate protected him/her against late onset disease (8). There is need for a phase III randomized trial recording neonatal disease events (1,9). Vaccination is the only strategy that would have the potential to protect against late-onset disease, which current strategies do not cover.

Universal Maternal Treatment

There is insufficient data to evaluate universal treatment of all women during birth.

Prenatal Maternal Screening and Prelabor Maternal Treatment

Antibiotics should not be used before the intrapartum period to treat asymptomatic maternal GBS colonization, except if GBS is present in the urine (2–4% of pregnancies). Asymptomatic women with <10,000 CFU of GBS in the urine culture at 27 to 31 weeks gestation have decreased preterm birth (PTB) <37 weeks when treated with penicillin 1 million IU three times per day for six days compared to placebo (10). GBS bacteriuria during pregnancy should be treated at the time of diagnosis. In fact, every urine specimen sent in pregnancy should be labeled "pregnant," so to alert the laboratory to report any isolation of GBS. GBS identified in urine is a marker for heavy maternal colonization, is associated with a higher risk for early-onset GBS sepsis, and is also an indication for intrapartum antibiotic prophylaxis (1). Antibiotic therapy (with erythromycin) does not prevent PTB or affect stillbirths in women with GBS colonization (11).

No Prenatal Maternal Screening and Intrapartum Treatment Based on Risk Factors

Risk factors used for this strategy are delivering <37 weeks, intrapartum temperature ≥100.4°F (≥38°C), or ROM ≥18 hours (7). Over 20% of neonates with early-onset GBS sepsis are born to women without risk factors. As shown below, while this was a popular strategy in the past, it is less effective than a screening-based strategy (10,12). A risk factor–based

Table 37.1 Early- Vs. Late-Onset GBS Characteristics

	Early onset	Late onset
Definition	Occurs <1 wk	≥1 wk
Usual timing of manifestation after birth	24–48 hr	≥1 wk
Incidence (of all neonatal GBS sepsis)	80% (natural); 50% (screen and treat)	20% (natural); 50% (screen and treat)
Most common/predominant clinical signs/ symptoms	Sepsis, pneumonia (meningitis 10–30%)	Meningitis, localized infections (ears, eyes, breasts, bone, joints, skin, etc.)
Serotype		III (95%)
Case-fatality ratio	Overall = 5% Full-term = 2–3% <33 wk = 30%	<2%
Long-term morbidity		If meningitis—15–50% can have neurologic sequelae

strategy is still common in the United Kingdom and other European countries. Intrapartum treatment for chorioamnionitis is recommended regardless of GBS maternal status.

Universal Prenatal Maternal Screening and Intrapartum Treatment (Fig. 37.2)
A screening-based strategy is >50% more effective than a risk factor–based strategy (13). This is the protocol with the most evidence for efficacy (1,14). After the Center for Disease Control (CDC) recommended this screening strategy compared to either the risk factor–based strategy in 2002, the incidence of early-onset GBS sepsis declined from 0.47/1000 live births (1999–2001) to 0.32–0.34/1000 (2004–2008) (1). A screening-based strategy involves an incidence of intrapartum antibiotic prophylaxis similar (24%) to that of the risk-factor approach (12); thus, the treatment risks should be similar. This approach of screening for GBS colonization and intrapartum treatment **does not affect incidence of late-onset GBS sepsis**. A screen-

ing-based strategy is recommended in the United States (1,15) (see section "Screening" below for more details).

Neonatal (Screening and) Treatment Only
Screening and/or treatment of just the neonate without some form of in utero prophylaxis is a much inferior approach than the maternal screening approaches just described (screening or risk factor–based). Neonatal treatment only is "too little too late," as 40% of neonates with GBS are already bacteremic at birth. Evaluation of neonates born to GBS-positive mothers who were not treated or to mothers with risk-factors is imperative (16).

Screening/Diagnosis (Fig. 37.2)
Detection
Detecting vaginal GBS colonization of pregnant women is a way of detecting women at high risk for early-onset GBS infection. Because colonization can be intermittent, a swab

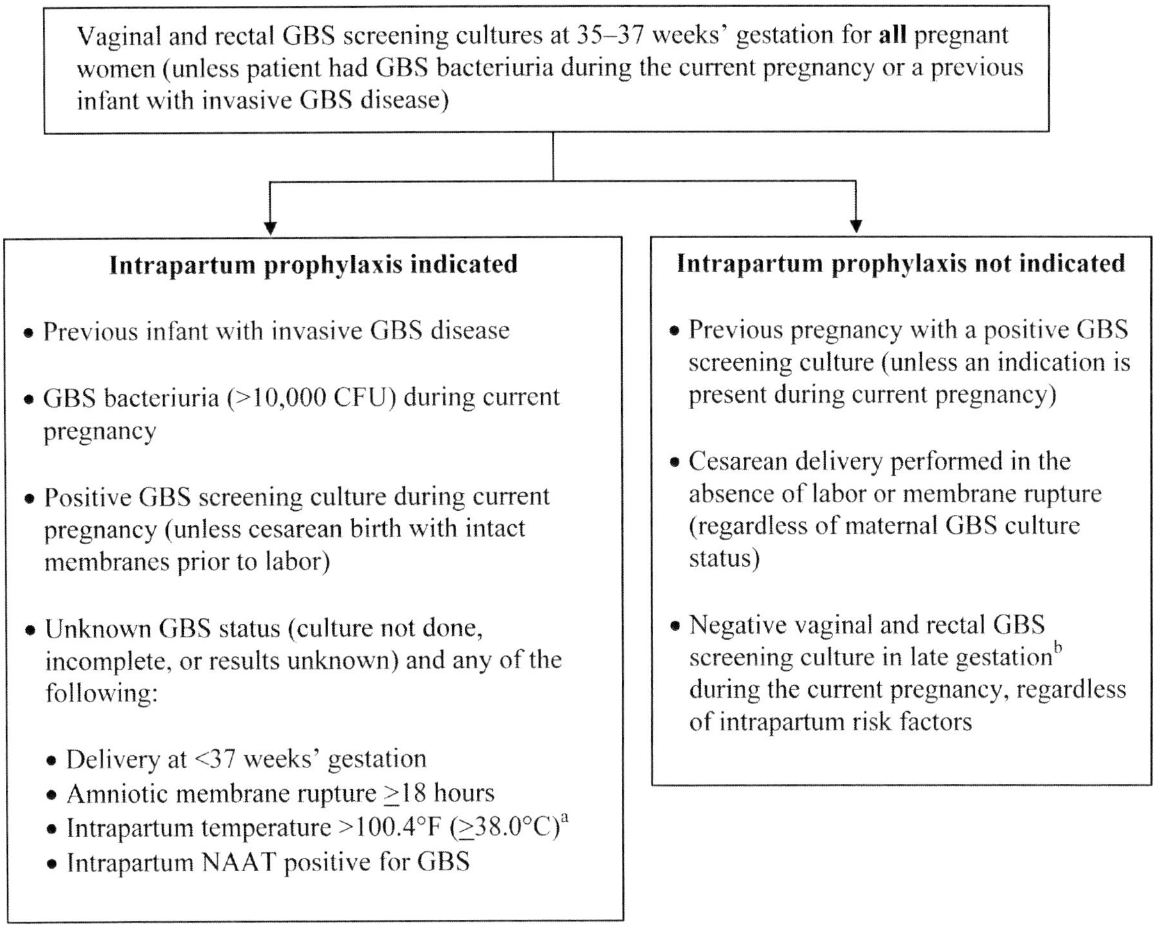

Vaginal and rectal GBS screening cultures at 35–37 weeks' gestation for **all** pregnant women (unless patient had GBS bacteriuria during the current pregnancy or a previous infant with invasive GBS disease)

Intrapartum prophylaxis indicated

- Previous infant with invasive GBS disease

- GBS bacteriuria (>10,000 CFU) during current pregnancy

- Positive GBS screening culture during current pregnancy (unless cesarean birth with intact membranes prior to labor)

- Unknown GBS status (culture not done, incomplete, or results unknown) and any of the following:

  - Delivery at <37 weeks' gestation
  - Amniotic membrane rupture ≥18 hours
  - Intrapartum temperature >100.4°F (≥38.0°C)[a]
  - Intrapartum NAAT positive for GBS

Intrapartum prophylaxis not indicated

- Previous pregnancy with a positive GBS screening culture (unless an indication is present during current pregnancy)

- Cesarean delivery performed in the absence of labor or membrane rupture (regardless of maternal GBS culture status)

- Negative vaginal and rectal GBS screening culture in late gestation[b] during the current pregnancy, regardless of intrapartum risk factors

If Nucleic Acid Amplification Test (NAAT) is negative and any of the above risk factors are present, then intrapartum prophylaxis is indicated.
[a]If amnionitis is suspected, broad-spectrum antibiotic therapy that includes an agent known to be active against GBS should replace GBS prophylaxis.
[b]Optimal timing 35–37 weeks' gestation.

Figure 37.2 Indications for intrapartum antibiotic prophylaxis to prevent perinatal GBS disease under a universal prenatal screening strategy based on combined vaginal and rectal cultures collected at 35 to 37 weeks' gestation from all pregnant women. *Source*: From Ref. 1.

Table 37.2 Recommended Regimens for Intrapartum Antimicrobial Prophylaxis for Perinatal GBS Disease Prevention[a]

Recommended	Penicillin G, 5 million units IV initial dose, then 2.5–3 million units IV every 4 hr until delivery
Alternative	Ampicillin, 2 g IV initial dose, then 1 g IV every 4 hr until delivery
If penicillin allergic[b]	
Patients not at high risk for anaphylaxis	Cefazolin, 2 g IV initial dose, then 1 g IV every 8 hr until delivery
Patients at high risk for anaphylaxis[c]	
GBS susceptible to clindamycin and erythromycin[d]	Clindamycin, 900 mg IV every 8 hr until delivery
GBS resistant to clindamycin or erythromycin or susceptibility unknown	Vancomycin, 1 g IV every 12 hr until delivery

[a]Broader-spectrum agents, including an agent against GBS, may be necessary for treatment of chorioamnionitis.
[b]History of penicillin allergy should be assessed to determine whether a high risk for anaphylaxis, angioedema, respiratory distress, or urticaria is present.
[c]If laboratory facilities are adequate, clindamycin and erythromycin susceptibility testing should be performed on prenatal GBS isolates from penicillin-allergic women at high risk for anaphylaxis.
[d]Resistance to erythromycin is often, but not always, associated with clindamycin resistance. If a strain is resistant to erythromycin, but appears susceptible to clindamycin, it may still have inducible resistance to clindamycin. Treatment with erythromycin is not recommended. *Source*: From Ref. 1.

done earlier in pregnancy is less predictive of intrapartum status and early-onset GBS disease than a culture performed near term. The recommended time frame for performing the culture is 35 to 37 weeks gestation (1). The negative predictive values of GBS cultures performed at 35 to 37 weeks (prevalence about 20%) are 95% to 98% (1). **Women with GBS bacteriuria** in the current pregnancy or who had a **prior infant with GBS sepsis** are candidates for **intrapartum antibiotics prophylaxis,** and **should not be screened** (1).

Collection of Screening Specimen
A vaginal-rectal swab, collected at 35 to 37 weeks' gestation. Sampling the lower vagina, followed by the anorectal area gives highest yield for GBS (1). Vaginal-rectal swabs, during which >70% of women report at least mild pain, do not

increase GBS detection rates compared to vaginal-perianal swabs (17). The swab is transported in special medium (e.g., Amies or Stuart's without charcoal), which maintains GBS viability for up to one to four days. It is labeled "penicillin allergy" when applicable. The swab is cultured using a selective enrichment broth media (e.g., Todd-Hewitt with antibiotics) over 18 to 24 hours. For penicillin-allergic patients, clindamycin and erythromycin disk susceptibility is done (1).

Definitive microbiologic identification is done by serologic detection of group B antigen or PCR (10). **PCR test** has sensitivity 97%, specificity 100%, and positive predictive value 100% when compared with conventional vaginal-rectal cultures, but is not widely available, and PCR universal screening has not been sufficiently tested in clinical studies (10).

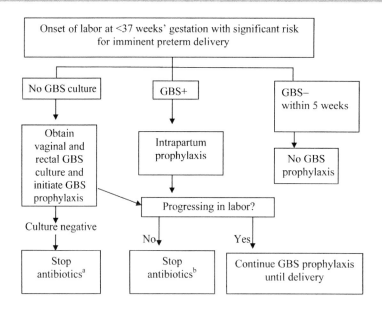

[a]If delivery has not occurred within 4 weeks, a vaginal and rectal GBS screening culture should be repeated and the patient should be managed as described, based on the result of the repeat culture.
[b]GBS prophylaxis at onset of true labor.

Figure 37.3 Algorithm for GBS prophylaxis for women with threatened preterm delivery. This algorithm is not an exclusive course of management. Variations that incorporate individual circumstances or institutional preferences may be appropriate. *Source*: From Ref. 14.

The availability of a sensitive rapid screening test to accurately detect women in labor who are colonized with GBS would make prevention strategies more efficient, but the available **rapid tests still lack acceptable performance characteristics**. A rapid and sensitive test with appropriate therapy could further decrease the incidence of GBS sepsis.

Intrapartum Prophylaxis (Table 37.2)

The incidence of early-onset GBS infection is reduced with use of intrapartum antibiotic prophylaxis in women colonized with GBS. Treatment is associated with a 90% decreased incidence of infant colonization and 83% decreased incidence of early-onset neonatal infection with GBS (18). The rate of infant

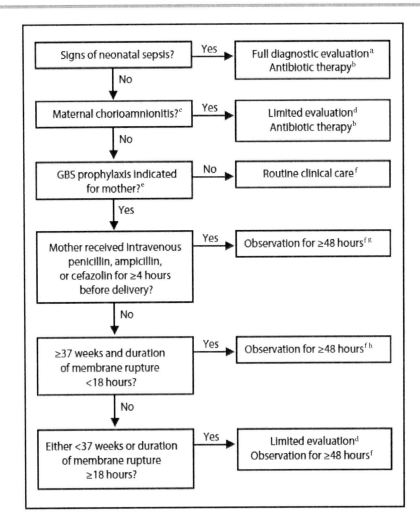

[a]Blood culture, a complete blood count (CBC) with white blood cell differential and platelet counts, chest radiograph (if respiratory abnormalities are present), and lumbar puncture (if patient is stable enough to tolerate procedure and sepsis is suspected).

[b] Directed toward the most common causes of neonatal sepsis, including intravenous ampicillin for GBS and coverage for other organisms (including *Escherichia coli* and other gram-negative pathogens) and should take into account local antibiotic-resistance patterns.

[c] Consultation with obstetric providers is important to determine the level of clinical suspicion for chorioamnionitis.

[d] Blood culture (at birth) and CBC with differential and platelets (at birth and/or at 6–12 hours of life).

[e] See Table 37.2 for indications for intrapartum GBS prophylaxis.

[f] If signs of sepsis develop, a full diagnostic evaluation should be conducted and antibiotic therapy initiated.

[g] If ≥37 weeks' gestation, observation may occur at home after 24 hours if other discharge criteria have been met, access to medical care is readily available, and a person who is able to comply fully with instructions for home observation will be present. If any of these conditions is not met, the infant should be observed in the hospital for at least 48 hours and until discharge criteria are achieved.

[h] Some experts recommend a CBC with differential and platelets at age 6–12 hours.

Figure 37.4 Algorithm for secondary prevention of early-onset GBS disease in the newborn. *Source*: From Ref. 1.

GBS sepsis in the control groups of the studies where this outcome was reported ranged from 2% to 9%. This is higher than the overall infection rates of 1% to 3% that are reported in babies whose mothers are colonized with GBS, raising questions as to how representative the populations studied were.

Penicillin is the first-line agent for intrapartum GBS prophylaxis (Table 37.2). When antibiotics are given ≥2 hours before delivery, early-onset sepsis is minimized (1). For women with penicillin allergy not at high risk for anaphylaxis, cefazolin is recommended. For the woman at high risk for anaphylaxis to penicillin and a cultured isolate sensitive to both clindamycin and erythromycin, treatment with clindamycin is indicated. If the culture is resistant to either clindamycin or erythromycin or the results are unknown, then treatment with vancomycin is recommended (1). If intrauterine infection is diagnosed, broad-spectrum antibiotic therapy (e.g., ampicillin and gentamicin) is recommended.

Adverse consequences of prophylaxis are anaphylaxis to penicillin (4–40/100,000), drug resistance, and neonatal infection from agents different than GBS. Penicillin is the preferred antibiotic to decrease emerging resistance. Early-onset sepsis from pathogens other than GBS requires continuous surveillance.

Newborns of women undergoing **cesarean delivery** before labor or ROM have an extremely low risk for early-onset GBS disease. Antibiotic prophylaxis is not recommended in this circumstance. However, women planning to be delivered by cesarean should still undergo screening for GBS at 35 to 37 weeks, in case they present in labor or with ROM.

For women with **threatened preterm delivery**, see Figure 37.3.

Vaginal chlorhexidine is associated with a statistically significant 28% reduction in GBS colonization of seven-day-old neonates, but is not associated with reductions in other outcomes, including neonatal early-onset GBS infection, pneumonia, sepsis, or mortality (19). The lack of efficacy may be due to insufficient data (type II error).

Antepartum testing
No specific indication for GBS carriers.

Delivery
Intrapartum antibiotic prophylaxis is described in Figure 37.2 and Table 37.2. There is insufficient evidence to assess whether digital vaginal examinations or intrauterine fetal monitoring affect incidence of GBS sepsis (1). There seems to be no increase in GBS sepsis in pregnancies undergoing stripping of membranes (20), but none of the studies reported screening or results for GBS.

NEONATAL MANAGEMENT
See Figure 37.4 (1).

REFERENCES
1. Verani JR, McGee L, Schrag SJ. Prevention of perinatal group B streptococcal disease—revised guidelines from CDC, 2010. Division of Bacterial Diseases, National Center for Immunization and Respiratory Diseases, Centers for Disease Control and Prevention (CDC). MMWR Recomm Rep 2010; 59(RR–10):1–3. [Review/guideline; Accessible at: http://www.cdc.gov/groupbstrep]
2. Regan JA, Klebanoff MA, Nugent RP. The epidemiology of GBS colonization in pregnancy. Vaginal infections and prematurity study group. Obstet Gynecol 1991; 77(4):604–610. [II-2]
3. Anthony BF, Okada DM, Hobel CJ. Epidemiology of group B *Streptococcus*: longitudinal observations during pregnancy. J Infect Dis 1978; 137:524–530. [II-3]
4. Dillon HC Jr., Gray E, Pass MA, et al. Anorectal and vaginal carriage of group B streptococci during pregnancy. J Infect Dis 1982; 145:794–799. [II-3]
5. Boyer KM, Gadzala CA, Kelly PD, et al. Selective intrapartum chemoprophylaxis of neonatal group B streptococcal early-onset disease. II. Predictive value of prenatal cultures. J Infect Dis 1983; 148:802–809. [II-2]
6. Rouse DJ, Goldenberg RL, Oliver SP, et al. Strategies for the prevention of early-onset neonatal group B streptococcal sepsis: a decision analysis. Obstet Gynecol 1994; 83:483–494. [Decision analysis]
7. Paoletti LC, Mafoff LC. Vaccines to prevent neonatal GBS infection. Semin Neonatal 2002; 7(4):315–323. [Review]
8. Lin FY, Philips III JB, Azimi PH. Level of maternal antibody required to protect neonates against early onset disease caused by group B *Streptococcus* type Ia: a multicenter, seroepidemiology study. J Infect Dis 2001; 184:1022–1028. [II-2]
9. Law MR, Palomaki G, Alfiveric Z, et al. The prevention of neonatal group B streptococcal disease: a report by a working group of the medical screening society. J Med Screen 2005; 12:60–68. [III]
10. Thompsen AC, Morup L, Hansen KB. Antibiotic elimination of group-B streptococci in urine in prevention of preterm labour. Lancet 1987; 591–593. [RCT; *n* = 69]
11. Klebanoff MA, Regan JA, Rao AV, et al. Outcome of the vaginal infections and prematurity study: results of a clinical trial of erythromycin among pregnant women colonized with group B streptococci. Am J Obstet Gynecol 1995; 172:1540–1545. [RCT; *n* = 938; vaginal-cervical GBS at 23–26 weeks: Erythromycin 333 mg tid or placebo for 10 weeks or up to 35 6/7 weeks, whichever came first]
12. Gibbs RS, Schrag S, Schuchat A. Perinatal infections due to group B streptococci. Obstet Gynecol 2004; 104:1062–1076. [Review]
13. Schrag SJ, Zell ER, Lyndfield R, et al. A population-based comparison of strategies to prevent early-onset group B streptococcal disease in neonates. N Engl J Med 2002; 347:233–239. [II-1]
14. Locksmith GJ, Clark P, Duff P. Maternal and neonatal infection rates with three different protocols for prevention of group B streptococcal disease. Am J Obstet Gynecol 1999; 180:416–422. [II-1]
15. American College of Obstetrics and Gynecologists. Prevention of early-onset group B streptococcal disease in newborns. Committee Opinion No. 485. Obstet Gynecol 2011; 117. [III, guideline]
16. Puopolo KM, Madoff LC, Eichenwald EC. Early-onset group B streptococcal disease in the era of maternal screening. Pediatrics 2005; 115(5):1240–1246. [II-2]
17. Jamie WE, Edwards RK, Duff P. Vaginal-perianal compared with vaginal-rectal cultures for identification of group B *Streptococcus*. Obstet Gynecol 2004; 104:1058–1061. [II-2]
18. Ohlsson A, Shah VS. Intrapartum antibiotics for known maternal group B streptococcal colonization. Cochrane Database Syst Rev 2009; (3):CD007467. [Three RCTs, *n* = 488 infants. Overall poor-quality RCTs]
19. Stade BC, Shah VS, Ohlsson A. Vaginal chlorhexidine during labour to prevent early-onset neonatal infection. Cochrane Database Syst Rev 4, 2008. [Meta-analysis; five RCTs, *n* = 2190]
20. Boulvain M, Stan CM, Irion O. Membrane stripping for induction of labor. Cochrane Database Syst Rev. Jan 20, 2010. [Meta-analysis]

38

Vaccination

Edward M. Buchanan, Christina M. Hillson, and Joshua H. Barash

KEY POINTS

- Evaluation of a woman's immune status should occur in the preconception period. Optimally, immunization with indicated vaccines should occur prior to pregnancy.
- Immunity to **rubella, varicella, influenza, hepatitis B, tetanus, and pertussis** should be checked and administered as necessary in the **preconception period.**
- Nonetheless, in most cases, vaccines should be administered to pregnant women believed to be at high risk for acquiring a vaccine-preventable illness, as there is **no vaccine** that is **more dangerous to a pregnant woman or her fetus than the disease it is designed to prevent.**
- Recombinant, inactivated, and subunit vaccines, as well as toxoids, and immunoglobulins pose no threat to a developing fetus.
- **Inactivated Influenza vaccine should be given (by injection, as killed virus) to all pregnant women during the influenza season. The live attenuated form of the vaccine (intranasal spray) should not be given during pregnancy.**
- **Hepatitis B** vaccine can be safely given in pregnancy.
- Td (tetanus-diphtheria) vaccination can be deferred during pregnancy and **Tdap vaccination given before postpartum discharge** from the hospital. For pregnancies at high risk for neonatal tetanus or pertussis, Tdap may be used during pregnancy.
- **Live, attenuated vaccines are contraindicated in pregnancy** because of the theoretical concern for fetal infection. However, if inadvertent vaccination occurs during pregnancy, no adverse fetal outcomes have been described with rubella, varicella, or BCG vaccination.
- **Rubella and varicella immunity should be determined in all women of childbearing age.** MMR (measles-mumps-rubella) and varicella vaccination should be avoided in pregnancy as they are live attenuated vaccines, and administered to all nonimmune women in the preconception or postpartum period.
- Breast-feeding does not adversely affect immunization and is not a contraindication for any vaccine, with the exception of smallpox vaccine.
- No vaccine is 100% safe and 100% effective in nonpregnant or pregnant adults.

HISTORICAL NOTES

Vaccination is one of the most cost-effective and clinically successful medical interventions available. The incidence of vaccine-preventable diseases drops precipitously upon initiating an effective vaccination program within a population (1). Although traditionally targeted for children, adult vaccination programs are critically important to prevent disease in pregnant women and their offspring.

PREGNANCY AND VACCINE-PREVENTABLE DISEASES

Pregnancy is an important part of the life cycle when certain infections can play a particularly destructive role. Pregnancy creates a relative immune suppression, which places a woman at greater risk of complications from illnesses such as influenza and varicella. Likewise, maternal infections with such viruses as varicella and rubella can cause a spectrum of fetal effects including congenital anomalies, fetal morbidities, and even fetal death. Finally, neonates are highly susceptible to complications from vaccine-preventable diseases at a time when they do not receive full protection from vaccination themselves. By **immunizing close contacts of a newborn**, the risk of exposure is reduced, a strategy known as "**cocooning**." **Maternal vaccination also provides protection of the neonate through passive immunization**, in which maternal antibodies (IgG) are transmitted transplacentally, particularly in the last four to six weeks of gestation (2). An additional benefit may occur with the passage of antibodies (IgA) via breast milk.

GENERAL GUIDELINES FOR VACCINATION AND PREGNANCY
Preconception

Evaluation of a woman's immune status should occur in the preconception period. Optimally, immunization with indicated vaccines should occur prior to pregnancy. For the reproductive age female, immunity to **rubella, varicella, influenza, tetanus, pertussis, and hepatitis B** are particularly beneficial for the health of the woman and her offspring (Tables 38.1–38.3). **If live, attenuated vaccines are administered, the patient should avoid pregnancy for four weeks** because of the theoretical concern for transplacental infection of the fetus (3).

In addition, **family members of a newborn should be immunized against influenza and pertussis**. Although vaccination does not have to occur preconception as is optimal for the mother, these vaccinations should be administered to family members before or during a woman's pregnancy to provide a protective barrier to disease from the moment of birth.

Pregnancy

If a woman is pregnant at the time of evaluation, careful selection of appropriate vaccinations should be made on the basis of the clinical situation to reduce morbidity from high-risk infections. Recombinant, **inactivated, and subunit vaccines, as well as toxoids and immunoglobulins, pose no threat to a developing fetus** (4–6). These medications may be administered at any time in pregnancy although delaying until the second trimester will avoid false associations with adverse events in the first trimester.

Table 38.1 Recommended for All Women of Childbearing Age (Preconception, Postpartum, and Considered Safe in Pregnancy)

Vaccine	Vaccine type	Dosing regimen	Indications/Comments

Influenza (7,8)
  Trivalent inactivated
  vaccine (TIV)
	Inactivated subunit
	  (IM injection)
		Annually	Vaccinate all adults and children > 6 mo. Pregnant women should be immunized during the influenza season at any gestation. Do not administer live vaccine (LAIV,FluMist) during pregnancy.

Tetanus/diphtheria Td (9)	Toxoids	Booster every 10 yr after primary series completed	Uncertain history or incomplete primary series, administer three-dose primary series (Td): • Vaccines given at 0, 4 weeks, and 6–12 months • Tdap should replace one dose of Td, preferably during the late second or third trimester of pregnancy (10)
Tdap (9)	Toxoids/acellular	Single dose of Tdap to replace one Td booster (see Indication/Comments for details)	No history of prior Tdap vaccination: • Tdap should be administered as a one-time booster regardless of interval since the last tetanus- or diphtheria-toxoid containing vaccine. Tdap and pregnancy: • Women who have not received Tdap should receive it during pregnancy, preferably after 20 weeks gestation. Immediately postpartum is an alternative option (10).
Hepatitis B (11)	Recombinant	*Pre-exposure prophylaxis*: • Three-dose series: 0,1, and 4 mo[a] • Third dose at least 2 mo after second dose AND at least 4 mo after initial dose *Postexposure prophylaxis*: • Either vaccinate, give HBIG or both *(depends on exposure type, vaccine status, time from exposure)*	Exposure to blood in workplace, dialysis/ESRD patients, current or history of injection drug use, more than 1 sexual partner in the past 6 months, other sexually transmitted infections, hepatitis C, household contact or sexual partner of person with chronic Hepatitis B, health care personnel, travel to area of high prevalence for >6 mo[b]
Human papilloma (HPV) (12,13)	Recombinant	Three-dose series • Second dose 1–2 mo after the first dose • Third dose 6 mo after the initial dose	Although HPV vaccine has not been causally associated with adverse outcomes during pregnancy (category B), it is not recommended during pregnancy If a woman becomes pregnant after starting the series, the remainder of the series should be delayed until after delivery No interventions are needed if a dose is inadvertently administered during pregnancy

[a]Special dosing required for dialysis and immunocompromised patients.
[b]Diseases related to travel, available at: http://wwwnc.cdc.gov/travel/content/diseases.aspx.

Table 38.2 Recommended for Pregnant Women at Significant Risk for Exposure

Vaccine	Subtype	Dosing regimen	Indications/*Comments*
Hepatitis A (14,15)	Inactivated	*Pre-exposure prophylaxis*: • Two-dose vaccine series, second dose 6–18 mo after the first dose *Postexposure prophylaxis*: • Either vaccinate, give IG or both depending on exposure type, age, health status[a]	Chronic liver disease, clotting disorders requiring clotting factor precipitates, illicit drug users (both injection and noninjection), men who have sex with men, travel/ live/ work in endemic areas Unvaccinated persons in contact with an infected person (both sexual and household contacts), members of child care centers with an infected employee or child, to be considered for hospital workers in close contact with infected patients
Pneumococcal (16)	Polysaccharide	Single dose	Smoking (adults 19 yr and older), chronic pulmonary disease including smoking, asthma, chronic liver disease, chronic alcoholism, chronic cardiovascular disease, chronic renal failure or nephrotic syndrome, functional or anatomic asplenia (e.g., sickle cell disease or splenectomy), diabetes mellitus, immunosuppressive conditions (e.g., HIV)
		One time revaccination after 5 yr	Chronic renal failure or nephrotic syndrome, functional or anatomic asplenia (e.g., sickle cell disease or splenectomy), chronic high-dose steroids, immunosuppressive conditions
Rabies (17–19)	Inactivated	*Pre-exposure prophylaxis:* • Three doses: day 0,7,21, or 28 • Test Ab titer every 6 mo for continuous exposure or every 2 yr for intermittent exposure • Booster vaccination if titer < acceptable level *Postexposure prophylaxis:* • *Not previously vaccinated*: single dose of rabies immune globulin (RIG) + four doses of vaccine on days 0,3,7, and 14[c] • *If previously vaccinated*: one dose of vaccine immediately, and repeat 3 days later	Veterinary workers, persons having frequent contact with animal species at risk for rabies,[b] spelunkers, travelers to areas where dog rabies is enzootic and rapid access to medical care may not be available Indicated for any wound/scratch/bite caused by a possibly rabid animal[b] Multiple studies on the vaccine and RIG in pregnant women failed to show an elevated risk, vaccine felt to be overall safe in pregnancy (17,18).
Meningococcal (20–23)	Polysaccharide, Conjugate	Single dose, revaccination after 5 yr recommended if continued high risk for infection	Anatomic or functional asplenia, terminal complement component deficiency, military recruits, boarding school or college students, travel or reside in endemic or epidemic area *(MCV4 is safe and immunogenic among nonpregnant persons aged 11–55 years, but no data are available on the safety of MCV4 during pregnancy).*
Polio (IPV, *inactivated polio vaccine*) (24)	Inactivated	Three-dose primary series if not previously completed • Second dose 1–2 mo after first dose • Third dose 6–12 mo after second dose Booster—if risk of exposure and primary series completed more than 10 yr previously: • Single dose of IPV	Travel to or live in areas where polio is endemic or epidemic, lab worker who might handle poliovirus, health care workers who might care for polio infected persons, unvaccinated adults whose children will receive OPV • IPV is used exclusively for routine vaccination in the United States and other nations where polio is not endemic. OPV is still used for outbreaks (24). • *Pregnancy*: Vaccination should be avoided on theoretical grounds, but if at increased risk for infection, IPV can be administered. No adverse effects have been found in pregnant women or their fetuses.

Table 38.2   Recommended for Pregnant Women at Significant Risk for Exposure (*Continued*)

Vaccine	Subtype	Dosing regimen	Indications/*Comments*
Polio (OPV, *oral polio vaccine*)	Live	If less than 4 wk available to immunize, a single dose of OPV may be given (24) Three-dose primary series and booster recommendations are same as above	[d]OPV has a risk of causing *vaccine-related paralytic poliomylitis*. It is used in countries endemic for polio where the superior secretory immunity in the gastrointestinal tract induced by OPV is an advantage. OPV is the only product available in many developing nations and should be used in pregnancy as indicated. No adverse effects have been found to mother/fetus
Anthrax (25)	Inactivated, acellular vaccine	***Pre-exposure:*** 5 IM doses (0 wk, 4 wk, 6 mo, 12 mo, and 18 mo (IM)) + annual booster to maintain immunity ***Postexposure:*** three doses SC (0, 2, 4 wk) with 60-day antimicrobial postexposure prophylaxis	***Pre-exposure:*** Military personnel in high risk areas, persons who perform high risk laboratory work, handle animal product/hides and unable to adhere to standards of prevention ***Postexposure*** Given to persons exposed including pregnant and breast-feeding women, children <18 yr decided case by case
Japanese encephalitis (26)	Inactivated	Three-dose series • 0,7, and 30 days	Travelers with significant risk of exposure based on destination, duration of travel, season, and activities (27)
Typhoid Oral TY21a	Live attenuated	Oral: three-dose series • One dose every 2 days Injection Vi:	Given to those at high risk: travel to or live in area where typhoid is endemic, close contact of typhoid carrier, lab exposure to *Salmonella typhi* bacteria. Information on safety in pregnancy is not available, on theoretical grounds avoid vaccination in pregnancy
Injectable Vi Whole-cell vaccine	Polysaccharide Inactivated	• Single dose Inactivated injection: • Two doses 4 wk apart	
Yellow fever (28–30)	Live virus	Single dose Booster every 10 yr for continued risk/exposure	Given to those at high risk: live in or travel to area where yellow fever is endemic, or lab exposure to the virus. Not well studied in pregnancy, pregnant women who must travel to areas where risk of yellow fever infection is high should be vaccinated

[a]Recommendations for hepatitis A postexposure prophylaxis: http://www.cdc.gov/mmwr/preview/mmwrhtml/mm5641a3.htm#box.
[b]Animals at high risk for carrying rabies: http://www.cdc.gov/mmwr/preview/mmwrhtml/rr57e507a1.htm
[c]For persons with immunosuppression, rabies post-exposure prophylaxis should be administered using all five doses of vaccine on days 0,3,7,14, and 28.
[d]Diseases related to travel: http://wwwnc.cdc.gov/travel/content/diseases.aspx. *Abbreviation*: IG, immunoglobulin.

Live, attenuated vaccines are contraindicated in pregnancy because of the theoretical concern for fetal infection. However, if inadvertent vaccination occurs during pregnancy, no adverse fetal outcomes have been described with rubella, varicella, or BCG vaccination (31–36).

SPECIFIC VACCINES
Influenza
Inactivated influenza vaccine should be administered in any trimester during the flu season because of the risk that infection poses to a pregnant woman (37) (Table 38.1). Pregnant women and young infants are at significant increased risk for serious consequences of influenza. During pregnancy, women have a fourfold increased rate of serious illness and hospitalization (38). The increased morbidity related to influenza during pregnancy is related to physiologic changes that include decreased pulmonary volume, increased cardiac output, and suppression of cell-mediated immunity (39). A randomized controlled trial of 314 mothers and infants demonstrated immunization benefits to both mother and child. Immunized pregnant women had 30% less respiratory febrile illnesses. Infants less than six months old born to immunized mothers had 63% fewer cases of influenza (40). Influenza

vaccine has been routinely administered during pregnancy since 1957. No study to date has shown an adverse consequence of inactivated influenza vaccine in pregnant women or their offspring (7,8,41) (see also chap. 24).

Td/Tdap
Td (tetanus toxoid, reduced inactivated **diphtheria** toxoid) is a tetanus vaccine containing diphtheria toxoid as well (Table 38.1). Tetanus in newborn infants, once common, is prevented if the mother has been immunized, because the immune mother passes antibodies to the baby across the placenta. The mother is immune if she has been immunized before becoming pregnant or during pregnancy. Maternal tetanus toxoid vaccination has been shown to be up to 98% effective in preventing neonatal tetanus (42).

Td effectiveness in preventing neonatal deaths was 62% (9). The WHO estimates that 1.5 million cases of neonatal tetanus have been prevented since a 1989 initiative to eliminate maternal and neonatal tetanus. **An expectant mother whose tetanus immunization status is uncertain or whose last immunization was more than 10 years ago should be immunized against tetanus.**

Table 38.3 Not Recommended in Pregnancy

Vaccine	Type	Dosing regimen	Comments
Varicella	Live attenuated	Two-dose series: • Second dose 4–8 wk after first	Not given to pregnant women or women planning to become pregnant within 4 wk **Initiate series in the immediate postpartum period to those women determined to be varicella nonimmune** on prenatal evaluation

		Postexposure prophylaxis:
		• Varicella zoster immune globulin (VZIG) within 96 hr of exposure to varicella or herpes zoster
		• If VZIG is not available:
		  • IVIG can be used at a dose of 400 mg/kg given IV as a single dose
		  OR
		  • Closely monitor for development of disease and treat with acyclovir if disease develops.
			VZIG and IVIG are safe in pregnancy and breast-feeding
			
			Acyclovir in Pregnancy Registry was completed in 1999. Data on 1246 exposures in pregnancy did not find an association with any adverse pregnancy outcome (43)

MMR (measles-mumps-rubella)	Live attenuated	Single dose	Not given to pregnant women or women planning to become pregnant within 4 wk **Administer this MMR vaccine in the immediate postpartum period to those women determined to be rubella nonimmune** on prenatal evaluation
BCG	Live attenuated	Single dose	Consider giving to health care workers in areas where drug resistant strains of TB persist. No harmful fetal effects have been associated with BCG, but its use is not recommended in pregnancy (31)
Smallpox (44,45)	Live attenuated	Single inoculation Immunity decreases 3–5 yr after vaccination	Pregnant women, or women planning to become pregnant within 4 wk should not be vaccinated in the absence of exposure to active disease
		Postexposure prophylaxis: Vaccination within 3 days of exposure will completely prevent or significantly modify smallpox in the vast majority of persons. Vaccination 4–7 days after exposure likely offers some protection from disease or decreases severity	Close contacts of pregnant women or women planning to become pregnant within 4 wk should not be vaccinated unless exposed to active disease—exposure to the resulting lesion can cause vaccinia viral infection in the pregnant woman and/or fetus

CDC's Advisory Committee on Immunization Practices does not recommend preventive use of vaccinia immune globulin (VIG) for pregnant women. However, if a woman has a complication from smallpox vaccine that could be treated with VIG, she should receive it while pregnant (45).

Tdap (**tetanus** toxoid, reduced inactivated **diphtheria** toxoid, and **acellular pertussis**) was licensed in 2005 for persons aged 11 to 64 in the United States (Table 38.1). The addition of **pertussis** occurred because family members with pertussis are the source of infection in 75% of cases in early infancy, when complications and fatalities are high (46). Infants less than 12 months old account for most of the morbidity and mortality related to pertussis (42).

Ideally, Tdap immunization should be recommended preconception. Pregnancy is not a contraindication to Tdap immunization. Theoretically, when Tdap is administered during pregnancy, transplacental maternal antibodies might protect the infant against pertussis in early life. However, these same antibodies could also interfere with the infant's immune response to infant doses of DTap, and leave the infant less well protected against pertussis (42). **Pertussis vaccination, when indicated, should not be delayed, even if it means vaccination during pregnancy. Tdap should be administered postpartum regardless of interval since the last tetanus or diphtheria toxoid-containing vaccine.** While longer intervals between Td and Tdap vaccination could decrease the occurrence of local reactions, the benefits of protection against pertussis outweigh the potential risk for adverse events (47) (Table 38.1). In settings of low risk for neonatal tetanus, Td vaccination can be deferred until after pregnancy. For pregnant women who need tetanus or diphtheria protection during pregnancy, and have not received a dose of Tdap, replacement of Td with Tdap is recommended. Tdap may be given during pregnancy, preferably in the third or late second (after 20 weeks gestation) trimester (10).

Hepatitis B

Hepatitis B is a serious problem in pregnancy because of the possibility of vertical transmission to the neonate (see chap. 30) (Table 38.1). Vertical transmission occurs in up to 90% of infected women depending on their viral status, and 90% of the children who become infected develop chronic infection (48). Nonimmune women at high risk for HBV infection during pregnancy should be immunized. This includes women who have had more than one sexual partner in the past six months, illicit drug users (both injection and noninjection), those with an HBsAg-positive sex partner, and those being evaluated or treated for a sexually transmitted disease (11). Women at risk should also be counseled on safe sexual practices to prevent HBV infection. Although reports are limited, this vaccine has not been shown to have any adverse effects on the developing fetus (49).

Pneumococcal

Indications for pneumococcal vaccine are presented in Table 38.2. In pregnancy the evidence is often insufficient to get enough statistical power for effectiveness, but pneumococcal vaccination during pregnancy reduces the risk of neonatal infection (RR 0.51; 95% CI 0.18–1.41), and pneumococcal colonization in infants by 16 months of age (RR 0.33; 95% CI 0.11–0.98) (16).

CONTRAINDICATIONS TO VACCINATION

The only true contraindication applicable to all vaccines is a history of a *severe* allergic reaction after a prior dose of vaccine or to a vaccine component, unless the recipient has been desensitized. An extensive listing of vaccine components, their use, and the vaccines that contain each component is available from CDC's National Immunization Program Web site at http://www.cdc.gov/nip.

REFERENCES

1. Roush SW, Murphy TV; Vaccine-Preventable Disease Table Working Group. Historical comparisons of morbidity and mortality for vaccine-preventable diseases in the United States. JAMA 2007; 298(18):2155–2163.[III, Review]
2. Insel RA. Maternal immunization to prevent neonatal infection. N Engl J Med 1988; 319(18):1219–1220. [III, Review]
3. Centers for Disease Control and Prevention. Guidelines for vaccinating pregnant women. Available at: http://www.cdc.gov/vaccines/pubs/preg-guide.htm. Accessed September 1, 2011. [Guideline]
4. Kroger AT, Sumaya CV, Pickering LK, et al. General recommendations on immunization—recommendations of the Advisory Committee on Immunization Practices (ACIP). MMWR Recomm Rep 2011; 60(2):1–61. [Guideline]
5. Grabenstein JD. Pregnancy and lactation in relation to vaccines and antibodies. Pharm Pract Manag Q 2001; 20(3):1–10. [III, review]
6. Koren G, Pastuszak A, Ito S. Drugs in pregnancy. N Engl J Med 1998; 338(16):1128–1137. [III, review]
7. Munoz FM, Greisinger AJ, Wehmanen OA, et al. Safety of influenza vaccination during pregnancy. Am J Obstet Gynecol 2005; 192(4):1098–1106. [II-2]
8. Fiore AE, Uyeki TM, Broder K, et al., Centers for Disease Control and Prevention (CDC). Prevention and control of influenza with vaccines: recommendations of the Advisory Committee on Immunization Practices (ACIP). MMWR Recomm Rep 2010; 59 (RR-8):1–62. [Guideline]
9. Demicheli V, Barale A, Rivetti A. Vaccines for women to prevent neonatal tetanus. Cochrane Database Syst Rev 2005; (4): CD002959. [Meta-analysis; two RCTs, n = 10,560]
10. Center for Disease Control and Prevention: ACIP Provisional Recommendations for Pregnant Women on Use of Tetanus Toxoid, Reduced Diphtheria Toxoid and Acellular Pertussis Vaccine (Tdap). Posted August 2011. Available at: http://www.cdc.gov/vaccines/recs/provisional/default/htm. Accessed September 1, 2011.
11. Mast EE, Weinbaum CM, Fiore AE; CDC. A comprehensive immunization strategy to eliminate transmission of hepatitis B virus infection in the United States: recommendations of the Advisory Committee on Immunization Practices (ACIP). MMWR Recomm Rep 2006; 55(RR16):1–25. [Guideline]
12. Garland S, Ault K, Gall S, et al. Pregnancy and infant outcomes in the clinical trials of a human papilloma virus type 6/11/16/18 vaccine: a combined analysis of five randomized controlled trials. Obstet Gynecol 2009; 114:1179–1188. [Meta-analysis; five RCTs, n = 25,551]
13. Centers for Disease Control and Prevention. Quadrivalent human papillomavirus vaccine: recommendations of the Advisory Committee on Immunization Practices (ACIP). MMWR Recomm Rep 2007; 56(RR-2):1–32. [Guideline]
14. Fiore AE, Wasley A, Bell BP, Advisory Committee on Immunization Practices (ACIP). Prevention of hepatitis A through active or passive immunization: recommendations of the Advisory Committee on Immunization Practices (ACIP). MMWR Recomm Rep 2006; 55(RR-7):1–23. [Guideline]
15. Duff B, Duff P. Hepatitis A vaccine: ready for prime time. Obstet Gynecol 1998; 91(3):468–471. [Review]
16. Chaithongwongwatthana S, Yamasmit W, Limpongsanurak S, et al. Pneumococcal vaccination during pregnancy for preventing infant infection. Cochrane Database Syst Rev 2006; (1):CD004903. [Meta-analysis; three RCTs, n = 280]
17. Chabala S, Williams M, Amenta R, et al. Confirmed rabies exposure during pregnancy: treatment with human rabies immune globulin and human diploid cell vaccine. Am J Med 1991; 91(4):423–424. [II-3]
18. Sudarshan MK, Madhusudana SN, Mahendra BJ. Post-exposure prophylaxis with purified vero cell rabies vaccine during pregnancy—safety and immunogenicity. J Commun Dis 1999; 31(4):229–236. [Review]
19. Manning SE, Rupprecht CE, Fishbein D, et al.; Advisory Committee on Immunization Practices Centers for Disease Control and Prevention (CDC). Human rabies prevention—United States, 2008: recommendations of the Advisory Committee on Immunization Practices (ACIP). MMWR 2008; 57(RR-3):1–28. [Guideline]
20. Bilukha OO, Rosenstein N; National Center for Infectious Diseases, Centers for Disease Control and Prevention. Prevention and control of meningococcal disease: recommendations of the Advisory Committee on Immunization Practices (ACIP). MMWR Recomm Rep 2005; 54(RR-7):1–21. [Guideline]
21. Adam I, Abdalla MA. Is meningococcal polysaccharide vaccine safe during pregnancy? Ann Trop Med Parasitol 2005; 99(6):627–628. [Review]
22. Shahid NS, Steinhoff MC, Roy E, et al. Placental and breast transfer of antibodies after maternal immunization with polysaccharide meningococcal vaccine: a randomized, controlled evaluation. Vaccine 2002; 20(17–18):2404–2409. [II-2, RCT; n = 157]
23. Leston GW, Little JR, Ottman J, et al. Meningococcal vaccine in pregnancy: an assessment of infant risk. Pediatr Infect Dis J 1998; 17:261–263. [II-3]
24. CDC. Poliomyelitis prevention in the United States: updated recommendations of the Advisory Committee on Immunization Practices (ACIP). MMWR Recomm Rep 2000; 49(RR05):1-22. [Guideline]
25. CDC. Use of anthrax vaccine in the United States: recommendations of the Advisory Committee on Immunization Practices (ACIP). MMWR Recomm Rep 2000; 49(RR-15):1–20. [Guideline]
26. Fischer M, Lindsey N, Staples JE, Hills S; Centers for Disease Control and Prevention (CDC). Japanese encephalitis vaccines: recommendations of the Advisory Committee on Immunization Practices (ACIP). MMWR Recomm Rep 2010; 59(RR-1):1–27. [Guideline]
27. CDC. Inactivated Japanese encephalitis vaccine: recommendations of the Advisory Committee on Immunization Practices (ACIP). MMWR 2010; 50(RR-01):1–27. [Guideline]
28. Tsai TF, Paul R, Lynberg MC, et al. Congenital yellow fever virus infection after immunization in pregnancy. J Infect Dis 1993; 168(6):1520–1523. [II-3]
29. Nasidi A, Monath TP, Vandenberg J, et al. Yellow fever vaccination and pregnancy: a four-year prospective study. Trans R Soc Trop Med Hyg 1993; 87(3):337–339. [II-2]
30. Nishioka Sde A, Nunes-Araujo FR, Pires WP, et al. Yellow fever vaccination during pregnancy and spontaneous abortion: a case-control study. Trop Med Int Health 1998; 3(1):29–33. [II-2]
31. CDC. The role of BCG vaccine in the prevention and control of tuberculosis in the United States. A joint statement by the Advisory Council for the Elimination of Tuberculosis and the Advisory Committee on Immunization Practices. MMWR Recomm Rep 1996; 45(RR-4):1–18. [Guideline]
32. Bar-Oz B, Levichek Z, Moretti ME, et al. Pregnancy outcome following rubella vaccination: a prospective controlled study. Am J Med Genet 2004; 130A:52–54. [II-1]

33. Bart SW, Stetler HC, Preblud SR, et al. Fetal risk associated with rubella vaccine: an update. Rev Infect Dis 1985; 7(suppl 1):S95–S102. [III, review]

34. Centers for Disease Control and Prevention (CDC). Rubella vaccination during pregnancy—United States, 1971–1988. MMWR Morb Mortal Wkly Rep 1989; 38(17):289–293. [III, review]

35. Sheppard S, Smithells RW, Dickson A, et al. Rubella vaccination and pregnancy: preliminary report of a national survey. Br Med J (Clin Res Ed) 1986; 292(6522):727. [Survey]

36. Wilson E, Goss MA, Marin M, et al. Varicella vaccine exposure during Pregnancy: data from 10 years of the pregnancy registry. J Infect Dis 2008; 197(suppl2): S178–S184. [II-2]

37. Mak TK. Influenza vaccination in pregnancy: current evidence and selected national policies. Lancet Infect Dis 2008; 8(1):44–52. [III, review]

38. MacDonald NE, Riley LE, Steinhoff MC. Influenza immunization in pregnancy. Obstet Gynecol 2009; 114(2 pt 1):365–368. [III, review]

39. Tamma PD, Ault KA, del Rio C, et al. Safety of influenza vaccination during pregnancy. Am J Obstet Gynecol 2009; 201(6):547–552. [III, review]

40. Zaman K, Roy E, Arifeen SE, et al. Effectiveness of maternal influenza immunization in mothers and infants. N Engl J Med 2008; 359(15):1555–1564. [I, RCT, *n* = 340]

41. American College of Obstetricians and Gynecologists **Committee** on Obstetric Practice. Influenza vaccination during pregnancy. ACOG Committee Opinion No. 468: Obstet Gynecol 2010; 116(4):1006–1007. [III, review]

42. Murphy TV, Slade BA, Broder KR, et al; Advisory Committee on Immunization Practices (ACIP) Centers for Disease Control and Prevention (CDC). Prevention of pertussis, tetanus, and diphtheria among pregnant and postpartum women and their infants: recommendations of the Advisory Committee on Immunization Practices (ACIP). MMWR Recomm Rep 2008; 57(RR-4):1–51. [Guideline]

43. Stone KM, Reiff-Eldridge R, White AD, et al. Pregnancy outcomes following systemic prenatal acyclovir exposure: conclusions from the international acyclovir pregnancy registry, 1984–1999. Birth Defects Res A Clin Mol Teratol 2004; 70(4):201–207. [II-2]

44. CDC. Smallpox vaccination and adverse reactions. MMWR Recomm Rep 2003; 52(RR04):1-28. [Guideline]

45. CDC. Smallpox vaccination information for women who are pregnant or breastfeeding. Available at: http://www.bt.cdc.gov/agent/smallpox/faq/pregnancy.asp, 2009. Accessed September 1, 2011. [Guideline]

46. Bisgard K, Pascual FB, Ehresmann KR, et al. Infant pertussis: who was the source? Pediatr Infect Dis J 2004; 23:985–989. [II-3]

47. Centers for Disease Control and Prevention. Updated recommendations for use of tetanus toxoid, reduced diphtheria toxoid and acellular pertussis (Tdap) vaccine from the Advisory Committee on Immunization Practices, 2010. MMWR 2011; 60:13–15. [Guideline]

48. Gupta I, Ratho RK. Immunogenicity and safety of two schedules of hepatitis B vaccination during pregnancy. J Obstet Gynaecol Res 2003; 29(2):84–86. [II-2]

49. Levy M, Koren G. Hepatitis B vaccine in pregnancy: maternal and fetal safety. Am J Perinatol 1991; 8:227–232. [Review]

39

Trauma

Lauren A. Plante and Keren Lerner

KEY POINTS

- Trauma during pregnancy is a common complication, and accounts for a significant fraction of maternal deaths as well as perinatal mortality.
- Changes in physiology related to pregnancy must be borne in mind when managing trauma care.
- Care of the pregnant trauma patient:
  - **There is no reliable evidence** to dictate the initial care of the traumatized pregnant patient, the type and duration of monitoring, the type of testing required, or the follow-up care of ongoing pregnancy after trauma.
  - **Initial maternal stabilization takes priority over fetal assessment.**
  - Transfer to a trauma center should be considered for severe cases. This decision is usually made at the scene.
  - **Multidisciplinary** approach is important, as obstetrician, maternal-fetal specialist, trauma surgeon, intensivist, anesthesiologist, neonatologist and others may need to be involved.
  - **Maternal stabilization: "ABCs"** (airway, breathing, circulation).
  - **Appropriate studies should not be withheld because of pregnancy.**
  - Blunt abdominal trauma: FAST ultrasound (Figs. 39.2 and 39.3).
  - Ultrasound, fetal monitoring, tocodynamometer (contraction) monitoring and Kleihauer–Betke (KB) test can be considered in the management of the pregnant woman with trauma.
- After hospital discharge following trauma, there remains an increased probability of worse perinatal outcome. Ongoing fetal assessment may be indicated, although the exact type of surveillance has not been established.

DEFINITION

Trauma consists of intentional harm and accidents. Intentional harm includes assault, blunt force trauma, and penetrating trauma. Accidents include predominantly motor vehicle crashes and falls.

INCIDENCE

Incidence of trauma in pregnancy is unclear. Estimates vary widely from up to 8% (any physical trauma) (1) to 0.2% to 2% (evaluation for trauma) to 0.4–2/10,000 (hospitalization for trauma) (2–4). The incidence of hospital admission parallels increasing gestational age (5). Domestic violence against pregnant women ranges from 4% to 9% (6). These ranges may be due to reporting bias, and undercounting of the total number of injuries. Not all cases of maternal trauma are seen at a trauma center, or even referred to a hospital; hospital-acquired data are biased toward more serious injuries. No ongoing national data collection incorporates mention of pregnancy. Among motor vehicle crashes involving pregnant women, 25% occur in the first trimester, 39% in the second, and 34% in the third (7).

ETIOLOGY/BASIC PATHOPHYSIOLOGY

Causes of trauma in pregnancy are shown in Figure 39.1 (2):

- 71% motor vehicle accident (MVA; nearly 3% of all MVA involve a pregnant woman) (8)
- 12% assault
- 9% fall
- 2% bicycle
- 2% auto versus pedestrian
- <1% suicide
- 3% other (unintentional)

PROGNOSTIC FACTORS

Factors that predispose injured women to a worse pregnancy outcome, defined as delivery, pregnancy loss, or hysterectomy, are as follows:

- Higher ISS > 9 (Injury Severity Score—http://www.trauma.org/index.php/main/article/383/)
- Lactate >2 mmol/L
- Altered mental status at admission (Glasgow Coma Score <8)
- Lack of proper seat-belt use
- Severe head injury
- Injury to thorax, abdomen, lower extremities, or spine

Drug use and shock at admission are less highly correlated, although an increased risk is noted (2,9). Individual risk factors associated with fetal demise include penetrating injury, severity of injury, and maternal hypotension (10).

In cases of minor trauma (ISS = 0), classically described risk factors such as KB, fibrinogen <200, contraction pattern by tocodynamomoter, direct abdominal trauma, placenta location, and abdominal pain are not reliable predictors of adverse pregnancy outcomes (11). While the evaluation of each patient should be individualized, extensive evaluation measures that are routine in practice may be reconsidered in cases of minor trauma.

COMPLICATIONS (3,4)

Complications are more common if there is severe injury (ISS ≥ 9) (3), or if the woman is delivered during the hospitalization for trauma (4). Delayed complications may occur even when

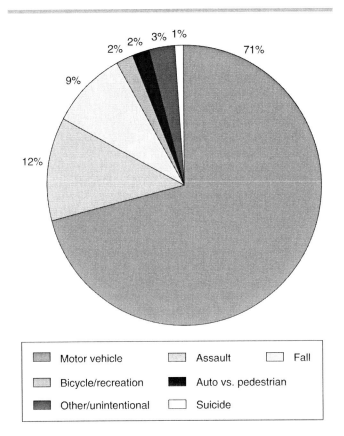

Figure 39.1 Causes of trauma in pregnancy. *Source*: From Ref. 2.

there is no injury diagnosed at the time of hospitalization and when the woman is discharged home undelivered.

Maternal Death

Maternal mortality associated with trauma is about 0.1% to 1.4% (2,4) (this is 10 to 100 times increased over the background U.S. maternal mortality ratio).

Among pregnant women hospitalized after trauma, the case fatality rate is about 4% (12–16).

Trauma is a leading cause of maternal death, as **about 27% of maternal deaths are injury related** (17). Of these deaths, the largest fraction is attributed to MVAs (44%), followed by homicide (31%), unintentional injuries (13%), and suicide (10%). Although the majority of pregnancy-associated homicides occur in the postpartum period, in 21% the woman dies undelivered (17). Trauma and other forms of violence are the leading cause of death in nonpregnant women of reproductive age.

Hospitalization

Women in the third trimester are more likely to be admitted to the hospital than women in the first or second trimester (7); 3% of all trauma admission is for pregnant patients (18).

Transfusion

0.6% to 4%.

Hysterectomy

0.5% to 2%. **May be indicated in cases of penetrating injury to the uterus or in cases of uterine rupture, resulting from blunt force trauma when surgical repair is not reasonable (19); or in cases where coagulopathy follows placental abruption.**

Fetal/Neonatal Outcomes

Nonreassuring fetal testing: 5% to 20%; **preterm birth (PTB)** <37weeks: 14% to 20% (3).

Abruptio Placentae

1% to 13%. Severity of maternal injury does not predict occurrence (20).

Fetal Injury

Very few cases have been reported of fetal injury from maternal gunshot or stab wounds, and of fetal fractures, visceral ruptures, and intracranial hemorrhage after blunt trauma. In cases of blunt force trauma, perinatal outcome measured by Apgar scores did not differ significantly than the general population (21).

Fetal Death

0.4% to 1.5%. The rate of fetal death for women *hospitalized* for trauma is about 11% (12–16). About 5/1000 fetal deaths can be attributed to trauma, or approximately 4 traumatic fetal deaths per 100,000 live births (22). The majority (>80%) of these fetal deaths are associated with MVA, while 6% are related to firearms and another 3% to falls. Less than half, however, include a designation of placental injury (42%), and 20% specify placental abruption. Fetal death is more likely in cases of maternal death, hemorrhagic shock, or no seat-belt use. The most significant factors for fetal death after blunt trauma are maternal ejection from a vehicle, maternal tachycardia (HR > 110), maternal ISS > 9, fetal bradycardia (FHR < 120), and maternal death (23).

Neonatal Death

0.4% to 1.5%.

SPECIAL CONSIDERATIONS FOR COMPLICATIONS FROM ASSAULT (24)

The rate of hospitalization for assault during pregnancy is 0.04%. Of all assaults, 46% were related to an unarmed fight, 12% to firearms or bomb, and 9% to stab injuries. Assaulted women had higher rates of preterm delivery, low birth weight, placental abruption, and uterine rupture compared to women who were never hospitalized for assault during pregnancy. Thirteen percent of women hospitalized after assault delivered during the hospitalization. These women had worse outcomes than either women who were not assaulted, or women who were assaulted but discharged undelivered.

Intimate-partner violence accounted for 20% of the assaults in women who were discharged undelivered and for 50% of the assaults in women who delivered during the hospitalization. In 2007, homicide was the second most common cause of mortality for women between 15 and 24 years of age (25).

PREGNANCY CONSIDERATIONS

Causes of trauma in pregnancy differ from nonpregnant trauma in that **more are attributed to motor vehicles** and fewer to other causes. Pregnancy is generally protective in relation to suicide. Compared to women of the same age who are not pregnant, pregnant women are younger, have **lower ISS and lower mortality** (1% vs. 4%), have shorter length of stay, and lower rates of alcohol and drug use; however, 12% had been drinking and 20% had been using drugs. A crash rate of 13/1000 person-years was calculated for pregnant women aged 15 to 39 (7), which is half the rate for nonpregnant women in this age group (26/1000) (7). Rate of seat-belt use is higher among pregnant patients than the comparison group (66% vs. 50%). Rate of interpersonal violence is similar among pregnant and nonpregnant women (12% vs. 10%). **In 11% of pregnancy trauma cases** (18), the **pregnancy status is unknown** at admission to the receiving trauma team, and in two-thirds of those the pregnancy was newly diagnosed by serum hCG screening—that is, the status had possibly not been known by the patient either. Of those pregnancies unknown to the trauma team at admission but presumably known to the patient (although she did not or could not communicate the status to the team), fetal mortality is >75%, including both spontaneous and elective abortion. Incidental pregnancies that were news to the trauma team although *not* to the patient carry a 25% probability of fetal mortality (18). One-third of the non-survivors in the newly diagnosed group were voluntary abortions, in which the women reported they were fearful of nonspecific damage because of either injury or radiation. It must be cautioned, however, that the stated rationale for elective abortion is not always true.

PREGNANCY MANAGEMENT
Prevention of Injury
Seat Belts

Three-point **seat belts should** always **be worn by pregnant women,** with the shoulder belt over the shoulder, collar bone, and across the chest, between the breasts, and the lap belt as low as possible under the abdomen and the uterus. Clearly, seat belts save maternal lives—by preventing ejection. **In one sample of 57 pregnant women involved in MVAs, acceptable fetal outcomes were four times more likely with proper maternal seat-belt restraint** (26). Seat-belt restraints also have a protective role in low-velocity collisions. Impact testing using a crash-test dummy modeled to represent a woman at 30 weeks of pregnancy has clearly demonstrated two to three times higher peak abdominal pressure when the dummy was unrestrained compared to properly belted (27). Fetal deaths after MVAs are nearly three times more likely in unrestrained women than in those who had been belted during the crash. In minor- or moderate-severity crashes, the risk of an adverse fetal outcome is strongly affected by the use of seat belts, increasing from 29% among women who were properly restrained, to 50% among women who were improperly restrained, to 80% among unrestrained women (26). However, severity of the crash is an independent predictor of poor fetal outcome: 85% of severe crashes (≥30 mph) in this convenience sample were followed by fetal death, direct fetal injury, uterine rupture, or preterm delivery. Fetal deaths were caused by placental abruption and maternal death, in equal numbers (26).

Air Bags

A cohort study in Washington State that cross-referenced State Patrol crash data with birth certificate (and fetal death certif-

icate) data found no significant differences in maternal or fetal outcomes among 198 women whose airbag deployed compared to 622 women whose airbag did not deploy (28). The authors caution, however, that rates of preterm labor and of fetal death were higher in the no-airbag group, and that the lack of statistical significance may be a function of small numbers.

A case series of 30 women past 20 weeks of pregnancy who were hospitalized after crashes in which their air bags deployed (67% were also restrained) showed that only 10% were free of obstetrical signs or symptoms at admission (contractions, abdominal pain, abnormal fetal heart rate, or vaginal bleeding,) but there was only one fetal death. The remaining 29 women were discharged home undelivered, after a mean length of stay of 24 hours, and largely lost to follow-up (29). On the basis of available evidence, no statement can be made as to the utility or safety of air bags in pregnancy.

Care of the Pregnant Trauma Patient

There are no trials to assess the effectiveness of the initial care and interventions for the traumatized pregnant patient, including the type and duration of monitoring, the type of testing required, or the follow-up care of ongoing pregnancy after trauma. Therefore, these recommendations are drawn from guidelines in the nonpregnant population (from Eastern Association for the Surgery of Trauma, EAST) (30).

Workup and Management (Figs. 39.2–39.4)
Stabilization

General principles from both the American College of Surgeons (31) and the American College of Obstetricians and Gynecologists (1) suggest that **maternal stabilization takes priority over fetal assessment.** The standard algorithm in ATLS (Advanced Trauma Life Support) requires, in order, assessment and stabilization as shown in Table 39.1. These are addressed briefly, in regard to pregnant patients especially, in the following subsections.

Airway. Airway edema is more common in pregnant women, so smaller endotracheal tube size is required. Airway reflexes are not changed in pregnancy, but longer gastric emptying times and diminished function of the lower esophageal sphincter leave pregnant women more prone to aspiration of gastric contents.

Breathing. In pregnancy, minute ventilation is increased, functional residual capacity is decreased, so periods of apnea or hypopnea lead more quickly to hypoxemia.

Circulation. Physiologic changes in pregnancy include increased cardiac output, expanded plasma volume, peripheral vasodilation, and a decrease in systolic and diastolic blood pressure. As a result, the signs of hypovolemia are seen later in pregnant women because of these compensatory mechanisms. Tachycardia and narrowed pulse pressure are late findings as pregnant women progress through the stages of hypovolemic shock. Fetal heart rate should be evaluated as an additional vital sign. A normal fetal heart rate suggests normal uterine perfusion, while an abnormal FHR may reflect compromised perfusion and function as an early warning sign of decreased circulatory volume. **Maintenance of left uterine displacement** is important in maintaining preload and cardiac output after mid-pregnancy because of the effect of the gravid uterus on compressing the inferior vena cava. If the patient is visibly pregnant to the prehospital provider, the supine position should be avoided.

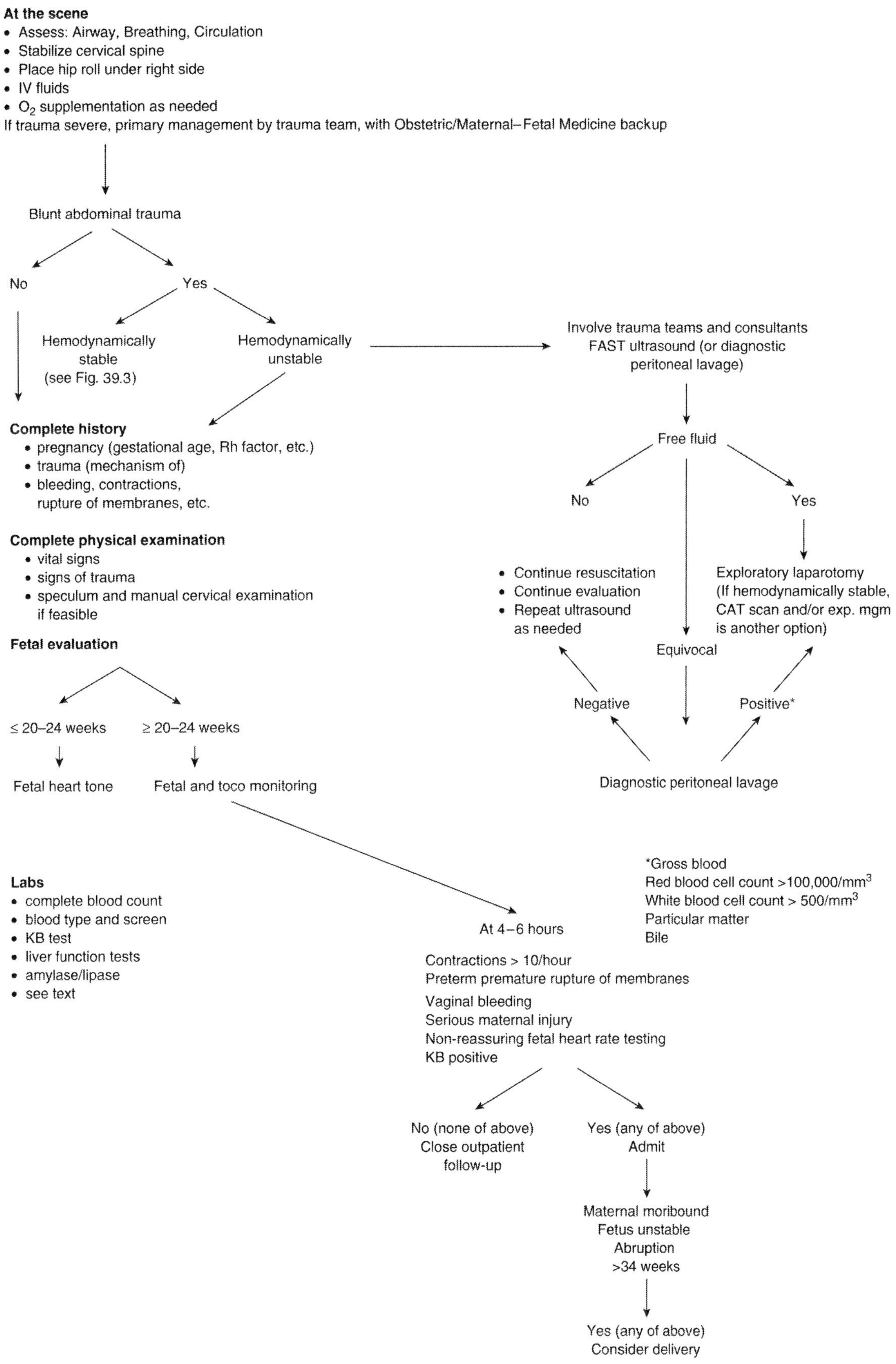

At the scene
- Assess: Airway, Breathing, Circulation
- Stabilize cervical spine
- Place hip roll under right side
- IV fluids
- O$_2$ supplementation as needed

If trauma severe, primary management by trauma team, with Obstetric/Maternal–Fetal Medicine backup

Blunt abdominal trauma

No → Yes

Hemodynamically stable (see Fig. 39.3)

Hemodynamically unstable → Involve trauma teams and consultants FAST ultrasound (or diagnostic peritoneal lavage)

Free fluid

No → Yes

- Continue resuscitation
- Continue evaluation
- Repeat ultrasound as needed

Exploratory laparotomy (If hemodynamically stable, CAT scan and/or exp. mgm is another option)

Equivocal

Negative ← → Positive*

Diagnostic peritoneal lavage

Complete history
- pregnancy (gestational age, Rh factor, etc.)
- trauma (mechanism of)
- bleeding, contractions, rupture of membranes, etc.

Complete physical examination
- vital signs
- signs of trauma
- speculum and manual cervical examination if feasible

Fetal evaluation

≤ 20–24 weeks   ≥ 20–24 weeks

Fetal heart tone   Fetal and toco monitoring

Labs
- complete blood count
- blood type and screen
- KB test
- liver function tests
- amylase/lipase
- see text

*Gross blood
Red blood cell count >100,000/mm^3
White blood cell count > 500/mm^3
Particular matter
Bile

At 4–6 hours

Contractions > 10/hour
Preterm premature rupture of membranes
Vaginal bleeding
Serious maternal injury
Non-reassuring fetal heart rate testing
KB positive

No (none of above) Close outpatient follow-up

Yes (any of above) Admit

Maternal moribound
Fetus unstable
Abruption
>34 weeks

Yes (any of above)
Consider delivery

Figure 39.2 Evaluation and management of trauma in pregnancy. *Abbreviations*: FAST, focused abdominal sonography for trauma; KB, Kleihauer–Betke; exp. mgm, expectant management.

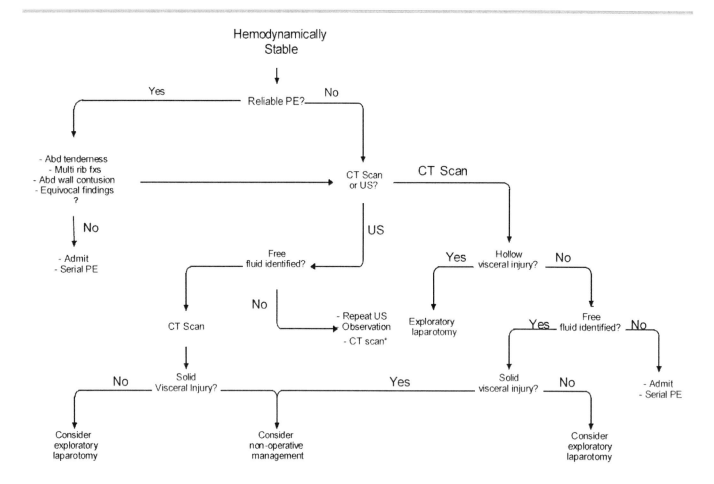

*CT scan may be elected based on institutional experience or clinical suspicion of intra-abdominal injury.

Figure 39.3 Evaluation and management of blunt abdominal trauma in the stable patient. *Abbreviations*: PE, physical exam; ABD, abdominal; Multi, multiple; fxs, fractures; CT, computed tomography; US, ultrasound. *Source*: From Ref. 30.

After maternal and fetal **stabilization**, complete **history** (pregnancy and gestational age, trauma, etc.), review of records (ultrasounds, laboratory test—Rh factor), and more extensive **physical** examination (vital signs, signs of trauma, uterine tenderness, speculum, and manual exam) should be performed. In severe trauma, history may be unobtainable as the patient's neurologic status is compromised. The mechanism of injury is an important part of the history. Uterine tenderness may be unreliable. Speculum/manual exam is often not feasible because the patient is in c-spine immobilization or has pelvic fractures.

Perimortem Cesarean Delivery
If efforts to resuscitate the pregnant patient are unsuccessful or if the patient expires, perimortem cesarean section should be performed for patients in the third trimester. While no controlled trials exist to establish optimal fetal and maternal outcomes, it has been reported that **the best fetal outcomes occur with delivery within five minutes** with higher fetal mortality rates occurring at greater than 10 minutes **of cardiopulmonary arrest** (32).

Evaluation and Diagnostic Studies
Appropriate studies should not be withheld because of pregnancy.

1. CT is recommended for evaluation of hemodynamically stable patients with associated neurological injury, multiple nonabdominal injury, or equivocal physical examination. Patients with a negative CT should nonetheless be admitted for observation (30) (radiation concerns, see below and Tables 39.2–39.4) (33).
2. **Blunt abdominal trauma** (Figs. 39.2 and 39.3)
   a. **FAST ultrasound:** The maternal abdomen can be evaluated for the presence of intraperitoneal blood with diagnostic peritoneal lavage (DPL) or with ultrasound; the FAST scan (focused abdominal sonography for trauma: 4-quadrant ultrasound to look for free fluid in abdomen or pelvis) has supplanted DPL in most institutions (30). FAST scan has 80% sensitivity and 100% specificity for intra-abdominal injury in the pregnant patient following blunt abdominal trauma (34). However, in penetrating injury, FAST scan is reported to have sensitivity of 28% to 100% and specificity of 94% to 100% in the general (nonpregnant) population (35). If DPL is elected, it is typically performed with an open technique in pregnancy. Both these techniques avoid ionizing radiation altogether.
   b. Exploratory laparotomy is indicated for a positive FAST (35) or DPL (30).

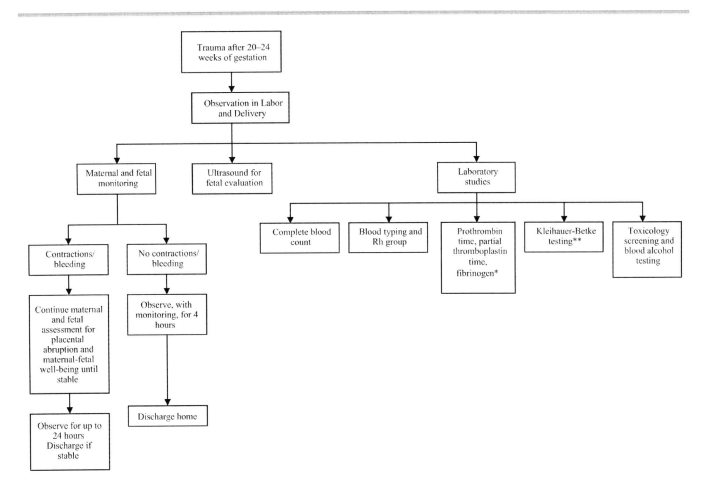

*not evidence-based, and not indicated in all cases; ** Detects maternal-fetal hemorrhage and allows calculation of immune globulin dosing in Rh-negative women (immune globulin 30 μg covers up to 15 mL. of red cells bleed)
Adapted from ref 19: Brown. Trauma in Pregnancy. Obstet Gynecol 2009.

Figure 39.4 Evaluation of common minor (not blunt) trauma in labor and delivery. *Source*: Adapted from Ref. 19.

Table 39.1 Maternal Stabilization After Trauma in Pregnancy: Advanced Trauma Life Support Principles

- **Airway**
- **Breathing**
- **Circulation**
- **Disability** (neurological evaluation)
- **Exposure**, environmental control (looking everywhere else for injuries, and keeping them warm)
- **Fetus**

Table 39.2 Estimates of Fetal Radiation Dose for the Following Examinations

Examination	Mean fetal dose (mGy)	Maximum fetal dose (mGy)
Skull	<0.01	<0.01
Chest	<0.01	<0.01
Abdomen	1.4	4.2
Thoracic spine	<0.01	<0.01
Lumbar spine	1.7	10
Pelvis	1.1	4
IVP	1.7	10

Source: From Ref. 33.

Table 39.3 Estimates of Fetal Radiation Exposure with Computed Tomography (CT)

CT examination	Mean fetal dose (mGy)	Maximum fetal dose (mGy)
Head	<0.005	<0.005
Chest	0.06	0.96
Abdomen	8.0	49
Lumbar spine	2.4	8.6
Pelvis	25	79
Pelvimetry	0.2	0.4

Source: From Ref. 33.

Table 39.4 Threshold Doses by Gestational Age for the Appearance of Embryo/Fetus Death or Congenital Malformation

Weeks from LMP	Embryo/fetus death	Congenital malformation
No threshold at conception		
4 to 7	250–500 mGy	200 mGy
7 to 9	500 mGy	500 mGy
9 to 23	>500 mGy	Very few observed
23 to term	>1000 mGy	Very few observed

Source: From Ref. 33.

3. In hemodynamically stable patients with positive FAST scan, follow-up CT scan should be considered.
4. **Penetrating abdominal wound: Single preoperative** dose of broad-spectrum **antibiotic** (30).
5. **Open fractures:** Preoperative prophylactic **antibiotics** with gram-positive coverage, administered as soon as possible after injury (30).
6. **Special pregnancy-specific evaluations/studies:**
    a. **Fetal ultrasound:** there is insufficient evidence to assess the effectiveness of performing a fetal ultrasound in the woman with trauma in pregnancy. Assessment of fetus, AFV, and placenta by ultrasound may be beneficial for management. Ultrasound detects placental abruption when this involves >50% of the placenta, so that negative ultrasound does not exclude abruption, especially since abruption may develop days after the initial trauma.
    b. **Fetal monitoring:** There is insufficient evidence to assess fetal monitoring and especially its duration in the woman with trauma in pregnancy. Assessment of fetal status may be beneficial as the fetus is often one of the most sensitive "organs" to be affected by maternal circulatory compromise. If done, continuous monitoring is suggested. More than one-third of third trimester women with trauma have ominous findings on monitoring (14). The fact that maternal and fetal outcomes are worse in women who do not have electronic monitoring in some reports (14) reflects the team priorities (more severely injured mothers require interventions that preclude fetal monitoring, or electronic monitoring is deemed of low priority).
    c. **Tocodynamometer or contraction monitoring:** At >20 weeks' gestation, >90% of women with trauma presenting for evaluation demonstrate some uterine contractions in first four hours, with uterine activity decreasing over time. Within the first hour, 64% were contracting with a frequency of every five minutes or more, declining to 29% by hour 4 (20). Patients without contractions or whose contractions never exceed q10 minute frequency were discharged at the end of four hours, and none had abruption (20). Those who had been contracting at more than q11 minute frequency were all kept for at least 24 hours. There was one placental abruption at six hours, resulting in emergent delivery for fetal distress, and among the patients hospitalized beyond 24 hours, there was a 40% delivery rate, with one stillborn infant. Total abruption rate was 8% (20). From these data comes the common recommendation for **monitoring at least four hours after maternal trauma.** Expert opinion (EAST Practice Management Guidelines) has alternatively recommended a minimum of six hours of monitoring, despite acknowledging that the best duration of monitoring is unknown (5). In nearly 5% of trauma in pregnancy cases, fetal compromise or placental abruption becomes evident only after prolonged monitoring (6–48 hours or more) (36).
    d. The **Kleihauer–Betke (KB)** test assesses presence of fetal red blood cells in the maternal circulation. This test is based on the premise that fetal hemoglobin (Hb F) is resistant to acid elution. KB is particularly helpful with Rh-negative women to determine dose of Rh immune globulin needed to prevent rhesus isoimmunization. While the test is inexpensive and simple to perform, it has been criticized for its subjectivity and lack of repro-

ducibility (37). Using known admixtures of fetal and maternal blood, KB testing overestimates the volume of fetomaternal hemorrhage and has been demonstrated to vary more than 10-fold with repeat testing of a single sample (37). Some have advocated substitution of flow cytometry (using a fluorescence-activated cell sorter) or monoclonal antibodies to Hb F as a test for fetomaternal hemorrhage; while these are both sensitive and more precise, they are expensive and not widely available. Twenty percent of pregnant trauma patients who had KB drawn had positive results, although the test proved neither sensitive nor specific for a poor outcome (36): 96% of traumatized women with a positive KB (defined as >0.01 mL of fetal blood in the maternal circulation) had preterm contractions, half of whom also had cervical change, while none of those with a negative test had any contractions during the period of surveillance, which encompassed a minimum of four hours. The likelihood ratio of a positive KB for predicting preterm labor was calculated at greater than 20. In addition, women who required delivery for fetal compromise shortly after admission all had a positive KB (38).
    e. **Coagulation studies** (e.g., fibrinogen, D-dimer, PT, and PTT): there is no evidence of benefit of coagulation studies, unless massive hemorrhage has occurred or is expected.
    f. **Admission:** admission to the hospital for **longer (≥24–48 hours) observation** should be considered for women with evidence of **persistent (>4/hour) contractions, preterm premature rupture of membranes, abruption on ultrasound, positive KB, bleeding, nonreassuring fetal heart rate tracing, or other abnormal fetal testing** with continuous fetal and uterine monitoring.

The indication for **tetanus prophylaxis** do not change during pregnancy (see chapter 38).

Radiation in the Pregnant Trauma Patient

Recent estimates of **fetal radiation dose** for the following examinations are shown in Table 39.2 (33).

Gray is the unit of measurement for absorbed dose; it is defined as 1 J of energy deposited in 1 kg of material. This has replaced the rad or roentgen-absorbed dose, which is defined as the dose delivered to an object of 100 ergs of energy per gram of material. One Gray = 100 rads (or, 1 rad = 10 mGy). **Teratologic effects start usually after 5 to 10 mGy.** Plain radiographs of the spine and chest can be performed in pregnancy with minimal radiation exposure to the fetus, with abdomen and pelvis shielding. With CT scanning, the total radiation dose to the fetus depends on the site imaged, the machine and technique used, and on the distance between cuts.

Recent estimates of fetal radiation exposure with **computed tomography** (CT) are shown in Table 39.3 (33).

Since the actual fetal dose given in a procedure may be as much as 10-fold higher than the published mean dose, depending on the patient's size and the technique used, **actual dose should be estimated** wherever possible **by contacting the institution's radiation physicists for dosimetry.** The proxy for fetal radiation dose is uterine dose.

Concerns about radiation effects on the embryo or fetus include **death, malformation, growth restriction, abnormal development of the brain with severe cognitive sequelae, and cancer.** No data are available for cellular effects per se, only for clinical effects. Threshold doses for the appearance of death or malformation are shown in Table 39.4 (33). Data for cognitive impairment (mental retardation), based on survivors of the atomic bomb exposed in utero, suggest no effect with exposure before 10 weeks or after 27 weeks. These data do raise the possibility of a dose-response (rather than threshold) model between 10 and 17 weeks, with a loss of 30 IQ points per Gy (1000 mGy). Diagnostic radiologic procedures are orders of magnitude below these limits. Even in the 10- to 17-week fetus in which a dose-response curve may be postulated for cognitive impairment, an 80-mGy study, such as CT of the pelvis, would have only minimal potential to compromise intellectual function, for example, 2 IQ points.

Concerns have also been raised about the possibility of cancer induction in children exposed to intrauterine radiation. Unlike death or malformation, the induction of cancers is believed to be a dose-response rather than threshold phenomenon. Because childhood cancers are rare events, even a doubling or quadrupling of the risk has little impact on cancer deaths. Excess risk of fatal childhood cancer attributed to fetal exposure with typical diagnostic procedures range from 1 in 30,000 to 1 in 1700. The derived risk is estimated at 1 excess case per 33,000 per mGy of exposure. The highest risks, which remain quite small on a population basis, are seen with the highest exposures, for example, CT of the pelvis (33). This concern is not a reason to routinely offer termination of pregnancy (33,39). Recent estimates of conceptus radiation dose with a single anteroposterior chest radiograph (assuming an average maternal size: dose increases with increasing maternal size) range from 0.0021 to 0.0028 mGy in the first trimester to 0.1 to 5.9 mGy in the second and 0.1 to 1.9 mGy in the third trimester (40). This corresponds to an excess risk of childhood cancer of approximately 10 per million.

Ultrasound and magnetic resonance imaging (MRI) do not utilize radiation energy and are not associated with adverse effects on the embryo or fetus. MRI, however, is used less in the setting of trauma. When indicated, however, mutagenic and teratogenic effects have not been reported with the use of gadolinium or iodinated contrast (41).

PRENATAL CARE

If the pregnant patient who had trauma can be discharged undelivered, she should be counseled that abruption, PTB, and other complications can occur even after discharge (even >10 weeks) of a stable woman after trauma. Even if they have been discharged from the hospital, women who suffered trauma in pregnancy should be aware that a normal baby outcome cannot be guaranteed. Therefore, education and written discharge instructions regarding fetal kick counts, signs of labor, and abruption (vaginal bleeding, uterine tenderness or persistent abdominal pain) should be given.

ANTEPARTUM TESTING

There is no trial to assess effectiveness of testing in this population.

DELIVERY

No specific recommendations.

ANESTHESIA

No specific recommendations.

POSTPARTUM/BREAST-FEEDING

No specific recommendations.

PENETRATING INJURIES IN THE PREGNANT PATIENT

Penetrating injuries in the pregnant patient are evaluated in a similar fashion as the nonpregnant patient, with some special considerations. Depending on gestational age and uterine size, the fetus may potentially be at risk of injury. The uterus remains within the pelvis until the twelfth week of gestation. As the uterus enlarges and constrains intraperitoneal organs restricting the intestines to the upper abdomen, it also protects these organs in the event of penetrating injury. Gunshot wounds tend to have a poorer prognosis than stab injuries. In the unstable patient, resuscitation and exploratory laparotomy are indicated. In the hemodynamically stable patient, attempt should be made to use noninvasive diagnostic modalities such as FAST or CT imaging. If a gunshot wound appears to have penetrated the uterus and the fetus is of viable gestational age, cesarean delivery may be indicated (10). Studies specifically addressing penetrating injuries in the pregnant patient are lacking.

REFERENCES

1. American College of Obstetricians (Webb) Gynecologists. Obstetric aspects of trauma management. ACOG Educational Bulletin No. 251, 1998, Washington DC: ACOG. [The American College of Obstetricians and Gynecologists quotes trauma rates of 1 in 12 pregnancies, but it is unclear how the figure was obtained.]

2. Ikossi DG, Lazar AA, Morabito D, et al. Profile of mothers at risk: an analysis of injury and pregnancy loss in 1195 trauma patients. J Am Coll Surg 2005; 200:49–56. [The American College of Surgeons maintains a National Trauma Data Bank (NTDB)—data collected from 130 trauma centers in the United States, including level I, level II, and level III facilities. Review of the NTDB between 1994 and 2001 compared 1195 female admissions that were additionally coded as pregnant to a control group of 76,126 injured women in the same age group. Since during this time there were approximately 27 million live births in the United States (NCHS), that equates to four trauma center admissions per 100,000 live births.]

3. Schiff MA, Holt VL. Pregnancy outcomes following hospitalization for motor vehicle crashes in Washington State from 1989 to 2001. Am J Epidemiol 2005; 161:503–510. [State of Washington hospitalizations for MVA in pregnancy from 1989 to 2001, n = 625]

4. El Kady D, Gilbert WM, Anderson J, et al. Trauma during pregnancy: an analysis of maternal and fetal outcomes in a large population. Am J Obstet Gynecol 2004; 190(6):1661–1668. [California large cohort: 10,316 women who sustained trauma during a pregnancy of at least 20 weeks' gestation identified via a statewide hospital discharge database from 1991 to 1999]

5. Barraco RD, Chiu WC, Clancy TV, et al.; EAST Practice Management Guidelines Work Group. Practice management guidelines for the diagnosis and management of injury in the pregnant patient: the EAST Practice Management Guidelines Workgroup. J Trauma 2010; 69(1):211–214. [III, review]

6. Saltzman LE, Johnson CH, Gilbert BC, et al. Physical abuse around the time of pregnancy: an examination of prevalence and risk factors in 16 states. Matern Child Health J 2003; 7 (1):31–43. [II-3]

7. Weiss HB, Strotmeyer S. Characteristics of pregnant women in motor vehicle crashes. Inj Prev 2002; 8:207–210. [1995–1999 National Automotive Sampling System Crashworthiness Data System, drawn from police-reported traffic accidents]

8. Hyde LK, Cook LJ, Olson LM, et al. Effect of motor vehicle crashes on adverse fetal outcome. Obstet Gynecol 2003; 102:279–286. [II-3]

9. Aboutanos SZ, Aboutanos MB, Dompokowski D, et al. Predictors of fetal outcome in pregnant trauma patients: a five-year institutional review. Am Surg 2007; 73(8):824–827. [II-3]

10. Petrone P, Talving P, Browder T, et al. Abdominal injuries in pregnancy: a 155-month study at two level 1 trauma centers. Injury. 2011; 42(1):47–49. [II-3]

11. Cahill AG, Bastek JA, Stamilio DM, et al. Minor trauma in pregnancy—is the evaluation warranted? Am J Obstet Gynecol 2008; 198:208.e1–208.e5. [II-2. Prospective cohort of 256 complete records of patients with minor trauma. Rate of positive KB at presentation 2.8%. Adverse pregnancy outcome in this cohort consisted of 19.2% with no statistically significant association of any single predictor variable or in combination.]

12. Corsi PR, Rasslan S, de Oliveira LB, et al. Trauma in pregnant women: analysis of maternal and fetal mortality. Injury 1999; 30:239–243. [II-3. Fetal death: Corsi's 315; Shah's 14% if you don't count elective abortions; Rogers was 9%; Warner's—a fairly small study—was 6%; and Theodorou's 18%. Maternal death: Corsi 12%, Shah 9%, Rogers 4%, and Warner 3%]

13. Shah KH, Simons RK, Holbrook T, et al. Trauma in pregnancy: maternal and fetal outcomes. J Trauma 1998; 45:83–86. [II-3]

14. Rogers FB, Rozycki GS, Osler TM, et al. A multi-institutional study of factors associated with fetal death in injured pregnant patients. Arch Surg 1999; 134:1274–1277. [II-3]

15. Warner MW, Salfinger SG, Rao S, et al. Management of trauma during pregnancy. ANZ J Surg 2004; 74:125–128. [II-3]

16. Theodorou DA, Velmahos GC, Souter I, et al. Fetal death after trauma in pregnancy. Am Surg 2000; 66:809–812. [II-3]

17. Chang J, Berg CJ, Saltzmann LE, et al. Homicide: a leading cause of injury deaths among pregnant and postpartum women in the United States, 1991–1999. Am J Public Health 2005; 95:471–477. [Pregnancy Mortality Surveillance System, established in 1989 by the Center for Disease Control, identified 7342 deaths among women who were pregnant or within one year postpartum]

18. Boccichio GV, Napolitano LM, Hann J, et al. Incidental pregnancy in trauma patients. J Am Coll Surg 2001; 192:566–569. [II-3]

19. Brown HL. Trauma in pregnancy. Obstet Gynecol 2009; 114 (1):147–160. [III, review]

20. Pearlman MD, Tintinalli JE, Lorenz RP. A prospective controlled study of outcome after trauma during pregnancy. Am J Obstet Gynecol 1990; 162:1502–1510. [II-2; *n* = 60. Recommendations for at least four hours of monitoring]

21. Weintraub AY, Levy A, Holcberg G, et al. The outcome of blunt abdominal trauma preceding birth. Int J Fertil Womens Med 2006; 51(6):275–279. [II-2]

22. Weiss HB, Songer TJ, Fabio A. Fetal deaths related to maternal injury. JAMA 2001; 286:1863–1868. [Fetal death certificates in 16 U.S. States, 1995–1997]

23. Curet MJ, Schermer CR, Demarest GB, et al. Predictors of outcome in trauma during pregnancy: identification of patients who can safely be monitored for less than 6 hours. J Trauma 2000; 49:18–24. [Eight years' experience at a large level I trauma center; 271 pregnant women who were admitted after blunt trauma; reviewed delivery outcomes in approximately half]

24. El Kady D, Gilbert WM, Xing G, et al. Maternal and neonatal outcomes of assaults during pregnancy. Obstet Gynecol 2005; 105:357–363. [II-3, *n* = 2070 pregnant women hospitalized following an assault]

25. Centers for Disease Control and Prevention. Web-based Injury Statistics Query and Reporting System (WISQARS). Available at: http://www.cdc.gov/injury/wisqars. August 23, 2011. [Review]

26. Klinich KD, Flannagan CAC, Rupp JD, et al. Fetal outcome in motor-vehicle crashes: effects of crash characteristics and maternal restraint. Am J Obstet Gynecol 2008; 198:450.e1–450.e9. [II-3]

27. MotozawaY, Hitosugi M, Abe T, et al. Effects of seat belts worn by pregnant drivers during low-impact collisions. Am J Obstet Gynecol 2010; 203:62.e1–62.e8. [II-3]

28. Schiff MA, Mack CD, Kaufman RP, et al. The effect of air bags on pregnancy outcomes in Washington State, 2002–2005. Obstet Gynecol 2010; 115:85–92. [II-2]

29. Metz TD, Abbott JT. Uterine Trauma in pregnancy after motor vehicle crashes with airbag deployment: a 30-case series. J Trauma 2006; 61:658–661. [II-3]

30. Hoff WS, Holevar M, Nagy KK, et al.; for the EAST Practice Management Guidelines Work Group. Practice management guidelines for the management of blunt abdominal trauma. 2001. Eastern Association for the Surgery of Trauma. Available at: http://www.east.org/tpg/bluntabd.pdf. Accessed September 10, 2005. [III, review]

31. American College of Surgeons. Advanced Trauma Life Support for Doctors (Student Course Manual). Chicago IL: American College of Surgeons, 1997. [III, review]

32. Katz VL, Dotters DJ, Droegemueller W. Perimortem cesarean delivery. Obstet Gynecol 1986; 68:571–576. [III]

33. Health Protection Agency, the Royal College of Radiologists and the College of Radiographers. Protection of pregnant patients during diagnostic medical exposures to ionizing radiation: advice from the Health Protection Agency, the Royal College of Radiologists and the College of Radiographers. 2009. Available at: http://www.hpa.org.uk/web/HPAwebFile/HPAweb_C/1238230848746. Accessed November 20, 2010. [III, review]

34. Brown MA, Sirlin CB, Farahmand N, et al. Screening sonography in pregnant patients with blunt abdominal trauma. J Ultrasound Med 2005; 24:175–179. [II-3]

35. Quinn AC, Sinert R. What is the utility of the Focused Assessment with Sonography in Trauma (FAST) exam in penetrating torso trauma? Injury. 2011; 42(5):482–487. [III, review]

36. Dahmus MA, Sibai BM. Blunt abdominal trauma: are there any predictive factors for abruption placentae or maternal-fetal distress? Am J Obstet Gynecol 1993; 169:1054–1059. [II-2; 1988–1991; 233 patients >20 weeks' gestation admitted after noncatastrophic abdominal trauma. Unusually, in this population assaults and falls each outnumbered motor vehicle accidents. Duration of monitoring ranged from 0 to 120 hours, with a mean of 13 hours]

37. Ochsenbein-Imhof N, Ochsenbein AF, Seifert B, et al. Quantification of fetomaternal hemorrhage by fluorescence microscopy is equivalent to flow cytometry. Transfusion 2002; 42:947–953. [II-3]

38. Muench MV, Baschat AA, Reddy UM, et al. Kleihauer–Betke testing is important in all cases of maternal trauma. J Trauma 2004; 57:1094–1098. [II-2]

39. ACOG. Guidelines for diagnostic imaging during pregnancy. ACOG Committee Opinion No. 299. Obstet Gynecol 2004; 104:647–651. [III]

40. Damilakis J, Perisinakis K, Prassopoulos P, et al. Conceptus radiation dose and risk from chest screen-film radiography. Eur Radiol 2003; 13:406–412. [II-2]

41. Webb JA, Thomsen HS, Morcos SK, Members of Contrast Media Safety Committee of European Society of Urogenital Radiology (ESUR). The use of iodinated and gadolinium contrast media during pregnancy and lactation. Eur Radiol 2005; 15:1234–1240. [III]

40

Critical care

Lauren A. Plante

KEY POINTS

- In the developed world, <1% of maternity admissions require admission to intensive care, but up to 5% require admission to intermediate care or high-dependency unit.
- Most maternal admissions to ICU are postpartum.
- Antepartum admission to ICU is associated with high rates of preterm birth.
- Best ventilator strategy in pregnant women with acute respiratory distress syndrome is unknown, but fetal monitoring may be useful in determining ventilator settings.
- Early recognition and appropriate treatment of sepsis reduces mortality.

BACKGROUND

The field of maternal critical care remains insufficiently researched. While many recommendations in critical care are based on good evidence, little is specifically focused on pregnant or postpartum women. Much of this chapter will, perforce, address general critical care, extrapolating to maternal critical care whenever possible.

INCIDENCE

In the developed world, between **1 and 8/1000 obstetric admissions are managed in an intensive care unit (ICU)** (1–11). Among this population, the risk of death ranges from 2% to 11%, a figure that, while better than average ICU mortality in a general population, is orders of magnitude higher than the maternal mortality ratio in the developed world.

Figures on ICU admission do *not* include women with similarly life-threatening conditions who are treated within the confines of a labor and delivery unit or specialized obstetric care unit. Another 1% to 5% of all women admitted for delivery require this type of care (12–14).

Audits of near-miss maternal mortality or severe acute maternal morbidity have been used to quantitate life-threatening conditions and therefore constitute a proxy for intensive care utilization. In Scotland, severe morbidity and near-miss events were recorded in 4/1000 deliveries, although only one-third of these ended up in ICU (8). Severe maternal morbidity also occurred in 4/1000 deliveries between 1991 and 2001 in Canada (15), but increased to 14/1000 between 2003 and 2007 (16). This increase in Canadian figures may represent differential classification, different datasets, or a real increase in severe acute maternal morbidity over time. Analysis of year-by-year data shows a steady increase in rates of acute renal failure, assisted ventilation, and major obstetrical hemorrhage in Canada (17). Admission to an ICU was reported in 2.4/1000 deliveries in the Netherlands, but only one-third of women with serious maternal morbidity were cared for in the ICU (18). Recent population-based estimates put rates of severe morbidity among delivering women at 5/1000 in the United States (19). Given four million births per year (20), a rate of 5/1000 would equate to 20,000 cases of severe morbidity among pregnant and postpartum women in the United States per year. **The need for maternal critical care appears to be increasing in the developed world**, influenced largely by an increase in both the rate of postpartum hemorrhage and the risk of adverse outcomes among women with postpartum hemorrhage (21,22). One may predict that the need will continue to rise in parallel with a rising cesarean rate (23,24).

ORGANIZATION OF CRITICAL CARE

The American College of Critical Care Medicine (ACCM) describes **three levels of adult ICUs**: (25).

> *Level I critical care*: Typically found in university medical centers; provide comprehensive, sometimes specialized, critical care. They require continuous availability of sophisticated technologies (Table 40.1), highly trained nursing staff, and physicians with critical care training immediately available at the bedside. Comprehensive support services are in place.
>
> *Level II critical care*: Although level II centers can provide comprehensive critical care, they lack resources for highly specialized subpopulations, such as cardiothoracic patients, and must have arrangements in place to transfer out patients who exceed their expertise.
>
> *Level III critical care*: Level III ICUs provide only initial stabilization of critically ill patients, followed by transfer for comprehensive critical care to a level I or II facility.

An alternative to the ICU is the **intermediate care or high-dependency unit (HDU)** (26). Patients who require frequent monitoring of vital signs or frequent nursing interventions but do not need specific ICU life-support treatments may be admitted to such a unit. The intermediate care unit is staffed at lower nursing levels and includes less complex technology than the ICU, which makes it less expensive to run, frees up beds in the ICU, and has been associated with greater family satisfaction. Intermediate care units include post-ICU step-down units, telemetry units for cardiac patients, etc.

Low-risk monitor patients are those predicted to be at low risk of requiring active life-saving treatment, such as mechanical ventilation or vasopressors. The most frequent monitoring services deployed in the care of such patients in the ICU are **ECG (>99%), intra-arterial BP monitoring (51%), and pulse oximetry (33%)**, and the most frequent labor-intensive nursing interventions were intake/output measurement, hourly vital signs, and hourly neurologic checks (27). When planning obstetric critical care services, the intermediate care unit is a good approximation of the type and acuity of services needed. However, recent experience in 2009 with novel

Table 40.1 Equipment and Support That an ICU Should Be Prepared to Provide

Continuous ECG monitoring (with high/low alarms), all patients
Continuous arterial pressure monitoring (invasive and noninvasive)
Central venous pressure monitoring
Transcutaneous oxygen monitoring or pulse oximetry for all patients receiving supplemental oxygen
Airway equipment, including laryngoscopes and endotracheal tubes
Ventilatory equipment: Ambu bags, ventilators, oxygen, compressed air
Emergency resuscitation equipment
Equipment to support hemodynamically unstable patients: infusion pumps, blood/fluid warmers, pressure bags, blood filters
Beds with removable headboard and adjustable position; various specialty beds
Adequate lighting for bedside procedures
Suction
Cooling/warming blankets
Scales
Temporary pacemakers (transcutaneous and transvenous)
Temperature monitoring devices
Pulmonary artery pressure monitoring
Cardiac output monitoring
Continuous and intermittent dialysis and ultrafiltration
Peritoneal dialysis
Capnography
Fiberoptic bronchoscopy
Intracranial pressure monitoring
Continuous EEG monitoring capability
Positive and negative pressure isolation rooms
Immediate access to information (medical books, journals; drug information, poison control; personnel phone and page numbers; patient lab and test data; medical record information)

Source: Adapted from Ref. 25

influenza should remind us that pregnant women are at higher risk of respiratory failure, and a contingency plan for epidemic flu (and other respiratory infections) must be made, including provision of mechanical ventilatory support (28–30).

ORGANIZATION OF OBSTETRIC CRITICAL CARE SERVICES

If the discipline of critical care is young, that of obstetric critical care is younger still. **There are no evidence-based recommendations published specifically for critical care in pregnancy.** The interested practitioner must extrapolate from the general critical care literature instead (31,32), or rely on expert opinion.

Hemorrhage and hypertension are, consistently, the **most common causes of admission from obstetrical services to intensive care** (1–11,15,18,33–47). The majority of these patients require monitoring and only simple interventions. The degree of nursing care involved, while higher-acuity than on most general wards, is well within the abilities of most labor and delivery nurses in a specialty or subspecialty care facility (perinatal care services level II and III) (48). The intermediate care unit or HDU is also designed to provide care of this type.

A smaller number of obstetrical patients have nonobstetric causes for ICU admission: these amount to 20% to 30% of the total (1,5,7,13). **Most obstetric patients who are admitted to ICU are sent there postpartum rather than undelivered** (5,6,36). The preponderance of postpartum over antepartum admissions may stem from postpartum vulnerability (e.g., postpartum hemorrhage, postpartum decompensation of cardiac disease) or to ascertainment bias: obstetricians may be

reluctant to transfer, or intensivists to accept, a patient whose fetus must be considered in management. In the rare case of an "obstetrical ICU" existing within a labor/delivery unit, there is a higher percentage of both antepartum admissions and primary medical (nonobstetric) admissions (7,41). This may reflect lower threshold for admission to the obstetrical ICU (as no transfer or travel is involved); a need to justify the continuation of the service; or a preference to transfer out postpartum patients: labor and delivery (L&D) beds are a scarce commodity, and a postpartum patient requiring intensive care ties up space and personnel when she could be adequately cared for outside of the obstetric unit.

Most obstetrical services would be unable to implement a full-service obstetrical ICU. Both the technology and the personnel mandated by ICU guidelines are impracticable. **The HDU or intermediate care unit, however, is a reasonable model for much of obstetric critical care.** Published experience, albeit limited, is encouraging. A high-volume public hospital in Dallas admitted 1.7% of maternity cases to a five-bed Obstetrics Intermediate Care Unit, usually postpartum (80%), with a mean length of stay less than 24 hours (13). Of these 500 women, 15% subsequently were transferred to a full-service medical or surgical ICU, most for mechanical ventilation. A referral maternity hospital in Dublin opened a "high-dependency" or intermediate care unit (12). Prior to debut of the HDU, patients requiring intensive care services (0.1% of maternity admissions) were transferred out to another hospital with a medical/surgical ICU. After the obstetric HDU was established, the referral rate to the offsite ICU dropped by 50%, but the HDU was busier than one might have expected: 1% of maternity patients were admitted thereto, a 10-fold increase in the percentage of patients who were managed as higher acuity. The question as to whether this represents underutilization of needed services before the advent of the obstetric intermediate care unit, or overutilization after, cannot be answered. In a large women's hospital in Birmingham without an on-site ICU, a three-bed HDU within the delivery suite accommodated between 1% and 5% of all obstetric patients: the percentage has steadily been increasing over time (14). Among women admitted to this HDU, 3.5% were then transferred out to intensive care.

The American College of Critical Care Medicine states, "The Physician Director should meet guidelines for the definition of an intensivist and the practice of critical care medicine." **The definition of an intensivist (49) is one few obstetricians or maternal-fetal medicine specialists would be able to meet,** including not only skills, interest, and availability but also completion of an approved training program in critical care medicine. Mabie has suggested several ways in which an obstetrician might obtain some critical care training (41): a critical care fellowship, a residency in internal medicine, or a maternal-fetal medicine fellowship. Having acquired formal training would, of course, be insufficient if there is not enough clinical material to **maintain skills and expertise**: this is an even higher hurdle. Zeeman et al. (13) mentioned only that a maternal-fetal medicine faculty member was director of the OB intermediate care unit, without mentioning, as it would have been preferable, whether this individual had any critical care qualifications or training. Despite the patient volume, it appears that no mechanical ventilation, pulmonary artery catheterization, or vasopressor therapy was carried out in this unit: this is appropriate for an intermediate care unit, but ensures that providers' skills decay. The Birmingham HDU, which also appears to exclude mechanical ventilation (14), is described only as "staffed by qualified midwives" with anesthetic and obstetric teams covering.

Recommendations for nursing care in an ICU (25,49) state that **all nurses working in critical care should**: complete a clinical and didactic course in critical care before taking on patient responsibilities; participate in continuing education; and assume nurse-to-patient ratios either 1:2 *or* based on patient acuity. High nurse-to-patient ratios are already recommended on labor/delivery units (48) and would, therefore, be rather easy to implement. As above, acquiring and maintaining critical care skills would be more difficult.

Competence in core procedural skills is expected of any physician practicing in critical care (50):

1. Maintenance of airway (nonintubated patient)
2. Ventilation (bag and mask)
3. Endotracheal intubation
4. Management of pneumothorax
5. Arterial puncture; insertion of an arterial line
6. Central venous cannulation
7. Pulmonary artery catheterization (insertion, maintenance, interpretation)
8. ECG interpretation
9. Cardioversion, defibrillation

Some critical care techniques are used less frequently now than in the past. **Utilization of the pulmonary artery catheter has dropped by two-thirds in the past decade** (51) **following demonstration that its use is not associated with improvement in outcomes**. Noninvasive methods of ventilation have replaced mechanical ventilation in some cases. As some techniques are phased out, new ones appear, such as transesophageal echocardiography. Thus, the list here can only be taken as a snapshot of current critical care practice. Skill maintenance may not be feasible unless alternative means are sought, perhaps simulation-based or supervised experience.

CONSIDERATIONS IN TRANSFER (INTERHOSPITAL)

Preterm delivery may occur concurrently with critical illness, because of underlying medical or obstetric conditions, spontaneous preterm labor, or iatrogenic interventions. One case-control study (6) puts at 36 weeks the mean gestational age achieved by antepartum patients admitted to ICU. For respiratory failure in pregnancy, median gestational age achieved is 31 to 32 weeks (52,53). The Mayo series of 93 antepartum admissions to ICU reported that one-third resulted in fetal losses and one-half in preterm births (54). Thus, it would appear prudent that **a pregnant woman requiring ICU services, after achieving a gestational age compatible with extrauterine viability, should be managed in a facility with both adult and neonatal ICU capability. Guidelines for perinatal transfer (48) advocate antenatal over neonatal transfer**. In the event that maternal transport is unsafe or impossible, alternative arrangements for neonatal transport must be made.

Transfer in cases of critical illness is more complex than the usual perinatal transfer. The transport process increases risk of morbidity and mortality for the critically ill (55), and therefore cannot be embarked upon lightly. Once the decision to transfer has been made and the patient (or her designated decision-maker) has consented, she should be transferred as expeditiously as possible to the receiving facility that has agreed to accept her. If the patient is unstable, she should be **stabilized and/or resuscitated to the best possible condition prior to transport**, albeit with the understanding that complete stabilization may not be possible outside of the receiving facility. Transport may be by ground or air, based on the urgency of the patient's condition, the distance between facilities, weather conditions, potential interventions during transport, and equipment or personnel available. **The minimum monitoring of a critically ill patient during transport includes continuous pulse oximetry and ECG as well as regular assessment of vital signs** (55). Patients who already have arterial or central lines should have those monitored as well. Women who are mechanically ventilated must have the endotracheal tube position confirmed and secured before transport and must be assessed for adequacy of oxygenation and ventilation. All critically ill patients must have secure venous access before transport.

Opinion, but no data, guides us as to additional monitoring during transport of the critically ill obstetrical patient. Patients at high risk of delivering en route should be held at the initial hospital until delivered, since there is unlikely to be access to both the patient's head and her vagina in tight transport quarters, most transport teams lack expertise in delivery and neonatal resuscitation, and a dedicated neonatal transport team can be summoned for the newborn. There is little benefit in tocodynamometry during the transport process. Fetal monitoring during transport may be feasible to perform but is of unproven utility. Because fetal monitoring equipment takes up space in tight quarters and there is little or nothing the transport team can do en route for an ominous tracing, it seems preferable to avoid fetal monitoring when transporting a critically ill obstetric patient. Simple measures such as left uterine displacement and supplemental oxygen should be routine during transport of the critically ill pregnant patient.

ADMISSION TO INTENSIVE CARE

The commonest reasons for transfer to ICU are, reliably, hemorrhage and hypertension, and most admissions are postpartum. Specialty and subspecialty perinatal centers (48) may be able to care for such patients on the labor and delivery unit, particularly if an intermediate care unit or HDU is located there. Level I centers (basic care facilities), however, should consider transfer either to a higher-level perinatal center or to the ICU at their own facility. In cases where both obstetric and critical care services are at the most basic level, transfer of such patients to another facility may be the best approach. A small number of OB-GYN specialty hospitals exist in the United States (56): these may have limited critical care support or consultation available and might therefore also have a low threshold for transfer. Obstetrics services in such hospitals should have a set of **site-specific guidelines established at the hospital level**.

The American College of Obstetricians and Gynecologists has suggested adoption of an objective parameters model (57,58) when deciding need for maternal critical care: see Table 40.2.

In any center, a decision to transfer to ICU should be made on the basis of need for site-specific care. An obstetric service should adopt guidelines for transfer based on the level of care required, modified by the level of care that could be provided on the labor floor or within an existing obstetric intermediate care unit.

LOGISTICS

Zeeman proposed a "blueprint" for obstetric critical care (13,59): an intermediate care unit in the obstetric setting. She lists as advantages the "concurrent availability of expert obstetric care and critical care management ... the option of continuous fetal

Table 40.2 Objective Parameters Model: Criteria for Admission to ICU

Vital signs
  Heart rate <40 or >150 bpm
  Blood pressure <80 mmHg systolic (or 20 mmHg below the
    patient's usual BP)
  Mean arterial pressure <60 mmHg
  Blood pressure >120 mm diastolic
  Respiratory rate >35/min
Laboratory values (new)
  Serum sodium <110 or >170 mEq/L
  Serum potassium <2.0 or >7.0 mEq/L
  PaO_2 <50 mmHg
  pH < 7.1 or > 7.7
  Serum calcium > 15 mg/dL
  Serum glucose > 800 mg/dL
  Toxic drug level in a hemodynamically or neurologically
    compromised patient
Imaging (new)
  Cerebrovascular hemorrhage, contusion or subarachnoid
    hemorrhage with altered mental status or focal neurologic
    findings
  Ruptured viscus or esophageal varices with hemodynamic
    instability
  Dissecting aortic aneurysm
ECG
  MI with complex arrhythmia, hemodynamic instability or
    congestive heart failure
  Sustained ventricular tachycardia or ventricular fibrillation
  Complete heart block with hemodynamic instability
Physical findings (new)
  Airway obstruction
  Anuria
  Burns > 10% of body surface area
  Cardiac tamponade
  Coma
  Continuous seizures
  Cyanosis
  Unequal pupils (unconscious patient)

Source: Adapted from Ref. 57.

monitoring with on-hand expertise in its interpretation ... the advantages of keeping mother and infant together combined with the improved continuity of antenatal and postnatal care" (59). This seems indisputable for units that are big enough to keep up expertise. For lower-volume centers, however, it is not always feasible, and for even the largest services, there will be patients who are best treated in a full-service ICU.

Better outcomes are demonstrated in a general medical/ surgical ICU population when specialized ICU physicians staff the unit. High-intensity ICU physician staffing (either a closed ICU model or mandatory intensivist consultation) is associated with lower ICU mortality, lower hospital mortality, and decreased length of stay in both ICU and hospital, compared to models in which intensivist consultation is optional (60). Although there are limited data specifically addressing the critical care obstetric patient, it would be odd indeed if intensivist input did not improve outcomes in this population as well (61,62).

If a patient who is still pregnant requires critical care services, the first question to answer is: where is she best cared for? **If the pregnancy is early or the duration of ICU services is anticipated to be lengthy, the labor floor is not likely the best location. If she is in active labor, the labor floor probably is the best choice. Most patients, however, will fall into**

neither of these categories; factors affecting the decision include degree of instability, interventions required, staffing and expertise available, anticipated duration of ICU stay, probability of delivery, access for family, etc.

The obstetrician transferring a patient to an ICU must be familiar with the types of units available, that is, general medical/surgical ICU or specialty unit (cardiothoracic, neurologic/neurosurgical, etc.), and understand whether the ICU is open, closed, or hybrid/transitional (63). In an open unit, any physician can write orders or perform procedures; management or consultation by an intensivist is not mandatory. **In a closed ICU, only the critical care staff writes orders and manages patients: the primary team gives over control. The hybrid or transitional model allows all physicians to write orders but requires an on-site critical care physician to consult, round on, or comanage all patients in the unit. As above, involving the intensivist improves outcome.**

Despite the need for expertise, it is acknowledged that critical care requires a multidisciplinary approach (49) to achieve best outcomes. The usual ICU team comprises physicians, nurses, pharmacists, and respiratory therapists. In the case of maternal critical care, the ICU team must also include obstetricians, obstetric/perinatal nurses, and pediatricians. Commonly, the physician cohort would be subspecialty-trained, for example, maternal-fetal medicine and neonatology.

When an undelivered patient is transferred to ICU, efforts should be made to map out the anticipated course of her condition or disease, look ahead to possible complications, and set parameters for delivery (except in cases of too-early gestational age). Modifications of physical and laboratory assessment related to pregnancy must be known and taken into account; the obstetrician will be more familiar with these than the intensivist. The plan should be clear to the medical team and to the patient's family, and to the patient herself if she is able to understand. The risk-benefit balance for a given intervention will change as pregnancy progresses, so it is important to revisit the care plan on a regular basis.

Fetal monitoring will often, but not always, be appropriate. If plans are made for fetal monitoring outside of the labor and delivery unit, the team should strategize about the type and frequency of monitoring as well as the expected interventions. It is not appropriate to commit to continuous fetal monitoring unless the strip can be interpreted in real time by someone qualified to read it and empowered to take corrective action. In some cases this will entail an obstetric or perinatal nurse at the bedside in ICU. Alternatively, remote access monitoring can be used to transmit the tracing to a display on the obstetrical unit. Changes in the fetal monitor tracing often reflect alterations in maternal physiology rather than in the fetal status per se, and thus may function as an early warning system for derangements in maternal end-organ status (acid-base balance, volume status, etc.). This means that the response, which is a reflex on the labor floor—in which the nonreassuring fetal tracing should be immediately evaluated for delivery—must be suppressed long enough to look for alternate explanations that would be better addressed by correcting maternal status.

The **plan for delivery** should be made long before delivery is imminent, and should address preferred location for delivery, mode of delivery, requirement for analgesia or anesthesia, and access for the neonatal team. It must also include alternatives in case matters do not go as anticipated.

The patient in an HDU or intermediate care unit on the labor floor can easily be delivered there. Many critically ill obstetric patients will, however, be elsewhere. Advantages of vaginal delivery in ICU include ready availability of critical care interventions and staff, plus avoidance of potentially destabilizing transport. Disadvantages include lack of space to conduct delivery, unfamiliarity of critical care personnel with obstetric management, space constraints for the pediatric team and equipment, and inadequate privacy. The alternative, transport to L&D, ensures familiarity with obstetric issues but unfamiliarity with critical care issues. The process of transport itself is risky for a critically ill patient (55).

When considering delivery in ICU, the increased likelihood of instrumental delivery must be kept in mind. Patients with translaryngeal intubation cannot close the glottis to push and therefore may have a prolonged second stage, often requiring delivery via vacuum or forceps. Patients with cardiac, respiratory or neuromuscular compromise are at risk of decompensation during labor, especially in second stage. Women with altered mental status may not tolerate pain or obstetric manipulation. Pain relief cannot be forgone in ICU even when a patient cannot verbalize discomfort, but patients may not qualify for regional analgesia techniques because of issues with positioning, hemodynamic instability, or coagulopathy. Intravenous analgesia is, of course, an alternative to epidural, but is not as effective in protecting a medically fragile patient from hemodynamic derangements associated with pain.

Cesarean delivery in ICU is fraught with hazards. The ICU does, on occasion, host surgical procedures performed under local anesthesia, such as tracheostomy, percutaneous gastrostomy, insertion of vena cava filters and, more recently, diagnostic laparoscopy (64–67). Some cardiothoracic units allow emergency re-exploration in ICU for bleeding or tamponade rather than re-transport back to the operating room (68). For the most part, however, surgical procedures are avoided in ICU when possible. Disadvantages of performing cesarean in the ICU include inadequate space for anesthetic and surgical equipment (to say nothing of required neonatal resuscitation gear), unfamiliarity of attendant personnel with the operation, the accumulation of a crowd of onlookers, and the risk of nosocomial infection with drug-resistant organisms: ICUs have the highest rates of health care–associated infections in a hospital (69,70).

ROLE OF OB-GYN

In an intermediate care unit on a labor/delivery floor, the lead physician will typically be an obstetrician-gynecologist (Ob-Gyn), with or without subspecialty maternal-fetal medicine training; sometimes this function will be fulfilled by an obstetric anesthesiologist. The team leader would coordinate and manage the patient's care, in addition to providing hands-on care as necessary. It is essential that the lead physician be immediately available to the critically ill obstetrical patient and that coverage arrangements are adequate, in order to avoid interference with prompt and timely delivery of care. When other specialty consultation is required, the lead physician must coordinate and integrate such consultation as appropriate. He/she must also be able to clearly decide when the patient's condition is no longer appropriate for intermediate care and then transfer up for intensive care or down for routine ward care.

When obstetric patients are transferred to the ICU, the obstetrician's role will depend on the ICU model (open or closed) and the patient's status (antepartum or postpartum). The Ob-Gyn's anxiety about having a patient in the ICU is easily matched by the ICU team's anxiety about having a fetus

in the uterus, and even in a closed unit, the obstetrician's input is welcomed. Decisions about care for a pregnant patient in the ICU should be made in concert by the multidisciplinary team and should involve the patient and her family insofar as this is feasible. No matter what the ICU model, the obstetrician should generally continue to see the patient and consult with the primary ICU team daily, offering pregnancy-specific knowledge necessary to give the best care to these complex patients.

If a patient is transferred to the ICU postpartum, the obstetrician's role becomes simpler medically, although the patient and family may have concerns regarding any obstetrical event that precipitated transfer. Anger, dissatisfaction, or legal action often follow a perceived bad outcome: in case of a postpartum complication or condition requiring critical care, the obstetrician may bear the brunt of questions. This is likely to be stressful even when there has been no evident error, as the fear of litigation is prominent in such cases (71).

The medical issues with a postpartum admission to the ICU typically relate to uncertainty (on the part of the primary ICU team) about vaginal bleeding, evaluation of fever, therapies such as magnesium, and feasibility of breast-feeding, especially compatibility with various medications. There may be surgical issues such as re-exploration or reclosure of incisions. Under some circumstances the Ob-Gyn will be the advocate for bringing together the critically ill mother and her new baby.

Fetal surveillance is often employed when a pregnant patient is admitted to ICU. The obstetrician who is used to reviewing fetal heart rate tracings as an indicator of fetal status should consider that the fetal heart rate tracing reflects maternal end-organ (uteroplacental) perfusion and maternal acid-base status as well. If baseline variability disappears or decelerations are seen, a reason should be sought in maternal physiology, such as hypotension, acidemia, or compression of the inferior vena cava by the gravid uterus in supine position. Correction of these factors may result in improvement of the tracing.

The potential for preterm delivery is high in the ICU (6,52–54). Attempts to suppress preterm contractions are ill-advised in the case of critical illness in pregnancy: aside from the equivocal efficacy of tocolytic drugs, preterm labor may represent an adaptive response. No drug is devoid of side effects, which must be carefully monitored in the setting of critical illness (tachycardia and decreased BP with beta-agonists, effects on platelet function and renal perfusion with indomethacin, magnesium's effects on cardiac function, etc.). But because of the potential for preterm birth, the threshold for administration of a course of antenatal corticosteroids to promote fetal lung maturity should be low. Corticosteroids are often given in an ICU setting for reasons such as to sepsis and spinal cord injury: it may be feasible to substitute to betamethasone or dexamethasone in these circumstances in order to obtain additional fetal benefit.

Physicians who deal with the critically ill are familiar with the difficulties of informed consent and with the frequent need to identify a designated decision-maker. This is not typically a problem with which obstetricians have much experience, but in critical care obstetrics the designated decision-maker must assume the role for both mother and fetus when the woman herself cannot. Even if a woman has previously made her wishes known with a living will or advance directive, state law varies: advance directives may be specifically invalidated if a patient is pregnant (72). The hospital ethics committee should be called upon for guidance as needed.

SPECIFIC CONDITIONS FOR WHICH CRITICAL CARE MAY BE REQUIRED

Reviews of severe acute maternal morbidity (1–11,15,18,33–47) suggest the following conditions are of most concern: **hemorrhage, eclampsia, cardiac arrest, pulmonary edema, respiratory failure, renal failure, sepsis, shock** (multiple types), **cerebrovascular event, coma, anesthetic complications** (e.g., aspiration, difficult/failed intubation), **and other cardiac conditions**. Most obstetricians will be familiar with hemorrhage, preeclampsia, and eclampsia—in fact, more familiar than most intensivists—and these conditions may be handled on a labor and delivery unit without transfer. The remainder of the chapter will address critical care topics with which the obstetrician is likely to be less familiar. With the understanding that critical care medicine, like any other branch of medicine, is constantly evolving, some current evidence-based practice in critical care is described below.

Acute Respiratory Distress Syndrome and Mechanical Ventilation

The **acute respiratory distress syndrome (ARDS)** is a nonspecific response of the lung to a variety of inciting events. It is the extreme form of a spectrum of **acute lung injury (ALI)** and is defined as "a syndrome of inflammation and increased permeability that is associated with a constellation of clinical, radiology, and physiologic abnormalities that cannot be explained by, but may coexist with, left atrial or pulmonary capillary hypertension" (73). In other words, **ARDS is** in general **noncardiogenic pulmonary edema**. Criteria for diagnoses of ALI and ARDS are shown in Table 40.3. The only difference between ALI and ARDS is the severity of oxygenation impairment. The lungs are poorly compliant and resist expansion. Positive-pressure ventilation risks barotrauma and further lung injury.

ARDS is an uncommon disorder in pregnancy, with an incidence estimated at between 1/3000 and 1/6000 deliveries (52,74). The mortality rate for ARDS among obstetrical patients was estimated to be 24% to 44% in older case series (52,74–76), and 33% in a more recent series (77), neither greatly different from the general population case-fatality rate of 38% (78). A review of Canadian hospital admissions between 1991 and 2002, however, found that the case-fatality rate among obstetric patients with ARDS in the absence of any major preexisting condition was only 6% (15). On the other hand, among pregnant women with H1N1 influenza, the rate of ARDS was nearly twice as high as among nonpregnant women (9.7% vs. 5.4%) (79); the difference in severity was demonstrated in a report from Australia and New Zealand in which extracorporeal membrane oxygenation was required in 45% of pregnant or postpartum women with severe H1N1 respiratory disease (80).

In managing ARDS in pregnancy, many authorities recommend maintaining maternal $SpO_2 > 95\%$, or $PaO_2 > 60$ mmHg, in an effort to promote fetal well-being, but it is

unclear what evidence supports this recommendation. The gradient between maternal and fetal oxygen content drives transfer. Because the oxygen content of fetal blood is quite low, the gradient is easily preserved: normal fetal umbilical venous pO_2 is only 31 to 42 mmHg (81). Oxygen delivery to the fetus and to fetal organs, as to the adult, is the product of blood flow and oxygen content. Adaptive strategies in the fetus include higher affinity of fetal hemoglobin for oxygen, and high cardiac output relative to size.

There is one experimental trial of deliberate hypoxia in human pregnancy (82). Ten women with normal pregnancies near term were exposed to a hypoxic gas mixture with an FIO_2 approximately 0.1 (50% room air, 50% nitrogen) for 10 minutes, during which time maternal oxygen saturation (SpO_2) decreased by 15%. Fetal heart rate baseline and variability, umbilical artery Doppler indices, and middle cerebral artery Doppler indices did not change during experimental maternal hypoxia. Direct sampling of fetal blood was not performed in this study.

In ARDS and ALI, the **use of lower tidal volumes in mechanical ventilation is associated with lower mortality and more ventilator-free days in nonpregnant adults** (83) in a randomized controlled trial in a general medical-surgical ICU population. This strategy allows hypercapnia and respiratory acidosis but minimizes inflation pressures and stretch-induced lung injury. There are no data on outcomes of a lung-protective or lower-tidal-volume-ventilation strategy for pregnant women with ARDS. In fact, **there are no randomized controlled trials of ventilator strategies in an obstetrical population**. Maternal acidemia does affect fetal acid-base status, which suggests that continuous fetal monitoring could be useful, specifically in determining the lower acceptable limits of maternal pH.

After the publication of the ARDSNet trial, which demonstrated better survival when low-tidal-volume ventilation was employed (83), strategies for mechanical ventilation swung away from normalizing arterial blood gases to limiting volutrauma. No trials have been performed on ARDS in pregnant patients. Few publications describe ventilator settings in the case of ARDS in pregnancy. In case series from the era preceding low-tidal-volume ventilation for ARDS, barotrauma rates were high in obstetric patients who were mechanically ventilated: 36% to 44% (52,74). This compares unfavorably with the background rate of barotrauma of 11% among nonobstetric patients ventilated with "traditional" tidal volumes in ARDS (83). There is, however, no head-to-head trial among pregnant patients with ARDS.

When contemplating a low-tidal-volume ventilation strategy for pregnant women with ARDS, the maternal $PaCO_2$ must also be considered. CO_2 transfer across the placenta also requires a gradient; in this case the higher PCO_2 of fetal blood diffuses across placental interface to the lower PCO_2 of maternal blood. High maternal PCO_2, as in permissive hypercapnia, might be expected to impede transfer and allow fetal acidemia. In a small trial of CO_2 rebreathing in 35 healthy pregnant women, a rise in the maternal end-tidal CO_2 as high as 60 torr was associated with a loss of fetal heart rate variability in 57% of fetuses monitored, this being a proxy for fetal acidemia; 90% of fetuses thus affected normalized the tracing posttest (84). A few case reports describe women with status asthmaticus during pregnancy in whom permissive hypercapnia was implemented so as to decrease the risk of barotrauma (85,86). In most cases, there appeared to be no immediate or long-term ill effects on the fetuses, but one of six exhibited a nonreassuring fetal heart rate tracing after

Table 40.3 Acute Lung Injury and Acute Respiratory Distress Syndrome: Criteria for Diagnosis

Acute onset
Bilateral infiltrates seen on chest X ray
Severe impairment of oxygenation
  PaO_2/FIO_2 ratio ≤ 300 = acute lung injury (ALI)
  PaO_2/FIO_2 ratio ≤ 200 = ARDS
Pulmonary capillary wedge pressure <18 mmHg (if measured) or
  absence of evidence of increased left atrial pressure

Source: Adapted from Ref. 73.

seven days' hypercapnia and was therefore delivered. There is also a small case series of airway pressure release ventilation (ARPV) in pregnancy, an alternative lung-protective strategy, in which the lungs were kept inflated to a high PEEP (28–33 cm H_2O), interrupted for brief periods with low PEEP (8–10 cm H_2O). This was well tolerated by mothers and fetuses, and maternal oxygenation immediately improved (87).

The author suggests that a **pregnant woman ventilated with a low tidal volume strategy should have the fetal heart rate tracing continuously monitored once viability has been reached, and if the tracing is suspicious for fetal acidemia, consider increasing tidal volume (to increase maternal pH, decrease PCO_2), or switch to airway pressure release ventilation.**

Delivery does not improve maternal survival in ARDS (52,53,88). Fetal survival, however, is tightly linked to gestational age at delivery: this would imply a fetal benefit to continuing rather than interrupting pregnancy, assuming maternal and fetal condition permits.

Sepsis

The diagnoses of systemic inflammatory response syndrome (SIRS), sepsis, severe sepsis, and septic shock are shown in Table 40.4. **There are no randomized trials on sepsis specific to the obstetric population**. In most trials, pregnant patients are explicitly barred from enrollment. Since severe sepsis and septic shock (aside from unsafe abortion) are not common in pregnancy, the epidemiology of sepsis in this population is not as well described as in a general medical-surgical population. The World Health Organization recently estimated 77,000 deaths worldwide per year from maternal sepsis, with up to 10% of all live births being complicated by maternal infection (90). In the United Kingdom, 0.04% of deliveries have been complicated by severe sepsis (91). The case-fatality rate for sepsis among obstetric patients was 7.7% in the Netherlands between 1993 and 2006 (92). The case-fatality rate for septic abortion is as high as 20% (93), but in the developed world, this condition is seen almost exclusively where abortion is illegal.

Sepsis may be obstetric or nonobstetric. Obstetric sepsis includes uterine infection, septic abortion, and wound infection; in addition, sepsis may follow invasive procedures such as amniocentesis, chorionic villus sampling, cervical cerclage, or percutaneous umbilical blood sampling. In an American case series of septic shock in pregnancy (94), half of cases had an obstetric cause, while of the 50% with nonobstetric causes,

the majority were urinary in origin. Figures are comparable in a larger Dutch study (92), with the 42% attributed to non-obstetric causes heavily influenced by urosepsis, pneumonia, and appendicitis.

The Surviving Sepsis Campaign (95) is a multiorganizational effort to improve outcomes in sepsis and septic shock, based on best available evidence. It proposes the following therapeutic goals. **Adherence to these goals has been shown to improve mortality in septic shock** (96). There is no evidence base for these guidelines in a pregnant or postpartum patient, but no evidence against them either.

1. *Early goal-directed resuscitation during the first six hours after admission.* This refers specifically to initial fluid resuscitation of a septic patient within the first six hours after diagnosis. Patients with sepsis-induced hypoperfusion (hypotension persisting after initial fluid challenge *or* blood lactate level $\geq$ 4 mmol/L) should be swiftly fluid resuscitated to central venous pressure 8 to 12 mmHg, mean arterial pressure $\geq$ 65 mmHg, and/or urine output $\geq$ 0.5 mL/kg/hr. Early goal-directed therapy should not wait for admission to ICU but should begin as soon as septic shock is diagnosed (95). **Broad-spectrum antibiotic therapy should be begun within one hour of diagnosis of severe sepsis or septic shock** (see below); cultures, including blood cultures, should be obtained as appropriate, providing this does not delay the start of antibiotics. Early goal-directed therapy for septic shock has been shown to decrease in-hospital mortality by 35% in a randomized controlled trial in a general medical/surgical population (97). A recent review of early goal-directed therapy for sepsis in pregnancy (98) acknowledges the absence of data in obstetrics but nonetheless advocates incorporating the strategy into obstetric critical care.

2. *Blood cultures before antibiotic therapy.* No theoretical reason this would not apply. One study in Finland described this specific policy for obstetric patients: 2% (of over 40,000) were cultured for fever and had broad-spectrum antibiotics instituted immediately. Bacteremia was confirmed in 5% of cases; only 1 of the 798 patients cultured developed septic shock, for an incidence of 0.1% (99).

3. *Imaging studies performed promptly to ascertain source of infection.* Pregnant women can indeed be imaged, although there are issues relating to ionizing radiation. The American College of Obstetricians and Gynecologists recommends limiting total radiation dose during pregnancy to 5 rads as no fetal effects are known this low; substitute nonionizing modality if feasible. If ionizing radiation is to be used, shield abdomen if possible. If ionizing radiation is required and the abdomen/pelvis is to be included in the field, modify technique to minimize dose delivered to fetus, and use dosimetry to tally fetal dose (100,101). Gadolinium has been used in a few pregnancies without evident fetal compromise, although numbers are limited (102–105). If iodinated contrast material is used during pregnancy, there is potential for depression of fetal and/or neonatal thyroid, so neonatal thyroid function should be checked within a few days after birth (106).

4. *Initiation of broad-spectrum antibiotic therapy within one hour of diagnosis of sepsis.* No reason this would not be feasible; however, the hemodynamic picture that characterizes normal pregnancy may result in overcalling of a sepsis diagnosis. The central hemodynamics of normal pregnancy, like those of sepsis, include increased cardiac

Table 40.4 Sepsis Definitions

Systemic inflammatory response syndrome (SIRS): characterized by any two of the following:
$T > 38°C$ or $< 36°C$
HR > 90/min
RR > 20/min
WBC > 12,000 cells/mm^3 **or** < 4000 **or** > 10% bands

Sepsis
SIRS resulting from infection

Severe sepsis
Sepsis PLUS organ dysfunction or evidence of hypoperfusion or hypotension (either systolic BP < 90 mmHg or more than a 40-mmHg drop from baseline)

Septic shock
Sepsis-induced hypotension persisting despite adequate fluid resuscitation

Unclear how these criteria should be modified for the physiologic changes of pregnancy. *Source*: Adapted from Ref. 89.

output, increased heart rate, decreased systemic vascular resistance, and a somewhat lower blood pressure (104). Broad-spectrum coverage is appropriate in OB patients: in a large study of peripartum sepsis, more than 40 organisms were cultured, including aerobic gram-positive and gram-negative as well as anaerobic bacteria (99).

5. *Reassessment of antibiotic therapy with clinical and microbiologic data to narrow antibiotic coverage when appropriate.* No data specific to pregnancy. When narrowing coverage, consideration should be given to whether transplacental coverage is needed; some drugs do not cross placenta well and result in inadequate fetal treatment, such as azithromycin in the treatment of syphilis (105).

6. *Seven to ten days of antibiotic therapy.* No evidence base specific to pregnancy. No reason to recommend alteration in this goal.

7. *Source control.* No data specific to pregnancy. About half of cases of sepsis in pregnant/postpartum women localize to the uterus (92,94), and would therefore require the uterus be emptied. *There are no data on antibiotics without delivery for women diagnosed with clinical sepsis attributed to intraamniotic infection.* Women with a diagnosis of *subclinical* intra-amniotic infection, treated with antibiotics alone in the hope of delaying delivery to a more favorable gestational age, have had pregnancy prolonged by days to weeks, with the only maternal morbidity a 3% rate of postpartum endometritis (106) but with an infant death rate of 33% and major infant morbidity >75%. It should be emphasized that patients with subclinical chorioamnionitis, who typically present with preterm labor or membrane rupture, are unlikely to come to the ICU; if these nonseptic patients cannot be managed without delivery, there is no argument for managing clinical chorioamnionitis without it. There is no evidence for deferring source control in pregnancy.

8. *Crystalloid or colloid fluid resuscitation.* No evidence to recommend one versus the other in pregnancy. Decreased oncotic pressure in pregnancy and decreased gradient between colloid oncotic pressure and pulmonary artery occlusion pressure (104) may increase risk of pulmonary edema in pregnancy when crystalloid resuscitation is chosen.

9. *Fluid challenge to restore circulating filling pressure.* No data specific to pregnancy; however, the gradient between colloid oncotic pressure and pulmonary artery occlusion pressure is lower in pregnancy (104), so there is more risk of inducing pulmonary edema.

10. *If filling pressures rise and tissue perfusion does not improve, reduction of rate of fluid administration.* Seems reasonable; no specific data in the pregnant population.

11. *Norepinephrine or dopamine to target initial mean arterial pressure >65 mmHg.* No data exist to recommend a lower limit of mean arterial pressure in pregnancy, but since mean arterial pressure is normally lower in pregnancy (107), a target MAP $\geq$ 65 may be too stringent. Although MAP is approximately 4 to 5 mmHg lower in pregnancy, one cannot extrapolate a target of 60 mmHg instead. The uteroplacental circulation does not autoregulate, and compromised placental perfusion is expected to affect the fetus. The electronic fetal heart rate tracing may allow individualization of target MAP. In a sheep model, dopamine at rates above 4 to 5 µg/kg/min increases resting uterine tone and decreases uterine blood flow (108,109), which would be expected to affect placental perfusion. However, cardiac output in these animal studies is

demonstrably increased with dopamine, which may overcome the specific effect on the uterus, and pregnant ewes show a greater increase in cardiac output (CO) than nonpregnant animals at a given dopamine infusion rate (110). Human data are limited. Dopamine has been used successfully in low doses in oliguric pregnant women (111,112), but the dose required for support of blood pressure is significantly higher than this. A small trial randomized women who were hypotensive (not septic) after administration of a spinal anesthetic for cesarean to either dopamine or ephedrine for blood pressure support, and demonstrated no difference in Apgar scores or cord pH in either compared to normotensive controls (113). Umbilical vein pO$_2$, however, was significantly lower in the ephedrine- or dopamine-treated group than in the control. In a dual-perfused single-cotyledon model of human placenta, no change in fetal arterial perfusion was seen with administration of norepinephrine (114). The clinical implications are unclear.

12. *Dobutamine when cardiac output remains low despite fluid and vasopressor therapy.* The normal cardiac output in pregnancy is increased and the systemic vascular resistance decreased (104); thus, it is unclear what would constitute a "low" cardiac output in pregnancy. It probably requires clinical assessment of both mother and fetus rather than a cutoff number. Dobutamine has little effect on resting uterine tone even at high doses, but like dopamine decreases uterine blood flow in gravid ewes (108). Human data are lacking.

13. *Stress dose steroid therapy if BP remains unresponsive to fluid and vasopressors.* In septic patients whose hypotension cannot be corrected despite fluid resuscitation and vasopressors, current guidelines suggest addition of intravenous hydrocortisone (95). The recommendation comes from a randomized controlled trial in which the subgroup of patients with septic shock refractory to fluids and vasopressors, who *also* had relative adrenal insufficiency, had a 50% lower risk of mortality after treatment with intravenous steroids (115). The larger CORTICUS trial has not, however, confirmed benefit to steroids in septic shock (116). As ever, there are no data in pregnancy. There are specific fetal benefits to a brief course of dexamethasone or betamethasone, which cross the placenta and stimulate earlier lung maturation (117). Hydrocortisone does not cross placenta and would be expected to confer no fetal benefit, although this is the steroid specifically recommended in the subgroup of septic patients without response to fluids and vasopressors; in the instance of unresponsive septic shock in pregnancy, one might consider using betamethasone or dexamethasone, rather than hydrocortisone.

14. *Recombinant activated protein C (rhAPC) in severe sepsis if clinical assessment of high risk for death.* Pregnant patients were specifically excluded from trials, so efficacy in this population is unknown. ICU prediction models overestimate risk of death in the obstetric patient, which creates difficulties in deciding whether rhAPC should be used. One case of placental abruption and hemorrhage with fetal death after rhAPC was reported to Eli Lilly in 2005 (personal communication). A handful of case reports describe rhAPC use in pregnancy, albeit with minimal information on the infant outcome (118–120). Bleeding is a known complication, which would limit use in pregnancy or puerperium.

15. *Intensive insulin therapy to achieve tight glucose control in critical illness.* Insulin infusion targeted to maintain glucose 80 to 115 mg/dL has been shown to decrease

mortality in a surgical ICU population (121), although not in a sicker medical ICU population (122). Although there are no data demonstrating benefit to this practice in obstetric critical care, obstetricians are already accustomed to targeting tight glucose control in diabetic pregnancy, frequently use insulin infusions in labor, and should find this an easy recommendation to adopt.

16. Randomized controlled trials confirm that the pulmonary artery catheter does not improve outcome in ALI or respiratory failure (123), sepsis (124), or pulmonary edema (125), although it does increase the complication rate. There are no RCTs addressing use in preeclampsia. It has become more difficult to justify use of the pulmonary artery catheter in critical care medicine generally and in critical care obstetrics specifically.

REFERENCES

1. Panchal S, Arria AM, Labhsetwar SA. Maternal mortality during hospital admission for delivery: a retrospective analysis using a state-maintained database. Anesth Anal 2001; 93:134–411. [II-2; case-control; *n* = 135]
2. Keizer JL, Zwart JJ, Meerman RH, et al. Obstetric intensive care admissions: a 12-year review in a tertiary care centre. Eur J Obstet Gynecol Reprod Biol 2006; 128:152–156. [II-3; case series; *n* = 142]
3. Umo-Etuk J, Lumley J, Holdcroft A. Critically ill parturient women and admission to intensive care: a 5-year review. Int J Obstet Anesth 1996; 5:79–84. [II-3; case series, *n* = 39]
4. Hazelgrove JF, Price C, Pappachan VJ, et al. Multicenter study of obstetric admissions to 14 intensive care units in southern England. Crit Care Med 2001; 29:770–775. [II-3; case series, *n* = 210]
5. Lapinsky SE, Kruczynski K, Seaward GR, et al. Critical care management of the obstetric patient. Can J Anaesth 1997; 44:325–329. [II-3; case series, *n* = 65]
6. Selo-Ojeme DO, Omosaiye M, Battacharjee P, et al. Risk factors for obstetric admissions to the intensive care unit in a tertiary hospital: a case-control study. Arch Gynecol Obstet 2005; 272:207–210. [II-2; case-control, 33 cases]
7. Munnur U, Karnad DR, Bandi VD, et al. Critically ill obstetric patients in an American and an Indian public hospital: comparison of case-mix, organ dysfunction, intensive care requirements, and outcomes. Intensive Care Med 2005; 31(8):1087–1094. [II-3; case series, 174 in Houston, 754 in Mumbai]
8. Brace V, Penney G, Hall M. Quantifying severe maternal morbidity: a Scottish population study. BJOG 2004; 111:481–484. [II-2; audit, *n* = 196]
9. Heinonen S, Tyrvainen E, Saarikoski S, et al. Need for maternal critical care in obstetrics: a population-based analysis. Int J Obstet Anesth 2002; 11:260–264. [II-3; case series, *n* = 22]
10. Baskett TF, O'Connell CM. Maternal critical care in obstetrics. J Obstet Gynaecol Can 2009; 31:218–221. [II-3; case series, *n* = 117]
11. Pollock W, Rose L, Dennis CL. Pregnant and postpartum admissions to the intensive care unit: a systematic review. Intensive Care Med 2010; 36:1465–1474. [Review, 40 studies, *n* = 7887 patients]
12. Ryan M, Hamilton V, Bowen M, et al. The role of a high-dependency unit in a regional obstetric hospital. Anaesthesia 2000; 55:1155–1158. [II-3; case series, *n* = 123]
13. Zeeman GG, Wendel GD, Cunningham FG. A blueprint for obstetric critical care. Am J Obstet Gynecol 2003; 188:532–536. [II-3; case series, *n* = 483]
14. Saravanakumar K, Davies L, Lewis M, et al. High dependency care in an obstetric setting in the UK. Anaesthesia 2008; 63:1081–1086. [II-3; case series, 3551]
15. Wen SW, Liston R, Heaman M, et al.; for the Maternal Health Study Group, Canadian Perinatal Surveillance System. Severe maternal morbidity in Canada, 1991–2001. CMAJ 2005; 173:759–764. [II-2; population database, *n* = 11,066]
16. Joseph KS, Liu S, Rouleau J, et al. Severe maternal morbidity in Canada, 2003–2007: surveillance including routine hospitalization data and ICD-9 codes. J Obstet Gynaecol Can 2010; 32:837–846. [II-2; administrative database of 1.3 million]
17. Liu S, Joseph KS, Bartholomew S, et al. Temporal trends and regional variations in severe maternal morbidity in Canada, 2003 to 2007. J Obstet Gynaecol Can 2010; 32:847–855. [II-2; administrative database]
18. Zwart JJ, Dupuis JRO, Richters A, et al. Obstetric intensive care unit admission: a 2-year nationwide population-based cohort study. Intensive Care Med 2010; 36:256–261. [II-2; cohort study, *n* = 847]
19. Callaghan WM, MacKay AP, Berg CJ. Identification of severe maternal morbidity during delivery hospitalizations, United States, 1991–2003. Am J Obstet Gynecol 2008; 199:133.e1–e8. [II-2; administrative database, 423,480 records with 2235 qualifying cases]
20. Martin JA, Hamilton BE, Sutton PD, et al. Births: final data for 2005. Nat Vital Stat Reports 2007; 56:1–104. Available at: http://www.cdc.gov/nchs/data/nvsr/nvsr56/nvsr56_06.pdf. Accessed March 3, 2008. [Epidemiologic data]
21. Roberts CL, Ford JB, Algert CS, et al. Trends in adverse maternal outcomes during childbirth: a population-based study of severe maternal morbidity. BMC Pregnancy Childbirth 2009; 9:7. Available at http://www.biomedcentral.com/1471-2393/9/7. Accessed November 20, 2010. [II; administrative dataset, *n* = 6242]
22. Knight M, Callaghan WS, Berg C, et al. Trends in postpartum hemorrhage in high resource countries: a review and recommendations from the International Postpartum Hemorrhage Collaborative Group. BMC Pregnancy Childbirth 2009; 9:55. Available at http://www.biomedcentral.com/1471-2393/9/55. Accessed November 20, 2010. [II-2; multiple datasets]
23. Plante LA. Public health consequences of cesarean on demand. Obstet Gynecol Surv 2006; 61:807–815. [III; decision analysis]
24. Galyean AM, Lagrew DC, Bush MC, et al. Previous cesarean section and the risk of postpartum maternal complications and adverse neonatal outcomes in future pregnancies. J Perinatol 2009; 29:726–730. [II-3; database, *n* = 17,406]
25. Haupt MT, Bekes CE, Brilli RJ, et al. Guidelines on critical care services and personnel: recommendations based on a system of categorization of three levels of care. Crit Care Med 2003; 31:2677–2683. [III; expert opinion]
26. Nasrawat SA, Cohen IL, Dennis RC, et al. Guidelines on admission and discharge for adult intermediate care units. Crit Care Med 1998; 26:607–610. [III; expert opinion]
27. Zimmerman JE, Wagner DP, Sun X, et al. Planning patient services for intermediate care units: insights based on care for intensive care unit low-risk monitor admissions. Crit Care Med 1996; 24:1626–1632. [II-2; cohort study, *n* = 8040]
28. Seppelt I, for ANZIC writing committee. Critical illness due to 2009A/H1N1 influenza in pregnant and postpartum women: population based cohort study. BMJ 2010; 340:c1279. [II-2; cohort study, *n* = 64]
29. Louie JK, Acosta M, Jamieson DJ, et al.; for the California Pandemic (H1N1) Working Group. Severe 2009 H1N1 influenza in pregnant and postpartum women in California. N Engl J Med 2010; 362:27–35. [II-2; cohort, *n* = 102]
30. Siston AM, Rasmussen SA, Honein MA, et al. for the Pandemic H1N1 Influenza in Pregnancy Working Group. Pandemic 2009 influenza A (H1N1) virus illness among pregnant women in the United States. JAMA 2010; 303:1517–1525. [II; public health surveillance dataset, *n* = 788]
31. Martin SR, Foley MR. Intensive care in obstetrics: an evidence-based review. Am J Obstet Gynecol 2006; 195:673–689. [III; review]
32. Galvagno SM, Camann W. Sepsis and acute renal failure in pregnancy. Anesth Analg 2009; 108:572–575. [III; review]
33. Afessa B, Green B, Delke I, et al. Systemic inflammatory response syndrome, organ failure, and outcome in critically ill obstetric patients treated in an ICU. Chest 2001; 120:1271–1277. [II-3; case series, *n* = 74]

34. Bouvier-Colle M-H, Salanave B, Ancel P-Y, et al. Obstetric patients treated in intensive care units and maternal mortality. Eur J Obstet Gynecol Reprod Biol 1996; 65:121–125. [III; population-based survey, n = 435]

35. Collop NA, Sahn SA. Critical illness in pregnancy: an analysis of 20 patients admitted to a medical intensive care unit. Chest 1993; 103:1548–1552. [II-3; case series, n = 20]

36. Gilbert TT, Smulian JC, Martin AA, et al. Obstetric admissions to the intensive care unit: outcomes and severity of illness. Obstet Gynecol 2003; 102:897–903. [II-3; case series, n = 233]

37. Graham SG, Luxton MC. The requirement for intensive care support for the pregnant population. Anaesthesia 1989; 44:581–584. [II-3; case series, n = 23]

38. Karnad D, Guntupalli KK. Critical illness and pregnancy: review of a global problem. Crit Care Clin 2004; 20:555–576. [III; review]

39. Kilpatrick SJ, Matthay MA. Obstetric patients requiring critical care: a five-year review. Chest 1992; 101:1407–1412. [II-3; case series, n = 32]

40. Kwee A, Bots ML, Visser GHA, et al. Emergency peripartum hysterectomy: a prospective study in the Netherlands. Eur J Obstet Gynecol Reprod Biol 2006; 124:187–192. [III; survey; 48 reports]

41. Mabie WC, Sibai BM. Treatment in an obstetric intensive care unit. Am J Obstet Gynecol 1990; 162:1–4. [II-3; case series]

42. Mahutte NG, Murphy-Kaulbeck L, Le Q, et al. Obstetric admissions to the intensive care unit. Obstet Gynecol 1999; 94:263–266. [II-3; case series, n = 131]

43. Monaco TK, Spielman FJ, Katz VL. Pregnant patients in the intensive care unit: a descriptive analysis. South Med J 1993; 86:414–417. [II-3; case series, n = 38]

44. Say L, Pattinson RC, Gulmezoglu AM. WHO systematic review of maternal morbidity and mortality: the prevalence of severe acute maternal morbidity (near miss). BMC Reproductive Health 2004; 1:3. Available at: http://www.reproductive-health-journal.com/content/1/1/3. Accessed August 8, 2006. [Systematic review, 30 studies]

45. Soubra SH, Guntupalli KK. Critical illness in pregnancy: an overview. Crit Care Med 2005; 33(suppl):S248–S55. [III; review]

46. Sriram S, Robertson MS. Critically ill obstetrics patients in Australia: a retrospective audit of 8 years' experience in a tertiary intensive care unit. Crit Care Resusc 2008; 10:120–124. [II-3; case series, n = 56]

47. Zhang W-H, Alexander S, Bouvier-Colle M-H, et al. Incidence of severe preeclampsia, postpartum haemorrhage and sepsis as a surrogate marker for severe maternal morbidity in a European population-based study: the MOMS-B survey. BJOG 2005; 112:89–96. [III; survey, 1734 responses]

48. American Academy of Pediatrics and American College of Obstetricians and Gynecologists. Guidelines for Perinatal Care. 6th ed. Elk Grove Village, IL: AAP; Washington DC: ACOG, 2007. [III; guidelines]

49. Brilli RJ, Spevetz A, Branson RD, et al.; the members of the American College of Critical Care Medicine Task Force on Models of Critical Care Delivery, the members of the American College of Critical Care Medicine Guidelines for the Definition of an Intensivist and the Practice of Critical Care Medicine. Critical care delivery in the intensive care unit: defining clinical roles and the best practice model. Crit Care Med 2001; 29:2001–2019. [III; task force, expert report]

50. Dorman T, Angood P, Angus DC, et al. Guidelines for critical care medicine training and continuing medical education. Crit Care Med 2004; 32:263–272. [III; task force, expert opinion]

51. Soylemez Weiner R, Welch HG. Trends in the use of the pulmonary artery catheter in the United States, 1993 to 2004. JAMA 2007; 298:423–429. [II-3; administrative database]

52. Catanzarite V, Willms D, Wong D, et al. Acute respiratory distress syndrome in pregnancy and the puerperium: causes, courses, and outcomes. Obstet Gynecol 2001; 97:760–764. [II-3; case series, n = 28]

53. Tomlinson MW, Caruthers TJ, Whitty JE. Does delivery improve maternal condition in the respiratory-compromised gravida? Obstet Gynecol 1998; 91:92–96. [II-3; case series, n = 10]

54. Cartin-Ceba R, Gajic O, Iyer V, et al. Fetal outcomes of critically ill pregnant women admitted to the intensive care unit for nonobstetric causes. Crit Care Med 2008; 36:2746–2751. [II-2; cohort study, n = 153]

55. Warren J, Fromm RE, Orr RA, et al. Guidelines for the inter- and intrahospital transport of critically ill patients. Crit Care Med 2004; 32:256–262. [III; expert opinion]

56. American Hospital Association. AHA Hospital Statistics 2008. Chicago IL: Health Forum LLC, 2008. [Epidemiologic data]

57. Egol AB, Fromm RE, Guntupalli KK, et al. Guidelines for ICU admission, discharge, and triage. Crit Care Med 1999; 27:633–638. [III; expert opinion]

58. American College of Obstetricians and Gynecologists. Critical care in pregnancy. ACOG Practice Bulletin No. 100, 2009. Washington DC: ACOG 2009 Compendium of Selected Publications. [III; expert opinion]

59. Zeeman GG. Obstetric critical care: a blueprint for improved outcomes. Crit Care Med 2006; 34(suppl):S208–S214. [III; review]

60. Pronovost PJ, Angus DC, Dorman T, et al. Physician staffing patterns and clinical outcomes in critically ill patients: a systematic review. JAMA 2002; 288:2151–2162. [Systematic review, 26 observational studies]

61. Jenkins TM, Troiano NH, Graves CR, et al. Mechanical ventilation in an obstetric population: characteristics and delivery rates. Am J Obstet Gynecol 2003; 188:549–552. [II-3; case series]

62. Plante LA. Mechanical ventilation in an obstetric population [letter]. Am J Obstet Gynecol 2003; 189:1516. [III]

63. Chang SY, Multz AS, Hall JB. Critical care organization. Crit Care Clin 2005; 21:43–53. [III; review]

64. Barba CA. The intensive care unit as an operating room. Surg Clin N Am 2000; 80:957–973. [III; review]

65. Kelly JJ, Puyana JC, Callery MP, et al. The feasibility and accuracy of diagnostic laparoscopy in the septic ICU patient. Surg Endosc 2000; 14:617–621. [II-3; case series, n = 16]

66. Pecoraro AP, Cacchione RN, Sayad P, et al. The routine use of laparoscopy in the intensive care unit. Surg Endosc 2001; 15:638–641. [II-3; case series, n = 11]

67. Jaramillo EJ, Trevino JM, Berghoff KR, et al. Bedside diagnostic laparoscopy in the intensive care unit: a 13-year experience. JSLS 2006; 10:155–159. [II-3; case series, n = 13]

68. Charalambous C, Zipitis CS, Keenan DJ. Chest reexploration in the intensive care unit after cardiac surgery: a safe alternative to returning to the operating theater. Ann Thorac Surg 2006; 81:191–194. [II-2; cohort study, n = 240]

69. Weber DJ, Sickbert-Bennett EE, Brown V, et al. Comparison on hospitalwide surveillance and targeted intensive care unit surveillance of healthcare-associated infections. Infect Control Hosp Epidemiol 2007; 28:1361–1366. [III; surveillance data]

70. Edwards JR, Peterson KD, Andrus ML, et al. National Healthcare Safety Network (NHSN) Report, data summary for 2006. Am J Infect Control 2007; 35:290–301. [III; surveillance data]

71. American College of Obstetricians and Gynecologists. Coping with the stress of medical professional liability litigation. ACOG Committee Opinion No. 309, 2005. Washington DC: ACOG 2008 Compendium of Selected Publications. [Review]

72. Sperling D. Do pregnant women have (living) will? J Health Care Law Policy 2005; 8(2):331–342. [III; review]

73. Bernard GR, Artigas A, Brigham KL, et al. Report of the American-European consensus conference on ARDS: definitions, mechanisms, relevant outcomes and clinical trial coordination. Intensive Care Med 1994; 20:225–232. [III; expert opinion, consensus]

74. Mabie WC, Barton JR, Sibai BM. Adult respiratory distress syndrome in pregnancy. Am J Obstet Gynecol 1992; 167:950–957. [II-3; case series, n = 16]

75. Smith JL, Thomas F, Orme JF, et al. Adult respiratory distress syndrome during pregnancy and the puerperium. West Med J 1990; 153:508–510. [II-3; case series, n = 14]

76. Perry KG, Martin RW, Blake PG, et al. Maternal mortality associated with adult respiratory distress syndrome. South Med J 1998; 91:441–445. [II-3; case series, n = 41]

77. Vasquez DN, Estenssoro E, Canales HS, et al. Clinical characteristics and outcomes of obstetric patients requiring ICU admission. Chest 2007; 131:718–724. [II-3; cohort study, n = 161]

78. Rubenfeld GD, Caldwell E, Peabody E, et al. Incidence and outcomes of acute lung injury. N Engl J Med 2005; 353:1685–1693. [II-2; cohort study, n = 1113]

79. Creanga AA, Johnson TF, Graitcer SB, et al. Severity of 2009 pandemic influenza A (H1N1) virus infection in pregnant women. Obstet Gynecol 2010; 115:717–726. [II-3; case series, n = 62]

80. Davies AR, Jones D, Bailey M, et al.; for the Australia and New Zealand Extracorporeal Membrane Oxygenation (ANZ ECMO) Influenza Investigators. Extracorporeal membrane oxygenation for 2009 influenza A (H1N1) acute respiratory distress syndrome. JAMA 2009; 302:1888–1895. [II-3; case series, n = 68]

81. Nicolaides KH, Economides DL, Soothill PW. Blood gases, pH, and lactate in appropriate- and small-for-gestational-age fetuses. Am J Obstet Gynecol 1989; 161:996–1001. [II-3; cross-sectional study, n = 404]

82. Erkkola R, Pirhonen J, Polvi H. The fetal cardiovascular function in chronic placental insufficiency is different from experimental hypoxia. Ann Chir Gynaecol Suppl 1994; 208:76–79. [III; experimental trial, n = 10]

83. The Acute Respiratory Distress Syndrome Network (ARDSNet). Ventilation with lower tidal volumes as compared with traditional tidal volumes for acute lung injury and the acute respiratory distress syndrome. N Engl J Med 2000; 342:1301–1308. [I; RCT, n = 861]

84. Fraser D, Jensen D, Wolfe LA, et al. Fetal heart rate response to maternal hypocapnia and hypercapnia in late gestation. J Obstet Gynaecol Can 2008; 30(4):312–316. [III; experimental trial, n = 35]

85. Siddiqi AK, Gouda H, Multz AS, et al. Ventilator strategy for status asthmaticus in pregnancy: a case-based review. J Asthma 2005; 42:159–162. [II-3; case series, n = 2]

86. Elsayegh D, Shapiro JM. Management of the obstetric patient with status asthmaticus. J Intensive Care Med 2008; 23(6):396–402. [II-3; case series, n = 5]

87. Hirani A, Marik PE, Plante LA. Airway pressure release ventilation in pregnant patients with acute respiratory distress syndrome: a novel strategy. Respir Care 2009; 54:1405–1409. [II-3; case series, n = 2]

88. Grisaru-Granovsky S, Ioscovich A, Hersch M, et al. Temporizing treatment for the respiratory-compromised gravida: an observational study of maternal and neonatal outcome. Int J Obstet Anesthesia 2007; 16:261–264. [II-3; case series, n = 3]

89. No authors listed. American College of Chest Physicians/Society of Critical Care Medicine Consensus Conference: definitions for sepsis and organ failure and guidelines for the use of innovative therapies in sepsis. Crit Care Med 1992; 20:864–874. [III; expert opinion]

90. Dolea C, Stein C. Global burden of maternal sepsis in the year 2000. Evidence and information for policy, World Health Organization, Geneva 2003. Available at: http://www.who.int/healthinfo/statistics/bod_maternalsepsis.pdf. Accessed December 1, 2010. [Systematic review]

91. Waterstone M, Bewley S, Wolfe C. Incidence and predictors of severe obstetric morbidity: case-control study. BMJ 2001; 322:1089–1093. [II-2; case-control study; n = 588]

92. Kramer HM, Schutte JM, Zwart JJ, et al. Maternal mortality and severe morbidity from sepsis in the Netherlands. Acta Obstet Gynecol Scand 2009; 88:647–653. [II-3; population-based dataset]

93. Finkielman JD, De Feo FD, Heller PG, et al. The clinical course of patients with septic abortion admitted to an intensive care unit. Intensive Care Med 2004; 30:1097–1102. [II-3; case series, n = 63]

94. Mabie WC, Barton JR, Sibai BM. Septic shock in pregnancy. Obstet Gynecol 1997; 90(4 pt 1):553–561. [II-3; case series, n = 18]

95. Dellinger RP, Levy MM, Carlet JM, et al.; for the International Surviving Sepsis Campaign Guidelines Committee. Surviving Sepsis Campaign: international guidelines for the management of sepsis and septic shock: 2008. Crit Care Med 2008; 36:296–327. [III; report of expert committee]

96. Lefrant JY, Muller L, Raillard A, et al. Reduction of the severe sepsis or septic shock associated mortality by reinforcement of the recommendations bundle: a multicenter study. Ann Fr Anesth Reanim 2010; 29:621–628. [II-3; time series, n = 445]

97. Rivers E, Nguyen B, Havstad S, et al. Early goal-directed therapy in the treatment of sepsis and septic shock. N Engl J Med 2001; 345:1368–1377. [I; RCT, n = 263]

98. Guinn DA, Abel DE, Tomlinson MW. Early goal directed therapy for sepsis during pregnancy. Obstet Gynecol 2007; 34:459–479. [III; review]

99. Kankuri E, Kurki T, Hiilesma V. Incidence, treatment and outcome of peripartum sepsis. Acta Obstet Gynecol Scand 2003; 82:730–735. [II-2; cohort study, n = 41]

100. American College of Obstetricians and Gynecologists. Guidelines for diagnostic imaging during pregnancy. ACOG Committee Opinion No. 299, 2004. Washington DC: ACOG 2008 Compendium of Selected Publications. [III; expert opinion]

101. Wall BF, Meara JR, Muirhead CR, et al. Protection of pregnant patients during diagnostic medical exposures to ionising radiation. Advice from the Health Protection Agency, the Royal College of Radiologists, and the College of Radiographers. RCE 9. 2009. Available at: http://www.hpa.org.uk/web/HPAwebFile/HPAweb_C/1238230848746. Accessed November 24, 2010. [III; expert opinion]

102. Webb JA, Thomsen HS, Morcos SK; members of Contrast Media Safety Committee of European Society of Urogenital Radiology (ESUR). The use of iodinated and gadolinium contrast media during pregnancy and lactation. Eur Radiol 2005; 15:1234–1240. [III; expert opinion]

103. DeSantis M, Straface G, Cavaliere AF, et al. Gadolinium periconceptional exposure: pregnancy and neonatal outcome. Acta Obstet Gynecol Scand 2007; 86:99–101. [II-2; cohort study, n = 26]

104. Clark SL, Cotton DB, Lee W, et al. Central hemodynamic assessment of normal term pregnancy. Am J Obstet Gynecol 1989; 161:1439–1442. [II-3; cross-sectional study, n = 10]

105. Zhou P, Qian Y, Xu J, et al. Occurrence of congenital syphilis after maternal treatment with azithromycin during pregnancy. Sex Transm Dis 2007; 34:472–474. [II-3; case series, n = 5]

106. Miyazaki K, Furuhashi M, Matsuo K, et al. Impact of subclinical chorioamnionitis on maternal and neonatal outcomes. Acta Obstet Gynecol Scand 2007; 86:191–197. [II-2; cohort study, n = 100]

107. Macedo ML, Luminoso D, Savvidou MD, et al. Maternal wave reflections and arterial stiffness in normal pregnancy as assessed by applanation tonometry. Hypertension 2008; 51:1047–1051. [II-3; cross-sectional study, n = 193]

108. Fishburne JI, Meis PJ, Urban RB, et al. Vascular and uterine responses to dobutamine and dopamine in the gravid ewe. Am J Obstet Gynecol 1980; 137:944–952. [III; experimental trial, n = 6]

109. Santos AC, Baumann AL, Wlody D, et al. The maternal and fetal effects of milrinone and dopamine in normotensive pregnant ewes. Am J Obstet Gynecol 1992; 167(4 pt 1):11794–18480. [III; experimental trial, n = 7]

110. Blanchard K, Dandavino A, Nuwayhid B, et al. Systemic and uterine hemodynamic responses to dopamine in pregnant and nonpregnant sheep. Am J Obstet Gynecol 1978; 130:669–673. [Experimental trial]

111. Gerstner G, Grunberger W. Dopamine treatment for prevention of renal failure in patients with severe eclampsia. Clin Exp Obstet Gynecol 1980; 7:219–222. [II-2; cohort study, n = 9]

112. Kirshon B, Lee W, Mauer MB, et al. Effects of low-dose dopamine therapy in the oliguric patient with preeclampsia. Am J Obstet Gynecol 1988; 159:604–607. [II-2; cohort study, n = 6]

113. Clark RB, Brunner JA. Dopamine for the treatment of spinal hypotension during cesarean section. Anesthesiology 1980; 53:514–517. [II-1; nonrandomized trial, n = 68]

114. Mintzer BH, Johnson RF, Paschall RL, et al. The diverse effects of vasopressors on the fetoplacental circulation of the perfused human placenta. Anesth Analg 2010; 110:857–862. [II-1; controlled trial]

115. Annane D, Sebille V, Charpentier C, et al. Effect of treatment with low doses of hydrocortisone and fludrocortisone on mortality in patients with septic shock. JAMA 2002; 288:862–871. [I; RCT, *n* = 300]

116. Sprung CL, Annane D, Keh D, et al. Hydrocortisone therapy for patients with septic shock. N Engl J Med 2008; 358:111–124. [I; RCT, *n* = 499]

117. Roberts D, Dalziel S. Antenatal corticosteroids for accelerating fetal lung maturation in women at risk of preterm birth. Cochrane Database Syst Rev 2006; 3:CD004454. [Systematic review]

118. Medve L, Csitari IK, Molnar A, et al. Recombinant activated protein C treatment of septic shock syndrome in a patient at 18th week of gestation: a case report. Am J Obstet Gynecol 2005; 193:864–865. [III; case report]

119. Michalska-Krzanowska G, Czuprynska M. Recombinant factor VII (activated) for haemorrhagic complications of severe sepsis treated with recombinant protein C (activated). Acta Haematol 2006; 116:126–130. [II-3; case series, *n* = 2]

120. Barraclough K, Leone E, Chiu A. Renal replacement therapy for acute kidney injury in pregnancy. Nephrol Dial Transplant 2007; 22:2395–2397. [II-3; case report]

121. Van den Berghe G, Wouters P, Weekers F, et al. Intensive insulin therapy in critically ill patients. N Engl J Med 2001; 345:1359–1367. [I; RCT, *n* = 1548]

122. Van den Berghe G, Wilmer A, Hermans G, et al. Intensive insulin therapy in the medical ICU. N Engl J Med 2006; 354:449–461. [I; RCT, n-1200]

123. The National Heart, Lung and Blood Institute Acute Respiratory Distress Syndrome (ARDS) Clinical Trials Network (ARDSNet). Pulmonary-artery versus central venous catheter to guide treatment of acute lung injury. N Engl J Med 2006; 354:2213–2224. [I; RCT, *n* = 1000]

124. Harvey S, Harrison DA, Singer M, et al. Assessment of the clinical effectiveness of pulmonary artery catheters in management of patients in intensive care (PAC-Man): a randomized controlled trial. Lancet 2005; 366:472–477. [I; RCT, *n* = 1041]

125. The ESCAPE Investigators and ESCAPE Study Coordinators. Evaluation study of congestive heart failure and pulmonary artery catheterization effectiveness: the ESCAPE trial. JAMA 2005; 294:1625–1633. [I; RCT, *n* = 433]

41

Cancer

Elyce Cardonick

KEY POINTS
Cancer Diagnosed in Pregnancy

- **Avoid delay in diagnosis**, by performing necessary diagnostic studies in a timely and adequate fashion as in nonpregnant adults, with rare exceptions.
- Avoid unnecessary radiologic studies unless results will alter cancer treatment or patient decisions during pregnancy.
- Avoid iatrogenic preterm deliveries.
- When choosing a particular **chemotherapeutic regimen** for a particular cancer, **choose based on the one with the most experience of use and proven safety during pregnancy**, as long as it will offer a **similar chance of cure** for the patient. **Administer the same doses of chemotherapy as given to nonpregnant women.** Send **placental pathology** for all cancers, especially in cases of melanoma.
- Close multidisciplinary management, especially with **an oncologist and maternal-fetal specialist knowledgeable in cancer and pregnancy special considerations**, is vital to optimize outcomes.

Cancer Diagnosed Before Pregnancy

- **Women who have been treated for childhood cancer with chemotherapy, radiation therapy, or both are not at increased risk of having children with congenital or chromosomal anomalies.**
- **The available data do not support an adverse effect of prior chemotherapy on the risk of miscarriage, fetal demise, or birth weight.**
- Pregnancy in women who have received **prior pelvic irradiation appears to be associated with complications such as miscarriage, preterm labor and delivery, low birth weight, and placenta accreta.**
- Unless the cancer suffered by the patient was part of an inherited syndrome, such as retinoblastoma, the offsprings of cancer survivors are not at increased risk for cancer.
- With the possible exception of gestational trophoblastic disease, pregnancy does not affect the risk of recurrence of any type of cancer.
- **We suggest that women with a history of prior thoracic radiation therapy or who received anthracyclines** (daunorubicin, doxorubicin, idarubicin, epirubicin, and mitoxantrone) **undergo cardiac evaluation prior to pregnancy.**

CANCER DIAGNOSED IN PREGNANCY
Incidence/Epidemiology

Cancer complicates approximately 1/1000 pregnancies, and 1 out of every 118 malignancies is associated with pregnancy (1).

There is no increased incidence of malignancy in pregnant women. Upon reviewing the literature, almost 500 pregnant women have been diagnosed and treated for cancer during pregnancy. The most common cancers that occur during pregnancy are breast, cervical, leukemia, lymphoma, thyroid, and melanoma (2).

General Cancer in Pregnancy Considerations

There are no specific trials regarding the management of cancer in pregnancy. **Delay in diagnosis should be avoided** by performing necessary diagnostic studies in a timely and adequate fashion as in nonpregnant adults. **Diagnostic measures should not be delayed when a pregnant patient presents with a suspicious sign or symptom. The safest diagnostic studies should be employed, for example, an MRI in place of CT if similar diagnostic information can be obtained. Staging measures, however, can often be delayed until after delivery if the results would not change the course of treatment or** patient decisions during pregnancy. **Chemotherapy regimens should be comparable to those used in nonpregnant patients; however, using the newest agents is not recommended in absence of safety data even if favored for nonpregnant patients.** For example, nonpregnant women may be treated for breast cancer with adriamycin/cytoxan, idarubicin/cytoxan, or epirubicin/cytoxan. Although the latter may be better tolerated in nonpregnant patients, the first regimen has the most reported cases in the pregnancy literature, so this regimen with the most experience of use during pregnancy should be chosen, until more information accumulates. The second regimen has been associated with transient cardiomyopathy in infants exposed in utero (3–5). Different drugs in the same class of chemotherapy agents may have different properties that allow more placental transfer. **Once the regimen is chosen, the pregnant woman should be given the same doses of chemotherapy as given to nonpregnant women with the same cancer type and stage**, to ensure best treatment and outcomes. If dosage is based on patient weight, the woman's changing weight during pregnancy should be used, not ideal body weight. This recommendation may change if pharmacokinetic studies are performed in the future on pregnant women receiving chemotherapy as free drug levels may not be the same as in nonpregnant women due to the many physiologic changes during pregnancy which affect drug metabolism. **Close multidisciplinary management, especially with oncologist and maternal-fetal specialist knowledgeable in cancer and pregnancy special considerations, is vital to optimize outcomes**. Obstetrical management rarely needs to be altered, and evidence-based interventions proven beneficial in pregnancy should be available to all women with cancer in pregnancy. Moreover, nonproven interventions such as iatrogenic preterm deliveries should be avoided. **Placental pathology** should be sent for all cancers, especially in cases of melanoma. **For most cancers, termination of pregnancy does not improve or affect outcome**. If the patient wishes to continue the pregnancy, cancer treatment is discussed if treatment cannot be delayed until postpartum without compromising the woman's chance of cure. This concept brings into conflict what is best for maternal survival yet not harmful to the developing fetus.

General Chemotherapy Considerations

Chemotherapy often cannot and should not be delayed solely due to pregnancy if such a delay would decrease maternal chance of cure and there have been reassuring reports of using the intended chemotherapy regimen in pregnant women before. Chemotherapy given during the first trimester has the highest chance of causing malformations, as the majority of organogenesis occurs between three and eight weeks postconception. Many chemotherapeutic agents are relatively safe for the fetus, especially after 12 to 14 weeks of pregnancy, even though the brain continues to develop for the remainder of the pregnancy (6). **If one controls for the gestational age at delivery, fetal growth restriction does not appear to be increased in most cases, especially with solid tumors**. Patients with systemic disease such as leukemia are at risk for increased perinatal morbidity and mortality including an increased risk for growth restriction and intrauterine fetal demise.

Transplacental studies of different chemotherapy agents during pregnancy are very few, and at times conflicting. Doxorubicin was not detectable in amniotic fluid, placental tissue, fetal brain, or GI tract but detectable in fetal liver, kidney, and lung 15 hours after IV administration (7,8). Umbilical blood sampling two and five weeks post multiagent chemotherapy for maternal leukemia showed that fetal hematopoesis was normal each time (9).

Long-term follow-up of children exposed to chemotherapy is limited. A case series of neurodevelopmental follow-up for a mean of 18 years on 84 children exposed in utero to various types of chemotherapy for maternal hematologic malignancy shows that their clinical health status is comparable to their unexposed siblings. No cancer has been diagnosed in any of the children, and 12 children exposed in utero have now had their own children. All second-generation children were normal in appearance but did not undergo the same rigorous testing as their parents (10). According to a different author, a single case of malignancy has been diagnosed in a child exposed in utero to chemotherapy. Papillary thyroid cancer at age 11 and neuroblastoma at age 14 were diagnosed in a 14-year-old exposed in utero to multiple chemotherapeutic agents for maternal leukemia. His fraternal twin (exposed to the same agents) was healthy (11). He was also born with congenital anomalies including esophageal atresia, abnormal IVC, right-arm deformity.

Breast Cancer

Breast cancer is one of the most common cancers complicating pregnancy. During pregnancy, 7% to 15% of premenopausal cases occur. The histology of breast cancer diagnosed during pregnancy is no different from the nonpregnant patient population. There is no survival difference between women diagnosed with breast cancer during pregnancy and stage-matched nonpregnant women (1,12–14). Pregnant women may be more likely to be diagnosed at stage II compared to nonpregnant women (74% vs. 37%), and less likely to be diagnosed with early-stage disease (21% vs. 54%) (15). Women younger than 40 are more likely to be diagnosed with stage-II disease

compared to women older than 40. When matched for stage of disease, women younger than 40 have a statistically worse five-year survival compared to women older than 40 years of age at diagnosis (55% vs. 75%). According to these data, **it may be the age of reproductive age women which has a stronger influence on survival than pregnancy** (15). Nodal status is a highly significant predictor, whereas pregnancy is not (14).

Delay in Diagnosis
Studies show both patients and physicians follow a breast mass longer in pregnant women before performing a biopsy. Other factors contributing to a possible delay in diagnosis is that masses found on exam are ascribed to "normal breast changes" of pregnancy and malignancy is not suspected. Pregnant women, therefore, are often diagnosed with larger tumors at later stages than nonpregnant women. A **delay in diagnosis obviously worsens prognosis, and is inexcusable**.

Diagnostic Tests and Safety in Pregnancy
Mammography has less sensitivity for screening in pregnancy, due to the increased overall density, vascularity, cellularity, and water content, which leads to less contrast during pregnancy. The fetal exposure to mammography is not a concern (0.4 rads). **During pregnancy, breast ultrasound has a better accuracy than mammography and should be performed for palpable masses**. The workup of a solitary mass should continue as in nonpregnant women, with **fine-needle aspiration**, or excision. False positive cytological findings can occur in pregnancy due to the highly proliferative state of the breast (16). As in premenopausal nonpregnant women, most tumors in pregnant women are estrogen receptor negative (17). Receptor assays for estrogen and progesterone should be done with immunohistochemistry, not competitive binding assays, the latter of which may give false-negative results due to the saturation with endogenous steroid hormone during pregnancy (18).

Effects on the Pregnancy
Breast cancer itself (excluding therapy) does not directly affect perinatal outcome.

Termination of Pregnancy and Breast Cancer
Routine termination of pregnancy does not appear to offer a survival advantage for pregnant women diagnosed with breast cancer of any stage (15,19,20). It is difficult to determine from studies comparing survival for women who terminate their pregnancies to women who carry to term, if women with advanced or aggressive disease were more likely to be encouraged to terminate their pregnancy and therefore had a worse outcome than women with earlier-stage disease who continued their pregnancies. This has been called "the healthy mother effect." Stage of disease at diagnosis is not reported in these studies, but rather survival for the group who terminated the pregnancy is compared to women who continued beyond 24 weeks. In no study was an improved survival shown for women who terminated the pregnancy.

Staging During Pregnancy
Mammography is indicated once breast cancer is diagnosed during pregnancy, to exclude multifocal disease in the affected breast or cancer in the contralateral breast. A chest X ray (with abdominal shielding) is recommended to exclude pulmonary metastasis and can be safely performed with fetal exposure of 0.06 mrad. A chest CT scan is not warranted as the dose to the fetus is greater. If further evaluation is necessary, MRI of the

thorax is recommended (21). The risk of bony metastasis with stage I or II breast cancer is 3% to 7%. A bone scan can be safely deferred until after pregnancy for asymptomatic patients with early-stage disease. If a patient is symptomatic, or has advanced-stage disease, a bone scan can be performed with a Foley catheter in place and intravenous hydration to promote washout of the excreted radiopharmaceutical from patient's bladder. An exposure of 10 mCi rather than 20 mCi of Technitium-99m (Tc-99m) methylene diphosphonate (MDP) and doubling the imaging time can reduce fetal radiation exposure (22). MRI of the skeleton can detect 80% of metastatic deposits. Brain scan is of little yield unless patient has neurologic symptoms and physical findings. An abdominal MRI is recommended as an alternative to contrast-enhanced CT. Abdominal ultrasound is no longer recommended as it is insensitive to detect metastasis compared to CT or MRI. In the liver function tests, alkaline phosphatase is physiologically increased in pregnancy and therefore not reliable for management decisions.

Surgery During Pregnancy

Breast conservation surgery or mastectomy can be safely performed at any gestational age during pregnancy, with attention paid to avoid the supine position after 20 weeks' gestation. One must consider that after breast-conservation surgery, radiation therapy is standard after chemotherapy is concluded. This is not mandatory after a full mastectomy. The time delay between completing chemotherapy and beginning radiation therapy that will not compromise the woman's prognosis is unknown; however, there is usually not a prolonged delay for nonpregnant women. Therefore, if a patient is diagnosed early in pregnancy and would complete chemotherapy by 30 weeks of gestation (usually four cycles given 2–3 weeks apart), at least 6 weeks of delay would occur before radiation therapy would start without an iatrogenic preterm delivery before 36 weeks. For patients who are diagnosed early in pregnancy, consider mastectomy rather than breast conservation so to avoid an extended period of time between completing chemotherapy during pregnancy, and starting radiation postpartum.

Radiation has been safely given during pregnancy for other cancers, but not usually for breast cancer. Other than this concern about the time delay between finishing chemotherapy and local radiation to the chest wall postpartum, there is no contraindication to breast-conservation surgery for pregnant women diagnosed with breast cancer. It is recommended for all pregnant patients to delay reconstruction after mastectomy until postpartum because of the inherent changes that will occur in the unaffected breast due to pregnancy, postpartum atrophy, and possibly breast-feeding. Cosmetic results will be better if one delays reconstruction until after the postpartum period to match the unaffected breast.

Sentinel Node Biopsy

Sentinel node mapping and biopsy is commonly used for young nonpregnant women to avoid the complications of lymphedema after complete axillary lymphadenectomy. Sentinel node biopsy can be safely performed in pregnancy with Tc-99m sulfur colloid, which identifies the first draining node (s) relative to the site of the primary invasive tumor (20). For sentinel node imaging, only a minimal dose (500–600 μCi) of double-filtered Tc-99m sulfur colloid is injected at the site of the breast tumor. The entire radioisotope stays trapped at the sight of injection or within the lymphatics until decay occurs (half-life = six hours), not traveling throughout the body to expose the fetus (21,23). There is limited information on the use of blue dyes such as lymphazurin for sentinel node map-

ping in pregnancy and this carries a risk of anaphylaxis. The current recommendation is to use Tc-99 rather than any dye injection.

Treatment During Pregnancy

The majority of women reported in the literature were treated with cytoxan, doxorubicin with or without 5-fluourouracil (5FU). To date, 253 cases of breast cancer treated with chemotherapy have been published. Currently, doxorubicin is the preferred anthracycline to use during pregnancy, given its safety and use in over 140 cases during pregnancy for various types of cancer. Another anthracycline, epirubicin, was used in 49 cases with two fetal deaths, and one neonatal death. An IUFD occurred at 30 weeks of gestation after second-trimester exposure to epirubicin, vincristine, and prednisone, and another after exposure to epirubicin with cyclophosphamide. One neonate died at eight days of life after third-trimester exposure to epirubicin, cyclophosphamide, and fluorouracil (6). From this data it is suggested that, **when doxorubicin therapy is as efficacious as idarubicin or epirubicin in selected cases of malignancy, doxorubicin be preferred in pregnancy**, even if epirubicin has lower myelotoxic and cardiotoxic properties compared with doxorubicin. Transient neonatal cardiomyopathy has been reported after idarubicin exposure and the use of this anthracycline is not recommended during pregnancy. Nonpregnant women with positive nodes are treated with taxane therapy, simultaneously or after completing cytoxan and an anthracycline, with or without 5FU. Only 15 cases of taxane use in human pregnancy have been published (24–32). The only demonstrated increase in this group was growth restriction. Herceptin/trastuzumab use is contraindicated in pregnancy as its use has been found to be associated with oligohydramnios and pulmonary hypoplasia (33–38).

Hodgkin's Disease

The mean age of diagnosis for Hodgkin's disease (HD) is 32 years (39). Pregnant women are not more likely to be diagnosed at a higher stage compared to nonpregnant women (40). Pregnancy does not adversely affect survival rate. ABVD regimen (adriamycin/bleomycin/vincristine/dacarbazine) has been used safely during pregnancy (41). Chemotherapy during organogenesis in the first trimester will increase the risk for malformations (see treatment below). If patients require treatment during the first trimester, consider single-agent treatment with vinblastine followed by full regimen during second and third trimesters.

Diagnostic Tests and Safety in Pregnancy

The clinical behavior of HD during pregnancy does not appear to differ from nonpregnant women. Pregnant women can present with a cough, night sweats, and weight loss. A patient with such complaints should have a complete physical exam and clavicular adenopathy can be safely biopsied during pregnancy. A chest X ray can be performed safely with minimal fetal exposure. An abdominal shield is still indicated for all radiologic studies during pregnancy. A bone marrow biopsy can also be safely performed. Surgeons should be advised of the safety of narcotic use for pregnant women undergoing surgical procedures to avoid patient discomfort.

Effects on Pregnancy

HD's disease does not directly affect perinatal outcome. Infants born to women with HD do not have a higher risk for prematurity or intrauterine growth restriction (40).

Termination of Pregnancy
Therapeutic termination of a pregnancy does not improve the course of disease (42).

Surgery During Pregnancy
At times, histologic examination of a clavicular lymph node is inconclusive. In such cases, if mediastinal adenopathy is evident on X ray or CT of the chest, a guided biopsy may be indicated to confirm a diagnosis.

Staging of Disease in Pregnancy
The staging of lymphoma is based on history and physical examination, hematologic and biochemical testing, bone marrow biopsy and radiologic imaging. A staging laparotomy and splenectomy are no longer routinely performed in nonpregnant patients. Gallium scanning is not routine anymore, even in nonpregnant patients.

Currently, women with stages I and II receive combination modality treatment, so full staging during pregnancy is unlikely to change the recommended treatment during the course of pregnancy, and can be delayed to the postpartum period. Image staging in nonpregnant patients includes a chest X ray and CT. In the pregnant woman, a two-view chest X ray is suggested. Fetal exposure is negligible with abdominal shielding. A chest MRI can assess lymphadenopathy, and the information gained is comparable to a CT (21). MRI can also evaluate the bone marrow and detect splenic involvement that may be undetectable with CT.

Treatment of HD During Pregnancy
The ABVD regimen for Hodgkin's lymphoma has been reported to be safe in pregnancy, although dacarbazine is the least studied agent. Similar doses should be given to the pregnant patient with adjustment for weight gain during pregnancy.

Radiotherapy During Pregnancy
Radiotherapy for HD during pregnancy has been reported to be tolerable for the fetus at certain gestational ages (43). Exposure of the fetus to radiation is determined by the internal scatter, leakage from the tube head, and scatter from the collimator. Internal scatter depends on the source of radiation, the distance of the fetus from the source, and the size of treatment fields. Blocks are not recommended in pregnancy because of the additional scatter they create. Exposure of the fetus can be estimated with simulated measurements, which have shown that treatment with a 6 MV linear accelerator exposes the fetus to less radiation than treatment with Cobalt 60 (43). The highest risk of brain damage and mental retardation is between 8 and 15 weeks' gestation (44). Radiation for HD is usually reserved for cases progressing despite chemotherapy, lymphocyte predominant type, or if chemotherapy is not an option.

Non–Hodgkin's Lymphoma

Non–Hodgkin's lymphoma (NHL) is rarely reported during pregnancy as this generally occurs in an older age group (mean age at diagnosis is 42 years). Pregnant women present with an aggressive histology (39,45), but the response to treatment, failure and progression rates are similar to nonpregnant patients. Symptoms can vary widely, with many complaints similar to symptoms in normal pregnancy, which can lead to a delay in diagnosis of NHL in pregnancy.

Avoid Delay in Diagnosis
Pregnant women with NHL can present with breast or ovarian masses, misleading the initial diagnosis to a gynecologic malignancy. When masses are bilateral and massive in size, one should suspect NHL (see sections "Effects of Cancer on the Pregnancy" and "Treatment of NHL During Pregnancy" below).

Effects of Cancer on the Pregnancy and Vice Versa
NHL does not directly affect pregnancy. However pregnancy can affect the presentation of NHL, and some authors report a progression of NHL postpartum (46–48). In some cases, such as lymphoproliferative T-cell lymphoma, a component of Epstein–Barr virus in the etiology of NHL may explain, given the immunosuppression of pregnancy, why some cases of NHL seem to progress more rapidly in pregnant women. The number of cases however is too small to determine if termination of the pregnancy would improve prognosis. NHL can present with lymphadenopathy, as with nonpregnant patients; however, pregnant patients can have involvement of the breasts, ovaries, and uterus. A hormonal influence of pregnancy on the progression of NHL is suggested by the frequent and massive involvement of such organs during pregnancy, which are otherwise unusually involved with lymphoma in nonpregnant patients (45).

Treatment of NHL During Pregnancy
Thirty-five cases of NHL were treated during pregnancy with multiple regimens, most including doxorubicin, cyclophosphamide, and vincristine. No malformations occurred, even with first trimester treatment in 11 cases. Breast or ovarian masses should *not* be removed after biopsy confirms lymphoma. The masses will respond to systemic chemotherapy. Rituximab is often used in nonpregnant patients in addition to CHOP chemotherapy. It is a chimeric IgG1antibody, which can cross the placenta and interact with fetal B cells. It is unlikely that rituximab has any mutagenic potential. Infants exposed to rituximab in pregnancy initially had a period of low IgG, but B-cell counts normalized by four months after birth and the period with low IgG might not have been longer than average.

Leukemia: Acute and Chronic

Leukemia is rarely diagnosed during pregnancy as affected women usually have amenorrhea. Acute leukemia, which usually occurs in young women, is more common than chronic leukemia during pregnancy.

Avoid Delay in Diagnosis
Pregnant women with leukemia can present with severe anemia, thrombocytopenia, infection or sepsis, fever, bone pain, or bleeding.

Diagnostic Tests and Safety in Pregnancy
Bone marrow biopsy can be safely performed during pregnancy.

Termination of Pregnancy Issues
Termination of pregnancy has not been shown to improve prognosis. Patients newly diagnosed with acute leukemia are too ill to safely undergo a dilatation and curettage procedure when termination is elected. If a patient elects termination, induction chemotherapy should still be given during the pregnancy to induce remission so that the procedure can be safely performed. The patient is otherwise at too high a risk for the

complications of sepsis, hemorrhage, and disseminated intravascular coagulation (DIC).

Effects of Cancer on the Pregnancy
Acute leukemia is one of the cancers which can affect perinatal outcome. The earlier the diagnosis in pregnancy, the higher the perinatal mortality. Pregnancies complicated by acute leukemia are at higher risk for complications such as miscarriage, intrauterine fetal demise, preterm labor, and fetal growth restriction, unrelated to cancer treatment (48,49). Suspected etiologies include maternal anemia, DIC, or leukemia cells affecting blood flow and nutrient exchange in the intervillous spaces of the placenta, and decreased oxygen transport to the fetus (49). When intensive chemotherapy is given in pregnancy, complete remission is achieved in 75% of patients (49).

Treatment of Cancer During Pregnancy: Surgery, Chemotherapy, Radiation Therapy
Aggressive hematologic and obstetric management is advocated when acute leukemia is diagnosed. The prognosis for both mother and fetus is poor when acute leukemia is not treated during pregnancy. Without therapy, maternal death may occur within two months time (49). Chemotherapy treatment during pregnancy is associated with higher maternal and fetal/neonatal survival compared to postponing chemotherapy until postpartum (49). All cases with anomalies occurred with first-trimester exposure to cytarabine or 6-thioguanine, alone or in combination with an anthracycline. Cytarabine and 6-thioguanine should be avoided in the first trimester if possible. Combinations including vincristine, 6-MP, doxorubicin or daunorubicin, cyclophosphamide, prednisone and methotrexate were used in all trimesters without anomalies. Transient myelosuppression can occur in neonates, especially if delivered within three to four weeks of chemotherapy (50). More rarely, transient neonatal cardiomyopathy has been reported. Cardiomyopathy occurred mostly after use of idarubicin (4). Iatrogenic preterm deliveries or elective inductions should be avoided before remission is attempted, as the patient with acute leukemia is at risk for hemorrhage, DIC, and sepsis during labor and delivery if lacerations or endometritis occurs.

Chronic leukemia rarely occurs during pregnancy, as the average age at diagnosis is in the fifth or sixth decade. Hydroxyurea or busulfan appears safe for use during pregnancy if necessary, although in the majority of cases treatment can be delayed without consequence until after delivery. Leukophoresis can be a temporizing measure to reduce WBC and spleen size if necessary (51,52). Gleevec, the newest advance in the treatment of chronic leukemia in nonpregnant adults, has been shown to cause teratogenic effects in rats including exencephaly or encephalocele and absent or reduced frontal and absent parietal bones. Post implantation loss might occur as well. No teratogenicitiy has been shown in rabbits.

Melanoma
One-third of women diagnosed with malignant melanoma are of childbearing age (53). When pregnant patients are matched to nonpregnant controls for prognostic factors such as tumor thickness, there is **no significant difference in survival rates** for pregnant women with stage-I melanoma (54–57). One study reported that pregnancy at diagnosis was significantly associated with **metastatic disease** when controlling for tumor site, thickness, and Clark level, still with survival not significantly decreased for pregnant patients (58,59).

Avoid Delay in Diagnosis
Pregnant women are diagnosed with **thicker tumors** compared to nonpregnant women. This (as well as the increase in metastatic disease) has been ascribed in the literature to a delay in biopsy leading to delayed diagnosis when changes in mole's appearance are ascribed to pregnancy or the surgeon is hesitant to perform a biopsy during pregnancy. Hyperpigmentation can occur secondary to an increased secretion of melanocyte-stimulating hormone (MSH); however, the color of the mole should still be uniform. Maximum increases/decreases in the size of melanocytic nevi in pregnancy is 1 mm (60,61). During pregnancy, one must still look for signs of melanoma, listed below, which should *not* be ascribed to normal changes in pregnancy. These include the ABCD signs: A for asymmetry; B for notched, irregular, or indistinct borders; C for an uneven color; D for diameter greater than 6 mm. Itching of a mole can also be an early sign of malignant melanoma.

Effects of Cancer on the Pregnancy
Melanoma is one of the rare cancers that can **metastasize to the placenta**. Eighty seven cases of placenta/fetal metastasis have been reported. The largest percentage (31%) was in cases of maternal melanoma (62). Patients with placental metastases also had widespread disease. The placenta should be sent for pathologic evaluation in all cases of melanoma diagnosed during pregnancy. If melanoma is found in the placenta, the neonate should be followed closely for one year with frequent skin evaluations.

Termination of Pregnancy Issues
No advantage in prognosis or survival has been demonstrated with elective pregnancy termination in patients with stage-I melanoma.

Surgery During Pregnancy
Wide local excision is the only cure for melanoma, and can be safely performed during pregnancy at any gestational age. Patients should be positioned with uterine displacement after 20 weeks' gestation. See sentinel node biopsy below for safety information.

Staging and Sentinel Node Biopsy
Wide local excision is the only cure for melanoma, and should be done after a biopsy is suspicious for melanoma. Sentinel node mapping can be safely performed during pregnancy, with Tc-99 sulfur colloid. Intradermal injection of Technitium-labeled sulfur colloid causes negligible ionizing radiation to the fetus. The majority of the dose stays localized to the injection site or within the lymphatics until decay occurs. For stage-I or -II melanoma, a chest X ray is indicated for staging if the melanoma is greater than 1.0-mm thick. No other staging radiologic studies are required. For stage-III disease, an MRI of the chest, abdomen with or without the pelvis is recommended in addition to the chest X ray for evaluation of lymphadenopathy or evidence of liver metastases. MRI of the brain and skeleton is also recommended.

Treatment of Melanoma During Pregnancy
Surgery is the only effective treatment for melanoma, and chemotherapy has not been shown to significantly prolong survival. Postpartum, patients with advanced disease can enroll in clinical trials using interferon or melanoma vaccinations (see also chap. 42).

Invasive Cervical Cancer

Invasive carcinoma of the cervix occurs in approximately 1 out of 2200 pregnancies, but this incidence is declining due to widespread and improved Papanicolau screening (63,64). Tumor characteristics and maternal survival are not adversely affected by pregnancy (64). Unlike nonpregnant patients, presenting symptoms are more likely to be abnormal Papanicolau screens rather than bleeding. The predominant histologic type is squamous cell. Prognosis is comparable to nonpregnant patients (64–67).

Avoid Delay in Diagnosis
Pregnant women are more likely to be diagnosed with earlier-stage disease as cervical screening is routine during prenatal care (64).

Diagnostic Tests and Safety in Pregnancy
The cytobrush can be safely used during pregnancy to obtain an adequate Pap smear during prenatal care. Pregnant patients should be warned of the possibility of bleeding afterward.

Effects of Cancer on the Pregnancy
Cervical cancer does not adversely affect pregnancy directly; however, cancer treatment affects future fertility if hysterectomy is indicated.

Termination of Pregnancy Issues
A spontaneous loss of the pregnancy may occur when treatment for cervical cancer is initiated for patients diagnosed prior to 18 weeks' gestation.

Considerations Regarding Therapy During Pregnancy for Cervical Cancer
The gestational age at diagnosis determines the choices for the pregnant patient. For stages IB-IIA diagnosed before 18 weeks, immediate treatment is recommended. Nonpregnant patients with stages IB/IIA can have surgery or radiotherapy for cervical cancer. For early stage (IB/IIA), a radical hysterectomy or radiotherapy can be performed with the fetus in situ. Often a spontaneous miscarriage will occur within a short time after radiotherapy. For patients with advanced-stage disease, external radiotherapy and chemotherapy with fetus in situ is suggested. Spontaneous abortion often follows radiotherapy; however, hysterotomy may be required to facilitate brachytherapy if this does not occur (66).

Patients diagnosed after 18 weeks' gestation can consider delaying surgical treatment of cervical cancer in order to improve fetal maturity and survival. Neoadjuvant chemotherapy for invasive cervical disease may be given during the second and third trimesters of pregnancy so as to buy time for delivery of a viable fetus and postpartum radical treatment.

Surgery for Cervical Cancer Diagnosed During Pregnancy
The survival outcomes for pregnant women and their children when surgical treatment for cervical cancer is intentionally delayed for 6 to 17 weeks is very good, with fetal outcomes markedly improved, and maternal survival not adversely affected (68–72). Approximately 50 patients have been reported with this intentional delay to reach fetal viability and maturity. Radical treatment consists of radical hysterectomy with nodal dissection or radiotherapy for stages I-IIA and chemoradiotherapy for stages IIB-IVA tumors. If the fetus is viable, a prompt cesarean section is advised with radical hysterectomy performed simultaneously. A classical cesarean delivery is recommended to avoid extension into the lower uterine segment (72). At the time

of cesarean section pelvic and para-aortic nodes should be sampled, and an oophoropexy can be performed to move the ovaries out of the radiation field. Episiotomy site recurrences of cervical cancer have been reported after vaginal delivery (73).

Staging of Cervical Cancer During Pregnancy
Imaging for staging includes evaluation of regional lymph node chains as lymphadenopathy has prognostic and therapeutic implications. MRI can detect depth of stromal invasion and evaluate the parametria. MRI can also identify a dilated collecting system and enlarged lymph nodes. A two-view chest X ray with proper shielding can be performed if indicated clinically.

Treatment of Cancer During Pregnancy: Surgery, Chemotherapy, Radiation Therapy
Treatment for invasive cervical cancer involves either surgery, radiation or both, depending on the stage at diagnosis. The safe use of neoadjuvent platinum-based chemotherapy has been reported (74,75). See also chapter 31, *Obstetrics Evidence Based Guidelines*.

Thyroid Cancer

The mean age of diagnosis for thyroid cancer is between 30 and 34 years of age, with most cases in pregnancy presenting as a solitary nodule (76). There is no evidence that pregnancy changes the clinical course of the disease, and no evidence that thyroid cancer adversely affects pregnancy outcome. The prognosis of differentiated thyroid cancer is the same in pregnant and nonpregnant women (77). No endocrine association between maternal hormonal changes and thyroid cancer has been found. Treatment depends on histologic subtype, degree of differentiation, stage, and gestational age at diagnosis.

Avoid Delay in Diagnosis
The thyroid can enlarge during normal pregnancy, but solitary nodules should be evaluated.

Diagnostic Tests and Safety in Pregnancy
Biopsy of a solid nodule can be safely performed during pregnancy at any gestational age.

Termination of Pregnancy Issues
No survival advantage is known for elective termination of pregnancy for thyroid cancer.

Surgery During Pregnancy
The type of thyroid cancer and the gestational age at diagnosis determine if thyroidectomy is necessary during pregnancy, or can be safely postponed until postpartum. See section "Treatment of Thyroid Cancer During Pregnancy."

Treatment of Thyroid Cancer During Pregnancy
Differentiated types of thyroid cancer such as papillary, follicular, or mixed types are slow growing and surgery can be postponed until postpartum for patients diagnosed after 12 weeks' gestation. Prior to 12 weeks, a subtotal thyroidectomy is recommended (78). If a nodule is noted (77) to enlarge during pregnancy, if the surrounding tissues are fixed, or lymphatic invasion is seen on the original biopsy, surgery should not be delayed to postpartum, regardless of the gestational age at diagnosis. Patients who delay treatment due to pregnancy should be advised to undergo surgery within 1 year of diagnosis (78).

Medullary or anaplastic types of thyroid cancer are more aggressive, and surgery should not be postponed. A total thyroidectomy may be necessary. If the lesion is compromising the airway, radiotherapy may be necessary during pregnancy. During total thyroidectomy, parathyroid tissue is often inadvertently removed as well. For the remainder of the pregnancy and during preterm or term deliveries, calcium balance should be watched carefully. Magnesium for preterm labor or preeclampsia should be used with caution for this reason.

FOR ALL CANCERS
Complications of Cancer Therapy During Pregnancy

During chemotherapy, side effects such as nausea and vomiting can occur, and can compound the nausea related to the pregnancy. Patients should be well hydrated before, during, and after chemotherapy sessions. Odansetron, metoclopramide, kytril, and benadryl can be safely given for nausea. Decadron can also be given to enhance the effectiveness of antiemetics but should be given in the lowest effective dose (see section "Fetal Surveillance and Timing of Delivery"). Given the relative immunosuppression of pregnancy, combined with the bone marrow suppression with chemotherapy, pregnant women are at risk for infection, and therefore the fetuses are at risk for exposure as well. Case reports on the safety of neupogen use in pregnancy are scarce. Epogen is safe during pregnancy if anemia occurs. Another complication can be poor maternal weight gain due to either nausea and vomiting, or chemotherapy-induced stomatitis. Patients should increase caloric and protein intake in the weeks preceding and following chemotherapy. Nutritional supplementation is sometimes necessary. Theoretically antioxidants should not be supplemented with the prenatal vitamin as free radicals are supposed to be created by the chemotherapy and this may impede its therapeutic effect.

Maternal Surveillance
Prechemotherapy Studies
An echocardiogram is preferred over a multigated equilibrium radionuclide cineangiography (MUGA) to evaluate baseline cardiac function prior to anthracycline therapy. This can provide the necessary information regarding cardiac function and valvular disease. Patients who have any fevers during chemotherapy require comprehensive evaluations for presence of infection, especially during the nadir period. Monitor weight gain throughout pregnancy.

Fetal Surveillance and Timing of Delivery
Often decadron is given with chemotherapy to enhance the effectiveness of antiemetics. This is the intravenous form of dexamethasone. If the patient requires tocolysis for preterm labor, and has received IV decadron with chemotherapy after 24 weeks, steroids such as dexamethasone/betamethasone may not be necessary to stimulate fetal lung maturity. The fetal/neonatal safety of repeated doses of steroids has not been demonstrated and repeated courses of steroids are not currently recommended (see chap. 16, *Obstetrics Evidence Based Guidelines*).

The preterm infant cannot metabolize the chemotherapy agents as well as the term infant, therefore, iatrogenic preterm deliveries should be avoided in patients receiving chemotherapy, and preterm labor should be treated aggressively. Chemotherapy may need to be temporarily withheld/delayed if the patient has preterm labor. Growth ultrasounds in the late second and third trimesters (26–28 weeks) are suggested when women receive chemotherapy during pregnancy, especially for patients diagnosed with acute leukemia, given the increased risk of intrauterine growth restriction.

Transient bone marrow suppression of the neonate can occur if delivery is within three to four weeks of treatment. Delivery should be avoided during this nadir period if possible. Therefore, chemotherapy should not be given after 34 weeks as the patient could potentially go into spontaneous labor during the nadir period. If additional treatment is still required, one can consider early induction so that the interval between the last treatment in pregnancy and the postpartum treatment is not greater than six weeks (e.g., if treatment is 33 weeks, consider induction at 38 weeks so that 1 week afterward patient can continue with chemo with a 6-week interval between last treatment during pregnancy and postpartum treatment).

Fetal/Neonatal Evaluation After Chemotherapy During Pregnancy
The **placenta should be sent for pathology examination in all cases** of women diagnosed with cancer during pregnancy, regardless of cancer type or treatment. A complete blood count with differential is recommended on either the cord blood or the neonate when chemotherapy has been given during pregnancy. Additional long-term follow-up on the children exposed to cancer and its treatment in utero is necessary. A Cancer and Pregnancy Registry is established to follow all children of women diagnosed with cancer during pregnancy. The women are also followed yearly. Information about cancer diagnosis, treatment, pregnancy outcomes, and long-term neonatal health and maternal survival is collected and kept confidential. Contacting the **Cancer and Pregnancy Registry: 1-877-635-4499**; 856-757-7876, 856-342-2491, or **Cancerinpregnancy.com; Cancerandpregnancy.com**.

CANCER DIAGNOSED BEFORE PREGNANCY
General Principles
Pregnancy After Chemotherapy
The available data do **not support an adverse effect of prior chemotherapy on the risk of miscarriage, fetal growth and development, fetal demise, or uterine function** (79–81). The Childhood Cancer Survivor Study compared pregnancy outcome in five-year female cancer survivors who were less than 21 years old at diagnosis, with pregnancy outcomes in their sibling controls (79). The most frequently used agents were cyclophosphamide, doxorubicin, vincristine, dactinomycin, and daunorubicin. Over 1900 females reported 4029 pregnancies. There were no significant differences in pregnancy outcome between patients who had received chemotherapy and controls. Prior chemotherapy does not increase the risk of congenital malformations (82–85).

Chemotherapy-Induced Cardiac Toxicity
We suggest that **women who received anthracyclines** (daunorubicin, doxorubicin, idarubicin, epirubicin, and mitoxantrone) **undergo cardiac evaluation prior to pregnancy** (86).

Pregnancy After Radiation
Pregnancy in women who have received **prior pelvic irradiation appears to be associated with complications such as miscarriage, preterm labor and delivery, low birth weight, impaired fetal growth, placenta accreta, and stillbirth** (87–97). Hypotheses for these findings include changes in the uterine vasculature and its response to cytotrophoblast invasion, or

decreased uterine elasticity and volume from radiation-induced myometrial fibrosis. These responses to radiation, especially if before puberty, can affect fetoplacental blood flow or result in a small uterine size leading to preterm labor and delivery. In addition, radiotherapy may injure the endometrium and prevent normal decidualization, resulting in disorders of placental attachment, such as placenta accreta or percreta (92,93).

In the Childhood Cancer Survivor Study, compared with the children of survivors who did not receive any radiotherapy, the children of survivors treated with high-dose radiotherapy to the uterus (>500 cGy) were at significantly increased risk of preterm birth (50.0 vs. 19.6%), low birth weight (36.2 vs. 7.6%), and small for gestational age (18.2 vs. 7.8%). These risks were also noted at lower uterine radiotherapy doses (starting at 50 cGy for preterm birth and at 250 cGy for low birth weight) (79).

Radiation-Induced Cardiac Toxicity Due to Fibrosis
The clinical spectrum of cardiac injury resulting from radiation includes delayed pericarditis that can present abruptly or as chronic pericardial effusion or constriction; pancarditis, which includes pericardial and myocardial fibrosis with or without endocardial fibroelastosis; cardiomyopathy; coronary artery disease, and functional valve injury and conduction defects (98). Women with a history of **prior thoracic radiation therapy** (including left-sided breast cancer) **should undergo a baseline echocardiogram and electrocardiogram** prior to pregnancy to detect subclinical radiation-induced cardiac sequelae. Consultation with a cardiologist is advised if the echocardiogram is abnormal or an arrhythmia is noted.

Children of Cancer Survivors: No Increased Risk for Cancer
The offspring of cancer survivors are not at increased risk for cancer unless the tumor suffered by the parent was a component of an inherited syndrome, such as retinoblastoma (99,100).

Pregnancy After Cancer: Risk of Recurrence?
With the possible exception of gestational trophoblastic disease, **pregnancy does not affect the risk of recurrence of any type of cancer, although the diagnosis may be delayed because of the pregnancy**. In particular, recurrence of melanoma (101,102) and breast cancer (103–105) appear to be unaffected by a subsequent pregnancy.

Pregnancy After Breast Cancer
Some reports suggest that a subsequent pregnancy after treatment of early-stage breast cancer has a favorable impact on survival (106–109). **Prognosis is determined by nodal status and stage, not subsequent pregnancy** (110).

In one series, 94 women with early-stage disease who became pregnant after breast cancer were compared to 188 breast-cancer survivors without subsequent pregnancies matched for nodal status, tumor size, age, and year of diagnosis (108). The risk ratio for death was significantly lower (0.44) for women who became pregnant subsequent to the diagnosis of breast cancer compared to women with breast cancer who did not have a subsequent pregnancy. Sankila [RR 0.2 (0.1–0.5)] and Mueller [RR 0.54 (0.41–0.71)] also showed a decreased risk of death for women with subsequent pregnancy after breast cancer compared to controls matched for age, stage, and year of diagnosis (99,111).

How long to wait? One study linked data from three cancer registries to birth certificate data to evaluate survival of breast-cancer patients who had pregnancies subsequent to cancer treatment (111). A total of 438 women with invasive breast cancer were matched to 2775 controls for age at diagnosis, race, year of diagnosis, and stage. Among women who were lymph-node negative at diagnosis, younger than 35 years of age, or with only localized disease, pregnancy did not affect cancer mortality, even if conception occurred within 10 months of diagnosis. However, among women with positive lymph nodes at diagnosis, older than 35 years of age, or diagnosed with regional recurrence prior to pregnancy, there was a significant increase in cancer mortality if they conceived within 10 months of diagnosis. Women who conceived at least 10 months after diagnosis had lower mortality than women without births after breast cancer (RR 0.54, 95% CI 0.41–0.71). Decreased mortality was noted regardless of local/metastatic disease, maternal age, tumor size, or lymph-node status. For each year delay in conception after breast cancer, the relative risk of death was further decreased: two to three years after diagnosis, RR 0.49 (95% CI 0.27–0.86); three to four years after diagnosis, RR 0.30 (95% CI 0.12–0.71); and four to five years after diagnosis, RR 0.19 (95% CI 0.05–0.81). In general terms, women with a history of breast cancer should delay subsequent pregnancy at least 10 months after completing cancer treatment (not after diagnosis), realizing that the first two years after diagnosis carries the highest risk for recurrence.

There are also some concerns with regards to cancer treatment. As an example, the half-life of methotrexate [a commonly used agent in the CMF (cyclophosphamide, methotrexate, fluorouracil) regimen] is approximately 8 to 15 hours and it is retained for several weeks to months in the kidney and liver, respectively. Delaying conception at least 12 weeks after stopping methotrexate has been recommended (112).

Issue of tamoxifen. **Birth control should be strongly advised while survivors are taking tamoxifen**. There have been case reports of ambiguous genitalia and Goldenhar syndrome in children exposed to tamoxifen in utero (113,114). Animal studies show rib abnormalities, metaplastic and dysplastic changes in the epithelium of the uterus and reproductive tract similar to DES, growth restriction, and death (114–116).

Breast-feeding after treatment for breast cancer. Most women who have undergone irradiation for breast cancer are able to produce milk on the affected side, but the amount of milk produced may be less than that in a nonirradiated breast, particularly if the lumpectomy site was close to the areolar complex or transected many ducts (117). Even when breast milk is produced, **breast-feeding from the irradiated breast is not advised** because mastitis will be difficult to treat if it occurs (118,119).

REFERENCES

1. Donegan W. Cancer and pregnancy. CA Cancer J Clin 1983; 33(4):194–214. [Review, III]
2. Weisz B, Meirow D, Schiff E, Impact and treatment of cancer during pregnancy. Expert Rev Anticancer Ther 2004; 4(5):889–902. [II-2]
3. Siu BL, Alonzo MR, Vargo TA, et al. Transient dilated cardiomyopathy in a newborn exposed to idarubicin and all-trans-retinoic acid (ATRA) early in the second trimester of pregnancy. Int J Gynecol Cancer 2002; 12:399–402. [II-3]
4. Achtari C, Hohlfeld P. Cardiotoxic transplacental effect of idarubicin administered during the second trimester of pregnancy. Am J Obstet Gynecol 2000; 183:511–512. [II-3]
5. Reynoso EE, Hueta F. Acute leukemia and pregnancy—fatal fetal outcome after exposure to idarubicin during the second trimester. Acta Oncolog 1994; 33:703–716. [II-3]

6. Cardonick E, Iacobucci A. Use of chemotherapy during human pregnancy. Lancet Oncol 2004; 5(5):283–291. [Review; II-3]

7. Barni S, Ardizzoia A, Zanetta G, et al. Weekly doxorubicin chemotherapy for breast cancer in pregnancy. A case report. Tumori 1992; 78(5):349–350. [II-2]

8. D'Incalci M, Broggini M, Buscaglia M, et al. Transplacental passage of doxorubicin. Lancet 1983; 75:8314–8315. [II-2]

9. Morishita S, Imai A, Kawabata I, et al. Acute myelogenous leukemia in pregnancy: fetal blood sampling and early effects of chemotherapy. Int J Gynaecol Obstet 1994; 44(3):273–277. [II-2]

10. Aviles A, Neri N. Hematological malignancies and pregnancy: a final report of 84 children who received chemotherapy in utero. Clin Lymph 2001; 2(3):173–177. [II-2]

11. Zemlickis D, Lishner M, Erlich R, et al. Teratogenicity and carcinogenicity in a twin exposed in utero to cyclophosphamide. Terat Carcin Mutagenesis 1993; 13:139–143. [II-2]

12. Gallenberg MM, Loprinzi CL. Breast cancer and pregnancy. Semin Oncol 1989; 16:369–376. [Review; II-3]

13. Gemignani ML, Petrek JA. Breast cancer during pregnancy: diagnostic and therapeutic dilemmas. Adv Surg 2000; 34:272–286. [II-2]

14. Petrek JA, Dukoff R, Rogatko A. Prognosis of pregnancy-associated breast cancer. Cancer 1991; 67:869–872. [II-2]

15. Nugent P, O'Connell TX. Breast cancer and pregnancy. Arch Surg 1985; 120:1221–1224. [Review; II-3]

16. Finley JL, Silverman JF, Lannin DR. Fine-needle aspiration cytology of breast masses in pregnant in lactating women. Diag Cytopath 1989; 5:255–258. [II-3]

17. Barnavon Y, Wallack MK. Management of the pregnant patient with carcinoma of the breast. Surg Gynecol Obstet 1990; 171(4):347–352. [Review, II-3]

18. Elledge RM, Ciocca DR, Langone G, et al. Estrogen receptor, progesterone receptor, and HER-2/neu protein in breast cancers from pregnant patients. Cancer 1993; 71:2499–2506. [II-3]

19. Clark RM, Reid J. Carcinoma of the breast in pregnancy and lactation. Int J Radiation Oncol Biol Phys 1978; 4:693–698. [II-2]

20. Zemlickis D, Lishner M, Degendorfer P, et al. Maternal and fetal outcome after breast cancer in pregnancy. Am J Obstet Gynecol 1992; 166:781–787. [II-2]

21. Nicklas AH, Baker ME. Imaging strategies in the pregnant cancer patient. Semin Oncol 2000; 27(6):623–632. [II-3]

22. Baker J, Ali A, Groch MW, et al. Bone scanning in pregnant patients with breast carcinoma. Clin Nucl Med 1987; 12(7):519–524. [II-3]

23. Keleher A, Wendt R 3rd, Delpassand E, et al. The safety of lymphatic mapping in pregnant breast cancer patients using Tc-99m sulfur colloid. Breast J 2004; 10(6):492–495. [II-3]

24. Doi D, Boh Y, Takeshita T, et al. Combined chemotherapy with paclitaxel and carboplatin for mucinous cystadenocarcinoma of the ovary during pregnancy. Arch Gynecol Obstet 2009; 280:633–636. [II-2]

25. Mir O, Berveiller P, Goldwasser F, et al. Emerging therapeutic options for breast cancer chemotherapy during pregnancy. Ann Oncol 2008; 19:607–613. [II-3]

26. Potluri V, Lewis D, Burton G. Chemotherapy with Taxanes in breast cancer during pregnancy: case report and review of literature. Clin Breast Cancer 2006; 7(2):167–170. [II-3]

27. Gadducci A, Cosio S, Genazzani AR, et al. Chemotherapy with epirubicin and paclitaxel for breast cancer during pregnancy: case report and review of literature. Anticancer Res 2003; 23:5225–5230. [II-3]

28. Gonzalez-Angulo A, Walter RS, Carpenter RJ Jr., et al. Paclitaxel chemotherapy in a pregnant patient with bilateral breast cancer. Clin Breast Cancer 2004; 5(4):317–319. [II-3]

29. Gainford MC, Clemons M. Breast cancer in pregnancy: are taxanes safe? Clin Oncol (R Coll Radiol) 2006; 18(2):159. [II-3]

30. Nieto Y, Santisteban M, Aramendia JM, et al. Docetaxel administered during pregnancy for inflammatory breast carcinoma. Clin Breast Cancer 2006; 6(6):533–534. [II-3]

31. Modares Gilani M, Zarchi K, Behtash N, et al. Preservation of pregnancy in a patient with advanced ovarian cancer at 20 weeks of gestation: case report and literature review. Int J Gynecol Cancer 2007; 17:1140–1143. [II-3]

32. De Santis M, Lucchese A, De Carolis S, et al. Metastatic breast cancer in pregnancy: first case of chemotherapy with docetaxel. Eur J Cancer Care (Engl) 2000; 9(4):235–237. [II-3]

33. Sekar R, Stone PR. Trastuzumab use for metastatic breast cancer in pregnancy. Obstet Gynecol 2007; 110:507–509. [II-3]

34. Fanale MA, Uyei AR, Theriault RL, et al. Treatment of metastatic breast cancer with trastuzumab and vinorelbine during pregnancy. Clin Breast Cancer 2005; 6:354–356. [II-3]

35. Watson W. Herceptin (Trastuzumab) therapy during pregnancy: association with reversible anhydramnios. Obstet Gynecol 2005; 105:642–643. [II-3]

36. Bader AA, Schlembach D, Tamussino KF, et al. Anhydramnios associated with administration of trastuzumab and paclitaxel for metastatic breast cancer during pregnancy. Lancet Oncol 2007; 8:79–81. [II-3]

37. Shrim A, Garcia-Bournissen F, Maxwell C, et al. Favorable pregnancy outcome following trastuzumab use during pregnancy—case report and updated literature review. Reprod Toxicol 2007; 23:611–613. [II-3]

38. Waterston AM, Graham J. Effect of adjuvant trastuzumab on pregnancy. J Clin Oncol 2006; 24:321. [II-3]

39. Ward FT, Weiss RB. Lymphoma and pregnancy. Semin Oncol 1989; 16:397–409. [Review]

40. Lishner M, Zemlickis D, Degendorfer P, et al. Maternal and foetal outcome following Hodgkin's disease in pregnancy. Br J Cancer 1992; 65(1):114–117. [III]

41. Aviles A, Diaz-Maqueo JC, Talavera A, et al. Growth and development of children of mothers treated with chemotherapy during pregnancy: current status of 43 children. Am J Hematol 1991; 36:243–248. [II-2]

42. Nisce LZ, Tome MA, He S, et al. Management of coexisting Hodgkin's disease and pregnancy. Am J Clin Oncol 1986; 9(2):146–151. [II-3]

43. Woo SY, Fuller LM, Cundiff JH, et al. Radiotherapy during pregnancy for clinical stages IA-IIA Hodgkin's disease. Int J Radiat Oncol Biol Phys 1992; 23(2):407–412. [II-3]

44. Dekaban AS. Abnormalities in children exposed to x-radiation during various stages of gestation: tentative timetable of radiation injury to the human fetus. J Nucl Med 1968; 9:471–477. [II-3]

45. Ioachim HL. Non-Hodgkin's lymphoma in pregnancy. Arch Path Lab Med 1985; 109:803–809. [II-3]

46. Steiner-Salz D, Yahalom J, Samuelov A, et al. Non-Hodgkin's lymphoma associated with pregnancy. A report of 6 six cases, with a review of the literature. Cancer 1985; 56(8):2087–2091. [II-3]

47. Mavrommatis CG, Daskalakis GJ, Papageorgiou IS, et al. Non-Hodgkin's lymphoma during pregnancy—case report. Eur J Obstet Gynecol Reprod Biol 1998; 79(1):95–97. [II-3]

48. Reynoso EE, Shepherd FA,, Messner HA, et al. Acute leukemia during pregnancy: the Toronto leukemia study group experience with long-term follow-up of children exposed in utero to chemotherapeutic agents. J Clin Oncol 1987; 5:1098–1106. [II-2]

49. Catanzarite VA, Ferguson JE 2nd. Acute leukemia and pregnancy: a review of management and outcomes, 1972-1982. Obstet Gynecol Surv 1984; 39(11):663–677. [II-2]

50. Okun DB, Groncy PK, Sieger L, et al. Acute leukemia in pregnancy: transient neonatal myelosuppression after combination chemotherapy in the mother. Med Pediatr Oncol 1979; 7(4):315–319. [II-3]

51. Strobl FJ, Voelkerding KV, Smith EP. Management of chronic myeloid leukemia during pregnancy with leukapheresis. J Clin Apheresis 1999; 14:42–44. [II-3]

52. Fitzgerald D, Rowe JM, Heal J. Leukapheresis for control of chronic myelogenous leukemia during pregnancy. Am J Hematol 1986; 22:213–218. [II-3]

53. Colbourn DS, Nathanson L, Belilos E. Pregnancy and malignant melanoma. Semin Oncol 1989; 16:377–387. [Review, II-3]

54. McManamny DS, Moss AL, Pocock PV, et al. Melanoma and pregnancy: a long-term follow up. Br J Obstet Gynecol 1989; 96 (12):1419–1423. [II-2]

55. Wong DJ, Strassner HT. Melanoma in pregnancy. Clin Obstet Gynecol 1990; 33:782–791. [Review, II-3]

56. Mackie RM, Bufalino R, Morabito A, et al. Lack of effect of pregnancy on outcome of melanoma. Lancet 1991; 337:653–655. [II-2]

57. Lens MB, Rosdahl I, Farahmand BY, et al. Effect of pregnancy on survival of women with cutaneous malignant melanoma. J Clin Oncol 2004; 22(21):4369–4375. [II-2]

58. Slingluff CL Jr., Seigler HF. Malignant melanoma and pregnancy. Ann Plastic Surgery 1992; 28(1):95–99. [Review, II-2]

59. Slingluff CL Jr., Reintgen D. Malignant melanoma and the prognostic implications of pregnancy, oral contraceptives, and exogenous hormones. Semin Surg Oncol 1993; 9:228–231. [II-2]

60. Pennoyer JW, Grin CM, Driscoll MS, et al. Changes in the size of melanocytic nevi during pregnancy (see comment). J Am Acad Dermatol 1997; 36(3 part 1):378–382. [II-3]

61. Pennoyer JW, Grin CM, Driscoll MS, et al. Changes in size of melanocytic nevi during pregnancy. J Eur Acad Dermatol Venereol 2003; 17(3):349–351. [II-3]

62. Baergen RN, Johnson D, Moore T, et al. Maternal melanoma metastatic to the placenta: a case report and review of the literature. Arch Pathol Lab Med 1997; 121:508–511. [II-3]

63. Hacker NF, Berek JS, Lagasse LD, et al. Carcinoma of the cervix associated with pregnancy. Obstet Gynecol 1982; 59:735–745. [II-2]

64. Zemlickis D, Lishner M, Degendorfer P, et al. Maternal and fetal outcome after invasive cervical cancer in pregnancy. J Clin Oncol 1991; 9(11):1956–1961. [II-2]

65. Germann N, Haie-Meder C, Morice P, et al. Management and clinical outcomes of pregnant patients with invasive cervical cancer. Ann Oncol 2005; 16(3):397–402. [II-2]

66. Hopkins MP, Morley GW. The prognosis and management of cervical cancer associated with pregnancy. Obstet Gynecol 1992; 80(1):9–13. [II-2]

67. Method MW, Brost BC. Management of cervical cancer in pregnancy. Semin Surg Oncol 1999; 16(3):251–260. [Review, II-3]

68. Duggan B, Muderspach LI, Roman LD, et al. Cervical cancer in pregnancy: reporting on planned delay in therapy. Obstet Gynecol 1993; 82:598–602. [II-3]

69. Sood AK, Sorosky JI, Krogman S, et al. Surgical management of cervical cancer complicating pregnancy: a case control study. Gynecol Oncol 1996; 63(3):294–298. [II-2]

70. Prem KA, Makowski EL, McKelvey JL. Carcinoma of the cervix associated with pregnancy. Am J Obstet Gynecol 1966; 95:99–108. [II-2]

71. Greer BE, Easterling TR, McLennan DA, et al. Fetal and maternal considerations in the management of stage I-B cervical cancer during pregnancy. Gynecol Oncol 1989; 34(1):61–65. [II-2]

72. McDonald SD, Faught W, Gruslin A. Cervical cancer during pregnancy. J Obstet Gynecol Canada 2002; 24(6):491–498. [Review, II-3]

73. Cliby WA, Dodson MK, Podratz KC. Cervical cancer complicated by pregnancy: episiotomy site recurrences following vaginal delivery. Obstet Gynecol 1994; 84(2):179–182. [II-3]

74. Van Calsteren K, Vergote I, Amant F. Cervical neoplasia during pregnancy: diagnosis, management and prognosis. Best Pract Res Clin Obstet Gynecol 2005; 19(4):611–630. [Review, II-3]

75. Marana HR, de Andrade JM, da Silva Mathes AC, et al. Chemotherapy in the treatment of locally advanced cervical cancer and pregnancy. Gynecol Oncol 2001; 80(2):272–274. [II-2]

76. Morris PC. Thyroid cancer complicating pregnancy. Obstet Gynecol Clin North Am 1998; 25(2):401–405. [Review]

77. Moosa M, Mazzaferri EL. Outcome of differentiated thyroid cancer diagnosed in pregnant women. J Clin Endocrinol Metab 1997; 82(9):2862–2866. [II-3]

78. Vini L, Hyer S, Pratt B, et al. Management of differentiated thyroid cancer diagnosed during pregnancy. Eur J Endocrinol 1999; 140(5):404–406. [II-3]

79. Green DM, Whitton JA, Stovall M, et al. Pregnancy outcome of female survivors of childhood cancer: a report from the Childhood Cancer Survivor Study. Am J Obstet Gynecol 2002; 187:1070. [II-1]

80. Chiarelli AM, Marrett LD, Darlington GA. Pregnancy outcomes in females after treatment for childhood cancer. Epidemiology 2000; 11:161. [II-3]

81. Reulen RC, Zeegers MP, Wallace WH, et al. Pregnancy outcomes among adult survivors of childhood cancer in the British Childhood Cancer Survivor Study. Cancer Epidemiol Biomarkers Prev 2009; 18:2239. [II-1]

82. Dodds L, Marrett LD, Tomkins DJ, et al. Case-control study of congenital anomalies in children of cancer patients. Br Med J 1993; 307(6897):164–168. [II-2]

83. Blatt J, Mulvihill JJ, Ziegler JL, et al. Pregnancy outcome following cancer chemotherapy. Am J Med 1980; 69:828–832. [II-3]

84. Byrne J, Rasmussen SA, Steinhorn SC, et al. Genetic disease in offspring of long-term survivors of childhood and adolescent cancer. Am J Hum Genet 1998; 62(1):45–52. [II-3]

85. Li FP, Fine W, Jaffe N, et al. Offspring of patients treated for cancer in childhood. J Natl Cancer Inst 1979; 62(5):1193–1197. [II-3]

86. Bar J, Davidi O, Goshen Y, et al. Pregnancy outcome in women treated with doxorubicin for childhood cancer. Am J Obstet Gynecol 2003; 189:853. [II-3]

87. Hawkins MM, Smith RA. Pregnancy outcomes in childhood cancer survivors: probable effects of abdominal irradiation. Int J Cancer 1989; 43:399. [II-3]

88. Green DM, Peabody EM, Nan B, et al. Pregnancy outcome after treatment for Wilms tumor: a report from the National Wilms Tumor Study Group. J Clin Oncol 2002; 20:2506. [II-1]

89. Li FP, Gimbrere K, Gelber RD, et al. Outcome of pregnancy in survivors of Wilms' tumor. J Am Med Assoc 1987; 257:216. [II-3]

90. Sanders JE, Hawley J, Levy W, et al. Pregnancies following high-dose cyclophosphamide with or without high-dose busulfan or total-body irradiation and bone marrow transplantation. Blood 1996; 87:3045. [II-3]

91. Holm K, Nysom K, Brocks V, et al. Ultrasound B—mode changes in the uterus and ovaries and Doppler changes in the uterus after total body irradiation and allogeneic bone marrow transplantation in childhood. Bone Marrow Transpl 1999; 23:259. [II-3]

92. Pridjian G, Rich NE, Montag AG. Pregnancy hemoperitoneum and placenta percreta in a patient with previous pelvic irradiation and ovarian failure. Am J Obstet Gynecol 1990; 162:1205. [II-3]

93. Norwitz ER, Stern HM, Grier H, et al. Placenta percreta and uterine rupture associated with prior whole body radiation therapy. Obstet Gynecol 2001; 98:929. [II-3]

94. Winther JF, Boice JD Jr., Svendsen AL, et al. Spontaneous abortion in a Danish population-based cohort of childhood cancer survivors. J Clin Oncol 2008; 26:4340. [II-3]

95. Signorello LB, Cohen SS, Bosetti C, et al. Female survivors of childhood cancer: preterm birth and low birth weight among their children. J Natl Cancer Inst 2006; 98:1453. [II-3]

96. Lie Fong, S, van den Heuvel-Eibrink MM, Eijkemans MJ, et al. Pregnancy outcome in female childhood cancer survivors. Hum Reprod 2010; 25:1206. [II-3]

97. Signorello LB, Mulvihill JJ, Green DM, et al. Stillbirth and neonatal death in relation to radiation exposure before conception: a retrospective cohort study. Lancet 2010; 376:624. [II-3]

98. Stewart JR, Fajardo LF, Gillette SM, et al. Radiation injury to the heart. Int J Radiat Oncol Biol Phys 1995; 31:1205. [II-3]

99. Sankila R, Olsen JH, Anderson H, et al. Risk of cancer among offspring of childhood-cancer survivors. Association of the Nordic Cancer Registries and the Nordic Society of Paediatric Haematology and Oncology. N Engl J Med 1998; 338:1339. [III]

100. Mulvihill JJ, Myers MH, Connelly RR, et al. Cancer in offspring of long-term survivors of childhood and adolescent cancer. Lancet 1987; 2:813. [III]

101. Reintgen DS, McCarty KS Jr., Vollmer R, et al. Malignant melanoma and pregnancy. Cancer 1985; 55:1340. [II-3]

102. Grin CM, Driscoll MS, Grant-Kels JM. The relationship of pregnancy, hormones, and melanoma. Semin Cutan Med Surg 1998; 17:167. [II-3]

103. Peters MV. The effect of pregnancy in breast cancer. In: Forrest APM, Kunkler PB, eds. Prognostic Factors in Breast Cancer. Baltimore: Williams and Wilkins, 1968; 65. [II-3]

104. Velentgas P, Daling JR, Malone KE, et al. Pregnancy after breast carcinoma: outcomes and influence on mortality. Cancer 1999; 85:2424. [II-2]

105. Danforth DN Jr. How subsequent pregnancy affects outcome in women with a prior breast cancer. Oncology (Williston Park) 1991; 5:23. [II-3]

106. Cooper DR, Butterfield J. Pregnancy subsequent to mastectomy for cancer of the breast. Ann Surg 1970; 171:429. [II-3]

107. von Schoultz E, Johansson H, Wilking N, et al. Influence of prior and subsequent pregnancy on breast cancer prognosis. J Clin Oncol 1995; 13:430. [II-2]

108. Kroman N, Jensen MB, Melbye M, et al. Should women be advised against pregnancy after breast-cancer treatment? Lancet 1997; 350:319. [II-2]

109. Gelber S, Coates AS, Goldhirsch A, et al. Effect of pregnancy on overall survival after the diagnosis of early-stage breast cancer. J Clin Oncol 2001; 19:1671. [II-2]

110. Ariel IM, Kempner R. The prognosis of patients who become pregnant after mastectomy for breast cancer. Int Surg 1989; 74 (3):185–187. [II-3]

111. Mueller BA, Simon MS, Deapen D, et al. Childbearing and survival after breast carcinoma in young women. Cancer 2003; 98:1131. [II-1]

112. Donnenfeld AE, Pastuszak A, Noah JS, et al. Methotrexate exposure prior to and during pregnancy. Teratology 1994; 49:79. [II-3]

113. Tewari K, Bonebrake RG, Asrat T, et al. Ambiguous genitalia in infant exposed to tamoxifen in utero. Lancet 1997; 350:183. [II-3]

114. Cullins SL, Pridjian G, Sutherland CM. Goldenhar's syndrome associated with tamoxifen given to the mother during gestation. J Am Med Assoc 1994; 271:1905–1906. [II-3]

115. Wisel MS, Datta JK, Saxena RN. Effects of anti-estrogens on early pregnancy in guinea pigs. Int J Fertil Menopausal Stud 1994; 39:156–163. [II-3]

116. Diwan BA, Anderson LM, Ward JM. Proliferative lesions of oviduct and uterus in CD-1 mice exposed prenatally to tamoxifen. Carcinogenesis 1997; 18:2009–2014. [II-3]

117. Wobbes T. Effect of a breast saving procedure on lactation. Eur J Surg 1996; 162:419. [II-3]

118. Findlay PA, Gorrell CR, d'Angelo T, et al. Lactation after breast radiation. Int J Radiat Oncol Biol Phys 1988; 15:511. [III]

119. Higgins S, Haffty BG. Pregnancy and lactation after breast-conserving therapy for early stage breast cancer. Cancer 1994; 73:2175. [III]

42

Dermatoses of pregnancy

Dana Correale, Joya Sahu, and Jason B. Lee

BACKGROUND

Polymorphic eruption of pregnancy (PEP) comprises the only pregnancy-specific dermatosis. All other dermatoses mentioned herein may be encountered outside of pregnancy, but they have been traditionally grouped and discussed as dermatoses of pregnancy as they represent common and uncommon dermatoses encountered during pregnancy.

Stretch marks are the only dermatologic condition for which there are trials for interventions. Dermatoses of pregnancy as well as melanoma in pregnancy are not well studied, with no specific trials regarding treatment. Most evidence regarding pathogenesis and etiology, as well as typical disease presentation is based on case reports and case series. Dermatoses of pregnancy have been plagued by synonyms and eponyms in the past. However, more recent efforts have established a more unified nomenclature, which has improved communication among physicians regarding some of the rarer and more recently described entities. Atopic eruption of pregnancy (AEP), which comprises atopic dermatitis (eczema) of pregnancy, prurigo of pregnancy (PP), and pruritic folliculitis of pregnancy (PFP), is now accepted as a major category in dermatoses of pregnancy. The most common skin disorder in pregnancy is atopic dermatitis (eczema) of pregnancy. Table 42.1 provides a summary of the dermatoses of pregnancy. Multidisciplinary management involving a dermatologist expert in dermatologic conditions in pregnancy is of paramount importance.

STRIAE GRAVIDARUM
Key Points

* The **exact cause** of striae gravidarum (SG) is **unknown**, but the strongest associated risk factors for their development are presence of preexisting breast and thigh striae, and a family history.
* **There is no widely available product that has been shown to prevent the formation of SG.** Massage with either **Trofolastin cream** or **Verum ointment** is associated with a **decrease in the development of SG**.
* **Topical tretinoin and various types of laser therapy have been shown to be helpful in the treatment of SG.**

Diagnosis/Definition

Striae distensae (SD), or stretch marks, do not represent a disease, but rather they are a cosmetic problem for many people. They often occur for the first time during pregnancy and are referred to as SG. SD initially appear as linear patches that are red to purple in color and lack noticeable surface change (striae rubra). With time, their color fades to lighter than normal skin tone. They become atrophic or depressed with a fine, wrinkled surface (striae alba).

Symptoms

SD are largely asymptomatic. They may be slightly pruritic in their early stages.

Epidemiology/Incidence

The prevalence of SG ranges from 50% to 90% (1). The mean gestational age for the onset of SG is 25 weeks (1).

Genetics

There is no known clear genetic cause of SG; however, there may be a familial tendency to develop them (1).

Etiology/Basic Pathology

Many theories exist regarding the etiology of SG. Rapid weight gain, baseline weight, hormonal changes, and greater change in abdominal and hip girth during pregnancy have been associated in the past with SG (1,2). None of these theories have been supported by any recent studies. It is known, however, that elastin and fibrillin fibers, components of the dermal extracellular matrix, are reduced in SD (3).

Risk Factors/Associations

The factors most strongly associated with the development of SG are the **presence of breast or thigh striae**, having a **mother with SG**, having **additional family members with SG**, and belonging to a nonwhite race. In contrast, prepregnancy body mass index (BMI), mean weight gain during pregnancy, mean percent weight gain, and mean change in BMI seem not to be associated with the development of SG (1).

Management
Prevention
Massage with Trofolastin cream containing *Centella asiatica* extract, alpha tocopherol, and collagen-elastin hydrolysates applied daily is associated with a 59% **decrease in the development of SG** compared to massage with placebo (4). Overall, 56% of the placebo group developed SG compared with 34% of the Trofolastin group. **Massage with Verum ointment** containing tocopherol, essential fatty acids, panthenol, hyaluronic acid, elastin, and menthol is also associated with a 74% **decrease in the development of SG** compared to no treatment; so it is unclear in this study if the massage or the Verum ointment or the combination of the two were beneficial (4). In women with stretch marks from a previous pregnancy there is no benefit. It should be noted that neither of these compounds are widely available, nor is it known what their active ingredient, if any, might be. There is the suggestion from the second study that bland emollients and massage alone may be of benefit in preventing the formation of SG. Cocoa butter lotion

Table 42.1 A Summary of the Dermatoses of Pregnancy

Dermatosis	Course	Skin findings	Fetal risks	Treatment
PEP	Third trimester. Resolution postpartum	Urticarial lesions on the abdomen, often within striae with sparing of the periumbilical area. Extension to upper thighs and buttocks	None	High-potency topical steroids
ADP	First to third trimesters. Can persist postpartum	Hyperpigmented lichenified, excoriated patches and plaques on flexural surfaces in 80% and papules and/or prurigo nodules in 20%	None	Mid to high-potency topical steroids, emollients, and anthistamines; oral corticosteroids in severe cases
PFP	Second or third trimester. Resolution within 1–2 months postpartum	Follicular papules and pustules	None	Mid- to high-potency topical corticosteroids
PP	Second or third trimester. Resolution postpartum	Excoriated papules over extremities and occasionally abdomen	None	Mid to high-potency topical steroids
IH	Third trimester. Persists after delivery if untreated	Symmetric, erythematous patches with peripheral superficial sterile pustules on flexural skin	Placental insufficiency and fetal loss	Systemic corticosteroids

Abbreviations: IH, impetigo herpetiformis; PEP, polymorphic eruption of pregnancy (pruritic urticarial papules and plaques of pregnancy); PFP, pruritic folliculitis of pregnancy; PP, prurigo of pregnancy; ADP, Atopic dermatitis of pregnancy.

is not associated with reduction in the likelihood of developing SG (5).

Therapy
Once SG have formed, there are treatment options. *Topical tretinoin* 0.1% cream has been shown to reduce the appearance of SG/SD when used *on early lesions* (striae rubra) (6). It is important to note that once striae have become white and atrophic, topical tretinoin was shown to have no benefit in a double-blind, placebo-controlled study (7). Topical tretinoin (Retin A) works by binding to cytoplasmic proteins and nuclear receptors of keratinocytes and altering downstream gene transcription. The end biologic effect is to regulate the growth and differentiation of keratinocytes (8). In addition to regulating keratinocyte proliferation, topical retinoids have been shown to decrease fine wrinkling, increase dermal collagen, and repair elastin fiber formation (9). Improvement in the appearance of SD/SG is most likely the result of this particular biologic effect. Tretinoin is pregnancy category C. Its use is contraindicated during breast-feeding, which makes it difficult to use during the early stages of SG. The side effects of tretinoin therapy are erythema, desquamation, and photosensitivity limited to the application site.

In addition to tretinoin therapy, improvement in the appearance of SD/SG can be achieved with laser therapy. **Laser therapy** is a rapidly evolving field with new lasers and applications emerging on a regular basis. Two large, blinded studies using an objective grading system evaluating the treatment of SD using a 585-nm pulsed dye laser have shown improvement in their appearance (10). Both increases and decreases in collagen production have been shown posttreatment depending on the wavelength and energy density of laser used. An increase in dermal elastin content has also been shown in biopsies obtained after laser therapy (10). Again, newer, more erythematous striae respond more favorably to pulsed dye laser treatment. This may be a more reasonable treatment option during the postpartum period as laser therapy is believed to be safe in breast-feeding women. A more recent study evaluating the effects of a XeCl excimer ultraviolet B (UVB) laser and a UVB light device showed repigmentation of striae alba (2). Repigmentation was associated with an increase in melanin content, hypertrophy of melanocytes, and an increase in number of melanocytes 6 months after treatment.

POLYMORPHIC ERUPTION OF PREGNANCY (PRURITIC URTICARIAL PAPULES AND PLAQUES OF PREGNANCY)
Key Points

- Polymorphic eruption of pregnancy [pruritic urticarial papules and plaques of pregnancy (PUPPP)] is an extremely pruritic urticarial eruption occurring during the third trimester of pregnancy.
- There is no associated fetal morbidity or mortality.
- The mainstay of **treatment** is **topical steroids.**

Historic Notes
This entity was originally described by Lawley and colleagues in 1979 in a series of seven patients (11).

Diagnosis/Definition
PEP is characterized by urticarial lesions that **begin on the abdomen**, often within abdominal striae, and spare the periumbilical area (Fig. 42.1). Lesions frequently spread to the **upper thighs and buttocks and occasionally may affect the arms**. The face, palms, and soles are usually spared. Despite the severe pruritus, there is notable lack of excoriation. As its name implies, PEP is polymorphous. Clinical lesions may appear vesicular, targetoid, or purpuric. This eruption is seen mostly in primigravidas with onset in the third trimester of pregnancy. It resolves shortly after delivery, but there have been a few cases reported in which onset of the disease has occurred in the postpartum period (12–14). The diagnosis is primarily clinical. Histopathologic examination of affected skin most often yields nonspecific findings.

Symptoms
The eruption is accompanied by extreme pruritus. The itching is often so severe that it may interfere with sleep.

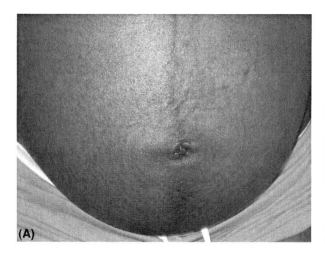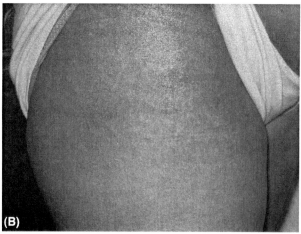

Figure 42.1 Polymorphous eruption of pregnancy (PEP). A 28-year-old primigravida with abrupt onset of extremely pruritic urticarial papules on the abdomen (A) and thighs (B) during her 39th week of pregnancy. Note the predilection for the abdominal striae with periumbilical sparing.

Epidemiology/Incidence

PEP is one of the most common dermatoses of pregnancy. It occurs in approximately 0.5% of pregnancies (15).

Genetics

There are no known genetic factors in PEP. In fact, some studies have looked for, but failed to document a human leukocyte antigen (HLA) association (16,17).

Etiology/Basic Pathology

To date, there are no widely accepted theories to explain the etiology of this disease. Associated factors include increased abdominal distension secondary to excessive maternal weight gain and fetal birth weight (13,17,18), increased incidence of multiple pregnancies (12,15,17,19), not autoimmune mechanisms (20), but decreased serum cortisol levels (21,22), and fetal DNA migration in PEP skin lesions (23).

Complications

There have been no consistent maternal or fetal complications associated with PEP, with newborns not affected with any related skin disease (14,17,21).

Management

Workup

The most important disease to exclude when diagnosing PEP is herpes gestationis (HG), which can present with urticarial lesions in the absence of more prototypical blisters. HG is usually a widespread eruption which begins on the abdomen but does not show a predilection for striae nor spares the periumbilical area. HG is rare, but it is associated with significant maternal and fetal morbidity and mortality (11,24). Exclusion of HG relies on the clinical presentation, but direct immunofluorescence (DIF) of affected skin may be required in equivocal cases. There are no consistent DIF findings in PEP (13,14,17,21,25). When positive DIF findings have been reported in PEP, they have been considered nondiagnostic for any particular disease (14,25). In contrast, HG is associated with very consistent and reliable DIF findings (24).

Preconception Counseling

The vast majority of cases of PEP do not recur with subsequent pregnancies (11,17,21) or oral contraceptive use (1,7). A few women affected by PEP have been reported to have episodes of transient hives while breast-feeding after the initial eruption resolved (11).

Therapy

The majority of cases of PEP can be effectively managed with **high-potency topical steroids** (11,17,21). This class of medication does not cause any known fetal complications when used properly. In rare cases of prolonged and widespread use, significant systemic absorption could occur. In severe and widespread cases, short courses of oral corticosteroids have been used effectively (11,17,21). The reader is referred to the guideline for impetigo herpetiformis for more detailed information on the use and safety of steroids in pregnancy. There is one reported case of severe PEP that required delivery by cesarean section at 35 weeks' gestation for intractable pruritus uncontrolled by topical and oral corticosteroids (26). In this case, the patient's symptoms were significantly improved within 12 hours of delivery.

ATOPIC DERMATITIS (ECZEMA) OF PREGNANCY
Key Points

- Atopic dermatitis of pregnancy (ADP) is an intensely pruritic eruption characterized by eczematous plaques or papular lesions involving the trunk and extremities.
- The mainstay of **therapy** is **topical steroids and emollients.**
- There is no associated maternal or fetal morbidity or mortality.

Diagnosis/Definition

ADP is characterized by intense itch accompanied by licheni-fied plaques or papular lesions in patients with a personal or family history of atopy and/or elevated IgE levels. The eruption most commonly presents before the third trimester of

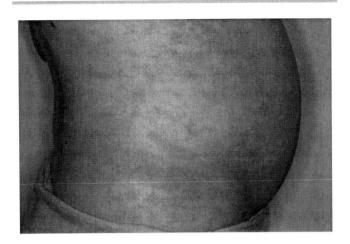

Figure 42.2 Atopic dermatitis (Eczema) of pregnancy. A 42-year-old G1P0 with multiple, lichenified, hyperpigmented patches and plaques on the abdomen and extremities.

pregnancy in 75% of patients, with onset occurring in all three trimesters, and is a diagnosis of exclusion (27). Recurrence in subsequent pregnancies is expected due to the background of atopy. The eruption consists of atopic dermatitis-like plaques and/or prurigo-like nodules accompanied by excoriations and secondary skin infections (Fig. 42.2). ADP classically involves the trunk and extremities in typical atopic sites such as the neck, décolletage, or flexural surfaces of extremities. Atopic dermatitis (Eczema) of pregnancy, PFP, and PP have been grouped into one category, AEP (28,29). Characteristic atopic clinical findings are key for diagnosis, as histopathologic findings are nonspecific and DIF reveals no immunoreactive deposition (30).

Symptoms
ADP is accompanied by intense pruritus which can lead to excoriations and secondary skin infections.

Epidemiology/Incidence
ADP is the most frequent dermatosis in pregnancy (22,27,31).

Etiology/Basic Pathology
Although causally linked to a personal or family history of atopy, there is no definitive evidence currently. One theory reflects a deterioration of existing atopic dermatitis or an exacerbation of a quiescent atopic state due to a TH2 shift in cytokine expression during pregnancy (22,31).

Pregnancy Considerations
There are no reports of adverse maternal or fetal outcomes in ADP.

Management
Workup. The diagnosis of ADP is made clinically due to the characteristic clinical atopic presentation. Other specific dermatoses of pregnancy must first be ruled out. Sparing of striae and time of onset differentiate from PEP. Elevated IgE levels may be present in 20% to 70% of cases but are not diagnostic (27). Total serum bile acid levels must be in the normal range. Histopathologic exam and DIF testing are not necessary for the diagnosis but may be performed in equivocal cases.

Therapy. Treatment strategies vary depending on the severity of the patient's clinical findings and symptoms. The mainstay of therapy for ADP is **mid- to high-potency topical steroids** accompanied by liberal use of emollients, with or without antihistamines (27,30). If necessary, first-generation antihistamines can safely be used in the first trimester of pregnancy, and second-generation antihistamines can be used in the second or third trimester of pregnancy (8). In severe cases, a tapered course of systemic corticosteroids (CS) may be required, in addition to treatment with phototherapy (UVB) (30).

PRURITIC FOLLICULITIS OF PREGNANCY
Key Points

- PFP is a **benign** eruption presenting in the second or third trimester.
- There is no underlying infectious etiology.
- There are no adverse maternal or fetal outcomes.
- The mainstay of **therapy** is **topical corticosteroids.**

Historic Notes
PFP was originally described by Zoberman and Farmer in 1981 in a series of six pregnant patients (32). It is now considered to be a part of the broad category of AEP (27,30).

Diagnosis/Definition
PFP is characterized by pruritic, follicular papules with some discrete pustules in a primarily truncal distribution (Fig. 42.3). The eruption occurs anywhere from the fourth to ninth month of gestation and resolves by one to two months postpartum. The rash may recur with subsequent pregnancies. Histopathological examination of affected skin shows a sterile folliculitis (32). Immunoreactive deposit is not detected in DIF in PFP (22,32,33).

Symptoms
PFP is usually accompanied by mild to moderate pruritus.

Epidemiology/Incidence
There are no formal data available that document the incidence of PFP, but estimated incidence ranges from 1:9 to 1:3000

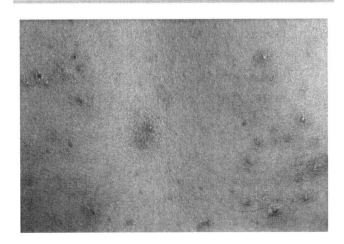

Figure 42.3 Pruritic folliculitis of pregnancy. A 28-year-old woman with erythematous, follicular papules on the abdomen.

pregnancies (22,34). This entity may be underreported because of frequent mistaken diagnoses of bacterial folliculitis (33,35,36).

Etiology/Basic Pathology

The underlying etiology of PFP is unknown. One case report suggests that pityrosporum yeast may be a causative agent (37). The vast majority of case reports fail to reveal any causative organism by special staining during histopathological examination or by culture (19,30,32,33,35,38). Some have proposed a hormone-related etiology based on the similarity of PFP to steroid acne (19,39), but a recent controlled, prospective study did not show any change in androgen levels in patients with PFP (22).

Pregnancy Considerations

There is one case report of premature delivery secondary to placental abruption at 32 weeks (38). There is a reported increase in the male to female birth ratio (22). Otherwise, there are no reports of adverse maternal or fetal outcomes in PFP.

Management

Workup. The diagnosis of PFP relies mostly on its clinical features. We advocate performing routine gram stain and culture on a primary pustule to rule out routine bacterial folliculitis. Skin biopsy for histopathology may be necessary for equivocal cases.

Therapy. The mainstay of therapy is **mid to high-potency topical corticosteroids** (22,30,32,35). The reader is referred to the guideline for PEP for a discussion on the use of topical corticosteroids during pregnancy. A recently reported alternative treatment in recalcitrant cases of PFP is narrowband UVB phototherapy (38). The mechanism of action of UVB is not entirely defined, but it is believed that ultraviolet radiation can depress certain components of the cell-mediated immune system and thereby exert beneficial effects in a wide variety of inflammatory skin diseases (40). UVB treatment is considered safe during pregnancy (40).

PRURIGO OF PREGNANCY
Key Points

- PP is an intensely pruritic eruption confined mostly to the extremities.
- The mainstay of **therapy** is **topical steroids**.
- There is no associated maternal or fetal morbidity or mortality.

Historic Notes

PP was first described by Nurse in 1968 (41). His case series of 31 patients is the largest group of women with PP to be described to date. A synonym for this skin disease is prurigo gestationis of Besnier. It is now considered to be part of AEP (27,30).

Diagnosis/Definition

PP is diagnosed by its clinical features. The eruption consists of pruritic papules occurring on the extensor surface of the extremities and occasionally the abdomen (Fig. 42.4). Excoriation is often present. The lesions appear between the 25th and 30th weeks of gestation. In the original description of this disease, there was no tendency toward recurrence in subsequent pregnancies. However, others have found that this is not

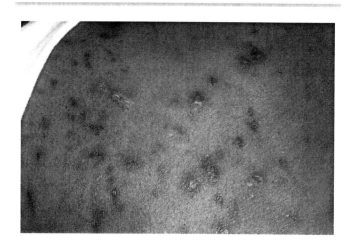

Figure 42.4 Prurigo of pregnancy. Grouped excoriated papules on the thigh of a 24-year-old primigravida with a prior history of asthma and seasonal allergies.

the case (34). The eruption resolves in the postpartum period, but there have been a few patients in which lesions have persisted for as long as three months after delivery (41). A skin biopsy shows nonspecific histopathological changes.

Symptoms

The papules are intensely pruritic.

Epidemiology/Incidence

In Nurse's original report, the incidence was calculated as 1 in 300 pregnancies. A more recent prospective analysis of pruritic eruptions during pregnancy yielded an incidence of PP of 1 in 450 pregnancies (34).

Etiology/Basic Pathology

There is no definitive evidence regarding the etiology of PP. One theory is that women who are affected have an underlying predisposition to atopy either by personal history or family history and that this predisposition is unmasked during pregnancy (42). Evidence to support this theory is that some women with PP have elevated serum IgE levels (22,42). Evidence for atopy by personal and/or family history has been present in some series (22,42) and absent in others (34). There have not been any significant changes detected in levels of beta-HCG, estradiol, or cortisol in women with PP versus controls (22,34).

Risk Factors/Associations

There may be an association between PP and a personal or family history of an atopic diathesis (atopic dermatitis, allergic rhinitis, asthma) (22,42).

Complications

There are no large-scale epidemiologic studies investigating maternal or fetal morbidity. No case series has ever reported any associated fetal or maternal complications (22,41,42) except for one patient who exhibited intrauterine growth restriction (34).

Management

Workup

The diagnosis of PP rests on the clinical features of the eruption. In all cases, DIF has been negative (22,34,42), and therefore is not indicated.

Therapy

The mainstay of therapy for PP is **mid to high-potency topical steroids** (22,30,34,39,41,42). This class of medication does not cause any known fetal complications when used properly. In rare cases of prolonged and widespread use, significant systemic absorption could occur. Oral antihistamines can be used in addition to topical corticosteroids if necessary (30).

IMPETIGO HERPETIFORMIS
Key Points

- Impetigo herpetiformis (IH) represents **pustular psoriasis** that occurs during pregnancy.
- Most patients have no prior history of psoriasis.
- There is an **increased risk of placental insufficiency and fetal loss.**
- Patients are at risk for recurrence of disease with subsequent pregnancies.
- The mainstay of **therapy** is **oral corticosteroids.**

Historic Notes

This disease was first described in 1872 by Von Hebra in a series of five pregnant women, 40 years before the first description of generalized pustular psoriasis (43).

Diagnosis/Definition

IH is characterized by symmetric, erythematous patches with peripheral superficial sterile pustules (Fig. 42.5). There is **no**

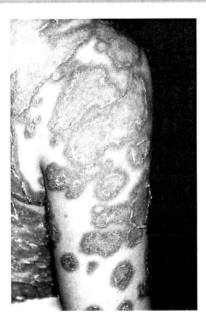

Figure 42.5 Impetigo herpetiformis. A 26-year-old pregnant woman with erythematous plaques bordered by tiny pustules on the trunk and extremities. There was no prior history of psoriasis. *Source*: From Ref. 47.

underlying infectious etiology despite the name this disorder was given. The eruption begins over the intertriginous and flexural skin and expands outward. Older lesions may become crusted or secondarily infected.

Symptoms

Patients may report very mild pruritus or burning at the sites of the lesions, however, most are asymptomatic. There may be accompanying fever, malaise, diarrhea, and vomiting.

Epidemiology/ Incidence

There are no formal epidemiological data. IH is very rare, with only about 100 cases being reported in the literature. The eruption most often occurs in the third trimester, but can occur as early as the first trimester. Most women do not have a prior history of psoriasis.

Genetics

Generalized pustular psoriasis is associated with HLA types B17 and Cw6 (2).

Etiology/Basic Pathology

IH is probably a **variant of pustular psoriasis** that occurs during pregnancy (24,44,45). The basic underlying etiology is unknown. Many theories exist including hormonal dysregulation and electrolyte imbalance, but these are based on a few case reports. Histopathology of the skin shows a characteristic sterile pustule containing polymorphonuclear neutrophils in the epidermis referred to as a spongiform pustule of Kogoj, which is indistinguishable from findings that are seen in pustular psoriasis. There may also be elongation of the rete ridges and overlying parakeratosis.

Risk Factors/Associations

Patients usually do not have a prior history of psoriasis and there is no evidence that having such a history increases the risk of IH in pregnancy (24).

Complications

The most important complication is **placental insufficiency and fetal death**, the etiology of which is unknown (24,44). There may be hypocalcemia or decreased vitamin D levels as a result of hypoparathyroidism or hypoalbuminemia (24,44,46). If severe, these changes may lead to tetany or seizure.

Management

Principles

Pregnancy is speculated to be a trigger for IH (24). The effect of the disease on the pregnancy is discussed above.

Workup

Workup includes **skin biopsy** for routine histopathology as well as a second specimen for DIF in order to rule out other pregnancy-specific dermatoses such as HG. When the presentation is accompanied by systemic symptoms, systemic infection must be ruled out with blood cultures as well as bacterial and viral cultures of one or more pustules. Serum calcium, vitamin D, and hypoparathyroid levels should be monitored. The patient should be questioned regarding the history of skin eruptions during any previous pregnancies.

Prevention
None.

Preconception Counseling
Any patient with a history of IH should be counseled that it may recur with subsequent pregnancies.

Therapy
The mainstay of therapy of IH is corticosteroids, usually in the form of prednisone at a dose of 15 to 30 mg/day. Doses as high as 60 to 80 mg/day may be required (24). Evidence for varying levels of effectiveness is based on case reports (43–45,47). Once the disease is under control, steroids may be tapered very slowly. Disease rebound is common with rapid tapering. The mechanism of action of corticosteroids is broad suppression of the immune system. They exert inhibitory effects on cell trafficking, as well as the humoral and cytotoxic portions of the immune system. Corticosteroids have well-documented side effects in humans including: hypothalamic pituitary axis (HPA) suppression, hyperglycemia, hyperlipidemia, cushingoid changes, osteoporosis, peptic ulcer disease, cataracts, and opportunistic infections. Fetal HPA suppression must be considered when corticosteroids are given near the time of delivery (8). Oral CS should be used with caution during lactation. They are excreted into human breast milk but do not have any known adverse reaction or potential in infants.

   When IH is insufficiently controlled with CS alone, the next therapeutic option is cyclosporine A (CsA). Doses of 3 to 10 mg/kg/day have been reported in the treatment of IH (47–49). Again, medication should be tapered to the lowest possible dose that results in control of the disease. The mechanism of action is inhibition of calcineurin with resultant decrease in interleukin 2 production by CD4+ T cells. CsA also inhibits interferon-γ production by T cells. CsA is pregnancy category C. The most serious adverse effects are renal dysfunction and hypertension (8). Renal function and blood pressure should be monitored during therapy. In a study of transplant recipients treated with CsA during pregnancy there was no evidence of teratogenicity (50). However, 44.5% of infants were born at less than 37 weeks' gestation and 44.3% weighed less than 2500 g at birth (50). CsA is excreted in human breast milk and breastfeeding should be avoided during therapy.

Antepartum Testing
Patients must be monitored closely with fetal ultrasound and fetal testing because of the risk of placental insufficiency (43).

CUTANEOUS MELANOMA
See chapter 41, "Cancer."

Key Points
- **Pregnancy** at the time of diagnosis or subsequent to the diagnosis of melanoma has **no impact on overall survival, tumor thickness, or disease-free survival.**
- **Pregnant women who are diagnosed with melanoma should not be counseled or managed any differently than a nonpregnant woman with a similar stage of disease.**

Diagnosis/Definition
Cutaneous melanoma is a malignant neoplasm of melanocytes that arises in the skin. Melanomas often display irregularities

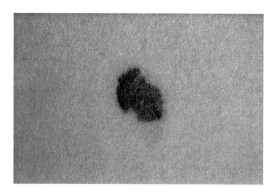

Figure 42.6 Melanoma. A 25-year-old G_2P_1 with a new, irregularly pigmented, asymmetric lesion in her back that had been gradually expanding over the past several months. Note the irregular borders.

in color, border, and symmetry, although these observations are neither sensitive nor specific (Fig. 42.6). Even the most experienced dermatologist may have difficulty differentiating a benign pigmented lesion from a malignant one. The gold standard for the **diagnosis** of melanoma is **excisional biopsy of the entire lesion** for tissue pathology. Biopsy specimens of all clinically pigmented lesions should be evaluated by an experienced dermatopathologist.

Symptoms
Melanomas are usually asymptomatic. They may rarely itch or bleed spontaneously.

Epidemiology/Incidence
The lifetime risk of melanoma for a Caucasian person born in the United States in 2001 is 1 in 75 (51). The estimated incidence of melanoma during pregnancy is between 2.8 and 5 in 100,000 (52).

Genetics
A rare group of patients with a family history of melanoma and many moles may carry inherited mutations in CDKN2A and CDK4. An individual who carries one of these mutations has a 60% to 90% lifetime risk of melanoma (53).

Classification
There are four main clinical types of melanoma. They are superficial spreading, acral lentiginous, lentigo maligna, and nodular melanoma. The clinical type bears no significance on the prognosis in melanoma. Rather, the **Breslow depth, which is a measure of tumor thickness, and ulceration** are the two major factors that have been shown to **impact prognosis** (54). In addition to Breslow depth, which is a measure of tumor thickness, ulceration, mitotic rate in thin melanomas, and although still controversial, sentinel lymph node status, are the major factors that have been shown more recently to impact prognosis (55,56).

Risk Factors
The major risk factors are fair skin, blue or green eyes, blond or red hair, inability to tan, intense intermittent sun exposure

(especially during childhood), use of tanning beds, and inherited mutations in CDKN2A or CDK4 (51,53).

Complications

Melanoma is a malignant neoplasm that can metastasize to regional lymph nodes as well as viscera. In general, the thicker the primary cutaneous melanoma, the higher the likelihood for metastasis at the time of diagnosis.

Pregnancy Considerations

For many years it was believed that pregnancy had an adverse impact on survival in patients diagnosed with malignant melanoma (MM). This belief was based on case reports and uncontrolled series in which confounding variables were not accounted for, namely, tumor thickness at the time of diagnosis (52,56). Several large, retrospective, controlled cohort studies of women who were diagnosed with melanoma during their pregnancy have confirmed that this is *not* the case (52, 57–59). In fact, these recent large cohort studies have shown that there is **no difference in overall survival or tumor thickness between pregnant and nonpregnant age- and disease stage-matched patients** (52,57–59). The **disease-free survival rate** is the **same** in pregnant and nonpregnant women (58,59). **Pregnancy in women who have been previously diagnosed with melanoma does not affect overall survival** (52,59). An important point related to pregnancy and melanoma is the concept that benign nevi may darken and change during pregnancy. There has been debate in recent years regarding this belief. In fact, there has been no study to date that has documented a significant change in size or color of benign nevi during pregnancy in normal, healthy women. The clinical lesions that are reported by patients to darken or change during pregnancy are usually nonpigmented lesions, such as dermatofibromas or skin tags (60). Photographic documentation and blinded comparison by physicians do not show any change in size of nevi between the first and third trimester of pregnancy (61). Women with the *dysplastic nevus syndrome* (DNS) may have an increased rate of change in clinically dysplastic nevi with pregnancy (62), but women with DNS represent only a very small portion of the population. Histopathologic study of nevi removed during pregnancy fails to detect a statistically significant difference in criteria for atypia (60). So, **any nevus that changes during pregnancy should be considered suspect and be carefully considered for excisional biopsy**, not observation. The belief that nevi may normally darken and change during pregnancy may lead to a false sense of security and a delay in the diagnosis of melanoma (56,60,61).

Management

Pregnancy Management

There is no difference in pregnancy outcomes including cesarean delivery, length of stay, risk of low birth weight, prematurity, or neonatal death (56). Pregnant women who are diagnosed with melanoma **should not be counseled any differently than nonpregnant women** with a similar stage of disease with respect to both pregnancy outcomes and their overall prognosis (56,59). There are approximately 22 cases of placental metastases of melanoma reported in the literature. Indeed, of all malignancies that tend to metastasize to the placenta, melanoma is the most common (56). However, metastasis to the fetus and/or placenta is an extremely rare event and has occurred exclusively in the setting of hematogenous dissemination of metastatic disease in the mother (63–65). **Placental involvement** implies a fatal prognosis for the mother and approximately 22% risk of metastasis to the fetus (65).

Workup

The extensiveness of the workup of primary cutaneous melanoma is primarily based on tumor thickness at the time of diagnosis. Initial diagnosis is made by tissue pathology. It is strongly recommended that all suspicious lesions be removed by **excisional biopsy with narrow margins** for diagnostic purposes (66). Once the diagnosis of melanoma is made, all patients should have a thorough review of systems and physical exam, with special attention given to the lymph nodes. There is no evidence that routine laboratory tests and imaging studies detect occult metastases in asymptomatic patients with tumors less than 4.0 mm in thickness (53,66). Therefore, **CXR, serum lactate dehydrogenase, and hemoglobin are reserved for patients who are symptomatic or have tumors that are thicker than 4.0 mm at the time of initial diagnosis**. Patients should be taught to give themselves monthly self-exams and should be seen one to four times per year for the first two years after the initial diagnosis and then one to two times yearly thereafter (66). The goal of follow-up is to detect recurrence or a new primary lesion. Screening tests should be ordered based on history and physical examination findings during follow-up care. **Sentinel lymph node biopsy** in melanoma is still a relatively controversial procedure at this date. It is used to detect occult nodal metastases at the time of diagnosis and is generally reserved for patients **with tumors that are 1.0 mm or greater in thickness** (53). Sentinel lymph node biopsy should be performed at the time of definitive excision. This procedure is considered safe to perform during pregnancy (56). For patients with microscopic or clinically apparent nodal disease, a full metastatic work up is indicated (3), including bloodwork and CT or MRI of the chest, abdomen, and pelvis. MRI is preferable in pregnant patients because it is the safer alternative (56).

Prevention

General preventative measures include the use of sun protection via sunscreens and protective clothing, especially during childhood and adolescence. Regular skin examination by a physician is recommended. Melanomas that are detected by a physician are diagnosed at an earlier stage than those detected by patients; however, a direct reduction in mortality has not been documented (54).

Preconception Counseling

Since melanomas tend to recur within the first two years after diagnosis, women should be counseled to wait this length of time before conceiving (51,56). Again, there is no evidence that pregnancy results in a higher rate of recurrence, but it seems unwise to conceive if there is *any* risk for recurrence of a potentially fatal disease. Additionally, in patients diagnosed with melanoma, future use of oral contraceptives and hormone replacement therapy has not been shown to enhance the risk for developing melanoma (59).

Therapy

The treatment of melanoma is primarily surgical. After the initial diagnostic biopsy, **excision of the primary lesion with 0.5 to 2 cm margins** depending on tumor thickness is recommended (53,66). Patients with evidence of metastasis can be considered for surgical debulking and/or adjuvant therapy (53).

REFERENCES

1. Chang ALS, Agredano YZ, Kimball AB. Risk factors associated with striae gravidarum. J Am Acad Dermatol 2004; 51:881–885. [III]
2. Goldberg DJ, Marmur ES, Schmults C, et al. Histologic and ultrastructural analysis of ultraviolet B laser and light source treatment of leukoderma in striae distensae. Dermatol Surg 2005; 31:385–387. [II-3]
3. Watson REB, Parry EJ, Humphries JD, et al. Fibrillin microfibrils are reduced in skin exhibiting striae distensae. Br J Dermatol 1998; 138:931–937. [II-3]
4. Young GL, Jewell D. Creams for preventing stretch marks in pregnancy. Cochrane Database Syst Rev 2005; 3. [Meta-analysis; 2 RCTs, n = 130]
5. Osman H, Usta IM, Rubeiz N, et al. Cocoa butter lotion for prevention of striae gravidarum: a double-blind, randomized and placebo-controlled trial. Br J Obstet Gynecol 2008; 115:1138–1142. [RCT, n = 175]
6. Kang S, Kim KJ, Griffiths CEM, et al. Topical tretinoin (retinoic acid) improves early stretch marks. Arch Dermatol 1996; 132:519–526. [I]
7. Pribanich S, Simpson FG, Held B, et al. Low-dose tretinoin does not improve striae distensae: a double-blind, placebo-controlled study. Cutis 1994; 54:121–124. [I]
8. Wolverton SE. Comprehensive Dermatologic Drug Therapy. Philadelphia: W.B. Saunders Company, 2007:625–641, 127–161. [III]
9. Kligman AM, Grove GL, Hirose R, et al. Topical tretinoin for photodamaged skin. J Am Acad Dermatol 1986; 15:836–859. [II-1]
10. McDaniel DH. Laser therapy of stretch marks. Dermatol Clin 2002; 20:67–76. [III]
11. Lawley TJ, Hertz KC, Wade TR et al. Pruritic urticarial papules and plaques of pregnancy. J Am Med Assoc 1979; 241:1696–1699. [III]
12. Roger D, Vaillant L, Lorette G. Pruritic urticarial papules and plaques of pregnancy are not related to maternal or fetal weight gain. Arch Dermatol 1990; 126:1517. [III]
13. Cohen LM, Capeless EL, Krusinski PA, et al. Pruritic urticarial papules and plaques of pregnancy and its relationship to maternal-fetal weight gain and twin pregnancy. Arch Dermatol 1989; 125:1534–1536. [III]
14. Aronson IK, Bond S, Fiedler VC et al. Pruritic urticarial papules and plaques of pregnancy: clinical and immunopathologic observations in 57 patients. J Am Acad Dermatol 1998; 39:933–939. [II-3]
15. Powell FC. Pruritic urticarial papules and plaques of pregnancy and multiple pregnancies. J Am Acad Dermatol 2000; 43:730–731. [II-3]
16. Weiss R, Hull P. Familial occurrence of pruritic urticarial papules and plaques of pregnancy. J Am Acad Dermatol 1992; 26:715–717. [III]
17. Yancey KB, Hall RP, Lawley TJ. Pruritic urticarial papules and plaques of pregnancy. J Am Acad Dermatol 1984; 10:473–480. [II-3]
18. Beckett MA, Goldberg NS. Pruritic urticarial papules and plaques of pregnancy and skin distension. Arch Dermatol 1991; 127:125–126. [III]
19. Kroumpouzos G, Cohen LM. Specific dermatoses of pregnancy: an evidence-based systematic review. Am J Obstet Gynecol 2003; 188:1083–1092. [Meta-analysis, n = 282]
20. Alcalay J, Ingber A, Kafri B, et al. Hormonal evaluation and autoimmune background in pruritic urticarial papules and plaques of pregnancy. Am J Obstet Gynecol 1988; 158:417–420. [II-3]
21. Callen JP, Hanno R. Pruritic urticarial papules and plaques of pregnancy (PEP). J Am Acad Dermatol 1981; 5:401–405. [II-3]
22. Vaughan Jones SA, Hern S, Nelson-Piercy C, et al. A prospective study of 200 women with dermatoses of pregnancy correlating clinical findings with hormonal and immunopathological profiles. Br J Dermatol 1999; 141:71–81. [II-2; n = 44]
23. Aractingi S, Berkane P, LeGoue' C, et al. Fetal DNA in skin of polymorphic eruptions of pregnancy. Lancet 1998; 352:1898–1901. [II-2]
24. Kroumpouzos GK, Cohen LM. Dermatoses of pregnancy. J Am Acad Dermatol 2001; 45:1–19. [III]
25. Alcalay J, Ingber A, David M, et al. Pruritic urticarial papules and plaques of pregnancy. J Reprod Med 1987; 32:315–316. [II-3]
26. Beltrani VP, Beltrani VS. Pruritic Urticarial papules and plaques of pregnancy: a severe case requiring early delivery for relief of symptoms. J Am Acad Dermatol 1991; 26:266–267. [III]
27. Ambros-Rudolph CM, Müllegger RR, Vaughan-Jones S, et al. The specific dermatoses of pregnancy revisited and reclassified: results of a retrospective two-center study on 505 pregnant patients. J Am Acad Dermatol 2006; 54:395–404. [II-2]
28. Cohen LM, Kroumpouzos G. Pruritic dermatoses of pregnancy: to lump or to split? J Am Acad Dermatol 2007; 56:708–709. [II-2]
29. Ambros-Rudolph CM, Jones SV, Black MM. Best serving the pregnant patient with pruritus. J Am Acad Dermatol 2008; 59:530–531. [II-2]
30. Roth MM. Pregnancy dermatoses: diagnosis, management, and controversies. Am J Clin Dermatol 2011; 1:25–41. [Review]
31. Ambros-Rudolph CM. Dermatoses of pregnancy. J Dtsch Dermatol Ges 2006; 9:748–759. [Review]
32. Zoberman E, Farmer ER. Pruritic folliculitis of pregnancy. Arch Dermatol 1981; 117:20–22. [III]
33. Kroumpouzos G, Cohen LM. Pruritic Folliculitis of pregnancy. J Am Acad Dermatol 2000; 43:132–134. [III]
34. Roger D, Vaillant L, Fignon A, et al. Specific pruritic diseases of pregnancy. A prospective study of 3192 pregnant women. Arch Dermatol 1994; 130:734–739. [II-2]
35. Fox GN. Pruritic folliculitis of pregnancy. Am Fam Physician 1989; 39:189–193. [III]
36. Kroumpouzos G, Cohen LM. Specific dermatoses of pregnancy: an evidence-based review. Am J Obstet Gynecol 2003; 188:1083–1092. [III]
37. Parlak AH, Boran C, Topcuoglu MA. Pityrosporum folliculitis during pregnancy: a possible cause of pruritic folliculitis of pregnancy. J Am Acad Dermatol 2005; 52:528–529. [III]
38. Reed J. Pruritic folliculitis of pregnancy treated with narrowband (TL-01) ultraviolet B phototherapy. Br J Dermatol 1999; 141:177–179. [III]
39. Black MM. Prurigo of pregnancy, papular dermatitis of pregnancy, and pruritic folliculitis of pregnancy. Semin Dermatol 1989; 8:23–25. [III]
40. British Photodermatology Group. An appraisal of narrowband (TL-01) UVB phototherapy. British photodermatology group workshop report. Br J Dermatol 1997; 137:327–330. [III]
41. Nurse DS. Prurigo of pregnancy. Australas J Dermatol 1968; 9:258–267. [III]
42. Holmes RC, Black MM. The specific dermatoses of pregnancy. J Am Acad Dermatol 1983; 3:405–412. [II-3]
43. Lotem M, Katzenelson V, Rotem A, et al. Impetigo herpetiformis: a variant of pustular psoriasis or a separate entity? J Am Acad Dermatol 1989; 20:338–341. [IIII]
44. Breier-Maly J, Ortel B, Breier F, et al. Generalized pustular psoriasis of pregnancy (impetigo herpetiformis). Dermatology 1999; 198:61–64. [III]
45. Chang SE. Impetigo herpetiformis followed by generalized pustular psoriasis: more evidence of the same disease entity. Int J Soc Dermatol 2003; 42:754–755. [III]
46. Ott F, Krakowski A, Tur E, et al. Impetigo herpetiformis with lowered serum level of vitamin D and its diminished intestinal absorption. Dermatologica 1982; 164:360–365. [III]
47. Imai N, Watanabe R, Fujiwara H, et al. Successful treatment of impetigo herpetiformis with oral cyclosporine during pregnancy. Arch Dermatol 2002; 138:128–129. [III]
48. Raddadi AA, Damanhoury ZB. Cyclosporin and pregnancy. Br J Dermatol 1999; 140:1197–1198. [III]
49. Finch TM, Tan CY. Pustular psoriasis exacerbated by pregnancy and controlled by cyclosporine A. Br J Dermatol 2000; 142:582–584. [III]
50. Lamarque V, Leleu MF, Monka C, et al. Analysis of 629 pregnancy outcomes in transplant recipients treated with sandimmun. Transpl Proc 1997; 29:2480. [II-3; n=629]
51. Lang PE. Current concepts in the management of patients with melanoma. Am J Clin Dermatol 2002; 3:401–426. [III]

52. Lens MB, Rosdahl I, Ahlbom A, et al. Effect of pregnancy on survival in women with cutaneous malignant melanoma. J Clin Oncol 2004; 22:4369–4375. [II-2]

53. Tsao H, Atkins MB, Sober AJ. Management of cutaneous melanoma. N Engl J Med 2004; 351:998–1012. [III]

54. Thompson JA. The revised American joint committee on cancer staging system for melanoma. Semin Oncol 2002; 29:361–369. [III]

55. Stebbins WG, Garibyan L, Sober AJ. Sentinel lymph node biopsy and melanoma: 2010 update Part I. J Am Acad Dermatol 2010; 62:723–734. [Review]

56. Katz VL, Farmer RM, Dotters D. From nevus to neoplasm: myths of melanoma in pregnancy. Obstet Gynecol Surv 2002; 57: 112–119. [III]

57. O'Meara AT, Cress R, Xing G, et al. Malignant melanoma in pregnancy. A population-based evaluation. Cancer 2005; 103:1217–1226. [II-2]

58. Daryanani D, Plukker JT, De Hullu JA, et al. Pregnancy and early-stage melanoma. Cancer 2003; 97:2248–2253. [II-2]

59. Gupta A, Driscoll MS. Do hormones influence melanoma? Facts and controversies. Clin Dermatol 2010; 28:287–292. [III]

60. Foucar E, Bentley TJ, Laube DW, et al. A histopathologic evaluation of nevocellular nevi in pregnancy. Arch Dermatol 1985; 121:350–354. [II-2]

61. Pennoyer JW, Grin CM, Driscoll MS, et al. Changes in size of melanocytic nevi during pregnancy. J Am Acad Dermatol 1997; 36:378–382. [II-2]

62. Ellis DL. Pregnancy and sex steroid hormone effects on nevi of patients with the dysplasctic nevus syndrome. J Am Acad Dermatol 1991; 25:467–482. [II-3]

63. Borden EC. Melanoma and pregnancy. Semin Oncol 2000; 27: 654–656. [III]

64. Altman JF, Lowe L, Redman B, et al. Placental metastasis of maternal melanoma. J Am Acad Dermatol 2003; 49:1150–1154. [IIII]

65. Alexander A, Harris RM, Grossman D, et al. Vulvar melanoma: diffuse melanosis and metastasis to the placenta. J Am Acad Dermatol 2004; 50:293–298. [III]

66. Sober AJ, Chuang T, Duvic M, et al. Guidelines of care for primary cutaneous melanoma. J Am Acad Dermatol 2001; 45:579–586. [III]

43

Multiple gestations

Edward J. Hayes and Michelle Broetzman

KEY POINTS

- **Determination of chorionicity by early (preferably first trimester) ultrasound** is of paramount importance for appropriate management of multiple gestations.
- **Preterm delivery** is the largest reason for the **increased morbidity and mortality associated with multiples.**
- No intervention has been shown to prevent **preterm birth in multiple gestations.** Although tests have been developed to determine ones risk for early delivery, since there is no proven intervention, screening cannot be recommended.
- **Multifetal pregnancy reduction** should be offered in higher-order gestations (quadruplets or higher) **to decrease the likelihood of a very premature delivery.**
- For noninvasive aneuploidy screening, nuchal translucency (NT) testing can be used in any multifetal gestation. Sequential screening (NT and serum analytes) can be used in twin gestations.
- The age-related risk of a mother having a child affected by trisomy must be adjusted depending on the number of fetuses; therefore, invasive testing may be considered for mothers of twins at age 33 and triplets at age 28.
- Discordant growth between multiples may be a marker for genetic or structural anomalies, infection, twin-to-twin transfusion, or placental issues; however, evidence of **FGR, not discordance, best predicts adverse neonatal outcome.**
- Multiples have **higher rates of preeclampsia** which tends to occur in an atypical fashion.
- A **single fetal death in multiple gestations** should **not mandate immediate delivery** for the risk of disseminated intravascular coagulation (DIC) is theoretical, and if they are monochorionic, adverse effects on the remaining fetus have already occurred.
- Routine antepartum testing has not been proven to be advantageous in multiple gestations without coexisting morbidity.
- **Monoamniotic twins** have a high rate of mortality that increases as gestational age increases, consequently **delivery should be considered at 32 to 34 weeks.**
- **Twin-to-twin transfusion syndrome** has significant mortality (>70%) if left untreated, particularly if diagnosed in the second trimester. While the evidence for effectiveness is still limited, laser coagulation appears to be the treatment of choice in advanced disease, but more research is needed to determine optimal therapy for milder stages.

DEFINITION

Multiple gestation is a gestation carrying more than one fetus. The overwhelming majority are twins. There are two types of twins:

- Monozygotic (MZ) twins are formed when a single fertilized ovum splits into two individuals who are almost always genetically identical, unless after their division there is a spontaneous mutation.
- Dizygotic (DZ) twins are formed when two separate ova are fertilized by two different sperms resulting in genetically different individuals.

EPIDEMIOLOGY/INCIDENCE

It is important to differentiate the natural from the actual incidence of multiple gestations.

The **natural incidence** of multiple gestations (Fig. 43.1) is as follows:

- MZ twining occurs at a constant rate of about 4 per 1000 (1/250).
- DZ twining rates vary with the individual's characteristics, such as race (low in Asians, high in blacks), age (increases with advanced maternal age), parity (increases with parity), and family history (especially on maternal side). The "natural" incidence of twins and triplets in the United States as reported in 1973 was 1 in 80 and 1 in 800, respectively (1).

The **actual incidence** of multiple gestations has been heavily influenced by the use of **assisted reproductive technologies (ART)** since the 1980s. Currently, >50% of multiple gestations in developed countries are from ART. The proportion of live births that are multiple gestations in the United States has increased significantly over the last two decades, with a 65% increase in twins and a 500% increase in triplets and higher-order births (2). This rise is associated with the increased use of ART treatments and the increasing maternal age at the time of pregnancy. The rate of multiple gestations in the United States, as recorded in 2007, was 3.2% of total births, with 3.2% twins and 0.1% triplets or higher-orders multiples (3). The vast majority of these pregnancies are DZ. MZ twin rates increase with ART to 3% to 5% (4). ART multiple pregnancies are associated with a higher incidence of fetal/neonatal and maternal complications.

ETIOLOGY

DZ twins are formed by two distinct fertilized ova and always have separate chorion and amnion (dichorionic/diamniotic, DC/DA).

MZ twin are formed from the division of one fertilized egg. The type is determined by the timing of the division of the fertilized ovum (Table 43.1).

DIAGNOSIS

The clinical signs for suspecting multiple gestations are a uterus larger than date, and a pregnancy that has resulted from ART. The accuracy of diagnosing twins on clinical criteria

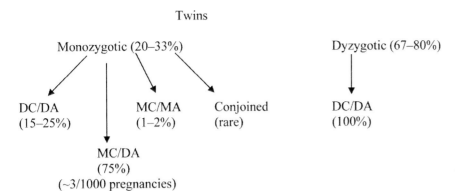

Twins

Monozygotic (20–33%)   Dyzygotic (67–80%)

DC/DA   MC/MA   Conjoined   DC/DA
(15–25%)   (1–2%)   (rare)   (100%)

MC/DA
(75%)
(~3/1000 pregnancies)

Figure 43.1 Natural incidence of multiple gestations. *Abbreviations*: MC, monochorionic; MA, monoamniotic; DC, dichorionic; DA, diamniotic.

Table 43.1 Timing of Zygote Division and Types of Twins

Timing of division	Type of twins	Characteristics	Picture
Day 1–3	Dichorionic/diamniotic (DC/DA)	Two placentas with two chorions and two amnions	
Day 3–8	Monochorionic/diamniotic (MC/DA)	Monochorionic placenta with two amnions	
Day 8–13	Monochorionic/ monoamniotic (MC/MA)	Monochorionic placenta with a single amniotic sac	
Day 13–15	Conjoined twins	Fused twins	

is poor, as 37% of women who do not undergo routine ultrasound screening will not have their twins diagnosed by 26 weeks, and 13% of multiples will only be diagnosed at the time of admission for delivery (5).

Ultrasound is 100% accurate in diagnosing multiple gestations (5). The best time for accurate diagnosis is the **first trimester**, as this is the **optimum time to determine** not only the fetal number, but also **chorionicity and amnionicity**. Determination of chorionicity and zygocity is paramount for correct risk assessment, counseling, and management of complications [e.g., twin-twin transfusion syndrome (TTTS), fetal

growth restriction (FGR), single fetal death]. In addition, this determination will help in future medical care of the babies for genetic component of diseases and organ-transplantation compatibility.

Determination of chorionicity and amnionicity in the first trimester is shown in Figure 43.2.

Determination of chorionicity and amnionicity status after first trimester is shown in Figures 43.3 and 43.4.

In the 30% to 40% of cases in which there are clearly two placentas, or differing fetal sex, the pregnancy is DC/DA, and DZ. In the majority of cases, the best ultrasound characteristic

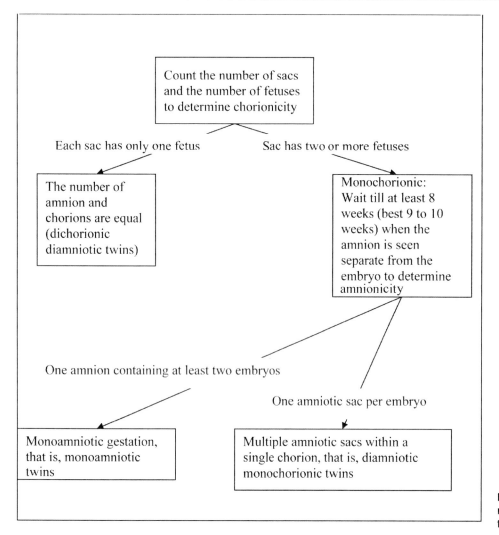

Figure 43.2 Determination of chorionicity and amnionicity in the first trimester.

to distinguish chorionicity and amnionicity is the **twin-peak sign**. Twin peak sign (also called lambda or delta sign) is a triangular projection of tissue with the same echogenicity as the placenta extending beyond the chorionic surface of the placenta (6). (Fig. 43.4)

DNA fingerprinting through polymorphisms or other means can also determine zygocity, but it is invasive and therefore associated with complications.

COMPLICATIONS

The incidence and severity of complications is related to chorionicity and amnionicity. Complications are more common in all types of multiple gestations compared to singleton gestations include:

Fetal

Spontaneous Reduction

A significant number of multiple gestations diagnosed in the first trimester undergo spontaneous reduction of one sac in the first trimester, referred to as the "**vanishing twin**." The rates of wastage of at least one gestation directly correlate with the initial number of gestational sacs, that is, about 20% to 50% of twins, 53% of triplets, and 65% of quadruplet (7). Since the

maternal serum alpha feto protein (MSAFP) and other analytes for aneuploidy and NTD screening can be elevated in pregnancies with vanishing twins, these tests are often not accurate for screening, and should not be performed subsequent to the diagnosis of vanishing twin.

Spontaneous Loss

The risk of miscarriage, especially in the first but also in the second trimester, is increased.

Higher Rates of Chromosomal and Congenital Anomalies

Because of the increased number of fetuses, particularly DZ, the risk of having one fetus affected by a trisomy is increased above the baseline risk of a singleton (8). Therefore the Down's syndrome risk of a 35-year-old singleton mother is obtained in twins at about age 31 to 33 (9), and for triplets this risk is obtained at about age 28 (10). Structural defects occur two to three times more commonly in live-born MZ twins than in DZ twins or singletons (11). Only in 5% to 20% are both MZ twins affected.

Fetal Growth Restriction and Discordant Growth

Discordant growth of multiples is usually defined as a 20% to 25% reduction in EFW of the smaller compared to the larger

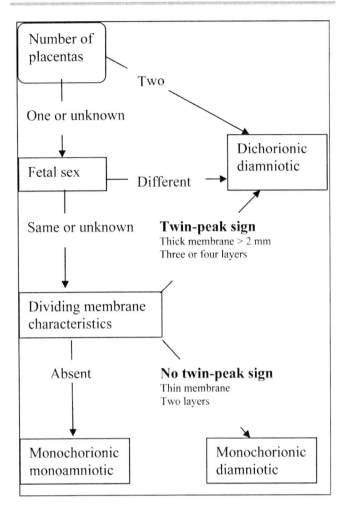

Figure 43.3 Determination of chorionicity and amnionicity after the first trimester.

fetus (difference of larger minus smaller EFW, divided by larger EFW). Discordance may be a marker for structural or genetic anomalies, infection, twin-to-twin transfusion syndrome, or placental issues. However, it is not the discordance per se, but evidence of **FGR of one fetus** that **predicts adverse neonatal outcome**. The risk of mortality or neonatal morbidity is higher among neonates in SGA-discordant twins than in AGA-discordant twins (20% vs. 6%) (12).

Single Fetal Demise in Multiple Gestations
Up to 5% of twins and 17% of triplets in the **second or third trimester** undergo spontaneous loss of one or more fetuses (13). This has been associated with a slight increase in risks of preterm birth (PTB) and growth restriction in the remaining fetus. Other impact on the remaining fetuses is dependent on chorionicity:

* DC twins: No significant neurologic morbidity in the remaining fetus after the death of one twin (10).
* Monochorionic (MC) twins: Because of vascular anastomoses, the remaining fetus is at significant risk of morbidity (about 25% neurologic) and mortality (about 10% perinatal) due to significant hypotension that occurs at the time of the demise.

Preterm Birth
Increasing numbers of fetuses are inversely associated with gestational age at birth, so that about 50% of twins are delivered preterm, most of the pregnancies with three or four fetuses have increased perinatal morbidity and mortality related to premature birth, and most of the pregnancies carrying more than four fetuses do not even reach viability (Table 43.2). PTB is mostly spontaneous from preterm labor (PTL) or preterm premature rupture of membranes (PPROM) but is also iatrogenic due to complications. **PTB is the main reason for the increased morbidity and mortality associated with multiples.** Twins conceived after in vitro fertilization are more likely delivered prior to 32 weeks than spontaneously conceived twins [OR 1.52 (1.18–1.97)] (14) Multiples are 10 times as likely to be very low birth weight than singletons (11.6% vs. 1.1%) (2), and account for nearly 20% of infant mortality (15), and significant morbidity evidenced by the rate of cerebral palsy, which is correlated to number of fetuses varying from 1.6 per thousand in singletons to 7.3 and 28 for twins and triplets, respectively (16).

Immaturity
Twins may have a higher rate of respiratory distress syndrome when matched with gestational–age-matched singletons (17).

Intrapartum Complications
These are more common especially in multiple gestations with first fetus nonvertex and trial of labor.

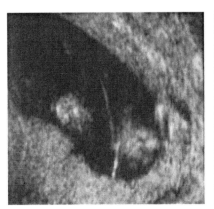 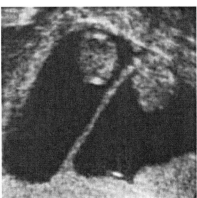

Figure 43.4 T-sign and twin-peak sign. On the left: T-sign (MC/DA gestation); always MZ. On the right: twin-peak sign (DC/DA gestation). *Abbreviations*: MC, monochorionic; MA, monoamniotic; DC, dichorionic; DA, diamniotic; MZ, monozygotic.

Table 43.2 Mean Gestational Age (GA) at Spontaneous Birth According to Number of Fetuses

Number of fetuses	Mean GA at birth (wk)
1	$\approx$ 40
2	$\approx$ 36
3	$\approx$ 33
4	$\approx$ 29–30
5	$\approx$ 24
$\geq$6	$\approx$ <20

Perinatal Neurologic Damage
It is related to some of the complications described above.

Perinatal Mortality
Twins have a higher rate (5% vs. 1%) of perinatal mortality compared to singletons. This risk comes mostly from MZ twins, since MZ twins have a higher (2.5–5 times) risk compared to DZ twins.

Maternal

In addition to the complications above: **Heartburn, hemorrhoids, tiredness, anxiety, hyperemesis gravidarum, maternal anemia**, as well as:

Preeclampsia
Multiples having a higher rate of developing hypertensive conditions associated with pregnancy, an incidence that is proportional to the total fetal number (singletons 6.5%, twins 12.7%, and triplets 20.0%) (18). Besides having a higher rate of preeclampsia, multiples are more likely manifest this disease in an atypical fashion (19).

Abruptio Placentae
Abruptio is more common in multiples and exhibits a correlation to the number of fetuses (1.2% of twins; 1.6% of triplets) (18).

Thrombocytopenia
Up to one third of triplet gestations can be complicated by thrombocytopenia, and unlike singletons where the number one cause of thrombocytopenia is gestational, severe preeclampsia is the most common cause in triplets (20).

Acute Fatty Liver
In contrast to singleton gestations where the rate of fatty liver is 1 in 10,000, the rate in triplets is up to 7% (21).

Gestational Diabetes
There is a mild correlation between twins and gestational diabetes when compared to singletons, although insulin requirements between these two groups are not significantly different (22). A significant association is demonstrated with triplets with a gestational diabetes rate of 22% (23).

Other maternal complications include **postpartum hemorrhage; peripartum hysterectomy**, with a significantly increased risk of emergent peripartum hysterectomy compared to singletons (24); **postpartum depression;** and **maternal death.**

COMPLICATIONS SPECIFIC TO MONOCHORIONIC GESTATIONS
Twin-twin Transfusion Syndrome

Incidence
This syndrome occurs in 10% to 15% of MC/DA pregnancies, and therefore in about 1/2500 pregnancies. Rare cases have been reported in monoamniotic (MA)/MC pregnancies.

Preterm Labor
All monochorionic pregnancies have one placenta only, with anastomoses of artery-to-artery (AA), vein-to-vein (VV), and artery-to-vein (AV) of the two twins. TTTS may not occur in MC/MA gestations because of more AA, and less AV anastomoses than in MC/DA gestations. An imbalance of arterial circulation of one twin (donor) to the venous circulation of another (recipient) probably through an AV anastomosis can lead to TTTS. Over 50% of TTTS placentas have $\geq$1 velamentous cord insertion, possibly associated with this imbalance. The donor twin develops anemia and resultant effects [e.g., IUGR (intrauterine growth restriction), oligohydramnios], while the recipient twin has polyhydramnios, becomes polycythemic, and can develop heart failure.

Diagnosis
The antepartum diagnosis requires ultrasound. The criteria are **MC/DA gestation** (see above) with **oligohydramnios** [maximum vertical pocket (MVP) < 2 cm] in one sac, and **polyhydramnios** (MVP > 8 cm) in the other. Supporting criteria can be the presence of same-sex twins with a single placenta, and significant discordance in fetal growth. It is important to rule out other etiologies for similar findings, such as FGR of just one twin with normal other twin, chromosomal or structural abnormalities, infection, etc. **Staging** is described in Table 43.3 (25).

Prognosis
The prognosis is poor, and depends mostly on gestational age at diagnosis and stage of disease. About 5% of TTTS, especially in early stages, can regress. Survival with diagnosis at <26 weeks without treatment is about 30% (26). Survival can often be with severe morbidity, including neurologic, cardiac, ischemia/necrosis of extremities, renal cortical necrosis, etc. Given this poor prognosis, support is important (e.g., http://www.tttsfoundation.org).

Monoamniotic Twins
Incidence is 1 in 10,000 pregnancies, but more common with in vitro fertilization using zona manipulation affecting up to 17% of multiples using this technique (27). Diagnosis is by ultrasound: Prior to eight weeks—one yolk sac and two fetal poles is diagnostic (28); if after eight weeks, then same sex, single placenta, and single amniotic sac with no dividing amniotic

Table 43.3 Staging for TTTS

Stage 1	MC/DA gestation with oligo (MVP < 2 cm) and polyhydramnios (MVP > 8 cm)
Stage 2	Absent (empty) bladder (in donor)
Stage 3	Abnormal Doppler[a]
Stage 4	Hydrops
Stage 5	Death of one twin

[a]Defined as either umbilical artery absent or reversed diastolic flow; ductus venosus absent or reversed diastolic flow; or umbilical vein pulsatile flow. *Abbreviations*: MC/DA, monochorionic/diamniotic; MVP, maximum vertical pocket. *Source*: From Ref. 25.

membrane allow diagnosis. Fetuses must be of the same sex. Demonstration of umbilical cord entanglement is also diagnostic of MA twins.

The rate of loss due especially to cord accidents in utero, and also to congenital anomalies, and very PTB in pregnancies beyond 22 weeks is up to 32% despite intensive care and monitoring at tertiary care centers (29). Perinatal mortality with aggressive inpatient monitoring (see below) and delivery at 32 weeks has been reported to be as low as 10%, with later delivery probably associated with continuing risk of mortality (30).

Acardiac Twin

Acardiac twin (also called twin reversal arterial perfusion— TRAP—syndrome) is a MZ, MC pregnancy characterized by a fetus lacking a normal developed heart and usually a head ("acardiac twin"). It occurs in 1% of MC twins, or about 1/ 35,000 pregnancies. This acardiac fetus survives in utero due to placental anastomoses shunting blood flow from the "pump twin." Diagnosis needs ultrasound Doppler confirmation of blood being pumped in from the "pump" twin. The "pump twin" can develop a high cardiac output state and subsequent failure, resulting in intrauterine or neonatal death of this normal twin in about 35% to 50% of cases (31).

Conjoined Twins

Conjoined twins are an anomaly linked to MZ twining with an incidence of 1 in 50,000 to 1 in 10,000 births (32). Classification is based on the site of connection with the suffix *pagus* added. Of those diagnosed in utero, 28% will die prior to delivery, 54% immediately after birth, with only an 18% survival rate (33). Diagnosis of shared anatomy is imperative to management and prognosis (31).

PREGNANCY CONSIDERATIONS

Compared to singleton gestations, physiologic changes in twins include a 50% to 60% increase in maternal blood volume (40–50% in singletons) leading to higher incidence of anemia, higher increase in cardiac output, slightly lower diastolic blood pressure, and more discomfort such as pressure, difficulty in ambulation, etc.

PREGNANCY MANAGEMENT
Nutrition

The recommended total weight gain for twin pregnancies starting with normal BMI is about 35 to 40 lb. Diet should include an increase in caloric intake by 300 kcal above singletons (600 kcal above nonpregnant state), folic acid 1 mg/day, iron 60 mg/day.

Prenatal Diagnosis

First trimester. In multiple gestations, **NT** alone has been shown to be as sensitive as in singletons, with an 88% detection rate for trisomy 21 with a 7.3 % screen positive rate (34). Serum-based screening in twins is possible, but less sensitive than in singletons. Serum-based screening is not available for triplets or higher-order multiple gestations. **Chorionic villus sampling** can be performed between 10 and 12 weeks. It has the same risks as amniocentesis in multiples (35), and has a 4% to 6% rate of twin-twin contamination (36).

Second trimester. Serum screening for neural tube defects with MSAFP using a cutoff of 4.5 MoM has a detection rate of 50% to 85% with a 5% false-positive rate.

Serum screening for Down syndrome is less sensitive in twins than in singletons. It is not available in triplets or higher-order multiple gestations, given poor detection rates, and high rates of false-positives and negatives (37). Genetic **amniocentesis** has been reported to have a loss rate with multiples similar to singletons (38). At sampling of the first sac, indigo carmine or Evan's blue can be injected; a clear sample obtained from the second sac with a second needle insures that two different sacs have been sampled. Methylene blue dye should not be used because of the risks of fetal hemolytic anemia, small intestinal atresia, and fetal demise. If gestation is MC, sampling of one sac is suggested for karyotype.

Prediction of PTB

Transvaginal measurement of cervical length performed between 16 and 24 weeks' gestation is a strong predictor of preterm delivery in asymptomatic women with twin gestations. A cervical length $\leq$20 mm increases the pretest probability of PTB prior to 32 weeks for 6.8% to 42.4%, whereas a length >20 mm decreased the risk to 4.5% (39). However, since there is currently no beneficial intervention if this screening test is positive, **routine screening with cervical length of multiples at risk for preterm delivery cannot be recommended**.

PREVENTION AND MANAGEMENT OF COMPLICATIONS
Selective Termination of an Anomalous Fetus

Selective termination of an anomalous fetus is usually performed in second trimester due to the time of diagnosis of the fetal anomaly.

In DC pregnancies, the procedure consists of injection of potassium chloride into the fetal heart transabdominally. The loss rate of the entire pregnancy is about 4% of those performed prior to 24 weeks, with a difference if twins were lower versus higher-order multiples (2.4% vs. 11.1%) and if more than one fetus is terminated (2.6% loss if one fetus vs. 42.9% if two) (40). In a review of twin DC pregnancies discordant for fetal anencephaly, there was no difference in survival of the nonaffected twin between those who elected selective termination versus expectant management; however, there was a statistically significant difference between both groups in mean gestational age at delivery (38.0 vs. 34.9 weeks) (41).

In MC pregnancies, potassium chloride should not be used, as it crosses to the other fetus through the placental anastomoses and therefore causes fetal death of both fetuses. Cord ligation, or occlusion with clips, diathermy, or other means have been used, with insufficient data for effective comparison.

Preterm Birth

See also chapters 16 to 18 in *Obstetric Evidence Based Guidelines*.

Prevention of Multiple Gestations

The incidence of multiple gestation is increased with both ovulation induction, which represent the majority of ART multiples, and IVF. Unfortunately it is difficult to prevent multiple gestations with ovarian stimulation. Excessive stimulation and insemination in the presence of excessive number of ripe follicles should be avoided. Transfer of one embryo almost guarantees avoidance of multiple gestation, and is associated with rates of successful pregnancy similar to transfer of >1 embryos with modern techniques. Many developed countries have laws that allow the transfer of only one, or maximum of two embryos. No more than three embryos should ever be transferred, even in the woman with poor prognosis (i.e., >40 years old). The successful outcome of ART should be based on the rate of healthy term singleton per cycle.

Multifetal Pregnancy Reduction
The goal of first trimester fetal reduction (safe only in DC gestations) is to decrease the number of fetuses in higher-order gestations thereby lessening the likelihood of a premature delivery and the associated morbidity and mortality. Although there have been no randomized controlled trials, several retrospective studies of higher-order gestations reduced to twins or singletons have shown significant prolongation of gestation when compared to those who did not undergo reduction (42). American College of Obstetricians and Gynecologists (ACOG) based on these findings states that "... **the risks associated with a quadruplet or higher pregnancy clearly outweighs the risks associated with fetal reduction.**" (43) There seems to be an increasing risk of IUGR with increasing fetal number. **Compared to triplets, triplets reduced to twins have a higher (about 9–6%) incidence of loss <24 weeks, but lower incidences of PTB < 32 weeks, maternal hospitalization, cesarean delivery (CD), and better neonatal outcome of the remaining twins after reduction compared to triplets**. As reduction involves termination of one triplet fetus, overall perinatal survival is not different, and might actually be slightly decreased, but improvement in morbidity and mortality is seen in "remaining" twin fetuses compared to nonreduced triplets and yield a higher rate of "intact" normal babies in the reduced-to-twins compared to the nonreduced triplets. Over 90% of women who underwent pregnancy reduction would opt for the procedure again.

Bed Rest
Bed rest, either prophylactic (before symptoms) or therapeutic (with symptoms of PTL) **does not prevent PTB** in multiple gestations (44). Compared to normal activity, prophylactic bed rest in the hospital has even been associated with increase in the rate of delivery before 34 weeks in some studies (44,45) in uncomplicated twin pregnancies. **There is no reduction in perinatal mortality with hospital bed rest in twins** (44) (see also chap. 16, *Obstetric Evidence Based Guidelines*).

Progesterone
Progesterone, administered either in injectable form (17-alpha-hydroxyprogesterone caproate, 17P) (46–49); or vaginally (50) does not prevent PTB in twin gestations.17P is also not beneficial in preventing PTB in triplet gestations (51,52).

Cerclage
Cerclage, either history-indicated (53) or ultrasound-indicated (54) does not prevent PTB in twins and triplet (55) gestations.

Home Uterine Activity Monitoring
Home uterine activity monitoring (HUAM) has not been proven to decrease the incidence of PTB in multiple gestations (56) and therefore this costly intervention should not be undertaken.

Prophylactic Tocolysis
Prophylactic tocolysis has no proven effect on the incidence of PTB, low birth weight, or neonatal mortality (all similar incidences with placebo) in twin gestations, and therefore this practice should be avoided (57).

Preterm Labor
Delivery should be offered if any of the following are present: ≥34 weeks' gestation, proven fetal lung maturity, chorioamnionitis, or nonreassuring testing.

If <34 weeks and none of the above criteria are present, evaluation of multiples presenting <34 weeks in threatened preterm labor may be based on cervical length, for this directly correlates with delivery within seven days in woman with regular painful contractions at 24 to 36 weeks:

a. More than 25 mm: 0%
b. 21–25 mm: 7%
c. 16–20 mm: 21%
d. 11–15 mm: 29%
e. 6–10 mm: 46%
f. 1–5 mm: 80% (58)

Corticosteroids (one course: betamethasone 12 mg q24h × 2 doses) should be administered to all patients who are between 24 and 33 6/7 weeks and at high risk (e.g., cervical length ≤20 mm) of delivery within seven days (59).

Tocolytics have not been sufficiently studied in multiple gestations (no specific trials) with PTL or PPROM to assess their efficacy in PTB prevention. They should be used judiciously due to higher incidence of side effects in multiple, that is, pulmonary edema, compared to singleton gestations (see chap. 17, *Obstetric Evidence Based Guidelines*).

PPROM
Delivery is suggested if any of the following are present: ≥34 weeks' gestation, proven fetal lung maturity, chorioamnionitis, or nonreassuring testing.

If <34 weeks and none of the above criteria are present, then expectant management with antibiotics, usually ampicillin and erythromycin, together with corticosteroids as above (see chap. 18, *Obstetric Evidence Based Guidelines*).

FGR/Discordant Twins

If neither fetus has growth restriction (EFW <10% for GA), no significant change in management needs to be done. If one fetus has FGR, then: review of all prenatal exposures, specialized ultrasound examination for anomalies, consider amniocentesis for karyotype (43); consider twice weekly NSTs and weekly umbilical artery (UA) Doppler velocimetry (see chap. 44). Consider delivery for reversed end-diastolic flow (REDF) of UA and >30 to 32 weeks.

Single Fetal Death

Management depends on chorionicity and gestational age.

Dichorionic Gestation
Less than 12 weeks: usually no consequences, so no intervention needed.

More than 12 weeks: Immediate delivery has no benefit for the remaining fetus and the often quoted maternal risk of DIC has not been demonstrated.

Monochorionic Gestation
Less than 12 weeks: associated with high risk of loss of other twin, with no intervention studied.

More than 12 weeks: associated with about 10% risk of intrauterine death and additional 25% risk of neurologic complications in other twin. These risks seem to occur from hypotension due to transfusion of blood from one to the already-demised twin. At the time the demise is discovered, the greatest harm has most likely already occurred in the remaining fetus, and there seems to be no benefit in immediate delivery, especially if the surviving fetus(es) is very preterm and otherwise healthy. In such cases, allowing the pregnancy to continue may provide the most benefit (43). The coagulopathy risk for the mother is minimal, probably <2%.

Twin-to-Twin Transfusion Syndrome

Workup
Upon diagnosis of TTTS, other possible etiologies should be ruled out, by obtaining detailed anatomy survey by ultrasound of both twins, including UA Doppler and echocardiography, fetal chromosomes by amniocentesis, infectious studies (e.g. CMV, parvovirus, toxoplasmosis) on amniotic fluid and maternal serum, and maternal glucose-tolerance testing.

Therapy
Amnioreduction involves removing with a 20 to 22 gauge needle excess fluid from the polyhydramniotic sac, so as to restore MVP <8. While in 20% of cases one amnioreduction is sufficient to resolve TTTS, in the other cases it might need to be performed serially, as often fluid quickly reaccumulates. The theory behind its efficacy is that it prevents preterm delivery due to polyhydramnios and also helps to stabilize the flow in arterial-venous connections and thereby slow the rate of blood transfer and fluid reaccumulation (60).

    Laser therapy involves direct coagulation of the placental vessels identified in the recipient twin and crossing the membrane to the other twin (semiselective), or of only those vessels thought to be responsible for the imbalance, such as AV anastomoses (selective). The techniques can therefore be more or less selective or nonselective of certain AV, AA, or VV anastomoses.

    Septostomy involves purposefully perforating the intertwine membrane under ultrasound guidance with a 22-gauge needle, thus allowing equalization of pressure in the two sacs.

    Treatment of choice for TTTS based on meta-analysis involving 213 women and 430 babies showed that there was no difference in perinatal outcome between amnioreduction and septostomy (61). However, laser coagulation of anastomotic vessels results in less death of both infants per pregnancy (RR 0.49; 95% CI 0.30–0.79), less perinatal death (RR 0.59; 95% CI 0.40–0.87), and less neonatal death (RR 0.29; 95% CI 0.14–0.61 adjusted for cluster), than in pregnancies treated with amnioreduction. These results are mostly based on just one positive RCT (62) in which there were 11 elective terminations (16%) in the amnioreduction group and none in the laser group; excluding these pregnancies, no differences in outcomes are present. The 41% perinatal survival rate of the amnioreduction group in this trial was much lower than the usual 60% to 65% reported in most series and another RCT. While some experts conclude that endoscopic laser coagulation of anastomotic vessels could be considered in all stages of TTTS, more research is needed to address those with milder forms (i.e., Quintero stage 1 and 2) (63).

    Selective fetocide via bipolar diathermy can allow the survival of one twin without neurologic complications (64). The most common indication for selective fetocide in TTTS is one of the twins has an anomaly or hydrops with impending fetal death. There are no trials available. The rate of loss or PPROM within two to three weeks of the procedure of the remaining twin is about 20%.

Other Interventions
There is insufficient evidence to evaluate the efficacy of other interventions reported for TTTS, such as transfusion therapy, indomethacin, digoxin, etc.

    Multiple treatment options for the **acardiac twin** have been described. In a systemic review, intrafetal radiofrequency ablation was determined to be the treatment of choice (65).

Monoamniotic Twins

Because of the rarity of the condition, there are no trials available. Several controlled series have suggested: first trimester screening with NT measurement; fetal echocardiography at 22 to 24 weeks; ultrasound every 3 to 4 weeks until 24 weeks to assess cord entanglement; corticosteroids in the standard dose at 24 to 26 weeks; daily nonstress tests initiated at viability; admission at 24 to 26 weeks with continuous monitoring (allow bathroom and shower privileges); after 24 weeks, serial ultrasound performed every two weeks for fetal biometry, size discordance and amniotic fluid volume, and umbilical cord Doppler performed weekly. In the presence of a persistent nonreactive fetal heart tracing (once documented as reactive) or abnormal biophysical profile, poor or discordant growth, and/or abnormal UA Doppler velocimetry, in-hospital continuous monitoring should be initiated.

Timing of Delivery
Consider delivery for obstetric indications including abnormal fetal testing or impaired fetal growth <32 weeks, or schedule around 32 to 34 weeks.

Single Intrauterine Death
If gestational age is less than 28 to 30 weeks, can continue to monitor. If gestational age is >30 weeks, urgent delivery can be considered.

Mode of Delivery
Cesarean section at 32 to 34 weeks is the preferred mode of delivery due to the risk of fetal interlocking and cord entanglement and to avoid the risk of inadvertently clamping and dividing the cord of the second twin during the delivery of the first twin, premature placental separation, and cord prolapse.

Acardiac Twin

Because of the rarity of the condition, there are no trials available. As cardiac failure is more common when the EFW of the acardiac twin is >70% of EFW of pump twin, interventions to "terminate" the acardiac twin in utero have been proposed for EFW of acardiac >70% together with "pump" twin compromise. Of all the proposed techniques, **ultrasound-guided laser coagulation or radiofrequency ablation** of intrafetal vessels seem to be the first line of treatment in centers experienced with these techniques. Cord ligation and occlusion have also been reported with some success (66).

Conjoined Twins

Because of the rarity of the condition, there are no trials available. Termination should be considered if cardiac (thoracopagus) or cerebral (craniopagus) fusion are present, due to poor outcome (32), or if the pregnancy outcome due to the level of deformity is unacceptable. If pregnancy is continued, planned cesarean at term is recommended.

ANTEPARTUM TESTING
Ultrasound

An ultrasound should be performed in the **first trimester** assessing viability, gestational age, and chorionicity.

    An ultrasound should be performed between **18 and 22 weeks** assessing gestational age, chorionicity (if not done previously), placental cord insertion sites, fetal anatomic surveys, and fetal gender.

Fetal Growth

Twins grow at the same rate as singletons up to 28 to 32 weeks, and then the growth of twins slows, so that fetal twin charts are best used for management. Sonographic assessment can be performed about every 4 weeks from 18 to 20 weeks until delivery. If discordance or IUGR is diagnosed, then frequency can be increased to every three weeks.

Amniotic Fluid

Multiple methods to access amniotic fluid by ultrasound in multiples has been described, including subjective assessment, total amniotic fluid index (AFI), individual AFI, single deepest pocket (SDP, aka MVP), two-diameter pocket, and others. The SDP technique, using <2 cm for polyhydramnios and >8 cm for polyhydramnios, is preferred, as it is accurate in assessing amniotic fluid volume in normal pregnancies. This technique is not very accurate in detection of oligohydramnios (see also chap. 56).

Fetal Surveillance

Routine antepartum testing has not been proven to be valuable in the management of multiple gestations. Therefore, antepartum fetal surveillance in multiple gestations is recommended in all situations in which surveillance would ordinarily be performed in a singleton pregnancy (e.g., FGR, maternal disease, decreased fetal movement) (43). Some start NSTs in all twin gestations at around 34 weeks, but there is no firm evidence for or against this intervention. Doppler flow studies are not routinely beneficial (67), but probably have the same benefit in fetal morbidity and mortality in cases of twin FGR as in cases of singleton FGR.

DELIVERY
Assessment of Fetal Lung Maturity

As disparity in lung maturity occurs usually in only 5% of twins, just one gestational sac may be sampled for assessment of lung maturity. In certain circumstances, such as diabetes or growth discordance, a bigger difference in maturity discordance may necessitate sampling both sacs.

Timing of Delivery

Fetal and neonatal morbidity and mortality begin to increase in twins at 37 completed weeks and triplets at 35 completed weeks. There are **insufficient data available** to assess any effect of scheduled delivery at around 37-week gestation for women with an otherwise uncomplicated twin pregnancy (68). If the fetuses are AGA with evidence of sustained growth, with normal AFI and reassuring testing without maternal disease, then the pregnancy can be delivered at **37 or 38 weeks**, with the woman being allowed to influence this decision. If the woman is experiencing morbidities, which would not usually mandate delivery (e.g., dyspnea, inability to sleep, severe edema, painful varicosities), delivery may be considered at these gestational ages (43).

Route of Delivery

Twins
There is insufficient evidence to assess the best mode of delivery for twins. Trial of labor after CD is associated with similar risks with twin as with singleton gestations (see chap. 14, *Obstetric Evidence Based Guidelines*).

There are **no trials for twins presenting vertex/vertex** (40% of twin pregnancies), with trial of labor usually suggested as this has been shown to be safe.

For vertex/non-vertex twins (about 34% of twin pregnancies), compared to trial of labor, planned CD had no benefit in neonatal outcome with increased maternal febrile morbidity in one small trial (69). However, when all twins at 36 weeks or beyond, not just those with a noncephalic second twin, were examined, it has been reported that the term second twin has a higher rate of perinatal mortality when delivered vaginally as opposed to scheduled CD (70). The rate of low 5-min Apgar score is less frequent in twins delivered by CD (66). Attempt at vaginal twin delivery has been supported especially for twins with EFW of >1500 g, and can only be performed with an adequately experienced obstetrician, and continuous availability of expert anesthesia, usually in or very close to an operating room. Interval between first and second twin deliveries is not critical, as long as the second twin is monitored continuously and accurately. Oxytocin may need to be (re)started as contractions often diminish, and amniotomy should be performed only when presenting part is engaged. The total breech extraction is associated with shorter maternal stay and lower neonatal pulmonary disease, infection, and intensive care nursery stay compared to podalic version in retrospective studies (71,72). One trial has recently completed recruitment and will be reported probably in 2012 or after.

There are no trials for twins presenting with **first twin nonvertex** (about 26%), with recommendation for CD made based mostly on data from singleton gestations.

Triplets and higher-order multiples. Because vaginal delivery of triplets is usually associated with an increased risk for stillbirth, neonatal and infant deaths as compared to CD (73), **cesarean section is the route of choice**. Some centers have recently reported similar outcomes for trial of labor or CD for triplets, but these series are small and not RCTs.

Delayed Interval Delivery

Preterm labor or PPROM can result in the delivery of only one twin or other multiple-gestation fetus. Delaying the delivery of the remaining fetus(es) may result in decreased morbidity and mortality of these remaining fetuses, with no trials to fully assess the effect of this intervention. Delayed delivery should not be attempted if MC gestation, abruption, preeclampsia, chorioamnionitis, need of CD, or other indications for delivery are present, making **only about 25% of multiple deliveries in the second trimester candidates for this attempt**. Delayed delivery is not very successful and does not result in significant improvements at >28 weeks (delay <2 weeks even with success). While tocolytics, antibiotics, and cerclage are often used, there is no firm evidence of their benefit. Delayed delivery is associated with decreases in perinatal and infant mortality, with averages gain of about two to five weeks if successful. The interval between deliveries is inversely correlated with gestational age of first delivery (74).

NEONATAL

There is probably no significant difference between multiples and singletons in odds of death and long-term outcomes (intraventricular hemorrhage, retinopathy of prematurity, necrotizing enterocolitis) at a given gestational age in those unaffected by FGR (75).

REFERENCES

1. Benirschke K, Kim CK. Multiple pregnancy. 1. N Engl J Med 1973; 288(24):1276–1284. [Level II-3]
2. Martin JA, Hamilton BE, Sutton PD, et al. Births: final data for 2002. Natl Vital Stat Rep 2003; 52(10):1–102. [Level II-3]

3. Available at: www.MarchofDimes.com/peristats. [Epidemiologic data]

4. Wenstrom KD, Syrop CH, Hammitt DG, et al. Increased risk of monochorionic twinning associated with assisted reproduction. Fertil Steril 1993; 60:510–514. [Level III]

5. LeFevre ML, Bain RP, Ewigman BG, et al. A randomized trial of prenatal ultrasonographic screening: impact on maternal management and outcome. RADIUS (Routine Antenatal Diagnostic Imaging with Ultrasound) Study Group. Am J Obstet Gynecol 1993; 169(3):483–489. [Level I]

6. Finberg HJ. The "twin peak" sign: reliable evidence of dichorionic twinning. J Ultrasound Med 1992; 11(11):571–577. [Level II-3]

7. Dickey RP, Taylor SN, Lu PY, et al. Spontaneous reduction of multiple pregnancy: incidence and effect on outcome. Am J Obstet Gynecol 2002; 186(1):77–83. [Level II-2]

8. Meyers C, Adam R, Dungan J, et al. Aneuploidy in twin gestations: when is maternal age advanced? Obstet Gynecol 1997; 89:248–251. [Level II-2]

9. Rodis JF, Egan JFX, Craffey A, et al. Calculated risks of chromosomal abnormalities in twin gestations. Obstet Gynecol 1990; 76(6):1037–1041. [Level II-2]

10. Malone FD, D'Alton ME. Multiple Gestation Clinical Characteristics and Management. Maternal-Fetal Medicine Principles and Practice. 5th ed. Philadelphia: Saunders, 2004. [Level III]

11. Jones KL. Smith's Recognizable Patterns of Human Malformation. 5th ed. Philadelphia: WB Saunders, 1997:654. [Level III]

12. Yinon Y, Mazkereth R, Rosentzweig N, et al. Growth restriction as a determinant of outcome in preterm discordant twins. Obstet Gynecol 2005; 105:80–84. [Level II-3]

13. D'Alton ME, Simpson LL. Syndromes in twins. Semin Perinatol 1995; 19(5):375–386. [Level II-3]

14. Kallen B, Finnstrom O, Lindam A, et al. Selected neonatal outcomes in dizygotic twins after IVF versus non-IVF pregnancies. Br J Obstet Gynecol 2010; 117:676–682.

15. Magee BD. Role of multiple births in very low birth weight and infant mortality. J Reprod Med 2004; 49(10):812–816. [Level II-2]

16. Petterson B, Nelson KB, Watson L, et al. Twins, triplets and cerebral palsy in births in Western Australia in the 1980s. Br Med J 1993; 307:1239–1243. [Level II-2]

17. Chasen ST, Madden A, Chervenak FA. Cesarean delivery of twins and neonatal respiratory disorders. Am J Obstet Gynecol 1999; 181(5 pt 1):1052–1056. [Level II-2]

18. Day MC, Barton JR, O'Brien JM, et al. The effect of fetal number on the development of hypertensive conditions of pregnancy. Obstet Gynecol 2005; 106:927–931. [Level II-2]

19. Sibai BM, Hauth J, Caritis S, et al. Hypertensive disorders in twin versus singleton gestations. National Institute of Child Health and Human Development Network of Maternal-Fetal Medicine Units. Am J Obstet Gynecol 2000; 182:938–942. [Level I]

20. Al-Kouatly HB, Chasen ST, Kalish RB, et al. Causes of thrombocytopenia in triplet gestations. Am J Obstet Gynecol 2003; 189 (1):177–180. [Level II-2]

21. Malone FD, Kaufman GE, Chelmow D, et al. Maternal morbidity associated with triplet pregnancy. Am J Perinatol 1998; 15:73–77. [Level II-3]

22. Schwartz DB, Daoud Y, Zazula P, et al. Gestational diabetes mellitus: metabolic and blood glucose parameters in singleton versus twin pregnancies. Am J Obstet Gynecol 1999; 181(4):912–914. [Level II-2]

23. Silvan E, Maman E, Homko CJ, et al. Impact of fetal reduction on the incidence of gestational diabetes. Obstet Gynecol 2002; 99:91–94. [Level II-3]

24. Francois K, Ortiz J, Harris C, et al. Is peripartum hysterectomy more common in multiple gestations? Obstet Gynecol 2005; 105 (6):1369–1372. [Level II-3]

25. Quintero RA, Morales WJ, Allen MH, et al. Staging of twin-twin transfusion syndrome. J Perinatol 1999; 19:550–555. [II-2]

26. Berghella V, Kaufmann M. Natural history of twin-twin transfusion syndrome. J Reprod Med 2001; 46(5):480–484. [Level II-3]

27. Slotnick RN, Ortega JE. Monoamniotic twining and zona manipulation: a survey of U.S. IVF centers correlating zona manipulation procedures and high-risk twinning frequency. J Assist Reprod Genet 1996; 13:381–385. [Level II-3]

28. Bromley B, Benacerraf B. Using the number of yolk sacs to determine amniocity in early first trimester monochorionic twins. J Ultrasound Med 1995; 14:415–419. [Level II-2]

29. Demaria F, Goffinet F, Kayem G, et al. Monoamniotic twin pregnancies: antenatal management and perinatal results of 19 consecutive cases. Br J Obstet Gynecol 2004; 111(1):22–26. [Level II-3]

30. Roque H, Young BK, Lockwood CJ. Perinatal outcomes in monoamniotic gestations. J Matern Fetal Neonatal Med 2003; 13(6):414–421. [Level II-3]

31. Van Gemert MJ, Umur A, van den Wijngaard JP, et al. Increasing cardiac output and decreasing oxygenation sequence in pump twins of acardiac twin pregnancies. Phys Med Biol 2005; 50(3): N33–N42. [Level II-3]

32. Spitz L, Kiely EM. Conjoined twins. J Am Med Assoc 2003; 289(10):1307–1310. [Level II-3]

33. Mackenzie TC, Crombleholme TM, Johnson MP, et al. The natural history of prenatally diagnosed conjoined twins. J Pediatr Surg 2002; 37(3):303–309. [Level II-3]

34. Sebire N, Snijders R, Hughes K, et al. Screening for trisomy 21 in twin pregnancies by maternal age and fetal nuchal translucency thickness at 10-14 weeks of gestation. Br J Obstet Gynaecol 1996; 103(10):999–1003. [Level II-2]

35. Wapner RJ, Johnson A, Davis G. Prenatal diagnosis in twin gestations: a comparison between second trimester amniocentesis and first trimester chorionic villus sampling. Obstet Gynecol 1993; 82(1):49–56. [Level II-2]

36. Wapner RJ. Genetic diagnosis in multiple pregnancies. Semin Perinatol 1995; 19:351. [Level III]

37. O'Brien J, Dvorin E, Yaron Y. Differential increases in AFP, hCG and uE3 in twin pregnancies: impact on attempts to quantify Down syndrome screening calculations. Am J Med Genet 1997; 73(2):109–112. [Level II-1]

38. Ghidini A, Lynch L, Hicks C, et al. The risk of second-trimester amniocentesis in twin gestations: a case-control study. Am J Obstet Gynecol 1993; 169(4):1013–1016. [Level II-2]

39. Conde-Agudelo A, Romero R, Hassan SS, et al. Transvaginal sonographic cervical length for the prediction of spontaneous preterm birth in twin pregnancies: a systematic review and metaanalysis. Am J Obstet Gynecol 2010; 203:128.e1–12.

40. Eddleman KA, Stone JL, Lynch L, et al. Selective termination of anomalous fetuses in multifetal pregnancies: two hundred cases at a single center. Am J Obstet Gynecol 2002; 187:1168–1172. [Level II-3]

41. Lust A, De Catt L, Lewi L, et al. Monochorionic and dichorionic twin pregnancies discordant for fetal anencephaly: a systematic review of management options. Prenat Diagn 2008; 28:275–279.

42. Miller V, Ransom S, Shalhoub A, et al. Multifetal pregnancy reduction: perinatal and fiscal outcomes. Am J Obstet Gynecol 2000; 182(6):1575–1579. [Level II-3]

43. Multiple gestation: complicated twin, triplet, and higher-order multifetal pregnancy. ACOG Practice Bull Number 56, 2004. [Level III]

44. Crowther CA, Han S. Hospitalization and bed rest for multiple pregnancies. Cochrane Database Syst Rev 2010; (7):CD000110, 8. [Meta-analysis; 7 RCTs, 731 women. Mostly in Harare, Zimbabwe]

45. Crowther CA, Neilson JP, Verkuyl DAA, et al. Preterm labour in twin pregnancies: can it be prevented by hospital admission? Br J Obstet Gynaecol 1989; 96:850–853. [RCT, $n = 139$]

46. Rouse D, Caritis S, Peaceman A, et al. A trial of alpha-hydroxyprogesterone caproate to prevent prematurity in twins. N Engl J Med 2007; 357:454–461. [RCT, $n = 655$]

47. Briery CM, Veillon EW, Klauser CK, et al. Progesterone does not prevent preterm births in women with twins. South Med J 2009; 102:900–904. [RCT, $n = 30$]

48. Hartikainen-Sorri AL, Kauppila A, Tuimala R. Inefficacy of 17 a-hydroxyprogesterone caproate in the prevention of prematurity in twin pregnancy. Obstet Gynecol 1980; 56(6):692–695. [RCT, $n = 77$]

49. Combs CA, Garite T, Maurel K, et al. for the Obstetrix Collaborative Research Network. 17-hydroxyprogesterone caproate for twin pregnancy: a double-blind, randomized clinical trial. Am J Obstet Gynecol 2011; 204:221.e1–8. [RCT, n = 240]

50. Norman J, Mackenzie F, Owen P. Progesterone for the prevention of preterm birth in twin pregnancy (STOPPIT): a randomized, double-blind, placebo-controlled study and meta analysis. Lancet 2009; 373:2034–2040. [RCT, n = 500]

51. Caritis SN, Rouse DJ, Peaceman AM, et al. for the Eunice Kennedy Shriver National Institute of Child Health and Human Development (NICHD), Maternal-Fetal Medicine Units Network (MFMU). Prevention of preterm birth in triplets using 17 alpha-hydroxyprogesterone caproate: a randomized controlled trial. Obstet Gynecol 2009; 113(2):285–292. [RCT, n = 134]

52. Combs CA, Garite T, Maurel K, et al. for the Obstetrix Collaborative Research Network. Failure of 17-hydroxyprogesterone to reduce neonatal morbidity or prolong triplet pregnancy: a double-blind, randomized clinical trial. Am J Obstet Gynecol 2010; 248.e1–9 [RCT, n = 56]

53. Dor J, Shalev J, Mashiach S, et al. Elective cervical suture of twins pregnancies diagnosed ultrasonically in the first trimester following induced ovulation. Gynecol Obstet Invest 1982; 13(1):55–60. [RCT, n = 50]

54. Berghella V, Odibo AO, To MS, et al. Cerclage for short cervix on ultrasonography: meta-analysis of trials using individual patient-level data. Obstet Gynecol 2005; 106(1):181–189. [Meta-analysis; 4 RCTs, n = 49 twin gestations]

55. Rebarber A, Roman AS, Istwan N, et al. Prophylactic cerclage in the management of triplet gestations. Am J Obstet Gynecol 2005; 193:1193–1196 [Level II-2]

56. Reichmann J. Home uterine activity monitoring; an evidence review of its utility in multiple gestations. J Reprod Med 2009; 54:559–562. [Review]

57. Yamasmit W, Chaithongwongwatthana S, Tolosa JE, et al. Prophylactic oral betamimetics for reducing preterm birth in women with a twin pregnancy. Cochrane Database Syst Rev 3, 2009. [Meta-analysis; 5 RCTs, n = 344]

58. Fuchs I, Tsoi E, Henrich W, et al. Sonographic measurement of cervical length in twin pregnancies in threatened preterm labor. Ultrasound Obstet Gynecol 2004; 23:42–45. [Level II-3]

59. Effect of corticosteroids for fetal maturation on perinatal outcomes. NIH Conses Statement 1994; 12:1–24. [Level III]

60. Bower SJ, Flack NJ, Sepulveda W, et al. Uterine artery blood flow response to correction of amniotic fluid volume. Am J Obstet Gynecol 1995; 173:502–507. [Level II-3]

61. Moise KJ Jr., Dorman K, Lamvu G, et al. A randomized trial of amnioreduction versus septostomy in the treatment of twin-twin transfusion syndrome. Am J Obstet Gynecol 2005; 193(3 pt 1):701–707. [RCT, n = 73]

62. Senat M, Deprest J, Boulvain M, et al. Endoscopic laser surgery versus serial amnioreduction for severe twin-to-twin transfusion syndrome. N Engl J Med 2004; 351(2):136–144. [RCT, n = 142]

63. Roberts D, Neilson JP, Kibly M, et al. Interventions for the treatment of twin-twin transfusion syndrome. Cochrane Database Syst Rev 2008; (1):CD002073. DOI:10.1002/14651858.CD002073.pub2.

64. Taylor MJ, Shalev E, Tanawattanacharoen S, et al. Ultrasound guided umbilical chord occlusion using bipolar diathery for stage III/IV twin-twin transfusion syndrome. Prenat Diagn 2002; 22:70–76. [Level II-3]

65. Tan TY, Sepulveda W. Acardiac twin: a systemic review of minimally invasive treatment modalities. Ultrasound Obstet Gynecol 2003; 22(4):409–419. [Review of II-2 and II-3 studies]

66. Wong AE, Sepulveda W. Acardiac anomaly: current issues in prenatal assessment and treatment. Prenat Diagn 2005; 25:796–806. [Level II-3]

67. Giles W, Bisits A, O'Callaghan S, et al. The Doppler assessment in multiple pregnancy randomized controlled trial of ultrasound biometry versus umbilical artery Doppler ultrasound and biometry in twin pregnancy. Br J Obstet Gynecol 2003; 110(6):593–597. [Level I]

68. Dodd JM, Crowther CA. Elective delivery of women with a twin pregnancy from 37 weeks gestation. Cochrane Database Syst Rev 2010; (1):CD003582. DOI: 10.1002/14651858.CD003582.

69. Rabinovici J, Barkai G, Reichman B, et al. Randomized management of the second twin: vaginal delivery or cesarean section. Am J Obstet Gynecol 1987; 156:52–56. [RCT, n = 60]

70. Smith GC, Pell JP, Dobbie R. Birth order, gestational age, and risk of delivery related perinatal death in twins: a retrospective cohort study. Br Med J 2002; 325(7371):1004. [Level II-2]

71. Hogle KL, Hutton EK, McBrien KA, et al. Cesarean delivery for twins: a systematic review and meta-analysis. Am J Obstet Gynecol 2003; 188:220–227. [Meta-analysis; 4 studies—only 1 RCT, ref. 69—n = 1932]

72. Maudin JG, Newman RB, Mauldin PD. Cost-effective delivery management of the vertex and non-vertex twin gestation. Am J Obstet Gynecol 1998; 179:864–869. [II-2]

73. Vintzileos AM, Ananth CV, Kontopoulos E, et al. Mode of delivery and risk of stillbirth and infant mortality in triplet gestations: United States, 1995 through 1998. Am J Obstet Gynecol 2005; 192:464–469. [Level II-3]

74. Oyelese Y, Ananth CV, Smulian JC, et al. Delayed interval delivery in twin pregnancies in the United States: impact on perinatal mortality and morbidity. Am J Obstet Gynecol 2005; 192:439–444. [Level II-3]

75. Garite TJ, Clark RH, Elliot JP, et al. Twins and triplets: the effect of plurality and growth on neonatal outcome compared with singleton infants. Am J Obstet Gynecol 2004; 191:700–707. [Level II-2]

44

Fetal growth restriction

Shane Reeves and Henry L. Galan

KEY POINTS

- A fetus is defined as growth restricted (fetal growth restriction, FGR) when the estimated fetal weight (EFW) is <10th percentile for gestational age. So both screening and diagnosis of FGR are based on ultrasound biometry, and they rely on accurate dating by an early ultrasound (preferably first trimester).
- FGR may be due to normal genetic (constitutional) reasons in about 70% of the cases, or to pathologic reasons in about 30% of the cases.
- Umbilical artery (UA) Doppler ultrasound is not helpful for screening, but most effective in differentiating between pathologic FGR (abnormal UA Doppler) and a constitutionally small fetus.
- Risk factors associated with FGR are numerous, and include maternal, fetal, and placental factors (Table 44.1).
- Complications of FGR occur in utero and in later life (Table 44.2):
  - Fetus: oligohydramnios, nonreassuring fetal heart testing (NRFHR), and death.
  - Neonate: preterm birth and its consequences [respiratory distress syndrome (RDS), intraventricular hemorrhage (IVH), necrotizing enterocolitis (NEC), sepsis, etc.), hypoglycemia, electrolyte disturbances, hyperviscosity syndrome, NEC, neurodevelopmental delay, and death].
  - Infant and child (as well as later in life): impaired gross motor development, cerebral palsy, lower intelligence quotient, mental retardation, speech/reading disabilities, learning deficits, poor academic achievement, and suicide.
  - Adult: hypertension, coronary artery disease, diabetes, obesity, social and financial problems.
- Effective prevention strategies for FGR include the following:
  - Early (<20 weeks) ultrasound.
  - Identification and treatment of modifiable risk factors (e.g., smoking and other toxic exposures, medical disorders, etc.).
  - A low-dose aspirin reduces the incidence of recurrent FGR by 10%, especially (decrease up to 56%) if >75 mg and started before 16 weeks.
- Workup of FGR should include the following:
  - Review of risk factors (Table 44.1).
  - Fetal anatomy, placenta, amniotic fluid ultrasound.
  - Pulsed-wave Doppler of the UA.
- Workup of FGR may also include the following:
  - Infectious workup, including maternal serum IgG and IgM of cytomegalovirus (CMV), toxoplasmosis, and possibly herpes simplex virus (HSV). Rubella immunity should be ascertained.
  - Amniocentesis to rule out aneuploidy (karyotype) and infection (PCR for CMV, toxoplasmosis, and possibly HSV).
  - Antiphospholipid antibodies may be checked, but there is no intervention, if they are positive, proven to alter outcome.
  - Maternal workup for preeclampsia, or evaluation for any disease possibly associated with FGR, should be done.
- Fetal therapy is limited, since interventions studied have not been shown to be beneficial or have been insufficiently studied. Control or elimination of risk factors (e.g., stop drug abuse or smoking, control maternal disease) should be performed.
- Doppler of the UA is the cornerstone of FGR follow-up and management, since it is associated with a decreased risk of perinatal mortality.
- Steroids should be given if there is anticipated need for delivery of FGR at 24 to 34 weeks within the next two to seven days.
- The timing of delivery should be individualized and based on gestational age and all antepartum tests.
  - Delivering early at <32 weeks for hypothetical avoidance of fetal hypoxia (e.g., in presence of abnormal fetal Doppler studies) has not been associated with improved outcome.
  - Reversed end-diastolic flow (REDF) in the UA Doppler at ≥32 weeks: consider delivery.
  - Absent end-diastolic flow (AEDF) in the UA Doppler at ≥34 weeks: consider delivery.

DEFINITIONS/DIAGNOSES

FGR is diagnosed when the EFW is <10th percentile for gestational age on a standardized population growth curve. So both screening and diagnosis of FGR are based on ultrasound biometry, and they rely on accurate dating by an early ultrasound (preferably first trimester).

Intrauterine growth restriction (IUGR) refers to FGR with a small placenta and oligohydramnios. We will preferentially use the term FGR in this chapter as the diagnosis management mainly involves the fetus.

Small for gestational age (SGA) is a term used for the neonate (1), defined as a birth weight <10th percentile.

The categorization of FGR as <10th percentile has often been criticized secondary to the inclusion of many fetuses that are constitutionally small and not at risk for poor perinatal outcome (2). In fact, 70% of infants with a birth weight <10th percentile are normally grown and not at risk for adverse perinatal outcome, while the remaining 30% truly have pathologic SGA (and, in utero, FGR), and these fetuses (and neonates) are most at risk (3). It is also possible to have a fetus that

Table 44.1 Risk Factors Associated with FGR

Maternal
Hypertension (20–30%)
  Preeclampsia
  Chronic hypertension
  Secondary hypertension
Pregestational Diabetes
Autoimmune disease
Antiphospholipid syndrome
Lupus
Maternal cardiac disease
Congenital heart disease
Heart failure
Pulmonary disorders
  Cystic fibrosis
  COPD
  Uncontrolled asthma
Renal disease
  Chronic renal insufficiency
  Nephrotic syndrome
  Chronic renal failure
Gastrointestinal disease
  Ulcerative colitis
  Chron's disease
  Malabsorptive disorders
  Gastric bypass
Toxic exposure
  Smoking
  Alcohol
  Cocaine
  Stimulants
Malnutrition
Living at high altitudes
Low socioeconomic status
Race
Extremes of maternal age
Fetal
Genetic diseases[a]
Aneuploidy[a]
Fetal malformations (1–2%)
Multiple gestation (3%)
Fetal infection (5–10%)
  CMV
  Toxoplasmosis
  Rubella
  Malaria
  HSV
Placental
Abruption
Placental mosaicism
Placenta accreta
Chorioangioma
Implantation abnormalities with abnormal analytes on serum
  screening

[a]Incidence of genetic diseases or aneuploidy is about 5% to 20%.
Abbreviations: FGR, fetal growth restriction; COPD, chronic obstructive pulmonary disease; CMV, cytomegalovirus; HSV, herpes simplex virus.

Table 44.2 Complications Associated with FGR

Fetal
- **Oligohydramnios**
- **Nonreassuring fetal heart rate testing (NRFHR)**
- **Fetal death**

Neonate
- Iatrogenic or spontaneous **preterm birth**
  - Its consequences (**RDS, IVH, NEC, sepsis**, etc.)
- **Low Apgar score**
- **Hypoglycemia**
- **Electrolyte disturbances, acidosis**
- **Hyperviscosity syndrome**
- **Seizures**
- **Death**

Child
- **Neurodevelopmental and cognitive delay**
- **Cerebral palsy, impaired gross motor development**
- **Lower intelligence quotient**
- **Speech/reading disabilities**
- **Learning deficits**
- **Poor academic achievement**
- **Short stature**

Adult
- **Hypertension**
- **Coronary artery disease**
- **Stroke**
- **Type 2 diabetes mellitus**
- **Obesity**
- **Low socioeconomic status**
- **Suicide**
- **Financial problems**

Mother
- Cesarean delivery

Abbreviations: RDS, respiratory distress syndrome; IVH, intraventricular hemorrhage; NEC, necrotizing enterocolitis.

Low birth weight (LBW) is defined as <2500 g. For SGA or FGR in a multiple gestation, please refer to chapter 43.

EPIDEMIOLOGY/INCIDENCE

By definition, 10% of fetuses will be diagnosed by FGR by population growth charts.

SGA complicates about 4% to 8% of pregnancies in developed countries and up to 25% of pregnancies in undeveloped countries (6). Birth weight <3rd percentile carries the highest risk for perinatal morbidity [UA blood pH < 7.0, grade 3 or 4 IVH, respiratory distress, NEC, and sepsis] and mortality when compared against other cut-offs (7).

Approximately 35% of infants identified as FGR have abnormal UA Doppler evaluation (8). An additional percentage (about 20%) will have only an abnormal middle cerebral artery (MCA) Doppler, but normal UA Doppler flow. These fetuses are also at an increased risk of poor perinatal outcome (9). So >30%, and possibly up to 50%, of FGR cases are at risk for poor perinatal outcome.

GENETICS/INHERITANCE/RECURRENCE

Since there are multiple risk factors associated with IUGR (Table 44.1), the recurrence risk is largely linked to the underlying etiology in the affected pregnancy. When looking at unselected pregnancies affected by LBW, the recurrence risk of another small child is increased (10–14). When the prior neonate was SGA, the risk of SGA in a subsequent singleton

is above the 10th percentile on a population growth curve who is still at risk for poor perinatal outcome secondary to not meeting its individualized growth potential (4). Severe FGR can be defined as that associated with fetal weight <3rd percentile; the majority of these cases are associated with pathologic reasons for FGR.

UA Doppler ultrasound is not helpful for screening, but most effective in differentiating between pathologic FGR (abnormal UA Doppler) and a constitutionally small fetus (5).

pregnancy is about 24%, and it is about 17% if the subsequent pregnancy is a twin gestation (14). Recurrence of FGR in cases associated with aneuploidy is low, but the risk of aneuploidy in subsequent pregnancies is higher than the risk of maternal age alone. In fact, the risk of aneuploidy recurrence is approximately 1% in women who have aneuploidy in the first pregnancy at a maternal age of <30 years (15–17). The majority of FGR fetuses do not have a genetic change that can help predict inheritance and recurrence, but if a genetic syndrome is discovered as the cause, proper counseling regarding recurrence is indicated. When the cause of IUGR is an intrauterine infection from a viral source, the recurrence risk is low, as the patient will have attained immunity prior to her subsequent pregnancies. In summary, the risk of recurrence is situation-dependent, and counseling regarding future risks will need to be based on the individual circumstances for each case.

CLASSIFICATION

FGR has been classified as asymmetric or symmetric. Asymmetric FGR refers to a reduction in abdominal circumference (AC) relative to other measures, such as head circumference (HC). Often, an HC/AC ratio >95th percentile is used as a cutoff. Symmetric IUGR is characterized by a similar reduction in all biometric measurements. Usually, the etiology is present from the beginning of the pregnancy, and it can include aneuploid or euploid genetic diseases, viral infection, drug/toxic exposure, and/or placental causes.

This classification has been traditionally used as a tool to distinguish between etiologies, with asymmetry pointing to a placental cause; however, early onset of placental disease may also lead to symmetric FGR, making the classification less helpful. The classification system has been predictive of outcome as asymmetric FGR has a stronger association with major anomalies, hypertensive disorders of pregnancy, cesarean delivery, lower birth weight, perinatal mortality, earlier gestational age at delivery, and poor postnatal outcome compared to symmetric FGR (18,19). However, the value of the classification system is often criticized since both types are at risk for poor perinatal outcome, and Doppler velocimetry and antenatal monitoring are better predictors of pregnancy outcome in either form of FGR (19). Although the segregation into asymmetric and symmetric FGR may help to stratify risk, **the clinical use of such a classification system has yet to be determined.**

ETIOLOGY/BASIC PATHOPHYSIOLOGY

There are two scenarios that can lead to an FGR baby, and it is very important to distinguish them. The so-called "**constitutional**" FGR fetus is the one with an EFW below the 10th percentile for gestational age, but otherwise healthy. This baby characteristically grows at a constant speed that usually parallels a specific percentile throughout the pregnancy. More importantly, this baby is not prone to develop any fetal or perinatal complications, has a normal postnatal outcome, and does not need therapy. Ultrasound shows normal amniotic fluid and UA Doppler patterns. Some ethnic groups are more likely to show FGR babies if race-adjusted charts are not used.

Some FGR fetuses are **not healthy** because of one or more disorders (Table 44.1) contributing to the FGR weight. While the causes of FGR are diverse, many of them lead to a common pathway: **compromise of the uteroplacental perfusion.** Over time, the supply of nutrients and oxygen mismatch

the fetal requirements that the normal process of growth entails. Then, the normal accretion of tissue decreases, and components of fetal structure and physiology are removed from the tissue to undertake abnormal biochemical paths (proteolysis, gluconeogenesis, and beta-oxidation), which are the results of an adaptive attempt to maintain a supply of energy substrates to support vital functions in an adverse environment, giving up on fetal growth. Placental apoptosis is increased. Such biochemical phenomena translate into sonographically recognizable traits, such as decreased growth. Often altered fetal proportion is evident, since places of normal fat accretion such as abdominal wall will show lack of it, with the resultant small AC at ultrasound. At the same time, in an attempt to maintain blood supply to critical tissues (brain, heart, adrenals), the fetal circulation decreases in some not-so-critical organs such as the splanchnic circulation and fetal kidneys, often generating oligohydramnios. This pattern of redistribution of the fetal blood flow is detected by Doppler analysis showing less diastolic flow (increased impedance) in the UA. At times, increased diastolic flow in the MCA develops as "brain-sparing" changes try to maintain adequate oxygenation and nutrition to the fetal brain circulation. Compared to an adequate for gestational age (AGA) fetus, metabolic changes associated with the FGR fetus are **lower pH, pO_2, glucose, LDH, cholesterol, fatty acids, triglycerides, growth factors (e.g., insulin-like GF), insulin, most aminoacids, and increased pCO_2, lactic acid, and bilirubin.** Finally, the process may be so severe that **heart failure** ensues and the fetus can die in utero.

The causes of FGR can be divided into three basic categories: maternal factors, fetal factors, and placental factors (Table 44.1). While the pathophysiology of each factor is different, maternal factors (e.g., maternal medical disease) and placental factors may have a common final pathway of decreased placental perfusion and transfer of nutrients across the placenta to the fetus. Fetal factors describe scenarios where growth is reduced secondary to genetic, chromosomal, or infectious causes. Details of how each of these contribute to FGR is outlined below.

Maternal Factors

Several maternal characteristics including age, weight, height, race, and parity contribute to fetal growth (20). These factors would largely be considered constitutional determinants of growth, and fetuses that are labeled FGR secondary to normal inheritable maternal characteristics would not be at risk for adverse pregnancy outcome. However, multiple other maternal factors have been associated with pathological growth inhibition. These include factors listed in Table 44.1 (1).

Many maternal medical conditions can lead to FGR, with one of the leading causes being maternal hypertension in pregnancy (chronic hypertension, preeclampsia, and chronic hypertension with superimposed preeclampsia) (21). Auto-immune disorders, chronic renal disease, pregestational diabetes, and chronic lung disease are other maternal factors that have been associated with FGR (22–24).

In addition to maternal medical disorders, substance abuse, malnutrition, and pharmacotherapy have been associated with FGR. **The leading cause of preventable FGR is tobacco consumption,** where approximately 13% of growth restriction can be attributed to this drug (25). Other illicit drug use such as alcohol, cocaine, and narcotics has been associated with FGR (26–29). Not only is substance abuse associated with FGR, but poor nutritional status can inhibit growth. Longitudinal data from women who conceived and gave birth during times of famine suggests an association between FGR and maternal malnutrition (30,31). Additionally, factors generally associated with poor nutritional status such as low maternal weight, poor weight gain, and obesity can all lead to pathological growth of the fetus (32,33). Also, multiple maternal medications have been associated with growth restriction, and a complete list would be out of the scope of this chapter. However, antineoplastic medications, antiepileptic drugs, and repeat courses of glucocorticosteroids that can cross the placenta have all been implicated as agents that increase the risk of FGR (34).

Fetal Factors

Multiple fetal factors affect growth. Between **4%** and **25%** of fetuses with growth restriction will have an **abnormal karyotype** (35,36). Trisomy 18 is particularly at risk for FGR as 35% of these fetuses will measure <10th percentile (37). Other chromosomal anomalies, particularly trisomies, triploidy, translocations, and sex chromosome abnormalities are also at high risk for FGR. Other than chromosomal aberrations, genetic disorders such as uniparental disomy and imprinting disorders are rare causes of FGR (34). Many genetic disorders can lead to major structural malformations, and the findings of these on ultrasound will increase the risk of growth abnormalities to 22% (38). **Fetal infection** has been associated with FGR, but data on the exact incidence of fetal infection in FGR are scant. Known infections that have been associated include cytomegalovirus, varicella, herpes simplex virus, malaria, human immunodeficiency virus, rubella, and syphilis (1). Malaria is the most common cause of FGR worldwide.

Placental Factors

Placental risk factors for FGR include placental abruption, maternal floor infarct, placental mosaicism, velamentous cord insertion, and placenta accreta (1).

COMPLICATIONS

FGR is associated with morbidity and mortality to the fetus and infant (Table 44.2) (18,39–42). In utero, 53% of preterm stillbirths and 26% of term stillbirths are growth restricted. Perinatal death may be increased up to 100 times compared to normally grown babies. Additionally, intrapartum asphyxia has been reported to complicate 50% of pregnancies with FGR (43). In addition to stillbirth, FGR increases the risk of preterm birth, NEC, and RDS (44,45). Preterm infants with birth weight <3rd percentile carry the highest perinatal morbidity and mortality risk. When matched for gestational age at both term and preterm gestations, the smallest infants are at the highest risk for low Apgar score, acidosis, intubation, seizures, and death in the first 28 days of life (7).

FGR goes beyond the neonatal period, where children who were born with growth restriction have a higher risk of cerebral palsy, short stature, and cognitive delay (46).

In later life, adults who had FGR have a higher incidence of hypertension, coronary artery disease, stroke, type 2 diabetes mellitus, and obesity (47). Other than medical diseases, there is an increased risk of low socioeconomic status, suicide, and financial distress in later life (39). Clearly, the implications of IUGR are grand, and rather than having complications limited to the peripartum period, the effects of IUGR may be lifelong.

The primary risk to the mother is cesarean section with a reported cesarean section rate of 43% if induction is performed in fetuses that have an EFW <5th percentile (48).

MANAGEMENT
Prevention
Gestational Age Determination
Since gestational age is the primary component dictating if a fetus is measuring FGR, **accurate determination of an estimated date of confinement (EDC) is paramount. First-trimester ultrasound between 7 and 11 weeks** is the most precise method to determine the EDC, where a crown-rump length (CRL) will be within two to three days of the true gestational age when using in vitro fertilization as the standard (49). A first-trimester (up to 13 6/7 weeks) CRL two to six days less than expected is associated with an increased risk for LBW (50). Uncommonly, first-trimester FGR can be diagnosed, and this is also associated with complications (51). Beyond 11 weeks, the CRL can be used up to 14 weeks with an accuracy of up to five days (49). Second-trimester ultrasound between 16 and 20 weeks also has accuracy in determining the true gestational age, but the error rate is up to 10 days (52) (see also chap. 4, *Obstetric Evidence Based Guidelines*). After about 14 weeks, biometric measurements such as biparietal diameter, head circumference, AC, and femur length are used for estimation of fetal weight. AC is the single sonographic measurement most predictive of fetal growth. Using ultrasound to establish an accurate EDC prior to 20 weeks will help in identifying fetuses that are truly FGR and at risk for poor perinatal outcome. Early dating ultrasound probably decreases both false-positive and false-negative cases of FGR.

Pregnancy Interval
A short interpregnancy interval has been associated with FGR. If conception occurs less than six months from a delivery, there is a 30% increase in FGR (53,54). The **optimal timing to decrease rates of FGR is an interpregnancy interval of 18 to 23 months** (54).

Substance Cessation
Cessation of maternal substance abuse should be strongly encouraged. Women who quit smoking prior to 16 weeks will have the risk of FGR similar to women who never smoked at all (55). **Smoking cessation interventions reduce LBW** (RR 0.83, 95% CI 0.73–0.95) and preterm birth (RR 0.86, 95% CI 0.74–0.98) (56). Cessation of other substances in pregnancy or prior to conception also help to reduce the risk of pathological FGR.

Nutrition
In low-risk women, significant dietary management does not prevent FGR. In this population, ineffective methods include individualized nutritional advice (57); increased fish, low-fat meats, grains, fruits, and vegetables (58); low-salt diet (59); iron supplementation (60); and calcium supplementation (61). Dietary supplements that may be beneficial include magnesium (62) and vitamin D (63), but the evidence is still limited, and they cannot be recommended for clinical use.

In high-risk women with nutritional deficiencies, increasing caloric intake with low-protein supplementation reduces the risk of FGR by 32% (64). High protein supplementation may lead to higher rates of FGR and should be avoided (64).

Control of Maternal Medical Disorders
Modification of maternal risk factors for FGR can be performed as a primary preventative factor. Hypertension has been associated with an increased risk of FGR, but placing women on antihypertensive medication when the blood pressure is between 140–169/90–109 will not improve the rate of

preeclampsia, FGR, preterm birth, or stillbirth (65). However, it does decrease the rates of severe hypertension. Controlling diabetes, autoimmune disorders, and other medical illnesses is important for both maternal and fetal health.

Aspirin

Aspirin therapy has been shown to be effective for reducing the risk of FGR in women determined to be at moderate to high risk for this disorder (e.g., those with hypertensive disorders or prior FGR). The benefit of aspirin seems to be largest in early gestational ages. Low-dose (e.g., 81 mg) aspirin is associated with a 56% decrease (RR 0.44, 95% CI 0.30–0.65) in FGR when initiated prior to 16 weeks, and it has no effect (RR 0.98, 95% CI 0.87–1.10) when initiated after this gestational age (66). A dose of >75 mg is associated with the largest benefit (67). Aspirin prophylaxis reduced the recurrence of FGR in subsequent pregnancies in mothers who have had a prior FGR pregnancy (66).

Screening for FGR

Serum Analytes

Abnormalities of trophoblastic invasion have also been suggested by many to be involved in abnormal fetal growth, and clues to aberrant placental cellular processes may be elucidated through investigating maternal serum screening for aneuploidy.

First-trimester analytes have been shown to be associated with abnormal fetal growth and abnormal pregnancy outcomes as **low PAPP-A** levels significantly increase the risk of FGR (68–76). Despite the association, if the PAPP-A level is below the fifth percentile, the sensitivity of detecting birth weight <10th percentile is only 10.4%, and the positive predictive value is only 18.7%. The negative predictive value is at 91.3% (73).

With second-trimester quadruple marker screening, factors associated with FGR are an **AFP > 2.0 multiple of the medians (MoMs), uE3 < 0.5 MoMs, and an inhibin A > 2.0 MoMs** (77). The risk of birth weight <10th percentile increases as the number of abnormal markers increases (78). However, like PAPP-A, the sensitivity and positive predictive value of combining second-trimester markers to screen for FGR is low, questioning its clinical use as a screening test.

Fundal Height

The evidence that fundal height can be used as an effective screening tool for FGR is mixed, with some studies showing it is a good predictor (79–82) and others failing to find benefit (83–87). Maternal central adiposity and leiomyomata uteri will be factors that significantly affect the use of fundal height as a screening tool. However, fundal height measurement is an inexpensive tool (see also chap. 2, *Obstetric Evidence Based Guidelines*). When the risk of FGR is high, **ultrasound should be the primary modality used to screen for fetal growth abnormalities.**

The Growth Curve

The identification of a population at risk for poor perinatal outcome depends largely upon the screening tool used. The tool most often used to determine if a fetus has FGR is the growth curve. Standardized population growth curves can be created in a multitude of ways. Ideally, the optimal growth standard will be able to identify fetuses that are at the highest risk for adverse neonatal and fetal outcome. Data exist showing that race and regional differences affect mean birth weight (88–91). In fact, individual regional differences in birth weight parallel

the nadir of newborn mortality in those regions. In other words, one region in Europe will have a modal birth weight of 3446 g with the lowest perinatal mortality occurring at 3888 g. Another region will have a modal birth weight of 3622 g, with a perinatal mortality nadir at 4305 g (92). This suggests that an "ideal birth weight" exists, and this weight is dependent upon unique population characteristics. **Creating a growth standard that is population specific will better identify fetuses that fall out of the range of "normal" for that population.**

A birth weight standard is created using cross-sectional data of newborn birth weight per gestational age strata. This has been criticized secondary to the known association between FGR and preterm gestations (93). Fetal weight can be determined using linear regression of measurable parameters, and this mathematical modeling has been used to generate multiple in utero fetal weight standards (94–97). Studies indicate that using birth weight data, rather than EFW data, to generate fetal growth standards, will underestimate the amount of FGR fetuses and overestimate the number of large for gestational age (LGA) fetuses (98–100). Additionally, fetal weight standards have been shown to better predict perinatal outcomes of preterm delivery, RDS, bronchopulmonary dysplasia, IVH, and retinopathy of prematurity (44,101). However, a birth weight derived growth curve is more predictive of neonatal mortality (101). The difference in predictive ability for each standard probably lies in the fact that the fetuses identified as SGA by a birth weight standard are the smallest neonates using either schema, and these would be the ones at highest risk for demise and adverse perinatal outcome. However, a growth curve created from birth weight alone will miss a significant portion of infants at risk for poor outcome, and **evidence supports using a standardized growth curve generated from EFW by ultrasound.**

The creation of a **customized growth curve** using factors that are known to affect birth weight including **maternal height, weight in early pregnancy, parity, and ethnic group** has been proposed (4). Using coefficients of variation, and a log polynomial equation, a growth curve is generated for each individual pregnancy, and deviation from this curve identifies fetuses with abnormal growth. When comparing this growth standard to ones created using birth weight data, **the customized growth model is better able to predict poor perinatal outcome** including stillbirth, neonatal death, Apgar score of less than four at five minutes, cesarean section, admission to the neonatal intensive care unit, and neurologic morbidity (102–105).

The effect of the use of these personal customized growth charts, with the diagnosis of FGR based on a change in an already established preexisting growth pattern, has not been assessed in any trial. Race/gender-specific nomograms of weight for gestational age make the diagnosis of FGR more accurate, but there are no trials to show change in outcome. The Royal College of Obstetricians and Gynecologists have adopted the customized standard to identify fetuses at risk for poor perinatal outcome (106). However, **comparing an in utero standard to the customized growth model showed that they were similar in their ability to predict stillbirth and neonatal death**, and both were better at predicting these outcomes than a birth weight standard (107). **Evidence supports the use of either the customized growth model or an in utero EFW standard by ultrasound** to identify fetuses at risk for poor perinatal outcome secondary to FGR.

Uterine Artery Doppler

Uterine artery Doppler interrogation has been used to stratify the risk of subsequent growth abnormalities in pregnancies at high and low risk for the development of FGR. Measurement of the uterine artery blood flow is determined through interrogation of uterine vessels bilaterally at the bifurcation from the internal iliac artery. The presence of a protodiastolic notch or an abnormal index of resistance [systolic/diastolic (S/D) ratio, pulsatility index (PI), or resistive index (RI)] has been used to predict the onset of IUGR.

Abnormal first-trimester uterine artery Doppler waveforms have shown a correlation with aberrant growth. In the first trimester, notching is seen in the majority of all patients with 55% to 63% having bilateral notching, and an additional 18% with unilateral notching (108–110). Therefore, this characteristic pattern is not as helpful. When using an abnormal PI in the first trimester, the sensitivity for IUGR is only 12% (108), while the sensitivity for severe FGR requiring delivery at <34 weeks is only 24% (108,109). Despite its poor performance as a screening tool in the first trimester, using the information to initiate preventative measures may be beneficial. In women with abnormal uterine artery Doppler evaluation, giving low-dose aspirin prior to 16 weeks significantly reduced the incidence of FGR. Similar to data without using uterine artery Doppler, the benefit was not seen after this gestational age (66). This is obviously not clinically effective if one offers low-dose aspirin to women based on risk factors such as hypertension, prior preeclampsia, prior FRG, as discussed above.

Screening at a later gestational age improves the test characteristics. When comparing first- and second-trimester results, uterine artery Doppler notching or elevated PI was more predictive of FGR in the second trimester (111). Timing in the second trimester is also important, as investigators have shown that the test characteristics are better at 22 week than at 18 weeks (112). When the uterine artery Doppler PI is >1.55 between 22 and 24 weeks, 47% of these pregnancies will develop preeclampsia, FGR, or fetal death (113). When using Doppler as a screening tool in a population with abnormal serum analytes (AFP > 3.5 MoMs, or HCG > 5.3 MoMs), the sensitivity increases to 94% with a positive predictive value of 67% (114). However, it is rare for patients to have these abnormal AFP or HCG values, and the use of combining serum markers and uterine artery Doppler has been less predictive in other studies (115,116). There certainly is a relationship between abnormal uterine artery Doppler blood flow and FGR. **The test performs best at gestational ages between 22 and 24 weeks in populations determined to be at high risk for preeclampsia and FGR.** However, **the sensitivity, negative predictive value, and positive predictive value for predicting FGR may be too low to be clinically useful.**

Additionally, **no therapeutic measure has been shown to be useful at this gestational age**. An argument can be made to initiate low-dose aspirin therapy prior to 16 weeks in all women at high risk for the development of preeclampsia and FGR. Use of uterine artery Doppler to determine the optimal management of surveillance of growth has yet to be determined.

UA Doppler
UA Doppler is predictive of FGR in the second trimester, where abnormal values in a high-risk population will increase the development of FGR later in pregnancy (5). Nonetheless, UA Doppler cannot be used for screening for FGR due to its poor sensitivity and positive predictive value.

Diagnosis
When using ultrasound as a screening tool, **the diagnosis of FGR is made when the EFW is <10% for gestational age** (see section "Definitions/Diagnoses").

Workup
For all fetuses presenting as FGR, **the first step is to confirm the gestational age and ensure that the fetus is truly measuring small**. As knowing the appropriate gestational age is key in making the diagnosis, it is particularly difficult when a patient presents for her first ultrasound later in pregnancy and is found to have a fetus measuring small for the proposed gestational age. In these instances, the cerebellar diameter can be used to assist in stratifying risk. In both FGR and LGA fetuses, the cerebellar diameter is largely conserved, and this can help identify a fetus that is measuring small when gestational age is uncertain (117). For biometry, particular attention should be paid to AC, and to the HC/AC ratio. Asymmetric growth with a lagging AC (<5th percentile) should increase the suspicion for early growth abnormalities, as this is often the first clue to pathological growth inhibition (118).

Identification of risk factors, especially modifiable risk factors, can be obtained by review of the medical history (Table 44.1). Maternal blood pressure can be obtained, and if abnormal, exclusion of preeclampsia is warranted. Any substance abuse should be discussed, and cessation of these substances should be encouraged. The identification of maternal diseases that increase the risk for FGR is helpful since optimal management of those disorders may improve growth in the fetus for the remainder of the pregnancy.

Detailed ultrasound evaluation should be performed by a center skilled in such assessments with special attention paid to identify fetal anomalies. Additionally, evaluation of the fetus for evidence of chromosomal abnormalities and intrauterine infection should be performed. The placenta, placental umbilical cord insertion, amniotic fluid, and biometry should be scrutinized. **UA Doppler evaluation should be performed**. Depending on these results, Doppler assessment of other vessels including the MCA, ductus venosus (DV), and umbilical vein may be considered, but there is not enough information to justify routine use of these Doppler studies. A fetal echocardiogram should be considered if inadequate heart views (four chamber and outflow tracts) are obtained (119).

Amniocentesis should be offered to rule out aneuploidy (karyotype) and infection (PCR for CMV, toxoplasmosis, and HSV), especially if no other causes are identifiable and the **FGR is severe (e.g., EFW <5%), diagnosed at early gestational age such as <24 weeks, and/or associated with fetal anomalies or hydramnios**. If the placental image on ultrasound is abnormal, placental biopsy (late CVS) may be considered to evaluate for placental mosaicism, which is present in up to 15% of placentas in cases of FGR (120).

An **infectious workup** including maternal serum IgG and IgM for CMV, toxoplasmosis, and HSV may be offered. Rubella immunity should be ascertained by checking IgG from earlier prenatal care or new testing if this is unavailable. If amniotic fluid is available, PCR for CMV, toxoplasmosis, and HSV can be performed. History should dictate any other further infectious workup for agents associated with FGR.

There is insufficient evidence to recommend a thrombophilia workup, because an association between inherited thrombophilia is not proven in the better studies, and there is no intervention proven to be beneficial (121) (see chap. 27) Antiphospholipid antibodies (anticardiolipin IgG and IgM, lupus anticoagulant, and beta-2 microprotein IgM and IgG) may be checked, especially for counseling regarding etiology and a future pregnancy.

Counseling

Prognosis, complications, options regarding pregnancy termination, thresholds for delivery, when antenatal corticosteroids would be administered in anticipation of preterm birth, and the planned frequency and type of antenatal surveillance should be discussed with the patient with FGR and her family members as available. Recommendations resulting from these discussions should be documented in the patient's chart (119). Prognosis depends largely upon the underlying etiology. **Aneuploidy, fetal malformations, and intrauterine infection are associated with a worse prognosis**. In instances where these factors are absent, gestational age at delivery, amniotic fluid volume, absent/reversed end-diastolic flow of the UA, and birth weight are independent predictors of adverse neonatal outcome (40). More specifically, **gestational age is one of the best predictors of outcome**, where prior to 29 weeks and 2 days, it is the leading predictor of intact survival. Beyond this age, birth weight above 600 g, DV Doppler, and cord artery pH were the strongest predictors of intact survival and neonatal mortality in one study (122).

Complications of FGR include preterm delivery, and in the newborn that was born small, the risk of the diseases of prematurity are higher than in age-matched controls (123). Additionally, birth weight has been linked to fetal and newborn mortality and multiple neonatal morbidities (7). Counseling should include a detailed discussion regarding weighing the **risks of prematurity secondary to an iatrogenic delivery against the risks of stillbirth while remaining in utero**. Multiple tools are available to help distinguish when the risk of remaining in utero is higher than the risk of delivery, or vice versa, and these are discussed below.

Interventions for FGR Pregnancies

Avoidance of Toxins

Discontinuation of toxins known to be associated with FGR should be stressed. When the toxins are the result of substance abuse, such as in smoking, strong counseling should be performed to **encourage cessation of the substance** associated with FGR (Table 44.1). If the toxin is a pharmacotherapy, weighing the potential risks of cessation of the medication with continued exposure to the fetus should be performed. Discussion of alternative therapies should be considered. However, once the fetus is identified as FGR, data is lacking on whether cessation of the offending agent will improve growth during the remainder of pregnancy, but biological plausibility exists, and cessation should still be encouraged.

Therapy for Medical Conditions

Proper treatment of chronic hypertension, preeclampsia, diabetes, or other medical condition is important, but there are no trials to prove a beneficial effect on IUGR.

Bed Rest

Bed rest has long been used by obstetricians as a tool for improving pregnancy outcome, even though data is lacking to support its use. One nonrandomized study looking at women hospitalized for preterm labor showed that bed rest decreased the rate of developing FGR (RR 0.38, 95% CI 18–84) (124). Alternatively, another nonrandomized study reported a higher incidence of SGA in patients prescribed bed rest (125). The only one RCT showed **no difference** in fetal growth parameters (RR 0.43, 95% CI 0.15–1.27) and neonatal outcomes when bed rest was compared to ambulation in patients with FGR (126). Currently, there is insufficient evidence to support the use of bed rest to treat patients with FGR. Hospitalization for bed rest is **possibly dangerous** (associated with venous thromboembolism, etc.), expensive, and inconvenient for the pregnant woman.

Nutrient Therapy

Improving nutrient delivery to the fetus by increasing maternal intake of these nutrients has been widely studied. **Some nutrient supplementation may be beneficial in preventing FGR, while others are not**. Docosahexenoic acid has been shown in a large RCT to result in larger birth weights if patients continue with the supplementation in pregnancy (127). Maternal micronutrient therapy with the UNICEF/ WHO/UNO international multiple micronutrient preparation has been shown to increase birth weight in regions where nutritional supplementation is rare (128). Long-chain polyunsaturated fatty acid supplementation has not been shown to improve birth weight (129). Although supplementation may improve birth weight prior to the development of FGR, **once there is FGR, there is insufficient evidence that supplementing the mother** with amino acids, minerals, vitamins, glucose, or energy supplements improves birth weight (130).

Betamimetics

The theoretical basis for using betamimetic therapy for impaired fetal growth is promoting fetal growth by increasing the availability of nutrients and by decreasing vascular resistance. In fetuses diagnosed with FGR, the administration of betamimetics is not associated with improvement in birth weight or neonatal morbidity and mortality (131). Betamimetics are associated with several complications, and therefore **should not be used for this indication**.

Calcium Channel Blockers

There is currently **insufficient evidence** to promote the use of calcium channel blockers for FGR. Calcium channel blockers may theoretically increase uteroplacental perfusion, and, therefore, improve nutrient and oxygen delivery to a fetus that is at risk or currently growth restricted. Only one study has been published which randomized 100 smoking women to either flunarizine or placebo. The treatment group had a higher mean birth weight, but no other significant differences were seen (132).

Aspirin

In high-risk populations, **such as in women with a first-trimester uterine artery Doppler PI that is abnormal, low-dose aspirin has been shown to decrease the incidence of FGR when initiated prior to 16 weeks** (66,67). After this gestational age, and once FGR is established, aspirin has no proven benefit.

Oxygen

There is **insufficient evidence** to evaluate the benefits and risks of maternal oxygen therapy for suspected impaired fetal growth. A Cochrane analysis showed that oxygen administration to pregnancies with suspected FGR **decreased the rates of perinatal mortality (33% vs. 65%; a 50% reduction) compared to no oxygenation** (133). In all studies birth weights were higher in the oxygen group, despite similar (average range: 10–20 days) intervals to delivery. No significant side-effects or adverse outcomes have been reported. Higher gestational age in the oxygenation groups may have accounted for the difference in mortality rates. Also, two of the studies did not use placebos, there was no blinding, and the small number of patients does not allow a thorough assessment of effect (133).

Plasma Volume Expansion

There is **insufficient evidence** to assess the effect of increase in maternal fluid intake (either IV or orally) on FGR. In pregnancies complicated by FGR, maternal volume expansion is lower than in pregnancies with normally grown fetuses (134). Expanding maternal plasma volume once FGR has been identified was evaluated in only one very small trial in patients with absent end-diastolic flow (AEDF) of the UA. Compared to no volume expansion, volume expansion in women with FGR fetuses with AEDF of UA was associated with a decrease (2/7 vs. 6/7) in perinatal mortality. There was no difference in the gestational age at delivery and mean birth weight (135).

Abdominal Decompression

There is **insufficient evidence** to assess the effect of this intervention, as all trials are old, and they contain serious bias. Abdominal decompression consists of a rigid dome placed about the abdomen and covered with an airtight suit, with the space around the abdomen decompressed to −50 to −100 mmHg for 15 to 30 seconds out of each minute for 30 minutes once to thrice daily, or with uterine contractions during labor. This is thought to "pump" blood through the intervillous space. Therapeutic abdominal decompression is associated with reductions in persistent preeclampsia; "fetal distress" in labor; low birth weight; Apgar scores less than six at one minute; and perinatal mortality (7% vs. 40%) (136).

Nitric Oxide Donors

There is **insufficient evidence** to recommend the use of nitric oxide donors to fetuses with FGR. L-Arginine is a precursor to nitric oxide, and may play a role in placental blood flow. In one randomized study evaluating pregnancies with FGR, administration of this compound did not increase mean birth weight or duration of pregnancy (137). Alternatively, two other nonrandomized studies showed improvement in fetal growth when L-arginine was given, either orally or intravenously, to pregnancies with suspected FGR (138,139).

ANTEPARTUM TESTING

See also chapter 55, "Antepartum Testing."

Ultrasound

Intervals of Growth Assessment

Repeated in utero growth assessments through ultrasound have been used to monitor pregnancies complicated by FGR. Most growth curves are derived from cross-sectional data on large populations, and this gives the appearance of a continuous, smooth pattern of fetal growth. In truth, fetuses do not demonstrate growth in this fashion. Data on child growth through 22 months of age shows that infants will have long periods of stasis punctuated by short bursts of growth (140). Fetuses show a similar **saltatory pattern of growth**, where EFW and anthropometric measures will show no demonstrable change over multiple intervals of assessment. In fact, when assessing growth every two to three days in normal fetuses, measures of femur length, AC, and biparietal diameter will show no growth for periods greater than two weeks, and all measures will have some growth by four weeks (141). **Absence of growth in two weeks is therefore a normal phenomenon**. Additionally, mathematical modeling has shown that due to the error inherent to ultrasound, the false-positive rate of diagnosing FGR when assessing a fetus at two-week intervals is significantly higher than at three-week intervals. The error

rate is also gestational age dependent. As gestational age advances, when assessing every 2 weeks, the false-positive rate increases from 12% at 28 weeks to 24% at 38 weeks (142). The optimal timing for repeat assessment of fetal growth has yet to be determined, but based on available data, **repeat assessment should be performed no earlier than every three weeks, and only rarely every two weeks**.

Doppler

Ultrasound evaluation of fetal blood vessels using pulsed-wave **Doppler velocimetry is the cornerstone of management and follow-up of FGR**. The UA Doppler flow patterns are predictive of fetal outcome. UA end-diastolic velocity can decrease, and can progress to first absent (AEDF) and then reversed end-diastolic flow (REDF) as placental resistance increases (143). Fetuses with absent or reversed end-diastolic flow (AREDF) of the UA have higher incidences of preterm delivery, stillbirth, neonatal mortality, low arterial pH, bronchopulmonary dysplasia, NEC, and severe neurologic morbidity (144,145). Thus, UA Doppler surveillance in a fetus that has FGR will help to identify the fetus that has FGR and is at risk, rather than one which is constitutionally small. In women with normal Dopplers and AF volume, twice weekly nonstress tests (NSTs) are associated with higher incidence of labor induction at an earlier gestational age with no difference in infant morbidity or composite perinatal outcome compared to UA Doppler fortnightly in a small RCT (146). **Doppler (mostly UA) assessment of pregnancies at high risk for placental insufficiency (such as those with FGR) reduces the incidences of perinatal deaths** (1.2% vs. 1.7%, a 29% decrease), **inductions of labor** (11% decrease), **and cesarean sections** (10% decrease) compared to no Doppler or other mode of testing (e.g., CTG and/or biophysical profile, BPP) (147).

During instances of placental dysfunction, blood flow resistance in the fetal brain is decreased. **MCA** Doppler evaluation has been used as an adjunct to UA blood-flow assessment, where fetuses that show evidence of decreased resistance to flow in the brain are at higher risk of poor perinatal outcome. In fact, prior to 34 weeks, the prediction of poor perinatal outcome is improved over UA Doppler assessment alone when the MCA PI is decreased (148,149). This will help to further identify fetuses at risk and separate them from fetuses that are constitutionally small. Unfortunately, unlike the UA Doppler, there is insufficient evidence (no RCT) to assess the effect of using MCA Doppler in FGR.

Doppler assessment of the **fetal venous system** can also help to identify fetuses at risk for poor perinatal outcome. In FGR, when the NST is nonreactive, absent a-wave flow in the DV has better predictive ability for acidemia and significant neonatal morbidity than a contraction stress test (150). In the presence of AREDF of the UA, pulsations of the umbilical vein or absent/reversed flow of the a-wave of the DV increase the risk of acidemia, IVH, neonatal death, and perinatal death (151–153). There is **insufficient evidence (no RCT) to assess the effect of using venous Doppler in FGR**, but results from a RCT will soon be available.

In summary, **UA Doppler assessment is beneficial in managing pregnancies that have FGR** (147). Most data suggest, **once FGR is diagnosed, weekly UA Doppler surveillance**. However, the exact UA Doppler flow pattern that should initiate timing of delivery has yet to be fully elucidated in the literature (Fig. 44.1). MCA Doppler can be used as an adjunct to identify fetuses at risk for poor outcome, but the optimal timing of delivery when MCA PI is abnormal has yet to be determined. When venous Doppler is assessed,

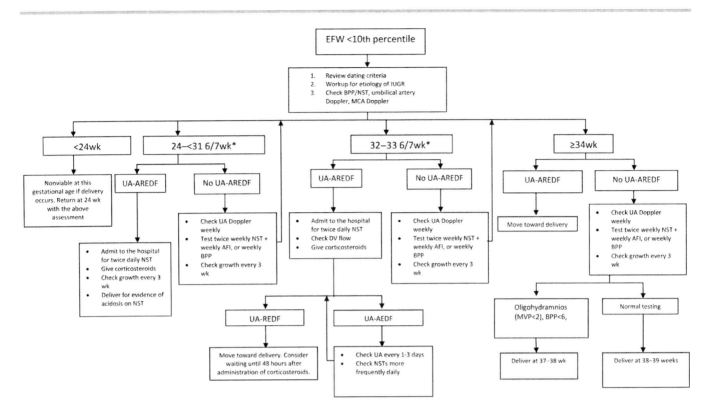

Figure 44.1 Algorithm for the management of the IUGR fetus. *Indicates at >24 weeks, deliver for category III NST/CTG. *Abbreviations*: wk, weeks; EFW, estimated fetal weight; BPP, biophysical profile; NST, nonstress test; MCA, middle cerebral artery Doppler; UA, umbilical artery; AREDF, absent or reversed end diastolic flow; REDF, reversed end diastolic flow; AEDF, absent end diastolic flow; DV, ductus venosus; MVP, maximum vertical pocket (of amniotic fluid).

abnormalities in flow can identify fetuses with the worst outcomes. Further research is needed to evaluate the optimal timing of delivery with the above abnormalities in fetal blood flow.

Fetal Kick Counts

There is insufficient evidence (no trials) to assess the effect of fetal kick counts specifically for FGR fetuses.

NST/Cardiotocography

Monitoring of the fetal heart rate is commonly referred to as NST, or as cardiotocography (CTG). CTG has not been well-evaluated with high-quality studies in FGR. When comparing CTG with no CTG, there is no difference in the prediction of perinatal mortality, preventable deaths, or cesarean sections (154). Computerized CTG may improve perinatal mortality when compared to traditional CTG (154). However, this analysis was not limited to FGR fetuses, and the benefit of antenatal CTG has yet to be fully investigated in this population. In many management schemas, CTG has been cited as a standard monitoring tool, despite the lack of rigorous studies proving its efficacy (1). Nonreactive and abnormal CTG has been associated with acidosis and hypoxemia, (155,156) and this justifies its use as a screening tool for fetal well-being.

Biophysical Profile

Evidence from RCTs does not support the use of BPP as a test of fetal well-being in high-risk pregnancies (157). In high-

risk pregnancies (including FGR, post-term pregnancies, hypertensive disorders, or other conditions), when comparing a BPP to other tests of fetal well-being, there is no difference in perinatal deaths or low Apgar scores (157). Although the overall incidence of adverse outcomes was low, there is no significant differences between the groups in perinatal deaths (RR 1.33, 95% CI 0.60–2.98) or in Apgar score <7 at five minutes (RR 1.27, 95% CI 0.85–1.92). Combined data from the two high-quality RCTs suggest an increased risk of cesarean section in the BPP group (RR 1.60, 95% CI 1.05 to 2.44) (157). The impact of the BPP on other interventions, length of hospitalization, serious short-term and long-term neonatal morbidity and parental satisfaction requires further evaluation. In FGR alone, **RCTs are lacking to prove the value of the BPP**, but it is still mentioned as a surveillance tool in these pregnancies (1). This is justified in that fetal death within one week of a normal score on BPP testing is rare, estimated at about <0.1% in one study (158).

Estriol Levels

Compared to concealed levels, knowledge of plasma estriol levels does not affect perinatal mortality (3% in each group) in women with FGR, hypertension, or adverse obstetric history (159).

Interval of Fetal Testing

Testing should start usually on the diagnosis of FGR. On the basis of the evidence above, **UA Doppler evaluation is** recommended, usually initially on a weekly basis, with the option of increased Doppler frequency in the presence of abnormal UA Doppler flow.

The other testing modalities and their testing interval are not supported by level 1 evidence. Some experts suggest monitoring with NSTs twice a week with once weekly amniotic fluid assessment, or BPPs weekly in pregnancies with FGR and normal UA Doppler. In the presence of abnormal UA Doppler, more frequent testing with NST/AFV and/or BPP can be considered. The NST will not show reactivity usually before 32 weeks, so a category III tracing may be used as criteria for delivery. The data on BPP screening are mostly from term pregnancies, with very little data on the effectiveness of BPP monitoring on very preterm (e.g. <28 weeks) FGR.

Sequence of Deteriorization

During antepartum surveillance of a fetus with FGR, resistance to blood flow in the UA starts to increase prior to abnormalities in BPP testing (160). MCA resistance will decrease, and this can occur either before or after changes are seen in the UA Doppler flow. As a later finding, blood flow through the UA either becomes absent or reversed. DV a-wave flow then becomes absent or reversed, and this can occur prior to abnormalities on a BPP are observed (160,161). Not all fetuses follow this characteristic pattern, but abnormalities in Doppler imaging usually precede findings indicative of acidosis on CTG or BPP testing, and the use of these measures can help in timing of delivery.

DELIVERY
Preparation: Antenatal Steroids for Fetal Maturity
When fetal testing in the FGR fetus suggests need for delivery at 24 to 34 weeks in the next two to seven days, steroids for fetal maturity should be administered to the mother (162). Either betamethasone or dexamethasone can be used. Betamethasone 12 mg IM q24h × 2 doses (one course) is associated with decrease in RDS, IVH, NEC, and perinatal mortality (162). A single "rescue" course can be considered >14days from the first course, if pregnancy is still <30 to 32 weeks (163,164). Steroids can temporarily affect NST, BPP, and Doppler testing (see also chap. 16, *Obstetric Evidence Based Guidelines*). The evidence for safety and effectiveness of steroids specifically in FGR pregnancies is limited (165).

Timing
The timing of delivery of the FRG fetus should be based mostly on gestational age and all antepartum testing factors, and in general not just one test. A possible management algorithm is shown in Figure 44.1. Given the current state of the literature, and absence of strong data that specifically delineates the optimal timing of delivery, this proposed strategy for managing pregnancies complicated by FGR is subject to change as new evidence accumulates. Retrospectively, the largest predictors of perinatal outcome are gestational age at delivery, birth weight, AREDF of the UA, abnormal DV blood flow, nonreassuring CTG or BPP, and placental villitis (166,167).

Delivery timing has been investigated in one large trial, where 548 patients with FGR (>90% singletons, >70% with abnormal UA Doppler) at 24 to 36 weeks were randomized to

delivery after 48 hours of steroid administration versus expectant management (168,169). In the group randomized to expectant management, delivery criteria and surveillance strategies were not based on a protocol or described in detail. Patients moved toward delivery when the clinicians managing the pregnancy felt that pregnancy prolongation was no longer safe.

Immediate delivery after 48 hours of steroids was associated with similar incidence of perinatal death (10%) compared to delayed delivery (9%) (delayed delivery was an average of only four days later). Incidence of fetal (0.7% vs. 3.1%) and neonatal (7.7% vs. 4.1%) deaths, as well as death and disability at two years of age (19% vs. 16%) were similar in the two groups (168,169). Trends for ventilation >24 hours, IVH and NEC tended to favor delayed delivery. Disability in babies younger than 31 weeks was higher in those delivered immediately (13%) compared to those in the delayed group (5%) (169). At age 6 to 13 years, there was not a clinically significant difference between groups in standardized school-based evaluations of cognition, language, motor performance, and behavior (170). This trial has been criticized for several reasons, including the following: (*i*) there was no clearly defined surveillance strategy or explicit delivery indications described in the expectantly managed group; (*ii*) the expectant management group only gained an average of four days, which may explain the lack in differences shown; and (*iii*) the immediate delivery group average time to delivery was 0.9 days (range of 0.4–1.3 days), and thus, fetuses did not likely benefit from steroid administration. However, the trial provides benefit in showing that early delivery does not necessarily prevent neurodevelopmental damage from fetal metabolic deterioration inherent to FGR.

As no specific protocol based on fetal testing (either Doppler, CTG, or other) was followed, specific recommendations cannot be made from this important RCT, except that delivering early for hypothetical avoidance of fetal hypoxia might not improve outcome, with the authors recommending that the "obstetrician should delay." The following recommendations are based mostly on nontrial evidence.

At <24 weeks, FGR is associated with poor outcome, and counseling regarding termination can be offered in some states. Transfer to tertiary care center is recommended if pregnancy is continued. Delivery of a severe FGR fetus at <25 weeks is associated with a dismal prognosis (167), and delivery for nonreassuring testing at this gestational age is unlikely to improve survival.

At any gestational age, in particular after 23 to 24 weeks, NRFHR consistent with category III patterns (e.g., recurrent late decelerations or bradycardia with absent variability) on monitoring should prompt decision for delivery. Absent/minimal (<5 beats) variability from 32 weeks on in the presence of FGR should also be an indication for considering delivery. If BPP testing is employed, a BPP <6 is an indication for delivery. If the managing physician is not willing to deliver the fetus for a BPP of 4 or less (e.g. in cases of FGR <28 weeks), a BPP should not be performed.

At 24 to 31 6/7 weeks, FHR may not show accelerations or more than minimal variability even in normal fetuses, but delivery is always indicated for recurrent late decelerations or bradycardia on monitoring. It is unclear when in the progression of pathologic changes is delivery best indicated at this gestational age, since a very preterm delivery could prevent in utero deterioration or death but be associated with the morbidity and mortality of extreme prematurity.

Whenever possible (in the absence of recurrent late decelerations or bradycardia), **delivery should be postponed after 48 hours of steroids for fetal maturity.** At <30 weeks, gestational age and birth weight are the largest predictors of outcome, and antenatal surveillance tools may not contribute significantly to survival (167,171,172).

Between 24 and 34 weeks, weekly UA Doppler evaluation will be the mainstay of surveillance with either twice weekly NSTs with weekly amniotic fluid assessment or weekly BPPs. MCA Doppler velocimetry will help to identify fetuses that are pathologically FGR, and the patient with abnormal MCA blood flow should be counseled about the increased risks in pregnancy and the newborn period. If there is evidence of AREDF of the UA, DV Doppler evaluation can be performed, and the patient should be hospitalized for corticosteroid administration and daily monitoring.

At **32 to 33 6/7 weeks, REDF in the UA and BPP<6 are indications for delivery** 48 hours after steroids have been given (119). With AEDF, reversed flow of the a-wave of the DV is a strong predictor of fetal acidemia and poor perinatal outcome (151–153), and delivery should also be considered. Usually tocolysis should not be used for PTL or PPROM in the presence of FGR unless FHR tracing is reassuring and 48 hours are needed to obtain the benefit of steroid administration.

At **≥34 weeks, FGR** should probably be delivered if there is a **BPP <6, oligohydramnios with SDP < 2, AEDF or REDF in UA, or absent/reversed flow of the a-wave in the DV** (119).

If the UA S/D, PI, or RI are at or above the 95th percentile, but flow during diastole is still present, delivery should be considered at around 37 weeks. In singleton gestations with FGR at 36 to 41 weeks, induction at around 37 weeks was associated with similar maternal outcomes, incidences of cesarean delivery, and neonatal morbidity and mortality compared to expectant management (173). The incidence of FGR<3rd percentile is decreased from 31% with expectant monitoring to 13% with induction. **If the CTG and/or BPP remain reassuring, delivery at approximately 38 to 39 weeks can be performed for the remainder of FGR fetuses.** Some recommend delivery at 39 weeks (by EDC) of the FGR fetus with otherwise normal testing if dating is accurate (i.e., based on first-trimester ultrasound).

In DC/DA twin gestations, with FGR in one or both fetuses, similar suggestions can be made in the presence of abnormal UA Doppler or NST/CTG as in singletons with FGR. If fetal testing is reassuring, considerations should be given to delivery by 36 weeks when FGR is present in a DC/DA gestations. For more details, see also chapter 43, "Multiple Gestation."

Mode

There is insufficient evidence to assess the mode of delivery associated with the best outcomes for the FGR fetus. However, some evidence exists showing that **pregnancies with suspected FGR which necessitate delivery can be safely induced if there is a reassuring fetal tracing**, normal oxytocin contraction test (OCT), and normal BPP (174). Fetuses with abnormal UA Doppler velocimetry are more likely to fail the OCT and require a cesarean section, but vaginal delivery is possible in 40% to 60%% of these patients with FGR (48,175). When induction of labor is performed, especially at or after 36 weeks, the rate of cesarean section does not increase (173). The decision for either induction of labor or planned cesarean section should account for numerous variables like fetal hemodynamic status, monitoring, cervical ripening, and parent desires. A trial of labor for the vertex FGR fetus can only be attempted if fetal monitoring is reassuring. The placenta should be sent for pathologic evaluation after delivery of an FGR fetus.

NEONATOLOGY MANAGEMENT

FGR neonates frequently require assistance with ventilation and feeding, especially if born preterm. FGR neonates <32 weeks or <1500 g require special care, usually in a tertiary care center. Workup of the etiology of FGR should be completed if not already done prenatally. Hypoglycemia, polycythemia, and coagulopathies are common, and may need treatment. Involvement of the neonatology team on counseling the patient prior to delivery on expectations in the intensive care unit may be helpful for families.

FUTURE PREGNANCY PRECONCEPTION COUNSELING

Recurrence risks are dependent upon the etiology, but when the etiology is uncertain, the rate of recurrence is increased to as high as 24% (10–13). The next pregnancy is also at increased risk for fetal death if FGR necessitated PTB (176). When the first pregnancy had FGR, several interventions are available to prevent recurrence of FGR (Table 44.3) (177). The subsequent pregnancy should have initiation of low-dose aspirin prior to 16 weeks (unless the cause has been identified and is either non-recurrent or treatable otherwise) (66). In the subsequent pregnancy, screening for FGR with ultrasound surveillance of fetal growth should be performed at regular intervals.

Table 44.3 Intervention to Prevent Recurrent FGR

Preconception
- Adequate spacing of pregnancies (e.g., 18–24 mo between last delivery and next conception)
- Optimization of maternal medical conditions such as diabetes and rheumatologic disease, smoking cessation

Prenatal
- Accurate dating by first trimester sonography
- Low-dose aspirin (50–150 mg) started at ≤16 wk
- Women with nutritional deficiencies, especially in developing countries:
  - Supplementation of 500 to 1000 calories with low (<25%) protein content
- Women living in areas endemic for malaria:
  - Antimalarial prophylaxis

Source: Modified from Ref. 177.

REFERENCES

1. American College of Obstetrics and Gynecology Practice Bulletin No. 12:IUGR. January 2000. [III]
2. Favre R, Nisand G, Bettahar K, et al. Measurement of limb circumferences with three-dimensional ultrasound for fetal weight estimation. Ultrasound Obstet Gynecol 1993; 3:176–179. [III]
3. Ott WJ. The diagnosis of altered fetal growth. Obstet Gynecol Clin North Am 1988; 15:237. [II-2]
4. Gardosi J. New definition of small for gestational age based on fetal growth potential. Horm Res 2006; 65(suppl 3):15–18. [II-2]
5. Morris RK, Malin G, Robson SC, et al. Fetal umbilical artery Doppler to predict compromise of fetal/neonatal wellbeing in a high-risk population: systematic review and bivariate meta-analysis. Ultrasound Obstet Gynecol 2011; 37:135–142. [II-1]
6. De Onis M, Blossner M, Villar J. Levels and patterns of intrauterine growth retardation in developing countries. Eur J Clin Nutr 1998; 52(supp 1):S5–S15. [II-3]
7. McIntire D, Bloom S, Casey B, et al. Birth weight in relation to morbidity and mortality among newborn infants. N Engl J Med 1999; 340(16):1234–1238. [II-2]
8. McCowan LM, Harding JE, Stewart AW. Umbilical artery Doppler studies in small for gestational age babies reflect disease severity. Br J Obstet Gynecol 2000; 107:916–925. [II-2]
9. Hata T, Aoki S, Manabe A, et al. Subclassification of small-for-gestational-age fetus using fetal Doppler velocimetry. Gynecol Obstet Invest 2000; 49(4):236–239. [II-2]
10. Bakewell J, Stockbauer J, Schramm W. Factors associated with repetition of low birth weight: Missouri longitudinal study. Paediatr Perinat Epidemiol 1997; 11(suppl 1):119–129. [II-2]
11. Bakketeig L, Bjerkedal T, Hoffman H. Small for gestational age births and successive pregnancy outcomes: results form a longitudinal study of births in Norway. Early Hum Dev 1986; 14(3–4):187–200. [II-3]
12. Bratton S, Shoultz D, Williams M. Recurrence risk of low birth weight deliveries among women with a prior very low birth weight delivery. Am J Perinatol 1996; 13(3):147–150. [II-3]
13. Wang X, Zuckerman B, Coffman G, et al. Familial aggregation of low birth weight among whites and blacks in the United States. N Engl J Med 1995; 333(26):1772–1774. [II-3]
14. Ananth C, Kaminsky L, Getahun D, et al. Recurrence of fetal growth restriction in singleton and twin gestations. J Matern Fetal Med 2009; 22(8):654–661. [II-2]
15. Warburton D, Dallaire L, Thangavelu M, et al. Trisomy recurrence: a reconsideration based on north American data. Am J Genet 2004; 75:376–385. [II-2]
16. DeSouza E, Halliday J, Chan A, et al. Recurrence risks for trisomies 13, 18, and 21. Am J Med Genet A 2009; 149A:2716–2722. [II-2]
17. Morris JK, Mutton DE, Alberman E. Recurrences of free trisomy 21: analysis of data from the national Down dyndrome cytogenetic register. Prenat Diagn 2005; 25:1120–1128. [II-2]
18. Dashe J, McIntire D, Lucas M, et al. Effects of symmetric and asymmetric fetal growth on pregnancy outcomes. Obstet Gynecol 2000; 1996(3):321–327. [II-2]
19. David C, Gabriellie S, Pilu G, et al. The head-to-abdomen circumference ratio: a reappraisal. Ultrasound Obstet Gynecol 1995; 5(4):256–259. [II-2]
20. Bukowski R, Uchida T, Smith G, et al. Individualized norms of optimal fetal growth: fetal growth potential. Obstet Gynecol 2008; 111:1065–1076. [II-2]
21. Ounsted M, Moar V, Scott A. Risk factors associated with small-for-dates and large-for-dates infants. Br J Obstet Gynaecol 1987; 92:226–232. [II-2]
22. Cunningham F, Cox S, Harstad T, et al. Chronic renal disease and pregnancy outcome. Am J Obstet Gynecol 1990; 163:453–459. [II-3]
23. Duvekot J, Cheriex E, Pieters F, et al. Maternal volume homeostasis in early pregnancy in relation to fetal growth restriction. Obstet Gynecol 1995; 85:361–367. [III]
24. Duvecott J, Cheriex E, Pieters F, et al. Severely impaired fetal growth is preceded by maternal hemodynamic maladaptation in very early pregnancy. Acta Obstet Gynecol Scand 1995; 74:693–697. [III]
25. Bada H, Das A, Bauer C, et al. Low birth weight and preterm births: etiologic fraction attributable to prenatal drug exposure. J Perinatol 2005; 25(10):631–637. [II-2]
26. Shu X, Hatch M, Mills J, et al. Maternal smoking, alcohol drinking, caffeine consumption, and fetal growth: results from a prospective study. Epidemiology 1995; 6:115–120. [II-2]
27. Virji S. The relationship between alcohol consumption during pregnancy and infant birth weight. An epidemiologic study. Acta Obstet Gynecol Scand 1991; 70:303–308. [II-3]
28. Naeye R, Blanc W, Leblanc W, et al. Fetal complications of maternal heroin addiction: abnormal growth, infections and episodes of stress. J Pediatr 1973; 83:1055–1061. [III]
29. Fulroth R, Phillips B, Durand D. Perinatal outcome of infants exposed to cocaine and/or heroin in utero. Am J Dis Child 1989; 143:905–910. [II-3]
30. Anatov A. Children born during the siege of Leningrad in 1942. J Pediatr 1947; 30:250–250. [III]
31. Smith C. Effect of maternal undernutrition upon newborn infant in Holland. J Pediatr 1947; 30:29–243. [III]
32. World Health Organization. A WHO collaborative study of maternal anthropometry and pregnancy outcomes. Int J Gynecol Obstet 1997; 57:1–15. [II-2]
33. Nieto A, Matorras R, Serra M, et al. Multivariate analysis of determinants of fetal growth retardation. Eur J Obstet Gynecol Reprod Biol 1994; 53:107–113. [II-2]
34. Maulik D. Fetal growth restriction: the etiology. Clin Obstet Gynecol 2006; 49(2):228–235. [III]
35. Gersak K, Verdenik I, Antolic ZN. Karyotyping in symmetrically growth-restricted fetuses. Eur J Obstet Gynecol Reprod Biol 2009; 145(1):123. [II-3]
36. Snijders RJ, Sherrod C, Gosden CM, et al. Fetal growth retardation: associated malformations and chromosomal abnormalities. Am J Obstet Gynecol 1993; 168:547–555. [II-2]
37. Viora E, Zamboni C, Mortara G, et al. Trisomy 18: fetal ultrasound findings at different gestational ages. Am J Med Genet A 2007; 143(6):3–557. [III]
38. Khoury J, Erickson D, Cordero J, et al. Congenital malformations and intrauterine growth retardation: a population study. Pediatrics 1988; 82:83–90. [II-3]
39. Mittendorfer-Rutz E, Rasmusen F, Wassertman D. Restricted fetal growth and adverse maternal and psychosocial and socio-economic conditions as risk factor for suicidal behavior of offspring: A cohort study. Lancet 2004; 364:1135–1140. [II-2]
40. Craigo SD, Beach ML, Harvey-Wilkes KB, et al. Ultrasound predictors of neonatal outcome in intrauterine growth restriction. Am J Perinatol 1996; 13:465–471. [II-3]
41. Hack M, Taylor HG, Drotar D, et al. Chronic conditions, functional limitations, and special needs of school-aged children born with extremely low birth weight in the 1990's. J Am Med Assoc 2005; 294(3):318–325. [II-2]
42. Gembruch U, Gortner L. Perinatal aspects of preterm intrauterine growth restriction. Ultrasound Obstet Gynecol 1998; 11: 233–239. [II-3]
43. Hepburn M, Rosenburg K. An audit of the detection and management of small-for-gestational age babies. Br J Obstet Gynaecol 1986; 93:212–216. [II-2]
44. Lackman F, Capewell V, Richardson B, et al. The risks of spontaneous preterm delivery and perinatal mortality in relation to size at birth according to fetal versus neonatal growth standards. Am J Obstet Gynecol 2001; 184:946–953. [II-2]
45. Bernstein I, Horbar J, Badger G, et al. Morbidity and mortality among very-low-birth weight neonates with intrauterine growth restriction. Am J Obstet Gynecol 1999; 182(1):198–206. [II-3]
46. Pallotto E, Kilbride H. Perinatal outcome and later implications of intrauterine growth restriction. Clin Obstet Gynecol 2006; 49 (2):257–269. [II-2]
47. Barker D. Adult consequences of fetal growth restriction. Clin Obstet Gynecol 2006; 49(2):270–283. [III]
48. Maslovitz S, Shenhav M, Levin I, et al. Outcome of induced deliveries in growth-restricted fetuses: second thoughts about the vaginal option. Arch Gynecol Obstet 2009; 279:139–143. [II-3]

49. Daya S. Accuracy of gestational age estimation by means of fetal crown-rump length measurement. Am J Obstet Gynecol 1993; 168(3 pt 1):903–908. [II-2]

50. Smith GCS, Smith MFS, McNay MB, et al. First-trimester growth and the risk of low birth weight. N Engl J Med 1998; 339:1817–1822. [II-2]

51. Mook-Kanamori DO, Steegers EAP, Eilers PH, et al. Risk factors and outcomes associated with first trimester fetal growth restriction. J Am Med Assoc 2010; 303:527–534. [II-2]

52. ACOG practice bulletin No. 101:Ultrasonography in pregnancy. Obstet Gynecol 2009; 113(2):451–461. [III]

53. Smith G, Pell J, Dobbie R. Interpregnancy interval and risk of preterm birth and neonatal death: retrospective cohort study. Br Med J 2003; 327:313–319. [II-2]

54. Zhu B, Rolfs R, Nangle B, et al. Effect of the interval between pregnancies on perinatal outcomes. N Engl J Med 1999; 340:589–594. [II-2]

55. MacArthur C, Knox E. Smoking in pregnancy: effects of stopping at different stages. Br J Obstet Gynaecol 1988; 95:551–555. [II-2]

56. Lumley J, Chamberlain C, Dowswell T, et al. Interventions for promoting smoking cessation during pregnancy. Cochrane Database Syst Rev 2009; 3:CD001055. [Meta-analyis; 72 trials, *n* = 25,000]

57. Kfatos A, Vlachonikolis I, Codrington C. Nutrition during pregnancy: the effects of an educational intervention program in Greece. Am J Clin Nutr 1989; 50:970–979. [II-1]

58. Khoury J, Henriksen T, Christophersen B, et al. Effect of a cholesterol-lowering diet on maternal, cord, and neonatal lipids, and pregnancy outcome: a randomized clinical trial. Am J Obstet Gynecol 2005; 193:1292–1301. [RCT; *n* = 290]

59. Steegers E, Van Lakwijk HP, Jongsma H, et al. Pathophysiological implications of chronic dietary sodium restriction during pregnancy; a longitudinal prospective randomized study. Br J Obstet Gonecol 1991; 98:980–987. [RCT; *n* = 42]

60. Mohomed K. Iron supplementation in pregnancy. Cochrane Database Syst Rev 2007; 3:CD000117. [Meta-analysis; 20 trials]

61. Hofmeyr G, Lawrie T, Atallah A, et al. Calcium supplementation during pregnancy for preventing hypertensive disorders and related problems. Cochrane Database Syst Rev 2010; 9: CD001059. [Meta-analysis; *n* = 15,730]

62. Makrides M, Crowther C. Magnesium supplementation in pregnancy. Cochrane Database Syst Rev 2001; 4:CD000937. [Meta-analysis; 7 trials, *n* = 2689]

63. Mohomed K, Gulmezoglu A. Vitamin D supplementation in pregnancy. Cochrane Database Syst Rev 2000; 2:CD000228. [Meta-analysis; *n* = 232]

64. Kramer MS, Kakuma R. Energy and protein intake in pregnancy. Cochrane Database Syst Rev 2003; 4:CD000032. [Meta-analysis; 5 trials, *n* = 1134]

65. Abalos E, Duley L, Steyn D, et al. Antihypertensive drug therapy for mild to moderate hypertension during pregnancy. Cochrane Database Syst Rev 2007; 1:CD002252. [Meta-analysis; 19 trials, *n* = 2437]

66. Bujold E, Roberge S, Lacasse Y, et al. Prevention of preeclampsia and intrauterine growth restriction with aspirin started in early pregnancy: a meta-analysis. Obstet Gynecol 2010; 116(2):402–414. [Meta-analysis: RCT = 34, *n* = 11,348]

67. Knight M, Duley L, Henderson-Smart DJ, et al. Antiplatelet agents for preventing and treating pre-eclampsia. Cochrane Database Syst Rev 4, 2005. [Meta-analysis; 25 RCTs, *n* ≥ 20,000]

68. Irwin JC, Suen LF, Martina NA, et al. Role of the IGF system in trophoblast invasion and preeclampsia. Hum Reprod 1999; 14: S90–S96. [II-2]

69. Spencer K, Cowans NJ, Avgidou K, et al. First-trimester biochemical markers of aneuploidy and the prediction of small-for-gestational age fetuses. Ultrasound Obstet Gynecol 2008; 31:15–19. [II-2]

70. Spencer K, Cowans NJ, Molina F, et al. First-trimester ultrasound and biochemical markers of aneuploidy and the prediction of preterm or early preterm delivery. Ultrasound Obstet Gynecol 2008; 31:147–152. [II-2]

71. Spencer K, Cowans NJ, Avgidou K, et al. First trimester ultrasound and biochemical markers of aneuploidy and the prediction of impending fetal death. Ultrasound Obstet Gynecol 2006; 28:637–643. [II-2]

72. Spencer K, Cowans NJ, Nicolaides KH. Low levels of maternal serum PAPP-A in the first trimester and the risk of preeclampsia. Prenat Diagn 2008; 28:7–10. [II-2]

73. Dugoff L, Hobbins JC, Malone FD, et al. First-trimester maternal serum PAPP-A and free-beta subunit human chorionic gonadotropin concentrations and nuchal translucency are associated with obstetric complications: a population-based screening study (The FASTER Trial). Am J Obstet Gynecol 2004; 191:1446–1451. [II-2]

74. Krantz D, Goetzl L, Simpson JL, et al. Association of extreme first-trimester free human chorionic gonadotropin-beta, pregnancy-associated plasma protein A, and nuchal translucency with intrauterine growth restriction and other adverse pregnancy outcomes. Am J Obstet Gynecol 2004; 191:1452–1458. [II-2]

75. Goetzl L, Krantz D, Simpson JL, et al. Pregnancy-associated plasma protein A, free beta-hCG, nuchal translucency, and risk of pregnancy loss. Obstet Gynecol 2004; 104:30–36. [II-2]

76. Spencer K, Yu CK, Cowans NJ, et al. Prediction of pregnancy complications by first-trimester maternal serum PAPP-A and free beta-hCG and with second-trimester uterine artery Doppler. Prenat Diagn 2005; 25:949–953. [II-2]

77. Dugoff L. First- and second-trimester maternal serum markers for aneuploidy and adverse obstetric outcomes. Obstet Gynecol 2010; 115:1052–1061. [III]

78. Dugoff L, Hobbins J, Malone F, et al. Quad screen as a predictor of adverse pregnancy outcome. Obstet Gynecol 2005; 106(2):260–267. [II-2]

79. Westin B. Gravidogram and fetal growth. Acta Obstet Gynecol Scand 1977; 56:273–282. [II-2]

80. Grover V. Altered fetal growth: antenatal diagnosis by symphysis–fundal height in India and comparison with western charts. Int J Gynaecol Obstet 1991; 35(3):231–234. [II-2]

81. Cnattingius S, Axelsson O, Lindmark G. Symphysis–fundus measurements and intrauterine growth retardation. Acta Obstet Gynecol Scand 1984; 63(4):335–340. [II-2]

82. Belizan JM, Villar J, Nardin JC, et al. Diagnosis of intrauterine growth retardation by a simple clinical method: measurement of uterine height. Am J Obstet Gynecol 1978; 131:643–646. [II-3]

83. Lindhard A, Nielsen PV, Mouritsen LA, et al. The implications of introducing the symphyseal- fundal height-measurement: a prospective randomized controlled trial. Br J Obstet Gynaecol 1990; 97:675–680. [I]

84. Persson B, Stangenberg M, Lunell NO, et al. Prediction of size of infants at birth by measurement of symphysis fundus height. Br J Obstet Gynaecol 1986; 93:206–211. [II-2]

85. Rogers MS, Needham PG. Evaluation of fundal height measurement in antenatal care. Aust N Z J Obstet Gynaecol 1985; 25(2):87–90. [II-3]

86. Rosenberg K, Grant JM, Tweedie I, et al. Measurement of fundal height as a screening test for fetal growth retardation. Br J Obstet Gynaecol 1982; 89(6):447–450. [II-2]

87. Beazley JM, Underhill RA. Fallacy of the fundal height. Br Med J 1970; 4:404–406. [III]

88. Hulsey TC, Levkoff AH, Alexander GR, et al. Differences in black and white infant birth weights. South Med J 1991; 84:443–446. [II-2]

89. Goldenberg RL, Cliver SP, Cutter GR. Black white differences in newborn anthropometric measurements. Obstet Gynecol 1991; 78:782–788. [II-2]

90. Yip R, Li Z, Chong WH. Race and birth weight: the Chinese example. Pediatrics 1991; 87:688–693. [II-2]

91. Alver J, Brooke OG. Fetal growth in different racial groups. Arch Dis Child 1978; 53:27–32. [II-2]

92. Ott WJ. Intrauterine growth retardation and preterm delivery. Am J Obstet Gynecol 1993; 168:1710–1715. [II-2]

93. Graafmans WC, Richardus JH, Borsboom GJ, et al. Birth weight and perinatal mortality: a comparison of "optimal" birth weight

in seven Western European countries. Epidemiology 2002; 13:569–574. [II-2]

94. Warsof SL, Gohari P, Berkowitz RL, et al. The estimation of fetal weight by computer assisted analysis. Am J Obstet Gynecol 1977; 128:881–892. [II-3]

95. Hadlock FP, Harrist RB, Martinez-Poyer J. In utero analysis of fetal growth: a sonographic weight standard. Radiology 1991; 181:129–133. [II-3]

96. Shepard MJ, Richards VA, Berkowitz RL, et al. An evaluation of two equations for predicting fetal weight by ultrasound. Am J Obstet Gynecol 1982; 142:47–54. [II-3]

97. Persson P-H, Weldner B-M. Intra-uterine weight curves obtained by ultrasound. Acta Obstet Gynecol Scand 1986; 65:169–173. [II-2]

98. Bernstein IM, Meyer M, Capeless E. Fetal growth charts: comparison of cross-sectional ultrasound examinations with birth weight. J Matern Fetal Med 1994; 3:182–186. [II-2]

99. Bernstein IM, Mohs G, Rucquoi M, et al. Case for hybrid "fetal growth curves": a population-based estimation of normal fetal size across gestational age. J Matern Fetal Med 1996; 5:124–127. [II-3]

100. Salomon LJ, Bernard JP, Ville Y. Estimation of fetal weight: reference range at 20-36 weeks' gestation and comparison with actual birth weight reference range. Ultrasound Obstet Gynecol 2007; 29:550–555. [II-2]

101. Zaw W, Gagnon R, da Silva O. The risks of adverse neonatal outcome among preterm small for gestational age infants according to neonatal versus fetal growth standards. Pediatrics 2003; 111:1273–1277. [II-2]

102. Gardosi J. Customized fetal growth standards: rationale and clinical application. Semin Perinatol 2004; 28:33–40. [II-2]

103. Clausson B, Gardosi J, Francis A, et al. Perinatal outcome in SGA births defined by customized versus population-based birth weight standards. Br J Obstet Gynaecol 2001; 108:830–834. [II-2]

104. Ego A, Subtil D, Gilles G, et al. Customized versus population-based birth weight standards for identifying growth restricted infants: a French multicenter study. Am J Obstet Gynecol. 2006; 194:1042–1049. [II-2]

105. Figueras F, Figueras J, Meler E, et al. Customised birth weight standards accurately predict perinatal morbidity. Arch Dis Child Fetal Neonatal Ed 2007; 92:F277–F280. [II-2]

106. Royal College of Obstetricians and Gynaecologists. The Investigation and Management of the small-for-Gestational-Age Fetus. Guideline No. 31. London: RCOG, 2002. [III]

107. Hutcheon JA, Zhang X, Cnattingius S, et al. Customized birth weight percentiles: does adjusting for maternal characteristics matter? BJOG 2008; 115:1397–1404. [II-2]

108. Martin A, Bindra R, Curcio P, et al. Screening for pre-eclampsia and fetal growth restriction by uterine artery Doppler at 11-14 weeks of gestation. Ultrasound Obstet Gynecol 2001; 18:583–586. [II-2]

109. Gomez O, Martinez J, Figueras F, et al. Uterine artery Doppler at 11-14 weeks of gestation to screen for hypertensive disorders and associated complication in an unselected population. Ultrasound Obstet Gynecol 2005; 26:490–494. [II-2]

110. Pilalis A, Souka P, Antsakalis P, et al. Screening for preecmpsia and fetal growth restriction by uterine artery Doppler and PAPP-A at 11-14 weeks' gestation. Ultrasound Obstet Gynecol 2007; 29:135–140. [II-2]

111. Cnossen JS, Morris RK, ter Riet G, et al. Use of uterine artery Doppler ultrasonography to predict pre-eclampsia and intrauterine growth restriction: a systematic review and bivariable meta-analysis. Can Med Assoc J 2008; 178:701–711. [II-2]

112. Cooper S, Johnson J, Metcalfe A, et al. The predictive value of 18 and 22 week uterine artery Doppler in patients with low first trimester serum PAPP-A. Prenat Diagn 2009; 29:248–252. [II-2]

113. Palma-Dias RS, Fonseca MM, Brietzke E, et al. Screening for placental insufficiency by transvaginal uterine artery Doppler at 22-24 weeks of gestation. Fetal Diagn Ther 2008; 24:462–469. [II-2]

114. Alkazaleh F, Chaddha V, Viero S, et al. Second trimester prediction of severe placental complications in women with combined elevations in alpha-fetoprotein and human chorionic gonadotriphin. Am J Obstet Gynecol 2006; 94(3):821–827. [II-2]

115. Yu C, Khouri O, Onwudiwe N, et al. Prediction of preeclampsia by uterine artery Doppler imaging: relationship to gestational age at delivery and small-for-gestational age. Ultrasound Obstet Gynecol 2008; 31:310–313. [II-2]

116. Konchak P, Bernstein I, Capeless E. Uterine artery Doppler velocimetry in the detection of adverse obstetric outcomes in women with unexplained elevated maternal serum alpha-fetoprotein levels. Am J Obstet Gynecol 1995; 173:1115–1119. [II-2]

117. Chavez MR, Ananth CV, Smulian JC, et al. et al. transcerebellar diameter measurement for prediction of gestational age at the extremes of fetal growth. J Ulrasound Med 2007; 26(9):1167–1171. [II-2]

118. Niknafs P, Sibbald J. Accuracy of single ultrasound parameters in detection of fetal growth restriction. Am J Perinatol 2001; 18 (6):325–334. [II-2]

119. Publication Committee, SMFM. Early severe fetal growth restriction: evaluation and treatment. Cont Ob-Gyn 2011; 2:32–35. [III]

120. Wilkins-Haug L, Quade B, Morton CC. Confined placental mosaicism as a risk factor among newborns with fetal growth restriction. Prenat Diagn 2006; 26(5):428–432. [II-2]

121. Facco F, You W, Grobman W. Genetic thrombophilias and intrauterine growth restriction. Obstet Gynecol 2009; 113 (6):1206–1216. [II-2]

122. Baschat A, Cosmi E, Bilardo C, et al. Predictors of neonatal outcome in early-onset placental dysfunction. Obstet Gynecol 2007; 109(2 pt 1):253–261. [II-2]

123. Engineer N, Kumar S. Perinatal variables and neonatal outcomes in severely growth restricted preterm fetuses. Acta Obstet Gynecol Scand 2010; 89(9):1174–1181. [II-2]

124. Abenhaim H, Bujold E, Benjamin A, et al. Evaluating the role of bedrest on the prevention of hypertensive diseases of pregnancy and growth restriction. Hypertens Pregnancy 2008; f27(2):197–205. [II-2]

125. Maloni J, Alexander G, Schluchter M, et al. Antepartum bed rest: maternal weight change and infant birth weight. Biol Res Nurs 2004; 5(3):177–186. [II-3]

126. Laurin J, Persson P-H. The effect of bedrest in hospital on fetal outcome in pregnancies complicated by intra-uterine growth retardation. Acta Obstet Gynecol Scand 1987; 66:407–411. [I, RCT, n = 107. Allocation of treatment was by odd or even birth date.]

127. Ramakrishnan U, Stein A, Parra-Cabrera S, et al. Effects of docosahexaenoic acid supplementation during pregnancy on gestational age and size at birth: randomized, double-blind, placebo-controlled trial in Mexico. Food Nutr Bull 2010; 31 (2 suppl):S108–S116. [RCT, n = 1094]

128. Roberfroid D, Huybregts L, Lanou H, et al. MISAME Study Group. Effects of maternal multiple micronutrient supplementation on fetal growth: a double-blind randomized controlled trial in rural Burkina Faso. Am J Clin Nutr 2008; 88(5):1220–1240. [RCT, n = 1426]

129. Horvath A, Koletzko B, Szajewska H. Effect of supplementation of women in high-risk pregnancies with long-chain polyunsaturated fatty acids on pregnancy outcomes and growth measures at birth: a meta-analysis of randomized controlled trials. Br J Nutr 2007; 98(2):253–259. [Meta-analysis; 2 RCTs, n = 291]

130. Say L, Gulmezoglu AM, Hofmeyr GJ. Maternal nutrient supplementation for suspected impaired fetal growth. Cochrane Database Syst Rev 2010; (7):1–19. [4 RCTs, n = 165]

131. Say L, Gulmezoglu MA, Hofmeyr JG. Betamimetics for suspected impaired fetal growth. Cochrane Database Syst Rev 2009; (4):1–13. [2 RCTs, n = 118]

132. Janssens D. Prevention of low birth weight by flunarizine given to smoking mothers. Arch Gynecol 1985; 237(suppl 1):397. [RCT, n = 100]

133. Say L, Gulmezoglu AM, Hofmeyr GJ. Maternal oxygen administration for suspected impaired fetal growth. Cochrane Database Syst Rev 4, 2005:1–11. [I; 3 RCTs, n = 94]

134. Salas SP, Rosso P, Espinoza R, et al. Maternal plasma volume expansion and hormonal changes in women with idiopathic

fetal growth retardation. Obstet Gynecol 1993; 81(6):1029–1030. [II-2]

135. Karsdorp VHM, van Vugt JMG, Dekker GA, et al. Reappearance of end-diastolic velocities in the umbilical artery following maternal volume expansion: a preliminary study. Obstet Gynecol 1992; 80:679–683. [RCT, $n = 14$]

136. Hofmeyr GJ. Abdominal decompression for suspected fetal compromise/pre-eclampsia. Cochrane Database Syst Rev 4, 2005:1–13. [3 RCTs, $n = 367$]

137. Winer N, Branger B, Azria E, et al. L-Arginine treatment for severe vascular fetal intrauterine growth restriction: a randomized double-blind controlled trial. Clin Nutr 2009; 28(3):243–248. [I: RCT $n = 44$]

138. Sieroszewski P, Suzin J, Karowicz-Bilinska A. Ultrasound evaluation of intrauterine growth restriction therapy by a nitric oxide donors (L-arginine). J Matern Fetal Neonatal Med 2003; 13:115–118. [II-1]

139. Xiao XM, Li LP. L-Arginine treatment for asymmetric fetal growth restriction. Int J Gynaecol Obstet 2005; 88:15–18. [II-1]

140. Lampl MD, Veldhuis JD, Johnson ML. Saltation and stasis: a model of human growth. Science 1992; 258:801–803. [II-3]

141. Bernstein IM, Blake K, Wall B, et al. Evidence that normal fetal growth can be noncontinuous. J Matern Fetal Med 1995; 4:1997–1201. [II-3]

142. Mongelli M, Ek S, Tamyrajia R. Screening for fetal growth restriction: a mathematical model of the effect of time interval and ultrasound error. Obstet Gynecol 1998; 92(6):908–912. [II-3]

143. Todros T, Sciarrone A, Piccoli E, et al. Umbilical Doppler waveforms and placental villous angiongenesis in pregnancies complicated by fetal growth restriction. Obstet Gynecol 1999; 93:499–503. [II-2]

144. Hartung J, Kalache K, Heyna C, et al. Outcome of 60 neonates who had ARED flow prenatally compared with a matched control group of appropriate-for gestational age preterm neonates. Ultrasound Obstet Gynecol 2005; 25:566–572. [II-2]

145. Shand A, Hornbuckle J, Nathan E, et al. Small for gestational age preterm infants and relationship of abnormal umbilical artery Doppler blood flow to perinatal mortality and neurodevelopmental outcomes. Aust N Z J Obstet Gynaecol 2009; 49:52–58. [II-2]

146. McCowan L, Harding J, Roberts A, et al. A pilot randomized controlled trial of two regimens of fetal surveillance for small-for-gestational age fetuses with normal results of umbilical artery Doppler velocimetry. Am J Obstet Gynecol 2000; 182 (1):81–86. [I: RCT $n = 167$]

147. Alfirevic Z, Stampalija T, Gyte G. Fetal and umbilical Doppler ultrasound in high-risk pregnancies. Cochrane Database Syst Rev 2010; 1:CD007529. [I, meta-analysis, 18 RCTs, $n = 10,000$]

148. Bahado-Singh R, Kovanci E, Jeffres A, et al. The Doppler cerebroplacental ratio and perinatal outcome in intrauterine growth restriction. Am J Obstet Gynecol 1999; 180:750–756. [II-2]

149. Odibo A, Riddick C, Are E, et al. Cerebroplacental Doppler ratio and adverse perinatal outcomes in intrauterine growth restriction. J Ultrasound Med 2005; 24:1223–1228. [II-2]

150. Figueras F, Martiniz J, Puerto B, et al. Contraction stress test versus ductus venosus Doppler evaluation for the prediction of adverse perinatal outcome in growth-restricted fetuses with non-reassuring non-stress test. Ultrasound Obstet Gynecol 2003; 21:250–255. [II-2]

151. Baschat A, Gembruch U, Weiner C, et al. Qualitative venous Doppler waveform analysis improves prediction of critical outcomes in premature growth-restricted fetuses. Ultrasound Obstet Gynecol 2003; 22:240–245. [II-2]

152. Schwarze A, Gembruch U, Krapp M, et al. Qualitative venous Doppler flow waveform analysis in preterm intrauterine growth-restricted fetuses with ARED flow in the umbilical artery-correlation with short-term outcome. Ultrasound Obstet Gynecol 2005; 25:573–579. [II-2]

153. Alves S, Fancisco R, Miyadahira S, et al. Ductus venosus Doppler and postnatal outcomes in fetuses with absent or reversed end-diastolic flow in the umbilical artery. Eur J Obstet Gynecol Reprod Biol 2008; 141:100–103. [II-2]

154. Grivell R, Alfirevec Z, Gyte G, et al. Antenatal cardiotocography for fetal assessment. Cochrane Database Syst Rev 2010; 1: CD007863. [I, 4 studies, $n = 1627$]

155. Visser G, Sandovsky G, Nicolaides K. Antepartum fetal heart rate patterns in small-for-gestational-age third-trimester fetuses: correlations with blood gas values obtained at cordocentesis. Am J Obstet Gynecol 1990; 162:698–703. [II-2]

156. Donner C, Vermeylen D, Kirkpatrick C, et al. Management of the growth-restricted fetus: the role of noninvasive tests and fetal blood sampling. Obstet Gynecol 1995; 85:965–970. [II-3]

157. Lalor JG, Fawole B, Alfirevic Z, et al. Biophysical profile for fetal assessment in high risk pregnancies. Cochrane Database Syst Rev 2008; 1:CD000038. [Meta-analysis; 5 RCTs; $n = 2974$]

158. Dayal A, Manning F, Berck D, et al. Fetal death after normal biophysical profile score: an eighteen year experience. Am J Obstet Gynecol 1999; 181:1231. [II-3]

159. Duenhoelter JH, Whalley PJ, MacDonald PC. An analysis of the utility of plasma immunoreactive estrogen measurements in determining delivery time of gravidas with a fetus considered at high risk. Am J Obstet Gynecol 1976; 125:889–898. [I, RCT, $n = 622$ women with high risk pregnancies, including fetal growth restriction, hypertension, adverse obstetric history. RCT by hospital # to plasma estriol level either revealed or concealed]

160. Baschat AA, Gembruch U, Harman CR. The sequence of changes in Doppler and biophysical parameters as severe fetal growth restriction worsens. Ultrasound Obstet Gynecol 2001; 18:571–577. [II-2]

161. Ferrazzi E, Bozzo M, Rigano S, et al. Temporal sequence of abnormal Doppler changes in the peripheral and central circulatory systems of the severely growth-restricted fetus. Ultrasound Obstet Gynecol 2002; 19:140–146. [II-2, $n = 26$]

162. Roberts D, Dalziel S. Antenatal corticosteroids for accelerating fetal lung maturation for woman at risk for preterm birth. Cochrane Database Syst Rev 2006; 3:CD004454. [Meta-analysis; 21 RCTs, $n = 3885$]

163. Garite T, Kurtzman J, Maurel K, et al. Impact of a 'rescue course' of antenatal corticosteroids: a multicenter randomized placebo-controlled trial. Am J Obstet Gynecol 2009; 200:248.e1–e9. [RCT; $n = 437$]

164. McLaughlin K, Crowther C, Walker N, et al. Effects of a single course of corticosteroids given more than 7 days before birth: a systematic review. Aust N Z J Obstet Gynecol 2003; 43:101–106. [Meta-analysis; 7 trials; $n = 862$]

165. Vidaeff AC, Blackwell SC. Potential risks and benefits of antenatal corticosteroid therapy prior to preterm birth in pregnancies complicated by severe fetal growth restriction. Obstet Gynecol Clin N Am 2011; 38(2):205–214. [III]

166. Torrance H, Bloemen M, Mulde E, et al. Predictors of outcome at 2 years of age after early intrauterine growth restriction. Ultrasound Obstet Gynecol 2010; 365:171–177. [II-2]

167. Baschat AA, Cosmi E, Bilardo C, et al. Predictors of neonatal outcome in early-onset placental dysfunction. Obstet Gynecol 2007; 109:253–261. [II-2]

168. The GRIT study group. A randomized trial of timed delivery for the compromised preterm fetus: short term outcomes and Bayesian interpretation. Br J Obstet Gynecol 2003; 110:27–32. [RCT, $n = 588$]

169. The GRIT study group. Infant well being at 2 years of age in the Growth Restriction Intervention Trial (GRIT): multicentered randomized controlled trial. Lancet 2004; 364:513–520. [RCT follow-up, $n = 588$]

170. Walker D, Marlow N, Upstone L, et al. The growth restriction intervention trial: long-term outcomes in a randomized trial of delivery in fetal growth restriction. Am J Obstet Gynecol 2011; 204:34e1–34e9. [RCT follow-up, $n = 302$]

171. Sameshima H, Kodama Y, Kaneko M, et al. Clinical factors that enhance morbidity and mortality in intrauterine growth restricted fetuses delivered between 23 and 30 weeks of gestation. J Matern Fetal Neonatal Med 2010; 23:1218–1224. [II-2]

172. Mari G, Hanif F, Treadwell M, et al. Gestational age at delivery and Doppler waveforms in very preterm intrauterine growth-restricted fetuses as predictors of perinatal mortality. J Ultrasound Med 2007; 26:55–59. [II-2]

173. Boers KE, Vijgen SMC, Bijlenga D, et al. Induction versus expectant monitoring for intrauterine growth restriction at term: randomized equivalence trail (DIGITAT). Br Med J 2010; 341:c7087. [RCT, $n = 650$]

174. Ben-Haroush A, Yogev Y, Glickman H, et al. Mode of delivery in pregnancies with suspected fetal growth restriction following induction of labor with vaginal prostaglandin E2. Acta Obstet Gynecol Scand 2004; 83(1):52–57. [II-1]

175. Li H, Gudmundsson S, Olofsson P. Prospect for vaginal delivery of growth restricted fetuses with abnormal umbilical artery blood flow. Acta Obstet Gynecol Scan 2003; 82:828–833. [II-2]

176. Surkan PJ, Stephansson O, Dickman PW, et al. Previous preterm and small-for-gestational-age births and the subsequent risk of still births. N Engl J Med 2004; 350:777–785. [II-2]

177. Berghella V. Prevention of recurrent fetal growth restriction. Obstet Gynecol 2007; 110(4):904–912. [III]

45

Fetal macrosomia

Melissa I. March and Suneet P. Chauhan

KEY POINTS

- Though **clinical and sonographic estimated fetal weight (EFW)** can identify newborns with weight ≥4000 g, both methods **are poor at detecting neonates who will weigh ≥4500 g.**
- **Prevention of macrosomia** is obtained, in women with gestational diabetes (GDM), with the following:
  - **Diet and glucose monitoring with insulin if needed,** compared to no treatment or diet only.
  - **Postprandial blood glucose monitoring,** compared to preprandial, in GDM requiring insulin therapy.
  - **Strict glucose control, with fasting blood sugar <90 and two hours postprandial <120.**
- Among uncomplicated pregnancies, **induction for suspected macrosomia is not indicated**, as it has not been shown to reduce the risk of cesarean section, instrumental delivery, or shoulder dystocia.
- There is insufficient evidence to recommend best management of suspected macrosomia among pregnancies complicated by diabetes mellitus, prior cesarean delivery, or shoulder dystocia, because of the lack of randomized trials and the inaccuracy of predicting birth weight. The American College of Obstetricians and Gynecologists (ACOG) suggests a planned cesarean for women with no diabetes and an EFW of >5000 g, and for those with diabetes and an EFW of 4500 g, but these suggestions are not based on level 1 evidence.

DEFINITION

A fetus with EFW ≥4000 g can be presumed to be macrosomic. Macrosomic newborns can be classified as grades I (birth weight 4000–4499 g), II (4500–4999 g), and III (≥5000 g) (1). This classification is clinically relevant because the grades are associated with different types of complications.

EPIDEMIOLOGY/INCIDENCE

The prevalence of macrosomia has decreased significantly in the United States (2), though it is increasing in other countries, like Denmark. The rate of neonates in the United States weighing ≥4000 g was 10.2% in 1996, 9.2% in 2002, and 7.6% in 2008, continuing to decrease over 12 years. For newborns weighing ≥5000 g, the decrease in the prevalence has been notable as well (from 0.16% in 1996 to 0.13% in 2002 and 0.10% in 2008) (2,3). In some countries, such as Denmark, however, macrosomia is increasing. From 1998 to 2008, that country's rate of macrosomia (live births weighing >4000 g) has increased from 5.2% to 5.8% (4). The rate of macrosomia in other countries has ranged from 1% in Thailand (5) to 5% in Antigua and Barbuda (6) and 20% in the Republic of Croatia (7).

RISK FACTORS

Hispanic women, maternal obesity, maternal birth weight >8 lb, grand multiparity (≥5 deliveries), prior macrosomic fetus, abnormal 50-g glucose screen but normal three-hour glucose test, diabetes (pre- or gestational diabetes), gestational age ≥40 weeks, excessive weight gain during pregnancy are well-known risk factors (8). Intrapartum hydramnios (9) and second stage of labor >120 minutes (10) are other risk factors for macrosomia. The majority of newborns with birth weights ≥4500 g do not have any known risk factors (8).

COMPLICATIONS

The *maternal* complications with macrosomic fetuses include **prolonged labor, operative vaginal delivery, cesarean delivery, postpartum hemorrhage, and vaginal lacerations** (8).

Compared to newborns with birth weights of 3000 to 3999 g, *neonatal* complications for grade I macrosomia include **breech presentation, induction, meconium staining, dysfunctional/prolonged labor, cephalopelvic disproportion, and cesarean delivery**. For grade II macrosomia, the complications are **also Apgar scores ≤3 at 5 minutes, assisted ventilation >30 minutes, birth injuries, meconium aspiration, and hyaline membrane disease**. For grade III macrosomia, there is also a significantly higher likelihood of **neonatal and infant mortality** (1).

MANAGEMENT
Prevention of Macrosomia

A **significant decrease in the rate of macrosomia** can be obtained in women with GDM with the following:

- **Diet and glucose monitoring with insulin** if needed compared to no treatment or diet only (11).
- **Postprandial** versus preprandial **blood glucose monitoring in GDM requiring insulin therapy** (12).
- **Continuous glucose monitoring** compared to standard antenatal care with intermittent self-monitoring (13).
- **Management of GDM with fasting blood sugar <90 and 2 hour postprandial <120,** versus modified blood sugar goal based on whether the abdominal circumference is <75% versus ≥75% for gestational age (if abdominal circumference ≥75% the fasting blood sugar should have been in this study <80 and 2 hour postprandial <100) (14).
- **Treatment, including nutrition instruction, diet, glucose testing, and insulin if necessary, of mild or borderline GDM,** defined by abnormal one-hour glucose challenge test but normal two-hour glucose tolerance test (15,16).

The rate of macrosomia was **not** significantly decreased with

- pre- and gestational diabetes, administering insulin twice daily versus four times daily (17);

- use of insulin or glyburide in the management of GDM not controlled adequately on diet (18);
- use of glyburide or metformin as alternatives to insulin therapy (19);
- induction of labor versus expectant management for pregnancy at >41 weeks (20).

Screening

During labor, the detection of neonates weighing at least 4000 g is similar with clinical or sonographic EFWs, though the likelihood ratio with clinicians' estimate was 15, while with measurements of biometric parameters it was 42 (i.e., better) (21).

Neither clinical nor sonographic EFW can accurately identify neonates that weigh 4500 g or more (22,23). The posttest probability of detecting macrosomia ranges from 15% to 79% by ultrasound and 40% to 52% with clinical estimates (2).

Management of Suspected Macrosomia

Whenever macrosomia is suspected, the pregnancy should be classified into one of the following groups: (*i*) uncomplicated, (*ii*) pre- or gestational diabetes, (*iii*) prior cesarean delivery, or (*iv*) history of shoulder dystocia.

Uncomplicated

Induction of labor for suspected fetal macrosomia in nondiabetic women has not been shown to alter the risk of maternal or neonatal morbidity, but the power of the included studies to show a difference in rare neonatal morbidity is limited. Compared to expectant management, **induction of labor for suspected macrosomia has not been shown to reduce the risk of cesarean section** (RR 0.96, 95% CI 0.67–1.38) **or instrumental delivery** (RR 1.02, 95% CI 0.60–1.74). **Shoulder dystocia is not statistically different between groups** (RR 1.06, 95% CI 0.44–2.56); one trial reported, however, two cases of brachial plexus injury and four cases of fracture in the expectant management group (24). Labor induction for suspected macrosomia results in an increased rate of cesarean delivery without an improved outcome (25). Thus, there is no indication for induction for suspected macrosomia among uncomplicated pregnancies.

While the ACOG practice bulletin on fetal macrosomia (8) suggests that planned cesarean delivery should be considered if the EFW is at least 5000 g, there is insufficient evidence to assess this intervention, and there are insufficient reports on the peripartum outcomes when the fetus is suspected to have grade III macrosomia (2).

Diabetes

In insulin requiring diabetic pregnancies, **induction at 38 weeks**, compared to expectant management until 42 weeks, is associated with a significant decrease in the rate of macrosomic fetuses, but the limited sample size does not permit drawing "firm conclusions" (26,27).

A retrospective study concluded that a protocol involving induction for EFW ≥90% but <4250 g and cesarean delivery for sonographic weight ≥4250 g decreases the rate of shoulder dystocia by 50% but increases the rate of cesarean delivery by 16% (28). While the ACOG practice bulletin on fetal macrosomia (8) suggests that cesarean delivery among diabetics is indicated if the EFW is ≥4500 g, others have set the threshold at ≥4000 g (26,28) or at ≥4250 g (28) (see also chap. 4).

Prior Cesarean Delivery

The majority of patients attempting vaginal birth after cesarean delivery (VBAC) can successfully deliver a macrosomic fetus (29–31). The rate of uterine rupture may be higher (3.6%) for a macrosomic trial of labor with prior cesarean delivery, if the patient has not delivered vaginally before (32). Thus, obstetric factors (prior deliveries, need for induction, etc.) should be considered when attempting VBAC with suspected macrosomia (see chap. 14, *Obstetric Evidence Based Guidelines*).

Prior Shoulder Dystocia

Women with prior shoulder dystocia are at much higher risk (about 12%) of recurrence (33,34) (see chap. 23, *Obstetric Evidence Based Guidelines*). In the general obstetric population, the likelihood of brachial plexus injury is 1.4/1000 births, but among women who had prior shoulder dystocia and deliver vaginally, it is 13/1000 if there is no recurrent dystocia. If there is recurrent shoulder dystocia, the likelihood of brachial plexus injury is 45/1000 (34).

There are no randomized trials (2) on how to manage these pregnancies, but it is reasonable to discuss cesarean delivery at term when managing a patient with a prior shoulder dystocia because the likelihood of recurrent shoulder dystocia is quite high (12% vs. 1% in general population) as is the risk of neurologic injury (see chap. 23, *Obstetric Evidence Based Guidelines*).

REFERENCES

1. Boulet SL, Alexander GR, Salihu H, et al. Macrosomic birth in the United States: determinant, outcomes, and proposed grades of risk. Am J Obstet Gynecol 2003; 188:1372–1378. [Level II-1]
2. Chauhan SP, Grobman WA, Gherman RA, et al. Suspicion and treatment of the macrosomic fetus: a review. Am J Obstet Gynecol 2005; 193:332–346. [Level III]
3. Martin JA, Hamilton BE, Sutton PD, et al. Births: Final Data for 2008. Natl Vital Stat Rep 2010; 59. [Epidemiologic data]
4. Statistics Denmark. Live births and stillbirths by weight of birth. 1998 and 2008 data. Available at: http://www.statbank.dk. [Epidemiologic data]
5. Serirat S, Deerochanawong C, Sunthornthepvarakul T, et al. Gestational diabetes mellitus. J Med Assoc Thai 1992; 75:315–319. [Level II-3]
6. Martin TC, Clarke A. A case control study of the prevalence of perinatal complications associated with fetal macrosomia in Antigua and Barbuda. West Indian Med J 2003; 52:231–234. [Level II-3]
7. Mikulandra F, Stojnic E, Perisa M, et al. Fetal macrosomia—pregnancy and delivery. Zentralbl Gynakol 1993; 115:553–561. [Level II-3]
8. American College of Obstetricians and Gynecologists: Fetal macrosomia. ACOG Practice Bulletin No. 22. Washington DC: ACOG, 2000. [Level III]
9. Chauhan SP, Martin RW, Morrison JC. Intrapartum hydramnios at term and perinatal outcome. J Perinatol 1993; 13:186–189. [Level II-2]
10. Myles TD, Santolaya J. Maternal and neonatal outcomes in patients with a prolonged second stage of labor. Obstet Gynecol 2003; 102:52–58. [Level II-2]
11. Crowther CA, Hiller JE, Moss JR, et al. Effect of treatment of gestational diabetes mellitus on pregnancy outcomes. N Engl J Med 2005; 352:2477–2486. [RCT, *n* = 1000. Impaired glucose tolerance (defined following 75-g OGTT as fasting <7.0 mmol/L, 2 hour between 7.8 mmol/L and 11.0 mmol/L). Diet, glucose monitoring, and insulin as needed vs. routine care]
12. de Veciana M, Major CA, Morgan MA, et al. Postprandial versus preprandial blood glucose monitoring in women with gestational diabetes mellitus requiring insulin therapy. N Engl J Med 1995; 333:1237–1241. [RCT, *n* = 66]

13. Murphy H, Rayman G, Lewis K, et al. Effectiveness of continuous glucose monitoring in pregnant women with diabetes: randomised clinical trial. Br Med J 2008; 337:a1680. [RCT, *n* = 71]

14. Bonomo M, Cetin I, Pisoni MP, et al. Flexible treatment of gestational diabetes modulated on ultrasound evaluation of intrauterine growth: a controlled randomized clinical trial. Diabetes Metab 2004; 30:237–244. [RCT, *n* = 229]

15. Bonomo M, Corica D, Mion E, et al. Evaluating the therapeutic approach in pregnancies complicated by borderline glucose intolerance: a randomized clinical trial. Diabet Med 2005; 1536–1541. [RCT, *n* = 300]

16. Landon M, Sponge C, Thom E, et al. A multicenter, randomized trial of treatment for mild gestational diabetes. N Engl J Med 2009; 361:1339–1348. [RCT, *n* = 958]

17. Nachum Z, Ben-Shlomo I, Weiner E, et al. Twice daily versus four times daily insulin dose regimens for diabetes in pregnancy: randomised controlled trial. Br Med J 1999; 319:1223–1227. [RCT, *n* = 392]

18. Langer O, Conway DL, Berkus MD, et al. A comparison of glyburide and insulin in women with gestational diabetes mellitus. N Engl J Med 2000; 343:1134–1138. [RCT, *n* = 404]

19. Nicholson W, Bolen S, Witkop CT, et al. Benefits and risks of oral diabetes agents compared with insulin in women with gestational diabetes: a systematic review. Obstet Gynecol 2009; 113:193–205. [Meta-analysis; 9 studies of which 4 RCTs, *n* = 1229]

20. No authors. A clinical trial of induction of labor versus expectant management in postterm pregnancy. The National Institute of Child Health and Human Development Network of Maternal-Fetal Medicine Units. Am J Obstet Gynecol 1994; 170:716–723. [RCT, *n* = 440]

21. Hendrix NW, Grady CS, Chauhan SP. Clinical vs sonographic estimate of birth weight in term parturients: a randomized clinical trial. J Reprod Med 2000; 45:317–322. [RCT, *n* = 758]

22. Gonen R, Spiegel D, Abend M. Is macrosomia predictable, and are shoulder dystocia and birth trauma preventable? Obstet Gynecol 1996; 88:526–529. [Level II-1]

23. Gonen R, Bader D, Ajami M. Effects of a policy of elective cesarean delivery in cases of suspected fetal macrosomia on the incidence of brachial plexus injury and the rate of cesarean delivery. Am J Obstet Gynecol 2000; 183:1296–1300. [Level II-1]

24. Irion O, Boulvain M. Induction of labour for suspected fetal macrosomia. Cochrane Database Syst Rev 2005; 4. [Meta-analysis; 3 RCTs, *n* = 372—includes ref. 19]

25. Sanchez-Ramos L, Bernstein S, Kaunitz AM. Expectant management versus labor induction for suspected fetal macrosomia: a systematic review. Obstet Gynecol 2002; 100:997–1002. [Meta-analysis; 11 studies, of which 2 RCTs; *n* = 3751]

26. Boulvain M, Stan C, Irion O. Elective delivery in diabetic pregnant women. Cochrane Database Syst Rev 2001; (2):CD001997. [Meta-analysis, *n* = 200]

27. Witkop C, Neale D, Wilson LM, et al. Active compared with expectant delivery management in women with gestational diabetes: a systematic review. Obstet Gynecol 2009; 113(1):206–217. [Meta-analysis; 5 studies of which 1 RCT, *n* = 200]

28. Conway DL, Langer O. Elective delivery of infants with macrosomia in diabetic women: reduced shoulder dystocia versus increased cesarean deliveries. Am J Obstet Gynecol 1998; 178:922–925. [Level II-1]

29. Phelan JP, Eglinton GS, Horenstein JM, et al. Previous cesarean birth. Trial of labor in women with macrosomic infants. J Reprod Med 1984; 29:36–40. [Level II-1]

30. Flamm BL, Goings JR. Vaginal birth after cesarean section: Is suspected fetal macrosomia a contraindication? Obstet Gynecol 1989; 74:694–697. [Level II-1]

31. Zelop CM, Shipp TD, Repke JT, et al. Outcomes of trial of labor following previous cesarean delivery among women with fetuses weighing > 4000 g. Am J Obstet Gynecol 2001; 185:903–905. [Level II-1]

32. Elkousy MA, Sammel M, Stevens E, et al. The effect of birth weight on vaginal birth after cesarean delivery success rates. Am J Obstet Gynecol 2003; 188:824–830. [Level II-1]

33. Lewis DF, Raymond RC, Perkins MB, et al. Recurrence rate of shoulder dystocia. Am J Obstet Gynecol 1995; 172:1369–1371. [Level II-2]

34. Bingham J, Chauhan SP, Hayes E, et al. Recurrent shoulder dystocia: a review. Obstet Gynecol Surv 2010; 65:183–188. [Level II-2]

46

Cytomegalovirus

Timothy J. Rafael

KEY POINTS

- Cytomegalovirus (CMV) is the most common cause of viral intrauterine infection, affecting **0.5% to 2.5% of all neonates.**
- In most of the cases, pregnant women acquire CMV by **exposure to children** in their home or from occupational exposure to children.
- Approximately **2% of immunoglobulin G (IgG)-negative women acquire CMV infection during pregnancy.** Approximately **1/3 (range 30–75%) of pregnant women with a primary infection transmit CMV infection to their fetus.** The rate of transmission increases with increase in gestational age (highest in the third trimester), but the severity of disease is instead inversely proportional to gestational age (the infant is most affected when maternal infection is in first trimester). Overall, about **15% to 20% of infected infants develop sequelae** (so about 5–8% of infants of infected mothers have sequelae).
- Complications of affected infants with congenital CMV infection include jaundice, petechiae ("blueberry muffin baby"), thrombocytopenia, hepatosplenomegaly, growth restriction, microcephaly, intracranial calcifications, non-immune hydrops, and preterm birth, as well as late complications such as hearing loss, mental retardation, delay in psychomotor development, chorioretinitis, optic atrophy, seizures, expressive language delays, and learning disabilities. Long-term mortality is about 10% to 30%.
- **Prevention (including avoiding intimate contact with children, frequent handwashing, and glove use) is associated with an 84% decrease in CMV seroconversion during pregnancy.**
- CMV screening in pregnancy is not routinely recommended in most countries, until an appropriate fetal intervention is proven to decrease neonatal disease in cases of maternal CMV infection.
- **Maternal diagnosis of CMV infection is by serum IgM+.**
- **Fetal diagnosis of CMV infection is by detection of virus in amniotic fluid (AF) by polymerase chain reaction (PCR) testing.**
- Presence or absence of **fetal abnormalities on ultrasound** can help counseling (Table 46.1), but ultrasound is very insensitive and poorly predictive of an affected (symptomatic) child.
- There are no trials to assess the effectiveness of any intervention aimed at preventing congenital CMV. Gancyclovir and CMV-specific hyperimmune globulin are not supported by sufficient evidence for recommendation, but are the most promising interventions reported so far.

PATHOGEN
CMV is a double-stranded DNA virus of the herpes family (1).

INCIDENCE/EPIDEMIOLOGY
CMV is the most common cause of viral intrauterine infection, affecting **0.5% to 2.5% of all neonates** in different parts of the world (2). The birth prevalence of symptomatic congenital CMV is about 1 in 1000 (3). The prevalence of CMV infection varies according to socioeconomic background. Overall in the United States, the seropositivity rate is approximately 50%; by background, it is 40% to 50% for women of middle and high, and 60% to more than 80% for women of lower socioeconomic background. The overall age-adjusted seroprevalence of CMV did not change significantly from 1988–1994 to 1999–2004 (4).

TRANSMISSION/RISK FACTORS/ASSOCIATIONS
Transmission usually occurs from close contact, with contamination from urine, saliva, blood, semen, and cervical secretions (3). Risk factors are low socioeconomic status, exposure to infective individuals, multiple partners, extremes of age, multiparity, and blood transfusion. Only cellular blood products that contain leukocytes are capable of transmitting CMV, and the risk factor is 0.1% to 0.4% per unit in immunocompetent recipients (5). The incidence of cases with congenital disease following maternal recurrent infection has been shown to be increased with immunodeficiency, hormonal exposure, nutritional deficiency, and genital tract infections (6). Although sexual transmission of CMV can occur, **in most cases pregnant women acquire CMV by exposure to children in their home or from occupational exposure to children**. Data extrapolated to the U.S. population estimate that every two years between 31,000 and 168,000 susceptible pregnant women will be exposed to CMV by an infected child (7).

SYMPTOMS
CMV is usually asymptomatic or with symptoms so mild that it goes undiagnosed. The symptoms might include a mononucleosis-like or flu-like syndrome, malaise, fatigue, lymphadenopathy, or persistent fever, and abnormal laboratory values (lymphocytosis, or increased aminotransferase levels). Rarely, hepatosplenomegaly, cough, headache, rash, and gastrointestinal symptoms can occur (8). The presence of symptoms or laboratory abnormalities is highly suggestive of primary infection (9).

PATHOPHYSIOLOGY/CLASSIFICATION
General
The CMV virus leads to infected large cells with intranuclear inclusions. It has a 4- to 8-week period of incubation, and 3- to 12-month-long viremia (infants can shed virus for up to 6 years). Serious disease occurs only in immunocompromised adults, or fetuses. The transmission of the virus to the fetus can

follow either a primary or recurrent infection. **Approximately 2% of immunoglobulin G (IgG)-negative women acquire CMV infection during pregnancy. Approximately 1/3 (range 30–75%) of pregnant women with a primary infection transmit CMV infection to their fetus** (Fig. 46.1) (10). Even periconception infection a week before or up to five weeks after the last menstrual period (LMP) is associated with this rate of transmission, although these rates may not be as high as previously thought (11). **The rate of transmission increases with increase in gestational age (highest in third trimester) but the severity of disease is instead inversely proportional to gestational age (infant is most affected when maternal infection is in first trimester)**. In fact, one series reported no affected neonates if fetuses were infected after 26 weeks, if the ultrasound findings are normal (12). The risk of congenital CMV disease at birth is mainly associated with maternal primary infection, but the presence of maternal antibodies before conception does not prevent transmission in all cases, even if it is protective in most cases.

Primary Infection

Fetal infection generally (99.5%) occurs following maternal primary infection, and rarely following recurrent CMV infection (Fig. 46.1). Of the women who are not immune (IgG–, IgM–) for CMV at the beginning of pregnancy, about 2% acquire maternal infection. Transplacental transmission may occur weeks or months after primary maternal CMV infection, and can be isolated from the AF by a PCR DNA technique to positively identify intrauterine transmission of CMV. **Overall, about 15% to 20% of infected infants develop sequelae (so about 5–8% of infants of infected mothers have sequelae)**.

Recurrent Infection

Recurrent infections can occur with immunosuppression and during pregnancy. Recurrent infections during pregnancy are most often asymptomatic and primarily caused by the reactivation of the endogenous virus, but can also be caused by a low-grade chronic infection or reinfection by a different strain of CMV (13). The risk of vertical transmission with recurrent infection is about 1.4% (range 0.5–2%) (10). Recurrent infection is responsible for only 0.5% of CMV congenital infections. Neonates infected from recurrent maternal infection have no symptoms at birth, do not have CMV in urine, and have a <10% risk of sequelae (hearing loss and chorioretinitis) (8).

Clinical Neonatal Findings and Complications

Clinical findings of symptomatic congenital CMV infection include jaundice, petechiae (blueberry muffin baby), thrombocytopenia, hepatosplenomegaly, growth restriction, microcephaly, intracranial calcifications, nonimmune hydrops, and preterm birth (1,14). CMV disease has late complications such as hearing loss, mental retardation, delay in psychomotor development, chorioretinitis, optic atrophy, seizures, expressive language delays, and learning disabilities (2). CMV is the most common cause of congenital sensorineural hearing loss (15). Long-term mortality is about 10% to 30%.

PREGNANCY MANAGEMENT
Counseling/Prognosis

Counseling should include at least the natural history of the disease, the chances of vertical transmission, prognosis, and complications (Fig. 46.1, and Table 46.1). A quantitative PCR count of $\geq 10^3$ genome equivalents/mL of AF is a certain sign of congenital infection, and $\geq 10^5$ genome equivalents/mL can predict symptomatic infection (16) (Fig. 46.2). In cases of severely injured fetuses on ultrasound, there is a high likelihood of sequelae, and pregnancy termination can be offered as a management option (17). When no ultrasonographic abnormalities are detected, the incidence of postnatal neurologic abnormalities is about 15% to 20% (16,18).

Prevention
Hygiene

Compared with no prevention, **prevention (including avoiding intimate contact with children, frequent handwashing, and glove use) is associated with an 84% decrease in CMV seroconversion during pregnancy**, especially in women in contact with children in day care facilities (19). Following the administration of oral and written hygienic information to susceptible pregnant women, seroconversion rates during pregnancy have been reported to be as low as 0.26% (20).

Vaccine

A live-attenuated CMV vaccine is available, but may be reactivated, and safety issues have not been resolved. In a trial including CMV-seronegative women of childbearing age, a **glycoprotein B vaccine demonstrated a 50% efficacy in preventing CMV infection**. One congenital infection occurred in the vaccine group, and three infections occurred in the placebo group, although the sample size was not large enough to test the efficacy in reducing congenital infection (21). While this vaccine may have the potential to decrease incident cases of congenital CMV infection, it is likely that a CMV vaccine will not be available clinically for several years.

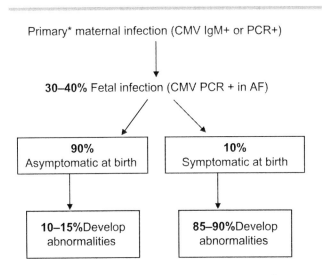

Figure 46.1 Natural history of CMV perinatal infection. *Abbreviations*: CMV, cytomegalovirus; PCR, polymerase chain reaction; IgM, immunoglobulin M; AF, amniotic fluid.

Table 46.1   Chance of Affected (i.e., Symptomatic) Neonate Depending on Clinical Scenario of CMV Infection

Maternal	Fetal	Ultrasound	Affected infant (%)
Confirmed infection (e.g., seroconversion, with positive IgM)	Unknown	Normal	5–7% (3)
	Unknown	Abnormal	35% (24)
	Confirmed infection (e.g., positive AF PCR)	Normal	14% (3)
	Confirmed infection (e.g., positive AF PCR)	Abnormal	78% (24)

Abbreviations: AF, amniotic fluid; PCR, polymerase chain reaction.

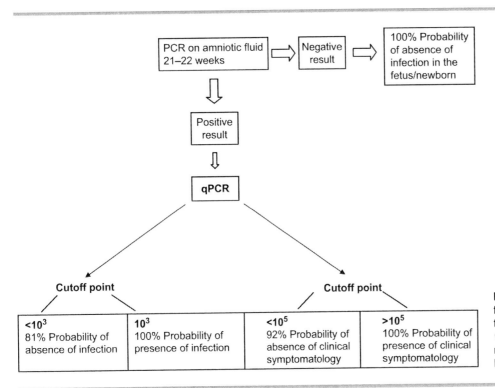

Figure 46.2   Assessment of chance of fetal infection and long-term complications by quantitative PCR in AF. *Abbreviations*: PCR, polymerase chain reaction; AF, amniotic fluid. *Source*: From Ref. 16.

Screening

Serum

CMV screening in pregnancy is not routinely recommended in most countries, even in women who are seronegative, mainly given the lack of proven intervention if seroconversion is detected (6).

If an appropriate fetal intervention is proven to decrease neonatal disease in cases of CMV, screening with IgM and IgG levels should be performed on all pregnant women between 8 and 12 weeks. IgM is 75% sensitive, and persists for four to eight months. Seronegative women should be provided with basic information on how to avoid infection (20). A second and possibly a third antibody control at 18 to 20 weeks and at 30 to 32 weeks could be recommended. IgG-positive and IgM-negative women with high IgG avidity index (e.g., >65%) could be assured of no risk of primary infection, which causes the majority of sequelae in the fetus (22). No further controls would be necessary (2).

Ultrasound Fetal Findings

These findings are growth restriction, ventriculomegaly, oligohydramnios, echogenic bowel, choroid plexus cyst (unilateral), pleural effusion, brain and liver calcification, and hydrops fetalis (16). Microcephaly, hydrocephaly, and intracranial calcifications are signs of high risk for neonatal

sequelae (2). A fetal cerebral periventricular "halo" seen on ultrasound examination is also suggestive of fetal infection, and may be associated with white-matter lesions (23). The limitations of ultrasound are well known. Fetal abnormalities may become evident late, change or disappear during pregnancy, **and not all symptoms of congenital inclusion disease are detectable by ultrasound**. Ultrasound detects fetal abnormalities in only 8.5% of women with primary CMV infection, and in 15% of congenitally CMV-infected fetuses. If fetal ultrasound abnormalities are detected, symptomatic CMV infection is present in 35% of neonates of primary-infected mothers, and 78% of congenitally infected neonates (Table 46.1) (24).

Investigations/Diagnosis/Workup

Maternal primary CMV infection is diagnosed by IgM+ serum, which persists for four to eight months. Although seroconversion is a reliable method for diagnosing primary CMV infection, the diagnosis can be problematic. The rise in CMV-specific antibodies may be delayed for up to four weeks, and the presence of CMV-specific IgM can be found in up to 10% of women with recurrent disease. Although CMV can be transmitted to the fetus both by primary and secondary (recurrent) infection, invasive prenatal diagnosis should be offered to women with primary infection, as they are at higher risk for fetal infection. In recurrent infection, the presence of maternal CMV IgG offers good protection, and fetal infection occurs only in 0.5% to 1% of cases (25).

At present, **detection of virus in AF by PCR testing is the most accurate means of diagnosis for CMV infection in the fetus**, with sensitivities ranging from 80% to 100% (18). Amniocentesis provides a direct method of diagnosing intrauterine CMV infection because the infected fetus excretes the virus via urine into AF. The sensitivity of detecting a true infection by sampling the AF increases after 21 weeks gestation and after a minimum of 6 weeks interval following maternal primary infection, so that if an amniocentesis is performed before this interval, it should be repeated later (6,18). It does not appear that amniocentesis, in and of itself, is implicated in iatrogenic CMV infection of the fetus (26).

CMV DNA detected in AF reveals a history of viremia but it does not directly demonstrate the current fetal condition (15). Quantitative PCR in amniotic fluid can help predict infection and later sequelae (Fig. 46.2). Infected fetuses may also have abnormal ultrasound findings. Normal fetal ultrasound does not rule out severe neurological damage. Percutaneous umbilical blood sampling (PUBS) should be avoided, and has been used in the past to diagnose the fetus with a high suspicion for CMV and negative PCR. The use of viral culture has decreased, also because it takes 2 to 6 weeks to obtain final results.

Neonatal diagnosis is based on detection of PCR in body fluids, in particular in urine.

Therapy

There has been no randomized trial on intervention to prevent maternal and/or fetal CMV infection in pregnancy. There is only one trial on treatment of proven fetal infection.

CMV-Specific Hyperimmune Globulin

There is insufficient evidence to recommend CMV-specific hyperimmune globulin for prevention or treatment of CMV congenital infection. In a nonrandomized study, CMV hyperimmune globulin IV 100 U/kg every month until delivery to the mother for prevention of vertical transmission in primary maternal CMV infection was associated with a decrease in the incidence of infected neonates from 40% in controls to 16% (27). Maternal CMV hyperimmune globulin 200 U/kg IV to the mother (with additional AF or umbilical cord infusions for persistent ultrasound findings) for therapy of known CMV DNA + fetuses was associated with a decrease in the incidence of symptomatic CMV disease at birth from 50% in controls to 3% (27). Follow-up to this study demonstrated a resolution of abnormal ultrasound findings in three treated fetuses, who subsequently had normal sensory, mental, and motor development at four to seven years of age (28). In the original study, almost all these women were infected in the first or second trimester, so efficacy in the third trimester is unknown. A case of resolution of hydrops secondary to CMV fetal infection with CMV-specific hyperimmune globulin has been reported (29).

Hyperimmune globulin appeared less effective for the prevention of fetal infection than for the treatment of fetuses already infected. An explanation to this outcome is that the mechanism of action of hyperimmune globulin differs in the prevention and in the therapy group. For the prevention of fetal infection, it presumably reduces maternal systemic or placental viral loads. Once the fetus is infected, hyperimmune globulin reduces placental or fetal inflammation, or both, resulting in increased fetal blood flow with enhanced fetal nutrition and oxygenation. Treatment with hyperimmune globulin acts by decreasing the number and percentage of both NK (natural killer) cells and HLA (human leukocyte antigen)-DR+ cells (27). Interestingly, this therapy is not effective in prevention of vertical transmission of HIV.

Ganciclovir and Valacyclovir

Ganciclovir inhibits viral DNA polymerase, and has been used successfully in adults, especially immunocompromised (AIDS, transplant, etc.) patients. A trial demonstrated reduction of hearing loss in neonates with proven congenital CMV infection with CNS involvement when treatment was begun within one month of birth (30). There are no controlled trials evaluating fetal therapy with ganciclovir. Ganciclovir administration into the umbilical vein and anti-CMV IgG injections into the fetal abdominal cavity have been reported in case reports (15), as has ganciclovir given orally to a pregnant woman with CMV DNA in the AF, but the evaluation of the prognosis is not well established; case reports have shown no teratogenicity of ganciclovir given in the early stages of pregnancy (31).

Valacyclovir (8g/day orally for 7 weeks) given to women with congenitally CMV-infected fetuses at about 30 weeks of gestations was associated with about a 50% normal child outcome at 1 to 5 years of age in one study (32).

Currently, there is a systematic review underway assessing both the benefits and harms of interventions used during pregnancy to prevent vertical transmission of CMV, as well as the efficacy of these interventions in reducing adverse outcomes in congenitally infected newborns/infants (33).

REFERENCES

1. ACOG Practice bulletin. Clinical Management Guidelines for Obstetrician-Gynecologists. No 20, Sept 2000. [Review]
2. Azam A-Z, Vial Y, Fawer CL, et al. Prenatal diagnosis of congenital CMV infection. Obstet Gynecol 2001; 97:443–448. [II-2]
3. Bhide A, Papageoghiou AT. Managing primary CMV infection in pregnancy. BJOG 2008; 115:805–807. [Review]
4. Lewis Bate S, Dollard SC, Cannon MJ. Cytomegalovirus seroprevalence in the United States: the national health and nutrition examination surveys, 1988-2004. Clin Infect Dis 2010; 50(11):1439–1447. [III]
5. Triulzi DJ. Transfusion transmitted cytomegalovirus. Available at: http://www.itxm.org/archive/tmu8-94.htm. [II-3; web document]
6. Henrich W, Meckies J, Dudenhausen JW, et al. Recurrent CMV infection during pregnancy: ultrasonographic diagnosis and fetal outcome. Ultrasound Obstet Gynecol 2002; 19:608–611. [II-3]
7. Marshall BC, Adler SP. The frequency of pregnancy and exposure to cytomegalovirus infections among women with a young child in day care. Am J Obstet Gynecol 2009; 200:163.e1–163.e5. [III]
8. Nigro G. Maternal-fetal cytomegalovirus infection: from diagnosis to therapy. J Matern Fetal Neonatal Med 2009; 22(2):169–174. [Review]
9. Nigro G, Anceschi MM, Cosmi EV. Clinical manifestations and abnormal laboratory findings in pregnant women with primary cytomegalovirus infection. BJOG 2003; 110:572–577. [II-3]
10. Kenneson A, Cannon MJ. Review and meta-analysis of the epidemiology of congenital cytomegalovirus (CMV) infection. Rev Med Virol 2007; 17:253–276. [Review]
11. Hadar E, Yogev Y, Melamed N, et al. Periconceptional cytomegalovirus infection: pregnancy outcome and rate of vertical transmission. Prenat Diagn 2010; 30:1213–1216. [II-3]
12. Gindes L, Teperberg-Oikawa M, Sherman D, et al. Congenital cytomegalovirus infection following primary maternal infection in the third trimester. BJOG 2008; 115:830–835. [II-2]
13. Boppana SH, Rivera L, Fowler KB, et al. Intrauterine transmission of CMV to infants of women with preconceptional immunity. N Engl J Med 2001; 344:1366–1371. [II-3]

14. Kylat RI, Kelly EN, Ford-Jones EL. Clinical findings and adverse outcome in neonates with symptomatic congenital cytomegalovirus (SCCMV) infection. Eur J Pediatr 2006; 165:773–778. [II-3]

15. Matsuda H, Kawakami Y, Furaya K, et al. Intrauterine therapy for a CMV infected symptomatic fetus. BJOG 2004; 111:756–757. [II-3]

16. Lipitz S, Achiron R, Zalen Y, et al. Outcome of pregnancies with vertical transmission of primary CMV infection. ACOG. Obstet Gynecol 2002; 100:428–433. [II-3]

17. Liesnard C, Donner C, Brancart F, et al. Prenatal diagnosis of congenital CMV infection: prospective study of 237 pregnancies at risk. Obstet Gynecol 2000; 95:881–888. [II-2]

18. Oshiro BR. CMV infection in pregnancy. Contemp Obstet Gynecol 1999; 11:16–24. [Review]

19. Adler SP, Finney JW, Manganello AM, et al. Prevention of child-to-mother transmission of cytomegalovirus among pregnant women. J Pediatr 2004; 145:485–491. [RCT, $n = 166$]

20. Picone O, Vauloup-Fellous C, Cordier AG, et al. A 2-year study on cytomegalovirus infection during pregnancy in a French hospital. BJOG 2009; 116:818–823. [II-3]

21. Pass RF, Zhang C, Evans A, et al. Vaccine prevention of maternal cytomegalovirus infection. N Engl J Med 2009; 360:1191–1199. [I, RCT, $n = 464$]

22. Kanengisser-Pines B, Hazan Y, Pines G, et al. High cytomegalovirus IgG avidity is a reliable indicator of past infection in patients with positive IgM detected during the first trimester of pregnancy. J Perinat Med 2009; 37:15–18. [II-3]

23. Simonazzi G, Guerra B, Bonasoni P, et al. Fetal cerebral periventricular halo at midgestation: an ultrasound finding suggestive of fetal cytomegalovirus infection. Am J Obstet Gynecol 2010; 202:599.e1–599.e5. [II-3]

24. Guerra B, Simonazzi G, Puccetti C, et al. Ultrasound prediction of symptomatic congenital cytomegalovirus infection. Am J Obstet Gynecol 2008; 198:380.e1–380.e7. [II-3]

25. Guerra B, Lazzarotto T, Quarta S, et al. Prenatal diagnosis of symptomatic congenital CMV infection. Am J Ostet Gynecol 2000; 183:476–482. [II-2]

26. Revello MG, Furione M, Zavattoni M, et al. Human cytomegalovirus (HCMV) DNAemia in the mother at amniocentesis as a risk factor for iatrogenic HCMV infection of the fetus. J Infect Dis 2008; 197:593–596. [II-3]

27. Nigro G, Adler SP, La Torre R, et al. Passive immunization during pregnancy for Congenital CMV infection. N Engl J Med 2005; 353:1350–1362. [II-1]

28. Nigro G, La Torre R, Pentimalli H, et al. Regression of fetal cerebral abnormalities by primary cytomegalovirus infection following hyperimmunoglobulin therapy. Prenat Diagn 2008; 28:512–517. [II-3]

29. Moxley K, Knudson EJ. Resolution of hydrops secondary to cytomegalovirus after maternal and fetal treatment with human cytomegalovirus hyperimmune globulin. Obstet Gynecol 2008; 111:524–526. [Case report; III]

30. Kimberlin DW, Lin C-Y, Sanchez PJ, et al. Effect of ganciclovir therapy on hearing in symptomatic congenital cytomegalovirus disease involving the central nervous system: a randomized, controlled trial. J Pediatr 2003; 143:16–25. [RCT, $n = 42$]

31. Adler SP, Nigro G, Pereira L. Recent advances in the prevention and treatment of congenital cytomegalovirus infections. Semin Perinatol 2007; 31(1):10–18. [Review]

32. Jacquemard F, Yamamoto M, Costa J-M, et al. Maternal administration of valacyclovir in symptomatic intrauterine cytomegalovirus infection. BJOG 2007; 114:1113–1121. [II-2]

33. McCarthy FP, Giles ML, Rowlands S, et al. Antenatal interventions for preventing the transmission of cytomegalovirus (CMV) from the mother to fetus during pregnancy and adverse outcomes in the congenitally infected infant. Cochrane Database Syst Rev 2010; (2):CD008371. DOI: 10.1002/14651858.CD008371. [Meta-analysis]

47

Toxoplasmosis

Timothy J. Rafael

KEY POINTS

- Maternal infection starts with **ingestion** (from food, water, hands, or insects) **of cysts from uncooked/undercooked meat of infected animals** *or* **contact with oocysts from infected cats or contaminated soil.**
- Fetal/neonatal disease is **more severe if maternal infection occurs in the first trimester**, and the **incidence of maternal-fetal transmission is directly proportional to gestational age** (low in first trimester, high in third trimester).
- **Prevention** has been shown to **decrease the incidence of the disease**, and remains the **most important of interventions.**
- **Prenatal and/or neonatal screening** is controversial and is not adopted in most countries, because of low incidence, concerns with poor/difficult diagnosis, availability of diagnostic and therapeutic services, population compliance, and high risk of terminating false-positive fetuses.
- The principle method used to diagnose and evaluate timing of congenital infection is based on detection of specific antibodies and by monitoring the immune response. *Maternal infection* is **diagnosed by sending maternal serology to a reference laboratory.** *Fetal congenital infection* is **diagnosed by amniotic fluid (AF) polymerase chain reaction (PCR).**
- **Correct interpretation** of serologic testing carried out in a reference laboratory **decreases unnecessary anxiety and even terminations.**
- **If maternal infection** is confirmed by a reference laboratory, **start spiramycin 3 to 4 g/day.**
- **If AF PCR is positive,** start **sulfadiazine, pyrimethamine,** and **folinic acid.**

PATHOGEN

Toxoplasma gondii (TG) is an obligate intracellular protozoan (parasite).

INCIDENCE/EPIDEMIOLOGY

The incidence of *primary acute maternal infection* is 0.01% to 0.1% in the United States and United Kingdom. The prevalence of past infection is approximately 10% to 15% in the United States (1), as high as 44% in France/Europe (2), 50% to 70% in Latin American countries, and 5% to 35% in Asia, China, and Korea. Once immune, immunity lasts for life (3).

The incidence of *congenital infection* is 1 to 5 cases per 10,000 live births in France/Europe (4), and 1 in 1000 to 1 in 10,000 live births in the United States (5).

SYMPTOMS

Most of the times (almost always) there are no maternal symptoms; occasionally flu/mononucleosis-like fever, fatigue, rash, and lymphadenopathy (around head and neck) can be associated with maternal infection. Rarely pregnant women will present with visual changes due to chorioretinitis from recently acquired infection or reactivation of chronic infection (6).

PATHOPHYSIOLOGY

TG can infect any mammal, which serves as an intermediate host. The definitive host is the cat (only one that can support both sexual and asexual reproduction). The parasite can exist as

1. Trophozoite (invasive form)
2. Cyst (latent form)
3. Oocyst (only in cats: result of sexual reproduction, which occurs in the small intestine of a cat who has eaten outside tissue cysts containing TG)

Only during this first exposure is the cat infectious, as these oocysts are produced for two weeks and contain infectious sporozoites; the oocysts require one to five days to become infected; after two weeks the cat becomes immune and not infectious. In soil, oocysts can remain infectious for years. Human infection starts with **ingestion** (from food, water, hands, or insects) **of cysts from uncooked/undercooked meat of infected animals** (e.g., lamb and mutton) *or* **contact with oocysts from infected cats** (who get it from infected mice, etc.) **or contaminated soil.** The infected oocysts become infective inside the pregnant woman in 4 to 10 (average 7) days, leading to parasitemia. Eventually, TG can infect and live forever in striated muscle or brain. Only a very few cases of congenital toxoplasmosis transmitted by mothers who were infected prior to conception have been reported; they can be attributed to either reinfection with a different strain or to reactivation of chronic disease. This reactivation is very rare, but can occur especially in an immunocompromised woman. Immunocompetent women with prior toxoplasmosis can be reassured that the risks to the subsequent fetus/neonate are miniscule, especially >9 months after infection (3).

MATERNAL-FETAL TRANSMISSION

Primary maternal TG infection in pregnancy can lead to fetal infection, with this rate highly dependent on gestational age of maternal infection (3) (Table 47.1) (Fig. 47.1).

Of the congenitally infected fetuses—PCR positive by amniocentesis—about 74% to 81% manifest only subclinical infection (only serologically positive), whereas 19% to 26% have fetal/childhood illness even if they received treatment (7,8). Overall, about 7% of fetuses of primary infected mothers are affected. **Fetal/neonatal disease is more severe if maternal infection occurs in the first trimester** (but fetus has a <1/1000 risk of getting affected if ≤4 weeks gestational age at time of maternal infection), but more common if maternal infection occurs in the third trimester.

Table 47.1   Likelihood of Congenital Infection by Timing of Maternal Infection

Maternal infection	Probability of congenital infection (%)
Preconception[a]	1
First trimester	10–25
Second trimester	30–55
Third trimester	60–80

[a]Usually within nine months of conception.

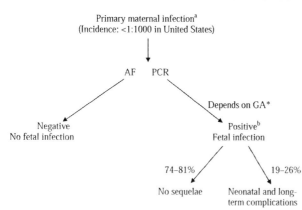

*See text for diagnosis.
[a]Start spiramycin.
[b]Stop spiramycin; start sulfadiazine, pyrimethamine, folic acid (except in first trimester).

Figure 47.1   Natural history of toxoplasmosis in pregnancy. *Abbreviations*: AF, amniotic fluid; PCR, polymerase chain reaction; GA, gestational age.

Table 47.2   Prevention of Congenital Toxoplasmosis

- Avoid raw or undercooked meat (or eggs) of any origin
- Avoid contact with raw meat or soil
- Wash fruits and vegetables before eating
- Cats: Avoid changing cat litter. Hand-wash after handling cat. Do not let cats outside the house (could eat infected mice). No stray cats in the house. No feeding raw meat to cats. Avoid raw milk.

needs to be provided to patients regarding avoidance of raw or undercooked meat, gardening, and washing fruits and vegetables (9). Prenatal education can effectively change pregnant women's behavior as it increases pet, personal, and food hygiene (10). There are no randomized trials on the effect of prenatal education on congenital toxoplasmosis rate, or toxoplasmosis seroconversion rate during pregnancy, but three observational studies consistently suggest that prenatal education might have a positive impact on these outcomes (11).

Screening
Serum
Routine toxoplasmosis screening programs for pregnant women have been established in some European countries such as France and Austria. In the United Kingdom and the United States no prenatal or neonatal screening for TG is formally recommended by appropriate medical societies, not without controversy (12). Prenatal maternal screening has not been recommended in the United States because of low incidence, concerns with poor/difficult diagnosis, availability of diagnostic and therapeutic services, population compliance, and high risk of terminating false-positive fetuses. If prenatal screening is implemented, it should start preconception or at least in the first trimester, and be repeated every month (or at least every trimester) in all IgG-negative mothers (Fig. 47.2). Neonatal screening in the United States would detect about one positive neonate for 12,000 screened mothers, with the possibility that treatment may prevent severe sequelae, but would probably not be cost-effective.

Ultrasound
Ultrasound findings associated with TG congenital infection can include intracranial calcifications, microcephaly, ventricular dilatation and hydrocephalus, ascites, hepatosplenomegaly, and increased placental thickness (13).

COMPLICATIONS
Fetal/neonatal complications (check by prenatal ultrasound) include ventriculomegaly (75%), increased placental thickness (32%), hepatomegaly (12%), ascites (15%), intracranial calcifications (18%), hydrocephalus (4%), microcephaly (5%), and hepatosplenomegaly (4%). Additionally, in the neonate, TG congenital infection is associated with neonatal chorioretinitis (26%) (8) (most prevalent consequence of TG), deafness, decreased IQ, and subsequent blindness, seizure disorders, and delay in neuropsychomotor development (3).

Congenital infection is also associated with an increased risk of preterm birth (PTB), but not intrauterine growth restriction (IUGR), when seroconversion occurs before 20 weeks. Stillbirth or neonatal death is rare.

PREGNANCY MANAGEMENT
Principles
Counseling regarding basic pathophysiology, maternal-fetal transmission, complications, and preventive/therapeutic management should be done. Termination can be offered, especially if the fetus is definitively positive (PCR-positive AF) and the infection occurred in the first trimester (worse prognosis).

Prevention
Prevention has been shown to decrease the incidence of the disease, and remains the most important of interventions (Table 47.2). While many U.S. obstetricians are counseling adequately regarding avoidance of cat litter, more information

Workup/Diagnosis
The principle method used to diagnose and evaluate the timing of congenital infection is based on detection of specific antibodies and monitoring the immune response (Fig. 47.2). *IgG antibodies* usually appear within two weeks of infection and persist in the body indefinitely. *IgM antibodies* are considered to be a sign of recent infection and can be detected by enzyme immunoassays (EIAs) or an immunosorbent agglutination assay test (IAAT) within two weeks of infection. They often remain positive for up to one to two years. **A positive IgM antibody test result** at any time **does not necessarily mean the infection was acquired recently; this needs to be confirmed at a reference laboratory**, in that only approximately 40% of positive IgM results obtained at nonreference laboratories in the United States are deemed to have had a recent acute infection (6). *IgA antibodies* may also persist for more than one year and their detection is informative mainly

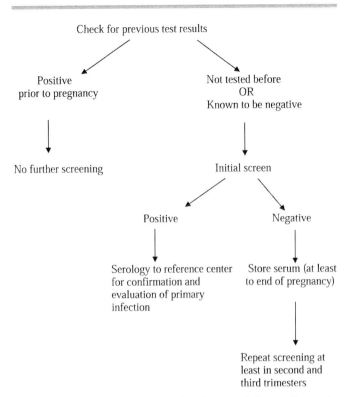

Figure 47.2 Laboratory diagnosis of congenital toxoplasmosis. *Source*: From Ref. 3.

for the diagnosis of congenital toxoplasmosis. *IgE antibodies* increase rapidly and remain detectable for less than four months after infection, which is a very short time to use them for a diagnostic test.

The **Sabin–Feldman dye test (SFDT) is still considered the "gold standard"** (3). It detects the presence of anti-TG-specific antibodies (total Ig). The absolute antibody titer is also important: values over 250 IU/mL are considered highly suggestive of recent infection. IgG avidity testing is based on the increase in functional affinity (avidity) between TG-specific IgG and antigen over time, as the host immune response evolves. Pregnant women with high avidity antibodies are those who have been infected at least three to five months earlier (14). Current testing cannot define which specific strain of TG caused the antibody response, so that reinfection with the same or different strains cannot be determined.

Maternal infection **is diagnosed by sending maternal serology to a reference laboratory** (in the United States: Jack Remington, Palo Alto: 650-853-4828; FAX 650-614-3292; http://www.pamf.org/serology/clinicianguide.html). It is best to make the diagnosis based on two different serum specimens collected at least four weeks apart. Usually, the reference laboratory reports many serologic results, with a high possibility of infection if there is

- seroconversion during pregnancy;
- increase in both specific IgG titer (>3-fold) and dye test titer (>3-fold);
- presence of specific IgM and dye test ≥300 IU/mL.

Correct interpretation of serologic testing done in a reference laboratory decreases unnecessary anxiety and even terminations (15).

Fetal congenital infection **is diagnosed by AF PCR**. The specificity and positive predictive value on AF samples are close to 100%; the sensitivity is around 70% to 80%, but is best when maternal infection occurs between 17 and 21 weeks of pregnancy. Real-time PCR appears to have a sensitivity of 92%, negative predictive value of 98%, and may not be as gestational-age dependent as conventional PCR (16). However, a negative AF PCR does not always completely rule out congenital infection. AF PCR should obviously be done after 15 weeks. Ultrasound can also aid in diagnosis of fetal infection (see section "Complications"), but it has very poor sensitivity and specificity.

Therapy

If maternal infection is detected, counsel regarding the risks, along with possibility of termination (especially in first trimester), and management.

If maternal infection is confirmed by a reference laboratory, start spiramycin 3 to 4 g/day (1 g every eight hours). This is available in the United States only by the Food and Drug Administration (FDA) when Palo Alto serology is positive. Spiramycin concentrates in the placenta, and therefore may not be reliable for treatment of infection in the fetus (6).

If AF PCR is positive, start **sulfadiazine** (initial dose of 75 mg/kg, followed by 50 mg/kg q12h with maximum of 4 g/day), **pyrimethamine** (50 mg po q12h for two days followed by 50 mg daily), and **folinic acid** (leucovorin) 10 to 20 mg with each dose of pyrimethamine (decreases bone marrow toxicity) and one week after completion of pyrimethamine therapy (6). Length of therapy is controversial, and has varied for a minimum of 28 days (with ½ dose until term), versus continuing therapy as is until term. Treatment with pyrimethamine and sulfadiazine to prevent fetal infection is contraindicated during the first trimester (pyrimethamine is teratogenic), but at this time sulfadiazine can be used alone (17,18). This treatment should be stopped in the last few weeks of pregnancy. This is the basic treatment protocol recommended by the WHO and CDC (3). Other drugs such as spiramycin (3–4 g/day × 3–4 weeks) are recommended in certain circumstances. Spiramycin is used to prevent placental infection; it is used in European countries, but in the United States it is not approved by the FDA. Treatment decreases complications of TG, but possibly not fetal infection. It is estimated that for every three congenitally infected fetuses that are treated, one case of serious neurological sequela is prevented (19). In one study, fetuses/neonates treated and subsequently followed for 12 to 250 months had a 17% rate of congenital TG, with 74% of the children asymptomatic, 26% developing chorioretinitis (72% peripheral and unilateral), and all except one child having age-appropriate neurological and intellectual development (8). Despite these encouraging findings, well-designed randomized controlled trials are needed to elucidate the optimal treatment regimen and duration in affected pregnancies, especially given the varying gestational ages at which fetuses can become infected.

REFERENCES

1. Jones JL, Kruszon-Moran D, Sanders-Lewis K, et al. *Toxoplasma gondii* infection in the United States, 1999-2004, decline from the prior decade. Am J Trop Med Hyg 2007; 77:405–410. [III]
2. Berger F, Goulet V, Le Strat Y, et al. Toxoplasmosis among pregnant women in France: risk factors and change of prevalence between 1995 and 2003. Rev Epidemiol Sante Publique 2009; 57(4):241–248. [III]

3. Rorman E, Zamir CS, Rilkis I, et al. Congenital toxoplasmosis—prenatal aspects of *Toxoplasma gondii* infection. Reprod Toxicol 2006; 21(4):458–472. Epub 2005. [Review]

4. Villena I, Ancelle T, Delmas C, et al. Toxosurv network and National Reference Centre for Toxoplasmosis. Congenital toxoplasmosis in France in 2007: first results from a national surveillance system. Euro Surveill 2010; 15(25):1–6. [III]

5. Feldman DM, Timms D, Borgida AF. Toxoplasmosis, parvovirus, and cytomegalovirus in pregnancy. Clin Lab Med 2010; 30:709–720. [Review]

6. Montoya JG, Remington JS. Management of *Toxoplasma gondii* infection during pregnancy. Clin Infect Dis 2008; 47:554–566. [Review]

7. SYROCOT (Systematic Review on Congenital Toxoplasmosis) study group, Thiébaut R, Leproust S, Chêne G, et al. Effectiveness of prenatal treatment for congenital toxoplasmosis: a meta-analysis of individual patients' data. Lancet 2007; 369:115–122. [Meta-analysis: no RCTs, 26 cohorts, *n* = 691 infected liveborn infants]

8. Berrébi MD, Assouline C, Bessiéres M-H, et al. Long-term outcome of children with congenital toxoplasmosis. Am J Obstet Gynecol 2010; 203:552.e1–552.e6. [II-3]

9. Jones JL, Krueger A, Schulkin J, et al. Toxoplasmosis prevention and testing in pregnancy, survey of obstetrician-gynaecologists. Zoonoses Public Health 2010; 57(1):27–33. [III]

10. Carter AO, Gelmon SB, Wells GA, et al. The effectiveness of a prenatal education programme for the prevention of congenital toxoplasmosis. Epidemiol Infect 1989; 103:539–545. [Cluster RCT, *n* = 432]

11. Di Mario S, Basevi V, Gagliotti C, et al. Prenatal education for congenital toxoplasmosis. Cochrane Database Syst Rev 2009; (1): CD006171. [Meta-analysis, one cluster RCT, *n* = 432]

12. Neto EC. Newborn screening for congenital infectious diseases. Emerg Infect Dis 2004; 10:1068–1073. [II-3]

13. El Ayoubi M, de Bethmann O, Monset-Couchard M. Lenticulostriate echogenic vessels: clinical and sonographic study of 70 neonatal cases. Pediatr Radiol 2003; 33:697–703. [II-3]

14. Montoya JG, Liesenfeld O, Kinney S, et al. VIDAS test avidity of Toxoplasma specific immunoglobulin G for confirmatory testing of pregnant women. J Clin Microbial 2002; 40:2505–2508. [II-3]

15. Liesenfeld O, Montoya JC, Tathinemi NJ, et al. Confirmatory serologic testing for acute toxoplasmosis and rate of induced abortions among women reported to have positive Toxoplasma immunoglobulin M antibody titers. Am J Obstet Gynecol 2001; 184:140–145. [II-2]

16. Wallon M, Franck J, Thulliez P, et al. Accuracy of real-time polymerase chain reaction for *Toxoplasma gondii* in amniotic fluid. Obstet Gynecol 2010; 115:727–733. [III]

17. WHO Model Prescribing Information. Drugs Used in Parasitic Diseases, 2nd ed. Geneva: World Health Organization, 1995. [Review]

18. Chin J. Toxoplasmosis. In: Control of Communicable Disease Manual. 17th ed. Washington DC: American Public Health Association, 2000:500–503. [Review]

19. Cortina-Borja M, Tan HK, Wallon M, et al. Prenatal treatment for serious neurological sequelae of congenital toxoplasmosis: an observational prospective cohort study. PLoS Med 2010; 7(10): e1000351. [II-3]

48

Parvovirus

Timothy J. Rafael

KEY POINTS

- **The incidence of acute primary maternal parvovirus B19** infection during pregnancy is about **1% to 1.5%**.
- The major means of infection is by **contact with young infected children**. The infection is usually **asymptomatic** in the adult (and pregnant woman).
- About **25% to 30% of fetuses of mothers with primary parvovirus B19 infection become infected themselves by vertical transmission**.
- Perinatal complications of fetal infection occur in about 10% of fetuses, and include **fetal anemia, and myocarditis**, leading to **hydrops (2–6%), and** occasionally **fetal death** if infection occurs <20 weeks.
- Screening is not recommended, since 1/5000 screened women would be at risk for fetal hydrops from parvovirus B19.
- **Maternal infection is usually diagnosed by IgM+ or by IgG seroconversion**.
- **Fetal ultrasound** can screen for development of anemia and/or hydropic changes in the infected mother by increased **peak systolic velocity (PSV) of the middle cerebral artery (MCA)** using a **threshold of ≥1.50** multiples of the median (**MoM**). If MCA PSV values are <1.50 MoM, it is suggested to **continue weekly ultrasound scans for 10 to 12 weeks after the exposure**.
- **If MCA PSV is ≥1.50 or fetal hydrops** is seen on ultrasound, **fetal transfusion is indicated**, even though the incidence of spontaneous resolution of hydrops is about 30%, since survival with transfusion is >90%.
- Even in cases of fetuses transfused in utero for parvovirus B19-induced hydrops, some, but not all studies, report long-term outcome similar to normal controls. Patients should be counseled that there are differing data regarding long-term neurodevelopmental outcome among survivors.

PATHOGEN

Human parvovirus B19 is a single-stranded DNA virus. Parvovirus B19 is the only known parvovirus which is a human pathogen.

INCIDENCE/EPIDEMIOLOGY

The **incidence of acute primary maternal parvovirus B19** infection during pregnancy in susceptible women is about **1% to 1.5%** (1,2). The parvovirus B19-specific immunoglobulin G (IgG) seroconversion incidence in susceptible pregnant women (primary infection) goes from 1% to 1.5% during endemic to 13% to 13.5% during epidemic periods (2). Approximately 50% to 75% of women of reproductive age are IgG+ (immune) for parvovirus B19, with approximately 25% to 50%

of women being susceptible to parvovirus B19 infection during pregnancy (1).

RISK FACTORS/ASSOCIATIONS

The infection is more common in the winter and spring. The risk of infection is associated with the level of **contact with young infected children**. The highest infection rates occur in schoolteachers, day care workers, and women with nursery or school-aged children in the home. Around 50% to 80% of susceptible household members and 20% to 30% of individuals exposed in a classroom acquire acute infection from an infected child. Adverse prognostic factors are older maternal age, maternal immunity and seroconversion, raised maternal serum alpha-fetoprotein (MSAFP), and ultrasound findings.

SYMPTOMS

In adults at least half of the infections are **asymptomatic** (2). About 30% may have flulike symptoms, arthralgias, and adenopathy. Parvovirus B19 causes a common exanthematous disease in children 5 to 14 years old, called fifth disease or erythema infectiosum. Children have symptoms such as low-grade fever and "slapped-cheeks" rash, and are usually diagnosed just based on these symptoms.

PATHOPHYSIOLOGY

Parvovirus B19 is mainly transmitted by respiratory droplets. The incubation period for erythema infectiosum is 13 to 18 days, and infectivity is greatest 7 to 10 days before the onset of symptoms. The major target cells for parvovirus B19 are erythroid progenitors bearing the main cellular parvovirus B19 receptor P blood group antigen globoside on their surface (Fig. 48.1). The virus is believed to cause arrest of maturation of red blood cell (RBC) precursors at the late normoblast stage and causes a decrease in the number of platelets. The virus causes infection and lysis of erythroid progenitor cells by apoptosis, leading to hemolysis and transient aplastic crisis. Subsequent fetal anemia is thought to be responsible for the development of skin edema and effusions. Hepatitis, placentitis, and myocarditis leading to heart failure may contribute to the development of fetal hydrops (2–4). Parvovirus B19 has been demonstrated to carry an apoptosis-inducing factor and to induce cell-cycle arrest. Cells in the S-phase of DNA mitosis are particularly vulnerable to parvovirus B19 and the fetus is at risk because of the vast number of cells in active mitosis, shorter half-life of RBCs, and immature immune system.

MATERNAL-FETAL TRANSMISSION

About **25% to 30% of fetuses of mothers with primary parvovirus B19 infection become infected themselves by vertical transmission** (Fig. 48.2). About 90% have no sequelae

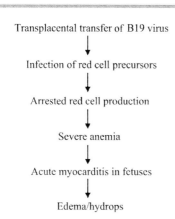

Figure 48.1 Pathophysiology of parvovirus B19 fetal infection.

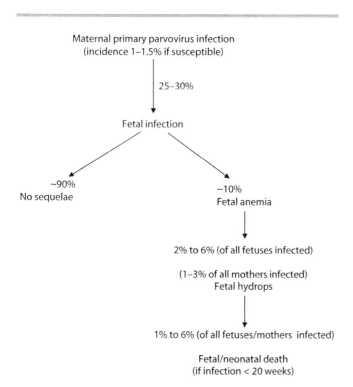

Figure 48.2 Natural history of parvovirus infection in pregnancy.

from this intrauterine infection (2). Although it is not easy to determine the exact timing of transmission of parvovirus B19 infection to the fetus, it is likely that parvovirus B19 infects the fetus during or immediately after maternal viremia, even in the early stages of gestation. Parvovirus B19 can persist until term or after birth, even when infection occurs early in gestation.

COMPLICATIONS
Of the infected fetuses, about 5% to 20% can develop **anemia**, of which 30% to 50% develop **hydrops fetalis** (about 2–6% of all infected fetuses), with some series showing hydrops rates as high as 66% of anemic fetuses (5) (Fig. 48.2). Some have reported a rate of 1% to 3% for fetal hydrops in infected mothers (3). The risk of **fetal death** is 1% to 6% of all infected fetuses (6). Fetal death occurs almost exclusively in hydropic

cases diagnosed at <20 weeks, especially if cases >20 weeks are treated with timely transfusion (90% survival) (6). Early embryonic/fetal death may manifest as miscarriage (about 10% of infected mothers <20 weeks). Although acute parvovirus infection may occur relatively commonly during pregnancy, an adverse fetal outcome is an uncommon complication (4,7,8). Rarely, parvovirus has been detected in fetuses with hydrocephalus (possibly from vasculitis), but it is unclear if malformations seen with parvovirus are just coincidental, and not related to the viral infection. Parvovirus B19 may be an important cause of fetal death, not always associated with fetal hydrops. **All cases of fetal death should be considered for testing for parvovirus B19 by polymerase chain reaction (PCR)**. Maternal serology might be a less sensitive determinant for parvovirus B19-associated fetal death, since immunoglobulin M (IgM) response generally lasts for two to four months, and parvovirus B19 infection can already be persistent in fetuses during the early stages of pregnancy, eventually leading to fetal death months later (see also chap. 54). The more mature immune response in older fetuses could delay any pathogenic consequences of parvovirus B19 infection, resulting in a lower rate of hydrops than in younger fetuses (9,10).

ULTRASOUND FETAL FINDINGS
Sonographically detectable markers of fetal compromise include pericardial or pleural effusion, ascites, abdominal wall/skin edema, bilateral hydroceles, oligohydramnios or hydramnios, increased (>95th percentile) cardiac biventricular outer diameter, and, rarely, hydrocephalus, microcephaly, and intracranial and hepatic calcifications (3,4).

PREGNANCY MANAGEMENT
Counseling/Prognosis
Counseling should include the natural history of the disease, including vertical transmission, chances of fetal disease (anemia and hydrops), prognosis, and possible interventions. The long-term outcome of fetuses affected after 20 weeks is very good.

Prevention
Avoidance of contact with infected children—or (better) children in general—is the best prevention. This is not always feasible. No specific antiviral therapy or vaccine is available for parvovirus B19 infection. Frequent hand washing is effective in preventing disease transmission (2). Intravenous immunoglobulin (IVIG) prophylaxis is reasonable to consider for documented exposures in immunocompromised patients, although it is not currently recommended for prophylaxis in pregnancy.

Screening
Universal screening is not recommended, as the risk of fetal hydrops from parvovirus infection is about 1/5000 screened pregnancies, making screening not warranted. Screening may be warranted in pregnant women who take care of young children, especially during epidemics (3).

Workup/Diagnosis
Workup includes determination of serum IgG and IgM. **Maternal infection is usually diagnosed by IgM+ or by IgG seroconversion.** IgM appears by 3 days of an acute infection, peaks at 25 to 30 days, and disappears by 4 months. Serum IgG appears a few days after IgM, and coincides with resolution of

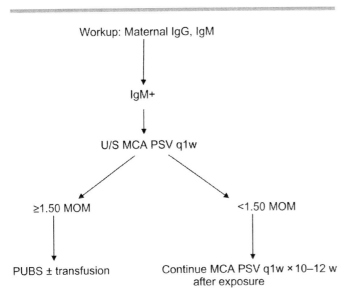

Figure 48.3 Management of parvovirus infection in pregnancy. *Abbreviations:* MCA, middle cerebral artery; IgG, immunoglobulin G; IgM, immunoglobulin M; PSV, peak systolic velocity; MoM, multiples of the median; PUBS, percutaneous umbilical blood sampling.

maternal symptoms. The detection of viral DNA by PCR is another means of diagnosis. Electron microscopy (EM) is also possible, whereas virus culture usually fails. Increased MSAFP has also been used as a prognostic factor for poor outcome (11), although this has been questioned in recent studies (5).

Once maternal infection has been diagnosed, **fetal ultrasound** can screen for development of anemia and/or hydropic changes. Anemia can be detected by increased **PSV of the MCA** prior to the appearance of sonographically detectable markers of hydrops (12). This is based on the observation (first in rhesus immunization, where the mechanism leading to anemia is different) that with fetal anemia there is an increase of fetal cardiac output to maintain adequate oxygen delivery to tissues, leading to increased blood flow velocities also in anemic fetuses with hydrops from parvovirus B19. MCA PSV using a **threshold of ≥1.50 MoM** has a high sensitivity (100%) and specificity (100%) for detecting fetal anemia (12). If MCA PSV values are <1.50 MoM, it is suggested to **continue weekly ultrasound scans for 10 to 12 weeks after the exposure** to follow those fetuses that potentially are at high risk for anemia and hydrops (Fig. 48.3). The peak incidence of hydrops is at about four to six weeks after maternal infection. Fetal surveillance should be initiated no later than four weeks after the onset of illness or estimate of seroconversion (2). In cases of elevated MCA PSV but no hydrops, surveillance should be increased with ultrasound scans two to three per week to detect any sign of hydrops, or umbilical cord sampling performed.

Fetal diagnosis is by amniotic fluid (AF) PCR+. There is at present no need for percutaneous umbilical blood sampling (PUBS) for diagnosis.

Therapy

There are **no trials** evaluating therapeutic interventions. **No antiviral therapy is available.**

Treatment should be directed at fetuses with abnormal MCA PSV and/or hydropic changes. In these fetuses, anemia

and even hydrops can resolve spontaneously over four to six weeks (about **30% spontaneous resolution for hydrops**) (13). Resolution is more common in older (>20 weeks) fetuses because of a more mature immune system.

Intervention for anemic and/or hydropic fetuses is gestational-age dependent:

- Between 24 and 33 6/7 weeks, steroids for fetal lung maturity should be given. Fetal cordocentesis to document anemia and transfusion as necessary improve outcome in anemic and/or hydropic fetuses. Frequently, one transfusion is sufficient (2,5).
- Before 24 weeks, with severe hydrops, termination may be offered, but transfusion can be beneficial, with apparently minimal to no significant sequelae if successful.
- After 34 weeks, delivery should be considered.

If cordocentesis is performed, anemia could be detected before a critical decrease of hemoglobin of <6 g/dL and before the development of severe hydrops. Blood sampling can allow testing for fetal hemoglobin/hematocrit and leukocyte and platelet counts. **Once sonographic signs of hydrops are present, transfusion is indicated using erythrocytes. Platelets** should also be ready at the time of PUBS, as multiple series have demonstrated a concomitantly high incidence of fetal thrombocytopenia at the time of transfusion (14,15). Several nonrandomized but controlled studies suggest a significant benefit of transfusion of fetuses with anemia and/or hydrops from parvovirus infection compared with conservative treatment (4,6,16). Intracardiac transfusion is a last resort alternative to intraumbilical cord transfusion, particularly when intraumbilical cord transfusion is not possible, because of risks of bradycardia and cardiac arrest of this procedure (17).

NEONATE AND LONG-TERM FOLLOW-UP

Infants born to IgM+ mothers are born IgG+ (mostly maternal), and 25% stay IgG+ at one year, as they were infected and have become immune. Regarding long-term outcome, while general health status of survivors is no different compared with the general population, there is conflicting evidence regarding incidences of developmental delay. Some trials illustrate an incidence of developmental delay similar to the general population even in cases of fetuses transfused in utero for parvovirus B19-induced hydrops (18,19). More recent data of survivors aged six months to eight years demonstrated a 32% incidence of psychomotor developmental delay, independent of pretransfusion hemoglobin, platelet, or blood pH values (20). **Patients need to be counseled regarding the overall uncertainty regarding long-term neurodevelopmental outcome among survivors.** Two phases of the infantile infection are described: a first phase of viremia of two to three days, accompanied by fever and myalgia; a second phase that can last several weeks, with dermatological signs such as erythema infectiosum, vasculitis, arthralgias, or arthritis. Long-term persistence of the virus in the neonate may be responsible for chronic manifestations.

REFERENCES

1. Mossong J, Hens N, Friederichs V, et al. Parvovirus B19 infection in five European countries: seroepidemiology, force of infection and maternal risk of infection. Epidemiol Infect 2008; 136:1059–1068. [II-3]
2. Lamont RF, Sobel JD, Vaisbuch E, et al. Parvovirus B19 infection in human pregnancy. BJOG 2011; 118:175–186. [Review]

3. Van Gessel PH, Gayvant MA, Vossen ACTM, et al. Incidence of parvovirus B19 infection among an unselected population of pregnant women in the Netherlands: a prospective study. Eur J Obstet Gynecol Reprod Biol 2006; 128:46–49. [II-3]

4. Von Kaisenberg CS, Jonat W. Fetal parvovirus B19. Ultrasound Obstet Gynecol 2001; 18:280–288. [II-3]

5. Simms RA, Liebling RE, Patel RR, et al. Management and outcome of pregnancies with parvovirus B19 infection over seven years in a tertiary fetal medicine unit. Fetal Diagn Ther 2009; 25:373–378. [II-3]

6. Enders M, Weidner A, Zoellner I, et al. Fetal morbidity and mortality after acute human parvovirus B19 infection in pregnancy: prospective evaluation of 108 cases. Prenatal Diagn 2004; 24:513–518. [II-2]

7. Sarfraz AA, Samuelsen SO, Bruu AL, et al. Maternal human parvovirus B19 infection and the risk of fetal death and low birthweight: a case-control study within 35,940 pregnant women. BJOG 2009; 116:1492–1498. [II-2]

8. Riipinen A, Väisänen E, Nuutila M, et al. Parvovirus B19 infection in fetal deaths. Clin Infect Dis 2008; 47:1519–1525. [II-2]

9. Tolfvenstam T, Papadogiannakis N, Norbeck O, et al. Frequency of human parvovirus B19 infection in intrauterine fetal death. Lancet 2001; 357:1494–1497. [II-2]

10. Skjoldbrand Sparre L, Tolfvenstam T, Papadogiannakis N. Association with the third trimester intrauterine fetal death. BJOG 2000; 107:476–480. [II-2]

11. Bernstein IM, Capeless IL. Elevated maternal serum alphafetoprotein and hydrops fetalis in association with fetal parvovirus B19 infection in the human fetus. BJOG 1989; 74:456–457. [II-2]

12. Cosmi E, Mari G, Delle Chiaie L, et al. Noninvasive diagnosis by Doppler ultrasonography of fetal anemia resulting from parvovirus infection. Am J Obstet Gynecol 2002; 187:1290–1293. [II-2]

13. Rodis JF, Borgida AF, Wilson M, et al. Management of parvovirus infection in pregnancy and outcomes of hydrops: a survey of members of the Society of Perinatal Obstetricians. Am J Obstet Gynecol 1998; 179:985–988. [II-3]

14. Segata M, Chaoui R, Khalek N, et al. Fetal thrombocytopenia secondary to parvovirus infection. Am J Obstet Gynecol 2007; 196:61.e1–61.e4. [II-3]

15. de Haan TR, van den Akker ESA, Porcelijn L, et al. Thrombocytopenia in hydropic fetuses with parvovirus B19 infection: incidence, treatment and correlation with fetal B19 viral load. BJOG 2008; 115:76–81. [II-3]

16. Schild RL, Bald R, Plath H, et al. Intrauterine management of fetal parvovirus B19 infection. Ultrasound Obstet Gynecol 1999; 13:161–166. [II-2]

17. Galligan BR, Cairns R, Schifano JV, et al. Preparation of packed red cells suitable for intravascular transfusion in utero. Transfusion 1989; 29(2):179–181. [II-3]

18. Dembinsky J, Haverkamp F, Maara H, et al. Neurodevelopmental outcome after intrauterine red cell transfusion for Parvovirus B19-induced fetal hydrops. BJOG 2002; 109:1232–1234. [II-2]

19. Rodis JF, Rodner C, Hansen AA, et al. Long-term outcome of children following maternal human parvovirus B19 infection. Obstet Gynecol 1998; 91:125–128. [II-2]

20. Nagel HT, de Haan TR, Vandenbussche FP, et al. Long-term outcome after fetal transfusion for hydrops associated with parvovirus B19 infection. Obstet Gynecol 2007; 109:42–47. [III]

49

Herpes

Timothy J. Rafael

KEY POINTS

- Around **20% to 30% of pregnant women have immuno-globulin G (IgG) for herpes simplex virus (HSV)-2 (prior infection) and are therefore infected with it, with inter-mittent shedding from the vaginal mucosa.** About **2% to 4% of IgG-negative women seroconvert (acquire HSV and convert to IgM+) during pregnancy,** and **90% of these women are undiagnosed because they are asymp-tomatic.**

- Most neonatal infections result from contact with infected maternal genital secretions during delivery. **Primary first-episode infection**, defined as HSV confirmed in a person without prior HSV-1 or HSV-2 antibodies, **can lead to a 25% to 50% vertical transmission rate if delivery occurs vaginally** during this episode, and therefore represents the most important clinical scenario to avoid.

- Vaginal delivery during **recurrent infection is associated with a <1% incidence of neonatal HSV infection.** Trans-placental HSV vertical transmission is rare.

- Neonatal HSV causes **disseminated or CNS disease** (seizures, lethargy, irritability, tremors, poor feeding, tem-perature instability, and bulging fontanelles) **in approxi-mately 55% of cases. Up to 30% of infants will die and more than 50% can have neurologic damage despite antiviral therapy.**

- **Prevention of maternal infection** is the most important management strategy.
  - ○ Universal maternal screening with HSV-1 and HSV-2 specific serology has not been tested in a trial and is controversial.
  - ○ If the woman is seronegative, the partner should be tested. If he is seropositive, avoidance of direct oro-genital contact, use of condoms, the possibility of abstinence, and medical suppression of the partner should be discussed.
  - ○ If the woman is seropositive, education, suppression with acyclovir or valacyclovir from 36 weeks until delivery, examination for lesions in labor with cesar-ean delivery (CD) if they are present, and avoidance (if possible) of artificial rupture of membranes (AROM), scalp electrodes, vacuum extractors, and forceps should be recommended.
  - ○ **If any genital lesion suspicious for HSV is seen at the time of labor, a CD should be performed.**

- Diagnosis of genital herpes is most sensitive with poly-merase chain reaction (**PCR**) **assay** of genital lesions (typed to determine whether HSV-1 or HSV-2 is the cause of the infection). Type-specific (**HSV-1 and HSV-2**) glycoprotein G-based **serologic testing** should also be sent.

- **Women with primary or first-episode genital HSV in pregnancy** should receive **acyclovir 400 mg po tid × 7–10 days**, or **valacyclovir (Valtrex) 1 g po bid × 7–10 days** (treatment can be extended in case of incomplete healing), and receive suppression with acyclovir **400 mg po tid or valacyclovir 500 mg po bid at 36 weeks until delivery.**

- **Women with reactivation (recurrent) symptomatic HSV** should receive either **acyclovir 400 mg po tid × five days**, or **valacyclovir (Valtrex) 500 mg po bid × three days**, and receive suppression with acyclovir or valacyclovir at 36 weeks until delivery.

PATHOGENS

HSV-1 and HSV-2 are both DNA viruses.

INCIDENCE/EPIDEMIOLOGY

Genital herpes is an infection (HSV-1 or HSV-2) causing ulcer-ation in the genital area. **Approximately 22% of pregnant women have IgG for HSV-2 (1) (prior infection) and are therefore infected with it, with intermittent shedding from the vaginal mucosa;** 63% are HSV-1 seropositive, 13% have both HSV-1 and HSV-2, and 28% are seronegative (1). Approx-imately 12% to 20% of couples in early pregnancy are discor-dant for HSV status, with the woman at risk to get primary infection from her partner (2). **About 2% to 4% of IgG-negative women seroconvert (acquire HSV) during pregnancy (3), and 75% to 90% of HSV-2 infected people are not aware of having the infection** (2). Approximately 0.1% to 1% of pregnant women carry HSV in their genitalia. The incidence of neonatal herpes is 1/60,000 live births annually in the United Kingdom and 12–60/ 100,000 live births annually in United States (2).

RISK FACTORS/ASSOCIATIONS

Risk factors for maternal HSV infection are immunocompro-mise, other sexually transmitted diseases (STDs), and risk factors for STDs. Risk factors for neonatal HSV infection are HSV in the genital tract at the time of delivery, primary HSV infection, and invasive obstetrical procedures (2).

SYMPTOMS

About 70% of newly acquired HSV infections among pregnant women are asymptomatic, and 30% of women have clinical presentations that range from minimal lesions to widespread genital lesions associated with severe local pain, dysuria, sacral paresthesia, tender regional lymph node enlargement, fever, malaise, and headache (rarely meningitis).

CLASSIFICATION/PATHOPHYSIOLOGY

HSV infection causes intranuclear inclusion bodies and multi-nucleated giant cells. Overall, HSV-1 causes about 90% of oral infections, and 10% of genital infections, while HSV-2 causes

10% of **oral and 90% of genital infections**, although among college-age populations, **the majority of new cases of genital HSV are caused by HSV-1 (2)**. Types of infection include the following:

Primary First Episode

Primary first episode infection is **defined as herpes simplex virus confirmed in a person without prior HSV-1 or HSV-2 antibodies**. About 2% to 4% of these seronegative women seroconvert to HSV-1 or HSV-2 during pregnancy (only 30% have symptoms—if symptoms are present, they are severe—and 50% have recurrence within 6 months), with no fetal consequences unless they convert shortly before labor and deliver vaginally; viral shedding is very high with primary infection, with 50% to 80% of cases of neonatal HSV infection resulting from women who acquire genital HSV-1 or HSV-2 infection near term (4).

Nonprimary First Episode

Nonprimary first-episode infection is HSV-2 confirmed in a person with prior findings of HSV-1 antibodies, or vice versa. About 1.5% to 2% of HSV-1 IgG+ women seroconvert to HSV-2+, whereas the risk of conversion from HSV-2 IgG to HSV-1+ is <1%. If symptoms are present, they are usually milder than first-episode primary infection.

Reactivation (Recurrent) Genital Herpes

Reactivation (recurrent) genital herpes is caused by **reactivation of latent HSV, usually HSV-2**. If symptoms are present, they last 7 to 10 days, are mild, with low viral load shedding for three to five days. Some clinicians distinguish another category within this one, called first-recognized recurrence, which is HSV-1 (or HSV-2) confirmed in a person with prior findings of HSV-1 (or HSV-2) antibodies, but this is not clinically different from reactivation disease.

Over 90% of HSV episodes in pregnancy are either recurrent or nonprimary first-episode HSV. Intimate contact between a susceptible person (without antibodies against the virus) and an individual who is actively shedding the virus or with body fluids containing the virus is required for HSV infection to occur. Contact must involve mucous membranes or open or abraded skin. HSV invades and replicates in neurons as well as in epidermal and dermal cells. Virions travel from the initial site of infection on the skin or mucosa to the sensory dorsal root ganglion, where latency is established. Viral replication in the sensory ganglia leads to recurrent clinical outbreaks. These outbreaks can be induced by various stimuli, such as trauma, ultraviolet radiation, extremes in temperature, stress, immunosuppression, or hormonal fluctuations. Viral shedding, leading to possible transmission, occurs during primary infection, during subsequent recurrences, and during periods of asymptomatic viral shedding.

Maternal-Fetal Transmission

Maternal-fetal transmission of HSV usually occurs at delivery from contact with infected genital secretions. Women with a history of HSV can have viral shedding at the time of delivery. HSV-2 is detected in genital secretions at term by PCR assay in 8% to 15% of HSV-2 seropositive women, most of whom have no clinically detectable lesions at the time (4). **Vaginal delivery during** *first-episode primary infection* **is associated with a 25% to 50% incidence of neonatal HSV infection**. Vaginal delivery during *recurrent* infection

is associated with a <1% incidence of neonatal HSV infection (2). The infant of the mother with primary HSV in the third trimester lacks the protection of transplacental type-specific antibodies (which take 6 to 12 weeks to fully protect the infant), and is at risk of exposure during delivery when viral shedding could be of greatest load. The major sites of intrapartum viral entry are the neonatal eyes, nasopharynx, or a break in skin.

Transplacental infection is rare. First-episode primary infection during pregnancy can lead to microcephaly, ventriculomegaly, spasticity, echogenic bowel, hepatosplenomegaly, and flexed extremities (5).

COMPLICATIONS

In the mother, primary infection can lead to severe symptoms, and occasionally to disseminated disease, hepatitis, and encephalitis.

Factors that influence the risk of fetal infection include primary maternal infection, gestational age, delivery mode, status of membranes, and maternal antibodies. Primary, rather than recurrent genital HSV, is the main risk factor for neonatal HSV. In the first episode, if genital herpes lesions are present at the time of delivery and the baby is delivered vaginally, the risk of **neonatal herpes** is 25% to 50%, calculated in different studies. The risk of neonatal infection in women with established infection and recurrence at term is <1% (4). The risk of neonatal infection from postnatal transmission without prevention is 15% (6). Neonatal HSV causes **disseminated or CNS disease (seizures, lethargy, irritability, tremors, poor feeding, temperature instability, and bulging fontanelles) in approximately 55% of cases. Up to 30% of infants will die and more than 50% can have neurologic damage despite antiviral therapy (4)**. Prenatal ultrasonography can detect **microcephaly, hydrocephaly, intracranial calcification, and placental calcifications** that result from a chronic fetal infection (5).

PREGNANCY MANAGEMENT
Pregnancy Considerations

The course of HSV infection in pregnancy is similar to that in nonpregnant women.

Counseling/Prognosis

Prevention, natural history, incidence of vertical transmission and sequelae, prognosis, and therapeutic options should all be reviewed with the pregnant woman with maternal HSV infection, especially if primary.

Prevention

Prevention of maternal infection includes avoidance of sexual contact with infected individuals. A **preventive strategy for maternal infection** involving universal screening has been proposed (Fig. 49.1) (7). Condoms can usually prevent infection from infected male partners, if the condom covers the lesion(s). For prevention of fetal/neonatal infection, **avoidance of vaginal delivery at times of primary infection is most important. If any genital lesion suspicious for HSV is seen at time of labor, a CD should be performed**. About 46% of these lesions test positive by PCR. Clinical diagnosis by visual exam fails to identify all women with HSV in their genital secretions (8). No scalp electrode, forceps, or vacuum should be used if viral shedding is possible. **Prevention of neonatal infection is critical, as neonatal treatment is poorly effective at avoiding long-term CNS complications** (see also section "Therapy").

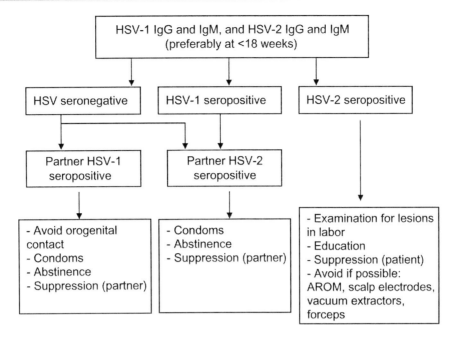

Figure 49.1 Testing and counseling women regarding HSV. *Abbreviations*: HSV, herpes simplex virus; IgG, immunoglobulin G; IgM, immunoglobulin M; AROM, artificial rupture of membranes. *Source*: Adapted from Ref. 7.

Screening

Universal screening is not generally offered to pregnant women, but has been recently proposed (Fig. 49.1). There has been no evidence that screening women to identify pregnancies at risk of new infections will effectively decrease incidence of infection at term, as such a study would require thousands of women. Screening to identify pregnant women with asymptomatic herpes infections may have no value at present without any known safe and effective interventions to prevent an already unlikely neonatal transmission. **All pregnant women should be asked about their own and their partner's histories of genital (and oral) herpes and examined for evidence of active herpes at delivery.** Asymptomatic pregnant women with positive partners, as well as HIV-positive pregnant women, should be offered type-specific serologic testing.

Workup/Diagnosis

Diagnosis of genital herpes relies on laboratory confirmation with **HSV culture** or **PCR assay** of genital lesions (typed to determine whether HSV-1 or HSV-2 is the cause of the infection). Type-specific (**HSV-1 and HSV-2**) glycoprotein G–based **serologic testing** should also be sent. **PCR assays are more sensitive**, and are now preferred, but lack of HSV detection by PCR does not indicate lack of HSV infection, because viral shedding is intermittent. HSV culture should be done within 48 to 72 hours of appearance of the lesion. If the serology type-specific result is discrepant from the culture or PCR result, a new infection is diagnosed (2). If a new infection is suspected and the virus is not isolated from the lesion, serologic testing should be repeated in six weeks. HSV antibodies appear during the first weeks after infection, and persist for life (7). Tzanck smear (Wright's stain with material from the vesicle) is diagnostic with multinucleated giant cells and viral inclusions.

Therapy (9)
Antiviral Drugs

Acyclovir and the other HSV antivirals have, as mechanism of action, the specific inhibition of viral thymidine kinase. They cross the placenta but do not accumulate in the fetus. All these antivirals are safe for the fetus (category B), as exposure to acyclovir and valacyclovir do not appear to increase the risk of birth defects (10).

Valacyclovir (Valtrex) is the prodrug of acyclovir and requires hepatic metabolism to become active. As for famciclovir, valacyclovir has better absorption, longer half-life, and decreased duration of pain and shedding compared to acyclovir.

Famciclovir is the prodrug of penciclovir and also requires hepatic metabolism to become active. As there are no adequate and well-controlled studies in pregnant women taking famciclovir, **acyclovir and valacyclovir are preferred**.

Trials in nonpregnant adults show no differences in outcomes with any of these drugs for primary HSV.

Primary or First-Episode HSV

Women with primary or first-episode genital HSV in pregnancy should be treated with the following:

- Analgesia (topical and systemic)
- Hygienic support to avoid secondary yeast and bacterial infection
- Antiviral therapy (hastens lesion healing and decreases viral shedding) with either:
  ○ **Acyclovir 400 mg po tid** × **7–10 days**, or
  ○ **Valacyclovir** (Valtrex) **1 g po bid** × **7–10 days**

Either regimen duration may be extended if healing is incomplete after 10 days.

These women should receive suppression with **acyclovir 400 mg po tid or valacyclovir 500 mg po bid** at 36 weeks until delivery. Suppression decreases the incidence of recurrent genital lesions at term, viral shedding, and therefore the need for CD. There is insufficient evidence to justify suppression based on neonatal HSV, since this outcome is so rare.

Complicated HSV Infection

Women with **disseminated genital HSV, pneumonitis, hepatitis, or CNS complications** should receive the following:

- **IV acyclovir 5 to 10 mg/kg body weight q8h until clinical improvement, followed by oral antiviral therapy for 10 days of total therapy.**

History of HSV

Women with a history of HSV with **reactivation (recurrent) symptomatic HSV** during pregnancy should be treated with the following:

- Analgesia (topical and systemic) as needed
- Hygienic support to avoid secondary yeast and bacterial infection as needed
- Antiviral therapy (hastens lesion healing, and decreases viral shedding) with either:
  - ◌ **Acyclovir 400 mg po tid × five days** or
  - ◌ **Valacyclovir** (Valtrex) **500 mg po bid × three days, or 1 g po qd for five days.**

These women should receive suppression with acyclovir or valacyclovir at 36 weeks until delivery, or starting even earlier if there are frequent recurrent episodes. **In women with recurrent genital herpes, antiviral suppressive medication initiated from 36 weeks until delivery reduces viral shedding and recurrences at delivery, and reduces the need for CD.** There is insufficient evidence, given the rarity of this outcome, to assess if antiviral prophylaxis reduces the incidence of neonatal HSV (11).

There is insufficient evidence to assess suppression in women with **history of genital HSV and no recurrence during pregnancy**, but suppression might be a reasonable option after counseling (7). Four out of seven RCTs evaluating suppression included women with history of genital HSV but not necessarily a recurrence during the index pregnancy (11).

Mode of Delivery

- **For active genital lesions, or prodromal symptoms of HSV (either primary or reactivation), especially in women presenting with first-episode genital herpes lesions at the time of delivery, cesarean section is recommended (9).** Some clinicians advocate CD even for

women with primary HSV within six weeks of delivery, despite maternal therapy (2).

- A reactivation/**recurrent episode** of genital herpes occurring **during pregnancy** is not an indication for delivery by cesarean section. In women with a history of **genital HSV** but without active genital lesions or prodromal symptoms at the time of labor, CD is not indicated.

Postpartum/Neonate

Seventy percent of mothers of HSV-infected neonates are asymptomatic. Neonates with infection manifest symptoms at the end of the first week of life with skin lesions, cough, tachypnea, cyanosis, jaundice, seizures, and disseminated intravascular coagulation (DIC). The classic triad is skin lesions, chorioretinitis, and CNS abnormalities. Severe HSV neonatal infection can lead to a 30% incidence of death and more than 50% incidence of mental problems/neurologic damage in survivors despite antiviral therapy (4).

Mothers with HSV at the time of delivery should wash their hands but can handle their neonate. Acyclovir is compatible with breast-feeding.

REFERENCES

1. Xu F, Markowitz LE, Gottlieb SL, et al. Seroprevalence of herpes simplex virus types 1 and 2 in pregnant women in the United States. Am J Obstet Gynecol 2007; 196:43.e1–43.e6. [III]
2. Gardella C, Brown Z. Prevention of neonatal herpes. Br J Obstet Gynecol 2011; 118:187–192. [Review]
3. Brown ZA, Selke SA, Zeh J, et al. Acquisition of herpes simplex virus during pregnancy. N Engl J Med 1997; 337:509–515. [II-2]
4. Corey L, Wald A. Maternal and neonatal herpes simplex virus infections. N Engl J Med 2009; 361:1376–1385. [Review]
5. Lanouette JM, Duquette DA, Jacques SM, et al. Prenatal diagnosis of fetal herpes simplex infection. Fetal Diagn Ther 1996; 11:414–416. [II-3]
6. Jungmann E. Genital herpes. Clinical evidence. Br Med J 2004; 11:2073–2088. [II-2]
7. Brown ZA, Gardella C, Wald A, et al. Genital herpes complicating pregnancy. Am Coll Obstet Gynecol 2005; 106:845–856. [Review]
8. Gardella C, Brown ZA, Wald A, et al. Poor correlation between genital lesions and detection of herpes simplex virus in women in labor. Obstet Gynecol 2005; 106:268–274. [II-2]
9. ACOG Practice Bulletin. Clinical management guidelines for obstetrician-gynecologists. No. 82 June 2007. Management of herpes in pregnancy. Obstet Gynecol 2007; 109:1489–1498. [Review]
10. Pasternak B, Hviid A. Use of acyclovir, valacyclovir, and famciclovir in the first trimester of pregnancy and the risk of birth defects. J Am Med Assoc 2010; 304(8):859–866. [II-2]
11. Hollier LM, Wendel GD. Third trimester antiviral prophylaxis for preventing maternal genital herpes simplex virus (HSV) recurrences and neonatal infection. Cochrane Database Syst Rev 2008; (1):CD004946. [Meta-analysis: 7 RCTs, *n* = 1249]

50

Varicella

Timothy J. Rafael

KEY POINTS

- As about 90% of pregnant women are immune (VZV IgG+) to varicella, **primary maternal varicella zoster virus (VZV) infection (chickenpox)** occurs in **about 0.5–3/1000 pregnancies.**
- **Pneumonia** can occur in up to **10% of pregnant women with chickenpox.**
- **Congenital varicella syndrome (CVS)** occurs in 0.4% to 2% of all maternal infections, **usually if maternal VZV infection occurs at <20 weeks of gestation.**
- CVS includes congenital limb hypoplasia, dermatomal skin scarring, rudimentary digits, intrauterine growth restriction (IUGR), and occasionally damage to the eyes (chorioretinitis, cataracts) and central nervous system (microcephaly, cortical atrophy, leading to mental retardation).
- All pregnant (and reproductive-age) women should be asked at their first prenatal visit if they have had a chickenpox infection. **All women who have not had chickenpox in the past or are unsure should have VZV IgG and IgM serology. VZV IgG-negative women should receive the vaccine postpartum.**
- Diagnosis of **maternal chickenpox** is usually made based on clinical findings alone, and confirmed by **VZV IgM.**
- **Ultrasound** can help in the diagnosis and estimation of the probability of CVS. **At least five weeks should be allowed between the onset of maternal symptoms and fetal ultrasound.** Fetal infection can be diagnosed by VZV DNA in amniotic fluid, but this does not predict risk of CVS.
- **VZV-seronegative pregnant women exposed to VZV** should receive **VZV IgG** (also known as **VariZIG**™).
- Pregnant women who develop **chickenpox** should receive oral [or intravenous (IV) if severe] **acyclovir** within 24 hours of rash, and should avoid contact with susceptible individuals such as other pregnant women or children. Varicella zoster immune globulin (VariZIG™) has no therapeutic effect once chickenpox has developed.
- **Delivery should be delayed until five days after the onset of maternal illness,** to allow for passive transfer of maternal IgG. **Neonates born to women who develop chickenpox between five days before and two days after delivery should receive VZV IgG.** If neonatal infection occurs, the neonate should receive acyclovir.
- Pregnant women who develop **pulmonary chickenpox** should be immediately hospitalized in isolation, and should receive **IV acyclovir.**
- **Maternal shingles is not a risk for the infant** who is protected from passively acquired maternal antibodies.
- **Nonimmune women should be offered postpartum varicella vaccination.** The vaccine is considered safe in breast-feeding women. Conception should be delayed until one month after the VZV vaccine was given (live attenuated vaccine).

PATHOGEN
VZV is a DNA virus of the herpes family.

INCIDENCE/EPIDEMIOLOGY
As about 95% of pregnant women are immune (VZV IgG+) to varicella, **primary maternal VZV infection (commonly called chickenpox, or VZD)** is uncommon, and estimated to **complicate about 0.5–3/1000 pregnancies.** Women from tropical areas are more susceptible (50% immunity only) to the development of chickenpox. VZV vaccine was licensed in 1995 and decreased the incidence of disease by 85% to 90% in the decade following licensure (1).

RISK FACTORS/ASSOCIATIONS
Maternal varicella infection is associated with contact with infected individuals, which usually are children, if not immunized. Risk factors for varicella pneumonia are cigarette smoking, >100 skin lesions, advanced gestational age, history of chronic obstructive pulmonary disease (COPD), immunosuppression, and household contact.

SYMPTOMS
Pruritic rash with maculopapular skin lesions in crops, which become vesicles and pustules, and later crust over, along with fever and malaise.

PATHOPHYSIOLOGY
VZV is highly contagious and transmitted by respiratory droplets and direct personal contact with vesicle fluid or indirectly via fomites. The incubation period is about 15 (10–21) days. The disease is infectious 48 hours before the rash appears, and continues to be infectious until the vesicles crust over (Fig. 50.1). The rash lasts 7 to 10 days. Chickenpox (or primary VZV infection) is a common childhood disease that usually causes a mild infection, leading to the 90% seropositivity of pregnant women. After the primary infection the virus remains dormant in sensory nerve root ganglia and can be reactivated to cause a vesicular erythematous skin rash known as herpes zoster (commonly called shingles).

MATERNAL-FETAL TRANSMISSION
Primary maternal infection leads to an about **8% vertical transmission,** causing primary fetal infection. Of these, about 10% develop CVS (**0.4–2% of all maternal infections**) **usually if maternal VZV occurs <20 weeks of gestation** (2).

COMPLICATIONS
Maternal
Although varicella infection is much less common in adults than in children, in adults it is more often associated with

Exposure → incubation period 10–21 days → viremia → 2 days → rash → 5 days →
IgM/IgG appear in blood, and vesicles crust over.

Figure 50.1   VZV infectious sequence. *Abbreviation*: VZV, varicella zoster virus.

pneumonia, hepatitis, and encephalitis. **Pneumonia can occur in up to 5% to 10% of pregnant women with chickenpox** and the severity seems increased in later gestation. Pulmonary symptoms start two to six days after the rash, with a mild cough leading to hemoptysis, chest pain, dyspnea, and cyanosis. The mortality rate with treatment for varicella pneumonia is now only <1%.

Fetal

Sequelae are dependent on fetal age at the time of infection. In up to 98% of cases of maternal infection, the fetus remains healthy without clinical signs of illness, but when infection occurs, it can result in **CVS**, neonatal varicella, or asymptomatic seroconversion.

The overall rate for CVS **when maternal infection occurs** *in the first 20 weeks of gestation* has been demonstrated to be about **0.4% to 2%** (1–5). CVS is characterized by **congenital limb hypoplasia, dermatomal skin scarring, rudimentary digits, IUGR, and occasionally damage to the eyes (chorioretinitis, cataracts) and central nervous system (microcephaly, cortical atrophy, leading to mental retardation)**. It is hypothesized that CVS may reflect disseminated infection in utero or consequences of failure of virus-host interaction to result in establishment of latency, as normally occurs in postnatal VZV infection (1). **Prenatal ultrasound findings** can include limb deformity, microcephaly, hydrocephalus, soft tissue calcification, and IUGR (6).

CVS with **maternal infection >20 weeks** is very rare, as it has only been reported in <10 case reports (<1/1000 risk) (3). Maternal infection after 20 weeks and up to 36 weeks may present as shingles in the first few years of infant life, as a reactivation of the virus after a primary infection in utero.

If maternal infection occurs **one to four weeks before delivery**, up to 50% of babies are infected and up to 23% of these develop clinical varicella. **Severe chickenpox occurs more often if the infant is born within seven days of onset the mother's rash** when cord blood VZV IgG is low. Both intrauterine and peripartum VZV infection predispose to

development of childhood zoster. Historically, neonates born to mothers who contract chickenpox between five days before delivery and two days after delivery have a 17% to 30% chance of developing **neonatal varicella** (7). Before VZV immunoglobulin was available, the risk of death among these neonates was as high as 31%, with current rates decreasing to 7% when the use of varicella immunoglobulin was introduced and neonatal intensive care improved (1).

There are no fetal consequences for herpes zoster, since the viral load is very low, and the mother has already VZV IgGs that cross the placenta and protect the fetus.

PREGNANCY MANAGEMENT
Pregnancy Considerations

Chickenpox is a more severe disease in the adult than in the child. In pregnant women, frequency of VZV, frequency of pneumonia, and mortality are not increased compared to nonpregnant adults. Pneumonia may be more severe in pregnant women, with up to 5% risk of maternal death even with therapy.

Counseling

Natural history, incidence of vertical transmission and sequelae (mostly occurring if maternal infection occurs <20 weeks), prognosis, and therapeutic options should all be reviewed with the pregnant woman with primary maternal VZV infection (Table 50.1).

Prevention

VZV-seronegative pregnant women should avoid exposure to individuals with chickenpox. A live attenuated varicella vaccine (Varivax®, Merck, New Jersey, U.S.) has demonstrated to be safe in preventing chickenpox in adults. In the United States and in some European countries seronegative women presenting for **preconception** counseling or women undergoing infertility treatment may be offered vaccination. The vaccine is not available in the United Kingdom for these indications.

Table 50.1   Counseling Advice for Pregnant Women at Risk

Maternal rash appears	Risk for varicella embryopathy	Counseling advice
First 20 wk	0.5% to 2% above the baseline risk	VZV IgG within 96 hr after contact if the woman is seronegative. Ultrasound 5 wk after maternal rash appears to detect defects.
21–28 wk	Rare	VZV IgG within 96 hr after contact if the woman is seronegative. Ultrasound 5 wk after maternal rash appears to detect defects.
After 28 wk	None	VZV IgG within 96 hr after contact if the woman is seronegative to prevent varicella complication. Explain baseline risk.
Five days before or two days after	None	If possible, delay the delivery until 5–7 days after the onset of maternal rash. Administer VZV IgG to neonate if exposed. IV Acyclovir is warranted for severe cases.
Maternal varicella pneumonia		IV Acyclovir 10–15 mg/kg every 8 hr for 5–10 days and antibacterial. Blood gas, mechanical ventilation, and supportive therapy as needed.

Abbreviation: VZV, varicella zoster virus. *Source*: From Ref. 3

Varicella vaccine is contraindicated in pregnant women. If a woman accidentally receives VZV vaccine within a month of conception or in pregnancy, the incidence of fetal infection and complications does not appear to be increased from baseline, and termination should not be recommended. In a recent registry, among 131 live births to VZV-seronegative women, there was no evidence of CVS, and the major birth defect rate was not statistically increased (8). Nonimmune health workers exposed to VZV should minimize patient contact from days 8 to 21 post contact.

Screening

Routine serologic screening of all pregnant women is currently not recommended. **All pregnant (and preconception repro-ductive-age) women should be asked at the first prenatal visit if they have had a prior chickenpox infection.** Over 97% of women who report a prior varicella infection have VZV IgG and are therefore immune. **All women who did not have chickenpox in the past or are unsure should have VZV IgG and IgM serology.** In the United States, of women who are uncertain or give negative histories, approximately 80% to 90% have VZV IgG (9). If testing is done in the preconception period, women can be offered two doses of varicella vaccine at least one month apart. Pregnancy should be delayed one month after vaccination. Based on a decision model, the above prenatal screening (selective serotesting) with postpartum vaccination of susceptibles would seem cost-effective (10).

Workup/Diagnosis

Diagnosis of **maternal chickenpox** is usually made based on clinical findings alone. Diagnosis can be confirmed by **VZV IgM** newly positive by ELISA (enzyme-linked immunosorbent assay), or by VZV antigen (Ag) in skin/vesicular lesions by immunofluorescence antibody (Ab) to membrane Ag. **Fetal infection can be diagnosed by VZV DNA** detected by polymerase chain reaction (PCR) in amniotic fluid, but its presence has a poor positive predictive value for both fetal disease or disease severity (1). The presence of fetal varicella-specific IgM, which remains in the blood for four to five weeks, is diagnostic (11). **Ultrasound** can help in diagnosis and estimation of probability of CVS. **At least five weeks should be allowed between the onset of maternal symptoms and fetal ultrasound**, to avoid false negative results. Initial PCR testing of amniotic fluid at 17 to 21 weeks may be negative with normal ultrasound findings, suggesting a low risk of CVS. Positive PCR at 17 to 21 weeks with normal ultrasound should lead to a repeat ultrasound at 22 to 26 weeks. A normal ultrasound at that stage makes CVS very unlikely. In contrast, an abnormal ultrasound suggests a high likelihood of CVS (12,13).

Therapy

Exposure

- **VZV-seronegative pregnant women exposed to VZV** should receive **VZV IgG (VariZIG™)** within 72 to 96 hours of exposure. VariZIG can be obtained 24 hours a day from the sole authorized U.S. distributor (FFF Enterprises, Temecula, California, U.S., tel. 1-800-843-7477 or online at http://www.fffenterprises.com). The recommended dose is 125 units/10 kg of body weight, up to a maximum of 625 units IM (five vials) (14). This may not prevent but may attenuate symptoms up to ten days after exposure. It probably does not affect fetal infection, and it is expensive.

Chickenpox

- **Pregnant women who develop chickenpox** should receive oral **acyclovir** within 24 hours of rash. Oral acyclovir reduces the duration of fever and symptoms of varicella infection in immunocompetent adults if commenced within 24 hours of developing the onset of rash (15). Administration of acyclovir does not appear to be teratogenic. Acyclovir is prescribed to treat extensive varicella at the high dose of 15 mg/kg of body weight or 500 mg/m^2 IV every eight hours. Major side effects often include local tissue irritation, transient elevation of hepatic transaminases, CNS toxicity, and renal dysfunction. Transplacental passage of acyclovir is prompt and therapeutic levels reach the placenta and fetal blood (11). **There is no information about whether giving acyclovir or valacyclovir to pregnant women with varicella reduces the already low risk for CVS** (1).
- **Pregnant women who develop chickenpox** should **avoid contact with susceptible individuals** such as other pregnant women or children.
- **Pregnant women who develop chickenpox** should undergo symptomatic treatment and maintain hygiene to avoid bacterial superinfection.
- VZV IgG has no therapeutic effect once chickenpox has developed.
- If maternal infection occurs at term there is a significant risk of varicella in the newborn. **Delivery should be delayed until five days after the onset of maternal illness**, to allow for passive transfer of maternal IgG. Infants delivered when maternal symptoms develop five days prior to two days after delivery are at 17% to 30% risk of getting neonatal varicella, and of these, about 7% can die. **Neonates born to women who develop chickenpox between five days before and two days after delivery should receive VZV IgG.** If neonatal infection occurs, the neonate should receive acyclovir.
- If there is neonatal exposure in the first seven days of life (e.g., from an infected sibling), no intervention is required if the mother is immune; however, the neonate should be given VZV IgG if the mother is not immune to varicella. Neonates who develop chickenpox in the first 14 days of life should receive IV acyclovir.
- Pregnant women who develop **pulmonary chickenpox** should be immediately hospitalized in isolation. They should receive **IV acyclovir** 10 to 15 mg/kg × 7 days within 72 hours of symptoms (decreases severity and mortality).

Maternal Shingles

Maternal shingles is **not a risk for the infant** who is protected from passively acquired maternal antibodies (4).

Nonimmune Women

Nonimmune women should be offered **postpartum varicella vaccination (two doses, one month apart)**. The vaccine is considered safe in breast-feeding women. Conception should be delayed until one month after the VZV vaccine was given (live attenuated vaccine).

Clinical Neonatal Findings of CVS (13)

- Skin scarring in a dermatomal distribution, 73%
- Neurological abnormalities (microcephaly, cortical atrophy, mental retardation), 62%
- Eye defects (microphthalmia, chorioretinitis), 52%

- Hypoplasia of the limbs, 46%
- Muscle hypoplasia, 20%
- Gastrointestinal abnormalities, 19%
- Genitourinary abnormalities, 12%
- Internal organs effects, 13%
- Developmental delay, 12%

REFERENCES

1. Smith CK, Arvin AM. Varicella in the fetus and newborn. Semin Fetal Neonatal Med 2009; 14:209–217. [Review]
2. Harger JH, Ernest JM, Thurnau GR, et al. Frequency of congenital varicella syndrome in a prospective cohort of 347 pregnant women. Obstet Gynecol 2002; 100:260–265. [II-3]
3. Tan MP, Koren G. Chickenpox in pregnancy: revisited. Reprod Toxicol 2006; 21(4):410–420. [Review]
4. Royal College of Obstet and Gynecol. Clinical Green Top Guideline: Chickenpox in pregnancy. January 17, 2005. [Guideline]
5. Sanchez MA, Bello-Munoz JC, Cebrecos I, et al. The prevalence of congenital varicella syndrome after a maternal infection, but before 20 weeks of pregnancy: a prospective cohort study. J Matern Fetal Neonatal Med 2011; 24(2):341–347. [II-3]
6. Pretorius DH, Hayward I, Jones KL, et al. Sonographic evaluation of pregnancies with maternal varicella infection. J Ultrasound Med 1992; 11:459–463. [II-3]
7. National Advisory Committee on Immunization update on varicella. Can Common Dis Rep 2004; 30:1–26. [Review]
8. Wilson E, Goss MA, Marin M, et al. Varicella vaccine exposure during pregnancy: data from 10 years of the pregnancy registry. J Infect Dis 2008; 197:S178–S184. [II-3]
9. Watson B, Civen R, Reynolds M, et al. Validity of self-reported varicella disease history in pregnant women attending prenatal clinics. Public Health Rep 2007; 122:499–506. [III]
10. De Moira AP, Edmunds WJ, Breuer J. The cost-effectiveness of antenatal varicella screening with post-partum vaccination of susceptibles. Vaccine 2006; 24:1298–1307. [III]
11. Mc Gregor JA. Varicella zoster infection in pregnancy. Contemp Obstet Gynecol 2002; 47–55. [Review]
12. Enders G, Miller E. Varicella and Herpes Zoster in Pregnancy and in Newborn. Cambridge: Cambridge University Press, 2000:317–347. [Review]
13. Koren G. Congenital varicella syndrome in the third trimester. Lancet 2005; 366:1591–1592. [Review]
14. Centers for Disease Control and Prevention (CDC). A new product (VariZIG) for postexposure prophylaxis of varicella available under an investigational new drug application expanded access protocol. MMWR Morb Mortal Wkly Rep 2006; 55:209–210. [Review]
15. Wallace MR, Bawler WA, Murray NB, et al. Treatment of adult varicella with oral acyclovir. A randomized placebo-controlled trial. Ann Intern Med 1992; 117:358–363. [RCT, non-pregnant adults]

51

Neonatal alloimmune thrombocytopenia

Jason K. Baxter

KEY POINTS

- Neonatal alloimmune thrombocytopenia (NAIT) is fetal/neonatal thrombocytopenia ($<150,000/\mu L$) due to **maternal sensitization to incompatible fetal platelet antigens**.
- The most significant complication of NAIT is fetal/neonatal 10% to 30% risk of **intracranial hemorrhage (ICH)**, of which 45% occurs antenatally, most often in the third trimester at around 30 to 35 weeks, but can occur as early as 20 weeks. There is also a 5% to 13% risk of **neonatal mortality.**
- Only **HPA-1a antigen** and **past history of ICH** predict a more severe thrombocytopenia.
- **Goal** of management is to **prevent ICH** in the fetus and neonate. Keeping fetal/neonatal platelets $>20,000/\mu L$ achieves this goal.
- Routine universal maternal screening is generally not recommended.
- **Intravenous immunoglobulin** (IVIG) is associated with a **75% response rate, and a very rare risk of ICH,** with half of the nonresponders showing improvement with the addition of a high dose of prednisone.
- **Fetal blood sampling (FBS)** is associated with a 1% to 2% risk of fetal loss per procedure, and 5% to 10% cumulative.
- **Management is usually based on IVIG therapy, with FBS as needed**, as determined by prior history of ICH and associated risk **(Fig. 51.1)**.

DEFINITION

NAIT is fetal/neonatal thrombocytopenia due to **maternal sensitization to incompatible fetal platelet antigens**. It is also called alloimmune thrombocytopenia (AIT), or fetal maternal alloimmune thrombocytopenia (FMAIT).

EPIDEMIOLOGY/INCIDENCE

1/1000 to 1/1500 births (1). NAIT is the most common reason for severe thrombocytopenia and/or ICH in term newborn.

ETIOLOGY/BASIC PATHOPHYSIOLOGY

Maternal alloimmunization occurs against fetal platelet antigen (Ag) lacked by mother's own platelets.

- **Platelet disease similar to RBC Rh disease**:
  - Similar to RBCs, platelets have specific surface proteins called antigens.
  - Mother lacks platelet antigen possessed by father.
  - Mother is exposed to antigen by fetal platelets.
  - **Maternal sensitization to incompatible fetal (platelet) antigens.**
  - Transplacental transfer of maternal antiplatelet antibody to the fetus.

  - Subsequent antibody-coating and sequestration of platelets in the fetal reticuloendothelial system.
- **Different from Rh disease**:
  - **Firstborn children are often affected** (primiparas account for 20–60% of cases).
  - Maternal antibody titers are not predictive of outcome.
  - Antiplatelet IgG production can occur in first pregnancy.

Maternal platelet count and function is normal (although 10% of women with NAIT may have gestational thrombocytopenia). **Most incompatibilities will not become sensitized** (1).

GENETICS/INHERITANCE/RECURRENCE

HPA-1b is due to a single base pair change of cytosine to thymine at position 196 (proline to leucine) in platelet glycoprotein IIIA (2).

CLASSIFICATION

There are five major biallelic systems of platelet-specific antigens (which differ by single amino acids). The **new nomenclature** is described in Table 51.1.

Whites: 97% HPA-1a+ : 68% homozygotes, 29% heterozygotes (HPA-1a/HPA-1b); 2% to 3% HPA-1b/HPA-1b.

HLA class II determinant DRW52a (HLA-DR3) or HLA-B8 are more likely to develop antibodies versus HPA-1a. One out of forty-two pregnancies have platelet Ag incompatibility, but only 1/30 of these get NAIT.

Other rare causes of NAIT are **HLA class I** (but not class II) antigens, which are also expressed by platelets. Gov (HPA-15) is unstable making serologic testing difficult.

NATURAL HISTORY/COMPLICATIONS

The fetus/neonate develops decreased platelets. This can lead to

- 90% affected neonates having diffuse petechiae
- 10% to 30% ICH
  - 45% occur antenatally, most often in third trimester at around 30 to 35 weeks, but as early as 20 weeks
  - Mostly intraparenchymal, leading to encephalomalacia
  - May result in porencephalic cysts (which may be seen by ultrasound)
  - Sometimes IVH, leading to arachnoiditis +/− hydrocephalus
- 5% to 13% **neonatal mortality**
- First case in family usually detected shortly after birth (due to petechiae, bleeding, or incidentally)

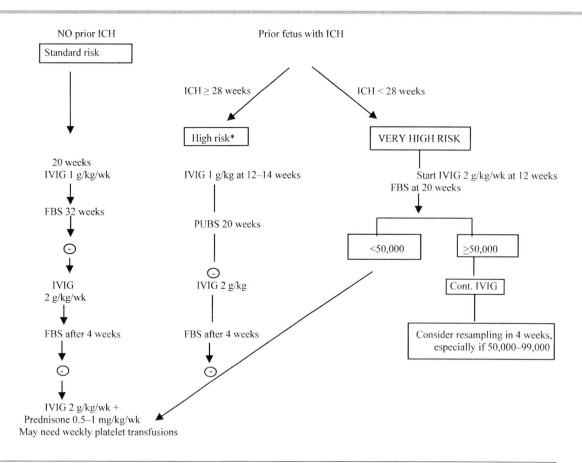

(-), fetal platelet count <50,000/µL; (+), fetal platelet count ≥50,000/µL.

*For cases in which the initial platelet count on the affected neonate was <20,000/µL, some experts suggest this management, or at least starting with the higher (2 g/kg/wk) IVIG dose at 20 weeks.

Figure 51.1 Suggested antenatal management for prior NAIT. *Abbreviations*: ICH, intracranial hemorrhage; IVIG, intravenous immuno-globulin therapy; FBS, fetal blood sampling.

Table 51.1 Nomenclature for NAIT

Old nomenclature	New nomenclature (in order of discovery)	
PI^A1, PLA-1, ZW^A	**HPA-1a**	Most common (>75%) (2% whites, 0.4% blacks, <0.1% Asians are negative)
PI^A2, PLA-2	**HPA-1b**	Worse severity
Ko^b	**HPA-2a**	
Ko^a	**HPA-2b**	
Bak^a, Lek^a	**HPA-3a**	Second most common (15% whites are negative)
Bak^b, Lek^b, PLA-3	**HPA-3b**	
Pen^a, Yuk^b	**HPA-4a**	
Pen^b, Yuk^a	**HPA-4b**	More common in Asians
Brb	**HPA-5a**	
Br^a, PLA-5	**HPA-5b**	Third most common (<1% whites are negative) Most common in Japan

[a]High-frequency antigen.
[b]Low-frequency antigen.
Abbreviation: NAIT, neonatal alloimmune thrombocytopenia.

RECURRENCE RISK

- Clinical history of affected sibling is the best indicator of risk in current/future pregnancy.
- **Recurrence** in subsequent pregnancy **is generally of greater severity**. It is about 100% for **HPA-1a** (usually **worst Ag**) (2).

- There is no correlation between platelet count at cordocentesis and degree of thrombocytopenia in previously affected infant. How severe NAIT was in the last pregnancy is not as predictive.
- Only **HPA-1a antigen** and **past history of ICH** predict a more severe thrombocytopenia.

- **Prior ICH**: greatest risk, only true predictor of severity.
- Fetal platelets in first-monitored pregnancy: **70% <50,000/ µL** at first percutaneous umbilical blood sampling (PUBS); 50% <20,000/µL, 50% <24 weeks. If the count is >50,000/ µL on first PUBS, it is still possible that it will decrease later (in HPA-1a, fetal platelets decrease as much as about 23,000/µL/wk) (2).

MANAGEMENT
Principles

- **Goal: prevent hemorrhage, specifically ICH, in fetus and neonate.**
- ICH is rare with platelets >20,000/µL, therefore **goal is to keep platelets >20,000/µL**. The normal platelet count of a fetus ≥18 weeks is ≥150,000/µL, as in an adult.
- FBS with direct measurement of fetal platelet count is the only method to assess disease severity.
- Optimal management of NAIT has not been determined, and no one therapy is proven to be 100% effective. There are some RCTs and several case series that can help guide management.

Prevention

Some have advocated routine universal maternal serologic screening for platelet antigens for identifying pregnancies at risk for NAIT, before it happens in the first pregnancy without warnings (3). Screening for HPA-1a alloimmunization detects about two cases in 1000 pregnancies. Severe NAIT occurs in about 31% of these immunized pregnancies, and perinatal ICH in about 10% (perhaps more) of pregnancies with severe NAIT. Therefore, the identification (for possible prevention) of 1 case of ICH would need the screening of about 15,000 pregnancies (4).

Rationale Against Routine Maternal Serologic Screening

- About 25% of NAIT is not caused by the most common antigen.
- Maternal immune response is influenced by other factors (e.g., HLA type).
- Only a minority of infants of mothers negative for platelet antigen will develop significant thrombocytopenia.
- Many false-negatives and false-positives.
- No adequate risk/benefit ratio or cost-effectiveness analyses have been performed. The incidence of ICH is low.

Screening by maternal ultrasound is futile, as fetal thrombocytopenia cannot be detected by ultrasound, and when it is so severe as to cause fetal ICH, it is too late for effective intervention.

Since there is no consensus regarding utility of screening unaffected women for alloimmune antiplatelet antibodies, active **management of the disease is usually confined to women who have had a previously affected fetus.**

WORKUP FOR SUSPECTED NAIT
Indications for Testing

- Neonate with petechiae and ecchymosis, unexplained thrombocytopenia.
- Fetus with unexplained ICH, hydrocephalus, or porencephalic cyst.
- Woman incidentally found to be HPA-1a negative.
- Family history of NAIT.

NAIT Serologic Testing

- Test parents in reference laboratory (e.g., Blood Center of Southeastern Wisconsin).
- Initial testing: Maternal platelet antibody. Paternal antigen typing (usually HPA-1,3,5) if maternal antibody positive.

DIAGNOSIS

- Mother is **antibody positive** (specific to father and fetal platelet antigen) and **antigen negative.**
- The **father's antigen zygosity** and **neonatal antigen** determines the risk of recurrence in subsequent pregnancies: 100% if father is homozygous, 50% if heterozygous.

This documentation of maternal, paternal, and neonatal serologic diagnosis should be always reviewed to guide management in the next pregnancy.

COUNSELING

Prognosis, natural history and complications, and management criteria should all be reviewed with the family. **All patients should be advised that the optimal management of NAIT has not been determined and that no one therapy has proven to be 100% effective.**

INVESTIGATIONS AND CONSULTATIONS

With heterozygous father, consider **amniocentesis to determine fetal antigen** status by PCR (CVS only if mother would terminate affected fetus). Multidisciplinary management should involve a hematologist and the blood bank.

FETAL THERAPY

There is insufficient data to assess different types of interventions for the pregnancy with NAIT.

There are two main antenatal treatment options:

1. **Intravenous immunoglobulin**
   - >$1000/dose.
   - Most common initial therapy in North America.
   - Pooled blood product, but risks of hepatitis and HIV transmission are minuscule (donor screening and viral inactivation procedures decrease risk).
   - Usually given as **weekly infusion** over 6 to 12 hours.
   - IVIG has unclear mechanism of action, but is theorized to work via
     - Fc-receptor **saturation in the placenta** with a reduction of antibody transfer across the placenta (most probable main mechanism)
     - Fc-receptor blockade on macrophages leading to inhibition of uptake of the antibody-coated platelets by fetal macrophages. Endothelial stabilization prevents damage by maternal platelet antibodies (low platelets not a cause of ICH)
     - Suppression of maternal IgG antibody production
   - IVIG can not only prevent/improve thrombocytopenia in the majority of cases, but it also prevents ICH. There are only very rare (possibly only two in the literature) reports of IVIG failures to prevent ICH (5).
   - Side effects: headaches and febrile reactions (pretreat with benadryl and acetaminophen).

- Only way to monitor efficacy of IVIG treatment is via FBS.
- **75% respond to weekly IVIG, half of the nonresponders improve with the addition of high-dose prednisone** (1 mg/kg = 60 mg/day) (6). Dexamethasone has been associated with oligohydramnios and FGR (6).
- When IVIG dose is 2 g/kg/wk, it can be infused at doses of 1 g/kg twice a week.
- If this fails, consider weekly in utero platelet transfusions via FBS until birth.

2. Repeated **intrauterine transfusion** of antigen-compatible platelets via FBS
   - More popular in Europe.
   - Weekly in utero transfusion of platelets via FBS may be required from 20 weeks until delivery.
   - Risk of increasing sensitization due to fetomaternal hemorrhage.
   - **Risk of fetal hemorrhage** is at least 1% to 2% per procedure, and 5% to 10% cumulative loss for each pregnancy (7–9). To minimize fetal hemorrhage at FBS, always begin transfusing platelets immediately after obtaining platelet sample (7–9).
   - Transfuse maternal platelets (antigen negative), obtained by plasmaphoresis a day or two earlier (packed, washed, and irradiated).

   - Volume infused

$$= \frac{(\text{estimated fetoplacental volume})(\text{desired increase in platelet})}{(\text{platelet infusion concentration})}$$

   (Table 51.2).
   - Goal: platelets >50,000/μL, and usually 200,000 to 400,000/μL.
   - Because of risk of emergent delivery, corticosteroids for fetal lung maturity before FBS are suggested at ≥24 weeks.
   - In fetuses with platelets >80,000/μL at first FBS and not treated, follow-up FBS showed decreases of at least 10,000/μL/wk.

Many centers use **IVIG as the initial treatment**, with FBS to monitor response, with the addition of oral steroids for refractory cases, as suggested in Figure 51.1. Management depends on history of prior ICH. This is an empiric approach, which tries to avoid a 20-week FBS, associated with significant complications as just discussed.

Table 51.2 Calculations for Fetal Platelet Transfusion for NAIT

Volume (in mL) to raise platelet count by 50, 000

$$= \frac{(\text{fetal weight in grams})(0.14)(50,000)(2)}{\text{Platelet count from lab expressed as per } \mu L^a}$$

Platelet goal	Volume to infuse
100,000	
150,000	
200,000	
250,000	
300,000	
350,000	
400,000	

[a]If volume is given in milliliters, just divide by mL volume × 1000; that is, if given total platelets is 6 million in 55 mL, then (6,000,000/55,000) = platelet count from lab.
   Then one can use the following chart to fill in, according to initial fetal platelet count obtained at PUBS.
Abbreviation: NAIT, neonatal alloimmune thrombocytopenia.

Previous Siblings Did Not Have In Utero ICH (Fig. 51.1)

A. **Begin IVIG at 1 g/kg/wk at 20 weeks**. Some also advocate adding prednisone 0.5 mg/kg/d, or using the higher dose of IVIG (2 g/kg/wk) (9); these two latter options were shown to be comparable in a RCT (8). Given the side effects of prednisone, we prefer to use IVIG only in these cases as initial therapy. One can consider starting at the higher dose (2 g/kg/w) if the initial platelet count of the affected neonate was <20,000/μL at birth.

B. Assess adequacy of therapy by FBS at about 32 weeks (10).
   - Have platelets ready at any FBS, with slow transfusion started after sampling even before platelet count (PC) is available.
   - Use compatible (mother's preferred) washed platelets.
   - Transfusion volume: aim for 200 to 400,000 platelets, by using the equation in Table 51.2.
   1. If adequate (platelet count ≥50,000/μL), continue IVIG weekly to term. If the first fetal platelet count is >20,000/μL while on IVIG, the chance of platelet count >20,000/μL at a later sampling is 89%, while if the first count is ≤20,000/μL, this chance is only 51% (11). Therefore, if the response is adequate (>20,000/μL, and especially >50,000 μL), a second FBS may not be required, provided IVIG is continued, given the risks of FBS (11).
   2. If inadequate, increase therapy to IVIG 2 g/kg/wk (some suggest adding prednisone at this point, too). The chance that this initial platelet count is <20,000 μL is <20%.
   3. Resample after four weeks of therapy. If inadequate, add prednisone 0.5 mg/kg/day to term.
   4. Resample after four weeks of therapy. If inadequate, intensify therapy to IVIG 2 g/kg/wk and prednisone 1.0 mg/kg/day and resample in two weeks. If response occurs, prednisone can be tapered.
   5. If above salvage therapy fails, continue IVIG, stop prednisone, and begin weekly in utero platelet transfusions and deliver ≥36 weeks.

C. Follow with serial (q2–4 week) ultrasound assessments.

Previous Sibling Had In Utero ICH (Fig. 51.1)

A. Begin IVIG at 1 to 2 g/kg/wk at 12 to 14 weeks (Fig. 51.1; If prior ICH <28 week: suggest IVIG 2 g/kg/wk).

B. Assess adequacy of therapy by FBS at 20 weeks.
   1. If adequate (>50,000/μL), (about 60% of cases) continue IVIG (platelet count falls if IVIG is stopped)
   2. If inadequate (<50,000/μL): IVIG 2 g/kg/wk and resample in four weeks. If still inadequate, add prednisone 0.5 to 1.0 mg/kg/day (Fig. 51.1).
      If medical management fails, offer weekly in utero platelet transfusions (half-life is 5–7 days), delivery at ≥36 weeks.

C. Follow with serial (q 2–4 week) ultrasound assessments.

Other Issues Regarding Therapy

- Patients should be instructed to avoid activities (i.e., sports) that could result in potential trauma.
- External cephalic versions and NSAIDs are contraindicated.
- Fetal IVIG therapy is not efficacious, since it increases antibody levels, but does not always increase the platelet count.

- There are **reported cases of ICH while receiving IVIG treatment** (5,9), so that IVIG should be considered a highly effective, but not perfect therapy to prevent ICH (and therefore FBS and possible transfusions are still necessary).
- Women with prior IVIG administration should have their serum checked for HTLV I+II and HepC antibodies.

FETAL MONITORING/TESTING

FBS is indicated as shown in Figure 51.1. Ultrasound can help detect ICH, but when this is detected it is too late for intervention to prevent severe sequelae.

ANESTHESIA

No special precautions, since maternal platelets are usually normal (10% of women with NAIT have gestational thrombocytopenia).

DELIVERY

- Avoid fetal trauma: avoid maternal abdominal trauma, external cephalic version, fetal scalp lead, vacuum, or forceps.
- There is no proven evidence that cesarean delivery prevents ICH.
- If platelet count is ≥50,000/μL, vaginal delivery can be suggested.
- If platelet count >100,000/μL at the 32 weeks FBS, and patient is compliant with the effective therapy, vaginal delivery can be allowed.
- Cesarean delivery is indicated if platelet count is <50,000/μL right before the time of delivery. Therefore, in cases with platelets at 50,000 to 99,000/μL at 32 weeks, one can consider FBS at around 37 weeks to confirm adequate platelet count (≥50,000/μL) which is safe for trial of labor and attempt at vaginal delivery (10).

NEONATOLOGY MANAGEMENT

- Maternal platelets (Ag negative, obtained by plasmaphoresis, plasma depleted, washed, irradiated, and packed) should always be available for transfusion after delivery.
- Neonatal treatment is with IVIG, IV steroids, and antigen-compatible platelets until platelet count recovers, usually by 7 to 10 days of age.
- The volume of platelets transfused can be calculated as blood volume × (desired platelet count − actual platelet count/platelet concentration). For a term neonate, this equates to 1 cc platelet = increase platelet count by 5000/μL (10 cc = 50,000; 20 cc = 100,000). Often neo-

natologists choose to transfuse 10 cc of platelets per kg of neonatal weight.

FUTURE PREGNANCY PRECONCEPTION COUNSELING

Management, events, and outcome of the pregnancy should be reviewed with the family postpartum (after discharge of the neonate). As stated above, the natural history of NAIT is that, if it recurs (depending on father's zygocity), it is more severe than in the previous pregnancy.

REFERENCES

1. Davoren A, McParland P, Crowley J, et al. Antenatal screening for human platelet antigen-1a: results of a prospective study at a large maternity hospital in Ireland. Br J Obstet Gynecol 2003; 110:492–496. [II-2]
2. Bussel JB, Zabusky MR, Berkowitz RL, et al. Fetal alloimmune thrombocytopenia. N Engl J Med 1997; 337:22–26. [II-3]
3. Tiller H, Killie MK, Skogen B, et al. Neonatal alloimmune thrombocytopenia in Norway: poor detection rate with nonscreening versus a general screening programme. Br J Obstet Gynecol 2009; 116:594–598. [II-3]
4. Kamphuis MM, Paridaans N, Porcelijn L, et al. Screening in pregnancy for fetal or neonatal alloimmune thrombocytopenia: systematic review. Br J Obstet Gynecol 2010; 117:1335–1343. [Systematic review]
5. Kroll H, Kiefel V, Giers G, et al. Maternal intravenous immunoglobulin treatment does not prevent intracranial haemorrhage in fetal alloimmune thrombocytopenia. Transfus Med 1994; 4 (4):293–296. [II-2]
6. Bussel JB, Berkowitz RL, Lynch L, et al. Antenatal management of alloimmune thrombocytopenia with intravenous gamma-globulin: a randomized trial of the addition of low dose steroid to intravenous gamma-globulin. Am J Obstet Gynecol 1996; 174 (5):1414–1423. [RCT, *n* = 54]
7. Paidas MJ, Berkowitz RL, Lynch L, et al. Alloimmune thrombocytopenia: fetal and neonatal losses related to cordocentesis. Am J Obstet Gynecol 1995; 172:475–479. [II-3]
8. Overton T, Duncan KR, Jolly M, et al. Serial aggressive platelet transfusion for fetal alloimmune thrombocytopenia: platelet dynamics and perinatal outcome. Am J Obstet Gynecol 2002; 186:826–831. [II-2]
9. Berkowitz RL, Kolb EA, McFarland JG, et al. Parallel randomized trials of risk-based therapy for fetal alloimmune thrombocytopenia. Obstet Gynecol 2006; 107:91–96. [RCT, *n* = 79]
10. Berkowitz RL, Lesser ML, McFarland JG, et al. Antepartum treatment without early cordocentesis for standard-risk alloimmune thrombocytopenia. Obstet Gynecol 2007; 110:249–255. [RCT, *n* = 73]
11. Gaddipatti S, Berkjowitz RL, Lembert AA, et al. Initial fetal platelet counts predict the response to intravenous gammaglobulin therapy in fetuses that are affected by PLA1 incompatability. Am J Obstet Gynecol 2001; 185:976–980. [II-2]

52

Hemolytic disease of the fetus/neonate

Jacques E. Samson and Giancarlo Mari

KEY POINTS

- The formation of maternal antibodies to fetal red blood cell (RBC) antigens is called **RBC alloimmunization** and can lead to hemolytic disease and anemia of the fetus/neonate.
- The most common antigens causing alloimmunization in the United States today are **Rh(D)** and Kell. Rh(D) alloimmunization occurs when a pregnant woman develops an immunological response to a paternally derived Rh(D) antigen foreign to the mother and inherited by the fetus. The IgG antibodies cross the placenta, bind to the antigens on the fetal RBCs, and can lead to hemolysis. Kell alloimmunization is usually caused by previous blood transfusions but may also occur by maternal-fetal hemorrhage during pregnancy.
- **Anti-D immune globulin** prophylaxis prevents >99% of cases of Rh(D) alloimmunization if given **both antepartum and postpartum**. It should be given to all Rh(D)-negative women with a negative antibody screen at 28 weeks, and if the neonate is Rh(D) positive, within 72 hours after birth. Anti-D immune globulin can be given as late as **28 days postpartum** if previously not given but indicated. Anti-D immunoglobulin prophylaxis is **300 μg** (1 μg = 5 IU) at 28 weeks, as well as after delivery if the neonate is Rh(D) positive. **A 100 μg dose administered at 28 and 34 weeks is also used. However, there are no trials to directly compare the different regimes. Mothers who are weak D positive (formerly called Du) do not need anti-D prophylaxis. A **Kleihauer–Betke (KB) test** should be done to determine the number of fetal cells that has entered the maternal circulation, and hence **the appropriate dose of anti-D immune globulin** in certain high-risk situations (abdominal trauma, abruption, manual extraction of the placenta, etc.), or when the 100 μg dose is used, after delivery of an Rh(D)-negative, nonalloimmunized woman.
- **Currently, there is no prophylactic immune globulin to prevent Kell alloimmunization.**
- If Rh(D) antibodies are detected in the maternal circulation on the antibody screen, the patient is considered alloimmunized. Management of the alloimmunized pregnancy is shown in **Figure 52.1**. This is based initially on genotyping of the fetus' father and, if necessary, fetal Rh(D) status determination, usually by polymerase chain reaction (PCR) from amniocytes. Maternal blood for fetal DNA testing is also available. **The critical titer for Rh(D) antibody should be determined in each laboratory.**
- **Ultrasound using the middle cerebral artery peak systolic velocity (MCA-PSV)** has 100% sensitivity for detecting significant fetal anemia (95% CI: 0.86–1.00), and is the screening method of choice in RBC alloimmunized pregnancies, if available and quality assurance can be confirmed. Compared with amniocentesis for delta OD450, the MCA-PSV assessment is associated with approximately 70% to 80% reduction in the number of invasive tests. Screening with MCA-PSV can be started as early as 15 weeks. If the **MCA-PSV is ≥1.5** multiple of the median **(MOM), fetal blood sampling (FBS) is indicated**. When a cordocentesis is performed at >24 weeks' gestation, corticosteroids for fetal lung maturation should be considered before the procedure. Blood transfusions should be initiated for fetal hemoglobin <5th percentile.
- If adequately trained sonographers are not available, screening for anemia should be done with amniocentesis using ΔOD_{450} values.
- In **Kell**-alloimmunized pregnancies, maternal titers do not correlate well with fetal disease. ΔOD_{450} levels also do not correlate with fetal anemia. However, MCA-PSV screening is predictive and accurate for the diagnosis of fetal anemia from Kell alloimmunization.

DEFINITION

RBC alloimmunization, formerly known as isoimmunization, or erythroblastosis fetalis, is the formation of maternal antibodies to fetal RBC antigens (1). Maternal RBC alloimmunization can cause hemolytic disease of the fetus/neonate.

EPIDEMIOLOGY/INCIDENCE

The most common antigen causing alloimmunization is Rh(D) followed closely by the Kell antigen (2,3). The Rh(D)-negative blood group is found in about 15% of whites, 3% to 5% of black Africans, and is rare in Asians. Spontaneous fetomaternal hemorrhages occur in increasing frequency and volume with advancing age. In 3%, 12%, and 46% of women, 0.01 mL or more of fetal cells in each of the three successive trimesters have been noted using the Kleihauer assay (4). The risk of Rh(D) alloimmunization during or immediately after a first pregnancy is about 0.7% to 1%. The risk of fetal anemia from RBC alloimmunization is about 0.35%, of which about 10% of cases require transfusion. Rh(D) alloimmunization affects 6.7 out of every 1000 live births (5).

The Kell (K1) antigen is found on red cells of 9% of Caucasians and 2% of people of African descent. Kell alloimmunization occurs in 1 to 3 per 1000 fetuses (6).

GENETICS

Rh(D)-negative pregnant women have a deletion of the sequence on both copies of the short arm of chromosome 1. The Kell glycoprotein is a type II membrane protein with homology to zinc endopeptidases (M13 family) (7).

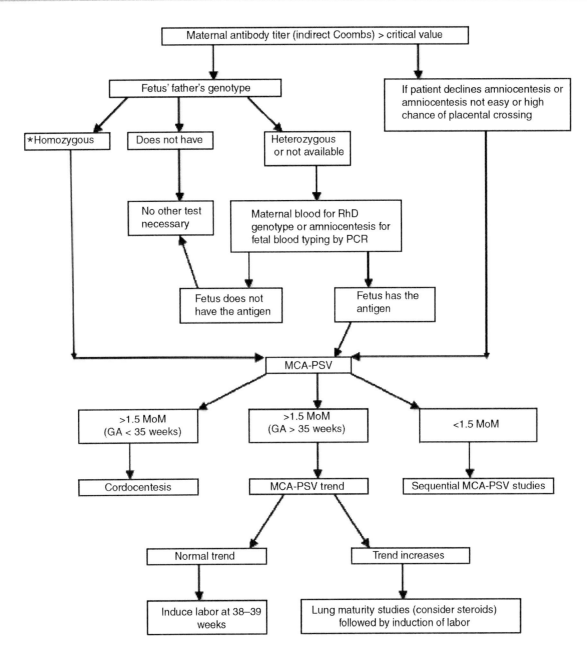

Maternal antibody titer (indirect Coombs) > critical value

Fetus' father's genotype

If patient declines amniocentesis or amniocentesis not easy or high chance of placental crossing

*Homozygous

Does not have

Heterozygous or not available

No other test necessary

Maternal blood for RhD genotype or amniocentesis for fetal blood typing by PCR

Fetus does not have the antigen

Fetus has the antigen

MCA-PSV

>1.5 MoM (GA < 35 weeks)

>1.5 MoM (GA > 35 weeks)

<1.5 MoM

Cordocentesis

MCA-PSV trend

Sequential MCA-PSV studies

Normal trend

Trend increases

Induce labor at 38–39 weeks

Lung maturity studies (consider steroids) followed by induction of labor

* Homozygous: Fetus will be Rh+

Figure 52.1 Algorithm for clinical management of RhD isoimmunization. *Abbreviations*: GA, gestational age; MCA, middle cerebral artery; MOM, multiples of the median; PCR, polymerase chain reaction; PSV, peak systolic velocity

ETIOLOGY/BASIC PATHOPHYSIOLOGY

Maternal Rh(D) alloimmunization occurs when a pregnant woman develops an immunologic response to a paternally derived RBC antigen—for example, Rh(D) that is foreign to the mother and inherited by the fetus. The immunoglobulin G (IgG) antibodies cross the placenta, bind to the antigens present on the fetal RBCs, and can cause hemolysis. Hemolysis then causes anemia which, if severe, leads to fetal cardiac failure, edema, hydrops, and eventually fetal death. Other antigens ("irregular antigens") than Rh(D) can cause RBC alloimmunization.

Alloimmunization of the Kell antigen may be caused by previous blood transfusion or by maternal-fetal hemorrhage

during the pregnancy with a fetus who is a Kell antigen carrier (8,9). The Kell glycoprotein is expressed very early in erythropoiesis (10). Antibody to Kell appears to inhibit erythropoiesis, suggesting another functional role for Kell in addition to its endopeptidase activity (11).

NATURAL HISTORY

About 17% of Rh(D)-negative women who do not receive prophylaxis become immunized. Over 90% of this immunization occurs from fetomaternal hemorrhage at delivery, and the majority of the remaining 10% occurs in the third trimester. Most of this immunization is caused by <0.1 mL of fetomaternal

Table 52.1   Risk of RBC Alloimmunization in Different Clinical Situations

Clinical situation	Risk of red blood cell alloimmunization (%)
Induced abortions	4–5
First-trimester losses	1–2
Chorionic villus sampling	14
Amniocentesis	7–15
External cephalic version	2–6
Threatened abortion	↑ (controversial)
Antepartum hemorrhage	↑↑
Placenta previa with bleeding	↑
Suspected abruption	↑
Blunt trauma to abdomen (including motor vehicle accidents)	↑
Fetal death	↑
Fetal blood sampling	↑
Fetal surgery	↑
Ectopic	↑
Partial molar pregnancy	↑

hemorrhage. Before anti-D immune globulin prevention, hemolytic disease of the fetus/neonate affected 9% to 10% of pregnancies, and was a major cause of perinatal mortality. The risk of RBC alloimmunization from different clinical situations is shown in Table 52.1.

Anti-K1 is responsible for severe neonatal anemia in approximately 40% of K1-positive babies of women with anti-K1 (12).

PREVENTION (ANTI-D IMMUNOGLOBULIN)

The ABO type, the Rh(D) status, and the antibody screen should be determined in all pregnant women at the initial prenatal visit. If the woman is Rh-negative and the antibody screen is negative, the patient should receive Rh(D) immune globulin. Anti-D immunoglobulin prophylaxis properly given prevents >99% of cases of alloimmunization. It is controversial whether the antibody screen should be repeated at 28 weeks before the administration of immune globulin. The advantage of this second screening test is the detection of those rare cases in which immunization occurs early in pregnancy. After delivery, if the neonate is Rh(D) positive, the patient should receive immune globulin. If the patient has never received immune globulin and the screening test is positive, the patient is at risk for having an anemic baby in the current pregnancy (if she has not delivered yet) or in a future pregnancy if she already has delivered. Usually, the effect of the immune globulin is not present 12 weeks after its administration.

Anti-D immune globulin prophylaxis properly given prevents the majority of cases of alloimmunization. Unfortunately, there is no immune globulin available for prevention of RBC antigens other than Rh(D). Anti-D immune globulin is extracted by cold alcohol fractionation from plasma of individuals with high-titer D IgG antibodies. The risk of transmission of viral infections or side effects is minimal to absent and clinically not a significant factor.

The accepted regimes of **anti-D immune globulin prophylaxis** are (i) 100 µg at 28 and 34 weeks and after delivery if the neonate is Rh(D) positive, or (ii) 300 µg at 28 weeks and after delivery if the neonate is Rh(D) positive and delivery occurs at least three weeks after the first administration. There are no trials to directly compare these two different regimes, but they probably both achieve >99% prevention of Rh(D) alloimmunization.

The half-life of anti-D immune globulin is 16 to 24 days. When the 300 µg dose is used and delivery does not occur within 12 weeks of injection, a second 300 µg dose of anti-D immunoglobulin should be given. The antibody titer obtained at term is occasionally still positive (1:1, 1:2 titer) after anti-D immunoglobulin at 28 weeks' gestation.

When indicated, a second dose of immune globulin is administered after delivery, even in cases of preterm delivery.

Mothers who are **weak D** positive with D present in reduced quantities (formerly called Du) **do not need anti-D prophylaxis**. Mothers who are **partial D** positive (lacking some epitopes of D) should receive anti-D immunoglobulin, since they are at risk for hemolytic disease (13). In those cases where the **father of the fetus/neonate is definitely known to be Rh(D) negative**, neither antepartum nor postpartum anti-D prophylaxis is administered.

Evidence for Dosing and Timing
After Birth (Postpartum)
Anti-D immune globulin given within 72 hours **after birth** is associated with a **96% decreased incidence** of Rh(D) alloimmunization six months after birth, and by a **88% decreased incidence** of Rh(D) alloimmunization in a subsequent pregnancy in Rh(D)-negative women who have given birth to an Rh(D)-positive infant (14). These benefits are seen regardless of the ABO status of the mother and baby. **Higher doses (up to 200 µg) are more effective than lower doses (up to 50 µg)** in preventing Rh(D) alloimmunization (14). Anti-D immune globulin can be given **as late as 28 days postpartum** if indicated but not previously given. **Anti-D immune globulin is given to all Rh(D)-negative women after confirmation from cord blood of Rh(D)-positive status of the neonate**.

Even when immune globulin is correctly administered and with higher doses, alloimmunization can still occur (antepartum) in up to 2% of these women if only postpartum anti-D is administered.

Before Birth (Antepartum)
The addition of anti-D immune globulin 100 µg (500 IU) prophylaxis at 28 and 34 week **lowers this risk (about 1–2%) to about 0.2%** without any adverse effects (15–17). When women receive anti-D immune globulin at 28 and 34 weeks' gestation, there is a trend for less immunization (i) for all women (RR: 0.42, 95% CI: 0.15–1.17); and (ii) for women giving birth to an Rh-positive infant (RR:0.41, 95% CI: 0.16–1.04), compared with no prophylaxis (15–17). In trials that used a 100 µg dose of anti-D immune globulin, there was a nonsignificant reduction in immunization at 2 to 12 months following birth of an Rh-positive infant in women who had received anti-D (RR: 0.14, 95% CI: 0.02–1.15). However, women receiving anti-D were significantly less likely to have a positive KB test (which detects fetal cells in maternal blood) both in pregnancy (RR: 0.60, 95% CI: 0.41–0.88) and at the birth of an Rh-positive infant (RR: 0.60, 95% CI: 0.46–0.79) (16). No data were available for the risk of Rh(D) alloimmunization in a subsequent pregnancy. No differences were seen for neonatal jaundice.

There are no trials using the 300 µg dose, or trials comparing just 28 week versus both 28 and 34-week prophylaxis.

Even with antepartum and postpartum prophylaxis, the risk of Rh(D) alloimmunization remains because of inadvertent antepartum or postpartum omission, failure to use the drug for other antenatal complications, and insufficient dosing at delivery in cases of large fetomaternal hemorrhage. **Practice guidelines in the United States** recommend that anti-D immune globulin be administered early in the third trimester: **300 μg at 28 weeks**. This practice reduces the incidence of antenatal alloimmunization from 2% to 0.1% (2,3). In the **United Kingdom, 100 μg** of anti-D immune globulin is given at 28 and 34 weeks (13). **In Canada, 100 to 120 μg** is administered at 28 and 34 weeks.

Special Clinical Situations

In addition to antepartum and postpartum prophylaxis, other indications for the use of anti-D immune globulin include those situations in which there is significant risk of fetomaternal hemorrhage. These indications are listed in Table 52.1. A repeat dose is unnecessary after prophylaxis if delivery occurs <3 weeks from the last dose.

Anti-D immune globulin 300 μg protects against 30 mL of fetal whole blood or 15 mL of fetal RBCs in the maternal circulation. In certain high-risk situations in which excessive fetomaternal bleeding may have occurred (e.g., abruption, manual removal of the placenta, abdominal trauma), this dose may be inadequate, and a **KB test** should be done **to determine** the amount of fetal cells that have entered the maternal circulation and, hence, **the appropriate dose of anti-D immune globulin** to be given. Some clinicians have advocated the KB test for all Rh(D)-negative women at delivery, since 50% of cases requiring more than the standard postpartum dose of anti-D immunoglobulin can be missed by high-risk situation screening only (18). **The risk of fetomaternal hemorrhage >30 mL is about 0.1% to 0.2%**.

The anti-D immunoglobulin available in the United States and other countries (RhoGAM, Rhophylac, WinRho, and BabyRho-D) are all very effective, with none shown to be significantly more effective in the prevention of hemolytic disease than the others. Thus cost and route of administration—intramuscular (IM) or intravenous (IV) —may be the only factors determining choice.

MANAGEMENT OF RBC ALLOIMMUNIZED PREGNANCIES
Counseling

If Rh(D) antibodies are detected in the maternal circulation, for example, positive indirect Coombs, the patient is considered alloimmunized. Among Rh(D) alloimmunized pregnancies, mild-to-moderate hemolytic anemia and hyperbilirubinemia occur in 25% to 30% of fetuses/neonates, and 25% of these can develop hydrops (19). With correct management, the **perinatal survival rate in cases of anemia is >90%**; when fetal hydrops is present, the survival rate is >80%. There is no trial that has assessed the best management for RBC alloimmunized pregnancies; however, fetal transfusion is probably the most beneficial of all the available therapies. Although it is reported that the risk of fetal demise is between 1% and 2% for each FBS, there are situations in which the risk is much higher, such as when cordocenteses and transfusions are performed at gestational ages (GAs) as early as 15 to 18 weeks.

Workup/Investigations Required

Management of the **alloimmunized** pregnancy is shown in Figure 52.1. In patients at risk for fetal anemia because of red cell alloimmunization, it is important to perform a first-trimester ultrasound to establish the GA. Assessment for risk of fetal anemia depends on history of previous Rh complications in pregnancies, titer of RBC antibodies, and MCA-PSV values (20,21).

The genotype of the fetus' father can be determined by zygosity testing. The most likely zygosity can also be predicted by evaluating the pattern of C, D, and E loci, since they are inherited together and some combinations are more common than others, but this is not 100% exact and not very useful clinically. If the father is Rh(D) negative, no further testing or intervention is necessary. If the father is heterozygous for the Rh(D) antigen, fetal Rh(D) testing is indicated. If the father is Rh(D) homozygous, the fetus is assumed to be Rh(D) positive and no fetal Rh(D) testing is necessary. Of course, the paternity should be certain; otherwise, fetal testing is indicated.

Fetal Rh(D) status can be determined by **PCR from amniocytes** with >95% accuracy (sensitivity and specificity). This is available in the United States in several centers. One of them is the Blood Center of Southwestern Wisconsin (http:// www.bloodcenter.com). This is also available for many other antigens, such as c, E, Kell, M, N, etc. Chorionic villus sampling (CVS) is not advised, as it results in high risk of worsening alloimmunization from fetomaternal hemorrhage. Determination of fetal Rh(D) status can **also** be obtained **noninvasively**, with fetal DNA analysis from maternal blood (22,23). This can be done through the International Blood Group Reference Laboratory in Bristol, United Kingdom (Molecular.Diagnostics@nhsbt.nhs.uk; http://ibgrl.blood.co. uk/), or, currently under a research basis, the Blood Center of Southeastern Wisconsin.

Rh(D) antibody titers correlate somewhat with risk of anemia/hydrops, with 1:16 = 10%, 1:32 = 25%, 1:64 = 50%, and 1:128 = 75% risk of anemia. **The critical titer should be determined in each laboratory**. Unfortunately large differences in titer can be seen in the same woman between laboratories. In most laboratories, the critical titer is ≥1:16 in albumin or ≥1:32 in indirect antiglobulin (indirect Coombs test). If the titer is less than 1:16, the fetus is not in jeopardy at that time. However, serial titers should be obtained every four weeks. If the patient has had a prior affected pregnancy, and the fetus is known to be Rh(D) positive, titers are not necessary. The MCA-PSV is used to detect those fetuses that are going to develop anemia (24). The presence of additional antibody(ies) with anti-D increases the need for intrauterine fetal transfusions (25).

Ultrasound is the screening method of choice for fetal anemia. With fetal anemia, decreased blood viscosity leads to increased venous return, consequent increase in cardiac output,

Table 52.2 Expected Peak Velocity of Systolic Blood Flow in the Middle Cerebral Artery as a Function of Gestational Age

Week of gestation	Multiples of the median			
	1.00	1.29	1.50	1.55
18	23.2[a]	29.9	34.8	36.0
20	25.5	32.8	38.2	39.5
22	27.9	36.0	41.9	43.3
24	30.7	39.5	46.0	47.5
26	33.6	43.3	50.4	52.1
28	36.9	47.9	55.4	57.2
30	40.5	52.2	60.7	62.8
32	44.4	57.3	66.6	68.9
34	48.7	62.9	73.1	75.6
36	53.5	69.0	80.2	82.9
38	58.7	75.7	88.0	91.0
40	64.4	83.0	96.6	99.8

Mild anemia: MCA-PSV between 1.29 and 1.49 MOM; **moderate anemia**: MCA-PSV between 1.50 and 1.54 MOM; **severe anemia**: MCA-PSV ≥1.55 MOM.
[a]Data shown are in cm/sec (median).

Table 52.3 Reference Ranges for Fetal Hemoglobin Concentrations as a Function of Gestational Age

Week of gestation	Multiples of the median				
	1.16	1.00	0.84	0.65	0.55
18	12.3[a]	10.6	8.9	6.9	5.8
20	12.9	11.1	9.3	7.2	6.1
22	13.4	11.6	9.7	7.5	6.4
24	13.9	12.0	10.1	7.8	6.6
26	14.3	12.3	10.3	8.0	6.8
28	14.6	12.6	10.6	8.2	6.9
30	14.8	12.8	10.8	8.3	7.1
32	15.2	13.1	10.9	8.5	7.2
34	15.4	13.3	11.2	8.6	7.3
36	15.6	13.5	11.3	8.7	7.4
38	15.8	13.6	11.4	8.9	7.5
40	16.0	13.8	11.6	9.0	7.6

The values at 1.16 and 0.84 multiples of the median correspond to the 95th and 5th percentiles, respectively (the normal range). **Mild anemia**: hemoglobin concentration between 0.84 and 0.66 MOM; **moderate anemia**: hemoglobin concentration between 0.65 and 0.55 MOM; **severe anemia**: hemoglobin concentration <0.65 MOM.
[a]Data shown are in g/dL (median).

with increased blood flow velocity in all vessels. Degrees of blood velocity (Table 52.2) correlate with anemia (Table 52.3). The vessel to study is the **middle cerebral artery** (MCA). The main advantage of the MCA is that it is easy to measure at a $0°$ angle. In the biparietal diameter view, the MCA can be visualized with color Doppler. The MCA-PSV should be measured at its proximal point, after the origin from the internal carotid artery, at a $0°$ angle (avoiding angle correction). Measurement at this point allows the lowest intra- and interobserver variability as well as standardization of the measurement (26). Multiples of the median for the hemoglobin concentration and MCA-PSV correct for the effect of GA on the measurement. The MCA-PSV had a sensitivity of 100% (95% CI: 0.86–1.0) for detection of significant fetal anemia with a false-positive rate of 12% at 1.50 MOM in one study (21). Other studies have reported lower sensitivity, but in general above 85% to 90% (27). The number of false-positives increases following 35 weeks' gestation (28). The number of false-positive cases after 35 weeks may be decreased by looking at the trend of the MCA-PSV (24).

Compared with amniocentesis for ΔOD_{450}, the MCA-PSV assessment is associated with a 70% to 80% reduction in the number of invasive tests (21). The MCA-PSV is more accurate than amniocentesis in detecting fetal anemia (27,29–31).

The correction of fetal anemia with intrauterine transfusion decreases significantly and normalizes the value of fetal MCA-PSV (32,33) because of an increased blood viscosity and an increased oxygen concentration in fetal blood. The MCA-PSV may be used in fetuses previously transfused (34,35).

Accuracy with the MCA-PSV can only be achieved with appropriate training and quality assurance. If adequately trained sonographers are not available, screening for anemia should be done with amniocentesis (see below). Screening with MCA-PSV can be started as early as 15 weeks (36). The MCA-PSV can also be used for other causes of anemia, including parvovirus infection, nonimmune hydrops, fetal-maternal hemorrhage, and twin-twin transfusion syndrome.

The steps for the correct measurement of the MCA-PSV are the following: (*i*) An axial section of the head is obtained at the level of the sphenoid bones; (*ii*) Color Doppler evidences the circle of Willis; (*iii*) the circle of Willis is enlarged; (*iv*) the

color box is placed around the MCA; (*v*) the MCA is zoomed; and, (*vi*) the MCA flow velocity waveforms are displayed and the highest point of the waveform (PSV) is measured. The waveforms should be all similar. The above sequence is repeated at least three times in each fetus.

There should be an absence of fetal movement or fetal breathing during measurement of the MCA-PSV.

Severe intrauterine growth restriction also shows an increased MCA-PSV (37). Therefore, this should be taken into account when the MCA-PSV is used to diagnose fetal anemia. However, it is very unlikely that an anemic fetus is also a severe IUGR fetus.

Moderate to severe anemia may also be suggested by hydropic signs (at least two of pericardial or pleural effusion, ascites, or skin edema), an increase in the size of fetal liver or placental thickness, or tricuspid regurgitation.

Amniocentesis for ΔOD_{450} measurement is used if accurate MCA screening is not available. The ΔOD_{450} measurement can be evaluated using either the Liley (38) or Queenan (39) charts. There is controversy over which one is best before 27 weeks, the "extended" Liley curve or the Queenan curve (40). The guidelines for the amniocentesis are arbitrary and serial MCA-PSV measurements are superior in terms of sensitivity, specificity, and positive and negative predictive values to both the Liley and the Queenan curve (27).

If the MCA-PSV test cannot be done and the patient opts for an amniocentesis, the following are general guidelines for managing the Liley curve readings:

- Zone 1: repeat amniocentesis in two to four weeks. If zone 1, follow with ultrasound every one or two weeks until delivery.
- Zone 2 (low/middle third): repeat amniocentesis in about two weeks. If low zone 2, follow with ultrasound every week until delivery. If upper third zone 2, consider FBS.
- Zone 2 (upper third): consider FBS or repeat amniocentesis in 7 days. If again upper third zone 2 or higher, FBS.
- Zone 3: FBS.

The advantage of using Queenan's curve is that it can be used following 14 weeks' gestation. Amniocentesis is associated with a 2% to 3% (up to 15%) risk of fetomaternal hemorrhage. Following fetal transfusions the maternal antibody titer rises significantly.

Fetal Intervention

An IV transfusion is indicated **when the MCA-PSV is >1.5 MOM**. (Table 52.2). Other ultrasonographic signs of hydrops may also suggest fetal anemia, or, if ΔOD_{450} is being used for screening instead of the MCA-PSV, a value in the upper third of zone 2 or zone 3 is an indication for FBS.

Transfusion is performed at the umbilical vein either at the placental insertion or inside the abdomen. Intraperitoneal transfusion is rarely performed and it is contraindicated in the hydropic fetus because of the poor absorption of blood. **Corticosteroids for fetal maturation should be considered before the procedure when FBS is performed at or after 24 weeks**. Type O, Rh(D) negative, cytomegalovirus negative, washed, leukoreduced, irradiated packed RBCs cross-matched against maternal blood should be used. The blood usually contains 75% to 85% RBCs, to allow minimal blood volume for the transfusions (41).

The procedure is performed under continuous ultrasound guidance. Prophylactic antibiotics can be given, although no trial has evaluated their efficacy. Following

24 weeks, the procedure should be performed in a location close to the OR and the anesthesiologist consulted should an emergency occur. Tubing and syringes should be heparinized. Maternal skin can be anesthesized with 1% lidocaine at the point of needle entry. A 20- or 22-gauge needle is used for the procedure. After entering the umbilical vein, a sample of fetal blood is withdrawn and the hemoglobin immediately (within one or two minutes) determined. Fetal blood is confirmed by a mean corpuscular volume (MCV) >110 μm^3. Then the fetus is given a paralytic agent (e.g., pavulon 0.1 mg/kg) to stop fetal movements (42).

If the hematocrit is below the fifth percentile (0.84 MOM) for GA, blood is transfused in a sterile fashion. A computer program (e.g., http://www.perinatology.com/protocols/rhc.htm) can be used to estimate the amount of blood to transfuse based on the initial fetal hematocrit, the estimated fetal weight and the concentration of the blood transfused (43,44). The following formula is used:

$$V_{transfused\,(mL)} = \frac{V_{fetoplacental\,(mL)}(Hct_{final} - Hct_{inital})}{Hct_{transfused\,blood}}$$

A final fetal blood sample is taken a few seconds after the transfusion has been completed. If the fetus is hydropic, it is better to perform more than one transfusion at a distance of three to five days to increase the hematocrit to the median hematocrit value for GA. At and after 24 weeks, the fetal heart rate should be monitored for the next two to three hours until fetal movements resume. The risk of fetal death is 1% to 2% even with ultrasound guidance, expert operators, and accurate management.

Thrombocytopenia, even at levels <100,000/mm^3, can be found in about 9% of Rh(D) alloimmunized fetuses at times of fetal sampling (45). Thrombocytopenia is associated with fetal hydrops, and with perinatal mortality (45).

Intravenous immunoglobulin in addition to fetal transfusion has been studied insufficiently, and is not currently recommended (46).

Hematocrit decreases about 1 point per day posttransfusion in the anemic alloimmunized fetus, and this knowledge helps to assess when to repeat the transfusion. If the fetus is nonhydropic, the second transfusion is often necessary 14 days after the first, but after the second/third transfusion, longer intervals of three weeks may be possible as the fetal RBCs are replaced by adult RBCs. Following three transfusions, 99% of the fetal blood is represented by the adult transfused blood. Maternal phenobarbital 30 mg three times per day for 7 to 10 days to enhance fetal liver maturity and ability to conjugate bilirubin is still unconfirmed by large studies (47).

Fetal Monitoring/Testing

Fetal testing with nonstress tests (NSTs) or biophysical profiles (BPPs) is started around 32 weeks or earlier if indicated. Its benefit has not been confirmed in a specific trial. Fetuses with very severe anemia (hemoglobin ≤2 g/dL) due to RBC alloimmunization may develop brain injury (e.g., intracerebellar hemorrhage). Therefore, clinicians have advocated fetal neuroimaging by ultrasound and/or MRI (48).

The surfactant/albumin ratio for fetal lung maturity (FLM) cannot be used since high amniotic fluid bilirubin can affect this result. The other tests for FLM are reliable (see also chap. 57).

Delivery

See Figure 52.1 for the timing of delivery. The mode of delivery depends on obstetrical indications. If fetal anemia is suspected during a trial of labor, procedures such as scalp FHR monitoring, scalp pH, and operative delivery should be avoided if possible.

Anesthesia

There are no specific anesthesia precautions.

Neonatology Management

Anemic neonates are usually treated with transfusions or exchange transfusions as necessary. They often need light therapy for hyperbilirubinemia. Breast-feeding is not contraindicated. A hearing screening test is indicated during the neonatal period and at two years of age given that hyperbilirubinemia can cause sensorineural hearing loss. Children who survive severe hemolytic disease (even with hydrops and/or necessitating transfusions) often have a normal neurologic outcome (49).

OTHER "ATYPICAL" ANTIBODIES

There are many atypical (irregular) blood group antibodies that are capable of producing hemolytic disease. Given their rarity, and the absence of large studies or any trial, the management of antibodies known to cause hemolytic disease other than Rh(D) is based on poor evidence. Many aspects of management are unknown or similar to Rh(D) alloimmunization, except for the details below. It should be acknowledged that the critical titer for antibodies other than Rh(D) has not been well-established.

Kell Alloimmunization

The incidence of Kell alloimmunization is about 0.1% to 0.3% in pregnant women. Kell alloimmunization is usually caused by prior transfusion. Over 90% of partners of Kell-immunized women are Kell negative. In the white population, only 9% of fathers are Kell positive, and only 0.2% are homozygous. **Maternal titers do not correlate well with fetal alloimmune disease.** Severe anemia can be diagnosed in fetuses whose mothers had a titer as low as 1:2. **ΔOD_{450} levels also do not correlate with fetal anemia.** This is because fetal anemia is not caused by hemolysis, but by suppression of erythropoiesis at the progenitor-cell level. Anti-Kell antibodies specifically inhibit the growth of Kell-positive erythroid burst-forming units and colony-forming units (11). In fact, anti-Kell anemic fetuses have lower reticulocyte counts and bilirubin levels compared to anti-D anemic fetuses. The Kell blood group is complex, consisting of over two dozen antigens. Kell 1 (Kell, or K1) and its allelic partner Kell 2 (Cellano, or K2) are strong immunogens. Poor fetal outcome occurs in about 1.5% to 3% of Kell-alloimmunized pregnancies, an incidence that is possibly higher than that of other RBC antigens. The management of Kell sensitization is somewhat controversial. Genotyping of the father of the baby (FOB) is extremely important. Most will be Kell negative, and, if paternity is certain, no further testing is necessary. The vast majority of Kell-positive FOBs are heterozygote, so the fetal Kell status needs to be determined, usually by amniocentesis PCR. **MCA-PSV screening is predictive and accurate for the diagnosis of fetal anemia from Kell alloimmunization** (21,50). MCA-PSV monitoring should start at 15 weeks, and be performed as suggested in Figure 52.1. **ΔOD_{450}** measurements from amniocentesis are inaccurate and should not be used.

Other CDE System Antigens

c (small): This antigen carries a 65% risk of hemolytic disease; 80% of FOBs are positive, of which half are homozygous, half heterozygous.

C (big): This antigen is associated with a 32% risk of hemolytic disease.

E (big): E-positive individuals have a 31% risk of hemolytic disease. Maternal titers do not correlate well with fetal hemolytic disease.

MNS Antigen System

Only 1% of titers ever rise to $\geq 1:64$. Only five cases of severe anemia from anti-M alloimmunization have ever been reported, such that, even if sensitized, the incidence of severe anemia is probably <1%.

Others

Other rare, but potentially lethal, antigens are **Duffy (Fya, Fyb, Fy3, etc.), and Kidd, as well as others**.

REFERENCES

1. Levine P, Katzin E, Burnham L. Isoimmunization in pregnancy: its possible bearing on the etiology of erythroblastosis fetalis. J Am Med Assoc 1941; 116:825–827. [II-3]
2. Landsteiner K, Weiner A. An agglutinable factor in human blood recognized by immune sera for Rhesus blood. Proc Soc Exp Biol Med 1940; 43:223. [II-3]
3. van Wamelen D, Klumper F, de Haas M, et al. Obstetric history and antibody titer in estimating severity of Kell alloimmunization in pregnancy. Obstet Gynecol 2007; 109(5):1093–1098. [II-3]
4. Bowman J, Pollock J, Penston L. Fetomaternal transplacental hemorrhage during pregnancy and after delivery. Vox Sang 1986; 51:117–121. [II-3]
5. Martin J, Park M, Sutton P. Births: preliminary data for 2001. Natl Vital Stat Rep 2002; 50(10):1–20. [II-3]
6. Geifman-Holtzman O, Wojtowycz M, Kosmas E, et al. Female alloimmunization with antibodies known to cause hemolytic disease. Obstet Gynecol 1997; 89:272–275. [II-3]
7. Castilho L, Rios M, Rodrigues A, et al. High frequency of partial Dilla and DAR alleles found in sickle cell patients suggests increased risk of alloimmunization to RhD. Transfus Med 2005; 15:49–55. [II-3]
8. Mayne K, Bowell P, Pratt G. The significance of anti-Kell sensitization in pregnancy. Clin Lab Haematol 1990; 12(4):379–385. [II-2]
9. Grant S, Kilby M, Meer L, et al. The outcome of pregnancy in Kell alloimmunisation. Br J Obstet Gynecol 2000; 107(4):481–485. [II-3]
10. Southcott M, Tanner M, Anstee D. The expression of human blood group antigens during erythropoiesis in a cell culture system. Blood 1999; 93(12):4425–4435. [II-2]
11. Vaughan J, Manning M, Warwick R, et al. Inhibition of erythroid progenitor cells by anti-Kell antibodies in fetal alloimmune anemia. N Engl J Med 1998; 338:798–803. [II-2]
12. Caine M, Mueller-Heubach E. Kell sensitization in pregnancy. Am J Obstet Gynecol 1986; 154:85–90. [III]
13. Lurie S, Rotmensch S, Glezerman M. Prenatal management of women who have partial Rh (D) antigen. Br J Obstet Gynecol 2001; 108:895–897. [Review]
14. Crowther C, Middleton P. Anti-D administration after childbirth for preventing Rhesus alloimmunisation. Cochrane Database Syst Rev 2000;(2):CD000021. PMID: 10796089. [Meta-analysis]
15. Crowther C, Keirse MJ. Anti-D administration in pregnancy for preventing rhesus alloimmunisation. Cochrane Database Syst Rev 2000; (2):CD000020. PMID: 10796088. [Meta-analysis]
16. Huchet J, Dallemagne S, Huchet C, et al. The antepartum use of anti-D immunoglobulin in rhesus negative women. Parallel evaluation of fetal blood cells passing through the placenta. The results of a multicentre study carried out in the region of Paris. Eur J Obstet Gynecol Reprod Biol 1987; 16:101–111. [RCT, n = 1882 primiparous Rh-D negative women. Administration of 100 μg (500 IU) anti-D immune globulin at 28 weeks and 34 weeks of pregnancy (n = 927). No placebo was given to the control group (n = 955)]
17. Lee D, Rawlinson V. Multicentre trial of antepartum low-dose anti-D immunoglobulin. Transfus Med 1995; 5:15–19. [RCT, n = 2541 Rh-D negative primigravidae. 50 μg (250 IU) anti-D intramuscularly at 28 and 34 weeks' gestation (n = 952). Control group had no placebo (n = 1068)]
18. Ness P, Baldwin M, Niebyl J. Clinical high-risk designations does not predict excess fetal-maternal hemorrhage. Am J Obstet Gynecol 1987; 156:154–158. [II-2]
19. ACOG. Prevention of Rh D alloimmunization. Obstet Gynecol 1999 (Practice Bulletin No. 4, May). [Review]
20. Mari G, Adrignolo A, Abuhamad A, et al. Diagnosis of fetal anemia with Doppler ultrasound in the pregnancy complicated by maternal blood group immunization. Ultrasound Obstet Gynecol 1995; 5:400–405. [II-2]
21. Mari G, Deter R, Carpenter R, et al. Noninvasive diagnosis by Doppler ultrasonography of fetal anemia due to maternal red-cell alloimmunization. Collaborative Group for Doppler Assessment of the Blood Velocity in Anemic Fetuses. N Engl J Med 2000; 342:9–14. [II-2]
22. Bianchi D, Avent N, Costa J, et al. Noninvasive prenatal diagnosis of fetal Rhesus D. Ready for prime(r) time. Obstet Gynecol 2005; 106:841–844. [Review]
23. Harper T, Finning K, Martin P, et al. Use of maternal plasma for noninvasive determination of fetal RhD status. Am J Obstet Gynecol 2004; 191:1730–1732. [II-3]
24. Detti L, Mari G, Akiyama M, et al. Longitudinal assessment of the middle cerebral artery peak systolic velocity in healthy fetuses and in fetuses at risk for anemia. Am J Obstet Gynecol 2002; 187:937–939. [II-2]
25. Spong C, Porter A, Queenan J. Management of isoimmunization in the presence of multiple maternal antibodies. Am J Obstet Gynecol 2001; 185:481–484. [II-2].
26. Mari G, Abuhamad A, Cosmi E, et al. Middle cerebral artery peak systolic velocity—technique and variability. J Ultrasound Med 2005; 24:425–430. [II-2]
27. Oepkes D, Seaward P, Vandenbussche F, et al. Doppler ultrasonography versus amniocentesis to predict fetal anemia. N Engl J Med 2006; 355:156–164. [II-1]
28. Zimmermann R, Durig P, Carpenter RJ, et al. Longitudinal measurement of peak systolic velocity in the fetal middle cerebral artery for monitoring pregnancies complicated by red cell alloimmunisation: a prospective multicentre trial with intention-to-treat. Br J Obstet Gynaecol 2002; 109:746–752. [II-2]
29. Mari G, Penso C, Sbracia M, et al. Delta OD 450 and Doppler velocimetry of the middle cerebral artery peak velocity in the evaluation for fetal alloimmune hemolytic disease. Which is the best? (1997, January) Proceedings, Society for Perinatal Obstetricians, Anaheim, CA. Am J Obstet Gynecol 1997; 176: S18. [II-3]
30. Nishie E, Brizot M, Liao A, et al. A comparison between middle cerebral artery peak systolic velocity and amniotic fluid optical density at 450 nm in the prediction of fetal anemia. Am J Obstet Gynecol 2003; 188(1):214–219. [II-2]
31. Pereira L, Jenkins T, Berghella V. Conventional management of maternal red cell alloimmunization compared with management by Doppler assessment of middle cerebral artery peak systolic velocity. Am J Obstet Gynecol 2003; 189((4)):1002–1006. [II-3]
32. Mari G, Rahman F, Oloffson P, et al. Increase of fetal hematocrit decreases the middle cerebral artery peak systolic velocity in pregnancies complicated by rhesus alloimmunization. J Matern Fetal Med 1997; 6:206–208. [II-3]
33. Stefos T, Cosmi E, Detti L, et al. Correction of fetal anemia and the middle cerebral artery peak systolic velocity. Obstet Gynecol. 2002; 99:211-5. [II-2]

34. Detti L, Oz U, Guney I, et al. Doppler ultrasound velocimetry for timing the second intrauterine transfusion in fetuses with anemia from red cell alloimmunization. Collaborative Group for Doppler Assessment of the Blood Velocity in Anemic Fetuses. Am J Obstet Gynecol 2001; 185:1048–1051. [II-3]

35. Mari G, Zimmermann R, Moise KJ, et al. Correlation between middle cerebral artery peak systolic velocity and fetal hemoglobin after 2 previous intrauterine transfusions. Am J Obstet Gynecol 2005; 193:1117–1120. [II-3]

36. ACOG. Management of alloimmunization. Obstet Gynecol 2006; 108 (Practice Bulletin No. 75):457–464. [Review]

37. Mari G, Hanif F, Kruger M, et al. Middle cerebral artery peak systolic velocity: a new Doppler parameter in the assessment of growth restricted fetuses. Ultrasound Obstet Gynecol 2007; 29:310–316. [II-3]

38. Liley A. Liquor amnii analysis in the management of the pregnancy complicated by rhesus sensitization. Am J Obstet Gynecol 1961; 82:1359–1370. [II-2].

39. Queenan J, Tomai T, Ural S, et al. Deviation in amniotic fluid optical density at a wavelength of 450nm in Rh-immunized pregnancies from 14 to 40 weeks' gestation: a proposal for clinical management. Am J Obstet Gynecol 1993; 168:1370–1376. [II-2]

40. Sikkel E, Vandenbussche P, Oepkes D, et al. Amniotic fluid Delta OD 450 values accurately predict severe fetal anemia in D-alloimmunization. Obstet Gynecol 2002; 100:51–57. [II-3]

41. El-Azeem S, Samuels P, Rose R, et al. The effect of the source of transfused blood on the rate of consumption of transfused red blood cells in pregnancies affected by red blood cell allimmunization. Am J Obstet Gynecol 1997; 177:753–757. [II-2]

42. Mouw R, Klumper F, Hermans J, et al. Effect of atracurium or pancuronium on the anemic fetus during and directly after intravascular intrauterine transfusion. Acta Obstet Gynecol Scand 1999; 78:763–767. [RCT, *n* = 24]

43. Nicolaides K, Soothill P, Clewell W, et al. Fetal haemoglobin measurement in the assessment of red cell isoimmunisation. Lancet 1988; 1(8594):1073–1075. [II-3]

44. Mandelbrot L, Daffos F, Forestier F, et al. Assessment of fetal blood volume for computer-assisted management of in utero transfusion. Fetal Ther 1988; 3:60–66. [II-3]

45. van den Akker E, de Haan T, Lopriore E, et al. Severe fetal thrombocytopenia in Rhesus D alloimmunized pregnancies. Am J Obstet Gynecol 2008; 199:387.e1–387.e4. [II-3]

46. Dooren M, van Kamp I, Scherpenisse J, et al. No beneficial effect of low-dose fetal intravenous gammaglobulin administration in combination with intravascular transfusions in severe Rh D haemolytic disease. Vox Sang 1994; 66:253–257. [RCT, *n* = 44]

47. Trevett T, Dorman K, Lamvu G, et al. Does antenatal maternal administration of Phenobarbital prevent exchange transfusion in neonates with alloimmune hemolytic disease? Am J Obstet Gynecol 2003; 189:s214. [II-3]

48. Ghi T, Brodelli L, Simonazzi G, et al. Sonographic demonstration of brain injury in fetuses with severe red blood cell alloimmunization undergoing intrauterine transfusions. Ultrasound Obstet Gynecol 2004; 23:428–431. [II-3]

49. Hudon L, Moise K, Hegemier S, et al. Long-term neurodevelopmental outcome after intrauterine transfusion for the treatment of fetal hemolytic disease. Am J Obstet Gynecol 1998; 179:858–863. [II-3]

50. Van Dongen H, Klumper F, Sikkel E, et al. Non-invasive tests to predict fetal anemia in Kell-alloimmunized pregnancies. Ultrasound Obstet Gynecol 2005; 25:341–345. [II-3]

53

Nonimmune hydrops fetalis

Ricardo Gómez, Juan Pedro Kusanovic, and Luis Medina

KEY POINTS

- Fetal hydrops is defined as the **accumulation of fluid in two or more fetal extravascular compartments**, including ascites, pleural effusion, pericardial effusion, and skin edema. These findings are commonly accompanied by polyhydramnios and placentomegaly.
- Nonimmune hydrops fetalis (NIH) is defined by the **absence of maternal antibodies against fetal cells** (negative indirect Coombs test in maternal serum).
- Because of the wide use of anti-Rh prophylaxis, currently **most cases (90%) of fetal hydrops are nonimmune** in origin. The frequency of NIH has been estimated between 1/2000 and 1/3000 births.
- The prognosis is often dismal, with an **overall perinatal mortality of 50% to 100%**, which is related to the etiology, gestational age at presentation, the presence of early and significant pleural effusions and the availability of treatment for certain conditions (e.g., parvovirus B19–induced NIH). Current data indicate that, among those who survive the neonatal period, 50% are free of long-term sequels at one year of age.
- NIH is a condition associated with a **large number of causes**. In general, **etiology may be suspected or confirmed prenatally in 50% to 80% of cases**. Chromosomal abnormalities account for a significant fraction of cases of NIH before 24 weeks, while structural abnormalities of the heart and infectious conditions are more frequently found after 24 weeks' gestation. After delivery, 5% of newborns remain classified as idiopathic. Following is a **simplified etiologic summary:**
  - Cardiovascular anomalies: 30%
  - Noncardiovascular anomalies: 20%
  - Chromosomal abnormalities: 20%
  - Infection: 10%
  - Hematologic disorders: 10%
  - Complications of monochorionic twins: 5%
  - Genetic syndromes: 1%
  - Metabolic syndromes: 1%
  - Overlapping of these conditions is frequent (e.g., a fetus with trisomy 21 and cardiac structural malformations)
- **Evaluation of cases with NIH** should be exercised according to local resources, and when required, cases must be transferred to a tertiary center where advanced diagnostic tests/procedures and potential treatments are available.
  - Always make sure that antibody screening (indirect Coombs) is negative (even in Rh-positive patients).
  - Because of the broad spectrum of the disease, efforts should be made to establish whether a treatable condition is present. Likewise, identification of recurrent causes of the disease is mandatory to provide appropriate counseling.

- Suggested evaluation may include the following:
  - **Detailed history** (recent flu-like symptoms, ethnic background, family history)
  - **Fetal, umbilical cord, and placental ultrasound,** with emphasis in fetal anatomy, echocardiogram and middle cerebral artery peak systolic velocity to search for cardiac and extracardiac malformations, arrhythmias and fetal anemia.
  - **Maternal laboratory tests:**
    - blood type and antibody screening to rule out immune-mediated anemia
    - CBC with red blood cell indices to look for thalassemias
    - serology for parvovirus, CMV, rubella
    - nontreponemal tests for syphilis (RPR)
    - Kleihauer–Betke to exclude fetal anemia for fetomaternal hemorrhage
    - Other tests may be necessary if there is a suggestive history (e.g., HSV, *Listeria monocytogenes*) or the etiology of the condition remains elusive. On the other hand, the workup may be concise or stopped if the etiology arises soon after initial evaluation of the patient
  - **Amniocentesis and/or fetal blood sampling** to perform fetal karyotype, hemoglobin concentration, PCR for parvovirus B19, toxoplasmosis and CMV as needed. It is a good practice to freeze and store amniotic fluid with the aim to test for rare conditions such as lysosomal storage disease.
  - Rarely, the mother may develop generalized edema, which could be life threatening (**mirror syndrome**).
- **Management of NIH is based on the etiology** and may include the following:
  - Treatment of conditions that benefit from maternal interventions (e.g., penicillin for syphilis-induced NIH) or fetal interventions (e.g., intrauterine blood transfusion for parvovirus B19–induced fetal anemia/ thrombocytopenia).
  - Termination of pregnancy in countries where this option is permitted.
  - Fetal monitoring: nonstress test, biophysical profile, Doppler studies of umbilical artery and middle cerebral artery, as well as heart and venous system as feasible and necessary.
  - Antenatal steroids to reduce the likelihood of neonatal complications associated with preterm delivery.
  - Delivery if there is evidence of fetal or maternal deterioration (e.g., mirror syndrome). Delivery may be preceded by interventions aimed to reduce the frequency of fetal cardiac failure, dystocia, and fetal trauma (e.g., aspiration of excessive pericardial, pleural

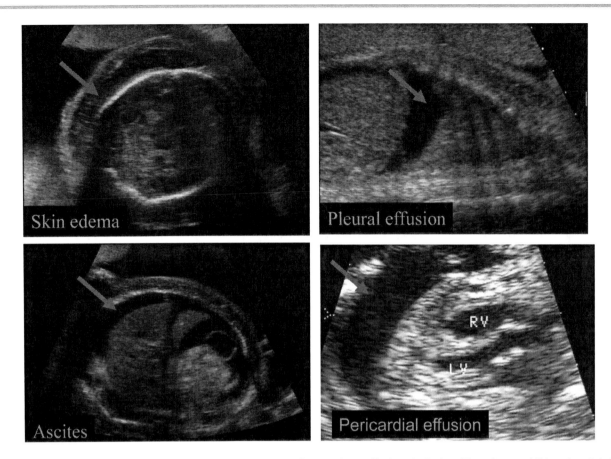

Figure 53.1 Diagnostic criteria for hydrops: need ≥2 of these four: (*i*) skin edema; (*ii*) pleural effusion, (*iii*) ascites, and (*iv*) pericardial effusion.

or peritoneal fluid). NIH increases the risk of postpartum hemorrhage and retained placenta.

DIAGNOSIS/DEFINITION

Hydrops fetalis is a severe fetal condition, end stage of many different disorders, leading to accumulation of fluid in body cavities or tissues. The diagnosis of NIH is established if **at least two** of the following conditions are present: **hydrothorax, ascites, pericardial effusion, and skin edema** (>5 mm measured at the level of skull or chest wall) (Fig. 53.1). These diagnostic findings can be associated with polyhydramnios (in 40–75% of cases) and placentomegaly. Immune hydrops is associated with isoimmunization to an RBC antigen (e.g., Rh disease) (see chap. 52), while nonimmune hydrops (NIH) includes all other etiologies except immune ones.

EPIDEMIOLOGY/INCIDENCE

The incidence of NIH ranges between **1/2000 and 1/3000 at birth**, and as high as 0.5% in tertiary referral centers. The incidence may be as high as 1/150 on ultrasound, since the high rate of intrauterine demise makes the hydrops incidence at birth an underestimation. NIH may account for up to 3% of perinatal mortality. When Potter described for the first time NIH in 1943, its incidence was very low compared to fetal hydrops for isoimmunization. After the introduction of anti-D prophylaxis, **NIH represents 90% of all hydrops cases**.

ETIOLOGY/BASIC PATHOPHYSIOLOGY

Pathophysiology of NIH is complex and basically related to three main mechanisms: impaired lymphatic flow, cardiac failure, and extravasation (either increased intravascular hydrostatic pressure, decreased intravascular osmotic pressure, or both) (Fig. 53.2). NIH is the final phenotype of hundreds of different disorders. Different etiologic factors and complex mechanisms convey to extra-accumulation of fluid in the fetal interstitial space, with 10% to 20% of hydrops causes still undetermined after workup (1). The complex physiopathology of hydrops makes it a challenge for the obstetrician to investigate its etiology and decide upon the management.

ASSOCIATIONS/POSSIBLE ETIOLOGIES/ DIFFERENTIAL DIAGNOSIS (TABLE 53.1) (2–4)
Cardiovascular Disorders (30–40%)

The main causal association of NIH is with fetal cardiovascular disease. The most common disorders involved are tachyarrhythmias (40%), cardiac structural malformations (20%), high-output cardiac failure (15%), and bradyarrhythmias (6%) resulting from congenital heart malformation or maternal connective disorders (antibody mediated).

Fetal arrhythmias are the leading cause of cardiac disorders associated with NIH (40% of these). Most of them are secondary to tachyarrhythmias and another fraction is the result of heart block. The most frequent tachyarrhythmia is supraventricular tachycardia, followed by atrial flutter and atrial fibrillation. Etiopathogenic disturbances induced by arrhythmias include reduction of the stroke volume,

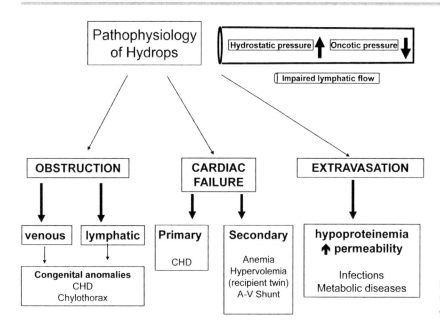

Figure 53.2 Possible pathophysiologic mechanisms for hydrops fetalis. *Abbreviations*: CHD, congenital heart disease; A-V, arterio-venous.

end-diastolic overload, and systemic venous congestion. These conditions are susceptible to in utero treatment with antiarrhythmic drugs administered to the mother or the fetus, which improve survival. The first-line drug is digoxin. Alternatives are flecainide, amiodarone, verapamil, and adenosine. Maternal administration of these drugs is frequently hampered by difficulties associated to an enlarged placenta. Therefore, direct administration to the fetus has been chosen as an alternative. Complete fetal heart block yields to fetal hydrops when the fetal heart rate is below 60 beats per minute or structural anomalies of the fetal heart are present. The presence of the latter is linked to a poor prognosis. Of cases of fetal heart block, 30% to 50% are associated with the presence of anti-Ro or anti-La antibodies in maternal blood (see chap. 25).

Structural abnormalities of the fetal heart typically include, but are not restricted to, atrioventricular septal defects (AV canal), hypoplastic left ventricle, hypoplastic right ventricle, large ventricular septal defects, atrial septal defects, Ebstein anomaly, and premature closure of the ductus arteriosus. The pathophysiology underlying the NIH associated with these conditions is diverse and complex, but is mainly attributable to an increase in the systemic venous pressure resulting from obstruction of right heart output as well as the transmission of systemic arterial pressure to the right heart by means of several pathologic shunts, including the primary or secondary closure of the foramen ovale. Other mechanisms involve obstruction to flow (cardiac tumors such as rhabdomyomas, which are associated in half of the cases to tuberous sclerosis) and the development of significant arteriovenous shunts with an increase in cardiac output, cardiac hypertrophy, and eventually heart failure (sacrococcygeal teratomas and placental chorioangiomas). Aneurysm of the great vein of Galen is a large cerebral arteriovenous malformation that conveys to right-to-left shunting through causing congestive heart failure and hydrops. With the exception of few case reports claiming successful outcomes, the presence of heart failure in these cases imposes a poor prognosis for the fetus.

Extracardiac Anomalies (15–25%)
Thoracic (5–10%) (5,6)

Cystic adenomatoid malformation (CAM), pulmonary sequestration, and congenital diaphragmatic hernia (CDH) are the most common causes of NIH in this category. CDH produces compression of venous return especially when liver is herniated in the chest and worse prognosis is expected when hydrops is found as associated factor. Primary hydrothorax is the accumulation of lymphatic fluid in the pleural cavity without any other demonstrated anomaly (mass or chromosomal abnormality). The most common cause of primary hydrothorax in neonates is chylothorax, characterized by a milky pleural fluid for the high concentration of lymphocytes. Prenatal diagnosis (i.e., lymphocytes count >80% in pleural effusion) is more difficult because of fetal physiologic leukocytosis.

Proposed pathophysiological mechanisms for these cases are the compression or deviation of the mediastinum with lymphatic or venous return obstruction as well as cardiac failure because of compression of the outflow tracts and polyhydramnios. Moreover, cases associated with substantial lung compression before 24 weeks are at risk for pulmonary hypoplasia. Other causes in this category are lymphangiectasia, bronchogenic cyst, and other thoracic tumors.

The most common sonographic finding of NIH of thoracic origin is the presence of a hypoechogenic area around the lungs. The use of a pleuroamniotic shunt in large effusions has been proposed in the management of the hydrothorax of fetuses with normal karyotype to alleviate the mediastinal compression, with an improvement in survival rate ranging from 25% to >60% (5). The same management has been proposed for fetuses with pulmonary sequestration and congenital pulmonary airway malformation (formerly known as cystic adenomatoid malformation) since the development of hydrops worsens the prognosis. Intrapleural injection of OK-432, a sclerosant product obtained from group A *Streptococcus pyogenes*, has been shown to have promising results in three studies reported so far (6). The practice of serial thoracocentesis (e.g., every 48 hours) is discouraged.

Genitourinary (3%)

Urinary tract anomalies may be associated with ascites, but rarely present generalized hydrops. Lower tract obstruction produces bladder overdistention that frequently leaks into the abdominal cavity. More rare causes of ascites are the rupture of a dilated renal pelvis or renal thrombosis. Congenital nephrotic syndrome of Finnish type, a rare fatal autosomal recessive disease, can be associated with fetal hydrops and diagnosed by serum or amniotic fluid α-fetoprotein.

Gastrointestinal (1%)

Intestinal perforation produces variable degrees of ascites (meconium peritonitis) not easy to differentiate from other kinds of intra-abdominal serum effusion. The presence of meconium seen as bright plaques or echo-poor cystic areas would lead to the diagnosis even in absence of dilated gut. When meconium peritonitis is not associated to generalized hydrops, the prognosis is good. Prenatal causes of bowel obstructions are atresias ("apple-peel" syndrome), and volvulus. Meconium peritonitis is associated with cystic fibrosis and a workup for this disorder is suggested during the neonatal period.

Skeletal Dysplasias (1%)

Many different skeletal dysplasias can be associated with hydrops, with severe thoracic hypoplasia impairing venous return leading to hydrops and polyhydramnios. Conditions for which NIH has been described include, but are not limited to, thanatophoric dysplasia, short rib-polydactily, osteogenesis imperfecta, achondrogenesis and hypophosphatasia. The outcome is uniformly poor.

Chromosomal Abnormalities (15–20%) (7–9)

The incidence of chromosome abnormalities is inversely proportional to GA at diagnosis of NIH, with 50% to 75% incidence when NIH is diagnosed <20 weeks (7). Turner and Down syndromes account for 90% of all aneuploidies associated with hydrops, although many other chromosomal abnormalities such as trisomy 18 and 13, 45X/46XX mosaicism, triploidy, and tetraploidy have been reported. The main features of Turner syndrome are cystic hygroma and tubular coartation of aorta, suggesting both lymphatic and cardiac etiology of hydrops (8). The mere finding of a cystic hygroma in the first trimester strongly suggests aneuploidy (60% of risk) (8), but it needs to be differentiated from an increased nuchal translucency (NT) because of other etiologies (e.g., congenital heart defects).

Congenital Infections (10–15%) (9,10)

Parvovirus B19 is the most common infective agent leading to severe anemia and NIH, representing about 5% of all cases of NIH. When congenital defects are excluded, parvovirus B19 infection accounts for about 25% to 50% of fetal hydrops. The key pathophysiological component of the disease is the fetal anemia, frequently severe, induced by the destruction of red blood cells, medullar hypoplastic changes (which explains the severe thrombocytopenia that sometimes may be present along with anemia), hepatitis, and myocarditis. The process is often self-limited, but the degree of anemia frequently requires intrauterine fetal transfusions until the pathologic process finally remits. **The sonographic landmark of the disease is a NIH fetus with a significant increase in the middle cerebral artery peak systolic velocity (MCS PSV)** (9,10) (see also chap. 48).

Syphilis is a rare cause of fetal hydrops, which is the consequence of anemia and hepatic dysfunction resulting in hypoproteinemia and portal hypertension. Other infections such as toxoplasmosis, coxsackie virus, herpes simplex virus, rubella and CMV have been shown to be occasionally associated with NIH. The pathophysiologic mechanisms involved in fetal hydrops because of infection are multiple and involve anemia (e.g., parvovirus B19, toxoplasmosis, and CMV), hepatitis with hypoproteinemia (e.g., CMV), and myocarditis (e.g., toxoplasmosis, rubella, and CMV). The diagnosis of these infections may be performed by demonstrating maternal seroconversion or through various specialized tests (mainly polymerase chain reaction, PCR). The treatment will vary according to the infectious agent involved. Infections because of CMV or toxoplasmosis have demonstrated to have little response to intrauterine treatment and the prognosis is poor (see chaps. 46 and 47). Sonographic landmarks of poor prognosis for NIH because of infections include fetal growth restriction (frequently early and severe), microcephaly, cerebral ventriculomegaly, and calcifications of various organs including the brain and the liver.

Hematological Disorders (5–15%)

Anemia is the most frequent cause of NIH from hematologic disorders. Fetuses with anemia develop hydrops because of the combination of high-output heart failure and endothelial damage secondary to hipoxia, leakage of proteins, and reduction in the oncotic pressure. The mechanisms leading to fetal anemia can be classified as follows:

Reduced Red Blood Cell/Hemoglobin Production

α-Thalassemia is a common cause for fetal hydrops in southeast Asia and European Mediterranean countries. This disease is characterized by a fetus that is unable to produce globin chains to form hemoglobin F in utero, leading to hypoxia and endothelial damage (see chap. 14). Other causes are congenital medullar aplasia secondary to fetal leukemia or parvovirus B19 infection.

Hemolysis

This has been observed in some cases of glucose 6 phosphate dehydrogenase deficiency and infection (CMV and toxoplasmosis).

Transfusion/Hemorrhage

Tissue damage secondary to hypoxia has been proposed in cases of twin-to-twin transfusion syndrome (donor) and as well as in cases of vascular overload (receptor) and twin reverse arterial perfusion (TRAP) sequence. The diagnosis of fetal anemia can be determined noninvasively through Doppler evaluation of the cerebral circulation, which has proven to be valuable in identifying anemia of both immune and nonimmune origins. Treatment includes intrauterine fetal transfusion, which has shown to be useful in cases with anemia secondary to parvovirus B19 infection. In cases of twin-to-twin transfusion syndrome (TTTS) and TRAP sequence, invasive therapy with fetoscopy and laser coagulation or umbilical cord ligation have been associated in some studies to improve fetal survival (see chap. 43). Fetomaternal hemorrhage may be significant enough to induce NIH and should be suspected after trauma and placental abruption. The diagnosis and assessment of the magnitude of the transfusion may be determined by performing a Kleihauer–Betke test.

Metabolic Diseases (1%) (11,12)

Even if metabolic diseases account for only 1% of NIH, up to 15% of the unexplained causes of NIH after negative basic workup include unknown metabolic disorders. Diagnosis is expensive, and investigation for metabolic diseases is justified only when the most frequent causes have been ruled out (6,7). Liver storage disease may cause hepatic cell damage with secondary hypoproteinemia, which may act as the etiopathogenic mechanism in these cases, as well as some degree of cardiac failure because of myocardial infiltration.

MATERNAL COMPLICATIONS

"Mirror syndrome," also known as "Ballantyne's syndrome," is a rare complication characterized by generalized maternal edema and a preeclampsia-like condition that sometimes requires the delivery of the fetus. However, the clinical phenotype is reversible if the fetal treatment is successful or a fetal demise occurs. Caution is advised for cases with polyhydramnios because of the risk of preterm labor, preterm prelabor rupture of membranes, placental abruption, and postpartum hemorrhage.

MANAGEMENT
Counseling/Prognosis

NIH is the end stage of many severe diseases whose outcome is related to the etiology, the severity, and the time of onset. **In general, perinatal mortality in pregnancies complicated by NIH ranges between 50% and 100%, depending on the etiology** (13). The worst prognosis is expected in cases of NIH before 24 weeks' gestation (high risk of chromosomal abnormalities), NIH and cystic hygroma (associated with 100% mortality), and NIH and chromosomal anomalies (very high mortality). Counseling should include the option of termination in countries where this is available. After 24 weeks of gestation, the survival rate, excluding aneuploidies, is nearly 50% when effective treatments are performed. Fetal anemia and fetal arrhythmia are two of the etiologies of NIH associated with >70% to 90% survival rate, if appropriate treatment is instituted (1).

Workup/Diagnosis (Fig. 53.3 and Table 53.1)

After the finding of hydrops by ultrasound, a systematic workup is mandatory. A thorough evaluation of cases with

fetal hydrops allows determination of their cause in up to 80% of cases. This is important to determine the therapeutic strategies that should be mounted as well as providing appropriate genetic counseling for future pregnancies.

Basic Workup

Demographic and clinical history. Ethnicity and race, consanguinity, work exposure to infections, genetic/metabolic diseases, congenital anomalies, autoimmune diseases, and events of the pregnancy, including previous infection screening and ultrasound findings.

Laboratory. Rule out Rh disease or any other cause of immune fetal anemia. Identifications of infectious diseases such as syphilis, parvovirus B19, toxoplasmosis, cytomegalovirus, rubella, coxsackie, HSV-1 and HSV-2, and *Listeria*. Perform the Kleihauer–Betke test and SSA and SSB antibody tests if patient has lupus.

Ultrasound. Include assessment of the following:

- Abdomen for ascites, thorax for pleural/pericardial effusion, and skin for edema
- Complete anatomy survey
- Fetal heart: arrhythmias (M-mode), structural anomalies, function (Doppler)
- Doppler analysis of umbilical artery, MCA PSV, ductus venosus, and possibly other arteries and veins
- Liver length, spleen size, AFI
- Placental thickness, malformations

MCA PSV is >90% sensitive and specific for fetal anemia, using MOM >1.50 (14,15). The most likely explanation for the observed increase in MCA PSV is the reduction of blood viscosity, leading to enhance venous return and preload with consequent increase in cardiac output.

Hydrothorax is an easily observable collection of fluid in the pleural space. It can be unilateral or bilateral, and when severe and presenting early in pregnancy, can lead to pulmonary hypoplasia. In the presence of severe-moderate *ascites*, liquid is evident all around the abdominal circumference and a thorough observation is necessary to differentiate real ascites from the hypoechogenic rime produced by dorsal and

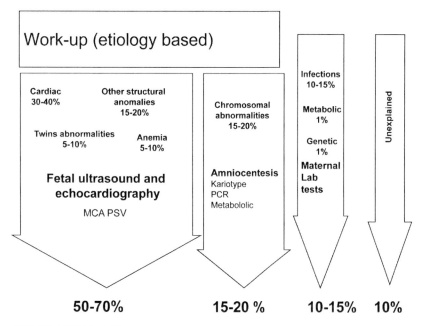

Figure 53.3 Etiology-based workup of hydrops. *Abbreviations*: MCA PSV, middle cerebral artery peak systolic velocity; PCR, polymerase chain reaction.

Table 53.1 Conditions Associated with Nonimmune Fetal Hydrops and Suggested Workup

Conditions associated with NIHF	Suggested workup
Cardiovascular *(30%)*	
Fetal arrhythmias	
Supraventricular tachycardia, atrial flutter, heart block with bradyarrhythmia, Wolff–Parkinson–White, nonconducted premature atrial contractions, others	Expert fetal **echocardiogram** for morphological and functional study, with 2D, M-mode, pulsed Doppler, color Doppler, including functional assessment of output tracts, ductus arteriosus and the fetal venous system (ductus venosus)
Structural	
Atrioventricular septal defects, hypoplastic left ventricle, hypoplastic right ventricle, large ventricular septal defects, atrial septal defects, Ebstein anomaly, premature closure of the ductus arteriosus, closure of the foramen ovale, tetralogy of Fallot and its variants, truncus, transposition of the great vessels, severe atrioventricular or arterial valve insufficiency, others	**Accurate fetal anatomical ultrasound**, including the umbilical cord and placenta.
Mass	
Cardiac rhabdomyoma, pericardial/intrapericardial/intracardiac teratoma	Color and pulsed Doppler of peripheral vessels including umbilical cord, placenta, cranial venous system (especially the base of the skull, under the hemispheres), and middle cerebral artery peak systolic velocity.
High cardiac output failure	
Chorioangioma (>5 cm), aneurysmal malformation of the vein of Galen, large sacrococcygeal teratoma, umbilical cord aneurysms, neuroblastoma, vena cava obstruction.	
Vascular disorders	
Cardiomyopathy, peripheral artery thrombosis	
Extracardiac anomalies (20%)	Accurate fetal anatomical ultrasound
Thorax	Consider thoracocentesis, or paracentesis, with biochemical, cytological, and microbiological analysis
Congenital pulmonary airway malformation (e.g., CCAM, pulmonary sequestration), congenital diaphragmatic hernia, pulmonary lymphangiectasia, chylothorax, bronchogenic cyst, any thoracic tumors.	
Urinary	
Posterior urethral valves, urethral stenosis/atresia, prune-belly syndrome, congenital nephrosis	
Gastrointestinal	
Volvulus-atresia, malrotation, duplication, meconium, peritonitis, hepatic fibrosis, cholestasis, billiary atresia, cloacal dysgenesis, hemochromatosis	
Skeletal dysplasias	
Thanatophoric dysplasia, short rib-polydactyly, osteogenesis imperfecta, achondrogenesis, hypophosphatasia	
Chromosomal abnormalities (20%)	**Amniocentesis**
45x (or mosaic 45X/46XX), trisomy 21, trisomy 18, trisomy 13, triploidy, others	
Infections (10%)	**RPR, serology for parvovirus B19, CMV, toxoplasmosis, rubella**, and others if suspected
Parvovirus B19, CMV, syphilis, toxoplasmosis, rubella, lysteria, adenovirus, coxsackie B, others	Amniocentesis: PCR (or culture) of fluid.
Hematologic (5–10%)	
Excessive red cells loss	
α-Thalassemia, G6PD-deficit, fetomaternal transfusion, TTTS, fetal hemorrhage, red cell enzyme deficiencies, congenital leukemia, others	
Underproduction	**Maternal testing**
Fetal liver and bone marrow replacement syndromes	• Indirect Coombs testing
Congenital leukemia	• Mean corpuscular volume
Parvovirus B19	• Hemoglobin electrophoresis
Red cell aplasia	• Maternal blood chemistry
	• Keihauer–Betke
	Ultrasound: MCA peak systolic velocity
	PUBS (if indicated by other workup)
	• Fetal complete blood cell count
	• Hemoglobin electrophoresis
	• Fetal albumin
Monochorionic twin pregnancy (5%)	Accurate fetal ultrasound with hemodynamic studies
Twin-to-twin transfusion syndrome (TTTS)	
TRAP sequence	

(continued)

Table 53.1 Conditions Associated with Nonimmune Fetal Hydrops and Suggested Workup (*Continued*)

Conditions associated with NIHF	Suggested workup
Genetic syndromes (1%) Myotonic dystrophy, arthrogryposis, multiple pterygium, Noonan syndrome (congenital lymphedema), skeletal (see above)	Accurate fetal ultrasound, genetic and tissue studies from AF
Metabolic (0.5–1%) Lysosomal storage disorders, Gaucher's disease (type2), Niemann–Pick disease, Tay–Sachs's, mucopolysaccharidosis, mucolipidosis, sialidosis, galactosialidosis, others	If indicated, **amniocentesis: enzymatic analysis of supernatant and cultivated amniocytes** (freeze AF if needed) **Maternal testing**

Abbreviations: NIHF, nonimmune hydrops fetalis; CCAM, congenital cystic adenomatoid malformation; AF, amniotic fluid.

abdominal musculature just beneath the abdominal wall. Pericardial effusion distends the pericardium without any motion during cardiac activity. Placental edema is diagnosed when its thickness is >6 cm, and polyhydramnios is conventionally defined as an amniotic fluid index above the 95th percentile for gestational age, or a maximal pocket of amniotic fluid >8 cm.

A detailed sonographic examination is important to determine anatomical defects associated to fetal hydrops. A systematic analysis should be performed to evaluate cardiac anatomy, fetal heart rate and rhythm, and signs of heart failure that can be secondary to extracardiac anomalies such as placental or fetal tumors (e.g., chorioangioma and teratoma), as well as arteriovenous shunts such as those of vein of Galen aneurysm and hepatic hemangioendothelioma. Also, signs of intrauterine infection should be evaluated, including the presence of brain or hepatic calcifications, ventriculomegaly or hydrocephalus, hyperechogenic bowel, and fetal growth restriction.

Fetal Doppler velocimetry, M-mode, and color mapping can be useful to diagnose and evaluate cases of fetal arrhythmia, as well as fetal anemia by evaluating the MCA PSV. Also, fetal Doppler studies are useful for the evaluation of the venous circulation (ductus venosus and inferior vena cava), to determine the prognosis of fetal hydrops of cardiovascular origin, and to evaluate fetal response to treatment. Along with other modalities to monitor fetal well-being, it plays an important role in defining the appropriate moment for a timely delivery.

An accurate **fetal echocardiography** aims first to examine position, size, function, and rhythm of the heart. The systematic observation of a four chambers view, outflow tracts, great arteries, and arches can rule out the majority of CHD associated to hydrops. The addition of color and pulse Doppler allows a more complete evaluation of heart function and flow across atrioventricular valves and arterial valves, while M-mode allows a more accurate study of heart squeezing, recording of wall thickness and rhythm. Color Doppler investigation can demonstrate atrioventricular valve regurgitation, and insonation of peripheral vessels can show venous abnormal pulsatility in ductus venosus or hepatic veins as signs of cardiac failure or provide information on right atrium pressure and heart function.

Amniocentesis. Different analyses in amniotic fluid permit the investigation of fetal karyotype, congenital infections, and metabolic diseases. FISH (fluorescence in situ hybridization) and QF-PCR (quantitative fluorescent polymerase chain reaction) can provide a rapid assessment of chromosome 13, 18, 21, X and Y, assessing about 70% of chromosomal anomalies. A full karyotype from culture of amniocytes rules out all chromosome anomalies.

For the investigation of infectious etiology, PCR in the amniotic fluid is the most sensitive test, although a negative result does not exclude the presence of the disease. Parvovirus B19, CMV, and toxoplasmosis are the most common infectious etiologies of NIH. Biochemical testing of enzymatic activity in cultured amniotic fluid allows the investigation of inborn errors of metabolism. Consider freezing amniotic fluid/extra fetal serum for future tests to study additional conditions when etiology remains unclear.

Cordocentesis and other invasive procedures. Cordocentesis should not be considered a routine procedure in the workup of NIH, but is strongly recommended when fetal anemia is suspected (i.e., elevated MCA PSV). The fragile hemodynamic condition of the fetus with NIH suggests exercising caution when the procedure is performed, especially in severely compromised fetuses with functional cardiac involvement. When performed, fetal blood tests should include full blood count, blood group and Coombs test, and serum biochemistry. In special cases, thalassemia screening, total IgM, and G6PD in male fetuses can be investigated. Peritoneal fluid, pleural fluid, and urine can be obtained with diagnostic and sometimes therapeutic purposes. Cytological and biochemical analysis of these fluids may incline toward a final etiology of NIH. Likewise, karyotype and microorganisms can be searched from these fluids.

Also consider magnetic resonance imaging (especially if ultrasound is suspicious but not diagnostic for certain anomalies); G6PDH deficiency; metabolic workup (e.g., lysosomal storage disorders and rare hemoglobinopathies), especially if positive family history, or recurrent NIH (Table 53.1).

Therapeutic Approach

Management, including fetal monitoring, treatment, and delivery, should follow the **appropriate guidelines for the specific etiology of the NIH.**

Fetal Monitoring/Testing

Doppler studies (especially umbilical artery and MCA Doppler interrogation), NSTs, and BPPs (at ≥28 weeks) can be performed at weekly intervals in the hydropic fetus to assess fetal status and determine the appropriate time for delivery.

Treatment

At 32 to 34 weeks, delivery and postnatal treatment should be considered. **Therapeutic approach depends on the differential diagnosis of the etiology of NIH.**

For parvovirus B19 and arrhythmias, treatment is feasible and effective. Intrauterine transfusion of fetuses with severe hydrops because of parvovirus B19 infection reduces the risk of fetal death. When heart failure and hydrops are associated with supraventricular tachycardia, the first-line drug is digoxin. Alternatives are flecainide, amiodarone, verapamil, and adenosine. Difficulties derived from placental enlargement may render maternal administration erratic and the direct administration to the umbilical cord is an alternative.

In severe pleural effusions, pulmonary compression may lead to lung hypoplasia and polyhydramnios because of mediastinal compression and obstruction of fetal swelling, increasing the risk of preterm labor. These conditions as well as low output cardiac failure may explain the poor prognosis of severe hydrothorax. In these cases, thoracoamniotic shunting may be indicated. Several series including the last 20 years suggest that this procedure may improve fetal and neonatal outcome. Amniodrainage may be considered in the case of severe polyhydramnios to reduce maternal respiratory dysfunction and provide the patient with comfort as well as potentially decreasing the risk of preterm delivery.

Obstetric Management
Steroids for fetal lung maturity may be considered between 24 and 33 6/7 weeks of gestation if delivery is expected within seven days. Tocolysis for preterm labor may not be advisable in all cases. Preeclampsia may develop in up to 50% of cases, adding another factor to consider when defining the time of delivery.

Delivery/Anesthesia
The delivery route will depend on the obstetrical conditions. However, the unique cardiovascular derangements usually present in hydropic fetuses, leading to nonreassuring fetal testing, may necessitate a cesarean section. Hemodynamically stable fetuses may be offered a vaginal delivery. These cases require a careful evaluation of fetal well-being as well as to determine if aspiration of excessive fluid from the pericardium, pleural and peritoneal cavities may be beneficial to facilitate delivery. At all times, the patient should be informed about the diagnosis, prognosis, and management of NIH in general and the specific characteristics of her case. So fetal monitoring results, size of effusions, need for procedures before delivery, and maternal consent procedures should all be taken into consideration. Written consent is mandatory, emphasizing the paucity of information about NIH.

NEONATOLOGY MANAGEMENT
All hydropic fetuses require intubation and mechanical ventilation. These neonates should be delivered in a tertiary care center, since they require expert, intensive, and multidisciplinary management. In cases of fetal or neonatal death, an autopsy should be performed to determine the cause of NIH and death. Long-term follow-up shows that the majority of hydropic neonates who are born and discharged alive have intact long-term survival (16).

MATERNAL POSTPARTUM
A separate outpatient visit should be set up to discuss a postpartum review of the possible etiology of the NIH, including recurrence risks. Recurrent NIH is very rare and mostly due to inborn errors of metabolism (e.g., lysosomal storage disorders, rare hemoglobinopathies, or other genetic disorders).

REFERENCES
1. Sohan K, Carroll SG, De La Fuente S, et al. Analysis of outcome in hydrops fetalis in relation to gestational age at diagnosis, cause and treatment. Acta Obstet Gynecol Scand 2001; 80(8):726–730. [II-3]
2. Machin GA. Hydrops revisited: literature review of 1,414 cases published in the 1980s. Am J Med Genet 1989; 34(3):366–390. [Review]
3. Hahurij ND, Blom NA, Lopriore E, et al. Perinatal management and long-term cardiac outcome in fetal arrhythmia. Early Hum Dev 2011; 87(2):83–87. [II-3]
4. Fukushima K, Morokuma S, Fujita Y, et al. Short-term and long-term outcomes of 214 cases of non-immune hydrops fetalis. Early Hum Dev 2011; 87(8):571–575. [II-3]
5. Aubard Y, Derouineau I, Aubard V, et al. Primary fetal hydrothorax: a literature review and proposed antenatal clinical strategy. Fetal Diagn Ther 1998; 13:325–333. [Review]
6. Yinon Y, Kelly E, Ryan G. Fetal pleural effusions. Best Pract Res Clin Obstet Gynaecol 2008; 22(1):77–96. [Review]
7. Iskaros J, Jauniaux E, Rodeck C. Outcome of nonimmune hydrops fetalis diagnosed during the first half of pregnancy. Obstet Gynecol 1997; 90(3):321–325. [II-3]
8. Ganapathy R, Guven M, Sethna F, et al. Natural history and outcome of prenatally diagnosed cystic hygroma. Prenat Diagn 2004; 24(12):965–968. [II-2]
9. Lamont RF, Sobel JD, Vaisbuch E, et al. Parvovirus B19 infection in human pregnancy. BJOG 2011; 118(2):175–186. [Review]
10. Tolfvenstam T, Broliden K. Parvovirus B19 infection. Semin Fetal Neonatal Med 2009; 14(4):218–221. [Review]
11. Stone DL, Sidransky E. Hydrops fetalis: lysosomal storage disorders in extremis. Adv Pediatr 1999; 46:409–440. [II-3]
12. Burin MG, Scholz AP, Gus R, et al. Investigation of lysosomal storage diseases in nonimmune hydrops fetalis. Prenat Diagn 2004; 24:653–657. [II-3]
13. Santo S, Mansour S, Thilaganathan B, et al. Prenatal diagnosis of non-immune hydrops fetalis: what do we tell the parents? Prenat Diagn 2011; 31(2):186–195. [Review]
14. Hernandez-Andrade E, Scheier M, Dezerega V, et al. Fetal middle cerebral artery peak systolic velocity in the investigation of non-immune hydrops. Ultrasound Obstet Gynecol 2004; 23(5):442–445. [II-3]
15. Cosmi E, Dessole S, Uras L, et al. Middle cerebral artery peak systolic and ductus venosus velocity waveforms in the hydropic fetus. J Ultrasound Med 2005; 24:209–213. [II-3]
16. Haverkamp F, Noeker M, Gerresheim G, et al. Good prognosis for psychomotor development in survivors with nonimmune hydrops. BJOG 2000; 107:282–284. [II-3]

54

Fetal death

Uma M. Reddy

KEY POINTS

- **Ultrasound examination** should be performed **for confirmation of fetal death.**
- Most informative exams **to find the etiology** of fetal death are **autopsy; examination of the placenta, cord, and membranes; and chromosomal analysis.**
- **Induction of labor** in patients with fetal death is recommended unless patient is already in labor.
- **For fetal death at about 14 to 28 weeks, misoprostol** (200–400 µg vaginally **every 4 hours**, 400 µg orally every 4 hours, or 600 µg vaginally every 12 hours) is the **most cost-effective method of delivery, with acceptable side effects.** After 28 weeks of gestation, drugs such as oxytocin and/or prostaglandins administered for induction of labor can be usually given according to standard obstetric protocols (see chap. 20, *Obstetric Evidence Based Guidelines*).

DEFINITIONS

Fetal death is defined by the U.S. National Center for Health Statistics (NCHS), a division of the Centers for Disease Control and Prevention, as

> *death prior to the complete expulsion or extraction from the mother of a product of human conception,* irrespective of the duration of pregnancy and which is not an induced termination of pregnancy. The death is indicated by the fact that after such expulsion or extraction, the fetus does not breathe or show any other evidence of life such as beating of the heart, pulsation of the umbilical cord, or definite movements of voluntary muscles. Heartbeats are to be distinguished from transient cardiac contractions; respirations are to be distinguished from fleeting respiratory efforts or gasps. (1)

The WHO definition of fetal death does not exclude spontaneous abortion at <12 weeks, which has different etiologies and management than fetal death occurring in the second or third trimester. There is not complete uniformity even among U.S. states regarding the birth weight and gestational age criteria for reporting fetal deaths. However, **NCHS** has recommended the reporting of **fetal deaths** at ≥**20 weeks of** gestation with known gestational age or weight ≥**350 g** if the gestational age is unknown (2). 350 g is the 50th percentile for weight at 20 weeks of gestation. Fetal losses because of terminations of pregnancy for lethal fetal anomalies and inductions of labor for previable premature rupture of membranes are excluded from these statistics and are classified separately as terminations of pregnancy. **Embryonic death** is defined as death occurring at ≤12 weeks. **Early fetal death** is defined as death occurring at 13 to 19 6/7 weeks of gestation. **Intermediate fetal death** is defined as death occurring at 20 to

27 weeks of gestation. **Late fetal death** is defined as death occurring at greater than 28 weeks of gestation.

Stillbirth is the term preferred by parent groups, and therefore has been increasingly used by the research community and by ACOG for fetal deaths ≥20 weeks of gestation or weight >350 g (3) and can be used as a synonym for fetal death. **Fetal demise** (often abbreviated **IUFD**, or intrauterine fetal demise) is often also used interchangeably with fetal death. **Unexplained fetal death** is defined as death before delivery with no identifiable cause after complete evaluation is performed.

DIAGNOSIS

The diagnosis of fetal death should be **confirmed by ultrasound**, with absence of heart movement.

EPIDEMIOLOGY/INCIDENCE

An estimated almost 3 million stillbirths occur annually worldwide; 98% of all stillbirths occur in low- and middle-income countries, with India, Nigeria, Pakistan, China, and Bangladesh being the five countries with the highest number of stillbirths (4). In the United States, in 2005, there were 25,894 reported fetal deaths at 20 weeks of gestation or more, resulting in a fetal death rate of 6.2/1000 live births plus fetal deaths in the United States (3). Close to one-half of these deaths occur in the third trimester. When compared to 1990 data, the rate of early fetal death remained stable at 3.2/1000 births, while the rate of late fetal death decreased from 4.3 to 3.1/1000 births (1). Over the last 15 years, the rate of late stillbirths has decreased by more than 25% in the United States (1).

ASSOCIATIONS/RISK FACTORS/POSSIBLE ETIOLOGIES

There are many maternal and fetal factors that have been associated with fetal death (Table 54.1). Up to 50% of fetal deaths are not associated with any of these risks, and are called "unexplained." Many classification schemes for assigning cause of stillbirth are currently used throughout the world. There are at least 35 different classification systems reported in the medical literature since 1954, and each system was created with a specific purpose by the investigators. The Stillbirth Collaborative Research Network (SCRN) Initial Causes of Fetal Death has been devised to provide a structured system so that the definitions used to assign the most likely cause of stillbirth are uniform and those reviewing the potential causes of stillbirth can communicate using a common language. An important goal of this system is to use the best available evidence and rigorous definitions determined before case review when assigning a cause of death (5). **Fetal death rate is an important marker of quality of health care.** Other factors associated with fetal demise are advanced maternal age,

Table 54.1 Associations/Risk Factors/Possible Etiologies of Fetal Death

Maternal risk factors	Fetal risk factors
Chronic hypertension	**Congenital malformations** (15–20%)
Preeclampsia	**Chromosomal/genetic abnormalities** (8–13%): monosomy X,
Diabetes mellitus, thyroid disorders	trisomy 21, trisomy 18, and trisomy 13
Renal disease	**Single gene disorders:** hemoglobinopathies (e.g., alpha-thalasse-
Systemic lupus erythematosus	mia); metabolic diseases (e.g., Smith–Lemli–Opitz syndrome)
Autoimmune disease	Glycogen storage diseases
Antiphospholipid syndrome	Peroxisomal disorders amino acid disorders
Cholestasis of pregnancy	Confined placental mosaicism (aneuploidy in placenta with a euploid
Alloimmunization	fetus)
Obesity	Placental abruption, placenta and vasa previa
Substance abuse (especially cocaine, alcohol, coffee:	Placental pathology
>3 cups/day, etc.)	Chronic villitis
Smoking	Massive chorionic intervillositis
Viral infections:	Complications of multifetal gestation (e.g., twin-twin transfusion, twin
Parvovirus B19	reversed arterial perfusion syndrome, and discordant growth)
Cytomegalovirus	Umbilical cord complications, fetomaternal hemorrhage
Enteroviruses (e.g., coxsackie virus)	Fetal growth restriction
Echoviruses	Uteroplacental insufficiency
HSV-1, HSV-2	Intrauterine asphyxia
HIV	Preterm labor or rupture of membranes
Bacterial infections:	Postterm
Listeria monocytogenes	
Escherichia coli	
Group B streptococci	
Ureaplasma urealyticum	
Treponema pallidum	
Parasitic infections:	
Toxoplasma gondii	
Uterine malformations	
Abdominal trauma	

In bold, most common associations.

non-Hispanic black race, nulliparity or multiparity (>5), unmarried status, low socioeconomic status, low education, multiple gestation, assisted reproductive technology, and past obstetric history (previous stillbirth, preterm delivery, or growth restriction) (6–16). **Obesity, smoking, drug, and alcohol abuse are common modifiable risk factors for fetal death.** Pesticides, radiation, and fertility drugs have also been associated with fetal death. In developing countries, the most common causes of stillbirths are complications of labor and infections. Basic emergency obstetric care, births in adequate facilities with option for safe cesarean delivery (CD), improvement in nutrition, and prevention and treatment of syphilis and malaria are the most feasible and cost-effective interventions in developing countries to decrease the incidence of stillbirth (17).

PREVENTION

Some of the risk factors listed in Table 54.1, in particular obesity, smoking, and drug and alcohol abuse, are modifiable, and should be avoided. As the vast majority of fetal deaths occur in developing countries, interventions should be focused on prevention in these settings, and include (18) the following:

- Periconception folate fortification
- Insecticide-treated bed nets or intermittent preventative treatment for malaria
- Syphilis detection and treatment
- Detection and treatment of hypertensive disorders
- Detection and management of diabetes in pregnancy
- Detection and management of FGR
- Induction at 41 weeks (prevention of postterm pregnancy)
- Skilled care at birth
- Basic and comprehensive emergency obstetric care

Table 54.2 Maternal and Fetal Investigation for Fetal Death

Predelivery
- Amniotic fluid for cytogenetics
- Screen for coagulopathy (only if fetal death > 4 wk from delivery)
- CBC, antibody screen, urine drug screen
- Kleihauer–Betke testing or flow cytometry
- Lupus anticoagulant, anticardiolipin antibodies (IgM, IgG) and anti-β_2-glycoprotein antibodies (IgM, IgG)
- Parvovirus B19 titers (IgM, and IgG)[a]
- Syphilis testing (RPR or VDRL)
- Thyroid-stimulating hormone
- Glucose screening (oral glucose tolerance test, hemoglobin A1C) (if glucose screening not done in pregnancy)
- Thrombophilia workup only to be considered in cases of severe placental infarcts, fetal growth restriction, or in the setting of a personal history of thrombosis (factor V Leiden mutation; G20210A prothrombin gene mutation; antithrombin III)

Postdelivery
- Cord blood for cytogenetics
- **Autopsy and placental examination**
- Protein C, protein S activity (in selected cases as described above for other thrombophilia workup)

[a]Consider workup for parvovirus especially in cases with fetal hydrops or other signs of this viral infection

PREGNANCY MANAGEMENT
Counseling

Counseling should include review of possible etiologies (Table 54.1), workup (Table 54.2), delivery options, as well as

Table 54.3 Management of Subsequent Pregnancy After Stillbirth

Preconception or initial prenatal visit
- Detailed medical and obstetrical history
- Evaluation/workup of previous stillbirth
- Determination of recurrence risk
- Discussion of increased risk of other obstetrical complications
- Smoking cessation
- Weight loss (back to normal BMI) in obese women
- Genetic counseling if family genetic condition exists
- Support and reassurance

First trimester
- Dating ultrasound by crown-rump length (first trimester)
- First-trimester screen—PAPP-A, hCG, and nuchal translucency[a]
- Diabetes screen
- Antiphospholipid antibodies
- Thrombophilia workup only if stillbirth associated with severe placental infarcts, fetal growth restriction, or in the setting of a personal history of thrombosis
- Support and reassurance

Second trimester
- Fetal anatomic survey at 18 to 20 wk
- Quadruple screen—MSAFP, hCG, estriol, and inhibin-A[a]
- Uterine artery Doppler studies at 22 to 24 wk[a]
- Support and reassurance

Third trimester
- Serial ultrasounds about every 4 wk to rule out fetal growth restriction, starting at 28 wk
- Fetal movement counting starting at 28 wk
- Antepartum fetal surveillance (e.g., nonstress tests or biophysical profiles) starting at 32 wk or 1 to 2 wk earlier prior to gestational age of previous stillbirth if occurred prior to 32 wk
- Support and reassurance

Delivery
- Planned induction at 39 wk, or before 39 wk if desired by the couple and lung maturity documented by amniocentesis

[a]Provides risk modification but does not alter management. *Source*: Adapted from Ref. 19.

possible complications. Grief counseling should be included, in addition to the option for referral to grieving help groups. Review of risk of recurrence, prevention of recurrence, and best management for a future pregnancy (Table 54.3) should be done postpartum.

Workup

Evaluation of the etiology of fetal death is essential to counsel regarding recurrence risks, facilitate the grieving process, and improve understanding to facilitate therapeutic measures (Table 54.2) (3,20–29). The evaluation can be emotionally difficult, and should be multidisciplinary (obstetrician, maternal-fetal specialist, pathologist, geneticist, radiologist, and neonatologist). Communication between all these members is important. Staff interacting with the family should refer to the stillborn baby by name, if one was given. Parents should be informed about the reasons for autopsy, procedures, and potential cost. **The most important components of the evaluation of a stillbirth are fetal autopsy; examination of the placenta, cord, and membranes; and karyotype analysis**. A complete evaluation (3) should include the following:

1. Review all relevant **maternal, perinatal, family history, and risk factors** to help identify specific possibilities (Table 54.1). See specific guideline if a specific factor is identified as probable cause. In family history particular attention should be paid to pregnancy losses, consanguin-

ity, mental retardation, diabetes, congenital anomalies with a three-generation pedigree. **All records** should be reviewed for any possible association.

2. Before delivery, **detailed ultrasound**, fetal echocardiogram, 3D ultrasound, and whole-body X rays, and/or MRI can be considered. These exams should be recommended especially if a detailed autopsy will not be available. Karyotypic analysis is not possible in 50% of cases because of cell culture failure. To increase the yield of cell culture, an **amniocentesis** (and/or CVS) should be offered for karyotype (30) and fetal infection workup. Even if 5% to 10% of cells from amniotic fluid of fetal deaths fail to grow, this yield is much higher than that obtained from postnatal study of karyotype (31).

3. Before delivery, **obtain consent for fetal autopsy**. If consent is not given for a full autopsy, ask the parents to consider a limited autopsy such as external examination by pathologist/clinical geneticist or internal examination limited to brain and/or spinal cord, chest organs or abdominal organs as appropriate; or an MRI (32).

4. At delivery, **examine baby and placenta carefully**. General exam immediately after delivery should include noting any dysmorphology/congenital abnormalities as well as obtaining weight, length, and head circumference. Foot length may be especially useful for earlier stillbirths that may have a few week lag between death and delivery to pinpoint gestational age at death. Photographs of the entire body; frontal and profile views of the face, extremities, and palms; and close-up photographs of specific abnormalities should be obtained (3). The placenta should be weighed and compared to the norms for gestational age. Clinical geneticist evaluation if available is often helpful.

5. Prior to autopsy, **karyotypic analyses should be performed on all stillbirths** after parental consent is obtained. Yield for abnormalities is higher if the following is present: fetus with growth restriction, anomalies or hydrops; or the parent is a balanced translocation carrier or has a mosaic karyotype (3). The most viable tissue for **cytogenetic and molecular genetic studies** is usually the **placenta** (1 × 1 cm block) taken from below the cord insertion site on the unfixed placenta or umbilical cord closest to the placenta, followed by fetal cartilage obtained from the costochondral junction or patella (3,24). **Placental tissue can be sent for karyotype to check for confined placental mosaicism.** Skin surface should be cleansed with betadine or hibiclens prior to obtaining specimen. Tissue should be placed in Hanks solution (pink), or normal saline, if Hanks solution is not available, not in formalin. Cytogenetic form should be completed with pertinent details. Attempts at cell culture, however, fail in half of cases. If culture is unsuccessful, **fluorescent in situ hybridization** to detect most common aneuploidies or **comparative genomic hybridization (cGH),** which detects small deletions or duplications, and termed copy number changes not detectable by karyotype, may be useful since both technologies do not require live cells (33). Testing for rarer causes of stillbirth such as single gene disorders should be guided by clinical suspicion or family history.

6. **Autopsy** is the **most useful** test in identifying the cause of fetal death. Not only are gross birth defects and morphologic abnormalities identified, but subtle findings of the autopsy may confirm infection, anemia, hypoxia, and metabolic abnormalities as the cause of death. Autopsy

reduces the number of unexplained fetal deaths by at least 10% (25). Autopsy findings altered counseling and recurrence risks autopsy in 26% of all cases at one institution (34). Autopsy should include X rays of the fetus, photographs, and follow College of American Pathologists guidelines (http://www.cap.org). Whole-body X ray with anterior-posterior and lateral views may reveal an unrecognized skeletal abnormality or further define an already visible abnormality. Estimation of the interval between intrauterine death and delivery should be performed. Clinical information, all records including ultrasound reports regarding case, and any specific requests, should be made available to the pathologist. **It is suggested for the obstetrician to call the pathology resident/attending assigned to autopsy for discussion**. A perinatal pathologist with experience in fetal death cases should perform the autopsy. Examination by a physician experienced in genetics and dysmorphology may increase the yield of autopsy. If autopsy is declined, it is important to consider a head-sparing autopsy, or at least **MRI** of the stillborn child (35).

7. Send **placenta, membranes, and umbilical cord for gross and microscopic pathologic examination**. Conditions causing or contributing to stillbirth may be diagnosed such as abruption, placental infarcts, umbilical cord thrombosis, velamentous cord insertion, and vasa previa. Placental evaluation can also yield important information regarding infection, genetic abnormalities, anemia, and thrombophilia. Umbilical cord knots and tangling should be noted but interpreted carefully as cord entanglement occurs in 30% of normal pregnancies (3,36). Examination of the placenta vasculature and membranes is particularly useful in multifetal gestations by establishing chorionicity and vascular anastomoses.

8. If autopsy, placental pathology, or history is suggestive of an infectious etiology, maternal or neonatal serology, special tissue stains, and/or testing for bacterial or viral nucleic acids may be undertaken. If clinical or histologic evidence is lacking, then routine testing for infection is of questionable benefit.

9. Maternal labs (3) (Table 54.2):
   a. Kleihauer–Betke testing or flow cytometry are sent to evaluate for fetal-maternal hemorrhage (prior to delivery is optimal).
   b. Lupus anticoagulant, anticardiolipin antibodies (IgM, IgG) and anti-β_2-glycoprotein antibodies (IgM, IgG) can be sent to test for antiphospholipid syndrome. Presence of lupus anticoagulant or anticardiolipin antibodies of moderate to high titer (>40 immunoglobulin M (IgM) binding/immunoglobulin G (IgG) binding or >99th percentile) or anti-β_2-glycoprotein antibody titer (>99th percentile) are all considered positive but should be confirmed with repeat testing 12 weeks later (37) (see also chap. 26).
   c. Parvovirus B19 titers (IgM, and IgG) can be considered, especially in cases in which there is suspicion for this infection, such as those with fetal hydrops or fetal anemia (38). CMV, toxoplasmosis and other viruses, and/or bacteria are not suggested for workup, unless clinical history or other factors (pathology findings) point to these infections.
   d. Syphilis testing can be sent with RPR or VDRL.
   e. Glucose screening (oral glucose tolerance test, hemoglobin A1c) (if glucose screening not done in pregnancy).
   f. Thrombophilia workup should be sent only in cases of severe placental pathology, fetal growth restriction, or

in the setting of a personal history or history in a first degree relative (e.g., parent or sibling) of thrombosis (factor V Leiden mutation; G20210A prothrombin gene mutation; deficiencies of antithrombin III, protein C, protein S) (see chap. 27). Routine testing is controversial and may lead to unnecessary interventions (3).

10. Consider any other workup, depending on risk factor identified in Table 54.1. For fetal demise before 20 weeks, consider individualized workup and refer to chapter on pregnancy loss (chap. 15, *Obstetric Evidence Based Guidelines*).

DELIVERY/ANESTHESIA

Once diagnosis is confirmed, and counseling and workup initiated, options for delivery should be discussed. **Options include expectant management, induction, or dilation and evacuation (D&E)**.

Expectant Management

Between **80% and 90% of women with fetal death will spontaneously enter labor within two weeks of fetal demise** (39). Duration of labor is shorter in patients with spontaneous labor (40). However, **endomyometritis** rate is higher in the spontaneous labor group (6% vs. 1%) compared to induction. There is no difference in the frequency of postpartum hemorrhage, retained placenta or need for blood transfusion. Retention of a dead fetus can cause chronic consumptive coagulopathy because of gradual release of thromboplastin from the placenta into the maternal circulation (24). This usually occurs after four weeks, but may occur earlier. Coagulation abnormalities occur in about 3% to 4% of patients with uncomplicated fetal deaths over the next four to eight weeks, and this number rises in the presence of abruption or uterine perforation (24). Another disadvantage of expectant management is a long interval between fetal death and spontaneous labor, limiting the amount of information that can be obtained about the cause of death from a postmortem examination or autopsy of the baby. Moreover, women with fetal death find it difficult psychologically to continue a pregnancy with a known fetal death. In patients opting for spontaneous labor (especially **with greater than four week interval between fetal death and time of delivery**), a **screen for coagulopathy** (fibrinogen level, platelet count, prothrombin time and activated partial thromboplastin measurement) should be obtained prior to administration of neuraxial anesthesia, as well as other invasive procedures (24).

Dilation and Evacuation

Comparing complication rates of patients who undergo D&E or medical induction **between 14 and 24 weeks of gestation**, D&E is a **safe** method in this time frame, especially **if done by experienced operators, under continuous ultrasound guidance** (41). Surgical termination of pregnancy between 14 and 24 weeks of gestation has a lower overall rate of complications (4%), as compared to 29% in women undergoing labor induction (41). Patients undergoing D&E are less likely to have failure of the initial method for delivery and retained products of conception. However, both groups are similar in the need for blood transfusion, infection, cervical laceration, maternal organ damage, or hospital readmission. Placement of **laminaria** is associated with a lower risk of complications from D&E, while **misoprostol** is associated with a lower complication rate in women undergoing medical termination (41). A recent Cochrane review (42) concluded that D&E is superior to instillation of prostaglandin $F_2\alpha$ and may be favored over mifepristone and misoprostol, although larger randomized studies are needed. Using decision analysis, a cost-effectiveness analysis concluded that D&E is less expensive and more effective than misoprostol induction of labor for second-trimester pregnancy termination (43). Studies do not show an increased rate of complications in subsequent pregnancies after D&E, although data are limited (44,45). Both methods for delivery are considered reasonably safe. Thus, **mode of delivery should usually be based on the patient's wishes**. However, patients should be counseled that **efficacy of autopsy is very limited with D&E** (3). In addition, **the availability of D&E may be limited by provider experience or gestational age**.

Induction

Induction of labor in women with fetal death is **usually recommended**, unless the patient is already in labor, given the problems mentioned with expectant management. Induction of labor is typically **initiated soon after diagnosis of fetal death**. Most of the data for management of fetal death is from randomized trials of second-trimester pregnancy termination.

Up to 28 Weeks

Options for induction of labor for fetal death at about 16 to 28 weeks (and in some cases up to about 31 weeks) include misoprostol (prostaglandin E1, PGE1); prostaglandins E2 (PGE2); high-dose oxytocin; and hypertonic saline. **Misoprostol and high-dose oxytocin are the two modalities with the best safety and effectiveness evidence.**

Available evidence from randomized trials do support the use of **vaginal misoprostol** as a medical treatment to terminate nonviable pregnancies before 24 weeks of gestation (46,47). On the basis of the limited data, the use of misoprostol between 24 to 28 weeks of gestation also appears to be safe and effective (46). **Therefore, for gestations less than 28 weeks, misoprostol is the most efficient method of induction**, regardless of Bishop score, although high-dose oxytocin infusion is an acceptable alternative (3). Typical dosages for misoprostol use are 200 to 400 μg vaginally every 4 to 12 hours (3). Examples of regimens for misoprostol dosing are **200 μg vaginally every 4 hours, 400 μg orally every 4 hours, or 600 μg vaginally every 12 hours. These result in successful expulsion (mostly within 24 hours) in 80% to 100% of cases** (3,48–53). **Misoprostol 400 μg given orally every 4 hours is more effective than misoprostol 200 μg given vaginally every 12 hours for the induction of second- and third-trimester pregnancy with intrauterine fetal death**, but is associated with more gastrointestinal side effects (48). Misoprostol 600 μg administered vaginally at 12-hour intervals is associated with fewer adverse effects and is as effective as dosing at 6-hour interval (53).

High-dose oxytocin (200 units in 500 mL saline at 50 mL/ hour) also may be used for induction of labor remote from term (54). **The mother should be observed for signs of water intoxication and maternal electrolyte concentrations should be monitored at least every 24 hours.** Nausea and malaise are the earliest findings of hyponatremia, and may be seen when the plasma sodium concentration falls below 125 to 130 mEq/L. This may be followed by headache, lethargy, obtundation and eventually seizures, coma, and respiratory arrest. Misoprostol 50 μg, with dose doubled every 6 hours until effective contractions, is associated with a success rate within 48 hours of induction of 100% compared to 96.7% to oxytocin infusion titrated on the basis of patient response, with **mean induction to delivery time significantly longer (almost double) in the oxytocin group compared with the misoprostol group** (23.3 vs.

12.4 hours). **Misoprostol is also cheaper (1/10th of the price of oxytocin)** (55).

Historically, **PGE2 suppositories**, with a dose of 20 mg inserted vaginally every four hours, were also utilized for labor induction before 28 weeks. Pretreatment with acetaminophen, compazine, and diphenoxylate is useful to minimize fever, nausea, vomiting, and diarrhea, which invariably occur. The PGE2 dose should be reduced to 5 to 10 mg if used at a more advanced gestation (off-label use) as uterine sensitivity and the risk of uterine rupture increase with gestational age (56). High-dose PGE2 suppositories are contraindicated >28 weeks gestation (57). Misoprostol is more efficacious, and at least as safe, and cheaper, than PGE2, and so the use of PGE2 for induction of fetal death before 28 weeks is not recommended, and of mostly historic importance only.

The efficacy and tolerance of **mifepristone** (RU 486), a progesterone antagonist, was investigated in a double-blind controlled multicenter study involving 94 patients with an intrauterine fetal death (58). Success of treatment was defined as the occurrence of fetal expulsion within 72 hours after the first drug intake. Mifepristone treatment (600 mg/day for two days) was considered to be effective in 29 of 46 patients (63%). There were only eight successes in 48 patients (17.4%) in the placebo group ($p = 0.001$). Tolerance was good in the mifepristone group. In the placebo group, disseminated intravascular coagulation occurred in one woman for whom the investigator waited several weeks for spontaneous expulsion. Mifepristone is of interest in the management of intrauterine fetal death, **with more studies needed to compare the above methods, in particular misoprostol, with mifepristone.**

To date, there are no studies evaluating **laminaria** for ripening of cervix in conjunction with other methods of induction for cases of fetal death.

After 28 Weeks

After 28 weeks of gestation, **drugs such as oxytocin and/or prostaglandins administered for induction of labor can be given according to standard obstetric protocols** (3) (see chap. 20, *Obstetric Evidence Based Guidelines*). Cesarean delivery for stillbirth is reserved for unusual circumstances (maternal indications) because it is associated with maternal morbidity without fetal benefit (3).

Women with Prior Uterine Scar

Women with a **prior uterine scar** represent a special group and treatment should be individualized. **For women with a previous low transverse incision and a uterus less than 28 weeks size, the usual protocols for misoprostol induction at less than 28 weeks may be used** (3,46). Several studies have evaluated the use of misoprostol at a dosage of 400 μg every six hours in women with a stillbirth up to 28 weeks of gestation and a prior uterine scar (59,60). There does not appear to be an increase in complications in those women. The risk of uterine rupture is about 0.4% with one prior low transverse CD, up to 9% with ≥2 prior CD, and up to 50% with prior vertical CD (61). Further research is required to assess effectiveness and safety, optimal route of administration, and dose (46).

For women with a previous low transverse incision, after 28 weeks of gestation, oxytocin protocols may be utilized and cervical ripening with Foley bulb may be considered (3,46). Patients may elect for a repeat CD in the setting of a stillbirth, but the risks and benefits should be discussed with the patient. Ideally, a cesarean should be avoided. Therefore, on the basis of limited data in patients with a prior low transverse CD, trial of labor remains a favorable option (3,46). There are limited data for patients with a prior classical uterine incision and the delivery plan should be individualized (3,46).

POSTPARTUM

Prior to discharge, the family needs to be counseled that results of all investigations may take two or three months for completion and that despite extensive evaluation a cause of death may not be found. Patients should be offered the **opportunity to see and hold their infant and be offered keepsake items such as photos, hand/footprints, or special blankets or clothing. Grief counseling** should be initiated prior to discharge from hospital. Referral to a bereavement counselor, religious leader, peer support group, or mental health professional may be advisable for management of grief and depression.

PREVENTION OF RECURRENCE AND MANAGEMENT IN A FUTURE PREGNANCY

A **special outpatient visit** should be set up to review the results of the complete workup, and discuss possible etiology and future management (Table 54.3). If a particular medical problem is identified in the mother, it should be addressed prior to next conception (see specific guidelines). For example, tight control of blood glucose prior to conception can substantially reduce the risk of congenital anomalies in the fetus. Preconception counseling is helpful if congenital anomalies or genetic abnormalities are found. In the future, comparative genomic hybridization, FISH, and other novel genetic techniques will provide better ways to workup the myriad genetic causes of fetal death. A woman with a prior fetal loss and either factor V or prothrombin heterozygocity, or protein S deficiency, might benefit from enoxaparin 40 mg SQ daily starting at eight weeks (62). In some cases, such as cord occlusion, the patient can be assured that recurrence is unlikely (36,63). Overall, there is an increased incidence of pregnancy complications, such as stillbirth (2.5- to 10-fold increase depending on the study) (15,64), preterm birth (OR 2.8, 95% CI 1.9–4.2), preeclampsia (OR 3.1, 95% CI 1.7–5.7) and placental abruption (OR 9.4, 95% CI 4.5–19.7) (65), in subsequent pregnancies (65). Most patients find increased fetal surveillance with the next pregnancy reassuring. **Fetal growth ultrasounds and kick counts starting at 28 weeks and antepartum surveillance starting at 32 weeks may be implemented** (3). Planned induction can be discussed with the patient in terms of risks and benefits, at 39 weeks, or earlier if fetal lung maturity has been proven (3).

REFERENCES

1. MacDorman MF, Kirmeyer S. Fetal and perinatal mortality, United States, 2005. Natl Vital Stat Rep 2009; 57:1–19. [II-2]
2. National Center for Health Statistics. Model state vital statistics act and regulations. 1992 revision. Hyattsville (MD):NCHS; 1994. Available at http://www.cdc.gov/nchs/data/misc/mvsact92b.pdf. Retrieved January 16, 2011. [Level III]
3. ACOG. Management of stillbirth. ACOG Practice Bulletin No. 102. Obstet Gynecol 2009; 113(3):748–761. [Level III]
4. Lawn JE, Blencowe H, Pattison R, et al. Stillbirths: where? when? why? how to make the data count? Lancet 2011; 377(9775):1448–1463. [II-2]
5. Dudley DJ, Goldenberg R, Conway D, et al. Stillbirth Research Collaborative Network. A new system for determining the causes of stillbirth. Obstet Gynecol 2010; 116(2 pt 1):254–260. [Level III]
6. Reddy UM, Ko CW, Willinger M. Maternal age and the risk of stillbirth throughout pregnancy in the United States. Am J Obstet Gynecol 2006; 195:764–770. [II-2]
7. Sharma PP, Salihu HM, Oyelese Y, et al. Is race a determinant of stillbirth recurrence? Obstet Gynecol 2006; 107:391–397. [II-2]
8. Vintzileos AM, Ananth CV, Smulian et al. Prenatal care black-white fetal death disparity in the United States: heterogeneity by high-risk conditions. Obstet Gynecol 2002; 99(3):483–489. [II-3]
9. Arias E, Anderson RN, Kung HC, et al. Deaths: final data for 2001. National Vital Statistics Reports; 52(3). Hyattsville, MD: National Center for Health Statistics. 2003. [Data review]
10. Froen JF, Arnestad M, Frey K, et al. Risk factors for sudden intrauterine unexplained death: epidemiologic characteristics of singleton cases in Oslo, Norway, 1986–1995. Am J Obstet Gynecol 2001; 184:694–702. [II-2]
11. Oron T, Sheiner E, Shoham-Vardi I, et al. Risk factors for antepartum fetal death. J Reprod Med 2001; 46(9):825–830. [II-2]
12. Nohr EA, Bech BH, Davies MJ, et al. Prepregnancy obesity and fetal death: a study within the Danish National Birth Cohort. Obstet Gynecol 2005; 106:250–259. [II-2]
13. Raymond EG, Cnattingius S, Kiely JL. Effects of maternal age, parity, and smoking on the risk of stillbirth. BJOG 1994; 101:301–306. [II-2]
14. Wisborg K, Ingerslev HJ, Henriksen TB. IVF and stillbirth: a prospective follow-up study. Hum Reprod 2010; 25:1312–1316. [II-2]
15. Surkan PJ, Stephansson O, Dickman PW, et al. Previous preterm and small-for-gestational-age births and the subsequent risk of stillbirth. N Engl J Med 2004; 350:777–785. [II-2]
16. Gardosi J, Kady SM, McGeown P, et al. Classification of stillbirth by relevant condition at death (ReCoDe): population based cohort study. BMJ 2005; 331:1113–1117. [II-2]
17. Mullan Z, Horton R. Bringing stillbirth out of the shadow. Lancet 2011; 377:1291–1292. [III]
18. Bhutta ZA, Yakoob MY, Lawn JE, et al. Stillbirths: what difference can we make and at what cost? Lancet 2011; 377:1523–1538. [II-2]
19. Reddy UM. Prediction and prevention of recurrent stillbirth. Obstet Gynecol 2007; 110:1151–1164. [Review]
20. Brady K, Duff P, Harlass FE, et al. The role of amniotic fluid cytogenetic analysis in the evaluation of recent fetal death. Am J Perinatol 1991; 8:68–70. [II-2]
21. Lockwood CJ, Rand JH. The immunobiology and obstetrical consequences of anti-phospholipid antibodies. Obstet Gynecol Surv 1994; 49:432–441. [II-3]
22. Laube DW, Schauberger CW. Fetomaternal bleeding as a cause for "unexplained" fetal death. Obstet Gynecol 1982; 60:649–651. [II-3]
23. Owen J, Stedman CM, Tucker TL. Comparison of predelivery versus postdelivery Kleihauer–Betke stains in cases of fetal death. Am J Obstet Gynecol 1989; 161:663–666. [II-2]
24. Maslow AD, Breen TW, Sarna MC, et al. Prevalence of coagulation abnormalities associated with intrauterine fetal death. Can J Anaesth 1996; 43(12):1237–1243. [II-3]
25. ACOG. Evaluation of stillbirths and neonatal deaths. ACOG Committee Opinion No. 383. Obstet Gynecol 2007; 110(4):963–966.[III]
26. Incerpi MH, Miller DA, Samandi R, et al. Stillbirth evaluation: what tests are needed? Am J Obstet Gynecol 1998; 178:1121–1125. [II-3]
27. Ahlenius I, Floberg J, Thomassen P. Sixty-six cases of intrauterine fetal death. A prospective study with an extensive test protocol. Acta Obstet Gynecol Scand 1995; 74(2):109–117. [II-2]
28. Langston C, Kaplan C, Macpherson T, et al. Practice guideline for examination of the placenta: developed by the Placental Pathology Practice Guideline Development Task Force of the College of American Pathologists. Arch Pathol Lab Med 1997; 121:449–476. [Review]
29. Silver RM, Varner MW, Reddy U, et al. Work-up of stillbirth: a review of the evidence. Am J Obstet Gynecol 2007; 196(5):433–444. [Review]
30. Korteweg FJ, Bouman K, Erwich JJ, et al. Cytogenetic analysis after evaluation of 750 fetal deaths: proposal for diagnostic workup. Obstet Gynecol 2008; 111(4):865–874. [II-2]

31. Khare M, Howarth E, Sandler J, et al. A comparison of prenatal versus postnatal karyotyping for the investigation of intrauterine fetal death after the first trimester of pregnancy. Prenat Diagn 2005; 25:1192–1195. [II-2]

32. Woodward PJ, Sohaey R, Harris DP, et al. Postmortem fetal MR imaging: comparison with findings at autopsy. AJR Am J Roentgenol 1997; 168(1):41–46. [II-2]

33. Reddy UM, Goldenberg R, Silver R, et al. Stillbirth classification—developing an international consensus for research: executive summary of a National Institute of Child Health and Human Development workshop. Obstet Gynecol 2009; 114(4):901–914. [III]

34. Faye-Petersen OM, Guinn DA, Wenstrom KD. Value of perinatal autopsy. Obstet Gynecol 1999; 94(6):915–920. [II-3]

35. Thayyil S, Cleary JO, Sebire NJ, et al. Post-mortem examination of human fetuses: a comparison of whole body high-field MRI at 9.4 T with conventional MRI and invasive autopsy. Lancet 2009; 374:467–475. [II-2]

36. Carey JC, Rayburn WF. Nuchal cord encirclements and risk of stillbirth. Int J Gynaecol Obstet 2000; 69(2):173–174. [II-2]

37. ACOG. Antiphospholipid syndrome. ACOG Practice Bulletin No. 118. Obstet Gynecol 2011; 117(1):192–199. [III]

38. Sarfraz AA, Samuelsen SO, Bruu AL, et al. Maternal human parvovirus B19 infection and the risk of fetal death and low birthweight: a case-control study with 35,940 pregnant women. BJOG 2009; 116:1492–1498. [II-2, plus commentary]

39. Goldstein DP, Reid DE. Circulating fibrinolytic activity—a precursor of hypofibrinogenemia following fetal death in utero. Obstet Gynecol 1963; 22:174–180. [III]

40. Salamat SM, Landy HJ, O'Sullivan MJ. Labor induction after fetal death. A retrospective analysis. J Reprod Med 2002; 47(1):23–26. [II-2]

41. Autry AM, Hayes EC, Jacobson GF, et al. A comparison of medical induction and dilation and evacuation for second-trimester abortion. Am J Obstet Gynecol 2002; 187(2):393–397. [RCT; n = 297]

42. Lohr PA, Hayes JL, Gemzell-Danielsson K. Surgical versus medical methods for second trimester induced abortion. Cochrane Database Syst Rev 2008; 1:CD006714. [Meta-analysis]

43. Cowett AA, Golub RM, Grobman WA. Cost-effectiveness of dilation and evacuation versus the induction of labor for second trimester pregnancy termination. Am J Obstet Gynecol 2006; 194:768–773. [II-3]

44. Jackson JE, Grobman WA, Haney E, et al. Mid-trimester dilation and evacuation with laminaria does not increase the risk for severe subsequent pregnancy complications. Int J Gynaecol Obstet 2007; 96:12–15. [II-2]

45. Schneider D, Halperin R, Langer R, et al. Abortion at 18–22 weeks by laminaria dilation and evacuation. Obstet Gynecol 1996; 88:412–414. [II-2]

46. ACOG. Induction of labor. ACOG Practice Bulletin No. 107. Obstet Gynecol 2009; 114(2 pt 1):386–397. [Review, III]

47. Neilson JP, Hickey M, Vazquez J. Medical treatment for early fetal death (less than 24 weeks). Cochrane Database Syst Rev 2006; 3:CD002253. [Review, III]

48. Bugalho A, Bique C, Machungo F, et al. Vaginal misoprostol as an alternative to oxytocin for induction of labor in women with late fetal death. Acta Obstet Gynecol Scand 1995; 74:194. [II-2]

49. Bugalho A, Bique C, Machungo F, et al. Induction of labor with intravaginal misoprostol in intrauterine fetal death. Am J Obstet Gynecol 1994; 171(2):538–541. [II-2]

50. Merrell DA, Koch MA. Induction of labour with intravaginal misoprostol in the second and third trimesters of pregnancy. S Afr Med J 1995; 85(10 suppl):1088–1090. [II-2]

51. Eng NS, Guan AC. Comparative study of intravaginal misoprostol with gemeprost as an abortifacient in second trimester missed abortion. Aust N Z J Obstet Gynaecol 1997; 37(3):331–334. [II-1]

52. Chittacharoen A, Herabutya Y, Punyavachira P. A randomized trial of oral and vaginal misoprostol to manage delivery in cases of fetal death. Obstet Gynecol 2003; 101(1):70–73. [RCT, n = 80]

53. Herabutya Y, Chanrachakul B, Punyavachira P. A randomized controlled trial of 6 and 12 hourly administration of vaginal misoprostol for second trimester pregnancy termination. BJOG 2005; 112(9):1297–1301. [RCT, n = 279]

54. Toaff R, Ayalon D, Gogol G. Clinical use of high concentration drip. Obstet Gynecol 1971; 37:112. [II-3]

55. Nakintu N. A comparative study of vaginal misoprostol and intravenous oxytocin for induction of labour in women with intra uterine fetal death in Mulago Hospital, Uganda. Afr Health Sci 2001; 1(2):55–59. [RCT, n = 120]

56. Kent DR, Goldstein AI, Linzey EM. Safety and efficacy of vaginal prostaglandin E2 suppositories in the management of third-trimester fetal demise. J Reprod Med 1984; 29:101. [II-2]

57. PROSTIN E2 Vaginal Suppository package insert. [III]

58. Cabrol D, Dubois C, Cronje H, et al. Induction of labor with mifepristone (RU 486) in intrauterine fetal death. Am J Obstet Gynecol 1990; 163(2):540–542. [II-2]

59. Dickinson JE. Misoprostol for second-trimester pregnancy termination in women with a prior cesarean delivery. Obstet Gynecol 2005; 105:352–6. [Level II-2]

60. Daskalakis GJ, Mesogitis SA, Papantoniou NE, et al. Misoprostol for second trimester pregnancy termination in women with prior caesarean section. BJOG 2005; 112:97–99. [II-2]

61. Berghella V, Airoldi J, O'Neill AM, et al. Misoprostol for second trimester pregnancy termination in women with prior caesarean: a systematic review. BJOG 2009; 116(9):1151–1157. [II-2]

62. Gris JC, Mercier E, Quere I, et al. Low-molecular-weight heparin versus low-dose aspirin in women with one fetal loss and a constitutional thrombophilic disorder. Blood 2004; 103(10):3695–3699. [RCT, n = 160]

63. Verdel MJ, Exalto N. Tight nuchal coiling of the umbilical cord causing fetal death. J Clin Ultrasound 1994; 22(1):64–66. [II-2]

64. Samueloff A, Xenakis EM, Berkus MD, et al. Recurrent stillbirth. Significance and characteristics. J Reprod Med 1993; 38(11):883–886. [II-3]

65. Black M, Shetty A, Bhattacharya S. Obstetric outcomes subsequent to intrauterine death in the first pregnancy. BJOG 2008; 115 (2):269–274. [II-2]

55

Antepartum testing

Christopher R. Harman

KEY POINTS

- There are no randomized trial data proving that antepartum testing reduces long-term neurologic deficits.
- Although entrenched in high-risk pregnancy management, most antenatal testing schemes are not supported by high-level evidence. Recommendations regarding which pregnancies to test and at what gestational age testing should start cannot be made given lack of sufficient evidence.
- Multiple parameter testing schemes have better correlation with fetal condition than do single-parameter tests.
- Compared to no testing, the nonstress test (NST) has been associated with a trend for a higher incidence of perinatal death (2.3% vs. 1.1%). The NST used alone is not adequate to exclude several important sources of perinatal injury; there is no increase in the incidence of interventions. Computerized cardiotocography may have significant benefit over standard NST, in high-risk cases.
- Biophysical profile score (BPS) surveillance may be beneficial in reducing cerebral palsy, with insufficient trial evidence. **Compared to other fetal testing (usually NST), biophysical profile increases the incidence of induction, but does not affect incidences of cesarean delivery, admission to ICN, or perinatal mortality**. Individual components have been compared in some trials, but the value of that evidence is limited.
- **Umbilical artery (UA) Doppler decreases perinatal mortality in antenatal management of FGR fetuses**, and should be routinely used in these pregnancies. Compared to no Doppler ultrasound, UA Doppler ultrasound in high-risk pregnancy (especially those complicated by hypertension or presumed FGR) is associated with a reduction in perinatal deaths, with fewer inductions of labor and fewer admissions to hospital.
- There are few studies comparing Doppler versus BPS. There are no management trials. BPS may correlate better with perinatal results, but this has not been shown to improve long-term neurologic outcomes.
- Testing frequency and complexity should be adjusted to reflect the stability of the clinical situation.
- Ancillary tests such as contraction stress test, oxytocin challenge test, and vibroacoustic stimulation, may have specific uses, but limited applicability.
- Formal maternal counting of fetal movement has been associated with differing results in trials, and has insufficient data to prove ability in preventing fetal death.

BACKGROUND

There are many motives underlying antepartum fetal assessment. **Preventing stillbirth by prompt intervention for proven fetal compromise is balanced by avoiding impacts of unnecessary intervention, for both fetus (iatrogenic pre-**maturity) and mother (surgical complications). Extending the pregnancy to reduce prematurity impact may increase the risk of unexpected stillbirth (because no test is perfect), but has measurable benefits in reduced long-term neurologic outcomes. Optimizing testing regimens means choosing methods, frequency, disease-specific components, while accounting for gestational-age influences, drug interactions, test variability, and even the interaction of test components.

Just as the reasons for testing, and the conditions surrounding testing, are complex, so too, are the endpoints that may inform us about the results of various testing modalities. If, for example, fetal testing is designed to prevent cerebral palsy, then the test best at predicting fetal acidosis (umbilical venous pH < 7.20) may be the test of choice, because of the high correlation between neonatal acidosis and long-term neurologic handicap (1). However, the large majority of children with cerebral palsy had normal cord gases, and normal Apgar score (2,3), so the impact of that test's correlation would be hard to prove in a population-based study. This weakness is found in almost all newborn criteria—the resilience of individual babies, the continuing improvements in the excellence of neonatal care, the profound influence of remote antenatal factors on fetal brain development, all mean that neonatal outcome factors are lightweight, at best (4). **If we want to choose the test that is best at reducing stillbirth, there is very little high-level evidence to inform us.** Two notable examples illustrate these difficulties.

Growth Restriction Intervention Trial (5–7)

The trial was designed to answer the question—can early intervention (immediate delivery) prevent fetal deterioration and avoid hypoxemic brain injury? Cases were allocated to immediate delivery or to delivery delayed until worsening testing results made caregivers certain of the need to proceed. Neonatal and two-year results are summarized in Table 55.1.

This study demonstrated that a policy of "automatic" delivery based on the risk (or fear) of fetal hypoxemia, did not prevent subsequent death or permanent neurologic sequelae. Perinatal mortality (PNM) was the same with either approach, because the stillbirth rate favoring immediate delivery (0.67% vs. 2.4%), was balanced by the neonatal death rate (9% vs. 6%). Delivering immediately avoided stillbirth, but produced more babies who died or had permanent injury later. **Gestational age, and not the severity of initial Doppler status, was the dominant factor deciding outcome.** The Growth Restriction Intervention Trial (GRIT) did not confirm the belief that early delivery based on UA Doppler and other risk factors produced better results. GRIT did parallel other delayed-intervention trials in suggesting that delaying to achieve more gestational time tended to improve the quality and health of the surviving babies (8,9) (see chap. 44).

Table 55.1 Results from the Growth Restriction Intervention Trial (GRIT)

Endpoint	Immediate delivery	Delayed delivery	Odds ratio
C/S rate	91%	79%	2.7 (CI 1.6–4.5)
Early PNM	10%	9%	1.1 (CI 0.61–1.8)
Late PNM	2%	2%	1.0
Cerebral palsy	5%	1%	Not calculated
All disabilities	8%	4%	Not calculated
Death or disability at 2 years	55/290 19%	44/283 15.5%	1.1 (CI 0.7–1.8)

Abbreviations: C/S, cesarean section; PNM, perinatal mortality; CI, 95% confidence interval.

Biophysical Profile Score and Cerebral Palsy Study (10)

At-risk pregnancies were all managed according to the BPS protocol, delivered by a single university-based team. Delivery was according to fixed fetal criteria, which do account for gestational age in some of the variables (11). The 26,290 monitored cases were compared to 58,657 nonmonitored controls delivered during the same five-year period in the same healthcare jurisdiction. Cerebral palsy and other neurologic injuries were determined by computerized review of healthcare records and secondary analysis of all index cases, at age 4. The diagnoses were proven in the acquired cases, but an unknown number of cases left the jurisdiction altogether or were unreported for other reasons. Neonatal data were available only on the BPS-monitored cases, and were not reported in this study (Table 55.2).

There was no significant difference in birth weight (2.09 kg vs. 2.28 kg) or mean gestational age at delivery (33.4 weeks vs. 34.4 weeks) between groups. Small differences in extremes included babies under 1.0 kg (14% vs. 6.7%) and births before 28 weeks (13.5% vs. 10.9%) reflecting a somewhat higher acuity, and a significantly higher rate of intervention, comparing monitored versus nonmonitored pregnancies.

Before accepting this management scheme as directly applicable to current high-risk practices, recall that this was a clinical study using a cohort of undocumented pregnancies. Referral indications included history of stillbirth, suspected FGR, and abnormal Doppler (all GRIT criteria) and also included postdate pregnancy and diabetic macrosomia. At the time of this study, many nonmonitored women had very limited ultrasound evaluation—the current high rate of detection of FGR, anomalies, malpresentation, and so on, may diminish the apparent advantage of ultrasound-based BPS. The frequency of abnormal scores prompting intervention (567/26,290, 2.2%) is likely not a solely sufficient explanation

Table 55.2 Comparison of Cerebral Palsy Rates in Pregnancies Managed and Not Managed by BPS Protocol

Endpoint	BPS monitored	Nonmonitored	Odds ratio
Cerebral palsy	1.33	4.74	3.6, $p < 0.001$
Cortical blindness	0.66	1.04	1.6, $p < 0.01$
Cortical deafness	0.90	2.2	2.4, $p < 0.005$
Mental retardation	0.80	3.1	3.9, $p < 0.001$
ADHD	4.7	28.1	6.0, $p < 0.001$
EDoC	1.2	1.0	1.2, NS

Rates are per 1000 live births.
Abbreviations: BPS, biophysical profile scoring; ADHD, attention-deficit hyperactivity disorder; EDoC, emotional disorders of childhood (control variable).

for the different rates of neurologic deficit—51% of those with cerebral palsy had normal BPS and had no intervention. It seems likely that the role of normal BPS in delaying delivery was also important. In summary, **biophysical profile scoring management appears associated with a significant reduction in long-term neurologic handicap, but the quality of the evidence merits reservation** (12).

PRINCIPLES OF FETAL MONITORING
The ideal antenatal testing regime should do the following:

- Identify impending fetal injury with near-perfect sensitivity, with warning advanced enough to allow effective intervention.
- Distinguish normal variation, benign abnormality, and degrees of significant abnormality, facilitating graded response.
- Identify normal fetal condition with near-perfect predictive value, reliably excluding stillbirth or injury for a clinically relevant interval.
- Exclude grievous fetal abnormality as the source of abnormal testing.
- Be applicable to a variety of common sources of fetal compromise, practicable in common prenatal settings, and reproducible between situations.
- Produce measurable benefits in reduction of perinatal death and long-term neurologic handicap.

FETAL-MONITORING METHODS
Fetal Heart Rate Testing (Also Called Nonstress Test or Cardiotocography [CTG])
This was first formalized as the NST, which was defined as "reactive" when there **are two or more accelerations of at least 15 beats per minute (bpm) above the baseline, that last for at least 15 seconds, in a 20-minute period** of combined fetal heart rate (FHR) and uterine activity monitoring—cardiotocography or CTG (Fig. 55.1). These criteria were adapted to premature fetuses <32 weeks, with the use of computerized CTG (CCTG), assigning reactivity to accelerations of at least 10 bpm for at least 10 seconds. This was incorporated in BPS (13) and integrated fetal testing (14) schemes, on the basis of correlation with biophysical and Doppler parameters of fetal well-being. This recognition of gestational age characteristics seems obvious, and indeed these criteria for interpretation <32 weeks have been endorsed in national guidelines (15,16). While the principle has broad consensus (17,18), a clinical basis for associating these smaller accelerations with fetal well-being has not been established. The concordance between fetal movement and accelerations in FHR is good evidence of fetal well-being, with a **negative predictive value against fetal demise within seven days of 99.5% to 99.8%** (19). However, in specific circumstances, such as FGR with abnormal placental resistance, the NST may give a false-positive reassurance against acidosis, as high as 15% (20). Missed anomalies and missed oligohydraminos are major contributors to fetal complications in patients with reactive tracings, when NST is used in isolation.

In practical monitoring terms, the false-alarming nonreactive NST is more problematic, occurring in up to 10% of tests at term (21), and up to 50% of the time at 24 to 28 weeks gestational age. When the subsequent confirmatory test [BPS, contraction stress test (CST), vibroacoustic stimulation (VAS),

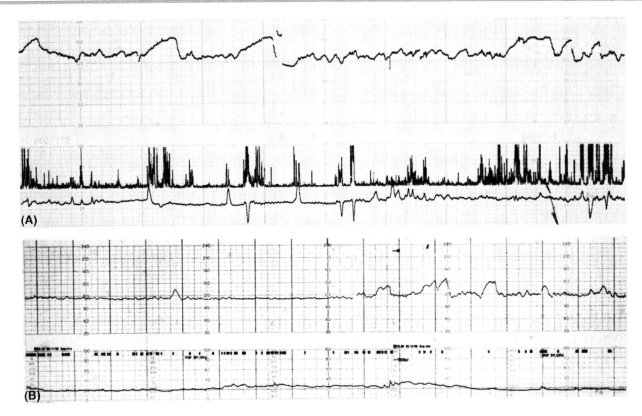

Figure 55.1 FHR monitoring. (**A**) A reactive nonstress test (NST), demonstrates multiple FHR accelerations associated with fetal movements. This external tracing, obtained at 37 weeks' gestation, is highly reassuring of fetal health, the absence of hypoxemia and the presence of a normal umbilical arterial pH. (**B**) Cyclic fetal behavior demonstrated by FHR tracing. For the first nine minutes the fetus was virtually inactive, with a nonreactive segment. When fetal movements resumed, an increase in variability and repetitive accelerations, demonstrates conversion to active sleep (a "state change" from 1F on the left, to 2F on the right. (**C**) Print out from Oxford Sonicaid computerized CTG interpretation system. *Abbreviations*: CTG, cardiotocography; bpm, beats per minute; FHR, fetal heart rate.

as examples] is performed, up to 85% will be normal. If performed, the NST should be done in the semi-Fowler ("sitting") position—this decreases the need for prolonged monitoring compared to the supine position (22,23).

Strong evidence, including randomized trial data, supports the position that nonstressed fetal heart testing should not be used as a solitary method of monitoring high-risk fetuses (24–27). **Compared to no CTG or concealment of information, knowledge of antenatal CTG results appears to have no significant effect on PNM or potentially preventable deaths**, with a worrying trend toward harm (RR 2.46, 95% CI 0.96–6.30). There was no significant impact on cesarean section rate, or on the occurrence of various secondary outcomes (26).

Computerized interpretation of FHR monitoring has evolved as a more specific, objective means of maximizing the information obtained from the CTG (28). The CCTG analyzes digitized epochs of FHR for numerical criteria, outputting objective data on short-term variability (mean of 4–8 milliseconds) and overall variability, recorded as mean minute variation. Values for short-term variability below three milliseconds show strong correlation with fetal acidosis. The CCTG is not as limited by gestational age, and does not require vigorous fetal activity to document a normal result, so it might be adopted as a better version of FHR analysis for a broader range of fetal indications. CCTG is superior to simple NST in performance time, positive and negative predictive accuracies, and fewer equivocal test results (29).

Computerized assessment is associated with lower PNM compared to traditional CTG interpretation (9/1000 vs. 4.2/1000, RR 0.20, 95% CI 0.04–0.88), **but the clinical significance of this difference is elusive, as there was no difference in potentially preventable deaths** (26).

Intrapartum FHR monitoring has advanced significantly because of advanced computerized analysis (30) (see chap. 10, *Obstetric Evidence Based Guidelines*). Access to computerized assessment improves intrapartum prediction of acidosis (31). ST-segment analysis enhances intrapartum monitoring when fetal EKG is obtained (32), but has not led to a significant decline in neonatal acidosis in a randomized study (33). *Antenatal* assessment using CCTG for high-risk premature fetuses may produce more accurate correlation with fetal condition (as compared to traditional NST) but has limited value as a stand-alone test (34).

Response to Abnormal Test Results
In specific circumstances, intervention may be based on FHR testing alone. At term, in a fetus previously documented as having reactive NST with normal variability, delivery should be considered if the tracing shows minimal or absent variability and/or repetitive late decelerations. In other uncommon cases, the first NST may detect a fetal arrhythmia, requiring prompt referral for fetal echocardiography and ultrasound examination. With these exceptions, nonreassuring CTG results should be followed immediately by full BPS or ultrasound and Doppler assessment as appropriate.

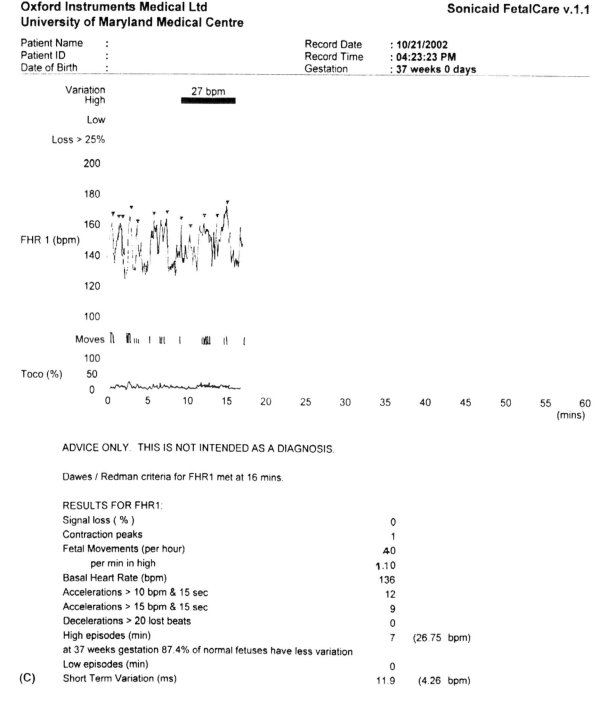

Oxford Instruments Medical Ltd
University of Maryland Medical Centre

Sonicaid FetalCare v.1.1

Patient Name	:	
Patient ID	:	
Date of Birth	:	

Record Date	: **10/21/2002**
Record Time	: **04:23:23 PM**
Gestation	: **37 weeks 0 days**

ADVICE ONLY. THIS IS NOT INTENDED AS A DIAGNOSIS.

Dawes / Redman criteria for FHR1 met at 16 mins.

RESULTS FOR FHR1:

Signal loss (%)	0	
Contraction peaks	1	
Fetal Movements (per hour)	40	
per min in high	1.10	
Basal Heart Rate (bpm)	136	
Accelerations > 10 bpm & 15 sec	12	
Accelerations > 15 bpm & 15 sec	9	
Decelerations > 20 lost beats	0	
High episodes (min)	7	(26.75 bpm)
at 37 weeks gestation 87.4% of normal fetuses have less variation		
Low episodes (min)	0	
(C) Short Term Variation (ms)	11.9	(4.26 bpm)

Figure 55.1 *(Continued)*

Biophysical Profile Scoring

This ultrasound-based modality uses five parameters of fetal behavior in a protocol-driven format (Table 55.3) to manage high-risk pregnancies (35). The parameters have different sensitivities for different fetal outcomes, but the combination of variables consistently gives the best prediction of fetal status, PNM, and neonatal complications (Fig. 55.2) (11,36,37).

Fetal Breathing Movements

These are rhythmic contractions of the fetal diaphragms, unrelated to fetal CO_2 levels, but related to diurnal rhythms, fetal cortisol levels, and demonstrating a maturational pattern.

In BPS, fetal hiccups are treated equivalently. Human fetuses are stimulated to breathe by maternal glucose levels, a response that contributes directly to the time-efficiency of outpatient BPS, which typically follows mealtimes. Fetal breathing movements are very sensitive to hypoxemia, first illustrating longer periods of fetal apnea between bursts, then being lost altogether (38).

Fetal Body Movements

Total fetal activity declines when hypoxemia begins, often associated with a gradual drop in amniotic fluid volume (39). The frequency of fetal movements is a maturational

Table 55.3 Interpretation of BPS Variables

Fetal variable	Normal behavior (score = 2)	Abnormal behavior (score = 0)
Fetal breathing movements	Intermittent, multiple episodes of more than 30-sec duration, within 30-min BPS time frame. Hiccups count. Continuous FBM for 30 min = R/O fetal acidosis	Continuous breathing without cessation. Completely absent breathing or no sustained episodes
Body or limb movements	At least four discrete body movements in 30 min. Includes fine motor movements, rolling movements, and so on, but not REM or mouthing movements	Three or fewer body/limb movements in a 30-min observation period
Fetal tone/posture	Demonstration of active extension with rapid return to flexion of fetal limbs and brisk repositioning/ trunk rotation. Opening and closing of hand, mouth, kicking, and so on	Low-velocity movement only. Incomplete flexion, flaccid extremity positions, abnormal fetal posture. Must score = 0 when FM completely absent
Cardiotocogram	At least two episodes of fetal acceleration of >15 bpm and of >15 sec duration. Normal mean variation (computerized FHR interpretation), accelerations associated with maternal palpation FM (accelerations graded for gestation), 20-min CTG	Fetal movement and accelerations not coupled. Insufficient accelerations, absent accelerations, or decelerative trace. Mean variation <20 on numerical analysis of CTG
Amniotic fluid evaluation	At least one pocket >3 cm with no umbilical cord. Also consider criteria for subjectively reduced fluid	No cord-free pocket >2 cm, or multiple elements of subjectively reduced amniotic fluid volume definite

Abbreviations: BPS, biophysical profile score; CTG, cardiotocogram; FBM, fetal breathing movements; FHR, fetal heart rate; FM, fetal movement; REM, rapid eye movement; R/O, rule-out.

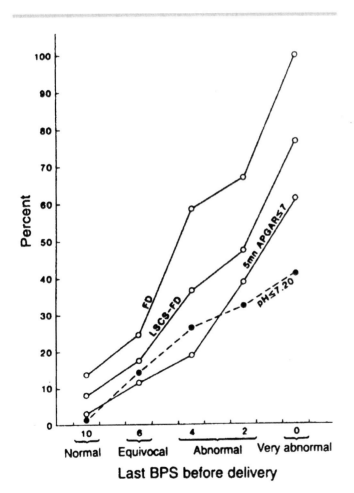

Figure 55.2 Biophysical profile score (BPS) has an exponential relationship to neonatal outcome. Declining scores strongly predict increasing frequency of fetal distress (FD), cesarean section for fetal distress (LSCS-FD), low five-minute Apgar score, and acidotic umbilical vein pH.

variable—many term fetuses will move during only 10 to 15 minutes in an hour of observation, while a 28-week fetus who did that would frequently prove abnormal.

Fetal Tone

The fetus must move to demonstrate tone—it is not simply a flexed posture. The spasm of fetal activity during startle motions provoked by acoustic stimulation does not constitute normal muscle tone and may give a misleading impression of well-being.

Amniotic Fluid Volume

This is discussed in detail in a separate guideline (see chap. 56). In BPS, the maximum single deepest pocket depth (SDP) is the standard (40,41). SDP > 2 cm meets criteria for BPS score of 2, while a number of criteria, including no SDP > 3 cm, meet criteria for subjectively reduced amniotic fluid volume (Table 55.4) (11). Reduced amniotic fluid volume is thought to represent reduced fetal urine production in the face of normal fetal swallowing. Hemodynamically mediated redistribution of fetal blood flow, not hypoxemic renal ischemia as once suggested, is the probable mechanism. The score is not modified for excessive amniotic fluid, while recognizing that the real-time ultrasound medium offers an ideal opportunity to investigate the many fetal factors associating polyhydramnios with increased PNM.

CTG

When fetal compromise occurs, the FHR is a sensitive indicator, with serial loss of NST reactivity, reduced variability, abolition of variability, and appearance of late decelerations.

Table 55.4 Subjectively Reduced Amniotic Fluid

Uterus tightly follows fetal contour
No single pocket >3 cm
No cord-free pockets of fluid
FHR decelerations with movements
FHR decelerations with transducer pressure
Restricted range of FM

Abbreviations: FHR, fetal heart rate; FM, fetal movements.

Table 55.5 Systematic Application of Biophysical Profile Scoring

BPS	Interpretation	Predicted PNM/1000[a]	Recommended management
10/10 8/8 8/10 (AFV—normal)	No evidence of fetal asphyxia present	Less than 1/1000	No acute intervention on fetal basis. Serial testing indicated by disorder-specific protocols
8/10-OLIGO	Chronic fetal compromise likely	89/1000	For absolute oligohydramnios, prove normal urinary tract, and disprove asymptomatic rupture of membranes
6/10 (AFV—normal)	Equivocal test, fetal asphyxia is not excluded	Depends on progression (61/1000 on average)	Repeat testing in about 6 hr, before assigning final value. If score is 6/10, then 10/10, in two continuous 30-min periods, manage as 10/10. For persistent 6/10, deliver the term fetus, repeat within 24 hr in the preterm fetus, then deliver if less than 6/10
4/10	Acute fetal asphyxia likely. If AFV-OLIGO, acute on chronic asphyxia very likely	91/1000	Deliver by obstetrically appropriate method, with continuous monitoring
2/10	Acute fetal asphyxia, most likely with chronic decompensation	125/1000	Deliver for fetal indications (usually needs cesarean section for intolerance to labor)
0/10	Severe, acute asphyxia virtually certain	600/1000	Deliver for fetal indications (usually needs cesarean section for intolerance to labor)

[a]Per 1000 live births, within one week of test result shown, without intervention. For scores of 0, 2, or 4, intervention should begin virtually immediately, provided the fetus is viable.

Abbreviations: AVF, amniotic fluid volume; PNM, perinatal mortality; OLIGO, oligohydramnios.

However, almost all fetuses show the first two of these during everyday normal cyclic behavior, so much so that a BPS of 8/8 is just as reliable in indicating normal well-being as a score of 10/10, and the NST can be used selectively—that is, NST is used sequentially, only in fetuses not demonstrating normal behavior in the ultrasound parameters done first (42).

Most fetuses score 8/8 for the ultrasound parameters and only 2.7% require addition of the NST, when the score is 6/8, mainly due to episodic absence of fetal breathing movements. As noted above, BPS applies prematurity criteria to CTG interpretation, but the three-tier classification of FHR patterns (normal, indeterminate, and abnormal) endorsed by NICHD (16) and recently shown to stratify neonatal outcome (43) has not yet been incorporated into BPS protocols.

BPS Management
Management by BPS follows a protocol that relates fetal condition, assumed perinatal risks, gestational age, and recommended action (Table 55.5). **If biophysical profile testing is performed, the managing physician should be willing to act on the test results.** Application of BPS has been shown to reduce PNM (historical controls, Table 55.6) (44–46), and long-term neurologic handicap (concurrent nonrandomized controls, as discussed above, Table 55.2). **Randomized trials of BPS versus no monitoring have not been done.** Randomized comparison of BPS versus NST alone (47) demonstrated BPS

superiority in composite adverse perinatal outcome and in excluding fetal growth restriction despite the small population studied (n = 652 high-risk pregnancies). Randomized trials comparing Doppler methods to BPS have been very small, and unable to evaluate such infrequent outcomes (48–52). Even current studies fail to meet standards of randomized trials—the lower quality evidence of cohort comparison continues to provide interesting information, however. In 315 high-risk pregnancies, BPS, umbilical Doppler, and uterine Doppler were performed in all subjects ≥36 weeks' gestation (52). In predicting nonreassuring fetal status, test sensitivity was BPS (60%), UA Doppler (50%), and uterine artery Doppler (30%). Sensitivity was optimized (70%) when BPS and umbilical Doppler were combined, reiterating the multivariable findings at earlier gestation (34). **Compared to other fetal testing (usually NST), biophysical profile may increase the incidence of cesarean section, but does not affect incidences of low Apgar scores, admission to ICN, or PNM (12). There are no randomized trials proving BPS alters perinatal outcome, compared to controls.**

Responses to Abnormal Test Results
Again, it should be emphasized that if biophysical profile testing is performed, the managing physician should be willing to act on the test results. In general, responses are as in Table 55.5, and are based on the differential survival rates in and out of the uterus (53). When BPS is persistently 8/10 on serial testing, that is, one variable is always missing, while the others are always present, specific inquiry should be made about cause. In some cases, that is obvious from the clinical context (e.g., oligohydramnios in preterm premature rupture of membranes with normal fetal status). In other cases, it is not so clear—in a fetus with persistent nonreactive NST despite always having normal ultrasound variables, neurologic anomalies, prior neurologic injury, fetal Down syndrome, or maternal drug ingestion may be underlying. As suggested by Table 55.7, equivocal results in the preterm fetus call for repeated testing, transfer to appropriate neonatal resources,

Table 55.6 Perinatal Mortality Changes with BPS Application

Program	n	PNM with BPS	PNM without BPS
Ireland (44)	3200	4.1	10.7
Nova Scotia (45)	5000	3.1	6.6
Manitoba (19)	56,000	1.9	7.7
California (46)	15,000	1.3	8.8

Abbreviations: BPS, biophysical profile score; n, number tested; PNM, perinatal mortality/1000.

Table 55.7 Risks of Stillbirth Vs. Neonatal Death Due to Prematurity

BPS	Stillbirth rate[a]	Equivalent neonatal death rate (wk)
0	560	25.4
2	153	28.3
4	91	29.1
6	61	30.0
8	0.5	Full term
10	0.5	Full term

[a]Death (per 1,000 births) within one week if the fetus remains undelivered. These figures change with time and differ between centers, including differences between inborn and transported babies.

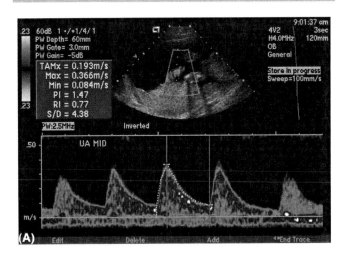

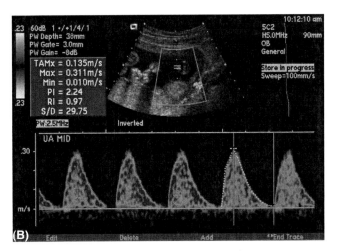

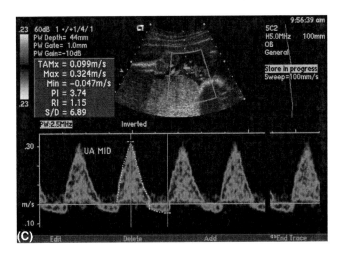

antenatal steroid administration, and so on, before moving to delivery. In high-risk fetuses, delivery can wait for valuable maturation time—the normal BPS of 8/8 or 10/10 is proof that the fetus is not acidotic (54). On the other hand, a BPS of 0–2/10 may justify delivery and neonatal management down to local thresholds of viability in absence of a transient cause (55).

Modified Biophysical Profile Score

Many modifications have been proposed. The most popular combination suggested has been the **AFI-NST combination** (56), including optional use of VAS (57,58), to shorten observation time. Full BPS (all five variables) was the backup test, required in 15% to 30% of cases. The simplified test reduced the time and complexity of BPS, without altering the false-negative rate, which is about 3 to 5 per 10,000 tests (57). However, in assessing differences in the false-positive rate, either the data are too few or the full BPS was superior to the restricted tests in avoiding unnecessary intervention.

The exceptions are trials of FGR management in which the modified BPS included Doppler information—in those cases, addition of Doppler assessment of umbilical arterial resistance both improved classification of fetal acidosis and reduced interference for false-alarm BPS (59,60). Shortening the BPS is not validated for high-risk fetuses with abnormal Doppler indices, preterm fetuses, postdate pregnancy, fetal anomalies, multiple gestation, or fetuses with arrhythmia, infection, anemia, or diabetic macrosomia.

Multivessel Doppler

Placental insufficiency has a large structural component, with tertiary stem villous deficiency and progressively smaller perfusion area leading to progressive rise in UA resistance (Fig. 55.3). Functional aspects, including placental volume flow, sequential placental flow distribution, and vascular responses to maternal hyperoxygenation, are interesting from the physiologic point of view, but too operator-dependent for clinical monitoring. UA Doppler assessment requires careful attention to technical detail, and is usually done in the midportion of the free umbilical cord (61). Although each mathematical expression of the Doppler arterial flow velocity waveform has some advantages, the pulsatility index (PI) has the advantage of infinite expression (remaining valid even when flow is reversed), and autocorrelation with the volume of the waveform itself. When UA PI reaches an individualized threshold, higher blood pressure leads to cardiac effects and systemic effects. Initial cardiac effects, including ejection fraction, wall velocity, transvalvular velocity, and so on, are measurable with sophisticated techniques, but the systemic effects are readily demonstrated in a shift toward more cerebral

Figure 55.3 Abnormalities in Doppler velocity wave forms of the umbilical artery depict increasing placental resistance. These Doppler examinations are from the same patient as pregnancy progresses. (**A**) The umbilical artery resistance is modestly elevated at 18 weeks (PI 1.47). By 24 weeks (**B**), end-diastolic velocities are absent in most cardiac cycles. By 28 weeks (**C**), reversal of end-diastolic flow occupies nearly one quarter of the cardiac cycle. Cesarean section was carried out on the basis of oligohydramnios at 29+ weeks, with umbilical venous pH 7.18. *Abbreviation*: PI, pulsatility index.

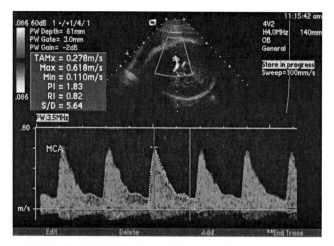

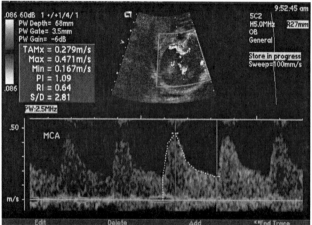

Figure 55.4 Serial MCA Dopplers demonstrate an increase in diastolic blood flow, termed centralization. Normally, the middle cerebral artery shows high resistance with low diastolic velocity (high PI 1.83, *upper image*). Diversion of blood flow toward the brain correlates with worsening umbilical artery depiction of increased placental resistance, with falling cerebrovascular resistance, increased end-diastolic velocities, and PI falling to 1.09 (*lower image*). *Abbreviations*: PI, pulsatility index; MCA, middle cerebral artery.

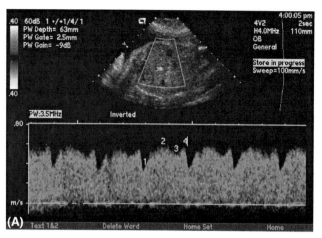

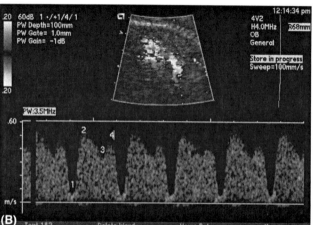

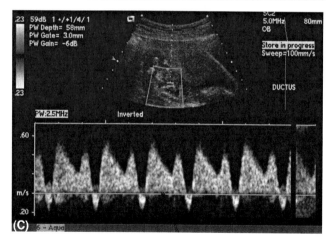

Figure 55.5 Progressive changes in venous return to the heart as depicted in the ductus venosus. (**A**) there are normally four phases in the wave form, consisting of (1) atrial contraction, (2) ventricular contraction, (3) restitution of the annulus, (4) diastole. Typically, the a-wave (1) shows the only significant downward deflection, a modest reduction in forward flow. (**B**) Increase afterload from placental resistance causes abnormal forward cardiac output, with the a-wave nearly retrograde. (**C**) Further progression in placental insufficiency is associated with cardiac malfunction, with severe retrograde a-waves, as well as distorted cardiac function, producing midwave depression as the annulus rises against an overfilled circulation.

perfusion using the Doppler waveform of the middle cerebral artery (MCA, Fig. 55.4). Initially present as a subtle change in the cerebral:placental ratio, this shift is later depicted as a significant decline in the MCA PI as diastolic blood flow rises (62). The initial change in proportional distribution has been termed centralization, and may simply be due to resistance-mediated diversion of flow away from an ailing placenta. The second change, which has been called brain sparing, may be mediated by hypoxemia-induced cerebral vasorelaxation.

As the hemodynamic and respiratory declines continue to interact, oxygen-sensitive interfaces between nutrient-rich and nonrich streams begin to dictate flow (63). Diversion through an opening ductus venosus (DV) is readily depicted as progressive changes in waveform pattern (DV, Fig. 55.5). Deep reversal of the atrial contraction wave, a-wave, indicates both cardiac impairment (forward volume flow insufficiency forcing the waveform more retrograde) and hypoxemia (dilating the DV itself). DV interrogation is easy to learn, as this vessel contains the highest venous velocities

Table 55.8 Abnormal Umbilical Artery Doppler Correlates with Neonatal Compromise

Cesarean section for fetal nonreassuring testing
Acidosis
Hypoxemia
Low Apgar-5
Ventilator required
Long-term oxygen
Bronchopulmonary dysplasia
Anemia
Increased NRBC
Thrombocytopenia
Prolonged NRBC release
Neutropenia
Transfusions required
IVH
NEC
Perinatal mortality

For all of these outcomes, their frequency rises exponentially from abnormal indices to absent end-diastolic velocities to reversed end-diastolic velocities. *Abbreviations*: BPD, bronchopulmonary dysplasia; NRBC, nucleated red blood cells; IVH, intraventricular hemorrhage; NEC, necrotizing enterocolitis.

in the fetal abdomen, but when the waveform is abnormal, it must be carefully differentiated from adjacent hepatic venous structures.

Doppler Application (64)
Worsening umbilical arterial Doppler correlates well with declining placental function and the emergence of hypoxemia and acidosis (62). Absent end-diastolic velocities denote an increasing risk of stillbirth, preterm delivery, birth weight below 10th percentile, and many neonatal complications (Table 55.8) (65) UA Doppler is useful in directing care—small fetuses with normal Dopplers probably do not need the same level of surveillance, and subsequently of intervention, as do those with abnormal umbilical flow (66). Perinatal outcome is superior when Doppler is utilized in decision-making, although interventions based on umbilical Doppler alone have a substantial risk of causing unnecessary prematurity (67,68). Compared with no Doppler ultrasound, **Doppler ultrasound in high-risk pregnancy (especially those complicated by hypertension or presumed fetal growth restriction) is associated with a reduction in perinatal death** (1.2% vs. 1.7%, RR 0.71, 95% CI 0.50–0.98). The use of Doppler ultrasound is also associated with **fewer inductions of labor** (RR 0.89) and **fewer cesarean sections** (RR 0.90) without reports of adverse effects. No difference is found for FHR abnormalities in labor or low Apgar scores (69) (see chap. 44).

Despite the strong correlations with fetal status, basing delivery decisions on UA Doppler alone, especially before 32 to 34 weeks and without the presence of absent or reversed diastolic flow, may lead to unnecessary mortality and morbidity due to extreme prematurity (2,70,71). Further, **routine application of UA and/or uterine artery Doppler in normal pregnancy is of no proven benefit**, even with the chance discovery of abnormality taken into account (72,73).

Evaluation of venous Doppler waveforms may be useful in correct prediction of morbidity and mortality in FGR. DV abnormality is a strong predictor of adverse perinatal outcome, surpassing all other predictors (74,75). However, the best outcomes occurred when BPS was used to maximize the safe prolongation of pregnancy (76). Even in the most compromised pregnancy, gestational age was the most influential

factor in determining outcome. These principles have been amplified further in recent nontrial observations. First, the most severe DV abnormality, absence or reversal of the a-wave (Fig. 55.5) is an accurate predictor of stillbirth when it exists >7 days (in fetuses with the most severe UA patterns) (77). Second, however, **when severe DV abnormality is found** *without* **abnormal UA Doppler, outcome may well be normal**. Again, the principle is emphasized: solitary Doppler abnormality, even a-wave reverse in the DV, is not sufficient for intervention (78).

Response to Abnormal Test Results
The literature includes several series where action solely on the basis of alarming Doppler findings led to iatrogenic prematurity, producing neonatal injury and death, at least partially avoidable if delivery had been postponed a little. With those experiences in mind, GRIT and other trials addressed the potential for adverse effects if delivery were delayed past the point of abnormal Doppler findings. Various steps may be taken during that extended time, including administration of antenatal steroids, transfer to a higher level of neonatal resource, stabilization of maternal conditions, evaluation for vaginal delivery, or retesting with additional Doppler parameters. These trials, constituting level I–II evidence, have shown no excess liability in the form of PNM, while adding significantly to intrauterine time. In virtually all Doppler-outcome trials, the single most critical influence on outcome has been gestational age at delivery and its determination of adverse impacts of prematurity. Safe extension of the pregnancy may be possible by adding other test parameters in sequence (79–81). An approach to sequential testing, Doppler establishing the appropriate level of intense surveillance, BPS indicating the timing of delivery, has been proposed by several independent teams. An example is shown in Table 55.9.

Doppler Surveillance and BPS: Integrated Fetal Testing

Fetuses at risk for placental insufficiency are best assessed with UA Doppler. However, elevated UA resistance may persist for months, and absent end-diastolic velocity for weeks, without fetal deterioration. Similarly, venous abnormalities may also persist for weeks, even at levels (>95th percentile for gestational age) used for intervention in one current trial (82). In this trial, timing of delivery using standard CTG (loss of

Table 55.9 Umbilical Artery Doppler Index Abnormality Suggests NST/SDP or BPS Surveillance

Abnormality[a]	NST/SDP or BPS frequency[b]	Decision to deliver (fetal)[c]
Decreased but present diastolic flow	Weekly	Abnormal BPS[d] or ≥36–37 wk
AEDV	Twice weekly	Abnormal BPS[d] or ≥34 wk
REDV	Daily	Abnormal BPS[d] or ≥32 wk

[a]Umbilical artery (UA) and precordial venous Doppler. MCA abnormalities confirm the elevated placental resistance, but do not directly alter management according to this scheme.
[b]*Minimum* frequency, increased on the basis of severity—maternal condition(s), degree of IUGR, gestational age.
[c]Neonatology consultation, maternal clinical factors, fetal blood sampling parameters, all will impact this collaborative decision.
[d]Any BPS≤4/10.
Abbreviations: NST, nonstress test; SDP, single deepest pocket; BPS, biophysical profile scoring.

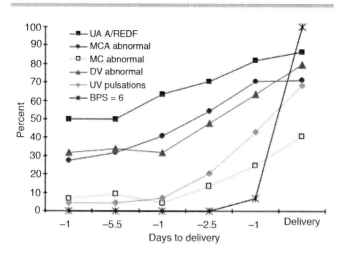

Figure 55.6 Progressive changes in multivessel Doppler occur in sequence before the BPS deteriorates, in many fetuses. Virtually all fetuses were delivered for abnormal BPS (*asterisks*). Most of these IUGR fetuses had reached the end of their Doppler progression before delivery. *Abbreviations*: A/REDV, absent or reversed diastolic velocity; MCA, middle cerebral artery; DV, ductus venosus; BPS, biophysical profile score; UA, umbilical artery; UV, umbilical vein.

variability) will be compared to two thresholds of DV abnormality [95th percentile (moderate) and a-wave reversal (severe)]. This study, TRUFFLE, is nearing its target accrual of nearly 600 patients for two-year follow-up, as this guideline is being written. However, a smaller study already published, suggests this computer-assisted Doppler method will not overcome the importance of gestational age. **In 113 pregnancies managed by combined UA and DV Doppler, with delivery triggered by BPS, gestational age and birth weight were "the predominant factors for poor neurodevelopment" assessed at age 2** (83). The rationale underlying the multivessel Doppler and BPS approach is the relationship of deterioration in vascular indices to the (later) decline in BPS (Fig. 55.6) (8). TRUFFLE may or may not resolve this issue, but current information suggests a-wave reversal should not be an instant trigger for delivery either—the international FGR registry suggests a-wave reversal may exist for many days before BPS deteriorates (79). Especially in the critical gestational ages before 32 weeks, such an interval may be crucial in reducing prematurity impacts.

For BPS, the underlying premise is that reduction in fetal activity reaches clinically detectable levels on a voluntary basis (i.e., responsive to the need for conservation rather than depressive due to a critical central decompensation). If the premise is valid, intervention on the basis of abnormal activity should allow the baby to recover, unharmed, in the neonatal period, if intervention is prompt and effective. If the premise is wrong, then waiting for the challenged fetus to become obtunded (i.e., without activity) would be associated with adverse long-term outcome, despite intervention. A high-level of evidence is now available, showing that waiting until the need for delivery is certain maximizes intrauterine time, optimizes reduction of prematurity, and at the same time, does not add morbidity or mortality by "delaying" intervention (9,74–77,79–81,8,84).

Testing is frequent, complex, and highly individualized, in the evaluation of these fragile FGR fetuses. Integrated fetal

testing is a framework, not a rigid scheme. The decision for delivery reflects not only the BPS parameters, but also the familiarity with fetal status arising from prolonged observation, up to several times every day by the same team. Subtle changes in serial Doppler pattern also play a role in determining intervention. This approach to surveillance in severe FGR (integrated fetal testing) is illustrated in Table 55.9 (14). For management of FGR, see also chapter 44, and in particular Figure 44.1.

Condition-Specific Testing

The specific example of FGR above demonstrates the potential interaction of multiple testing parameters to optimize management. Since other identifiable conditions have increased risks of fetal compromise, but may not have identical patterns of fetal deterioration, it may be necessary/beneficial to modify testing to fit the disorder.

Diabetic Vasculopathy

The subset of fetuses in diabetic pregnancy at highest risk of adverse outcome has elevated placental resistance as detected by UA Doppler. This includes women with hypertension, cardiac, renal, and other vascular diabetopathy, and fetuses with FGR. Doppler will correctly stratify the adverse outcomes better than BPS (85). Prospective randomized evaluation of management has not been reported.

Diabetic Fetal Macrosomia

Poor glycemic control as judged by maternal blood sugars, or as denoted by fetal macrosomia (estimated fetal weight >90th percentile and polyhydramnios), or both, requires increased surveillance. In the absence of Doppler abnormalities of placentation, management by BPS protocol using twice-weekly testing, achieves the same or better outcome (cord vein pH, mortality, neonatal morbidity) than euglycemic controls (86). The critical issue is glycemic control—when this is good, antenatal testing is less critical. When diabetic control is poor, identification and monitoring of the macrosomic fetus requires individualized care (87,88).

Obesity

The exponential rise in obesity and morbid obesity in pregnancy is alarming in many respects, including accelerated fetal risks (89). These associations include the effects of associated medical disorders such as hypertension and diabetes, but obesity itself has an independent impact on fetal macrosomia, stillbirth, and intrapartum complications that mandates heightened monitoring (90).

Postdate Pregnancy

Data are conflicting. Randomized trials indicate a policy of induction of labor before 42 weeks may reduce incidence of some key outcomes, but those trials have been criticized because they relied on NST alone, and did not take advantage of superior monitoring techniques, including CCTG, Doppler, and BPS (91). When women >41 weeks were randomly assigned to modern comprehensive fetal monitoring versus delivery, no differences were shown (92). Prior nonrandomized cohort studies have demonstrated superior results of full BPS compared to NST alone, and Doppler plus CTG versus CST/oxytocin challenge test (OCT) (93,94). At present, the best recommendation is made with moderate confidence: pregnancy beyond certain 41+ weeks should be evaluated for delivery, which we favor. Where delivery is not selected, twice-weekly monitoring should include amniotic fluid assessment using the single pocket depth method, CTG analysis and assessment of fetal activity (95) (see chap. 24, *Obstetric Evidence Based Guidelines*).

The "Small Normal" Fetus Near Term
Late third-trimester growth restriction is difficult to identify clinically. When serial sonography does show late growth delay, early placental senescence may be the cause, but such fetuses often have normal placental (umbilical and uterine artery) Doppler. Reduced MCA resistance ("centralization") was associated with increased frequency of intrapartum and neonatal complications (96). This observation may identify a testing correlate of late hemodynamic compensation, useful in determining which small fetuses should be monitored. There is emerging evidence that third-trimester subtle changes in growth, perfusion distribution, and long-term cognitive and focal brain abnormalities may be associated (97). Much more evidence on identification, monitoring management options, and impacts of intervention is required—although proceeding to delivery might seem to be an obvious solution, there is currently no evidence that this improves outcome (98).

Preterm Premature Ruptured Membranes
Infection may have an all or none effect on fetal behavior. When the NST was nonreactive and fetal breathing was absent, delivery produced superior neonatal and maternal infectious outcomes in one study—BPS management may be helpful in managing preterm premature ruptured membranes (PPROM) (99). This finding has not been replicated in other studies, and **fetal status is a poor predictor of culture results from amniocentesis**. Differentiation may be on the fetal effects of amniotic fluid infection—while BPS with CCTG did not predict culture results reliably, they did suggest which fetus was likely to show signs of infection (100). **Randomized comparison of BPS and NST alone in this setting did not resolve this issue—neither test has good sensitivity (25.0% and 39.1%, respectively) in predicting infectious morbidity**, but both had good predictive accuracy when abnormal (66.7% and 52.9%, respectively) (101). New evidence in neonates suggests that CCTG factors used to intervene for suspected fetal infection (decreased FHR variability and transient decelerations) are markers of advancing infection (102). This evidence seems to fortify the role of BPS with CCTG in monitoring pregnancies with chronic PPROM. Recommendation: monitoring in PPROM before 32 to 34 weeks should include meticulous daily assessment of markers of infection, preterm labor, and consideration for BPS or CTG. Delivery is indicated on reaching gestational age thresholds determined by local experience—passive waiting beyond that is not justified by the weak sensitivity of current antenatal testing. Although not studied in management trials to date, amniocentesis as a means of dictating delivery may be more effective than noninvasive methods.

Fetal Anemia
BPS deteriorates as an end-stage effect of visible hydrops, and gray-scale imaging is ineffective in predicting descent to severe anemia in alloimmune cases, so neither should be used alone in monitoring fetuses at risk for anemia. NST or CCTG do show correlation with anemia, based on a reduction in variability as anemia worsens, but this relationship is not early enough or reliable enough to dictate invasive management. **MCA Doppler velocimetry** is effective in determining the need for fetal transfusion, the timing between transfusions, and in differentiating degrees of fetal anemia (102). However, since there is a 1% to 10% failure rate in detecting severe anemia,

and a higher rate of missing mild anemia (which may progress rapidly) (103), MCA should form the core of a comprehensive approach that also includes fetal blood sampling by cordocentesis, and an experienced team familiar with fetal hematology (104) (see chap. 52).

Ancillary Testing Methods
Modified FHR recording methods utilize fetal stimulation to shorten the time to reach reactivity, to convert nonreactive FHR tracings to reactivity, as a confirmatory test for nonreactive NST, and in highest-risk populations, as a more precise test of fetal well-being.

In the **CST, and the OCT**, spontaneous and induced contractions, respectively, stress the fetoplacental unit, either by placental compression or by cord compression, producing decelerations in the abnormal test, no decelerations when the test is normal. These tests have higher negative predictive value than NST alone, similar to biophysical and Doppler methods (3–4 per 10,000 tests), but have high rates of equivocal results, and a high rate of false-alarming results. When BPS is used as the backup test for positive (abnormal) CST, at least 50% of pregnancies can safely continue for at least a week, for example (105). High cost, requirement of hospital facilities, disagreement on fundamental interpretation of the test, occasional complications resulting from the test methods, and the lack of superior practical performance (same time elapsed, more follow-up tests required) have marginalized these techniques. The OCT may have a role in determining the route of delivery when the need for intervention has already been determined (e.g., a positive OCT means proceed to cesarean section), but the data available do not justify any conclusion.

A second type of stimulation is **VAS** (106). The fetus is stimulated by external high-amplitude white noise applied to the maternal abdomen. This is capable of causing state change in most fetuses, including provoking conversion to 4F ("frantic fetus"), at term (11). Occasional side effects include conversion to fixed fetal arrhythmia, and serious concerns about delivery of high-pressure sound (up to 130 decibels) and effects on fetal hearing (11). Since premature fetuses typically require more sound pressure to elicit responses, and are more susceptible to hearing injury, use of VAS before 32 weeks should be very cautious.

Compared to no such stimulation, fetal VAS has been associated with a reduction in the incidence of nonreactive antenatal CTG test (RR 0.62, 95% CI 0.52–0.74) and reduced the overall mean CTG testing time by about 10 minutes (107). The focus on shortening time of testing has not been shown to increase the number of pregnancies that can be monitored to advantage, and comparison to multiple-component testing such as BPS is inconclusive. Applied to modified BPS testing, VAS is associated with a 67% false-alarm rate requiring performance of full BPS in any case (108). More critical, however, is the false-negative rate–55% of fetuses with subsequent FHR abnormalities had reassuring VAS-NST (109). Sound responsiveness is reduced in many high-risk groups (less than 32 weeks' gestation, hypertension, depression, severe IUGR, cocaine exposure, treatment with magnesium sulfate or antenatal steroids) (11). Specific trials have demonstrated superiority of multivariable testing including Doppler, NST, and biophysical variables over either CST or VAS in prolonged pregnancy and IUGR. Both trials concluded CST and VAS could be eliminated from fetal testing regimes (94,110). The proven effect of VAS to provoke fetal neurologic state change seems outweighed by its ability to generate false reassurance.

Table 55.10   Indications for Antenatal Surveillance

Primarily maternal conditions	Primarily placental conditions	Primarily fetal conditions	Miscellaneous conditions
Severe hyperthyroidism	Antiphospholipid syndrome	Decreased fetal movement	IVF pregnancy
Symptomatic hemoglobinopathy	Systemic lupus erythematosus	Oligohydramnios	Previous stillbirth
Cyanotic heart disease	Hypertensive disorders	Polyhydramnios	Previous recurrent abruption
Chronic renal disease	Marked placental anomalies	Intrauterine growth restriction	Teratogen exposure
Type I diabetes	Umbilical artery	Postdates pregnancy	
Marked uterine anomalies	Doppler abnormalities	Alloimmunization	
Uterine artery		Macrosomia	
		Fetal anomalies/aneuploidy	
		Multiple gestation	

Source: Modified from Ref. 117.

Routine application in high-risk fetal populations is not recommended.

Shining a bright halogen light on the mother's abdomen shortens the time to first acceleration on NST (111).

Compared to no administration, **antenatal maternal glucose administration** (20–50 mg orally, e.g., as orange juice) **does not decrease the incidence of nonreactive antenatal CTG tests**, regardless of prior fasting or nonfasting (112).

Compared to no manipulation, or to VAS, **manual fetal manipulation does not decrease the incidence of nonreactive antenatal CTG test** (113).

Fetal Movement Counting in Low-Risk Pregnancy

The largest randomized trial of maternal monitoring of fetal movement (114) failed to show any benefit over "informal inquiry about movement during standard antenatal care." This trial produced a noticeable effect on control subjects, whose experience in the trial led to improved perinatal performance compared to nontrial participants in the general population. It did not produce a benefit in treated patients, with the same PNM in both study and control patients. Many women do report reduced fetal activity prior to stillbirth, so why did this trial demonstrate no effect? First, decreased movement was not reported promptly by many subjects. Second, the "rescue" method was simple CTG, where false reassurance of a normal heart rate preceded a large proportion of fetal deaths. So, it may be that maternal awareness of fetal activity can be a useful adjunct in monitoring low-risk situations, if reporting is immediate, and if the rescue method is full BPS or even more complex assessment. While three additional small studies of movement counting provide some information, there are no apparent benefits in reduced adverse outcomes (115). **The "count to ten" method (count to ten movements, then resume normal activity)** versus counting for a specified length of time (e.g., 30 minutes of counting every six to eight hours) **was associated with better patient compliance** (116). Overall, data do not support reliance on fetal movement counting between episodes of formal fetal assessment in high-risk pregnancy (116).

Practical Antenatal Testing: Who, When, How, and Why?

No trial has conclusively proven that antenatal testing lowers long-term adverse neurologic outcomes, so recommendations might be rated as Level B or even C (i.e., consensus, expert opinion, but no clear evidence). Many trials have indicated that specific antenatal monitoring regimes have a possible impact on mortality and short-term outcomes—an inference is apparent. The standard of care, accordingly, can only be a

suggestion: women with any of the factors in Table 55.10 can be offered antenatal surveillance of appropriate intensity and precision.

Thresholds for viability, knowledge of the disease process, severity of individual cases, past history, all may indicate starting monitoring earlier than recommended by general guidelines (32–34 weeks for most at-risk fetuses, according to the ACOG) (Table 55.11). Routine application of testing methods such as NST or UA Doppler alone, pose substantial risk of iatrogenic prematurity in fetuses with abnormal testing—a blanket proposal of "testing early and testing often" is potentially more dangerous than helpful. Testing should be timed in recognition of the characteristics of the test and the fetal patient, in context.

The choice of test is determined not only by specific condition-related advantages above, but also by available personnel and equipment resources, cost, availability of effective treatment for abnormal results, and evidence of outcome impact of the management protocol. For disorders with placental/vascular components (FGR, hypertensive disorders, vascular disease), UA Doppler methods are necessary to optimize monitoring. In some situations, including determining delivery timing for FGR fetuses, multivariable BPS may offer significant benefits over single-variable testing (Table 55.11).

Testing interval will depend on severity (e.g., up to three times daily in FGR fetuses with the worst Doppler pattern, according to the integrated fetal testing protocol). There is no apparent high-level evidence supporting the widely practiced protocol of weekly BPS testing, as opposed to some other frequency of assessment—but the important role of maternal compliance with testing schedules should not be overlooked.

Pitfalls in Assessing Fetal-Monitoring Methods

- Pregnancy is usually uncomplicated. For instance, if pregnancy termination for lethal anomalies detected at 18 to 20 weeks were the only management maneuver, normal outcome would occur in >90%. In a population with a low incidence of the target outcome, predictive accuracies arising from large population-based studies, not sensitivity/specificity derived from small groups (even if randomized), are required (118).

- Monitoring is not performed in isolation. For ultrasound-based methods, detection of critical complications such as imminent cord prolapse, abruptio in progress, unsuspected twin complications, and so on, leads to important individual impacts not attributable to the testing scheme itself (11). Further, in the context of maternal participation, the interactive nature of monitoring likely benefits from detection of accelerated hypertension, polyhydramnios, or peripheral edema, heightening the acuity of monitoring

Table 55.11 Suggested Antenatal Surveillance for Specific Conditions

Condition[a]	Timing	Fetal surveillance
Preeclampsia	At diagnosis	UA Doppler
Chronic HTN	Usually 32 wk	Weekly NST/SDP or BPS
IUGR	At diagnosis	UA Doppler
	At 32 wk	Weekly NST/SDP or BPS
Gestational diabetes		
A1	38–40 wk	Weekly NST/SDP or BPS
A2	36 wk	
Pregestational DM	Usually 32 wk	Weekly NST/SDP or BPS
	Twice weekly ≥ 36 wk	
Postdates	41 wk	NST/SDP or BPS, twice weekly
Multiple gestation[b]		
Concordant, di-di	32–34 wk	Weekly NST/SDP or BPS
One twin IUGR, di-di	At diagnosis	UA Doppler
	At 32 wk	Weekly NST/SDP or BPS
Discordant, mono-di	At diagnosis	SDP, and UA Doppler at least weekly
Prior stillbirth	At 32 wk	Weekly NST/SDP or BPS
SLE, or renal disease	At 32 wk	Weekly NST/SDP or BPS
Maternal age ≥35 yr-old	At 36 wk	Weekly NST/SDP or BPS

[a]Patient care should be individualized. Some patients may require BPS, Doppler flow studies, or other testing in addition to the above. Specific examples are discussed in chapters 4, 5, 43, and 44, for instance.
[b]Knowledge of chorionicity is crucial; di-di, dichorionic diamniotic; mono-di, monochorionic diamniotic (shared placenta) (see chap. 43).

outside the test parameters. On the other hand, there appears no reciprocal benefit—high feedback during antenatal ultrasound did not reduce maternal anxiety or promote health behavior compared to scans with no narration and the screen not visible (119).

- Experience with new technologies influences results. For instance, as technical expertise with venous Doppler techniques improves, it seems quite likely that more detailed understanding of patterns of fetal disease will further influence monitoring patterns. Such effects undoubtedly occur *during* the performance of trials—the large numbers of subjects needed to answer research questions take time and often multiple sites—the testing regime may change significantly before results are finalized.
- Correlations do not prove impact. A large number of studies, including randomized trials, conclude method superiority based on statistical correlation with fetal or neonatal standards. Such correlations must exist if the testing regime has a significant chance of affecting outcome. Increasingly, attention should be paid to randomized management trials, not randomized studies limited to documentation of associations.
- Short-term outcome may be misleading. Focusing on umbilical cord pH at delivery, in relation to either Doppler or BPS testing, may not be informative. In the GRIT trial, any differences in pH for early intervention were clearly overbalanced by an excess of neurologic handicap at age three years in GRIT (Table 55.2), as the majority of BPS-monitored CP cases had normal BPS before delivery. In both these examples, the short-term outcome measures incompletely represented the (more important) long-term impacts. Newer management trials with funding for such long-term follow-up are likely to have much broader impact on practice (82,83).

- Low-level evidence or even nonmedical influences may be increasingly important in determining monitoring guidelines. If a professional society elevates nontrial data supporting BPS application (level II to III) to the highest reliability in a national guideline (I-A), practice patterns are likely to follow (15). If learned perinatal scholars recommend intensive regimens based on years of research and experience, these nontrial data will also likely change or reinforce practice (120,121).

Perhaps even more obvious in the North American setting are the interactions between monitoring guidelines and legal argument—this is not a one-way relationship (122).

Prenatal Care—the Final Frontier of Antenatal Monitoring

Absence of prenatal care is a risk factor for adverse outcome (123). The provision of adequate prenatal care, evaluation of risks, and institution of antenatal monitoring attending those risks will improve the frequency of preterm labor in adolescents (124), and in women in prison (125), and may facilitate maternal-fetal bonding, with important long-term implications (126). The means by which this happens is elusive, but there is strong evidence that reducing prenatal care for low-risk women is not without danger—an increase in PNM follows (127).

Standard prenatal care is unlikely to completely address the important issues of FGR and preterm labor. The identification of specific risk factors and specific mechanisms to address them likely will have measurable impact. An excellent example of the positive impact of focused care is seen in the application of UA Doppler in FGR. At the same time, cigarette smoking, teratogen exposure, the anemia of urban malnutrition, and social issues, including workspace hazards, all have proven impacts on perinatal health, opening major opportunities for public intervention.

A new focus on risk evaluation and target-specific prenatal care is required (128). This prenatal care may directly "treat" many of the causes of adverse outcome, focusing group or community resources and peer support on effective basic prenatal care. It will also form the basis of new monitoring plans for as yet unsolved issues such as the excess poor outcomes in mild maternal hypothyroidism, IVF pregnancy, and first-trimester bleeding. As prenatal care and antenatal monitoring have succeeded with many major perinatal problems to date, there are many more to be addressed (129).

REFERENCES

1. McCowan LM, Pryor J, Harding JE. Perinatal predictors of neurodevelopmental outcomes in small-for-gestational age children at 18 months of age. Am J Obstet Gynecol 2002; 186(5): 1069–1075. [II-3; Upgraded descriptive study due to neurodevelopmental follow-up, 282 subjects]
2. Nelson KB. The epidemiology of cerebral palsy in term infants. Ment Retard Dev Disabil Res Rev 2002; 8(3):146–150. [Review]
3. Schifrin BS. The CTG and the timing and mechanism of fetal neurological injuries. Best Pract Res Clin Obstet Gynecol 2004; 18(3):437–456. [Review]
4. Korst LM, Phelan JP, Wang YM, et al. Acute fetal asphyxia and permanent brain injury: a retrospective analysis of current indicators. J Maternal Fetal Med 1999; 8:101–106. [II-3; pre-trial survey]
5. GRIT study group. When do obstetricians recommend delivery for high-risk preterm growth-retarded fetus? Growth Restriction Intervention Trial. Eur J Obstet Gynecol Reprod Biol 1996; 67(2): 121–126. [II-3; pre-trial survey]
6. GRIT study group. A randomized trial of timed delivery for the compromised preterm fetus: short term outcomes and Bayesian interpretation. Br J Obstet Gynecol 2003; 110(1):27–32. [Multicenter RCT]
7. Thornton JG, Hornbuckle J, Vail A, et al. Infant well-being at 2 years of age in the Growth Restriction Intervention Trial (GRIT): multicentered randomized controlled trial. Lancet 2204; 364 (9433):513–520. [Multicenter RCT with neurodevelopmental follow-up]
8. Baschat AA, Gembruch U, Harman CR. The sequence of changes in Doppler and biophysical parameters as severe fetal growth restriction worsens. Ultrasound Obstet Gynecol 2001; 18:571–577. [II-2]
9. Cosmi E, Ambrosini G, D'Antona D, et al. Doppler, cardiotocography, and biophysical profile changes in growth-restricted fetuses. Obstet Gynecol 2005; 106(6):1240–1245. [II-2]
10. Manning FA, Bondaghi N, Harman CR, et al. Fetal assessment based on the fetal biophysical profile scoring VIII. The incidence of cerebral palsy in tested and untested perinates. Am J Obstet Gynecol 1998; 178(4):696–706. [II-2]
11. Harman CR. Antenatal assessment of fetal status. In: Creasy R, Iams J, Resnik R, eds. Maternal-Fetal Medicine. 6th ed. Toronto: WB Saunders, 2010. [Review]
12. Lalor JG, Fawole B, Alfirevic Z, et al. Biophysical profile for fetal assessment in high risk pregnancies. Cochrane Database Syst Rev 2008; 23(1):CD000038. [Meta-analysis]
13. Harman CR. Fetal biophysical variables and fetal status. In: Maulik D, ed. Asphyxia and Brain Damage. New York: Wiley-Liss, 1998:279–320. [Review]
14. Baschat AA. Integrated fetal testing in growth restriction: combining multivessel Doppler and biophysical parameters. Ultrasound Obstet Gynecol 2003; 21(1):1–8. [Review]
15. Liston R, Sawchuck D, Young D. Fetal health surveillance: antepartum and intrapartum consensus guideline. J Obstet Gynaecol Can 2007; 29(suppl 4):S3–S56. [III]
16. Macones GA, Hankins GD, Spong CY, et al. The 2008 national institute of child health and human development worksheet on electronic fetal monitoring: update on definitions, interpretation, and research guidelines. J Obstet Neonatal Nurs 2008; 37(5): 510–515. [III]
17. Snijders RJ, McLaren R, Nicolaides KH. Computer-assisted analysis of fetal heart rate patterns at 20-41 week's gestation. Fetal Diagn Ther 1990; 5(2):79–83. [II-2]
18. Park MI, Hwang JH, Cha KJ, et al. Computerized analysis of fetal heart rate parameters by gestational age. Int J Gynaecol Obstet 2001; 74(2):157–164. [II-2]
19. Manning FA. The fetal heart rate. In: Fetal Medicine Principals and Practice. Norwalk, CT: Appleton & Lange, 1995:13–111. [Review]
20. Visser GH, Sadovsky G, Nicolaides KH. Antepartum heart rate patterns in small-for-gestational-age third-trimester fetuses: correlations with blood gas values obtained at cordocentesis. Am J Obstet Gynecol 1990; 162(3):698–702. [II-2; Case control study of fetal heart rate patterns correlated with cordocentesis-derived blood gas values]
21. Lavin JP Jr., Miodovnik M, Barden TP. Relationship of nonstress test reactivity and gestational age. Obstet Gynecol 1984; 63: 338–344. [II-3]
22. Nathan EB, Haberman S, Burgess T, et al. The relationship of maternal position to the results of brief nonstress tests: a randomized trial. Am J Obstet Gynecol 2000; 182:1070–1072. [RCT, $n = 108$]
23. Alus M, Okumus H, Mete S, et al. The effects of different maternal positions on non-stress test: an experimental study. J Clin Nurs 2007; 16(3):562–568. [II-3]
24. Manning FA, Lange IR, Morrison I, et al. Fetal biophysical profile score and the nonstress test: a comparative trial. Obstet Gynecol 1984; 326–331. [RCT]
25. Keane MW, Horger EO III, Vice L. Comparative study of stressed and nonstressed antepartum fetal heart rate testing. Obstet Gynecol 1981; 57(3):320–324. [II-1; Sequential testing used each high-risk fetus ($n = 566$) as its own control. Only 24.8% of nonreactive NST had positive CST]
26. Grivell RM, Alfirevic Z, Gyte GM, et al. Antenatal cardiotocography for fetal assessment. Cochrane Database Syst Rev 2010; 20 (1):CD007863. [Meta-analysis; 6 RCTs, $n = 2105$]
27. Morrison I, Menticoglou S, Manning FA, et al. Comparison of antepartum results to perinatal outcome. J Matern Fetal Med 1994; 3:75–83. [II-2; All FGR fetuses underwent all tests: NST, BPS, umbilical artery Doppler and OCT. The best prediction of poor outcome used all tests. NST alone predicted only 32% of compromised fetuses]
28. Visser GH, Dawes GS, Redman CW. Numerical analysis of the normal human antenatal fetal heart rate. Br J Obstet Gynaecol 1981; 88(8):792–802. [III; Original development of the system 8000, with 196 fetal heart records]
29. Bracero LA, Morgan S, Byrne DW. Comparison of visual and computerized interpretation of nonstress test results in a randomized controlled trial. Am J Obstet Gynecol 1999; 181 (5 pt 1):1254–1258. [RCT, $n = 410$; computerized evaluation of fetal heart rate testing is superior to standard visual interpretation]
30. Roemer VM, Walden R. Sensitivity, specificity, receiver-operating characteristic (ROC) curves and likelihood ratios for electronic foetal heart rate monitoring using new evaluation techniques. Z Geburtshilfe Neonatal 2010; 214(3):108–118. [II-2]
31. Costa A, Santos C, Ayres-de-Campos D, et al. Access to computerized analysis of intrapartum cardiotocographs improves clinicians' prediction of newborn umbilical artery blood pH. Br J Ostet Gynecol 2010; 117(10):1288–1293. [II-2]
32. Ross MG, Devoe LD, Rosen KG. ST-segment analysis of the fetal electrocadiogram improves fetal heart rate tracing interpretation and clinical decision making. J Matern Fetal Neonatal Med 2004; 15(3):181–185. [II-3]
33. Westerhuis ME, Visser GH, Moons KG, et al. Cardiotocography plus ST analysis of fetal electocardiogram compared with cardiotocography only for intrapartum monitoring: a randomized controlled trial. Obstet Gynecol 2010; 115(6):1173–1180. [RCT]
34. Turan S, Turan OM, Berg C, et al. Computerized fetal heart rate analysis, Doppler ultrasound and biophysical profile score in

the prediction of acid-base status of growth-restricted fetuses. Ultrasound Obstet Gynecol 2007; 30(5):750–756. [II-2]

35. Manning FA, Platt LD, Sipos L. Antepartum fetal evaluation: development of a fetal biophysical profile. Am J Obstet Gynecol 1980; 136(6):787–795. [II-1; Blinded study of first clinical BPS application, $n = 216$]

36. Manning FA, Morrison I, Lange IR, et al. Fetal assessment based on fetal biophysical profile scoring: experience in 12,620 referred high-risk pregnancies. I. Perinatal mortality by frequency and etiology. Am J Obstet Gynecol 1985; 151(3):343–350. [III-3; Combined variables provided best indication of perinatal mortality]

37. Manning FA, Morrison I, Harman CR, et al. The abnormal fetal biophysical profile score. V. Predictive accuracy according to score composition. Am J Obstet Gynecol 1990; 162(4):918–924. [III-3; Different adverse outcomes are predicted better by different combinations of variables. This study included only fetuses with abnormal scores 131—6/10, 258—4/10, 113—2/10]

38. Bocking AD, Harding R. Effects of reduced uterine blood flow in electrocortical activity, breathing and skeletal muscle activity in fetal sheep. Am J Obstet Gynecol 1986; 154(3):655–662. [II-1; Controlled study of fetal sheep model showed increased sensitivity to hypoxia in abolishing FBM as gestation progresses]

39. Ribbert LS, Nicolaides KH, Visser GH. Prediction of fetal acidaemia in intrauterine growth retardation: comparison of quantified fetal activity with biophysical profile score. Br J Obstet Gynecol 1993; 100(7):653–656. [II-2; Comparative trial of multi-variable testing methods]

40. Magann EF, Doherty D, Field K, et al. Biophysical profile with amniotic fluid volume assessments. Obstet Gynecol 2004; 104 (1):5–10. [RCT demonstrates lower false-positive cases, fewer iatrogenic interventions, more accurate depiction of fetal status with single pocket method compared to AFI]

41. Naghan AF, Abdelmoula YA. Amniotic fluid index versus single deepest vertical pocket: a meta-analysis of randomized controlled trials. Int J Gynaecol Obstet 2009; 104(3):184–188. [Meta-analysis]

42. Manning FA, Morrison I, Lange IR, et al. Fetal biophysical profile scoring: selective use of the nonstress test. Am J Obstet Gynecol 1987; 156(3):709–712. [II-3]

43. Elliott C, Warrick PA, Graham E, et al. Graded classification of fetal heart rate tracings: association with neonatal metabolic acidosis and neurologic morbidity. Am J Obstet Gynecol 2010; 202(3):258.e1–258.e8. [II-3]

44. Chamberlain PF. Later fetal death—has ultrasound a role to play in its prevention? Irish J Med Science 1991; 160:251–254. [II-3; Application of biophysical profile score in an Irish healthcare region dropped PNM by more than 60%. Historical/concurrent nonrandomized controls]

45. Baskett TG, Allen AC, Gray JH, et al. Fetal biophysical profile and perinatal death. Obstet Gynecol 1987; 70:357–360. [II-2; Concurrent controls had PNM more than double those managed by BPS]

46. Miller DA, Rabello YA, Paul RH. The modified biophysical profile: antepartum testing in the 1990s. Am J Obstet Gynecol 1996; 174:812–817. [II-2; Large comparative trial of biophysical methodology demonstrated significant difference in outcome of cases managed or not managed by BPS]

47. Platt LD, Walla CA, Paul RH, et al. A prospective trial of the fetal biophysical profile versus the nonstress tests in the management of high-risk pregnancies. Am J Obstet Gynecol 1985; 153(6):624–633. [RCT]

48. Vintzileos AM, Campbell WA, Rodis JF, et al. The relationship between fetal biophysical assessment, umbilical artery velocimetry and fetal acidosis. Obstet Gynecol 1991; 77:622–626. [II-3; Clinical study showed BPS was superior and Doppler added nothing, in detection of fetal acidosis, $n = 62$]

49. Soothill PW, Ajayi RA, Campbell S, et al. Prediction of morbidity in small and normally grown fetuses by fetal heart rate variability, biophysical profile score and umbilical artery Doppler studies. Br J Obstet Gynaecol 1993; 100:742–745. [II-3; Prospective longitudinal study of 191 women studied with all three

methods. Doppler discriminated small "sick" fetuses from small normal fetuses, while the other tests did not]

50. Shalev E, Zalel Y, Weiner E. A comparison of the nonstress test, oxytocin challenge test, Doppler velocimetry and biophysical profile in predicting umbilical vein pH in growth-retarded fetuses. Int J Gynaecol Obstet 1993; 43:15–19. [II-3; Clinical series of 23 IUGR fetuses studied by all methods. NST, OCT, and BPS all had positive predictive values of 57%, while Doppler was only 14%]

51. Yoon BH, Romero R, Roh CR, et al. Relationship between the fetal biophysical profile score, umbilical artery Doppler velocimetry and fetal blood acid-base status determined by cordocentesis. Am J Obstet Gynecol 1993; 169:1586–1594. [II-2; Interventional cohort study. Doppler and BPS both had statistically significant association with acidemia and hypercarbia at cordocentesis, but Doppler scored higher in logistic regression, $n = 24$]

52. Bardakci M, Balci O, Acar A, et al. Comparison of modified biophysical profile and Doppler ultrasound in predicting the perinatal outcome at or over 36 weeks of gestation. Gynecol Obstet Invest 2010; 69(4):245–250. [II]

53. Dayal AK, Manning FA, Berck DJ, et al. Fetal death after normal biophysical profile score: an eighteen-year experience. Am J Obstet Gynecol 1999; 181(5 pt 1):1231–1236. [II-2, $n = 87,000$]

54. Manning FA, Snijders R, Harman CR, et al. Fetal biophysical profile score. VI. Correlation with antepartum umbilical venous fetal pH. Am J Obstet Gynecol 1993; 169(4):755–763. [II-2; Multicenter clinical trial demonstrates close relationship of multi-variable testing to fetal pH determined by antenatal cordocentesis, $n = 493$]

55. Manning FA, Harman CR, Morrison I, et al. Fetal assessment based on fetal biophysical profile scoring. III. Positive predictive accuracy of the very abnormal test (biophysical profile score = 0). Am J Obstet Gynecol 1990; 162(2):398–402. [II-2; A score of 0/10 is rare (9.2/10,000 tests), but has 100% positive predictive value for death or severe permanent handicap, justifying immediate delivery]

56. Nageotte MP, Towers CV, Asrat T, et al. Perinatal outcome with the modified biophysical profile. Am J Obstet Gynecol 1994; 170(6):1672–1676. [RCT; clinical trial valuating BPS (NST plus AFI) with randomized back-up testing (full BPS or CST) for abnormal values. MBPS discrimination well between adverse outcome (RR 2.0) and IUGR (RR 2.2) and those without these outcomes. CST was without benefit and led to iatrogenic morbidity compared to BPS]

57. Phattanachindakun B, Boonyagulsrirung T, Chanprapaph P. The correlation in antepartum fetal test between full fetal biophysical profile (FBP) and rapid biophysical profile (rBPP). J Med Assoc 2010; 93(7):759–764. [II-2]

58. Papadopoulos VG, Decavalas GO, Kondakis XG, et al. Vibroacoustic stimulation in abnormal biophysical profile: verification of facilitation of fetal well-being. Early Hum Dev 2007; 83 (3):191–197. [II-3]

59. Ott WJ, Mora G, Arias F, et al. Comparison of the modified biophysical profile to a "new" biophysical profile incorporating the middle cerebral artery to umbilical artery velocity flow systolic/diastolic ratio. Am J Obstet Gynecol 1998; 178(6):1346–1353. [RCT; the addition of Doppler studies enhances cesarean section rate in IUGR, but makes no other difference in outcome, compared to BPS alone]

60. Arabin B, Snyjders R, Mohnhaupt A, et al. Evaluation of the fetal assessment score in pregnancies at risk for intrauterine hypoxia. Am J Obstet Gynecol 1993; 169(3):549–554. [II-3; Fetal Apgar score including cerebral and placental Doppler was compared with standard BPS in 213 at-risk fetuses. Both tests correlated well with adverse outcome, but the addition of Doppler was a significant advantage in IUGR cases]

61. Harman CR, Baschat AA. Arterial and venous Dopplers in IUGR. Clin Obstet Gynecol 2003; 46(4):931–946. [Review]

62. Baschat AA, Gembruch R, Reiss I, et al. Relationship between arterial and venous Doppler and perinatal outcome in fetal

growth restriction. Ultrasound Obstet Gynecol 2000; 16:407–413. [II-3; Time sequence of Doppler in IUGR]

63. Bellotti M, Pennati G, De Gasperi C, et al. Simultaneous measurements of umbilical venous, fetal hepatic and ductus venosus blood flow in growth-restricted human fetuses. Am J Obstet Gynecol 2004; 190(5):1347–1358. [II-2; Case-control study depicting the progression of ductal opening and increased flow as condition deteriorated in 56 IUGR fetuses]

64. Harman CR, Baschat AA. Comprehensive assessment of fetal wellbeing: which Doppler tests should be performed? Curr Opin Obstet Gynecol 2003; 15(2):147–157. [Review; integration of arterial and venous vessel Dopplers]

65. Maulik D, Mundy D, Heitmann E, et al. Evidence-based approach to umbilical artery Doppler fetal surveillance in high-risk pregnancies: an update. Clin Obstet Gynecol 2010; 53 (4):869–878. [III]

66. Baschat AA, Weiner CP. Umbilical artery Doppler screening for the small for gestational age fetus in need of antenatal surveillance. Am J Obstet Gynecol 2000; 182:154–158. [II-2; Case-control trial. Umbilical artery Doppler differentiates small fetuses who do not need intensive surveillance, from those with serious IUGR]

67. Alfirevic Z, Neilson JP. Doppler ultrasonography in high-risk pregnancies: systemic review with meta-analysis. Am J Obstet Gynecol 1995; 172(5):1379–1387. [Meta-analysis; umbilical artery Doppler application reduces perinatal mortality and critical neonatal impacts in IUGR and pre-eclampsia]

68. Divon MY. Randomized control trials of umbilical artery Doppler velocimetry: how many are too many? Ultrasound Obstet Gynecol 1995; 6:377–379. [Review]

69. Alfirevic Z, Stampalija T, Gyte GM. Fetal and umbilical Doppler ultrasound in high-risk pregnancies. Cochrane Database Syst Rev 2010; 20(1):CD007529. [Meta-analysis; 18 RCTs, n ≥ 10,000]

70. Goffinet F, Paril-Llado J, Nisand I, et al. Umbilical artery Doppler velocimetry in unselected and low risk pregnancies: a review of randomized controlled trials. Br J Obstet Gynaecol 1997; 104:425–430. [Review]

71. Divon MY, Girz BA, Lieblich R, et al. Clinical management of the fetus with markedly diminished umbilical artery end-diastolic flow. Am J Obstet Gynecol 1989; 161(6 pt 1):1523–1527. [II-2; Case-control study of 51 fetuses with severe elevation of umbilical artery resistance. Immediate delivery may not be necessary. Combined surveillance can safely prolong the pregnancy]

72. Alfirevic Z, Stampalija T, Gyte GM. Fetal and umbilical Doppler ultrasound in normal pregnancy. Cochrane Database Syste Rev 2010; 4(8):CD001450. [Meta-analysis; 5 RCTs, n = 14,185]

73. Stampalija T, Gyte GM, Alfirevic Z. Utero-placental Doppler ultrasound for improving pregnancy outcome. Cochrane Database Syst Rev 2010; 8(9):CD008363. [Meta-analysis; 2 RCTs, n = 4993]

74. Baschat AA, Gembruch U, Reiss I, et al. Relationship between arterial and venous Doppler and perinatal outcome in fetal growth restriction. Ultrasound Obstet Gynecol 2000; 16(5):407–413. [II-2; Multicenter cohort study using multivessel Doppler to evaluate severe IUGR. Abnormal venous patterns denoted the worst outcomes, while prematurity retains a critical role]

75. Baschat AA, Gembruch U, Weiner CP, et al. Qualitative venous Doppler waveform analysis improves prediction of critical perinatal outcomes in premature growth-restricted fetuses. Ultrasound Obstet Gynecol 2003; 22(3):240–245. [II-2; Cohort study demonstrates combined arterial and venous Doppler maximized prediction of critical outcomes, n = 224]

76. Baschat AA, Cosmi E, Bilardo CM, et al. Predictors of neonatal outcome in early-onset placental dysfunction. Obstet Gynecol 2007; 109(2 pt 1):253–261. [II-2]

77. Turan OM, Turan S, Berg C, et al. The duration of persistent abnormal ductus venosus flow and its impact on perinatal outcome in fetal growth restriction. Ultrasound Obstet Gynecol 2011; 38:295–302. [II-2 Multicenter Study of FGR. Secondary analysis of 175 FGR fetuses with DV abnormality demonstrates that the duration of a-wave reversal is the factor predictive of stillbirth.]

78. Baschat AA, Harman CR. Discordance of arterial and venous flow velocity waveforms in severe placenta-based fetal growth restriction. Ultrasound Obstet Gynecol 2011; 37(3):369–370. [II-3]

79. Baschat AA, Galan HL, Bhide A, et al. Doppler and biophysical assessment in growth restricted fetuses: distribution of test results. Ultrasound Obstet Gynecol 2006; 27(1):41–47. [II-1; Multicenter study of combined Doppler and biophysical profile in IUGR suggests both should be used to maximize gestational age, n = 38]

80. Tyrrel SN, Lilford RJ, MacDonald HN, et al. Randomized comparison of routine vs. highly selective use of Doppler ultrasound and biophysical profile scoring to investigate high risk pregnancies. Br J Obstet Gynaecol 1990; 97(10):909–916. [RCT demonstrating combined Doppler and BPS reduced neonatal morbidity by directing intervention, but did not increase iatrogenic prematurity, n = 500]

81. Habek D, Hodek B, Herman R, et al. Fetal biophysical profile and cerebro-umbilical ratio in assessment of perinatal outcome in growth-restricted fetuses. Fetal Diagn Ther 2003; 18(1):12–16. [II-2; Clinical trial demonstrated the complimentary positive predictive values of biophysical profile and Doppler, n = 87 FGR fetuses]

82. Lees C. Protocol 02PRT/34 trial of umbilical and fetal flow in Europe (TRUFFLE): a multicentre randomized study. Available at: http://www.thelancet.com/protocol-reviews/02PRT-34. [III]

83. Baschat AA, Viscardi RM, Hussey-Gardner B, et al. Infant neurodevelopment following fetal growth restriction: relationship with antepartum surveillance parameters. Ultrasound Obstet Gynecol 2009; 33(1):44–50. [II-3]

84. Williams KP, Farwuharson DF, Bebbington M, et al. Screening for fetal well-being in a high-risk pregnant population comparing the nonstress test with umbilical artery Doppler velocimetry: a randomized controlled clinical trial. Am J Obstet Gynecol 2003; 188(5):1366–1371. [RCT; Randomized "high-risk" patients, beyond 32 weeks, to umbilical artery Doppler or nonstress testing as primary monitoring, amniotic fluid volume as secondary test]

85. Maulik D, Lysikiewicz A, Sicuranaza G. Umbilical arterial Doppler sonography for fetal surveillance in pregnancies complicated by pregestational diabetes mellitus. J Matern Fetal Neonatal Med 2002; 12(6):417–422. [Review]

86. Harman CR, Menticoglou SM. Fetal surveillance in diabetic pregnancy. Curr Opin Obstet Gynecol 1997; 9(2):83–90. [Review]

87. Graves CR. Antepartum fetal surveillance and timing of delivery in the pregnancy complicated by diabetes mellitus. Clin Obstet Gynecol 2007; 50(4):1007–1013. [II-2]

88. Zisser HC, Biersmith MA, Jovanovic LB, et al. Fetal risk assessment in pregnancies complicated by diabetes mellitus. J Diabetes Sci Technol 2010; 4(6):1368–1373. [II-3]

89. Davies GA, Maxwell C, McLeod L, et al. Obesity in pregnancy. J Obstet Gynaecol Can 2010; 32(2):165–173. [II-3]

90. Ehrenberg HM, Mercer BM, Catalano PM. The influence of obesity and diabetes on the prevalence of macrosomia. Am J Obstet Gynecol 2004; 191(3):964–968. [II-2]

91. Mandruzzato G, Alfirevic Z, Chervenak F, et al. Guidelines for the management of postterm pregnancy. J Perinat Med 2010; 38 (2):111–119. [III]

92. Heimstad R, Skogvoll E, Mattsson LA, et al. Induction of labor or serial antenatal fetal monitoring in postterm pregnancy: a randomized controlled trial. Obstet Gynecol 2007; 109(3):609–617. [RCT]

93. Weiner Z, Farmakides G, Schulman H, et al. Computerized analysis of fetal heart rate variation in post-term pregnancy: prediction of intrapartum fetal distress and fetal alkalosis. Am J Obstet Gynecol 1994; 171(4):1132–1138. [II-2; Cohort study evaluating multiple methods of assessing post-term pregnancy. CTG > BPS, Doppler did not help with management]

94. Arabin B, Becker R, Mohnhaupt A, et al. Prediction of fetal distress and poor outcome in prolonged pregnancy using Doppler ultrasound and fetal heart rate monitoring combined with stress tests (II). Fetal Diagn Ther 1994; 9(1):1–6. [II-2; CTG was

the only reliable prediction of acidemia in post-term pregnancy. Doppler, CST, and OCT were all irrelevant to predicting acidemia, while none were effective in predicting low Apgar scores]

95. Clinical Practice Obsetrics Committee; Maternal Fetal Medicine Committee, Delaney M, Roggensack A, Leduc DC, et al. Guidelines for the management of pregnancy at 41+0 to 42+0 weeks. J Obstet Gynaecol Can 2008; 30(9):800–823. [III]

96. Hershkovitz R, Kingdom JC, Geary M, et al. Fetal cerebral blood flow redistribution in late pregnancy: identification of compromise in small fetuses with normal umbilical artery Doppler. Ultrasound Obstet Gynecol 2000; 15(3):209–212. [II-3; MCA abnormality indicated an increased likelihood of perinatal complications in small fetuses with normal umbilical artery Doppler. However, indicators for delivery were multiple and unregulated. Physicians were not blinded to results (although none would know what the abnormal MCA meant), and cases were not controlled]

97. Baschat AA. Neurodevelopment following fetal growth restriction and its relationship with antepartum parameters of placental dysfunction. Ultrasound Obstet Gynecol 2011; 37(5):501–514. [II-3]

98. Boers KE, Vijgen SM, Bijlenga D, et al. DIGITAT study group. Induction versus expectant monitoring for intrauterine growth restriction at term: randomized equivalence trial (DIGITAT). Br Med J 2010; 341:c7087. [RCT]

99. Vintzileos AM, Bors-Koefoed R, Pelegano JF, et al. The use of fetal biophysical profile improves pregnancy outcome in premature rupture of the membranes. Am J Obstet Gynecol 1987; 157(2):236–240. [II-2]

100. Del Valle GO, Joffe GM, Izquierdo LA, et al. The biophysical profile and the nonstress test: poor predictors of chorioamnionitis and fetal infection in prolonged preterm premature rupture of membranes. Obstet Gynecol 1992; 80(1):106–110. [II-2]

101. Lewis DF, Adair CD, Weeks JW, et al. A randomized clinical trial of daily nonstress testing versus biophysical profile in the management of preterm premature rupture of membranes. Am J Obstet Gynecol 1999; 181(6):1495–1499. [RCT of two schemes of monitoring patients after PPROM. Both NST and BPS had good specificity, but detected less than half the babies who developed infectious complications]

102. Mari G. Middle cerebral artery peak systemic velocity: is it the standard of care for the diagnosis of fetal anemia? J Ultrasound Med 2005; 24(5):697–702. [Review]

103. Divakaran TG, Waugh J, Clark TJ, et al. Noninvasive techniques to detect fetal anemia due to red blood cell alloimmunization: a systemic review. Obstet Gynecol 2001; 98(3):509–517. [Meta-analysis suggests MCA Doppler lacks precision and the studies are incomplete]

104. Illanes S, Soothill P. Management of red cell alloimmunisation in pregnancy: the non-invasive monitoring of the disease. Prenat Diagn 2010; 30(7):668–673. [Review]

105. Nageotte MP, Towers CV, Asrat T, et al. The value of a negative antepartum test: contraction stress test and modified biophysical profile. Obstet Gynecol 1994; 84(2):231–234. [II-1; Controlled study, not randomized. New surveillance method, modified BPS was compared in a high risk population to CST. The authors agreed that CST was no longer first line]

106. Gagnon R, Patrick J, Foreman J, et al. Stimulation of human fetuses with sound and vibration. Am J Obstet Gynecol 1986; 155 (4):484–451. [II-3; Development of VAS]

107. Tan KH, Smyth R. Fetal vibroacoustic stimulation for facilitation of tests of fetal wellbeing. Cochrane Database Syst Rev 2010, 1. [Meta-analysis; 9 RCTs, $n = 4838$]

108. Kamel HS, Makhlouf AM, Youssef AA. Simplified biophysical profile: an antepartum fetal screening test. Gynecol Obstet Invest 1999; 47(4):223–228. [II-2; Although vibroacoustic stimulation shortened the testing time for normal results, 67% of the abnormal results were false-alarms]

109. Serafini P, Lindsay MP, Nagey DA, et al. Antepartum fetal heart rate response to sound stimulation: the acoustic stimulation test. Am J Obstet Gynecol 1984; 148(1):41–44. [II-2; Comparative study showed testing efficiency of VAS, but included 55% false-negative results for prediction of fetal distress]

110. Arabin B, Becker R, Mohnhaupt A, et al. Prediction of fetal distress and poor outcome in intrauterine-growth retardation—a comparison of fetal heart rate monitoring combined with stress tests and Doppler ultrasound. Fetal Diagn Ther 1993; 8(4):234–240. [II-2; IUGR fetuses ($n = 103$) were studied with NST/CST, VAS, and Doppler. The passive tests—Doppler and NST—were better predictors of adverse outcome. The authors recommended abolishing the stress test]

111. Caridi BJ, Bolnick JM, Fletcher BG, et al. Effect of halogen light stimulation on nonstress testing. Am J Obstet Gynecol 2004; 190 (5):1470–1472. [RCT fetal light perception shortens NST time]

112. Tan KH, Sabapathy A. Maternal glucose administration for facilitating tests of fetal wellbeing. Cochrane Database Syst Rev 2005; 4. [Meta-analysis; 2 RCTs, $n = 708$]

113. Tan KH, Sabapathy A. Fetal manipulation for facilitating tests of fetal wellbeing. Cochrane Database Syst Rev 2005; 4. [Meta-analysis; 3 RCTs, $n = 1100$]

114. Grant A, Chalmers I. Randomized trial of fetal movement counting. Lancet 1982; 2(8296):501. [RCT, $n = 68,000$]

115. Mangesi L, Hofmeyr GJ. Fetal movement counting for assessment of fetal wellbeing. Cochrane Database Syst Rev 2007; (1): CD004909. [Meta-analysis; 4 RCTs, $n = 71,370$]

116. Olesen AG, AVare JA. Decreased fetal movements: background, assessment, and clinical management. Acta Obstet Gynecol Scand 2004; 83(9):818–826. [Review]

117. American Congress of Obstetricians and Gynecologists. Practice Bulletin #9. Antepartum fetal surveillance. October 1999. [Review]

118. Mohide P, Grant A. Evaluating diagnosis and screening in pregnancy and childbirth. In: Chalmers I, Enkin M, Keierse MJNC, eds. Effective Care in Pregnancy and Childbirth. Vol. 1. Oxford: Oxford University Press, 66–80. [Review]

119. Nabhan AF, Faris MA. High feedback versus low feedback of prenatal ultrasound for reducing maternal anxiety and improving maternal health behavior in pregnancy. Cochrane Database Syst Rev 2010; (4):CD007208. [Meta-analysis]

120. Manning FA. Antepartum fetal testing: a critical appraisal. Curr Opin Obstet Gynecol 2009; 21(4):348–352. [III]

121. Freeman RK. Antepartum testing in patients with hypertensive disorders in pregnancy. Semin Perinatol 2008; 32(4):271–273. [II-3]

122. Dickens BM, Cook RJ. The legal effects of fetal monitoring guidelines. Int J Gynaecol Obstet 2010; 108(2):170–173. [III]

123. Vintzileos A, Ananth CV, Smulian JC, et al. The impact of prenatal care on postnatal deaths in the presence and absence of antenatal high-risk conditions. Am J Obstet Gynecol 2002; 187(5):1258–1262. [II-2; Population-based study identified significantly increased risks of post-term, pre-eclamptic, IUGR, and infectious complications in women with inadequate prenatal care]

124. Scholl TO, Hediger MO, Belsky DH. Prenatal care and maternal health during adolescent pregnancy: a review and meta-analysis. J Adolesc Health 1994; 15(6):444–456. [Meta-analysis]

125. Knight M, Plugge E. The outcomes of pregnancy among imprisoned women: a systematic review. Br J Obstet Gynecol 2005; 112 (11):1467–1474. [Meta-analysis, review]

126. Canella BL. Maternal-fetal attachment: an integrative review. J Adv Nurs 2005; 59(1):60–68. [Meta-analysis]

127. Doswell T, Carroli G, Duley L, et al. Alternative versus standard packages of antenatal care for low-risk pregnancy. Cochrane Database Syst Rev 2010; (10):CD000934.

128. Peck MG, Sappenfield WM, Skala J. Perinatal periods of risk: a community approach for using data to improve women and infants' health. Matern Child Health J 2010; 14(6):864–874. [II-3]

129. Haws RA, Yakoob MY, Soomro T, et al. Reducing stillbirths: screening and monitoring during pregnancy and labour. BMC Pregnancy Childbirth 2009; 9(suppl 1):S5. [III]

56

Sonographic assessment of amniotic fluid: oligohydramnios and polyhydramnios

Everett F. Magann and Suneet P. Chauhan

AMNIOTIC FLUID ASSESSMENT IN SINGLETON PREGNANCIES
Key Points

- Ultrasound estimates of amniotic fluid volume (AFV) correlate poorly with dye-determined or directly measured oligohydramnios and polyhydramnios.
- **The single deepest pocket (SDP) is the best ultrasound technique to estimate AFV** in both singleton and twin gestations, since the amniotic fluid index (AFI) overdiagnoses oligohydramnios.
- **AFI should be abandoned, and SDP should be used instead in most situations for clinical decisions, because AFI use leads to unnecessary inductions, operative deliveries, without concomitant neonatal benefit.**

Background

- Urine production: urethra patent at 8 to 9 weeks; 18 weeks: about 50 to 100 cc/day; term: 800 cc/day, or 5 cc/kg/hr. The primary component of amniotic fluid (AF) in the second half of pregnancy is fetal urine.
- AF swallowing: half of AF/day (about 0.5 L/day at term).
- Lungs also produce and absorb AF. Other systems involved include skin, saliva/nasal, membranes/placenta/cord.
- The fetus with in utero placental insufficiency will shunt blood flow to the brain, heart, and adrenal glands at the expense of the rest of the organ systems including the kidneys. Inadequate renal perfusion will result in decreased urinary output and oligohydramnios.

Indications
AFV can help in the assessment of the following:
In the second trimester,

- evidence of **fetal anomalies** (e.g., urinary obstruction or dysfunction),
- severe **FGR** (associated with fetal aneuploidy),
- assist in the confirmation of preterm premature rupture of the fetal membranes (**PPROM**).

In the late second and third trimester of pregnancy, as above, plus

- used along with the nonstress test (NST) or with the other components of the biophysical profile (BPP) in the **assessment of fetal well-being** in pregnancies at-risk for an adverse outcome.

Techniques
AFV can be precisely measured antepartum by a dye-dilution technique (the dye marker is placed into the uterine cavity by amniocentesis), and directly at the time of cesarean delivery.

These measurement techniques are invasive, time consuming, require laboratory support, and if measured at cesarean can only be done at the time of delivery. Because of these limitations, the AFV is estimated antepartum by ultrasound.

Following are three ultrasound methods of **estimating AFV** and identifying abnormalities of fluid:

- The subjective assessment evaluates the AFV without measurements and labels the observed volume as low, normal, or high. It is usually done at the time of the second trimester ultrasound, between 16 and 24 weeks (1).
- The **AFI**, divides the abdomen into four quadrants and measures the SDP in each quadrant without fetal small parts or cord and sums the measurements (2). AFI $\leq$ 5.0 is labeled as oligohydramnios, 5.1 to 20 as normal, and >20–25 as hydramnios (3). The AFI can also be evaluated more accurately by gestational age (GA)-specific charts that label AFV as oligohydramnios (<5th percentile), normal (5th–95th percentile), and hydramnios (>95th percentile) (4). AFI normal percentile values from two different U.S. populations are shown in Table 56.1 (4,5).
- The **SDP** technique (aka maximum vertical pocket, MVP) identifies the deepest vertical pocket of fluid that has a horizontal measurement of at least 1 cm and is without cord or fetal small parts (6). SDP $\leq$2 is labeled at oligohydramnios, 2 to 8 as normal, and >8 cm as hydramnios.

Originally, the pocket of fluid was measured if it did not have an aggregate of cord or small parts (3). There is a significantly greater number of low dye-determined AFVs identified using the "**to the cord**" measurement technique rather than "through the cord" and without any difference for normal and high dye-determined volumes (7). Therefore, the to "the cord" measurement is recommended.

Accuracy of Ultrasound to Identify Oligohydramnios
By direct measurements at the time of cesarean delivery or dye-determined fluid volumes, all three of the ultrasound techniques used to estimate AFV (subjective evaluation, AFI, SDP) can identify normal volumes but poorly identify oligohydramnios and hydramnios (8). The cumulative world's literature shows that the association between ultrasound measurements and normal actual volume is good (sensitivity of 70–98%), but in the clinically concerning area of oligohydramnios the association between an ultrasound-estimated AFV and the actual volume is poor (sensitivity of 6–18%) (1,8–16). A comparison of the third and fifth percentiles of the AFI and SDP adjusted for GA and the fixed cutoffs of an AFI of $\leq$ 5 and the SDP of $\leq$ 2, all compared to actual AFVs (17), showed that the percentiles were no better predictors of actual oligohydramnios. Additionally, the normal values and

Table 56.1 Amniotic Fluid Index Percentile Values

Week	5th	50th	95th
16	7.9 (3.6)	12.1 (5.8)	18.5 (9.6)
17	8.3 (4.1)	12.7 (6.3)	19.4 (10.3)
18	8.7 (4.6)	13.3 (6.8)	20.2 (11.1)
19	9.0 (5.1)	13.7 (7.4)	20.7 (12.0)
20	9.3 (5.5)	14.1 (8.0)	21.2 (12.9)
21	9.5 (5.9)	14.3 (8.7)	21.4 (13.9)
22	9.7 (6.3)	14.5 (9.3)	21.6 (14.9)
23	9.8 (6.7)	14.6 (10.0)	21.8 (15.9)
24	9.8 (7.0)	14.7 (10.7)	21.9 (16.9)
25	9.7 (7.3)	14.7(11.4)	22.1 (17.8)
26	9.7 (7.5)	14.7 (12.0)	22.3 (18.7)
27	9.5 (7.6)	14.6 (12.6)	22.6 (19.4)
28	9.4 (7.6)	14.6 (13.0)	22.8 (19.9)
29	9.2 (7.6)	14.5 (13.4)	23.1 (20.4)
30	9.0 (7.5)	14.5 13.6)	23.4 (20.6)
31	8.8 (7.3)	14.4 (13.6)	23.8 (20.6)
32	8.6 (7.1)	14.4 (13.6)	24.2 (20.4)
33	8.3 (6.8)	14.3 (13.3)	24.5 (20.0)
34	8.1 (6.4)	14.2 (12.9)	24.8 (19.4)
35	7.9 (6.0)	14.0 (12.4)	24.9 (18.7)
36	7.7 (5.6)	13.8 (11.8)	24.9 (17.9)
37	7.5 (5.1)	13.5 (11.1)	24.4 (16.9)
38	7.3 (4.7)	13.2 (10.3)	23.9 (15.9)
39	7.2 (4.2)	12.7 (9.4)	22.6 (14.9)
40	7.1 (3.7)	12.3 (8.6)	21.4 (13.9)
41	7.0 (3.3)	11.6 (7.8)	19.4 (12.9)

Source: Adapted from Refs. 4 and 5. Values in parenthesis are from Ref. 5.

percentiles for one specific patient population do not correlate with different patient populations, and, if percentiles are used, then normative values should be established for each patient population (4,5).

Despite the fact that subjective assessment of fluid is as accurate in identifying abnormalities of AFV as SDP or AFI, we recommend measurement of the deepest pocket (SDP) because it is linked with adverse outcome and its use in BPP has been shown to decrease the rate of perinatal mortality and cerebral palsy.

Use of Color Doppler to Estimate AFV

Color Doppler has been suggested to increase the detection of oligohydramnios by identifying pockets of fluid containing the umbilical cord that would not be detected by gray-scale. Both the measurements of the AFI and the SDP are decreased by approximately 20% with the use of color Doppler compared with gray-scale (18,19). In a study comparing color Doppler versus gray-scale to determine if the color Doppler identified more dye-determined oligohydramnios than gray-scale, color Doppler not only did not identify any more dye-determined oligohydramnios but labeled a number of normal pregnancies as having oligohydramnios (19). Because of the overdiagnosis of oligohydramnios and because its use has not been to correlate with peripartum outcomes, **the use of color Doppler cannot be recommended in the ultrasound estimate of AFV**.

Accuracy of the Ultrasound Estimates of AF to Predict Pregnancy Outcomes

Although the subjective estimation of AFV is as accurate as the AFI and SDP in the identification of dye-determined low, normal, and high AFVs (1), nearly all ultrasound evaluation and studies use either the AFI or the SDP technique.

The role of the AFI in classifying a pregnancy as high risk on antenatal testing remains uncertain. An AFI of ≤5 is

associated with an increased risk of nonreassuring fetal heart tracing (NRFHT) in labor, meconium-stained AF, cesarean delivery for NRFHT, and low Apgar scores at one and five minutes (3,20). Some investigators have found no association with a an AFI ≤5 and adverse pregnancy outcomes (21,22). Among diabetic patients, AFI < 5.0 cm is not associated with cesarean delivery for NRFHT (23). In postdate pregnancies and other high-risk pregnancies screened **comparing the SDP with the AFI, the AFI labels more pregnancies as having oligohydramnios (RR 2.39, 95% CI 1.73–3.28), resulting in more labor inductions (RR 1.92; 95% CI 1.50–2.46) and subsequent cesarean deliveries for NRFHT (RR 1.46; 95% CI 1.08–1.96), without a concomitant decrease in the likelihood of admission to neonatal intensive care unit (RR 1.04; 95% CI 0.85, 1.26) or in umbilical arterial pH < 7.10 (RR 1.10; 95% CI 0.74, 1.65)** (24).

Cesarean deliveries for NRFHT and Apgar scores of <7 at five minutes occurs in a significantly greater number of women if the AFI is ≤5 compared to controls (25). Both the Apgar score <7 at five minutes and cesarean delivery for NRFHT are subjective evaluations and can be influenced by a number of factors. The most objective assessment, umbilical arterial pH, has not been linked with an AFI ≤ 5.0 (25).

Do We Estimate AFV with the SDP or the AFI?

Both the AFI as a component of the modified BPP (NST + AFV estimation) and the SDP as part of the BPP (fetal movement, fetal breathing, fetal tone, NST, AFV estimation) are used extensively to monitor at-risk preterm pregnancies. While both fluid estimations have been linked with fetal intolerance of labor, cesarean deliveries for NRFHT, and low Apgar scores, **only the SDP as a component of the BPP has been correlated with the umbilical cord pH** (26). In addition **as a stand-alone test the SDP has been linked with perinatal morbidity and mortality** (27), while the AFI has never been evaluated as a stand-alone test for this outcome. No investigations have evaluated the AFI with the NST in the prediction of cerebral palsy. A low BPP is associated with antenatal asphyxial events, and may be of use in selected pregnancies to prevent poor pregnancy outcomes (28,29).

The AFI has been compared with the SDP as a component of the modified BPP (NST + AFI or SDP), the BPP (fetal movement, fetal tone, fetal breathing movement, NST, and AFI or SDP) in the antepartum evaluation of at-risk pregnancies, and as a fetal admission test. In high-risk pregnancies monitored using the BPP (30), **the AFI and SDP are similar in their predictability of adverse antepartum or intrapartum outcomes; however, the AFI labels twice as many women with low fluid compared to the SDP resulting in more interventions, without any improvement in outcome**. In high-risk pregnancies undergoing *modified* BPP, more women are labeled as having low fluid by the AFI with more interventions without any improvement in outcome compared to the SDP (31). As intrapartum screening tests, neither AFI nor SDP are found to be predictive of adverse intrapartum outcomes (32).

In summary, **both the AFI and the SDP poorly predict oligohydramnios**. The AFI + NST have been linked to perinatal morbidity and mortality, but not to umbilical cord pH at delivery. The AFI as a stand-alone test has not been linked to perinatal morbidity or mortality. The SDP as a component of the BPP has been correlated to perinatal morbidity and mortality, umbilical cord pH at delivery, and cerebral palsy, and as a stand-alone test the SDP has been independently linked with perinatal mortality (33). Directly compared, the AFI and SDP are similar in their prediction of outcomes but the AFI over-calls the diagnosis of oligohydramnios leading to increased interventions and more operative deliveries without any improvement in perinatal outcomes. For these reasons **the SDP appears to be the better ultrasound estimator of AFV to use with the NST or the BPP.**

Management

In pregnancies at-risk for an adverse pregnancy outcome, antenatal surveillance can be undertaken with either the **NST and SDP** technique **or the BPP using the SDP** technique to assess the AFV. If an estimation of the AFV is undertaken on admission to labor and delivery to identify those pregnancies that will have a greater risk of intrapartum complications, then the SDP techniques should also be used.

OLIGOHYDRAMNIOS
Key Points

- **Oligohydramnios** should be defined as **an SDP < 2 cm**. This definition **correlates with abnormal neonatal outcome, with the least false-positive rate.** Using the AFI (e.g., <5th percentile, or <5 cm) is not recommended to define oligohydramnios.
- **Question** the woman **concerning (P)PROM.**
- **Document** by ultrasound **normal fetal kidneys, bladder, and fetal weight.**
- **Suggest hydration** with 2 L of water orally.

At 16 to 24 weeks:

- Consider **amniocentesis.**
- Consider transabdominal amnioinfusion for better diagnostic visualization. The role of amnioinfusion as therapy for pregnancy prolongation and prevention of pulmonary hypoplasia has not been tested in a trial.

At 24 to 40 weeks:

- Consider intervention as for 16 to 24 weeks if severe oligohydramnios and fetal karyotype and anatomy have not been checked before.
- At ≥24 weeks, perform NST and/or BPP to assure fetal well-being. If reassuring, continue AFV/NST weekly/biweekly depending on fetal status.
- **At ≥36 weeks, consider induction/delivery if SDP < 2.0 cm and Bishop ≥ 9.**

At ≥40 weeks:

- Deliver.
- Transcervical amnioinfusion can be discussed and offered to women at or near term with oligohydramnios, but data are limited regarding safety and efficacy.

Diagnosis/Definition

Oligohydramnios should be defined as that low AFV that is linked with an adverse pregnancy outcome. Therefore, oligohydramnios can be defined as an SDP of <2 cm measured vertically.

Epidemiology/Incidence

The true incidence of oligohydramnios appears to be approximately 0.2% in the second trimester and 3% to 5% in the third trimester. The incidence depends on definition, being lower when defined as SDP <2 cm.

Etiology

ROM, renal hypofunction, urinary obstruction, placental insufficiency with/without FGR.

Complications

Fetal anomalies (up to 30% in second trimester, up to 50% if severe). Oligohydramnios, in particular SDP < 2 cm, has been associated with FGR, NRFHT, CD for NRFHT, endometritis, etc., but the true natural history is not well-known since many intervene for oligohydramnios.

Management (Fig. 56.1)

Question woman concerning (P)PROM, and perform clinical exam if (P)PROM suspected.

The ultrasound should document normal **fetal kidneys, bladder, stomach bubble and fetal weight.**

At 16 to 24 weeks: consider amniocentesis, if feasible. Also consider transabdominal amnioinfusion for better diagnostic visualization. The role of amnioinfusion as therapy for pregnancy prolongation and prevention of pulmonary hypoplasia has not been tested in a trial.

At 24 to 40 weeks, consider intervention as for 16 to 24 weeks if severe oligohydramnios and fetal karyotype and anatomy have not been checked before.

At ≥28 to <36 weeks, perform NST and/or BPP to assure fetal well-being. If reassuring, continue SDP/NST weekly/biweekly depending on fetal status.

a. if SDP is ≥2, follow with weekly NST/SDP.
b. if SDP <2, manage individually (suggest at least twice weekly NST/AFIs).
    Consider delivery only if there are substantial signs of fetal compromise such as abnormal BPP, UA Doppler flow, NST, etc.
c. If SDP normalizes in the consecutive ultrasounds, these patients can be followed with routine care.
d. **For any oligohydramnios, strongly encourage maternal hydration with 2-L water and reassess AFV.**

Maternal Hydration

The effects of maternal hydration on the AFV, as estimated by an increase in the AFI or an increase in fetal urine production, have been assessed in four randomized trials (34–37). The meta-analysis (38) of these four trials with 122 women concluded that **hydration (by drinking water or by intravenous route) increases AF, as assessed by pre- and posthydration AFI.** For oral hydration, the women were asked to **drink 2 L of water** before having a repeat ultrasound examination. Maternal hydration in women with and without oligohydramnios was associated with an increase in amniotic volume [mean difference (MD) for women with oligohydramnios 2.01, 95% confidence interval (CI) 1.43 to 2.60; and MD for women with normal AFV 4.50, 95% CI 2.92 to 6.08].

Intravenous hypotonic hydration in women with oligohydramnios was associated with an increase in AFV (MD 1.35, 95% CI 0.61–2.10). Isotonic intravenous hydration had no measurable effect. Most importantly, **no clinically important outcomes have been assessed** in these four trials (38). Thus, while oral hydration seems safe and helpful, additional trials assessing clinical benefits are warranted before hydration is recommended in the setting of oligohydramnios (38).

At ≥36 weeks, consider induction/delivery if Bishop ≥ 9. If SDP <2 cm and Bishop < 9, continue close monitoring if no other abnormal testing or significant fetal/maternal disease; consider delivery otherwise. If SDP ≥ 2 and Bishop < 9, follow with NST/AFI Q 3 days.

At ≥40 weeks, consider induction/delivery if SDP < 2.0 cm.

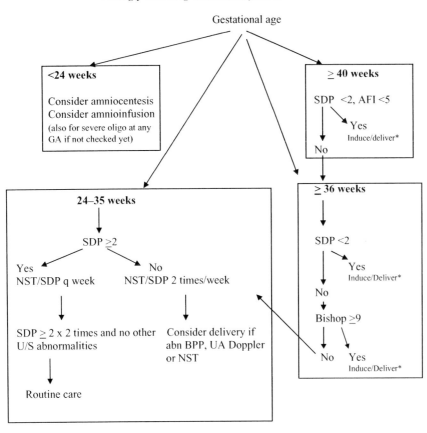

Oligohydramnios
Strongly encourage maternal hydration with 2–L water

Figure 56.1 Management of oligohydramnios. *Abbreviations*: SDP, single deepest pocket; AFI, amniotic fluid index; GA, gestational age; NST, nonstress test; BPP, biophysical profile; OLIGO, oligohydramnios.

*Amnioinfusion for labor at ≥34 weeks: Cesarean delivery for obstetrical indications.

Amnioinfusion

If oligohydramnios (without PROM) is detected just before or in **labor near or at term**:

- **Transabdominal amnioinfusion:** reduces NRFHT (from 42% to 5%) and CD for NRFHT (from 25% to 5%) (39).
- **Transcervical amnioinfusion:** in term women with oligo (usually AFI < 5 cm), amnioinfusion of usually about 500 cc normal saline and more as needed decreases CD for NRFHT by 77%, overall CD by 48%, umbilical artery pH < 7.20 by 60%, NRFHT by 76%, and low Apgar scores < 7 at five minutes by 48%. The rate of endometritis trended to be lower with amnioinfusion (40–42).

Given better results and a lot more data with this latter technique, prophylactic **transcervical amnioinfusion should be offered to women at or near term with oligohydramnios.**

POLYHYDRAMNIOS (AKA HYDRAMNIOS)
Key Points

- Polyhydramnios is defined as an **SDP ≥ 8**, or **AFI ≥ 95th percentile (AFI ≥ 24)** or ≥97.5 percentile (AFI > 25) **for GA** (Table 56.1). AFI > 24 or subjective assessment of increased fluid volume are all labeled as polyhydramnios at any GA. Severe polyhydramnios is a SDP ≥ 15, or AFI of ≥35.1 cm.
- **Major associations are diabetes and fetal malformation, but up to 50% of mild polyhydramnios is of unknown cause (idiopathic).**

- Risk of major anomaly at birth after normal ultrasound is 1% with AFI < 30, 2% with AFI 30 to 34.9, 11% with AFI ≥ 35 cm.
- Polyhydramnios is associated with higher rates of **macrosomia, malpresentation, cord prolapse, abruption, primary cesarean delivery, and uterine atony.**
- **Workup should include** (at least) a **glucose screening test**, antibody screen if not done in last four weeks, RPR, **and accurate fetal anatomy ultrasound.** Parvovirus, toxoplasma, and CMV IgM and IgG can be included. Amniocentesis should be strongly considered if there is severe polyhydramnios, hydramnios with fetal anomaly on ultrasound, polyhydramnios associated with FGR or detected <24 weeks.

Diagnosis/Definition

SDP ≥ 8, or **AFI ≥ 95th percentile (AFI ≥ 24)** or ≥97.5 percentile (AFI > 25) **for GA** (Table 56.1) or subjective assessment of increased AF. Any of these ultrasound measurements or if subjectively the AF is present then the AF would be labeled as polyhydramnios. Mild polyhydramnios AFI ≥ 25 to 30, moderate AFI 30.1 to 35, severe polyhydramnios AFI ≥ 35.1 (43). Severe polyhydramnios can also be defined as SDP ≥15.

Incidence/Epidemiology

1% to 5% of pregnancies depending on definition, but <1% severe polyhydramnios.

Etiology

Increased production (most commonly maternal diabetes) or decreased clearance (obstruction or poor swallowing). Most common causes are: (*i*) maternal diabetes (20–30%), (*ii*) fetal malformations (10–15%), (*iii*) multiple gestations (5%), Rh or other isoimmunization, "Mirror syndrome," others; unknown cause (about 50%, especially for mild polyhydramnios). Severe polyhydramnios is usually pathologic, not idiopathic.

Complications

Fetal anomalies may be present (risk of major anomaly on prenatal ultrasound: 8% with AFI < 30, 12% with AFI 30 to 34.9, 31% with AFI ≥ 35. **Risk of major anomaly at birth after normal ultrasound: 1% with AFI < 30, 2% with AFI 30 to 34.9, 11% with AFI ≥35**. Fetus may have chromosomal abnormality (risk of aneuploidy: ≤1% if normal ultrasound, about 10% if major anomaly present). Detailed ultrasound should detect about 60% to 80% of major anomalies associated with polyhydramnios. Perinatal mortality for normal anatomy fetuses is <5%. For anomalous fetuses is 10% to 80% depending on anomaly (44). Preterm birth (PTB) by preterm labor (PTL) or PPROM is increased especially with severe polyhydramnios. Polyhydramnios is associated with higher rates of **macrosomia, malpresentation, cord prolapse, abruption, primary cesarean delivery and uterine atony**. Idiopathic polyhydramnios is linked with fetal macrosomia, fetal labor intolerance, low five minute Apgar scores, greater risk for newborn intensive care unit admission, and **a two to fivefold increase in perinatal mortality** (45,46).

Workup (Differential Diagnosis)

History: **Diabetes mellitus**. Rh isoimmunization and diabetes insipidus. Family history of myotonic dystrophy or inborn errors of metabolism. Ask regarding maternal discomfort.

Ultrasound: Multiple gestation (in particular TTTS).

CNS/Neuro: Anencephaly, holoprosencephaly, Dandy Walker malformation, lissencephaly, agenesis of corpus callosum, NTD, etc.

Neuromuscular: Arthrogryposis.

Cardiac: Septal defects,[a] truncus arteriosus, aortic coartation, arch interruption, arrhythmias, etc.

Thoracic: CDH, CCAM, sequestration, chylothorax, tracheal atresia.

GI: Cleft lip/palate,[a] TE fistula,[a] esophageal or intestinal atresia, inperforate anus,[a] abdominal wall defects, annular pancreas.

Skeletal: Achondroplasia, thanatophoric dysplasia, campomelic dysplasia, OI, hypophosphatasia, etc.

Other: Cystic hygroma, neck masses, goiter, SCT (47). Rule out hydrops. Perform umbilical and middle cerebral artery (PI and PSV) Doppler.

Laboratory: One hour glucola and antibody screen if not done in last four weeks. Parvovirus IgM and IgG; Toxo IgM and IgG; CMV IgM and IgG; RPR (r/o syphilis).

Amniocentesis: Strongly consider if **severe polyhydramnios, hydramnios with fetal major or minor anomaly on ultrasound, polyhydramnios associated with IUGR, or detected <24 weeks**. Some advocate offering amniocentesis to all women with polyhydramnios given the 0.5% to 1% incidence of aneuploidy. If *amniocentesis* is done:

1. Karyotype (T21, T18, 45X: most common).
2. PCR for parvovirus, CMV, toxoplasmosis, syphilis.

---

[a]Most common anomalies with polyhydramnios.

3. Myotonic dystrophy study if positive family history or ultrasound evidence of hypotonia, for example, clubbed feet or positional abnormalities of the extremities (47).
4. Inborn errors of metabolism: Gaucher, gangliosidoses, mucopolysaccharidoses, etc. (consider especially if positive family history or above workup negative and severe polyhydramnios).

Labor Precautions

For appropriate management to decrease complications from polyhydramnios—associated macrosomia, malpresentation, cord prolapse, abruption, primary cesarean delivery and uterine atony, see appropriate chapters. Consider delaying or avoiding artificial ROM to avoid cord prolapse, or at least "needling" the membranes.

Management

- Appropriate **counseling** regarding complications as above.
- **Workup** as above.
- Manage anomaly/aneuploidy/maternal or fetal disease if detected during workup.
- GA < 24 weeks: consider amniocentesis.
- GA 24 to 40 weeks:
  - AFI < 30 cm: AFI/SDP every two to three weeks.
  - AFIs ≥ 30 cm: AFI/SDP and evaluations to rule out fetal hydrops weekly. Consider weekly NSTs or BPP. Consider amniocentesis.
  - AFI ≥ 40 cm, SDP ≥ 12, and/or maternal symptoms: as per severe polyhydramnios, plus consider the following options:
    - Amnioreduction: goal to normalize AFV; 1.5% complication rate, such as PPROM, chorioamnionitis, abruptio, membrane detachment. Associated with PTL/PPROM, and also abruptio if >2 L taken out at one time.
    - NSAID therapy.
      - Indomethacin: 75 to 200 mg/day (25–50 mg po q6–8h). Mechanism of action: decreases fetal urine production by increasing proximal tubular resorption of water and sodium. Side effects: Oligohydramnios and ductal closure (see chap. 16, *Obstetric Evidence Based Guidelines*). Only treat for 48 hours and <32 weeks to avoid/minimize side effects.
      - Sulindac: 200 mg q12h. Same mechanism of action and side effects as indomethacin.
    - For idiopathic hydramnios consider antenatal testing beginning at diagnosis or 28 weeks.
- GA ≥ 39 weeks: induction/delivery for maternal discomfort in severe polyhydramnios. Cesarean delivery for obstetrical indications only. Induction and delivery for idiopathic polyhydramnios.

AMNIOTIC FLUID ASSESSMENT IN TWIN PREGNANCIES
Background

In twin pregnancies the AFV of each sac is about the same (slightly exceeds) that for normal singleton pregnancies of similar third-trimester GA (48).

Technique

The most consistent method of estimating AFV in twin pregnancies is the **SDP** technique. The dividing membrane is identified and the SDP of AF in each amniotic sac is measured. Since the AFVs of twin pregnancies are similar to single pregnancies, **the same categories of oligohydramnios (SDP < 2), normal (2–8 cm) and hydramnios (>8 cm) can be used.** The summated AFI technique (49,50), which measures sums the four SDPs as have been identified in singleton pregnancies and without regard to membrane placement or fetal position, is inaccurate. When correlated to known AFVs in twin pregnancies, it has low sensitivity for intertwin differences in AFV and cannot identify twin pairs with either oligohydramnios or hydramnios (51). The subjective evaluation of the amount of AF surrounding each fetus, when correlated with dye-determined AFVs in diamniotic twins, has been found to be as accurate as the AFI and SDP in the identification of oligohydramnios (all of the ultrasound techniques poorly identify AFVs.) (52).

Management of Oligohydramnios and/or Hydramnios

In dichorionic, diamniotic twin pregnancies, workup and management of either oligohydramnios or hydramnios is similar to singleton gestations. If SDP > 2 or > 8 is found in a monochorionic gestation, the diagnosis of twin-twin transfusion syndrome should be considered, with workup and management covered in chapter 43.

REFERENCES

1. Magann EF, Perry KG, Chauhan SP, et al. The accuracy of ultrasound evaluation of amniotic fluid volume in singleton pregnancies. The effect of operator experience and ultrasound interpretive technique. J Clin Ultrasound 1997; 25:249–253. [II-2]
2. Phelan JP, Ahn MO, Smith CV. Amniotic fluid index measurements during pregnancy. J Reprod Med 1987; 32:601–604. [II-3]
3. Rutherford SE, Smith CV, Phelan JP, et al. The four quadrant assessment of amniotic fluid volume; an adjunct to antepartum fetal heart rate testing. Obstet Gynecol 1987; 87:353–356. [II-3]
4. Moore TR, Cayle TE. The amniotic fluid index in normal human pregnancy. Am J Obstet Gynecol 1990; 162:1168–1173. [II-2]
5. Magann EF, Sanderson M, Martin JN Jr., et al. The amniotic fluid index, single deepest pocket, and two-diameter pocket in normal human pregnancy. Am J Obstet Gynecol 2000; 182:1581–1588. [II-2]
6. Manning FA, Platt LD, Sipos L. Antepartum fetal evaluation: development of a fetal biophysical profile. Am J Obstet Gynecol 1980; 136:787–795. [II-3]
7. Magann EF, Chauhan SP, Washington W, et al. Ultrasound estimation of amniotic fluid volume using the largest vertical pocket containing umbilical cord: measure to or through the cord? Ultrasound Obstet Gynecol 2002; 20:464–467. [II-2]
8. Magann EF, Nolan TE, Hess LW. Measurement of amniotic fluid volume: accuracy of ultrasonography techniques. Am J Obstet Gynecol 1992; 167:1533. [II-2]
9. Croom CS, Banias BB, Ramos-Santos E. Do semiquantitative amniotic fluid indexes reflect actual volume. Am J Obstet Gynecol 1992; 167:995. [II-2]
10. Dildy GA, Lira N, Moise KJ. Amniotic fluid volume assessment: comparison of ultrasonographic estimates versus direct measurement with a dye-dilution technique in human pregnancy. Am J Obstet Gynecol 1992; 167:986. [II-2]
11. Horsager R, Nathan L, Leveno KJ. Correlation of measured amniotic fluid volume and sonographic predictions of oligohydramnios. Am J Obstet Gynecol 1994; 83:955. [II-3]
12. Sepulveda W, Flack NJ, Fisk NM. Direct volume measurement at midtrimester amnioinfusion in relation to ultrasonographic indexes of amniotic fluid volume. Am J Obstet Gynecol 1994; 170:1160–1163. [II-3]
13. Magann EF, Morton ML, Nolan TE, et al. Comparative efficacy of two sonographic measurements for the detection of aberrations in the amniotic fluid volume and the effect of amniotic fluid volume on pregnancy outcome. Obstet Gynecol 1994; 83:959–962. [II-2]
14. Magann EF, Nevils BD, Chauhan SP, et al. Low amniotic fluid volume is poorly identified in singleton and twin pregnancies using the 2×2 pocket technique of the biophysical profile. South Med J 1999; 92:802–805. [II-2]
15. Chauhan SP, Magann EF, Morrison JC, et al. Ultrasonographic assessment of amniotic fluid volume does not reflect actual volume. Am J Obstet Gynecol 1997; 177:291–297. [II-2]
16. Magann EF, Chauhan SP, Martin JN Jr. Oligohydramnios at term and pregnancy outcome. Fetal Matern Med Rev 2001; 12:209–227. [II-3]
17. Magann EF, Doherty DA, Chauhan SP, et al. How well do the amniotic fluid index and single deepest pocket indices (below the 3rd and the 5th and above the 95th and 97th percentiles) predict oligohydramnios and hydramnios? Am J Obstet Gynecol 2004; 190:164–169. [II-2]
18. Bianco A, Rosen T, Kuczynski E, et al. Measurement of the amniotic fluid index with and without color Doppler. J Perinat Med 1999; 27:245–249. [II-2]
19. Magann EF, Chauhan SP, Barrilleaux S, et al. Ultrasound estimate of amniotic fluid volume: Color Doppler overdiagnosis of oligohydramnios. Obstet Gynecol 2001; 98:71–74. [II-2]
20. Miller DA, Rabello YA, Paul RH. The modified biophysical profile: antepartum testing in the 1990s. Am J Obstet Gynecol 1996; 174:812–817. [II-3]
21. Magann EF, Chauhan SP, Kinsella MJ, et al. Antenatal testing among 1001 high risk women: the role of the ultrasonographic estimate of amniotic fluid volume. Am J Obstet Gynecol 1999; 180:1330–1336. [II-3]
22. Garmel SH, Chelmow D, Sha SJ, et al. Oligohydramnios and the appropriately grown fetus. Am J Perinat 1997; 14:359–363. [II-3]
23. Kjos SL, Leung A, Henry OA, et al. Antepartum surveillance in diabetic pregnancies: predictors of fetal distress in labor. Am J Obstet Gynecol 1995; 173:1532–1539. [II-2]
24. Nabhan AF, Abdelmoula YA. Amniotic fluid index versus single deepest vertical pocket as a screening test for preventing adverse pregnancy outcome. Cochrane Database Syst Rev 2008; (3): CD006593. [Meta-analysis; 5 RCT; $n = 3326$]
25. Chauhan SP, Sanderson M, Hendrix NW, et al. Perinatal outcome and amniotic fluid index in the antepartum and intrapartum periods: a meta-analysis. Am J Obstet Gynecol 1999; 181:1473–1478. [Meta-analysis; 18 studies, $n = 10,551$]
26. Manning FA, Harman CR, Morrison I, et al. Fetal assessment based on fetal biophysical profile scoring IV. An analysis of perinatal morbidity and mortality. Am J Obstet Gynecol 1990; 162:703–709. [II-2]
27. Chamberlain PR, Manning FA, Morrison I, et al. Ultrasound evaluation of amniotic fluid. I The relationship of marginal and decreased amniotic fluid volumes to perinatal outcomes. Am J Obstet Gynecol 1984; 150:245–249. [II-3]
28. Manning FA, Bondaji N, Harman CR, et al. Fetal assessment based on the fetal biophysical profile score: relationship of the last BPS result to subsequent cerebral palsy. J Gynecol Obstet Biol Reprod 1997; 26:720–729. [II-3]
29. Manning FA, Bondaji N, Harman CR, et al. Fetal assessment based on fetal biophysical scoring VIII. The incidence of cerebral palsy in tested and untested perinates. Am J Obstet Gynecol 1998; 178:696–706. [II-2]
30. Magann EF, Doherty DA, Field K, et al. Biophysical profile with amniotic fluid volume assessments. Obstet Gynecol 2004; 104:5–10. [II-3]
31. Chauhan SP, Doherty DA, Magann EF, et al. Amniotic fluid index vs. single deepest pocket technique during modified biophysical profile: a randomized clinical trial. Am J Obstet Gynecol 2004; 191:661–667. [RCT, $n = 1080$]
32. Moses J, Doherty DA, Magann EF, et al. A randomized clinical trial of the intrapartum assessment of amniotic fluid volume: amniotic fluid index versus the single deepest pocket. Am J Obstet Gynecol 2004; 190:1564–1569. [RCT, $n = 1000$]

33. Magann EF, Chauhan SP, Bofill JA, et al. Comparability of the amniotic fluid index and single deepest pocket measurements in clinical practice. Aust N Z J Obstet Gynaecol 2003; 43:75–77. [II-2]

34. Kilpatrick SJ, Safford SL. Maternal hydration increases the amniotic fluid index in women with normal amniotic fluid volume. Obstet Gynecol 1993; 81:49–52. [RCT, $n = 40$]

35. Kilpatrick SJ, Safford SL, Pomeroy T, et al. Maternal hydration increases the amniotic fluid index. Obstet Gynecol 1991; 78:1098–1102. [RCT, $n = 36$]

36. Doi S, Osada H, Seki K, et al. Effect of maternal hydration on oligohydramnios. A comparison of three volume expansion methods. Obstet Gynecol 1998; 92:525–529. [RCT, $n = 84$]

37. Yan-Rosenberg L, Burt B, Bombard AT, et al. A randomized clinical trial comparing the effect of maternal intravenous hydration and placebo on the amniotic fluid index in oligohydramnios. J Matern Fetal Neonatal Med 2007; 20(10):715–718. [RCT]

38. Hofmeyr GJ, Gülmezoglu AM, Novikova N. Maternal hydration for increasing amniotic fluid volume in oligohydramnios and normal amniotic fluid volume. Cochrane Database Syst Rev 2002; (1):CD000134. DOI:10.1002/14651858.CD000134. [Meta-analysis]

39. Vergani P, Ceruti P, Strobelt N, et al. Transabdominal amnioinfusion in oligohydramnios at term before induction of labor with intact membranes: a randomized clinical trial. Am J Obstet Gynecol 1996; 175:465–470. [RCT; $n = 79$]

40. Pitt C, Sanchez-Ramos L, Kaunitz AM, et al. Prophylactic amnioinfusion for intrapartum oligohydramnios: a meta-analysis of randomized controlled trials. Obstet Gynecol 2000; 96:861–866. [Meta-analysis of 14 RCTs; $n = 793/740$]

41. Amin AF, Mohammed MS, Sayed GH, et al. Prophylactic transcervical amnioinfusion in laboring women with oligohydramnios. Int J Gynecol Obstet 2003; 81:183–189. [RCT; $n = 160$; not included in Ref. 41]

42. Hofmeyr GJ, Justus G. Amnioinfusion for potential or suspected umbilical cord compression in labour. (Cochrane Review). Cochrane Database of Systematic Reviews. 8, 2010. [Meta-analysis; 14 RCTs, most with <200 women each—see also chap. 10, *Obstetric Evidence Based Guidelines*]

43. Lazebnik N, Many A. The severity of polyhydramnios, estimated fetal weight, and preterm delivery are independent risk factors for the presence of congenital anomalies. Gynecol Obstet Invest 1999; 48:28–32. [II-2]

44. Dashe JS, McIntire DD, Ramus RM, et al. Hydramnios: anomaly prevalence and sonographic detection. Obstet Gynecol 2002; 100:134–139. [II-3, $n = 672$, largest series of hydramnios]

45. Magann EF, Chauhan SP, Doherty DA, et al. A review of idiopathic hydramnios and pregnancy outcomes. Obstet Gynecol Surv 2007; 62:795–802. [II-2]

46. Magann EF, Doherty DA, Lutgendorf MA, et al. Peripartum outcomes of high risk pregnancies complicated by oligo-and polyhydramnios. A longitudinal prospective study. J Obstet Gynaecol Res 2010; 36:268–277. [II-2]

47. Esplin MS, Hallam S, Farrington PF, et al. Myotonic dystrophy is a significant cause of idiopathic polyhydramnios. Am J Obstet Gynecol 1998; 179:974–977. [II-3]

48. Magann EF, Whitworth NS, Bass JD, et al. Amniotic fluid volume of third-trimester diamniotic twins. Obstet Gynecol 1995; 85:857–860. [II-2]

49. Porter TF, Dildy GA, Blanchard JR, et al. Normal values for amniotic fluid index during uncomplicated twin pregnancy. Obstet Gynecol 1996; 87:699–702. [II-2]

50. Chau AC, Kjos SC, Kovacs BW. Ultrasonographic measurement of amniotic fluid volume in normal diamniotic twin pregnancies. Am J Obstet Gynecol 1996; 174:1003–1007. [II-2]

51. Magann EF, Chauhan SP, Whitworth NS, et al. Accuracy of the summated AFI in evaluating amniotic fluid volume in diamniotic twin pregnancies. Am J Obstet Gynecol 1997; 177:1041–1045. [II-2]

52. Magann EF, Chauhan SP, Whitworth NS, et al. Determination of amniotic fluid volume in twin pregnancies: ultrasonic evaluation versus operator estimation. Am J Obstet Gynecol 2000; 182:1606–1609. [II-3]

57

Fetal lung maturity

Sarah Poggi and Alessandro Ghidini

KEY POINTS

- Fetal lung maturity (FLM) testing is not necessary if delivery is indicated by accepted maternal and/or fetal obstetrical indications. Consideration for FLM testing is sometimes indicated in cases of **high chance for spontaneous preterm birth** from preterm labor, preterm premature rupture of membranes (PPROM), **or iatrogenic preterm delivery,** or the **need to plan delivery** in the presence of **unsure dates** or **obstetric complications affecting lung maturity.**
- The American College of Obstetricians and Gynecologists has recommended that **fetal pulmonary maturity should be confirmed before any planned nonindicated delivery at less than 39 weeks of gestation.**
- The probability for RDS should be calculated as **a function of gestational age** and the specific FLM test.
- **Lamellar body count** or **surfactant/albumin ratio** can be used as **the initial and only test** given their high negative predictive value, ease, and low cost. Lecithin/sphingomyelin **(L/S) ratio** can be used as a confirmatory test, if necessary.
- For diabetic pregnancies, positive phosphatidylglycerol (PG), surfactant/albumin ratio ≥ 70 mg/g, L/S >3, or a combination of these test have a high predictive value for maturity. Some experts, however, use the same threshold values of nondiabetic pregnancies for assessment of FLM in diabetic pregnancies.
- **Even with "mature" fetal lung profile, neonates delivered at less than 39 weeks can demonstrate morbidity associated with prematurity.**

HISTORIC NOTES

The L/S ratio for assessment of FLM was first introduced by Gluck and colleagues in 1971, and this test is still the standard to which others are compared (1).

DEFINITIONS

Surfactant is a complex substance containing phospholipids and apoproteins produced by the type II alveolar cells. It reduces surface tension throughout the lung, contributing to its compliance, leading to alveolar stability, and reducing the likelihood of alveolar collapse. Surfactant is "packaged" in lamellar bodies.

Neonatal respiratory distress syndrome (RDS) occurs when the lungs fail to produce adequate amount of surfactant. RDS is defined in many different ways, but in general involves mechanical ventilation and oxygen requirement at ≥ 24 to 48 hours of life, and radiographic chest findings (air bronchograms and reticulogranular appearance), without any other explanation for the respiratory insufficiency. The natural

(without steroids) incidence of RDS depends on gestational age: about 80% to 90% at 25 to 27 weeks, 55% to 65% at 28 to 30 weeks, 30% to 40% at 31 to 33 weeks, 13% at 34weeks, 6% at 35weeks, 3% at 36weeks, and 1% or less at ≥ 37 weeks. Therefore, **the probability for RDS should be calculated as a function of gestational age**. RDS affects approximately 1% of all live births. Complications of its treatment are associated with an increased risk of serious acute and long-term pulmonary and nonpulmonary morbidities. Although the frequency and severity of RDS are worse for delivery remote from term, the pulmonary system is the last organ systems to mature, and RDS can occur even near term.

INDICATIONS FOR ASSESSMENT OF FETAL PULMONARY MATURITY

There are no absolute indications for assessment of FLM. If an evidence-based, clear indication for delivery is present, the use of amniocentesis to assess FLM would not assist in guiding management. For example, FLM testing is not indicated if delivery is indicated by accepted maternal (e.g., severe preeclampsia after 34 weeks) and/or fetal (e.g., category III fetal heart rate monitoring after viability) indications. Because of the risk for HIV infection, risk of uterine rupture with prior uterine surgery with extensive myomectomy or vertical CD, and hemorrhage with placenta previa and/or accreta, proof of lung maturity before delivery is not necessary in these and other selected indications (see chap. 20, *Obstetric Evidence Based Guidelines*). Tests for FLM are not warranted before 33 weeks, because they are rarely positive this early in gestation. FLM testing in well-dated (e.g., by first-trimester ultrasound) singletons at ≥ 39 weeks or twins at ≥ 37 to 38 weeks is not indicated. As the probability of RDS depends on gestational age, gestational age estimation should be as accurate as possible, preferably based on first-trimester ultrasound (see chap. 4, *Obstetric Evidence Based Guidelines*).

Consideration for FLM testing is sometimes indicated in the following cases:

- High chance for **spontaneous preterm birth** from preterm labor, PPROM, **or iatrogenic preterm delivery**
- **Need to plan delivery in the presence of unsure dates or obstetric complications affecting lung maturity**

The American College of Obstetricians and Gynecologists has recommended that **fetal pulmonary maturity should be confirmed before any planned, nonindicated delivery at less than 39 weeks** (2).

TECHNIQUES FOR OBTAINING AMNIOTIC FLUID
Amniocentesis

Third-trimester amniocentesis performed under ultrasonographic guidance in experienced hands is associated with low rates of failure or of bloody fluid collection, and a <1% risk of complication, such as emergent delivery (3). The risk of complications (e.g., PTL, PROM, abruption, and fetomaternal hemorrhage) associated with amniocentesis for FLM performed under continuous ultrasound guidance has been estimated at about 0.7% (4,5).

Vaginal Pool Collection

The assessment of fetal pulmonary maturity can be obtained from vaginal pool specimens in the presence of premature rupture of membranes. Blood, meconium, and mucous can alter the results. In the absence of these contaminants, vaginally free-flowing collected fluid can be evaluated for determination of L/S ratio, surfactant/albumin ratio, PG, and lamellar body count yielding results similar to those observed with samples obtained with amniocentesis (Table 57.1). As obtaining a specimen via a sterile syringe is not always technically feasible, an alternative collection method using the commonly available "4 × 4" gauze sponge has been validated for both PG and TDx-FLM II analyses (see below). Essentially, the gauze is inserted into the vagina at the posterior fornix and then plunged into a 60-cc syringe to extract the vaginal pool specimen (6).

SPECIFIC TESTS FOR LUNG MATURITY (TABLE 57.1)
Lecithin/Sphingomyelin Ratio

The concentrations of these two substances are approximately equal until mid-third trimester of gestation, when the concentration of pulmonary lecithin (phosphatidylcholine, most common of surfactant compounds) increases significantly while the nonpulmonary sphingomyelin concentration remains unchanged.

Technique
Following amniocentesis, the sample should be kept on ice or refrigerated if transport to a laboratory is required. Thin-layer chromatography after centrifugation to remove the cellular component and organic solvent extraction is used.

Interpretation of Results
An L/S ratio of 2.0 or greater predicts absence of RDS in 98% of neonates. With a ratio of 1.5 to 1.9, approximately 50% of infants will develop RDS. Below 1.5, the risk of subsequent RDS increases to 73%.

Special Considerations
Maternal serum has an L/S ratio ranging from 1.3 to 1.9; thus, blood tinged samples could falsely lower a mature result. The presence of meconium can interfere with test interpretation, increasing the L/S ratio by 0.1 to 0.5, thus leading to an increase in falsely mature results.

Phosphatidylglycerol

PG is a minor constituent of surfactant that becomes evident in amniotic fluid several weeks after the rise in lecithin (7). Its presence indicates a more advanced state of fetal lung development and function, as PG enhances the spread of phospholipids on the alveoli.

Technique
The original PG testing was performed by thin-layer chromatography and required time and expertise. More recently, enzymatic assay or slide agglutinations have been used successfully to determine the presence of PG. Amniostat-FLM (Irvine Scientific, California, U.S.) is one such test.

Interpretation
The results are typically reported qualitatively as positive or negative, where positive represents >3% of total phospholipids, and an exceedingly low risk of RDS.

Special Considerations
PG determination is not generally affected by blood, meconium, or vaginal secretion.

Surfactant/Albumin Ratio

The fluorescence polarization assay uses polarized light to evaluate the competitive binding of a probe to both albumin and surfactant in amniotic fluid (8).

Technique
The TDx-FLM (Abbott, Illinois, U.S.) analyzer provides a quantitative and automated measurement of the amniotic fluid surfactant/albumin ratio (SAR). The test is simple, rapid, objective, reproducible, and can be performed with equipment commonly available in clinical laboratories. A recent commercial modification of the assay (TDx-FlxFLM II) allows simple, automated, and rapid results.

Interpretation
An SAR of 55 mg/g has been proposed as the optimal threshold to indicate maturity (9). Values of 35 to 55 are considered "borderline." As per other tests, **the probability for RDS should be calculated as a function of gestational age and the FLM test results** (Table 57.2). In other words, other pretest probabilities for maturity should be taken into account when interpreting these tests (10).

Special Considerations
As for L/S ratio, red blood cell phospholipids may falsely lower the TDx-FlxFLM II result, but a mature test can reliably predict pulmonary maturity.

Is a course of steroids indicated in face of an immature result at > 34 weeks? In a small RCT of patients over 34 weeks with "immature" TDX-FlxFLM II, results demonstrated a benefit to a single course of corticosteroids in terms of a progression to "mature" results with repeat amniocentesis one week later (50% vs. 27%, P = 0.002). However, as no actual neonatal outcomes were presented, this approach must be interpreted with some caution at this time (11).

Lamellar Body Counts

Lamellar bodies (LB) are produced by type II pneumocytes and are a direct measurement of surfactant production because they represent its storage form.

Technique
Lamellar bodies are quantified with a commercial blood cell analyzer, which takes advantage of the similar size between LB and platelets. The results can be obtained quickly, with a small fluid volume, and the test is less expensive than traditional phospholipids analysis. Although initial studies employed centrifugation, it is now agreed that the sample should be processed without spinning as centrifugation reduces the number of LB.

Interpretation
Values of 30,000 to 50,000/μL (least false-positives) generally indicate pulmonary maturity (12,13). Values of <15,000/μL are usually associated with immaturity. The test compares favorably with L/S and PG with a negative predictive value of a

Table 57.1 Characteristics of Fetal Lung Maturity Tests

Test	Technique	Threshold	Predictive value mature test (%)	Predictive value immature test (%)	Accurate with blood contamination	Accurate with meconium contamination	Accurate in vaginal pool	Difficulty	Cost
L/S ratio	Thin-layer chromatography	2/1	95–100	33–50	No	No	No	High	High
PG	Thin-layer chromatography	Present (usually means >3% of total phospholipids)	95–100	23–53	Yes	Yes	Yes	High	High
	Slide agglutination	Positive (>2%)						Low	Low
Surfactant/ albumin ratio (TDx-FLM)	Fluorescence polarization	≥55 mg (of surfactant)/g (of albumin)	96–100	47–61	No	No	Yes	Low	Moderate
LBC	Cell counter	30,000–50,000/μL	97–98	29–35	No	Yes	Yes	Low	Low
FSI	Ethanol dilution	≥47	95	51	No	No	No	Moderate	Moderate

Abbreviations: L/S, lecithin/sphingomyelin; PG, phosphatidylglycerol; LBC, lamellar body count; FSI, foam stability index.
Source: Adapted from Ref. 2.

Table 57.2 Probability of RDS on the Basis of Gestational Age and Surfactant/Albumin (S/A) Ratio (TDx-FLM)

S/A	Gestational age (wk)													
	27	28	29	30	31	32	33	34	35	36	37	38	39	40
0	72%	66%	59%	51%	44%	37%	30%	24%	19%	15%	12%	9%	7%	5.1%
10	67%	60%	53%	46%	39%	32%	26%	20%	16%	12%	9.6%	7.3%	5.5%	4.2%
20	62%	55%	48%	40%	33%	27%	22%	17%	13%	10%	7.8%	6%	4.5%	3.4%
30	57%	50%	42%	35%	29%	23%	18%	14%	11%	8.4%	6.4%	4.8%	3.6%	2.7%
40	51%	44%	37%	30%	24%	19%	15%	12%	9%	6.8%	5.2%	4%	3%	2.2%
50	46%	39%	32%	26%	21%	16%	13%	10%	7.4%	5.6%	4.2%	3.2%	2.4%	1.8%
60	40%	34%	27%	22%	17%	13%	10%	8%	6%	4.5%	3.4%	2.5%	1.9%	1.4%
70	35%	29%	23%	18%	14%	11%	8.5%	6.4%	4.9%	3.7%	2.7%	2%	1.5%	1.1%
80	31%	25%	20%	15%	12%	9.1%	7%	5.2%	4%	3%	2.2%	1.7%	1.2%	0.9%
90	26%	21%	16%	13%	10%	7.4%	5.6%	4.2%	3.2%	2.4%	1.8%	1.3%	1%	0.7%
100	22%	17%	14%	10%	8%	6%	4.6%	3.4%	2.6%	2%	1.4%	1%	0.8%	0.6%
110	19%	14%	11%	9%	6.5%	4.9%	3.7%	2.8%	2.1%	1.5%	1.2%	0.9%	0.6%	0.5%
120	15%	12%	9%	7%	5.3%	4%	3%	2.2%	1.7%	1.2%	1%	0.7%	0.5%	0.4%
130	13%	9.8%	7.5%	6%	4.3%	3.2%	2.4%	1.8%	1.3%	1%	0.7%	0.6%	0.4%	0.3%
140	10%	8%	6.1%	4.6%	3.5%	2.6%	2%	1.4%	1.1%	0.8%	0.6%	0.5%	0.3%	0.25%
150	9%	6.6%	5%	3.7%	2.8%	2.1%	1.6%	1.2%	0.9%	0.6%	0.5%	0.4%	0.3%	0.2%
160	7%	5.3%	4%	3%	2.3%	1.7%	1.3%	1%	0.7%	0.5%	0.4%	0.3%	0.2%	0.2%
170	5.7%	4.3%	3.2%	2.4%	1.8%	1.4%	1%	0.8%	0.6%	0.4%	0.3%	0.2%	0.2%	0.1%
180	4.7%	3.5%	2.6%	2%	1.5%	1.1%	0.8%	0.6%	0.4%	0.3%	0.2%	0.2%	0.2%	0.1%
190	3.8%	2.8%	2.1%	1.6%	1.2%	0.9%	0.7%	0.5%	0.4%	0.3%	0.2%	0.1%	0.1%	0.1%
200	3%	2.3%	1.7%	1.3%	0.9%	0.7%	0.5%	0.4%	0.3%	0.2%	0.1%	0.1%	0.1%	0.1%

mature cutoff of 97.7% versus 96.8% and 94.7%, respectively (14). A meta-analysis calculated receiver-operating characteristic curves based on data from six studies and showed the lamellar body count performed slightly better than the L/S ratio in predicting RDS (15).

Special Considerations
Meconium has a marginal impact on LB counts, increasing the count by 5000/μL. Bloody fluid can initially slightly increase the count because the platelets are counted as LB. Afterward, the procoagulant activity of AF produces an entrapment of both, platelets and LB, causing a decrease in LB counts. Because of variations in hematology analyzers, ideally laboratories should develop their own reference standards (16).

Foam Stability Index
The foam stability index (FSI) is a simple and rapid predictor of FLM based on the ability of surfactant to generate stable foam in the presence of ethanol.

Technique
After centrifugation, ethanol is added to a sample of amniotic fluid to eliminate the contributions of protein, bile salts, and salts of free fatty acids. The mixture is shaken for 30 second and will demonstrate generation of a stable ring of foam if surfactant is present in the amniotic fluid. Amniotic fluid samples should not be collected in silicone tubes as the silicone will produce "false foam."

Interpretation
The FSI is calculated by utilizing serial dilutions of ethanol to quantitate the amount of surfactant present. RDS is very unlikely with an FSI value of 47 or higher. A positive result virtually excludes the risk of RDS; however, a negative test often occurs in the presence of mature lung.

Special Considerations
Contamination of the amniotic fluid specimen by blood or meconium interferes with the FSI results.

SINGLE TEST, MULTIPLE TESTS, OR CASCADE?
Faced with different assays for FLM, some laboratories perform multiple tests simultaneously, leaving the clinician with the possibility of results discordant for pulmonary maturity from the same amniotic fluid specimen. In general, any mature test result is indicative of fetal pulmonic maturity given the high predictive value of any single test (5% or less of false mature rates). Conversely the use of a "cascade" approach has been proposed to minimize the risk of delivery of an infant with immature lungs, while avoiding unnecessary delay in delivery and costs. According to this approach, a rapid and inexpensive test is performed first, with follow-up tests performed only in the face of immaturity of the initial test (e.g., **lamellar body count or surfactant/albumin ratio as the initial and only test, and L/S ratio as the confirmatory test, as necessary**).

CLINICAL CONDITIONS AFFECTING RISK OF RDS AND PREDICTIVE VALUE OF PULMONARY MATURITY TESTS
Several maternal/fetal clinical or nonclinical circumstances can affect the risk of RDS and modify the predictive value of pulmonary maturity tests, including the following:

- African-American race is associated with FLM achieved at lower gestational ages and at lower L/S ratios (1.2 or greater) than in Caucasians.
- Female gender is associated with acceleration of lung maturation.
- Intrauterine growth restriction and preeclampsia are possibly associated with an acceleration of FLM.
- **Maternal diabetes** and Rh-isoimmunization are associated with a delay in fetal lung maturation. Some authors have recommended the use of higher thresholds of L/S ratio (e.g., a cutoff ratio of 3) to establish pulmonic maturity in these conditions. Presence of a lamellar body count 50,000/μL has similarly been recommended to indicate mature fetal lungs in diabetic women (17). Presence of PG is commonly considered as gold standard for documentation of FLM with

diabetes or Rh-isoimmunization. For diabetes, also a TDx-FLM value of ≥ 70 mg/g, or a L/S ≥ 3, or the combination of the two, have been associated with >95% predictive value for a mature test. Some experts, instead, use the same threshold values of nondiabetic pregnancies for assessment of FLM in diabetic pregnancies (2).

- Hydramnios is associated with lower levels of L/S ratio, lamellar body count, and PG test.
- In twin gestations it is commonly recommended that the sac of the male twin or the larger twin be sampled at amniocentesis. The reasoning is that if the sampled twin has mature pulmonic results, the co-twin is even more likely to be mature.

FINAL NOTE: FACTORS OTHER THAN LUNG MATURITY IMPACT FETAL OUTCOME

A recent retrospective cohort study compared the outcomes of neonates born between 36 and 38 6/7 weeks in the setting of mature fetal lung profile studies to those born at 39 0/7 to 40 6/7 weeks and found an increase in a composite adverse neonatal outcomes (RR = 2.4, 95% CI 1.7–3.5) with common complications including respiratory distress, hyperbilirubinemia, and hypoglycemia (18). It is **important to remember that there is more to fetal maturation than "just" the lungs and the decision to proceed with amniocentesis for the purposes of hastening delivery should always be carefully considered** (18).

REFERENCES

1. Gluck L, Kulovich MV, Boerer RC Jr, et al. Diagnosis of the respiratory distress syndrome by amniocentesis. Am J Obstet Gynecol 1971; 109:440. [II-2]
2. American College of Obstetricians and Gynecologists. Fetal lung maturity. ACOG Practice Bulletin No. 97. Washington, DC: ACOG, 2008. [Review]
3. Hodor JG, Poggi SH, Spong CY, et al. Risk of third-trimester amniocentesis: a case-control study. Am J Perinatol 2006; 23:177–180. [II-2]
4. Gordon MC, Narula K, O'Shaughnssy R, et al. Complications of third trimester amniocentesis using continuous ultrasound guidance. Obstet Gynecol 2002; 99:255–259. [II-3]
5. Stark CM, Smith RS, Lagrandeur RM, et al. Need for urgent delivery after third trimester amniocentesis. Obstet Gynecol 2000; 95:48–50. [II-3]
6. Gleaton KD, White JC, Koklanaris N. A novel method for collecting vaginal pool for fetal lung maturity studies. Am J Obstet Gynecol 2009; 201:408, e1–408.e4. [II-3]
7. Hallman M, Kulovich M, Kirkpatrick E, et al. Phosphatidylinositol and phosphatidylglycerol in amniotic fluid: indices of lung maturity. Am J Obstet Gynecol 1976; 125:613. [II-2]
8. Russell JC, Cooper CM, Ketchum CH, et al. Multicenter evaluation of TDx test for assessing fetal lung maturity. Clin Chem 1989; 35:1005. [II-2]
9. Kesselman EJ, Figueroa R, Garry D, et al. The usefulness of the TDx/TDxFLx fetal lung maturity II assay in the initial evaluation of fetal lung maturity. Am J Obstet Gynecol 2003; 188:1220–1222. [II-2]
10. Pinette MG, Blackstone J, Wax JR, et al. Fetal lung maturity indices—a plea for gestational age-specific interpretation: a case report and discussion. Am J Obstet Gynecol 2002; 187:1721–1722 [III]
11. Shanks A, Gross G, Shim T, et al. Administration of steroids after 34 weeks of gestation enhances fetal lung maturity profiles. Am J Obstet Gynecol 2010; 203:47, e1–e5. [I]
12. Dubin, SB. The laboratory assessment of fetal lung maturity. Am J Clin Pathol 1992; 97:836. [II-2]
13. Ghidini A, Poggi SH, Spong CY, et al. Role of lamellar body count for the prediction of neonatal respiratory distress syndrome in non-diabetic pregnant women. Arch Gynecol Obstet 2005; 271:325–328. [II-2]
14. Neerhof MG, Haney EI, Silver RK, et al. Lamellar body counts compared with traditional phospholipid analysis as an assay for evaluating fetal lung maturity. Obstet Gynecol 2001; 97:305–309. [II-2]
15. Wijnberger LD, Huisjes AJ, Voorbij HA, et al. The accuracy of lamellar body count and lecithin/sphingomyelin ratio in the prediction of neonatal respiratory distress syndrome: a meta-analysis. BJOG 2001; 108:585–588. [II-2]
16. Janicki MB, Dries LM, Egan JF, et al. Determining a cutoff for fetal lung maturity with lamellar body count testing. J Matern Fetal Neonatal Med 2009; 22:419–422. [II-2]
17. Ghidini A, Spong CY, Goodwin K, et al. Optimal thresholds of lecithin/sphingomyelin ratio and lamellar body count for the prediction of the presence of phosphatidylglycerol in diabetic women. J Matern Fetal Neonatal Med 2002; 12:95–98. [II-2]
18. Bates E, Rouse DJ, Mann ML, et al. Neonatal outcomes after demonstrated fetal lung maturity before 39 weeks gestation. Obstet Gynecol 2010; 116:1288–1295. [II-3]

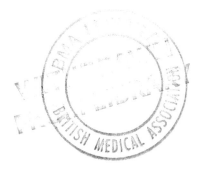